Dimond's Legal Aspects of Nursing

A Definitive Guide to Law for Nurses

Pearson

At Pearson, we have a simple mission: to help people make more of their lives through learning.

We combine innovative learning technology with trusted content and educational expertise to provide engaging and effective learning experiences that serve people wherever and whenever they are learning.

From classroom to boardroom, our curriculum materials, digital learning tools and testing programmes help to educate millions of people worldwide – more than any other private enterprise.

Every day our work helps learning flourish, and wherever learning flourishes, so do people.

To learn more, please visit us at **www.pearson.com**

Dimond's Legal Aspects of Nursing

A Definitive Guide to Law for Nurses

Ninth Edition

Richard Griffith

Iwan Dowie

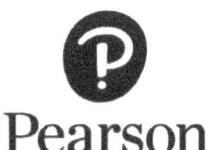

Harlow, England • London • New York • Boston • San Francisco • Toronto • Sydney • Dubai • Singapore • Hong Kong
Tokyo • Seoul • Taipei • New Delhi • Cape Town • São Paulo • Mexico City • Madrid • Amsterdam • Munich • Paris • Milan

PEARSON EDUCATION LIMITED
KAO Two
KAO Park
Harlow CM17 9NA
United Kingdom
Tel: +44 (0)1279 623623
Web: **www.pearson.com**

First published 1990 (print)
Eighth edition published 2019 (print and electronic)
Ninth edition published 2025 (print and electronic)

© Prentice Hall Europe 1990, 1995 (print)
© Pearson Education Limited 2002, 2005, 2008 (print)
© Pearson Education Limited 2011, 2015, 2019, 2025 (print and electronic)

The rights of Richard Griffith and Iwan Dowie to be identified as authors of this work have been asserted by them in accordance with the Copyright, Designs and Patents Act 1988.

The print publication is protected by copyright. Prior to any prohibited reproduction, storage in a retrieval system, distribution or transmission in any form or by any means, electronic, mechanical, recording or otherwise, permission should be obtained from the publisher or, where applicable, a licence permitting restricted copying in the United Kingdom should be obtained from the Copyright Licensing Agency Ltd, Barnard's Inn, 86 Fetter Lane, London EC4A 1EN.

The ePublication is protected by copyright and must not be copied, reproduced, transferred, distributed, leased, licensed or publicly performed or used in any way except as specifically permitted in writing by the publishers, as allowed under the terms and conditions under which it was purchased, or as strictly permitted by applicable copyright law. Any unauthorised distribution or use of this text may be a direct infringement of the authors' and the publisher's rights and those responsible may be liable in law accordingly.

Contains public sector information licensed under the Open Government Licence (OGL) v3.0. http://www.nationalarchives.gov.uk/doc/open-government-licence/version/3/

Contains Parliamentary information licensed under the Open Parliament Licence (OPL) v3.0. http://www.parliament.uk/site-information/copyright/open-parliament-licence/

Pearson Education is not responsible for the content of third-party internet sites.

ISBN: 978-1-292-46905-8 (print)
978-1-292-46942-3 (epub)
978-1-292-73711-9 (etext)

British Library Cataloguing-in-Publication Data
A catalogue record for the print edition is available from the British Library

Library of Congress Cataloging-in-Publication Data
Names: Griffith, Richard (Richard A.), author. | Dowie, Iwan, author. |
  Dimond, Bridgit. Legal aspects of nursing.
Title: Dimond's legal aspects of nursing : a definitive guide to law for
  nurses / Richard Griffith, Iwan Dowie.
Other titles: Legal aspects of nursing
Description: Ninth edition. | Harlow, England ; New York : Pearson, 2025. |
  Preceded by: Legal aspects of nursing / Bridgit Dimond. Seventh edition.
  2015. | Includes bibliographical references and index.
Identifiers: LCCN 2025002153 | ISBN 9781292469058 (paperback) |
  ISBN 9781292469423 (epub)
Subjects: MESH: Legislation, Nursing | United Kingdom
Classification: LCC RT41 | NLM WY 33 FA1 | DDC 610.73--dc23/eng/20250307
LC record available at https://lccn.loc.gov/2025002153

10 9 8 7 6 5 4 3 2 1
29 28 27 26 25

Cover image: © Pixtum/istock/Getty images
Cover design by Michelle Morgon

NOTE THAT ANY PAGE CROSS REFERENCES REFER TO THE PRINT EDITION

Brief Contents

Guided tour xiii
Table of cases xv
Table of statutes xix
Abbreviations xxviii
Preface to ninth edition xxxi
Acknowledgements xxxii

PART I General Principles Affecting all Nurses

Chapter 1	Professionalism, the Legal System and Human Rights	3
Chapter 2	Actions in the Criminal Courts and Defences to Criminal Charges	23
Chapter 3	Liability in a Civil Court Case for Negligence	48
Chapter 4	Specific Problem Areas in Civil Liability: Personal Liability of the Nurse, Vicarious Liability of the Employer and Managerial Issues	72
Chapter 5	Statutory Functions and Management of the NHS	104
Chapter 6	Progress of a Civil Claim: Defences and Compensation	149
Chapter 7	Consent to Treatment and Informing the Patient	176
Chapter 8	Data Protection: Confidentiality and Access	209
Chapter 9	Record Keeping, Statements and Evidence in Court	246
Chapter 10	The Nurse and Employment Law	266
Chapter 11	The Nurse as a Registered Professional	310
Chapter 12	Health and Safety and the Nurse	332

PART II Specialist Areas

Chapter 13	Children and Young Persons	395
Chapter 14	The Nurse and Gynaecology	437
Chapter 15	Acute Care	465

Chapter 16	Learning Disabilities and Safeguarding People	490
Chapter 17	Nurse Educator and Researcher	521
Chapter 18	Legal Aspects of the Care of Older People	542
Chapter 19	Nursing People with Mental Health Problems or Learning Disability	570
Chapter 20	Accident and Emergency, Outpatients, Genito-Urinary Departments and Day Surgery	605
Chapter 21	Human Fertility and Genetics	624
Chapter 22	Community and Primary Care Nursing	661
Chapter 23	Scope of Professional Practice, Clinical Nurse Specialist and Consultant Nurse	713

PART III General Areas

Chapter 24	Legal Aspects of Property	735
Chapter 25	Legal Aspects of Public Health	750
Chapter 26	Handling Complaints	774
Chapter 27	Legal Aspects of Medicines	798
Chapter 28	End-of-life Care and Death	831
Chapter 29	Complementary and Alternative Therapies	877
Chapter 30	The Future	892
Further Reading		894
Websites		898
Glossary		901
Index		903

Contents

Guided tour	xiii
Table of cases	xv
Table of statutes	xix
Abbreviations	xxviii
Preface to ninth edition	xxxi
Acknowledgements	xxxii

PART I General Principles Affecting all Nurses

1 Professionalism, the Legal System and Human Rights — 3
- Professionalism — 4
- Criminal liability — 5
- Professional liability — 7
- Civil liability — 8
- Accountability to employer — 9
- Professionalism and accountability — 9
- Sources of law — 9
- Differences between civil and criminal law — 11
- Civil actions — 11
- Judicial review — 12
- Legal personnel and legal complaints — 12
- Legal language — 13
- Human Rights Act 1998 — 13
- Freedom of Information Act 2000 — 19
- Devolved law-making powers — 19
- Conclusions — 19
- Further exercises — 20
- References — 20

2 Actions in the Criminal Courts and Defences to Criminal Charges — 23
- Initial stages of arrest and prosecution — 24
- Magistrates' courts — 27
- Plea and case management hearing — 29
- Crown court proceedings — 29
- Elements of a crime — 33
- Case of Beverley Allitt — 34
- Case of Sister Salisbury — 34
- Case of Nurse Patel — 35
- Case of Lucy Letby — 35
- Offence of ill-treatment or wilful neglect — 35
- Case of Nurse Amaro — 36
- Negligence as a crime — 36
- Administration of drug by epidural instead of intravenous injection — 39
- Defences — 39
- Criminal injuries compensation — 44
- Conclusions — 45
- Further exercises — 45
- References — 46

3 Liability in a Civil Court Case for Negligence — 48
- Duty of care — 49
- Standard of care — 53
- Causation — 60
- Liable for what? — 64
- Harm — 64
- Conclusions — 68
- Further exercises — 69
- References — 69

4 Specific Problem Areas in Civil Liability: Personal Liability of the Nurse, Vicarious Liability of the Employer and Managerial Issues — 72
- Negligence in communication — 73
- Inexperience — 74
- Team liability and apportionment of responsibility — 75

Taking instructions: refusal to obey	77		Compensation in civil proceedings for negligence	156
Nurse as manager	80		Defences to a civil action	160
Pressure on the manager	80		Clinical Negligence Scheme for Trusts (CNST)	
Vicarious liability of employer	82		and the NHS Litigation Authority (NHSLA)	170
In the course of employment	83		NHS Redress Act 2006	171
Liability for negligence of volunteers	87		Reforms to civil litigation	172
Duty of care and liability for independent contractors	87		Conclusions	172
Direct liability of employer	88		Further exercises	173
Indemnity from the employee at fault	90		References	173
Pressure from inadequate resources	91	**7**	Consent to Treatment and Informing the Patient	176
Public interest disclosure act 1998 and whistleblowing	96		Basic principles	177
Conclusions	101		Requirements of a valid consent	177
Further exercises	102		How should consent be given?	177
References	102		Right to refuse treatment	181
			Taking one's own discharge	184
5 Statutory Functions and Management of the NHS	104		Definition of mental capacity under the Mental Capacity Act 2005	185
National Health Service	105		Hunger strikes	187
White Paper Equity and Excellence: Liberating the NHS	105		Amputation of healthy limbs	188
Enforcement of statutory duties	109		Defences to an action for trespass to the person	188
Distinction between Statutory Duties and Guidance from the Department of Health and Social Care	113		Mental Capacity Act 2005	190
			Mental Health Act 1983	195
NHS England (the National Health Service Commissioning Board)	113		Giving information to a patient prior to consent being obtained	196
Clinical commissioning groups	116		Non-therapeutic procedures	200
The mandate	119		Giving information to the terminally ill patient	201
NHS foundation trusts	120		Notifying the patient of negligence by a colleague	203
NHS Improvement (formerly Monitor)	120			
Clinical governance	125		No decision about me, without me	204
Duty of quality	125		Conclusions	205
The Care Quality Commission	127		Further exercises	205
National Institute for Health and Care Excellence (NICE)	132		References	206
NHS 111 and walk-in clinics	135	**8**	Data Protection: Confidentiality and Access	209
NHS inquiries	136		General Data Protection Regulation (including Data Protection Act 2018)	209
Mid Staffordshire NHS foundation trust inquiry	138			
The NHS Constitution	142		Duty of confidentiality	217
NHS and the private sector	143		Caldicott Guardians	235
Conclusions	144		Freedom of Information Act 2000	236
Further exercises	145		DNA databases	240
References	145		Access to Medical Reports Act 1988	241
6 Progress of a Civil Claim: Defences and Compensation	149		Conclusions	241
			Further exercises	242
Civil proceedings	149		References	242
The hearing	154			

9	Record Keeping, Statements and Evidence in Court	246	Conclusions	386
			Further exercises	387
	Record keeping	246	References	387
	Statements	252		
	Evidence in court	257		
	Defamation	261		
	Internet and social media	263		
	Conclusions	264		
	Further exercises	264		
	References	265		

PART II Specialist Areas

13	Children and Young Persons		395
	Consent to treatment		396
	No absolutist test		409
	Referring the matter to court		410
	Permissive declarations		410
	Safeguarding children		411
	Parental care and the nurse		421
	Disciplining a child		423
	Adolescents		425
	Deprivation of liberty of children and young persons		426
	The National Deprivation of Liberty Court		429
	Authorising the deprivation of liberty of a child		429
	The inherent jurisdiction of the High Court		429
	Conclusions		431
	Further exercises		432
	References		432

10	The Nurse and Employment Law	266
	Human rights	267
	Contract of employment	268
	Statutory provisions covering employment	274
	Unfair dismissal	286
	Trade union rights	292
	Public and private employees	294
	Discrimination: The Equality and Human Rights Commission	294
	Equality Act 2010	295
	Conclusions	306
	Further exercises	306
	References	306

14	The Nurse and Gynaecology	437
	Abortion	437
	Sterilisation	452
	Female circumcision	458
	Conclusions	461
	Further exercises	462
	References	462

11	The Nurse as a Registered Professional	310
	Background to the establishment of the nursing and midwifery council	310
	Nursing and midwifery council	311
	Registration and removal	313
	Professional standards and codes of practice	324
	Education and training	324
	Post-registration revalidation and continuing professional development (CPD)	325
	Professional Standards Authority for Health and Social Care (PSA) (formerly the Council for Healthcare Regulatory Excellence (CHRE))	326
	Nursing associates	328
	Conclusions	328
	Further exercises	329
	References	329

15	Acute Care	465
	Civil liability procedures and practices in theatre	466
	The theatre nurse and the scope of professional practice	469
	Accidents in the theatre	469
	Consent in the theatre	471
	Recovery room nursing	473
	Transfusions and blood contamination	474
	Organ transplantation	475
	Intensive care units: resource pressures	482
	Review of critical care services	483
	Conclusions	484
	Further exercises	485
	References	486

12	Health and Safety and the Nurse	332
	Statutory provisions	332
	Corporate manslaughter and corporate homicide	360
	Common law duties: employer's duty	360
	Remedies available to an injured employee	363
	Special areas	365

16 Learning Disabilities and Safeguarding People — 490
- Acting in the best interests of a mentally incapacitated adult — 491
- Deprivation of Liberty Safeguards (DoLS) (Bournewood) — 494
- Carers — 499
- Court of Protection and Code of Practice — 501
- White Paper Valuing People — 504
- Safeguarding vulnerable adults — 507
- Sexual relations and related issues — 508
- Property — 511
- Direct payments — 511
- Registration and inspections — 515
- Conclusions — 516
- Further exercises — 517
- References — 517

17 Nurse Educator and Researcher — 521
- NMC and standards in education — 522
- Record keeping by teachers — 523
- Liability for instructing others — 524
- Hearing about unsound practices — 525
- Employment law — 526
- Legal aspects of research — 527
- Health Research Authority (HRA) — 531
- Confidentiality — 532
- Consent — 533
- Health Education England — 537
- Conclusions — 539
- Further exercise — 540
- References — 540

18 Legal Aspects of the Care of Older People — 542
- Rights to care — 543
- National Service Framework for Older People — 544
- Intermediate care — 546
- Consent to treatment — 547
- Force, restraint and assault — 549
- Medication and the confused older patient — 552
- Dementia — 553
- Standard of care — 557
- Risk management — 560
- Abuse of older people — 561
- Mental Capacity Act 2005 and decision making for the mentally incapacitated adult — 564
- Conclusions — 566
- Further exercises — 566
- References — 567

19 Nursing People with Mental Health Problems or Learning Disability — 570
- Informal patients — 571
- Patients detained under mental health legislation — 572
- Holding power of the nurse — 573
- Compulsory detention of an informal inpatient — 575
- Compulsory admission — 575
- Definition and role of nearest relative — 579
- Role of the approved mental health professional — 580
- Informing the patient and relatives — 582
- Consent to treatment provisions — 583
- Community provisions — 589
- Conclusions — 601
- Further exercises — 602
- References — 602

20 Accident and Emergency, Outpatients, Genito-Urinary Departments and Day Surgery — 605
- Accident and emergency department — 605
- Acting in the exercise of functions as an emergency worker — 609
- Aggravating factor for more serious offences — 610
- Assault on a nurse — 610
- Assaults continue to rise — 610
- Outpatients department — 615
- Genito-urinary medicine — 617
- Day surgery — 619
- Conclusions — 621
- Further exercises — 621
- References — 622

21 Human Fertility and Genetics — 624
- Artificial insemination — 626
- Human Fertilisation and Embryology Act 1990 as amended by 2008 Act — 629
- *In vitro* fertilisation (IVF) — 634
- Embryos — 636
- Confidentiality — 642
- Surrogacy — 642
- Conscientious objection — 646
- Genetics — 646
- Gene therapy and genetic diagnosis — 647
- Gender selection — 650
- Genetic screening and testing — 650

Cloning	653
Conclusions	655
Further exercises	656
References	656

22 Community and Primary Care Nursing — 661
- NHS and social services provision — 662
- Funding of long-term care — 666
- Care Act 2014 — 670
- Human rights and care homes — 681
- Delayed discharges — 684
- Carers — 687
- Negligence — 688
- Safety of the community professional — 691
- Consent to treatment — 695
- Protection of property — 697
- Disclosure of information — 698
- Criminal suspicion — 698
- Standards: care homes — 699
- Community matrons — 700
- The specialist community public health nurse — 700
- The school nurse — 701
- The clinic nurse — 703
- The practice nurse — 705
- Developments in technology and structure — 707
- Conclusions — 708
- Further exercises — 708
- References — 709

23 Scope of Professional Practice, Clinical Nurse Specialist and Consultant Nurse — 713
- Scope of professional practice — 714
- Delegation and supervision — 717
- Delegate tasks and duties that are within the other person's scope of competence — 718
- Confirm that the outcome of any task you have delegated to someone else meets the required standard — 719
- Nurse consultants — 720
- Clinical nurse specialists and specialist nurses — 720
- Concerns about developments in scope of professional practice — 722
- Scope of professional practice in primary care — 723
- Scope of professional practice in theatre nursing — 724
- Scope of professional practice in emergency nursing — 725
- Scope of professional practice and X-rays — 725
- NHS 111 (formerly NHS Direct) and walk-in clinics — 726
- Modern matrons — 727
- Agency nurses — 728
- Healthcare support workers — 728
- Conclusions — 730
- Further exercises — 731
- References — 731

PART III General Areas

24 Legal Aspects of Property — 735
- Principles of liability — 736
- Administrative failures — 737
- Exclusion of liability — 738
- Property of the mentally incapacitated patient — 739
- Mental Capacity Act 2005 — 740
- Day-to-day care of money — 740
- Power of attorney — 742
- Court of Protection — 743
- Protecting patients from relatives — 744
- Returning the patient's property — 745
- Staff property — 746
- Gifts — 747
- Conclusions — 748
- Further exercises — 748
- References — 749

25 Legal Aspects of Public Health — 750
- Public health legislation — 751
- Notifiable diseases — 752
- Cross-infection control — 755
- Health and Social Care Act 2008 — 757
- Health Protection Agency (now UK Health Security Agency) — 759
- Public Health England — 760
- Tuberculosis (TB) — 760
- Hepatitis — 761
- HIV-infected persons and AIDS patients — 761
- Vaccination — 764
- Coronavirus — 767
- Blood donors — 768
- Confidentiality — 768
- Conclusions — 769
- Further exercises — 770
- References — 770

26 Handling Complaints — 774
- Methods of complaining — 775

Handling complaints	777	**28**	End-of-life Care and Death	831
Hospital Complaints Procedure Act 1985			End-of-life care	832
and the Wilson Report	778		Definition of death	836
Complaints procedure 2004	779		Importance of exact time of death	838
Complaints procedure 2004 and 2006	780		Legality of switching machines off	840
Complaints procedure 2009	781		Not for resuscitation	845
The Health Service and Parliamentary			Patients refusing treatment	848
Ombudsman (HSC)	786		Relatives and treatment of the patient	850
The House of Commons Select Committee	788		Advance decisions to refuse treatment	
Healthwatch England	788		(living wills)	855
Local healthwatch (formerly LINKS)	789		Certification and registration of death	857
Independent Complaints Advocacy			Disposal of the body	860
Service (ICAS)	789		Post-mortems	861
Patient Advice and Liaison Services (PALS)	790		Deaths that have to be reported to the coroner	861
Other quality assurance methods	791		Inquests	862
Complaints relating to detained patients	791		Recommendations of the Shipman Inquiry	865
Secretary of State inquiries	792		The Coroners and Justice Act 2009: overview	869
The NHS Constitution	792		Property of the deceased	870
Review of NHS complaints system	793		Wills	870
Conclusions	794		Conclusions	872
Further exercises	795		Further exercises	873
References	796		References	873
27 Legal Aspects of Medicines	798	**29**	Complementary and Alternative Therapies	877
General principles	799		Definitions of complementary and	
Controlled drugs	801		alternative therapies	878
Problems in the administration of			The NMC practitioner as a complementary	
medicine	804		therapist	878
Management of errors or incidents in the			Liability for using complementary therapy	
administration of medicines	806		at work	879
Self-administration by patients	811		Patients receiving complementary therapies	881
Covert administration of medicines	811		House of Lords Select Committee	883
Nurse as prescriber	814		Herbal medicines and acupuncture	883
Group protocols or patient group			Complementary and Natural Healthcare	
directions	815		Council (CNHC)	884
Nurse prescribing: independent and			Conclusions	889
dependent (subsequently known as			Further exercises	889
supplementary) prescribers	817		References	890
Role of the pharmacist	820	**30**	The Future	892
Safety of medicines	820		References	893
Product liability and drugs	821			
Misuse of drugs	821	Further Reading		894
National Prescribing Centre	824	Websites		898
Availability of medicines within the NHS	824	Glossary		901
Conclusions	825	Index		903
Further exercises	826			
References	826			

Guided tour

This chapter discusses
- Initial stages of arrest and prosecution
- Magistrates' courts
- Plea and Case Management Hearing
- Crown Court proceedings
- Elements of a crime
- Cases of Beverley Allitt, Sister Salisbury, Nurse Patel and Nurse Amaro
- Offence of ill-treatment or wilful neglect
- Negligence as a crime
- Administration of drug by epidural instead of intravenous injection
- Defences
- Criminal injuries compensation

How can I get the most from my study?
This chapter discusses sections at the start of each chapter provide you with an instant point of reference that highlights what you can expect to learn within each chapter. You can use these as a checklist of key concepts during the course of your reading.

Will difficult concepts in law be presented in a manageable way?
Diagrams and **flowcharts** are used throughout to highlight complex legal processes.

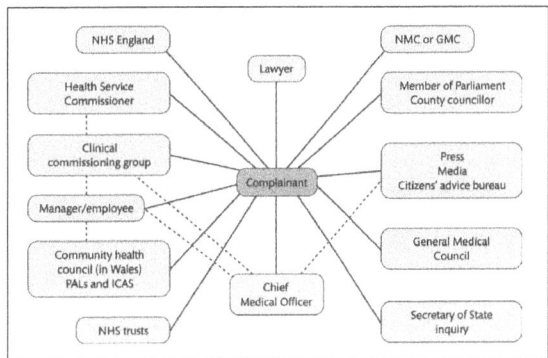

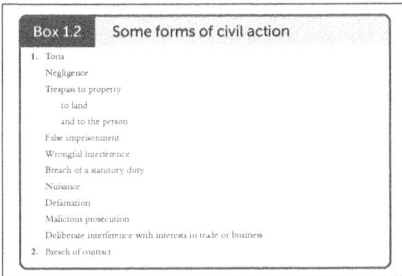

Summary information boxes pick out key points, examples and list the essential information and legal principles of a given topic. These can be found at regular intervals throughout chapters.

How can I contextualise all the theory I'll be learning?
Use the **practical dilemmas** located throughout the text to test that you understand the topics you are reading in relation to possible real life situations.

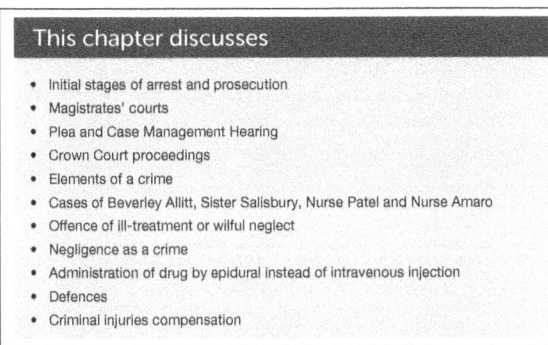

xiii

Guided tour

Case 4.5 Lister v Hesley Hall [2001]
Sexual abuse by warden[15]

The board of governors were sued by the victims of abuse by the warden at Hesley Hall, a children's home, because of its vicarious liability for his actions. The Home denied liability on the grounds that the abuse was not committed in the course of his employment. The House of Lords held that it was vicariously liable for the acts of the warden in abusing the claimants: the Home had undertaken the care of the children and entrusted the performance of that duty to the warden and there was therefore sufficiently close connection between his employment and the acts committed by him.

The House of Lords stated that the approach which was best when determining whether a wrongful act was to be deemed to be done by the employee in the course of his employment was to concentrate on the relative closeness of the connection between the nature of the employment and the particular wrongdoing. The defendant undertook to care for the claimants through the services of a warden, so there was a very close connection between the torts of the warden and the defendant. The torts were also committed at a time and place when the warden was busy caring for the claimants. The warden was carrying out his duties though in an unauthorised and improper mode.

How will I know which are the most relevant cases and statutes to be aware of?
Key case boxes explicitly highlight the key facts and related legal principle of the essential cases you need to know.

Key statute boxes identify some of the most important statutory provisions and articles to learn for your studies.

Statute 5.5
Section 13A of the NHS Act 2006

The mandate contents to be specified by Secretary of State

(a) the objectives that the Secretary of State considers the NHS Commissioning Board should seek to achieve in the exercise of its functions during that financial year and such subsequent financial years as the Secretary of State considers appropriate, and

(b) any requirements that the Secretary of State considers it necessary to impose on the Board for the purpose of ensuring that it achieves those objectives.

The Secretary of State must also specify in the mandate the amounts that the Secretary of State has decided to specify in relation to the limits on capital and revenue resource use. Also specified may be the ways in which the Secretary of State proposes to assess the Board's performance in relation to the first financial year to which the mandate relates.

The NHS Commissioning Board has the responsibility of seeking to achieve the objectives specified in the mandate, and complying with any specified requirements.

In preparing the mandate the Secretary of State must consult the NHS Commissioning Board, the Healthwatch Committee England of the Care Quality Commission and any other appropriate persons.

Reflection questions

1. Prepare guidelines for a new employee on the duty of confidentiality.
2. Do you consider that there is a breach of confidentiality if a nurse returns home and tells her husband that they are treating a patient with AIDS on the ward? She does not mention the patient's name.
3. Consider the exception to the duty of confidentiality entitled 'public interest' and consider examples from your own experience that may come under that heading. What justifications could you give for and against disclosure?
4. Do you consider that the patient should have an absolute right of access in law to health records? Justify your answer.
5. Hospitals are often seen as the most difficult institutions in which to keep personal matters secret. What action do you think could be taken to enforce the duty of confidentiality in practice?

How can I check I've understood what I've read?
Reflection questions at the end of each chapter can be used to test that you have followed and understood the key issues raised within the chapter.

How can I develop my understanding from the chapter?
Further exercises at the end of each chapter provide practical tasks that will help you apply what you have learnt and extend your knowledge.

Further Exercises

1. Why do you consider that causation is an important element in an action for negligence? Would it be fairer to the claimant if causation did not need to be proved?
2. New Zealand and Finland have a system of no-fault liability for personal injury claims. What are the advantages and disadvantages of introducing such a scheme into the UK?

References

[1] NHS Litigation Annual Report for 2013 July 2014, www.gov.uk/government/publications/the-nhs-litigation-authority-report-and-accounts-2013-to-2014
[2] Blackwater Law (2018) Report into Serious Incidents at NHS Trusts and Health Boards in England and Wales. Braintree, Essex.
[3] www.npsa.nhs.uk/
[4] News item, *The Times*, 24 June 2009
[5] News item, Cancer victim was told to suck ice cubes by the GP, *The Times*, 3 August 2013
[6] Kat Lay, Mother died after doctors took out ovary instead of appendix, *The Times*, 11 June 2013
[7] *Donoghue v Stevenson* [1932] AC 562
[8] *Kent v Griffiths and Others*, The Times Law Report, 23 December 1998; The Times Law Report, 10 February 2000; [2000] 2 All ER 474

Table of cases

AB (A Child) (Deprivation of Liberty: Consent) [2015] 429
AG v BMBC & SNH [2016] 813
A Health Authority v X 222
A Local Authority v JB [2021] 500, 508
A Local Authority v SY 187
A NHS Trust v Dr A 188
A NHS Trust v MB and Mr & Mrs B [2006] 410
Aintree University Hospitals Foundation Trust v James [2013] 844–6
Airedale NHS Trust v Bland [1993] 835, 841, 843, 844
AK (Adult Patient: Medical Treatment: Consent) Re [2001] 841
Alcock v Chief Constable of the South Yorkshire Police 66
Amanda Godfrey v Gloucester Royal Infirmary NHS Trust 168
Amanda Jenkinson 229
An asthma attack [2010] 702
An NHS Foundation Trust v P 398, 400
An NHS Trust v AW 842
An NHS Trust v DJ and others [2012] 843
An NHS Trust v Dr A [2013] 497
An NHS Trust v X [2021] 397
Atkin v Enfield Group HMC [1975] 290

B v Croydon Health Authority 587
Baby P 131, 416–18
Badger v The Home Office 162
Balamoody v UKCC 320
Barchester Healthcare Ltd v Tayeh [2013] 288
Barnett v Chelsea HMC [1968] 60
Becky Read 318
Bell & Anor v The Tavistock And Portman NHS Foundation Trust [2020] 397
Ben Silcock 591
Beverley Allitt 34, 229
Blyth v Bloomsbury Health Authority [1987] 197
Boag v Hounslow [1994] 373
Bodkin Adams 832
Bournewood 17, 493–5, 552, 571, 601
British Home Stores v Birchell [1978] IRLR 379 292
Burke 856

C v S [1987] 444
Camden LBC v R (A Minor) (Blood Transfusion) [1993] 409
Caparo Industries v Dickman Plc [1990] 50
Cassidy v Ministry of Health [1939] 89
Century Insurance Co. Ltd v Northern Ireland Road Transport Board [1942] 85
Cheshire West and Chester Council v P [2014] 426, 427, 812
Chester v Afshar [2002] 199–200
Christopher Clunis 591
Colclough v Staffordshire County Council 377
Coles v Reading HMC [1963] 73
Crawford v Charing Cross Hospital [1953] 59
Criminal proceedings against a retailer of Chinese herbal medicines 882

Daniel Pelka 418–19
Davis v Barking, Havering and Brentwood HA [1993] 180
Deacon v McVicar 93, 224, 250, 611
Debbie Purdy 849, 852
Diane Pretty 851–2
Donoghue v Stevenson 50
Doogan and Anor Re Judicial Review [2012] (Glasgow case) 440
Doogan and Another v Greater Glasgow and CLyde Health Board [2014] UKSC 68 440
Dr Arthur 408
Dr Simon Singh 262
Dwyer v Roderick [1984] 807

Early v Newham HA 56
Emeh v Kensington and Chelsea and Westminster Health Authority [1985] 453

Fatal diagnosis 858
Fenech v E. London and City Health Authority [2000] 168
Fitness to practise 808
Fraser v Winchester HA [1999] 364
Freeman v Home Office 177
Froom v Butcher [1975] 162

xv

G v E & Ors [2010] 497, 502
Gaynor and Vincent v Warrington HA and Liverpool HA 455
Gillick v West Norfolk and Wisbech AHA and the DHSS [1985] 402
GJ v the Foundation Trust 496
Glass v United Kingdom [2004] 410
Gold v Haringey Health Authority [1987] 200, 456
Gravil v Redruth Rugby Football Club 86
Gregg v Scott 64

H (A Healthcare Worker) v Associated Newspapers Ltd 228
Halfpenny v IGE Medical System Ltd [1999] 279
Hardman v Amin 455
Harold Shipman 835
Harris v Newcastle HA [1989] 2 All ER 273 152
Hart v Brown 479
Hawley v Luminar Leisure Ltd 88
Health and Social Care Trust v M and others 409
Hedley Byrne v Heller 262
Hefferon v Committee of the UKCC, Current Law 324
HL v United Kingdom (45508/99) [2005] 812
Hotson v Berkshire AHA [1987] 63

In re An Adoption (Surrogacy) [1987] 643
In re B (A Minor) [1981] 407, 408
In re B (A Minor: Wardship Sterilisation) [1987] 450, 452
In re C [1994] 587
In re D [1976] 404, 405
In re F (Adult: Court's Jurisdiction) [2000] 491
In re F v West Berkshire Health Authority 452
In re P (A Minor) [1981] 449
In re W 184
In re Walker Application [1987] 111
Isaghehi v NMC 321

J v DLA Piper 295
J (A Minor) (Child in Care: Medical Treatment) [1993] 409
Jolley v Sutton LBC [2000] 350
Jones v Manchester Corporation [1952] 90
Jones v Sandwell Metropolitan Borough Council 372

Kay v Ayrshire and Arran Health Board [1987] 61
Kay v Northumberland Healthcare NHS Trust [2001] 98–9
Kent v Griffiths 50–1, 612
Konzani 763

L v United Kingdom [2004] (The Bournewood Case) 494
LA v A 493
Lee v SW Thames RHA [1985] 223
Lister v Hesley Hall [2001] 85
Lister v Romford Ice and Cold Storage Co. Ltd [1957] 90

Local Authority X v MM [2007] 500
London Borough of Hillingdon v Neary [2011] 498
London Borough of Redbridge v G [2014] 548
Loveday v Renton and Another [1988] 766
Lucy Letby 35, 860

M v A Hospital [2017] 844
MAK and RK v the UK 420
Malette v Shulman [1991] 189, 472
Margaret Haywood 99
Martin 240
Maynard v West Midlands [1984] 54
McCormack v Redpath Brown [1961] 93
McDaid v NMC 318
McFarlane v Tayside Health Board 455, 456, 457, 458
McFarlane and Another v Tayside Health Board [1999] 454
McLoughlin v O'Brian [1982] 65
MD v Nottinghamshire Healthcare NHS Trust 583
MH v United Kingdom 498, 575
Michael Spence v Angela Naveda and Barking, Havering and Redbridge University Hospitals NHS Trust 156
Mid Staffordshire NHS Foundation Trust Inquiry 36, 138–42
Miss B 182
Montgomery v Lanarkshire [2015] 200
Morgan v Phillips 515
Ms B [2002] 183, 840

N v Chief Constable of Merseyside Police 86
Naomi Campbell 217
Nettleship v Weston [1971] 74
NHS Manchester v Fecitt and others 98
NHS Trust v Y [2017] 844
NHS Trust v Y [2018] 843, 844
Nicholson v Halton General Hospital NHS Trust [1999] 221
Nielsen v Denmark (33488/96) [2000] 428
North Glamorgan NHS Trust v Walters [2003] 67
Nottinghamshire Healthcare NHS Trust v RC 182, 588
Nunnerley and Another v Warrington Health Authority and Another 455
Nurse Amaro 36
Nurse Patel 35

P and Q v Surrey County Council 498
Parkinson v St James and Seacroft University Hospital NHS Trust 455, 457
Paton v Trustees of British Pregnancy Advisory Service [1978] 444
Pearce v United Bristol Healthcare NHS Trust [1998] 198
Penney, Palmer and Cannon v E Kent Health Authority [2000] 706
Phillip Simelane 595
PH v Local Authority 191

Prendergast v Sam Dee Ltd and Others [1989] 805
Pretty v *DPP* [2001] 835
Pretty v *United Kingdom* 381, 852
Professional Conduct proceedings against a GP practising ozone therapy 883
Property of the deceased 870
P (by his Litigation Friend the Official Solicitor) v *Cheshire West and Cheshire Council and Anor* [2014] 497

R v *Adomako* [1995] 37
R v *Bateman* [1925] 36
R v *Bodkin Adams* [1957] 834
R v *Broadmoor Special Hospital Authority* 493
R v *Brown* 178
R v *Cambridge HA* [1995] 111
R v *Cox* [1992] 834
R v *Dhingra* 447
R v *FHS Appeal Authority ex p Muralidhar* [1999] 690
R v *Gloucester CC and Another ex parte Barry* [1997] 663
R v *Hillingdon Health Authority ex parte Wyatt* [1977] 693
R v *Hinks* 748
R v *Hudson* 508
R v *Malcherek* 839
R v *Misra & Srivastava* [2004] 36
R v *Moor* [2000] 835
R v *N and E Devon Health Authority ex parte Coughlan* [2000] 663
R v *O* [2005] 834
R v *Patel* [2013] 141
R v *Portsmouth Hospitals NHS Trust ex p Glass* [1999] 405
R v *Rose* [2017] 37
R v *Salford Health Authority ex parte Janaway* [1988] 440
R v *Salisbury* [2005] 835
R v *Secretary of State for Health* [1979] 110
R v *Shipman* [2000] 835
R v *Steel* [1981] 839
R v *Strong* [2014] 141
R v *Woollin* [1999] 834
R v *Worcestershire Acute Hospitals NHS Trust* [2010] 382
R (adult: medical treatment) [1996] 846
R(Burke) v *GMC* [2005] 846
R (McDonald) v *Kensington and Chelsea Royal London Borough Council (ECHR)* [2014] 683
R (on the application of Gardner) v *SoS Health and Social Care* [2022] 12
R (on the application of Grogan) v *Bexley NHS care trust* [2006] 664
R (on the Application of Ireneschild) v *Lambeth* [2006] 699
R (Smeaton) v *Secretary of State for Health* 447
R (Quintavalle) v *HFEA* [2002-5] 648–9

RCN v *The Department of Health and Social Security* [1981] 441
Re A [1992] 510, 838
Ready-Mixed Concrete (South-East) Ltd v *Ministry of Pensions and National Insurance* [1968] 1 All ER 433 86
Re A-F (Children) (Care Orders: Restrictions on Liberty) [2018] 427
Re B [2017] 428
Re B (A Minor) (Treatment and Secure Accommodation) [1997] 429
Re C (An Adult: Refusal of Medical Treatment) [1994] 182, 184
Re C (HIV test) [1999] 762
Re D [1976] 509
Re D [2017] 430
Re D (a child) [2019] 428
Re E [2012] 400–1, 856
Re F 17, 189, 190, 509, 571
Re F [1989] 491
Re J (Deprivation of Liberty: Hospital) [2022] 430
Re K (A Child) (Secure Accommodation Order: Right to Liberty) [2001] 427
Re L 403
Re L [2000] 229
Re M (Medical Treatment: Consent) [1999] 478
Re MB [1997] 181, 182, 472, 588
Re P 451
Re R (A minor: wardship: consent to medical treatment) [1991] 4 All ER 177 CA 401
Re T [1992] 184
Re T (A Minor) (Wardship: Medical Treatment) [1997] 409
Re W 398, 400, 403
Re Wyatt (A Child) (Medical Treatment: Continuation of Order) [2005] 411
Re X [2016] 430
Rees v *Darlington Memorial Hospital NHS Trust* [2003] 456, 458
Roe v *Ministry of Health* [1954] 58
RT v *LT & Anor* 186

S (a child) v *Royal Bournemouth and Christchurch Hospital NHS Trust* [2012] 158–9
Shakoor (Deceased) v *Situ* [2000] 882
Sidaway v *Bethlem Royal Hospital Governors* [1985] 196
Sister Salisbury 34–5, 835, 836
Skinner v *Scottish Ambulance Service and others* [2004] 383
Slade v *Battersea HMC* [1955] 348
Slater v *United Kingdom Central Council for Nursing, Midwifery and Health Visitors* 324
Smith v *Leech Brain* [1961] 62–3
Smith v *Tunbridge Wells HA* [1994] 198
Smith (Jean) v *Northamptonshire County Council* [2008] 341

Staff Nurse Jarvis 24, 29, 32, 34, 39, 45
Stephens v *Avery and Others* 217
Steven Neary 684
St George's Healthcare Trust 183
Storck v *Germany ECHR 406* [2005] 427
Strunk v *Strunk* 479
Stubbings v *Webb* 167

T v *T* [1988] 450, 452
Tarasoff Case [USA 1976] 226–7
Thake v *Maurice* 457
Tracey v *Cambridge University Hospitals NHS Foundation Trust and others* [2014] 846, 847

W v *Egdell* [1989] Disclosure in the Public Interest 228
Walker v *Northumberland County Council* [1994] 370
Watkins v *Birmingham City Council* [1975] 87

Watling v *Gloucester County Council* [1995] 880
Watts 110
Waugh v *British Railway Board* 223
Weir v *Chief Constable of Merseyside Police* 86
White and Others v *Chief Constable of the South Yorkshire Police and Others* 66
Whitehouse v *Jordan* [1981] 53
Wilsher v *Essex Area Health Authority* [1986] 76, 89, 466
Wilsher v *Essex AHA* [1988] 61
Winspear v *City Hospitals Sunderland NHSFT* [2015] 847
Woolgar v *Chief Constable of Sussex Police* [1999] 233–4

X v *Y* [1988] 228, 619, 769
XM v *Leicestershire Partnership Trust* [2020] 719

ZH (A Protected Party) v *Commissioner of Police of the Metropolis, Liberty and Another Intervening* [2013] 493

Table of statutes

UK

Acts

Abortion Act 1967 4, 225, 437, 439, 440, 442, 444–8, 450, 451, 511, 630
   s. 1(1)(d) 439
   ss. 1(1) and 5(2) 438
   s. 4 440
   s. 5(1) 438
Access to Health Records Act 1990 239, 240
   s. 3(1)(f) 239–40
Access to Justice Act 1999 12
Access to Medical Reports Act 1988 209, 241
Administration of Justice Act 1982
   s. 1(1)(a) 157
   s. 2(a) 458
   s. 17 871
Adoption Act 1958
   s. 50 643
   s. 50(1) 643
Adoption and Children Act 2002 645
Adults with Incapacity (Scotland) Act 2000 564, 744
Aids Control Act 1987 763
Assaults on Emergency Workers (Offences) Act 2018 609
   s. 1 610
   s. 1(2) 609
   s. 2 610

Care Act 2014 142, 145, 204, 352, 499, 537, 559, 661, 669–81, 685, 688, 708, 709, 893
   Pt 1 597
   Pt 2 139
   s. 1 673–4
   s. 2 674, 682
   s. 3 119, 675
   s. 8 675–6
   s. 13 676–7
   s. 18 682
   ss. 18–20 687

   s. 19 682
   s. 20 682
   s. 24 677–8
   s. 25 678–80
   ss. 31–33 512–14
   ss. 35–37 680
   s. 38 682
   s. 42 741
   ss. 42–45 560–2
   ss. 42–47 560
   s. 46 697
   s. 47 697, 741, 742
   s. 48 682
   s. 51 682
   ss. 58–66 413
   s. 67(4) 680
   s. 73 558, 682
   s. 81 100, 142, 204
   s. 89 131
   s. 90 131
   s. 92 132
   s. 95 131, 729
   ss. 96–102 537
   s. 98 729
   s. 103–7 538
   s. 109–116 531
   s. 112(2) 531
   s. 248 132
   Sched. 2 560
   Sched. 3 685–7
   Sched. 5 537
   Sched. 6 538
Carers and Disabled Children Act 2000 504, 687, 688
Carer's Leave Act 2023 283
Carers (Recognition and Services) Act 1995 687
Care Standards Act 2000 275, 559, 699
   s. 5 122
   s. 82(4)(b) 275

Children Act 1989 224, 227, 395, 400, 402, 406, 412, 414, 450, 452, 509, 698, 705
  Pt V 412
  s. 1 767
  s. 3(5) 399, 401
  s. 20 502
  s. 23C(4) 413
  s. 25 429
Children (Leaving Care) Act 2000 412, 413
Children Act 2004 413, 414, 423, 431
  s. 11 415
  s. 58 424
Children (Equal Protection from Assault) (Scotland) Act 2019 425
Children (Abolition of Defence of Reasonable Punishment) (Wales) Act 2020 425
Children and Families Act 2014 277, 280, 414
  Pt 2 431
Children and Social Work Act 2017 413
Children and Young Persons Act 1933 424
  s.1 140, 419, 424
  s. 1(1) 411
Children, Schools and Families Act 2010
  Pt 2 431
Chronic Sick and Disabled Persons Act 1970 663
  s. 2(1) 664
Civil Evidence Act 1968 254
Civil Liability (Contribution) Act 1978 77, 807
Civil Partnership Act 2004 299
Community Care (Delayed Discharges) Act of 2003 668, 684, 685
Community Care (Direct Payments) Act 1997 511
Community Care (Residential Accommodation) Act 1998 664
  s. 1 664
Community Discharge (Delayed Discharges) Act 2003 547
Compensation Act 2006 361
Congenital Disabilities (Civil Liability) Act 1976 55, 642
  s. 1(5) 55
Consumer Protection Act 1987 167, 352–7, 363, 373, 479, 536, 814
  Pt 1 386, 821
  s. 3 352–3
  s. 4 352–3
Contracts (Rights of Third Parties) Act 1999 747
Coronavirus Act 2020 768
Coroners Act 1988 862
Coroners and Justice Act 2009 41, 831, 832, 840, 848–9, 859–60, 862, 869, 872
  s. 5(1) 863
  s. 7 864

s. 10(2) 863
s. 20 857
s. 54 41–3
Sched. 5 719, 865
Corporate Manslaughter and Corporate Homicide Act 2007 38, 113, 360, 756
Courts and Legal Services Act 1990 169
Crime and Disorder Act 1998 365
  s. 34 40
Crime and Justice Act 2013 822
Crimes Act 1958 442
Criminal Evidence (Witness Anonymity) Act 2008 869
Criminal Injuries Compensation Act 1995 44
Criminal Justice Act 1988 609
  ss. 23–28 253
Criminal Justice Act 2003 26, 29, 32
  Sched. 3 29
Criminal Justice and Courts Act 2015 892
  s. 20 7, 35, 140, 509
  s. 20(3) 140
  s. 21 140
  s. 21(1) 141
Criminal Justice and Public Order Act 1994 637
Criminal Law Act 1977
  Sched. 1 28

Damages Act 1996
  s. 1(2) 159
Data Protection Act 1998 209
Data Protection Act 2018 19, 209–17, 220, 248
Defamation Act 2013 261, 530, 537
Disability Discrimination Act 1995 516
  s. 49A 666
Disability Discrimination Act 2005 295
Domestic Violence Crime and Victims Act (DVCV Act) 2004 369, 563

Education Act 1996
  s. 2(5) 507
Emergency Workers (Obstruction) Act 2006 609
Emergency Workers (Offences) Act 2018 609
Employer's Liability (Compulsory Insurance) Act 1969 334, 361, 362
Employer's Liability (Defective Equipment) Act 1969 354, 355, 362, 363
Employment Act 1988 293
Employment Act 2002 277
  s. 47 283
Employment Act 2008 277
Employment Relations Act 1999 277, 280

Employment Relations Act 2004 277
Employment Rights Act 1996 96, 277, 347
   s. 117 288
Employment Rights (Flexible Working) Act 2023 283
Enterprise and Regulatory Reform Act 2013 96, 277, 287, 333
   s. 17 97
   s. 19 98
   s. 69 377
Environmental Protection Act 1990 339
Equality Act 2006 294, 516
   s. 35 572
Equality Act 2010 263, 266, 270, 277, 279, 280, 295–306, 379, 491, 543, 544
   s. 20 301
   s. 149 304–5, 511
   Sched. 1 763
European Communities Act 1972 9–10
European Union (Withdrawal) Act 2018 9, 10

Factories Acts 12
Family Law Reform Act 1969 397–9
   s. 8 396, 397, 399, 431
   s. 8(3) 403
   ss. 8(1) and (2) 397
Family Reform Act 1987
   s. 27 627
Female Genital Mutilation Act 2003 459, 460
   s. 1(1) 459
   s. 5A 460
   s. 5B 461
Financial Services (Banking Reform) Act 2013 169
Freedom of Information Act 2000 19, 98, 99, 209, 210, 216, 236–40, 283, 782
   Pt 2 236
   s. 31 238
   s. 36 238
   s. 40 216
   s. 41 239
   s. 42 224
   s. 50 238
   s. 57(2) 238
Freedom of Information Act 2013 431

Gender Recognition Act 2004 14

Health Act 1999 311, 681, 791
   s. 18 125
   s. 60 311
   s. 60A 318
   Sched. 3 311

Health Act 2006 802
   s. 4 38
   s. 16 760
Health Act 2009 108, 792
   s. 2 143
   s. 11 515
   s. 60 884
Health (Tobacco, Nicotine etc. and Care) (Scotland) Act 2016 345
Health and Care (Staffing) (Scotland) Act 2019 95
Health and Safety at Work Act 1974 (HASWA) 12, 296, 332–42, 361, 375, 382, 386, 485, 537, 691
   s. 2 333–4, 336, 376
   s. 2(4) 293
   s. 3 336, 338, 376
   s. (6) 293
   s. 7 334, 336
   s. 8 334, 338
   s. 20 337–8
   s. 47 377
Health and Social Care Act 2001
   Pt 3 125
   s. 12 789
   s. 61 532
   s. 63 817
Health and Social Care (Community Health and Standards) Act 2003 120
   Pt 2 780
   s. 45 125
   s. 46 125
   s. 53A 760
Health and Social Care Act 2008 108, 127, 129–31, 220, 225, 327, 328, 335, 343, 699, 741, 750–2, 757–9, 770
   Reg. 17(2)(c) 247
   ss. 2–5 127–8
   s 20 131, 142, 729
   s. 29 335
   s. 30 335
   s. 33 335
   s. 45 125, 126
   s. 45A 788
   s. 45B 788
   s. 45C 788
   s 46 131
   s. 46(4) 126
   s. 52 791
   s. 112 318
   s. 129 757
   s. 145 682
   s. 157 532

Health and Social Care Act 2012 88, 89, 104, 106–10, 113, 114, 116, 120–4, 144, 145, 204, 252, 328, 619, 662, 701, 707, 724, 752, 760, 763, 792
    Pt 3 120
    s. 3 143
    s. 9(1) 114
    s. 13 116
    s. 18 752
    s. 23 114, 143
    s. 26 118
    s. 27 118
    ss. 61–71 120
    s. 62 121
    s. 66 122–3
    ss. 81–110 124
    s. 179 120
    s. 181 788
    ss. 182–189 789
    s. 185 790
    s. 200 125
    ss. 232–234 133–4
    ss. 232–249 132
    s. 234 107, 115, 126
    s. 299 595
    Sched. 8 120
    Sched. 16 132
    Sched. A1 114
Health and Social Care (Quality and Engagement) (Wales) Act 2020 345
    s. 3 345
Health Protection Agency Act 2004 760
Health Service Commissioner Act 1993 782, 784–6
    s. 14(4) 787
Health Services and Public Health Act 1968
    s. 63 108
    s. 63(2) 537
Homicide Act 1957 41
Hospital Complaints Procedure Act 1985 774, 778–9
Human Fertilisation and Embryology Act 1990 438, 442, 511, 535, 624, 625, 627, 629, 630, 634–6, 638–40, 643, 649, 650
    s. 1 636
    s. 1(1) 636
    s. 3 535
    s. 3A 637
    s. 4(1)(a) 640
    s. 11 640
    s. 13(5) 634, 635
    s. 30 643, 644
    s. 31ZA 629
    s. 33 642
    s. 36(i) 643
    s. 37 448
    s. 38 646
    Sched. 2 650
    Sched. 3 640
    Sched. 3ZA 641
Human Fertilisation and Embryology Act 2008 406, 625, 629, 630, 634, 635, 637, 639–40, 642, 644, 650, 655
    s. 24 629
    s. 31ZA 642
    ss. 33–38 627
    s. 35 628
    s. 37 641
    s. 54 644
    s. 55 645
    s. 59 644
    Sched. 2 649
Human Fertilisation and Embryology (Deceased Fathers) Act 2003 639
Human Fertilisation and Embryology (Disclosure of Information) Act 1992 642
    s. 33 642
Human Organ Transplant Act 1989 479–80
Human Reproductive Cloning Act 2001 636
Human Rights Act 1998 9 , 10, 13–19, 112, 216, 241–2, 395, 420, 494, 572, 681, 682, 775, 841, 862, 863, 892
    s. 6 682
    Sched.1 10, 14206, 267, 420
Human Tissue Act 2004 406, 475, 476, 479, 482, 484, 485, 535, 861
    s. 27(4) 475–6
    s. 33 476
    s. 43 476
    s. 47 837

Infant Life Preservation Act 1929 437, 438, 442–4, 448
Interception of Communications Act 1985 217

Justice Act (Northern Ireland) 2015 277
Justice and Security Act 2013 19

Law Reform (Contributory Negligence) Act 1945
    s. 1 161
Legal Aid, Sentencing and Punishment of Offenders Act 2012
    s. 44 169
Limitation Act 1980 167
    s. 14 166–7
    s. 33 168
Local Government Act 1974 782, 784, 785

Local Government and Public Involvement in Health Act 2007 788, 789
  s. 221 788, 789
  s. 222(2) 128
  s. 223A 790

Marriage (Same Sex Couples) Act 2013 297
Medicinal Products (Prescription by Nurses) Act 1992 814
Medicines Act 1968 798–800, 817
  s. 4 820
  s. 52 34
  s. 53 799
  Sched. 1 820
Medicines Act 1971 800
Mental Capacity Act 2005 17, 128, 176, 178, 180, 184, 187–95, 205, 234, 248, 396, 398–400, 426, 450–3, 461, 472, 491–9, 501–3, 507, 509–11, 513, 516, 517, 534, 535, 539, 542, 547–53, 556, 563–5, 571, 587–9, 601, 683, 684, 695, 735, 740, 742–4, 748, 792, 831, 841–4, 847, 850, 851, 853, 855, 856
  s. 1 191
  s. 1(2) 177
  s. 1(4) 191
  s. 1(5) 843
  s. 2 177, 185–6, 744
  s. 2(1) 397, 500
  s. 2(2) 548
  s. 2(4) 177
  s. 2 177, 185–6, 744
  s. 4 192, 834, 844
  s. 4(5) 850
  s. 4(7) 848
  s. 5 844
  s. 9 564
  s. 15 501
  ss. 30–34 534
  s. 42 844
  s. 44 35, 140, 563
  s. 44(2) 509, 699
  Sched. A1 813
Mental Capacity (Amendment) Act 2019 509
Mental Health Act 1959
  s. 128 508
Mental Health Act 1983 66, 68, 127, 128, 130, 176, 182, 189, 195, 234, 248, 305, 352, 450, 451, 490, 491, 493–7, 550, 552, 556, 570, 572, 573, 579, 586–9, 595, 598, 599, 601, 695–7, 791
  Pt 4 552, 583, 792
  Pt 7 744
  s. 3 188, 862

  s. 5(2) 181
  s. 5(4) 574
  s. 7 590
  ss. 17A–17G 591–4
  s. 20A 594–5
  s. 20B 594–5
  s. 26(i) 579–80
  s. 37 33
  s. 41 33
  s. 57 584
  s. 58 584, 585
  s. 62A 585
  s. 63 584
  s. 73 571
  s. 115 696
  s. 117 134
  s. 118 572
  s. 127 140
  s. 129 696
  s. 130B 588
  s. 131 493
  s. 132 582
  s. 134 790
  s. 135 597–9, 697
  s. 135(1) 562, 596
  s. 135 (4) 596
  s. 135(3ZA) 596
  s. 136 597–9
  s. 136A 598
  s. 145 583
Mental Health Act 2007 400, 492, 494, 556, 570, 572, 573, 576, 577, 588–90, 595, 601, 695, 696
  s. 12 578–9
  s. 17 590
  s. 27 585
  s. 32 591
  s. 68 600
  s 135 596
Mental Health (Approved Functions) Act 2012 579
Mental Health (Discrimination) Act 2013 305
Mental Health (Patients in the Community) Act 1995 591
Mental Health Units (Use of Force) Act 2018 599
Mesothelioma Act 2014 158, 170, 766
Misuse of Drugs Act 1971 798–800, 802
  s. 4(1) 802
  s. 5(3) 802

National Assistance Act 1948 697
  s. 21(1)(a) 682
  s. 26 682

s. 22 591, 664
s. 47 670, 697
s. 48 697
National Health Service Act 1946 105
　s. 25 693
National Health Service Act 1977 88, 105, 110
　s. 1 110
　s. 11 760
National Health Service Act 2006 88, 105–9, 122, 134, 143, 225, 686
　s. 1 120
　s. 1(1) 122
　s. 1(3) 109
　s. 1A 110
　s. 1H 114
　s. 3 116, 120
　s. 7(A) 134
　ss. 12A–12D 515
　s. 13A 114, 119, 538
　s. 13B 114
　s. 13E 123
　s. 13N 121, 670
　ss. 14P–14Z24 118
　s. 14Z1 670
　s. 14Z8 135
　ss. 23G–23K 118
　s. 28 124
　ss. 30–65 120
　s. 31 120
　s. 77 125
　s. 251 532
　s. 258 120
　Sched. 1 109
　Sched. 7–10 120
National Health Service (Amendment) Act 1986
　s. 1 335
　s. 1 335
National Health Service and Community Care Act 1990 591
　s. 47 590
National Minimum Wage (NMW) Act 1998 284–5
NHS and Community Care Act 1990 120, 124, 662
　s. 47 562
　s. 60 272, 362
　Sched. 8 362
NHS Consequential Amendments Act 2006 105
NHS Redress Act 2006 149, 171–2
NHS Reform and Health Care Professions Act 2002 326, 327, 789
　s. 20 788
　s. 20(2) 788

Northern Ireland Disability Discrimination Act 1975 295
Northern Ireland (Executive Formation etc) Act 2019 443
Nurses, Midwives and Health Visitors Act 1979 310
Nurse Staffing Levels (Wales) Act 2016 95

Occupiers' Liability Act 1957 164, 347–52, 361, 536, 691
　s. 2(1) 347
　s. 2 (2) 347
　s. 2(3) 350
　s. 2(4)(a) 348
　s. 2(4)(b) 349
Occupiers' Liability Act 1984 165, 347–52
　s. 1(4) 351
Offences Against the Person Act 1861 178, 424, 447, 448
　s. 18 34, 424
　s. 20 34, 424
　s. 47 424
　s. 58 437, 442, 447
　s. 59 447
　s. 60 447

Personal Care at Home Act 2010 668
Police Act 1997
　Pt V 275
Police and Criminal Evidence Act 1984 24, 230, 241, 369, 448, 508, 574, 598, 614
　s. 17(e) 696
　s. 78 25
　Sched 1 231
　ss. 9, 12 and 14 230–1
Police Reform Act 2002 365
Policing and Crime Act 2017 596–9, 697
　s. 80 597, 598
　s. 81 598
　s. 82 598
　s. 83 598
　s. 136 597
Powers of Attorney Act 1971 742
Power of Attorney Act 1985 743
Presumption of Death Act 2013 839
Presumption of Death (Northern Ireland) Act 2009 839
Presumption of Death (Scotland) Act 1977 839
Prevention of Terrorism (Temporary Provisions) Act 1988 220
　s. 11 225
Prohibition of Female Circumcision Act 1985 458–9
Protection from Harassment Act 1997 86, 302, 378–80
Protection from Redundancy (Pregnancy and Family Leave) Act 2023 280

Protection of Children Act 1999 274, 275, 421
Protection of Freedoms Act 2012 240
  Pt 5 276
  s. 87(1) 276

Provisions of the Children Act 2004 415
Psychoactive Substances Act 2016 823
Public Health (Control of Disease) Act 1984 225, 751, 752, 757, 770
  s. 11 753
  s. 11(4) 755
  s. 45C 757–8
Public Interest Disclosure Act 1998 72, 96–101, 105, 204, 241, 287, 289, 347, 525, 529, 530, 690, 756

Regulation of Investigatory Powers Act 2000 224, 286
Rehabilitation of Offenders Act 1974 269
Road Traffic Act 1972 28
Road Traffic Act 1985 822
Road Traffic Act 1988 220, 703
  s. 170 225

Safeguarding Vulnerable Groups Act 2006 274, 276, 508, 563
  ss. 21–27 276
Serious Crime Act 2015
  s. 66 419
Sex Discrimination Act 1975 280, 305
Sexual Offences Act 1956
  s. 7 508
  s. 8 508
Sexual Offences Act 2003 508
Sexual Offenders Act 1997 274, 275
Sexual Offenders Act 2003 275
  Pt 1 275
Social Action, Responsibility and Heroism Act 2015 52
Social Services and Well-being (Wales) Act 2014 545, 670
  Pt 4 597
  s. 119 429
Social Work (Scotland) Act 1968
  s. 12/13A 682
Suicide Act 1961 11, 15, 848, 849, 851–2
  s. 2 855
  ss. 1 and 2(1) 848–9
Supreme Court Act 1981 224
  s. 32A 158
  s. 33 152, 224
  s. 34 224
Surrogacy Arrangements Act 1985 630, 643, 644

Tax Credits Act 2002 291
Terrorism Act 2000
  s. 44 18
Theft Act 1968
  s. 1(1) 34
Tobacco Advertising and Promotion Act 2002 381
Trade Union Reform and Employment Rights Act 1993 347
Traffic Act 1991 225

Unfair Contract Terms Act 1977 164–6, 173, 738, 880
  s. 11 738

Vaccine Damage Payments Act 1979 764

Wills Act 1837
  s. 9 871

Youth Justice and Criminal Evidence Act 1999 40

SIs
Abortion Regs 1968 448
Abortion (Northern Ireland) Regs, 2020, 2021 and 2022 443
Agency Workers Regs 2010 285

Care Quality Commission (Membership) Regs 2008 128
Children (Secure Accommodation) Regs 1991 429
Children Secure Accommodation (Wales) Regs 2015 429
Civil Procedure Rules (CPR) 27, 150, 151, 225, 254, 767
  Pt 7 153
  Pt 27 151
  Pt 28 151
  Pt 29 152
  Pt 31 152
  Pt 35 259
  Pt 36 153
  Pt 37 153
Commission on Human Medicine Regs 820
Conditional Fee Regs 2000 and 2003 169
Consumer Protection (Distance Selling) Regs 2000 356
Control of Substances Hazardous to Health (COSHH) Regs 1988 359
Control of Substances Hazardous to Health (COSHH) Regs 2002 383
Coroners' Investigations Regs 2013 860
Coroners (Inquest) Rules 2013 863, 864
CQC membership Amendment Regs 2013 128
Criminal procedure rules 2015 27

Damages-Based Agreements (DBA) Regs 169
Deprivation of Liberty Safeguards (DoLS) Regs 494–5
Duty of Candour Procedure (Scotland) Regs 2018 345

Environmental Information Regs 210

Fixed-term Employees (Prevention of Less Favourable Treatment) Regs 2002 291

General Data Protection Regs 2016 283
General Product Safety Regs 1994 356

Hazardous to Health 2002 359–60
Health and Personal Social Services (NI) Order 1972 (SI 1972/1265) 682
Health and Safety (Consultation with Employees) Regs 1996 338
Health and Safety (Display Screen Equipment) Regs 1999 339
Health and Safety (First Aid) Regs 1981 382
Health and Safety (Sharp Instruments in Healthcare) Regs 2013 383–5
Health and Social Care Act 2008 (Regulated Activities) Regs 2014 129–31, 247, 335, 343
Health and Social Care Act Regs 2009 699
Health Protection (Notification) Regs 2010 751, 753
   2010/657 751
   2010/658 751–2
   2010/659 752
Health Service (Control of Patient Information) Regs 2002 532
HIV Testing Kits and Services Regs 763
Human Medicines Regs 820

Information and Consultation of Employees Regs 2004 283, 291
Ionising Radiation (Medical Exposure) Regs 2017 725, 726

Lifting Operations and Lifting Equipment Regs 1998 (LOLER) 375

Management of Health and Safety at Work Regs 1999 339–40, 376, 383
Manual Handling Operations Regs 1992 376
Manual Handling Operations Regs 2002 339
Manual Handling Regs 373–5
Medicines for Human Use (Clinical Trials) Regs 2004 528, 529, 532, 535
Mental Health Act 1983 (Places of Safety) Regs 2017 598
Misuse of Drugs Regs 2001 798, 801–3, 817
Misuse of Drugs (Supply to Addicts) Regs 1997 225, 822

National Health Service (Venereal Diseases) Regs 1974 619
National Health Service Trust Development Authority Regs 124
NHS (Clinical Negligence Scheme) Regs 1996 171
Nursing and Midwifery Order 2001 311, 313, 314, 322, 326

Part-time Workers (Prevention of Less Favourable Treatment) Regs 2000 291
Personal Protective Equipment at Work Regs 1992 354, 382–3
Personal Protective Equipment at Work Regs 1999 339
Privacy and Electronic Communications Regs 210
Provision and Use of Work Equipment Regs 1998 339–41, 374, 375, 383

Quality and Safety of Organs intended for Transplantation Regs 2012 480

Reporting of Injuries, Diseases and Dangerous Occurrences Regs 1995 (RIDDOR) 342

Safety Representatives and Safety Committees Regs 1977 338, 382

Telecommunications (Lawful Business Practices) (Interception of Communications) Regs 2000 286
   2004 regulations 780

Working Time Regs 284, 291
Workplace (Health, Safety and Welfare Regulations) 1999 339, 341

EU

European Convention on Human Rights 1950 10, 110, 202, 238, 268, 277, 376, 426, 491, 529, 565, 571, 601
   Art 2 443, 445
   Art 3 112, 404, 423, 586
   Art 5 493–5, 497, 502, 552, 587, 601, 683, 812
   Art 5(1) 763
   Art 5.4 195
   Art 6 27, 275
   Art 8 10, 17, 112, 410, 420, 443, 586, 628, 682, 812, 813, 846, 855
   Art 8(1) 544
   Art 8(2) 228
   Art 10 99, 262
   Art 14 543, 544
   Protocol 1 18

Directives

Directive 2012/26/EU 820
Directive 65/66/EEC 528

EC Chemical Agents Directive 359
EC Directive
  2001/20/EC 528–9
  90/269 375
EC Framework Directive 373
EEC Directive 76/207 280
EU Organ Donation Directive 480
EU Part-Time Work Directive 285
European Directive 528
European Directive 97/43/Euratom 725

European Pregnant Workers Directive 278, 377
European Tissue Directive 482

Medical Devices Directives 357

Tissue and Cells Directive 650

Working Time Directive (WTD) 283–4

GLOBAL

UN Charter on the Rights of the Child 423
United Nations Convention on the Rights of the Child (1989) 19, 395

Abbreviations

The health services are awash with abbreviations and jargon. It would, however, be immeasurably tedious and unrealistic to ignore these and always use the full words. Some of the most commonly used abbreviations are therefore set out here. Where there is any possibility of confusion, words are spelt out in full.

ABI Association of British Insurers
ABPI Association of the British Pharmaceutical Industry
ACAS Advisory, Conciliation and Arbitration Service
ACGT Advisory Committee on Genetic Testing
ADR Adverse Drug Reaction
A&E accident and emergency department
AGMR Advisory Group on Medical Research
AID artificial insemination by donor
AIDS acquired immune deficiency syndrome
AIH artificial insemination by husband
AIP artificial insemination by partner
ALB arm's-length bodies
AMHP approved mental health professional
ARC AIDS-related complex
ASW approved social worker
AVMA Action for the Victims of Medical Accidents
BARNA British Anaesthetic and Recovery Nurses Association
BCA British Chiropractic Association
BID brought in dead
BMA British Medical Association
BMJ *British Medical Journal*
BNF *British National Formulary*
BP blood pressure
BPAS British Pregnancy Advisory Service
CAA Comprehensive Area Assessment
CAB Citizens' Advice Bureau
CAM complementary and alternative medicines
CCC Conduct and Competence Committee
CCETSW Central Council for Education and Training in Social Work
CCIAG Critical Care Information Advisory Group
CDRP crime and disorder reduction partnerships
CE Conformité Européenne (marking following EC directive 93/68/EEC)
CESDI Confidential Enquiry into Stillbirths and Deaths in Infancy
CESU Clinical Effectiveness Support Unit
CFA conditional fee agreement
CGWTs Care Group Workforce Teams
CHAI Commission for Healthcare Audit and Inspection (known as the Healthcare Commission)
CHC community health council
CHI Commission for Health Improvement (now CHAI)
CHRE Council for Healthcare Regulatory Excellence (formerly CRHCP) (now the PSA)
CICA Criminal Injuries Compensation Authority
CMI Chartered Management Institute
CMO Chief Medical Officer
CNHC Complementary and Natural Healthcare Council
CNR cell nuclear replacement
CNST Clinical Negligence Scheme for Trusts
COREC Central Office for Research Ethics Committees (replaced in 2007 by NRES)
COSHH Control of Substances Hazardous to Health (Regulations)
CPD continuing professional development
CPN community psychiatric nurse
CPPIH Commission for Patient and Public Involvement in Health
CPR cardiopulmonary resuscitation
CPS Crown Prosecution Service
CQC Care Quality Commission
CRHCP Council for the Regulation of Health Care Professionals (now *see* CHRE)
CSAG Clinical Standards Advisory Group
CSCI Commission for Social Care Inspection
CSIP Care Services Improvement Partnership
CSSD central sterile supply department
CTO Compulsory Treatment Order
D and C dilatation and curettage
DBERR Department for Business, Enterprise and Regulatory Reform
DBS Disclosure and Barring Service (replacing the Independent Safeguarding Service)
DCA Department for Constitutional Affairs

DCSF Department for Children, Schools and Families (formerly DfES)
DH Department of Health (now DHSC, Department of Health and Social Care)
DHA district health authority
DHSC Department of Health and Social Care
DHSS Department of Health and Social Security (now divided into DHSC, Department of Health and Social Care and DWP, Department for Work and Pensions)
DMD Drug Misuse Database
DNAR do not attempt resuscitation
DNR do not resuscitate
DoLS Deprivation of Liberty Safeguards
DPA Data Protection Act 1998
DPP Director of Public Prosecutions
DSS Department of Social Security (now DWP, Department for Work and Pensions)
DWP Department for Work and Pensions
EC European Community
ECC Ethics and Confidentiality Committee
ECHR European Court of Human Rights
ECJ European Court of Justice
ECL emergency care leads
ECP emergency care practitioner
ECT electroconvulsive therapy
EEA European Economic Area
EHR electronic health record
EHRC Equality and Human Rights Commission
EL executive letter (guidance from DH)
ELS Existing Liabilities Scheme
ENDPB executive non-departmental public body
EPR electronic patient record
ERG external reference group
eSET elective single embryo transfer
ET embryo transfer
EWC expected week of confinement
GDC General Dental Council
GIFT gamete intrafallopian transfer
GMC General Medical Council
GMS general medical services
GP general practitioner
GSL general sales list
GTAC Gene Therapy Advisory Committee
GUM genito-urinary medicine
GWC General Whitley Council
HAI hospital-acquired infection
HASC(CHS)A Health and Social Care (Community Health and Standards) Act 2003
HASWA Health and Safety at Work Act
HCPC Health and Care Professions Council (replacing HPC)
HCSS healthcare support staff
HEI higher education institution
HFEA Human Fertilisation and Embryology Authority
HGAC Human Genetics Advisory Commission
HGC Human Genetics Commission
HIV human immunodeficiency virus
HPA Health Protection Agency
HPC Health Professions Council (renamed HCPC)
HRA Health Research Authority (established 2011)
HSC Health and Safety Commission
HSC Health Service Commissioner
HSC health service circular
HSCIC Health and Social Care Information Centre
HSE Health and Safety Executive
HTA Human Tissue Authority
IAG Independent Advisory Group
IBB Independent Barring Board
ICAS Independent Complaints Advocacy Services
ICO Information Commissioner's Office
ICRS integrated care records service
IC(T)U intensive care (treatment) unit
IDMG inter-departmental ministerial group
IM and T information management and technology
IMCA independent mental capacity advocate
IMHA independent mental health advocate
ISA Independent Safeguarding Authority (replaced by DBS)
IUD intrauterine device
IV intravenous(ly)
IVF in vitro fertilisation
LA local authority
LBC liquid-based cytology
LCP Liverpool Care Pathway
LHB local health board (equivalent of PCT in Wales)
LINKS Local Involvement Networks
LOLER Lifting Operations and Lifting Equipment Regulations
LPA lasting power of attorney
LREC local research ethics committee
LSA Local Supervising Authority
LSC Legal Services Commission
LSP local service provider
MA maternity allowance
MCA Mental Capacity Act
MCA Medicines Control Agency (see MHRA)
MDA Medical Devices Agency (see MHRA)
MDU Medical Defence Union
MGN Mirror Group Newspapers
MHAC Mental Health Act Commission
MHRA Medicines and Healthcare products Regulatory Agency (since 1 April 2003)
MPP maternity period pay
MREC multi-centre research ethics committee
MRSA methicillin-resistant *Staphylococcus aureus*
MSW maternity support worker
NAI non-accidental injury

NAO	National Audit Office	**PPIFs**	patient and public involvement forums
NASP	national application service provider	**PREP**	post-registration education and practice
NCAA	National Clinical Assessment Authority	**PRN**	*pro re nata* (as required, whenever necessary)
NCAS	National Clinical Assessment Service	**PRSB**	Professional Records Standards Body
NCSC	National Care Standards Commission	**PSA**	Professional Standards Authority for Health and Social Care (replacing CHRE)
NFI	National Fraud Initiative		
NFR	not for resuscitation	**PUWER**	Provision and Use of Work Equipment Regulations
NHS	National Health Service	**PVS**	persistent vegetative state
NHSBT	NHS Blood and Transplant	**QA**	quality assurance
NHSTDA	NHS Trust Development Authority	**QC**	Queen's Counsel
NHSFT	NHS Foundation Trust	**QOF**	quality outcome framework
NHSLA	National Health Service Litigation Authority	**QSG**	Quality Surveillance Group
NHSU	National Health Service University	**QW**	qualifying week
NICE	National Institute for Health and Care Excellence	**RATE**	Regulatory Authority for Tissue and Embryos
NIGB	National Information and Governance Board for Health and Social Care	**RCM**	Royal College of Midwifery
		RCN	Royal College of Nursing
NIHR	National Institute for Health Research	**RCP**	Royal College of Psychiatrists
NMC	Nursing and Midwifery Council	**RCPCH**	Royal College of Paediatrics and Child Health
NMQP	non-medically qualified practitioners	**RCS**	Royal College of Surgeons
NMW	national minimum wage	**REC**	research ethics committee
NPEU	National Perinatal Epidemiology Unit	**RES**	Research Ethics Service
NPfIT	National Programme for Information Technology	**RIDDOR**	Reporting of Injuries, Diseases and Dangerous Occurrences Regulations
NPRB	National Pay Review Body		
NPSA	National Patient Safety Agency	**RMN**	registered mental nurse
NQB	National Quality Board	**RMO**	responsible medical officer
NRES	National Research Ethics Service (replaced COREC in 2007, now RES, the Research Ethics Service)	**RSI**	repetitive strain injury
		SAP	single assessment process
NRLS	National Reporting and Learning System	**SCIE**	Social Care Institute for Excellence
NRT	nicotine replacement therapy	**SCPHN**	specialist community public health nurse
NSDU	National Safeguarding Delivery Unit	**SCR**	summary care record
NSF	National Service Framework	**SEN**	state enrolled nurse
ODP	operating department practitioner	**SHA**	strategic health authority
OFV	opportunities for volunteering scheme	**SLA**	service level agreement
OOS	occupational overuse syndrome	**SMP**	statutory maternity pay
OPD	Outpatients department	**SOP**	standard operating procedures
OPSI	Office of Public Sector Information	**SPP**	statutory paternity pay
OTC	over the counter	**SRSC**	Safety Representative and Safety Committee
PALS	Patient Advice and Liaison Service	**SSI**	Social Services Inspectorate
PBC	prudential borrowing code	**SSP**	statutory sick pay
PCC	Professional Conduct Committee	**STD**	sexually transmitted disease
PCG	primary care group	**TB**	tuberculosis
PCMH	Plea and Case Management Hearing	**T+P**	temperature and pulse
PCT	primary care trust	**TUR & ER 93**	Trade Union Reform and Employee Rights Act 1993
PDR	personal development review		
PEP	post-exposure prophylaxis	**UKCC**	United Kingdom Central Council for Nursing, Midwifery and Health Visiting (now NMC, Nursing and Midwifery Council)
PGD	pre-implantation genetic diagnosis		
PGD	patient group directions		
PIAG	Patient Information Advisory Group	**UKCRC**	United Kingdom Clinical Research Collaboration
PMS	primary medical services	**UKECA**	United Kingdom Ethics Committee Authority
POM	prescription-only medicine	**ULTRA**	Unrelated Live Transplant Regulatory Authority
POVA	protection of vulnerable adults	**VBS**	Vetting and Barring Scheme
PPE	personal protective equipment	**VD**	venereal disease
		WDC	workforce development confederation
		WTD	Working Time Directives

Preface to ninth edition

It is now almost 30 years since the first edition of this book was published and there have been a number of changes and developments in the law since the last edition. The Supreme Court's decisions continue to impact of a nurses duty of care to patients and the Labour Government has announced new Acts of Parliament relating to health and care, for example the Supreme Court decision in *McCulloch* v *Forth Valley Health Board* [2023] clarifies the distinction between the professional practice standard and the advisory role of the nurse. The King's speech of 2024 set out the long awaited changes to the Mental health Act 1983 and a private member's bill on assisted dying has passed its second reading and might become law. Absent from the Kings Speech was any mention of the long awaited changes to the deprivation of liberty safeguards under the Mental Capacity Act 2005 or of a revised code of practice to the 2005 Act being introduced.

In terms of professional regulation, this edition undertakes a comprehensive review of the Nursing and Midwifery Council's fitness to practice procedures and considers the impact of the professional duty of candour on fitness to practice cases.

The High Court and Court of protection have had a number of cases that have considered the deprivation of liberty of minors. The family division of the High Court has established a deprivation of liberty Court to consider cases of children under 16 who are deprived of their liberty. The Court has also set out the interface between Gillick competence and the Mental Capacity Act 2005.

Knowledge of these developments is essential for nurses to ensure that they discharge their legal duties and meet the standards set out in the NMC Code.

Acknowledgements

I would like to thank Sharon for her help and support with this book.

– Richard Griffith

I'd like to thank first of all Professor Bridgit Dimond for being the author of this text from its inception to the present. Where we have changed, altered or updated the text we were mindful that we wanted to remain faithful to the ethos of this book; that it is clear, relevant and useful to all registered nurses and healthcare professionals. I also would like to thank my wife Nikki and my son James for supporting me in all that I do. I am also grateful to my work colleagues in particular Rachel and Maria for supporting me workwise during the past few years. Finally I'd like to thank Pearson for all their support and expertise.

– Iwan Dowie

Part I
General Principles Affecting all Nurses

Chapter 1

Professionalism, the Legal System and Human Rights

This chapter discusses

- Professionalism
- Criminal liability
- Professional liability
- Civil liability
- Accountability to employer
- Professionalism and accountability
- Sources of law
- Differences between civil and criminal law
- Civil actions
- Judicial review
- Legal personnel and legal complaints
- Legal language
- Human Rights Act 1998
- Freedom of Information Act 2000
- Devolved law-making powers

Introduction

This book is about the professionalism of the registered nurse. Professionalism can be defined as the competence, skills and values expected of a registered nurse, and a key theme of the Nursing and Midwifery Council (NMC) Code[1] emphasises the need to promote professionalism and trust. Registered nurses are required to uphold the reputation of the profession at all times by displaying a personal commitment to the standards of practice and behaviour set out in the Code, and to be law abiding and of good character. Registered nurses must be a model of integrity and leadership.

4 Chapter 1 Professionalism, the Legal System and Human Rights

This should lead to trust and confidence in the profession from patients, people receiving care, other healthcare professionals and the public.

Professionalism is underpinned by accountability, and registered nurses who fall below the legal or professional requirements imposed on them will be held to account for their acts and omissions.

Professionalism

This book is concerned with the law that underpins the professionalism and accountability of nurses. Four main fields of accountability in law are identified and discussed in detail. It might be considered that the most important has been omitted, i.e. accountability to oneself. Nurses often argue that they are accountable to themselves for their acts and omissions. Such an argument is characteristic of the altruistic nature of the profession. A nurse who harms a patient through their acts or omissions will often feel remorse and will reflect on their practice to prevent a recurrence. However, this cannot be regarded as a nurse truly holding themselves to account as they cannot apply sanctions or provide redress for the person who has been wronged.

Figure 1.1 illustrates the many areas of law that concern the nurse, and most of these topics are considered in Part I. Some of the more specialist areas such as the Abortion Act 1967, are considered in Part II of the book, which deals with different specialties. In this introductory

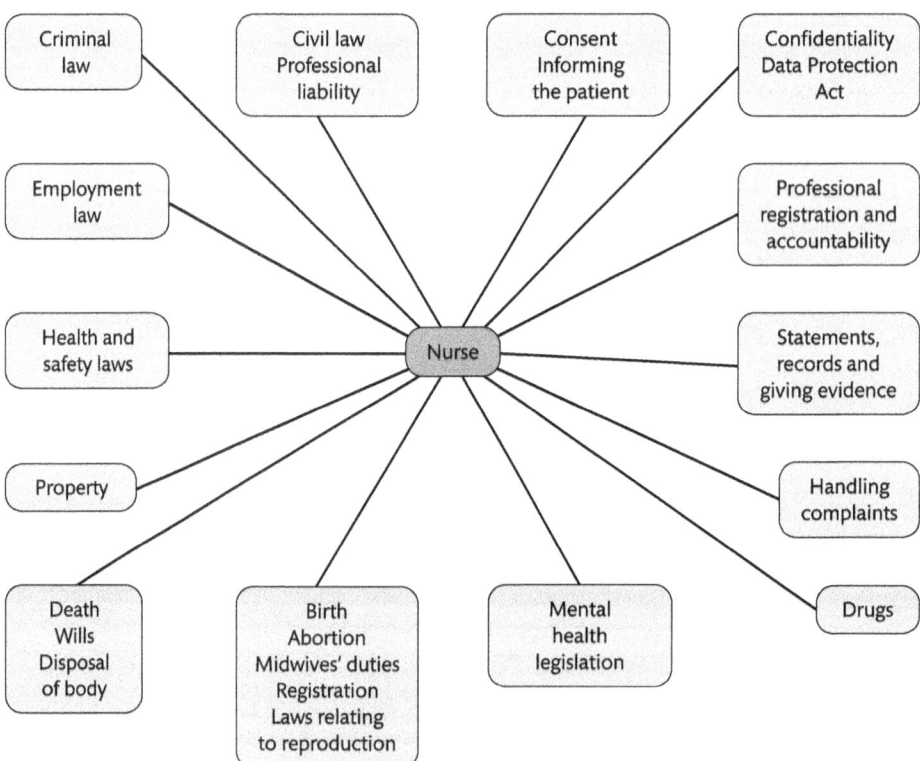

Figure 1.1 Areas that concern the nurse

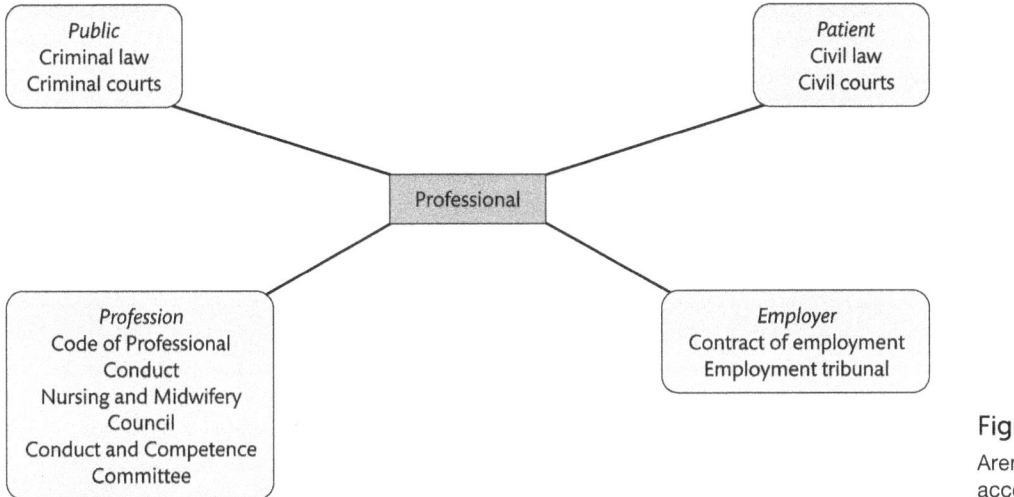

Figure 1.2
Arenas of accountability

chapter, the professionalism of nurses will be considered alongside the four fields of accountability that they face.

When a patient suffers harm or there is loss of or damage to property, the nurse may be called to account in four different courts and tribunals. Not all actions will be heard in all four, but they are rarely mutually exclusive and we shall give an example of an incident to illustrate the different procedures that could involve all four. Figure 1.2 illustrates the four arenas of accountability: accountability in the civil and criminal courts, in disciplinary proceedings and before the committees of the NMC.

A recent analysis of cases relating to nurses, the medical defence union (MDU) found that it was common for those nurses to have several different investigations launched into a single incident. This is known as multiple jeopardy (MDU 2022).[2]

Nurses' exposure to multiple jeopardy is founded on the multifaceted nature of the duty they owe to their patients and the nature of their accountability. Accountability underpins the professionalism, integrity and probity of nurses. It holds nurses answerable for their acts or omissions to a range of higher authorities and legally binds the nurse to their rules and regulations.

Criminal liability

Practical dilemma 1.1 The over generous vending machine

A thirsty nurse put money into a hospital vending machine to buy a can of lemonade and the machine dispensed 27 cans instead of one. The nurse kept 16 cans and gave the rest to her colleagues. Her actions were recorded on CCTV and her employer began their own investigation and reported the matter to the police.

In a case like this, it is highly likely that, after investigation by the police, a decision might be taken to prosecute the nurse for a criminal offence in connection to the taking of the extra cans of lemonade. Offences are classified as indictable or summary. An indictable offence is one that is heard before a judge and jury in the Crown Court, such as murder, manslaughter, rape and other very serious offences. A **summary offence** is one heard by the magistrates in a magistrates' court, such as driving without due care and attention and some parking offences. Many offences can be tried in either a magistrates' court or the Crown Court and are known as 'triable either way'. Theft is an offence that is triable either way. (For further discussion on this see chapter 2.)

Figure 1.3 shows the system of our criminal courts. Even where a case is to be heard in the Crown Court because it concerns an offence that can be tried only on **indictment**, a short appearance by the defendant will still take place before the magistrates. A date will be set for the Plea and Case Management Hearing (PCMH) (see chapter 2).

As an alternative to **prosecution** the police can issue a simple caution if the person admits the offence. This formal warning is not a conviction but will form part of a person's criminal

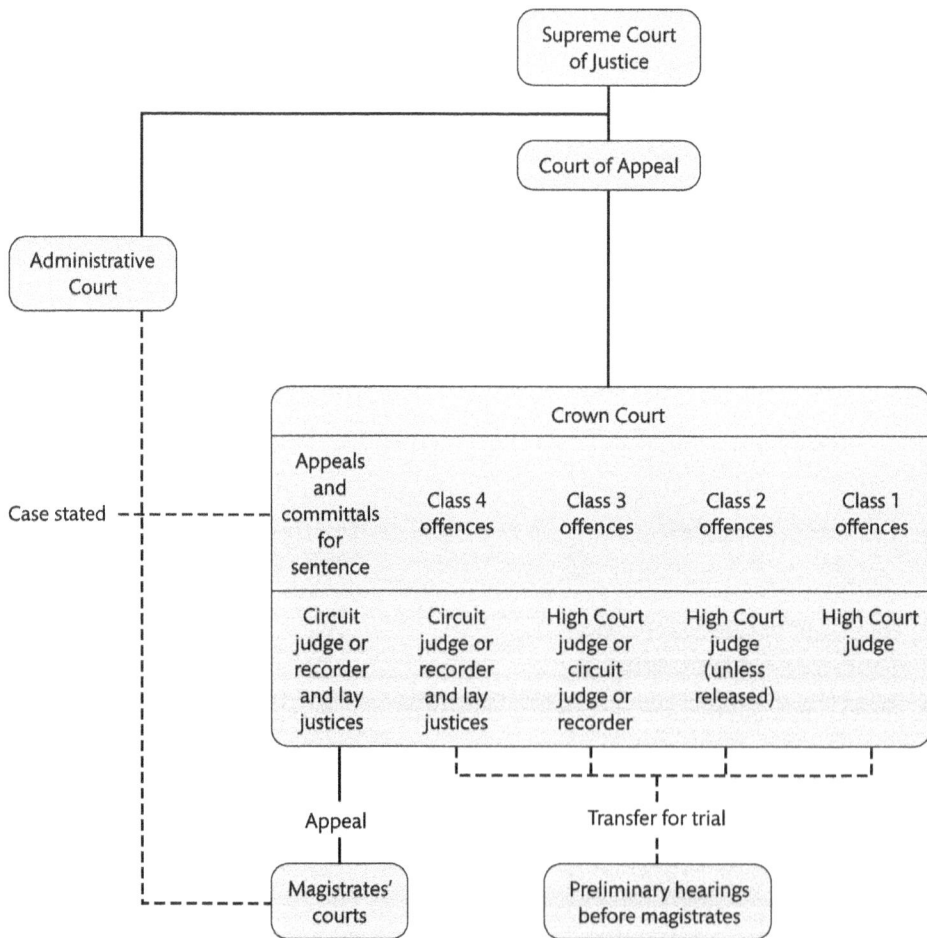

Figure 1.3
System of criminal courts

record and will be revealed in a Disclosure and Barring Service (DBS) check when a nurse seeks a new job. In the case set out above, the nurse accepted a police caution for theft.

Criminal charges in relation to the care of the patient were once rare, but following the public outcry arising from the findings of the inquiries into poor care and avoidable deaths of patients in Mid Staffordshire[3] and South Wales[4] the government sought to restore public confidence in their supervision and management of the National Health Service by making it a criminal offence for a care worker, which includes nurses, to ill-treat or wilfully neglect a patient in their care (Criminal Justice and Courts Act 2015, section 20).

(The nature of criminal proceedings is considered at greater length in chapter 2 and laws relating to death in chapter 28. Changes to the funding of defendants in criminal cases are also considered in chapter 2.)[5]

Professional liability

In Practical Dilemma 1.1, the nurse referred herself to the NMC once she had accepted a police caution for theft, as she recognised that her actions called into question her fitness to practice. After preliminary investigation had taken place, a Fitness to Practise Committee (FtPC) would hear the case to decide if the nurse was unfit to practice by reason of her misconduct and, if so, whether she should be removed from the Register. Information goes to the NMC from a variety of sources about the conduct of a nurse and in a case like this the police would also report it to the registration body. Non-criminal misconduct may also be reported. The nurse could argue that the special circumstances of the case do not warrant her being removed from the Register. (The full details of the powers and procedures of the FtPC are discussed in chapter 11.) The members who make up the constitute the FtPC are concerned with protecting the public from the unprofessional behaviour of a nurse; their intention is not to punish the nurse. The powers of the FtPC are set out in Box 1.1. Following any decision by the FtPC, an appeal on a point of law can be made to the High Court, which can instigate a **judicial review**.

Box 1.1 Powers of the fitness to practise commitee

Following investigation by the Investigating Committee and referral to the Fitness to Practise Commitee of the NMC, after a finding of unfitness to practise by the nurse the Fitness to Practise Commitee can take one of the following courses:

1. No action
2. Refer respondent to the Health Committee or to screeners
3. Postpone decision or issue interim order
4. Strike off the Register
5. Issue a caution (for 1–5 years) or condition of practice order (for 1–3 years)
6. Suspend from registration (for up to 1 year).

Civil liability

The financial loss to the vending machine company in the scenario set out in Practical Dilemma 1.1 can be recovered through the civil courts (Figure 1.4). In the civil courts, the **claimant** has to establish **liability** of the defendant on a **balance of probabilities**. This is an easier task than that facing the prosecution in the criminal courts, where **proof** is required beyond **reasonable doubt**.

It is unlikely that the nurse would try to defend an action for the recovery of the money due for the extra cans of lemonade and she would be more likely to offer a sum in compensation for the vending machine company's loss. (Civil claims are discussed in chapter 6.)

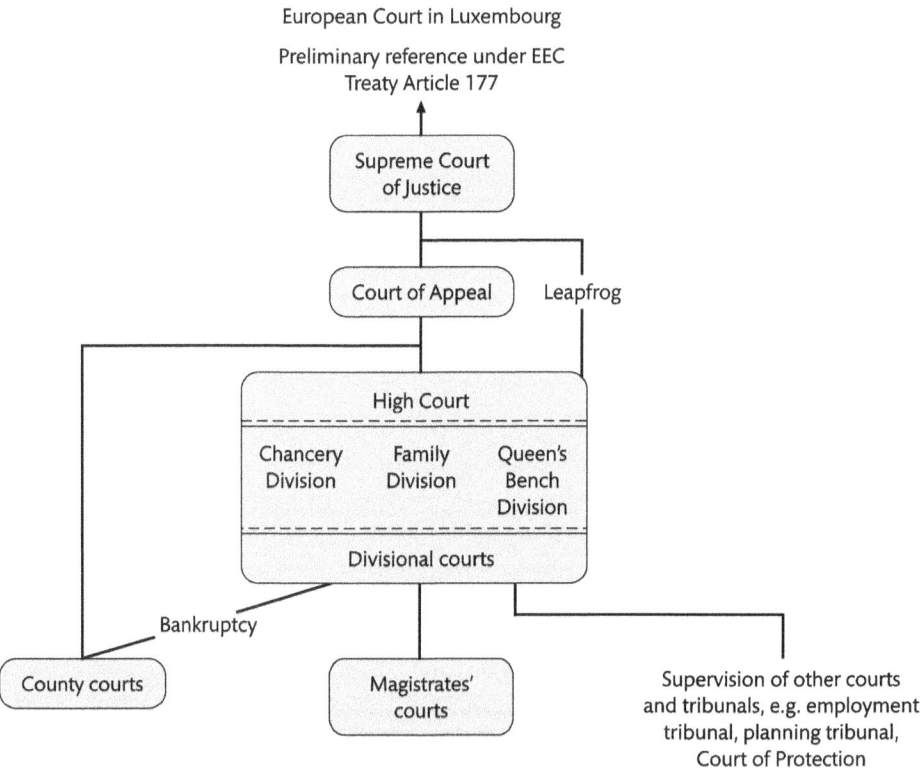

Figure 1.4 The civil courts

Accountability to employer

Finally, the nurse mentioned in Practical Dilemma 1.1 has to account to her employer. There is an implied term (i.e. a term that may never even be discussed or written down but which is assumed by the courts to exist unless there is evidence to the contrary) in every **contract** of employment that the employee will obey the reasonable instructions of the employer, use all care and skill in carrying out their duties and act with honesty and integrity. (See chapter 10 on implied terms in the contract of employment.) In a case such as this, where it is evident that the employee's behaviour has fallen below the standards of integrity expected of the employee, then that employee is in breach of contract and the employer can take appropriate disciplinary action. This might mean a warning – oral or written – demotion, suspension or even dismissal. (Disciplinary powers of the employer are considered in chapter 10.)

In the case discussed here, the employer initially suspended the nurse on full pay pending an inquiry and then, after all reasonable enquiries had been made and she had an opportunity to respond, they dismissed her. After an appeal, she was reinstated with a final written warning about her conduct.

Professionalism and accountability

The situation described in Practical Dilemma 1.1 is based on a real case and shows the high degree of professionalism and integrity required of nurses. Here, all four arenas of accountability were engaged, with the nurse accepting a simple caution from the police for theft; given a twelve-month caution by the NMC as a result of breaching the Code because of her unprofessional behaviour; dismissed from her job for gross misconduct; and required to pay compensation to the vending machine company. The initial actions of the nurse are not what many of us would consider to be particularly serious but that is not the issue. The actions of the nurse were unprofessional and she was held answerable for her actions – held legally accountable – in each of the four arenas.

However, this is not always the case and situations do arise where the employer dismisses the nurse, but the NMC keeps them on the Register, or where the employer does not dismiss the nurse, but they are removed from the Register (in which case, of course, the nurse would lose their registered post). In addition, a criminal charge may fail where a civil charge succeeds. The reason for the lack of consistency is that the four arenas are concerned with different aspects of the situation and have different standards of proof.

Sources of law

A brief word is appropriate on what is meant by the term 'law' and what its origin is. The law derives from two main sources:

1. Acts of Parliament *and* statutory instruments *that are enacted under the powers given by the former*: these are known as statutory sources, include the legislation of the European Union and take precedence over all other laws. Laws of the European Union automatically became part of the law of the United Kingdom (Figure 1.4). The Council and the Commission have law-making powers and this can be in the form of Regulations or Directives. The Human Rights Act 1998 is in a special position. When the United Kingdom left the European Union the European Union (Withdrawal) Act 2018 repealed the European

Communities Act 1972 and transferred existing European Union law across to domestic UK law to ensure certainty and avoid a legal vacuum. The 2018 Act gave ministers the authority to then amend, repeal or improve EU laws after Brexit.

2. **Common law** *(also known as case law or judge-made law)*: this is made up of the decisions by judges in individual cases that are often, but not always, interpretations of **statute law**. The judge, in deciding a particular case, is bound by a previous decision on the law made by judges in an earlier case if it is relevant to the facts before him and if that decision was made by a higher court than the one in which he is sitting. There is a recognised order of precedence so that, for example, a decision by the Supreme Court of Justice is binding on all other courts except itself, but would be subject to relevant **precedents** of the European Court of Justice. (In 2009 the judicial committee of the House of Lords was abolished and its powers transferred to a new Supreme Court. The House of Lords still remains as part of the parliamentary system.) The decisions of the courts are recorded by officially recognised reporters, so that in a case similar to a previous one the earlier decision can be put before the court. If the facts and the situation are comparable and the decision was made by a court whose decisions are binding, then the earlier precedent will be followed. If there are grounds for distinguishing the case then a different decision may follow.

Of vital importance to the system of precedence is a reliable procedure for recording the facts and decisions on any court case. Each court has a recognised system of reporting and the case is quoted by a reference that should enable the full report of the case to be found easily. (An example is given in the Glossary – see '**citation**'.)

Similarly, Acts of Parliament and Statutory Instruments have chapter numbers for each year, or a serial number.

There are recognised rules for interpreting Acts of Parliament and in relation to the following of precedents. Ultimately, however, if the law is unsatisfactory and fails to provide justice, the courts look to the Houses of Parliament to remedy the situation by new legislation. There is a right of appeal on matters of law to courts of higher jurisdiction. An appeal can be taken to the Court of Appeal and from there to the Supreme Court, if permission is granted. Until the Supreme Court has pronounced on a particular point of law, there may be considerable uncertainty as to what the law in a given situation is. A considerable number of medical law cases have been referred to the House of Lords, the predecessor to the Supreme Court, in recent years. In July 2014 the Supreme Court referred the issue of assisted suicide to Parliament since in a majority judgment it was not prepared to declare that the existing law was contrary to Article 8 of the European Convention on Human Rights (see chapter 28).[6]

Department of Health and Social Care (DHSC) circulars and other government memoranda and NMC Codes of Practice are not legally binding, but they are recommended practice and judges do use them to inform their decision making. Breach of these codes may be evidence of failure to follow the approved practice, but cannot in itself result in successful criminal or **civil action**.

The European Court of Justice and the European Court of Human Rights

A distinction must be drawn between these two courts. The European Court of Justice (ECJ) is part of the judicial machinery of the European Union, of which the UK is no longer a member following Brexit. The ECJ sits in Luxembourg. In contrast, the European Court of Human Rights is the judicial body for hearing cases on the European Convention on Human Rights. It meets in Strasbourg. The website for this book sets out Schedule 1 to the Human Rights Act 1998, listing the articles of the Convention.

Differences between civil and criminal law

What is the difference between civil law and criminal law? The only safe answer is that a breach of criminal law can be followed by prosecution in the criminal courts, whereas **liability** in civil law is actionable in the civil courts and may or may not be a crime. There is no necessary moral difference between the two. Prior to the Suicide Act of 1961 (which decriminalised an attempt to commit suicide), suicide and attempted suicide were crimes and, as such, the latter was subject to criminal proceedings. To many people, however, suicide may still be regarded as morally wrong irrespective of its non-criminal status, and it is still a criminal offence to assist someone in a suicide attempt. Some acts may be both **criminal** and **civil wrongs**: thus to drive without due care and attention and cause harm can be followed by both criminal and civil proceedings. How does one know if an act is a civil wrong? One way would be to consider previous cases to find out whether there is a precedent. The ultimate way would be to establish in the Supreme Court whether a particular action gives rise to civil liability. There is, for example, an increasing acceptance by the courts that information given in specific circumstances can give rise to an action for breach of confidence. Liability in civil law is thus a growth area.

Civil actions

A civil **action** for **negligence** will be the main one considered here in relation to the liability of the nurse or NHS trust, but there are other civil actions which will be considered briefly. The various forms of civil action are shown in Box 1.2. All these, except actions for breach of contract, are known as **torts**, i.e. civil wrongs.

Box 1.2   Some forms of civil action

1. Torts
   Negligence
   Trespass to property
      to land
      and to the person
   False imprisonment
   Wrongful interference
   Breach of a statutory duty
   Nuisance
   Defamation
   Malicious prosecution
   Deliberate interference with interests in trade or business
2. Breach of contract

The action for breach of a statutory duty arises when an Act of Parliament or Statutory Regulations place duties on organisations or individuals. In certain circumstances where an individual suffers harm as a result of the breach of these statutory duties, an action for compensation may ensue in the civil courts. For example, many of the provisions of the Factories Acts give rise to such actions. In contrast, a breach of the general duties under the Health and Safety at Work Act does not give rise to such an action, nor since October 2013 does a breach of the regulations made under the Health and Safety at Work Act (this is considered in chapter 12). The funding of civil cases and the no win, no fee system is considered in chapter 6.

Defamation is another tort that is considered in chapter 9. An action for breach of contract will be briefly considered in chapter 10 in connection with the nurse's contract of employment. An action for trespass to the person exists where a person alleges that they have been touched without their consent, and this is considered in chapter 7.

Judicial review

The legality of a judicial or administrative actions by a public body can be challenged by judicial review in which the High Court is asked to rule on the legality of the specified action.

Judicial review has long been a way for people to assert their rights by testing the lawfulness of decisions made by public bodies such as government departments and the NHS. People can use judicial review to seek a remedy when things go wrong.

In *R (on the application of Gardner)* v *SoS Health and Social Care* [2022][7] the children of two men who had died from COVID after being discharged from hospital into a care home sought judicial review of the lawfulness of the Department of Health and Social Care's guidance and discharge policy. The Court held that the guidance and policy was unlawful as each failed to consider the risk to elderly and vulnerable residents from non-symptomatic transmission of COVID. The Court further held that it was irrational for the DHSC not to have advised until mid-April 2020 that where an asymptomatic patient (other than one who had tested negative for COVID19) was admitted to a care home, he or she should, so far as practicable, be kept apart from other residents for 14 days.

Family Courts

All matters relating to a family including divorce, financial arrangements, adoption and care of children are dealt with by the Family Court. Care cases must be completed within six months by this single Family Court. Other changes include the requirement that separating couples attend a mediation awareness session before taking disputes over their finances or their children to court, and law students are being drafted in to set up advice centres and to assist in mediation. Expert evidence in cases involving children is only permitted when it is necessary to resolve the case justly.

Legal personnel and legal complaints

At present we have a divided legal profession: **solicitors** and **barristers** (counsel). There are over 128,000 solicitors and about 15,000 barristers. The former are the main link with the client. Thus, in Practical Dilemma 1.1, if the nurse wishes to defend her actions or ask for mitigation to be taken into account she would consult a solicitor, who would give advice. If the case were to proceed, she would probably instruct counsel (i.e. a barrister) to prepare the pleadings (see chapter 6) and represent the client in court.

Under Part III of the Access to Justice Act 1999, major reforms were made to the law on lawyers' rights of audience before the courts and rights to conduct **litigation**, and as a result all lawyers have full rights of audience before any court, subject only to meeting reasonable training requirements. The 1999 Act replaced the Lord Chancellor's Advisory Committee on Legal Education and Conduct with a new Legal Services Consultative Panel. The Act also made changes relating to complaints against lawyers. It gave additional powers to the Law Society and the Legal Services **Ombudsman** to strengthen the system for handling complaints against lawyers and created a Legal Services Complaints Commissioner to set targets for the handling of complaints by the professional bodies. Having completed its work in improving the speed, quality and consistency of complaints handling, the Office of the Legal Services Complaints Commissioner was abolished on 31 March 2010 and replaced by the Legal Services Board.[8] In October 2010, the Legal Ombudsman, an independent, lay organisation, was established to handle complaints. Unlike the former Legal Services Ombudsman, which was a last-stop appeal for people with complaints, the Legal Ombudsman is the frontline body handling complaints and there is no further appeal apart from judicial review.[9] The House of Lords decided that professional work in court is no longer immune from actions for negligence.[10]

These reforms may, in the long term, lead to a single legal profession. At present the initial training for both solicitors and barristers is the same (a law degree or Part 1 of the Common Professional Examination). Would-be solicitors then undertake practical training with a firm of solicitors, and then take the Law Society's Part 2 examination, called the Legal Practice Course, while would-be barristers study for the Bar to which they are 'called'. They must join one of the Inns of Court and must participate in twelve qualifying sessions of education and training including dining. The barrister must then undertake pupillage, where they are attached to a practising barrister. Barristers usually work together in chambers managed by a clerk who negotiates and collects the fees from solicitors. Fees are at present negotiated in advance and include a brief fee for accepting a case and a refresher fee, which is a daily fee for each day that the case is in court. Senior barristers and **solicitor-advocates** are eligible to 'take silk', i.e. they become **King's Counsel (KC)** appointed by the Lord Chancellor on the recommendation of an independent panel. The term 'lawyer' includes both solicitor and barrister.

Legal language

Lawyers, like any profession, have their own language, which can create barriers. In April 1999, new procedures for civil litigation were introduced together with a simplification of language to assist communication: thus the term '**plaintiff**' (used to describe a person bringing a civil action) was replaced by the word 'claimant'; '**writ**' (the document issued by the court which begins the civil case) is replaced by 'claim form'. A Glossary is provided to assist you with any specialist terms. It is the aim of this book to break down the barriers between the law and the nurse and to facilitate communication.

Human Rights Act 1998

The United Kingdom was a signatory of the European Convention for the Protection of Human Rights and Fundamental Freedoms in 1950. However, anyone who sought to bring an action for breach of their human rights, as set out in the Convention, was unable to take the case to the courts in this country but had to go to the European Court of Human Rights (ECtHR) in Strasbourg. It was estimated that to take a case to Strasbourg cost over £30,000 and took over five years. The Human Rights Act 1998 came into force on 2 October 2000. (It came into force in Scotland on devolution.)

It has three main effects: first, it is unlawful for a public authority (or organisation exercising functions of a public nature) to breach the rights set out in the Convention; second, from 2 October 2000 an allegation of a breach of the rights can be brought in the courts of this country; and third, judges can make a **declaration** that legislation that is raised in a case before them is incompatible with the articles of the Convention and the legislation will then be referred back to Parliament for reconsideration. The domestic courts are obliged to take into account the judgments of the ECHR under section 2(1) of the Human Rights Act 1998, but this does not apply on rare occasions when there are concerns as to whether the Strasbourg court's decision sufficiently appreciated or accommodated particular aspects of the domestic process.[11] Action can be brought against a public authority or an organisation exercising functions of a public nature for breach of the Convention articles in the courts of this country.

Human rights are universal rights that apply equally to everyone. So, the fact that a person is a paedophile does not mean that they have no human rights. In 2013 the Court of Appeal held that excessive detention of a convicted paedophile was contrary to his human rights even though he had been convicted of sex offences against school girls.[12]

An example of a declaration of the court of law incompatible with the articles of Human Rights is a declaration of the House of Lords,[13] which held that the then marriage laws in the country that prevented a transsexual marrying following his gender change (because the law did not recognise the change of gender) were incompatible with Human Rights articles; a Gender Recognition Act 2004 was passed and implemented, which enables applicants who meet specified criteria to apply for a replacement birth certificate and who are then allowed to marry in their adopted sex. It is possible for a person to take a case to the ECHR in Strasbourg if he or she is dissatisfied with the decision of the Supreme Court on a human rights issue.

The book's website sets out Schedule 1 to the Human Rights Act 1998. The alarmist prophecies of a huge increase in litigation were not realised, although there has been an increase in the number of cases alleging breach of the articles, often alongside another course of action. Some of the more significant articles will be considered below, but articles are also considered in relevant chapters. It is recommended that healthcare staff should undertake a proactive exercise in identifying possible breaches of the 1998 Act and be proactive in taking any necessary remedial action. Further information is available from the Ministry of Justice website[14], which took over the responsibilities on human rights from the Department for Constitutional Affairs (DCA) in 2007.[15] The Equality and Human Rights Commission also publishes practical guidance on human rights together with case reports.[16] (For further information see chapter 10.)

Right to Life

Statute 1.1

Article 2(1) European Convention for the Protection of Human Rights and Fundamental Freedoms

Article 2(1) of the Convention states that:

> Everyone's right to life shall be protected by law. No one shall be deprived of his life intentionally save in the execution of a sentence of a court following his conviction for a crime for which this penalty is provided by law.

(The sixth Protocol Article 1 states that 'The death penalty shall be abolished. No one shall be condemned to such penalty or executed.')

Claims have been made that this right to life could be used as the basis for legal action when resources are refused or when decisions are made for a person not to be resuscitated or treatment is withdrawn or withheld. For example, in a case where parents challenged a not for resuscitation (NFR) decision for their severely disabled baby,[17] the court held that the full palliative care recommended by the doctors, allowing the baby to die with dignity, was not a breach of either Article 2 or Article 3 (see below) of the European Convention for the Protection of Human Rights and Fundamental Freedoms. The President of the Family Division, Dame Elizabeth Butler-Sloss, held that the withdrawal of life-sustaining medical treatment was not contrary to Article 2 of the Human Rights Convention and the right to life, where the patient was in a persistent vegetative state. The ruling was made on 25 October 2000 in cases involving Mrs M, aged 49, who suffered brain damage during an operation abroad in 1997 and was diagnosed as being in a persistent vegetative state (PVS) in October 1998, and Mrs H, 36, who fell ill in America as a result of pancreatitis at Christmas 1999.[18] Diane Pretty failed in her attempt to have the Suicide Act 1961 (which made it an offence for her husband to aid and abet her suicide) declared incompatible with her right to a dignified death and therefore a breach of Articles 2, 3, 8 and 14.[19] She took her case to the ECtHR but failed.[20] Article 2 has also been relied upon by those who claim that there has been a miscarriage of justice in relation to a death in custody or near death. Thus, in one case[21] the claimant, who was assessed as a real suicide risk in prison, attempted to hang himself and was left severely brain damaged. A prison investigation took place but the report was not published. The Secretary of State proposed a private inquiry by the Prisons and Probation Ombudsman, but the claimant sought judicial review of this proposal, arguing that Article 2 rights implied an obligation on the State to carry out an effective investigation into the circumstances relating to a death. The judge upheld the claim, setting out the characteristics of an effective investigation. The Secretary of State appealed and the Court of Appeal held that any investigation should be held in public but that the claimant's representatives would not be entitled to cross-examine witnesses. In a subsequent case a young man attempted suicide in Feltham Young Offenders Institution and was left brain damaged. The Court of Appeal held that in such a situation, Article 2 rights required that there was a clear obligation on the Secretary of State to ensure that there was an effective inquiry into the near death.[22] A breach of Article 2 was successfully claimed when a witness for the prosecution who was known to be subject to intimidation did not receive police protection and was murdered before the **trial** took place.[23] Article 2 rights were also considered by the House of Lords when considering a **coroner's** refusal to resume an inquest[24] (see chapter 28). The Supreme Court held that an NHS trust was in breach of the Article 2 rights of an **informal** patient who committed suicide when on home leave to which the parents had objected in fear for her safety[25] (see chapter 19 Case 19.1).

Right not to be Subjected to Inhuman or Degrading Treatment

Statute 1.2
Article 3

Article 3 of the Convention states that:

> No one shall be subjected to torture or to inhuman or degrading treatment or punishment.

It could be argued that patients who spend six hours on a stretcher in a corridor outside the A&E department while a bed is being sought are being subjected to both degrading and inhuman treatment. The physical conditions in some hospitals or nursing or residential care homes may be seen to be an infringement of this right. Other examples could probably be given where patients are not treated with dignity or humanity. In the field of manual handling, there have been suggestions that to require a person to use a hoist is contrary to their human rights. However, it is thought that such an argument will not succeed, since if the alternative to a hoist is manual handling by another person, then that might be contrary to the rights of the other. This issue was considered in a manual handling case involving East Sussex County Council (see chapter 12).

The High Court has held that requiring an asylum seeker to sleep rough was inhuman and degrading treatment under Article 3. It was insufficient for the Home Office to provide a list of charities for the homeless.[26] In a case where a woman died after being imprisoned, her children won a case in the European Court of Human Rights (ECHR) that the conditions of her imprisonment prior to her death were inhuman and degrading and therefore a breach of Article 3. There were serious lapses of procedures to monitor her condition, especially her weight loss (from 50 kg to 40 kg) and her vomiting, and to arrange for earlier hospital admission.[27] The restraint of an autistic boy was held to be inhuman under Article 3[28] (see chapter 16 Case 16.2). Failure by the local authority (LA) to protect children from serious neglect and abuse (which was known to the LA) was held to be a breach of their Article 3 rights.[29] The ECHR held that mandatory life sentences for murder in the UK, without any real likelihood of reduction of period to be served amounted to a breach of Article 3 rights for the prisoners.[30]

Right to Liberty and Security

Statute 1.3
Article 5

Article 5 of the Convention states:

> Everyone has the right to liberty and security of person. No one shall be deprived of his liberty save in accordance with a procedure prescribed by law.

The use of common law powers (i.e. powers recognised by the courts as in the Re F[31] case) to detain mentally incapacitated adults in psychiatric hospitals was regarded as a breach of this article, since, although the article envisages the lawful detention of persons of unsound mind, a decision of the House of Lords did not lay down a procedure. This issue was raised in the Bournewood case[32] where the ECtHR ruled against the UK. (The case is discussed in chapters 7 and 16.) Amendments to the Mental Capacity Act 2005 to fill the gap revealed by the Bournewood case saw the introduction of the deprivation of liberty safeguards. (These are considered in chapter 16.) The Supreme Court held that disabled persons were deprived of their liberty and there was a breach of Article 5 in a case that has seen a dramatic tenfold increase in the use of the deprivation of liberty safeguards in hospitals and care homes (see chapter 16 Case 16.4).[33]

Right to a Fair Trial

> ### Statute 1.4
> #### Article 6
>
> Article 6 of the Convention states:
>
> > In the determination of his civil rights and obligations or of any criminal charge against him, everyone is entitled to a fair and public hearing within a reasonable time by an independent and impartial tribunal established by law.

This will apply to disciplinary hearings as well as courts and tribunals. Hearings must be independent and impartial. In criminal prosecutions, the accused is presumed innocent until proved **guilty**. A GP's claim that his suspension from his practice was a breach of Article 6 was not upheld since the suspension was an interim measure during which his pay was maintained. There was, however, a breach of the right to protection of property under Article 1 of the First Protocol to the Convention.[34]

Right to Respect for Private and Family Life, Home and Correspondence

> ### Statute 1.5
> #### Article 8
>
> Under Article 8 of the Convention:
>
> 1. Everyone has the right to respect for his private and family life, his home and his correspondence.
> 2. There shall be no interference by a public authority with the exercise of this right except such as is in accordance with the law and is necessary in a democratic society in the interests of national security, public safety or the economic wellbeing of the country, for the prevention of disorder or crime, for the protection of health or morals, or for the protection of the rights and freedoms of others.

It was argued by a father[35] whose wife wished to obtain an abortion that for it to be undertaken against the wishes of the father was contrary to Article 8. Failures to recognise confidential information or support the privacy of patients may lead to court action against hospitals and other organisations. In a case heard by the ECHR, it was held that the fact that the rights in law of an unmarried father differed from those of a married father were not a breach of Article 8 since there was an objective and reasonable justification for the difference in treatment.[36] The High Court held that restrictions on child visits to patients in high-security hospitals who had committed murder, manslaughter or certain sexual offences, unless the child was one of a permitted category, were lawful and were not in breach of Article 8 of the European Convention on Human Rights.[37] The onus of establishing family life lay on an applicant. The High Court also held that a prisoner serving a life sentence for murder did not have a right to his wife being artificially inseminated with his sperm. The right to found a family did not mean that an individual was guaranteed the right at all times to conceive children.[38] The appeal to the Court of Appeal failed.[39] However, the majority of the Grand Chamber of the ECHR found a breach of Article 8 when a prisoner was refused artificial insemination. There was a strong **dissenting judgment** that there was no breach[40] (see chapter 21). The Supreme Court held that there was a breach of Article 8 where sex offenders were denied a right of review of the notification provisions.[41] In 2009, Debbie Purdy sought clarification of the law relating to the offence of assisted suicide and claimed that the uncertainty relating to whether a prosecution would be brought against relatives who took terminally ill persons to Switzerland to end their lives was a breach of their Article 8 rights. She failed before the High Court and Court of Appeal but the House of Lords held unanimously that the Director of Public Prosecutions (DPP) should be required to promulgate a policy identifying the facts and circumstances he would take into account in considering whether to prosecute persons such as the claimant's husband for aiding and abetting an assisted suicide abroad. The lack of clarity on whether there would be a prosecution of relatives who took someone abroad to die was an infringement of Article 8 rights[42] (see chapter 28). The ECHR held that the order of deportation of a person of Pakistani heritage who had lived in the UK since the age of three years and had no connections with Pakistan was a disproportionate response to the offence of smuggling heroin. He had not reoffended since his release from prison in 2006.[43] In contrast, the ECtHR held, in the case of a man who alleged that there was secret surveillance of his removal business, that these measures did not interfere with his private life since there were sufficient safeguards in the UK's interception of communications regime to ensure that an individual's rights were not breached. There was no breach of Article 8.[44] In two further cases, breaches of Article 8 were established. In the first, the ECHR held that monitoring by prison authorities of medical correspondence between a convicted prisoner and his neuroradiology specialist violated his right for respect for his correspondence as guaranteed by Article 8.[45] In the second, the ECHR held in January 2010 that the police powers of stop and search were illegal as a breach of Article 8, holding that section 44 of the Terrorism Act 2000 violated individual freedoms guaranteeing the right to private life. The action was brought by Kevin Gillan and Pennie Quinton, who were awarded £30,400 in costs.[46]

The allegation that Kensington and Chelsea RLBC breached Article 8 rights when withdrawing a night service for disabled persons and the ECHR decision is considered in chapter 22.[47]

The Supreme Court held that hoteliers who refused to let a double room to a gay couple unlawfully discriminated against the couple on grounds of sexual orientation. The limitation on their religious beliefs that such relationships were sinful was justified as a proportionate means of achieving a legitimate aim of protecting the rights and freedoms of others. To rule otherwise would be to create a class of people who were exempt from the discrimination legislation.[48]

Article 2 of Protocol 1 of the European Convention on Human Rights recognises a right to education. The Supreme Court held that a delay of 18 months in providing special education for a severely disabled child while the local authority secured a place in a specialist school was not a breach of Article 2.[49]

It was held that there was no breach of Article 4(2) (no one shall be required to perform forced or compulsory labour) in the back to work scheme since it was a condition imposed for the payment of a claim for state benefit, i.e. jobseeker's allowance.[50]

Other significant articles include Article 9, freedom of thought, conscience and religion; Article 10, freedom of expression; and Article 14, prohibition of discrimination. As cases come before the courts, case law develops on the interpretation to be given to the various articles and the extent to which the NHS is recognising the rights of its staff and its patients. Further information on human rights and equalities can be found on the Equalities and Human Rights Commission website.[51] There are many other Conventions recognising the rights of specific groups. For example, the UN Convention on the Rights of the Child, while not directly enforceable in the UK, is observed, and compliance with it is monitored by a joint committee of the Houses of Parliament. The Convention and Protocol relating to the status of Refugees (1951 and 1967) was considered by the Supreme Court when it held that gay asylum seekers could stay in the UK if they feared that they would face persecution were they to live openly in their home countries.[52] The ECHR held in 2006 that the UK bereavement tax regime was discriminatory.[53]

Freedom of Information Act 2000

This Act, which gives a right of access to information held by public authorities, was brought into force in 2005. An Information Commissioner monitors both the Freedom of Information (FOI) Act and the Data Protection Act 2018, General Data Protection Regulations (GDPR), and Codes of Practice and Guidance have been issued. There are many exceptions to the right of access, including personal information, information provided in confidence and legal professional **privilege**. (Both Acts and the GDPR are considered in chapter 8.) Information on the GDPR, Data Protection Act and the FOI Act is available from the Information Commissioner's Office website.[54]

Devolved law-making powers

Increasingly, the four constituent parts of the UK are going their separate ways as law-making powers are devolved from Westminster. This book is of necessity focused on England. A fascinating analysis of the differences is provided by Nicholas Timmins[55] illustrating the difficulties in making any comparison of performance across the UK. The respective parliaments and assembly of Scotland, Wales and Northern Ireland have websites from which the specific laws and guidance for those countries can be accessed.[56] However, it is hoped that the general structure and content of this book will be relevant to readers across the UK.

Conclusions

The law and our legal systems are continually changing. It is essential that nurses keep up to date with the law that underpins their practice, but this can be difficult due to the secrecy of some court proceedings. Practice guidance issued by Sir James Munby, President of the Court of Protection, and in keeping with similar guidance issued for the family courts, has brought about an immediate and significant change in practice in relation to the publication of judgments in family courts and the Court of Protection, whose decisions are made more openly with case reports being much more readily available.[57] However, the Justice and Security Act 2013 extended closed material procedures (CMP) to civil cases with ministers now able to apply for a CMP to bar the public, media and claimant from the proceedings, usually on grounds of national security. There are likely to be major upheavals in the criminal courts system with plans to close more magistrates' courts and introduce privatisation.[58] Two recent reports recommend changes. The first, from the charity Transform Justice, is concerned that

magistrates are older and less diverse than 15 years ago. It recommends that recruiting should be changed to encourage diversity; recruiting through social media, changing the application process, giving recruitment to the Judicial Appointments Committee, targeting specific groups and considering positive discrimination. The second, from the Policy Exchange, outlines a new role for **justices of the peace (JPs)** who would dispense justice from new police courts in a drive to speed up the justice system. Offenders would be punished on the spot, with magistrates sitting in police stations at peak times including evenings and Saturdays.[59] Further changes to the legal system are proposed by the Secretary of State for Justice who is seeking to restrict the right to seek judicial review which is considered above.

In October 2013 the Court of Appeal was televised for the first time with the aim of opening up the workings of the appeal courts and making the justice system more transparent. Judges are being trained for such developments. The United Kingdom Supreme Court has its own YouTube channel where recordings of cases and summaries of judgments are publicly available.

Reflection questions

1. What is the difference between law that derives from a statute and the common law?
2. What is the difference between a solicitor and a barrister?
3. Look at the Glossary and identify those words with which you are not familiar.

Further exercises

1. Consider any situation you know of where a patient (almost) suffered harm as a result of a careless act by a professional and analyse the potential consequences as far as the civil and criminal courts, the FtPC and the employment tribunal are concerned. Refer to chapters 2, 3, 10 and 11 for more details.
2. Try to arrange a visit to one of the four arenas described here (Figure 1.2) or a coroner's court (see chapter 28) and draw up a plan for the procedure that you witness.
3. With colleagues, choose any Article in the Convention on Human Rights (see the book's website) that is relevant to your work and decide on the extent to which there are any infringements of that right. What action could you take?
4. If you work in Wales, Scotland or Northern Ireland, access the website of the relevant devolved assembly/parliament and obtain information on the statutes and regulations which have been enacted through their devolved powers.

References

[1] Nursing and Midwifery Council (2015) *The Code: Professional standards of practice and behaviour for nurses, midwives and nursing associates* London: NMC

[2] MDU (2022) Nurse practitioners face multiple investigations into single incident, according to MDU analysis available on the MDU Website at https://www.themdu.com/press-centre/press-releases/nurse-practitioners-face-multiple-investigations-into-single-incident-according-to-mdu-analysis

[3] House of Commons (2013) *Report of the Mid Staffordshire NHS Foundation Trust Public Inquiry (Chair Robert Francis QC) HC947* London: The Stationery Office
[4] Andrews J. and Butler M. (2014) *Trusted to Care An independent Review of the Princess of Wales Hospital and Neath Port Talbot Hospital at Abertawe Bro Morgannwg University Health Board Stirling*: University of Sterling
[5] www.acas.org.uk
[6] *Nicklinson and Anor R (on the application of) (Rev1)* [2014] UKSC 38
[7] *R (on the application of Gardner)* v *SoS Health and Social care* [2022] EWHC 967
[8] www.legalservicesboard.org.uk
[9] www.legalombudsman.org.uk
[10] *Arthur JS Hall and Co. (a firm)* v *Simons* [2000] 3 WLR 543 HL
[11] *R* v *Horncastle and Another; R* v *Marquis and Another*, The Times Law Report, 10 December 2009, Supreme Court
[12] Frances Gibb and Michael Savage, Paedophile who targeted schoolgirls can seek damages, *The Times*, 13 November 2013
[13] *Bellinger* v *Bellinger* [2003] UKHL 21; [2003] 2 WLR 1174
[14] www.equalityhumanrights.com/en
[15] Department for Constitutional Affairs, Study Guide on Human Rights Act 1998, 2nd edition, October 2002; now available from the Equality and Human Rights Commission: www.equalitycommission.com
[16] www.equalityhumanrights.com/en
[17] *National Health Service Trust A* v *D and Others* [2000] Lloyd's Rep Med 411
[18] *NHS Trust A* v *M; NHS Trust B* v *H* [2001] 1 All ER 801
[19] *R (on the application of Pretty)* v *DPP* [2001] UKHL 61, [2001] 3 WLR 1598
[20] *Pretty* v *UK* [2002] ECHR 427
[21] *R (on the application of D)* v *Secretary of State for the Home Department (Inquest intervening)* [2006] EWCA Civ 143; [2006] 3 All ER 946
[22] *R (on the application of JL)* v *Secretary of State for the Home Department* [2007] EWCA Civ 767
[23] *Van Colle and another* v *Chief Constable of Hertfordshire Police* [2006] EWHC 360 QBD; [2006] 3 All ER 963
[24] *R (on the application of Hurst)* v *London Northern District Coroner* [2007] UKHL 13; [2007] 2 All ER 1025
[25] *Rabone and another* v *Pennine Care NHS Trust* [2012] UKSC 2
[26] *R (Limbuela)* v *Secretary of State for the Home Department*, The Times Law Report, 9 February 2004
[27] *McGlinchey and Others* v *The United Kingdom* [2003] Lloyd's Rep Med 265
[28] *ZH (A protected party)* v *Commissioner of Police of the Metropolis, Liberty and another intervening* Court of Appeal 12 April 2013, The Times Law Report [2013] EWCA 69
[29] *Z* v *United Kingdom* (2002) 34 EHRR 3
[30] *Vinter and others* v *United Kingdom* [2013] ECHR 645
[31] *In re F (Mental Patient: Sterilisation)* [1990] 2 AC 1, [1989] 2 WLR 1025, [1989] 2 All ER 545
[32] *R* v *Bournewood Community and Mental Health NHS Trust ex p L* [1998] 3 All ER 289; *HL* v *United Kingdom* [2004] ECHR 471 Application no. 45508/99, 5 October 2004; The Times Law Report, 19 October 2004
[33] *P (by his litigation friend the Official Solicitor)* v *Cheshire West and Cheshire Council and Anor* [2014] UKSC 19
[34] *R (on the application of Malik)* v *Waltham Forest Primary Care Trust* (Secretary of State for Health, interested party) [2006] EWHC 487 admin, [2006] 3 All ER 71
[35] *Paton* v *UK* (1980) 3 EHRR 408

[36] *B* v *UK* [2000] 1 FLR 1 ECHR
[37] *R* v *Secretary of State for Health ex p Lally*, The Times Law Report, 26 October 2000; [2001] 1 FLR 406
[38] *R* v *Secretary of State for the Home Department ex p Mellor* [2000] 2 FLR 951
[39] *R* v *Secretary of State for the Home Department ex p Mellor* [2001] EWCA 472
[40] *Dickson* v *UK* [2007] ECHR 1050
[41] *F and another* v *Secretary of State for Home Department* [2010] UKSC 17
[42] *R (Purdy)* v *Director of Public Prosecutions*, The Times Law Report, 31 July 2009, HL; [2009] UKHL 45
[43] *Khan* v *United Kingdom*, Application no. 47486/06, The Times Law Report, 3 February 2010
[44] *Kennedy* v *United Kingdom*, Application no. 26839/05, The Times Law Report, 3 June 2010
[45] *Szuluk* v *United Kingdom,* Application no. 36936/05, The Times Law Report, 17 June 2009
[46] *Gillan and Quinton* v *United Kingdom,* Application no. 4158/05, The Times Law Report, 15 January 2010
[47] *McDonald* v *United Kingdom,* Application no. 4241/12 European Court of Human Rights, Times Law Report, 20 May 2014
[48] *Bull and Anor* v *Hall and Anor* [2013] UKSC 73
[49] *A* v *Essex County Council,* Supreme Court, The Times Law Report, 15 July 2010
[50] *R (Reilly and Another)* v *Secretary of State for Work and Pensions,* The Times Law Report, 18 November 2013 Supreme Court
[51] www.equalityhumanrights.com/en
[52] *HJ (Iran)* v *Secretary of State for the Home Department and HT (Cameroon)* v *Same Supreme Court,* The Times Law Report, 9 July 2010
[53] *Hobbs, Richards, Walsh, Goon* v *UK,* The Times Law Report, 27 November 2006
[54] www.ico.org.uk
[55] Nicholas Timmins, The four UK health systems, The King's Fund, London 2013
[56] https://gov.wales; www.scottish.parliament.uk; www.niassembly.gov.uk
[57] Practice Guidance (Transparency in the Court of Protection) 2014 EWHCB2 COP 16 January 2014
[58] Frances Gibb, Magistrates attack plans for more court closures, *The Times,* 29 May 2013
[59] Frances Gibb, Magistrates are older and less diverse than 15 years ago, *The Times,* 27 February 2014

Chapter 2
Actions in the Criminal Courts and Defences to Criminal Charges

This chapter discusses

- Initial stages of arrest and prosecution
- Magistrates' courts
- Plea and Case Management Hearing
- Crown Court proceedings
- Elements of a crime
- Cases of Beverley Allitt, Sister Salisbury, Nurse Patel and Nurse Amaro
- Offence of ill-treatment or wilful neglect
- Negligence as a crime
- Administration of drug by epidural instead of intravenous injection
- Defences
- Criminal injuries compensation

Introduction

In this chapter, we consider the course followed if criminal proceedings are brought against a nurse and the ways in which they could defend themselves. It must be emphasised that the burden is on the prosecution to establish the guilt of the accused beyond reasonable doubt. The accused still has a right of silence at all stages of the prosecution, but failure by the accused to answer questions or mention something they later rely on in court or failure to give evidence may allow adverse inferences to be drawn during the trial.

Practical Dilemma 2.1 — Theft

A discrepancy is found between the ward drug control records and the stock. An investigation is initiated and suspicion falls upon Staff Nurse Jarvis. The police are brought in and, after making their enquiries, they decide that Staff Nurse Jarvis should be charged with the offence of theft.

A situation such as this involves several kinds of investigation. The NHS trust will be concerned to determine whether there are grounds to discipline and possibly eventually dismiss the staff nurse. The fact that the police are brought in does not mean that the NHS trust can abandon its own investigation, but clearly its enquiries should not conflict with those of the police. The NHS trust must allow the staff nurse to give a full explanation of what has occurred and she should be allowed a representative. Disciplinary proceedings by the employer are discussed in chapter 10. There is also the possibility of a hearing before the Fitness to Practise Committee (FtPC) of the Nursing and Midwifery Council (NMC) (see chapter 11), but this may well be postponed pending the outcome of the police investigations and criminal charges. Here we are concerned only with the criminal proceedings.

Initial stages of arrest and prosecution

The staff nurse may well be asked to accompany the police to the station (see Figure 2.1). A Code of Practice (C 2023), prepared under the Police and Criminal Evidence Act 1984, provides guidance on the detention, treatment and questioning of persons by police officers. It is intended to provide clear and workable guidelines for the police, while strengthening safeguards for the public at the same time. The Codes of Practice were most recently revised in 2023 and are available on the UK government website.[1]

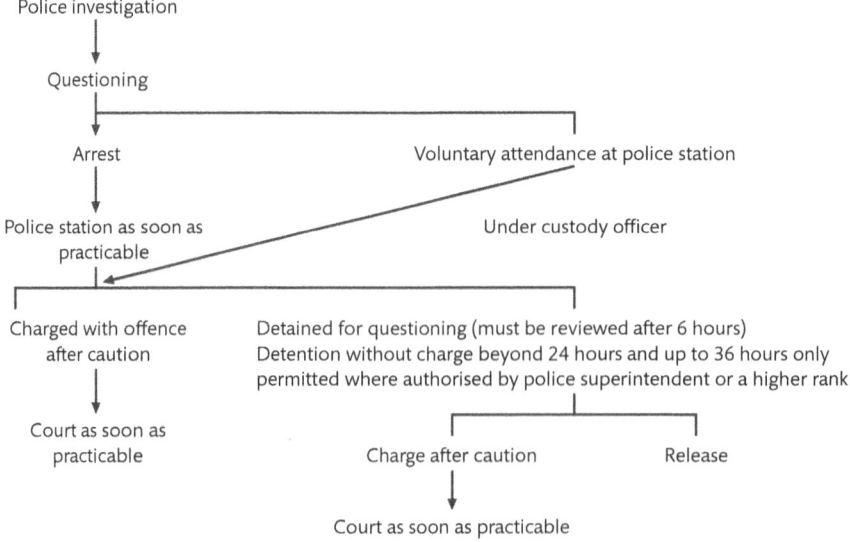

Figure 2.1 Initial stages of arrest and prosecution

The Codes of Practice must be readily available at all police stations. Code C2023 applies both to those who have been arrested and those who have voluntarily attended the police station. One of the most important safeguards is the right of the detained person to have access to free legal advice at the police station before and during any interview.

The staff nurse may have been arrested before she is taken to the police station or she may be arrested there. In either case, she should be given a caution as soon as there are grounds to suspect her of the offence and before she is questioned about it for the purpose of obtaining evidence that may be given to a court in a prosecution. The caution should be given in the following terms: 'You do not have to say anything but it may harm your defence if you do not mention when questioned something which you later rely on in court. Anything you do say may be given in evidence.'

Minor deviations may be a breach of the Code, but do not necessarily affect the fairness of the trial and make the evidence inadmissible under section 78 of the Police and Criminal Evidence Act 1984. The documentation that the police must retain is shown in Box 2.1. The Code sets out rules for the police in the interview. The usual procedure now is for the interview to be audio recorded and the guidelines and Code of Practice for audio recording should be followed. Visual recordings (which, unlike audio or secure digital recordings, are optional) can also be made digitally.[2]

Box 2.1 Documentation kept by the police

Custody records should be kept for each person who is brought to a police station under arrest or who is arrested at the police station after attending there voluntarily. They are entitled on request to be supplied with a copy when they leave the police station.

The information must be recorded as soon as practicable and should include the following:

1. Grounds for a person's detention.
2. Detained person's property.
3. Request made for a person to be informed and action taken; any letters or messages sent, calls made or visits received, and any refusal on the part of a person to have information about themselves or their whereabouts given to an outside enquirer.
4. Any request for legal advice and the action taken on it.
5. Replacement clothing and meals offered.
6. Medical examination by a police surgeon, or request for one and the arrangements made; any medication the detained person is on.
7. An interview record should record:
    - the times at which the detained person is not in the custody of the custody officer and why, and the reason for any refusal to deliver them out of that custody
    - any intoxicating liquor supplied to a detained person
    - any decision to delay a break in an interview
    - a written record of the interview (unless tape-recorded) signed by the detained person as correct.

8. Any action taken to call an interpreter and any agreement to be interviewed in the absence of an interpreter.
9. Grounds for and the extent of any delay in conducting a review.
10. Anything a detained person says when charged, any questions put after the charge and answers given relating to the offence shall be contemporaneously recorded in full on the forms provided and the record signed by the detained person.
11. Details of any intimate or strip search: which parts were searched, by whom, who was present, reasons and the result.
12. Grounds for any action in delaying the notification of an arrest or allowing access to legal advice.

When the officer considers that there is sufficient evidence to prosecute a detained person, they should be brought without delay before the custody officer, who will then be responsible for considering whether or not they should be charged. A further caution must then be given. In addition, a written notice should be given showing the particulars of the offence with which they are charged and including the name of the officer in the case, their police station and a reference number for the case. Questions relating to an offence may not be put to a person after they have been charged with that offence or after they have been informed that they may be prosecuted for it, unless they are necessary to prevent or minimise harm or loss to some other person or to the public, to clear up an ambiguity in a previous answer or statement or where it is in the interests of justice that they should have an opportunity to comment on some fresh information. Before these additional questions are put, the accused must be given another caution. Annex D to Code C2023 gives rules on written statements given under caution.

The Criminal Justice Act 2003 has introduced the power of a constable, investigating officer or person authorised by a relevant prosecutor to give a conditional caution provided five requirements are satisfied: evidence the offender has committed the offence; there is sufficient evidence to charge the person and a conditional caution should be given; the offender admits the offence; the effect of the conditional caution is explained; and the offender signs a document setting out specified details. The Secretary of State was required to prepare a Code of Practice in relation to conditional cautions covering specified topics (CJA 2003 ss. 22–25). It is accessible on the Crown Prosecution Service website.[3]

Role of the Crown Prosecution Service

Since the introduction of the Crown Prosecution Service (CPS), the responsibility for the conduct of most criminal proceedings is on the CPS, the head of which is the Director of Public Prosecutions (DPP), who acts under the Attorney General. They have the responsibility of instituting criminal proceedings and appearing for the prosecution. Victims are now able to appeal in specified circumstances when the Crown Prosecution Service decides not to pursue suspects.[4] This follows a Court of Appeal ruling in a case in 2007 where the CPS decided not to bring sexual assault charges. The decision was reversed in 2011 and Christopher Killick was jailed for three and a half years.[5] To prevent the CPS being swamped by appeals, strict criteria apply to the right to appeal including a requirement to show that the decision not to prosecute was wrong and needs to be reversed to maintain public confidence.

Magistrates' courts

If the staff nurse is charged with the offence of theft, she would probably be given police bail and told to appear at a magistrates' court. Almost all criminal cases begin in a magistrates' court and 98 per cent are dealt with completely there. The remaining cases go before the Crown Court before judge and jury. Revised criminal procedure rules for the criminal courts came into force in 2015[6] and are regularly updated.[7] They are comparable to the Civil Procedure Rules (see chapter 6) and, like the Civil Procedure Rules, set an overriding objective which is shown in Box 2.2 and give the courts case management powers.

Box 2.2 — Overriding objective of criminal court from the criminal procedure rules 2015

1.1

(1) The overriding objective of this new code is that criminal cases be dealt with justly.

(2) Dealing with a criminal case justly includes—

  (a) acquitting the innocent and convicting the guilty;

  (b) dealing with the prosecution and the defence fairly;

  (c) recognising the rights of a defendant, particularly those under Article 6 of the European Convention on Human Rights;

  (d) respecting the interests of witnesses, victims and jurors and keeping them informed of the progress of the case;

  (e) dealing with the case efficiently and expeditiously;

  (f) ensuring that appropriate information is available to the court when bail and sentence are considered; and

  (g) dealing with the case in ways that take into account—

    (i) the gravity of the offence alleged,

    (ii) the complexity of what is in issue,

    (iii) the severity of the consequences for the defendant and others affected, and

    (iv) the needs of other cases.

Participants in the conduct of a criminal case must prepare and conduct the case in accordance with the overriding objective and comply with procedure rules, **practice directions** and directions made by the court and inform the court if there is any significant failure to take any procedural step required by the rules, and so on.

Indictable-only offences can be heard only before a judge and jury in the Crown Court, summary offences can be heard only by magistrates, but many offences are triable either way. Box 2.3 shows the classification of the offences and Box 2.4 shows the course of a hearing.

Box 2.3 — Classification of offences

1. Offences triable only on indictment (i.e. by judge and jury): murder; genocide; infanticide; causing death by reckless driving; robbery; treason; wounding with intent; and many others.
2. Offences triable only summarily (i.e. by magistrates): drunk and disorderly; careless driving; assault on police; and other offences set down by statute, such as the Road Traffic Act 1972 and Schedule 1 of the Criminal Law Act 1977.
3. Offences triable either way (by judge and jury or by magistrates) – case can be heard by magistrates in summary trial or on indictment in the Crown Court. Offences include: theft; handling, obtaining property or pecuniary advantage by deception; assault occasioning actual bodily harm.

Box 2.4 — Course of a hearing in a magistrates' court

The magistrates' courts hear:

(a) offences that are triable only as summary offences, e.g. careless driving

(b) offences that are triable either way.

Hearing

1. Plea:

    a plea of guilty must be unequivocal

    a plea of guilty may be made by post, but only to summary non-imprisonable offences.

2. Summary trial where the defendant pleads not guilty:

    A. Prosecution:
    1. Opening speech by prosecution lawyer
    2. **Examination in chief** of prosecution witnesses
    3. Cross-examination by defence
    4. Re-examination by prosecution lawyer.

    B. Submission by defence of no case to answer (if appropriate). Prosecution have the right to reply and magistrates determine the question.

    C. Defence case:
    1. Defendant can remain silent or give evidence. (The court may in certain circumstances draw adverse inferences from silence.)
    2. Defence witnesses are called and can be cross-examined by the prosecution.
    3. Defence lawyer addresses the magistrates and the prosecution lawyer can make a closing speech.

    D. The finding: the magistrates determine the guilt or innocence and determine the sentence if a guilty verdict and if they feel their powers are adequate.

When the staff nurse is brought before the magistrates she will be asked to indicate a plea. If she indicates a plea of guilty to the summary offence, she will be sentenced by the magistrates. If she pleads not guilty, she will be tried by the magistrates.

If she is charged with an offence that is triable either way (i.e. as a summary offence before the magistrates or on indictment by a judge and jury) and she indicates a plea of guilty, then the magistrates will decide whether she should be sentenced by them; if they consider their powers are inadequate, they may then commit (**committal proceedings**) her to the Crown Court for sentencing. If she indicates that she intends to plead not guilty or declines to indicate a plea, the magistrate will then decide whether the trial should be before them or whether the case should be allocated to the Crown Court for trial. If the magistrates decide the case is suitable for trial before them, the defendant will be asked to consent to that procedure. The defendant has the right at that stage to elect trial by judge and jury at the Crown Court. Under the Criminal Justice Act 2003, magistrates can give an indication, if the accused were to plead guilty, of whether a custodial sentence would be imposed.

Plea and case management hearing

If, by the same token, Staff Nurse Jarvis elects to have the case heard in the Crown Court, the case will be referred directly to the Crown Court where a date for the Plea and Case Management Hearing (PCMH) will be agreed. Indictable-only cases are transferred to the Crown Court immediately (i.e. at first appearance before the magistrates), and sometimes before witness statements are taken. At this preliminary hearing, a timetable will be set for the service of the prosecution evidence, service of defence statements and a date for the Plea and Case Management Hearing (Criminal Justice Act 2003, schedule 3).

Crown court proceedings

Let us assume that Staff Nurse Jarvis's case is to appear in the Crown Court for trial, since it is an offence which is triable either way. (If she had been charged with an indictable-only offence, the case would have been transferred to the Crown Court.) The procedure followed is shown in Box 2.5. Changes have been made regarding the right to challenge the jury (see Box 2.6). Once the jury have been sworn in, the hearing follows the same path as that in a magistrates' court, but only counsel or a solicitor-advocate can represent the accused before the court, and a barrister may therefore have been briefed by Staff Nurse Jarvis's solicitor.

Box 2.5 Procedure in the Crown Court

1. Attendance of the defendant (in person or by video link if the defendant has been remanded in custody).
2. The indictment (the document embodying the charge(s) brought by the Crown against the defendant) is read by the clerk to the accused, who is asked whether they plead guilty or not guilty. This is known as the arraignment.

The accused can:

(a) plead guilty – if accepted, court proceeds to sentencing

(b) plead not guilty – see point 4, below

(c) stand silent – if mute of malice (this is determined by the jury), a plea of not guilty is entered – if mute by visitation of God, court will decide if accused is fit to plead (see insanity, p. 36)

(d) object on legal grounds – e.g. indictment is invalid and should be quashed.

3. Directions for smooth running of the trial: identification of all the issues.

4. Empanelling of the jury: if the defendant has pleaded not guilty to any count on the indictment, a jury must be empanelled. The jury is not usually present during the arraignment so that they are kept in ignorance if the accused has pleaded guilty to some offences and not guilty to others, unless the guilty pleas are admissible in the trial.

The jurors are called in after the arraignment and the names of 12 are called out. A list of the witnesses is read out to the jurors so that any jurors who know any witness can be excused from the jury. They can be challenged by defence or prosecution for cause (see Box 2.6). They are then sworn in and the clerk reads the indictment to them, tells them the defendant has pleaded not guilty and that their charge is to say, having heard the evidence, whether they be 'guilty' or 'not guilty'.

5. The hearing:

The judge will make introductory remarks telling the jury that they must base their decisions on the finding on the evidence given and they are not to use the internet.

A. Prosecution:

1. Opening speech by the prosecution
2. Prosecution evidence
   Examination in chief: prosecution witnesses questioned by the prosecution
3. Cross-examination – to discredit witnesses, leading questions can be used and earlier inconsistent statements by the witness can be put to them
4. Re-examination – to offset the effects of cross-examination. It cannot be used to produce new evidence, which should have been brought out in the examination in chief
5. Written statements of witnesses whose evidence the defence does not wish to dispute will be read out or summarised as agreed facts
6. Challenges to admissibility of evidence: the defence can (in the absence of the jury) challenge the admissibility of evidence. The judge will rule on the admissibility and, if they uphold the defence objections to the evidence, all reference to the evidence must be omitted.

B. Defence:

1. Defence submission: after the conclusion of the prosecution evidence, the defence can ask the trial judge to direct the jury as a matter of law that they should acquit the defendant:

    (a) either because the prosecution has failed to produce any evidence to establish some essential ingredient of the offence

    (b) or because the evidence produced is so weak or so discredited by cross-examination that no reasonable jury could convict. If the defence submission is upheld, an acquittal is directed.

    If this submission fails then the defence case is put.

2. Case for the defence: an opening speech can be made where the defendant and other witnesses are being called to give evidence as to facts (not where only the defendant is called or the other witnesses are only called as to character).

    Procedure as above

    Examination in chief

    Cross-examination

    Re-examination

C. Closing speeches: by prosecution and defence counsel.

D. Summing up by judge.

E. Verdict of jury.

F. Sentencing following finding of guilt.

Box 2.6 Challenging the jury

Prosecution: can ask for any would-be juror to 'stand by' until they have gone right through the panel. Can challenge for cause (e.g. ineligibility, disqualification, presumed or actual bias).

Defence: has lost the right to three peremptory challenges (i.e. challenging without having to give any reasons). Can challenge for cause (e.g. ineligibility, disqualification, presumed or actual bias). (There have been changes to the rules on ineligibility to sit as a juror, and now judges, barristers, police officers, prison officers and others who were formerly ineligible to sit can be summoned.)

The judge has a discretionary power to remove a juror.

The effect of challenging for cause is that if either side can show that a juror is personally concerned in the facts of the particular case or closely connected with a party to the proceedings or with a prospective witness they can be removed. A challenge for cause should not succeed if the only ground for bias is so insubstantial as to be unlikely to affect the jurors' approach to the case.

The challenging party says 'challenge' immediately before the juror takes the oath. They then have the burden of satisfying the judge on a balance of probabilities that their objection is well founded and producing ***prima facie*** evidence of this.

The charges on the indictment must be put to Staff Nurse Jarvis at the Plea and Case Management Hearing. If she pleads not guilty, directions will be given to ensure the smooth running of the trial and a trial date will be fixed. The trial will then proceed as set out in Box 2.5. There will be an opening address by the prosecution counsel, setting out the elements that the prosecution have to prove and the standard of proof. This has no evidential value, but can be an important scene-setting for the jury. The prosecution then calls its witnesses who are examined in chief, which means that the witness cannot be asked leading questions. The witness can be cross-examined by the defence and here leading questions, designed to show the irrelevance of this evidence or in some other way discredit it, can be asked (see chapter 9 on evidence in court). After the **cross-examination** has finished, the party calling that witness can re-examine the witness on points arising from the cross-examination. The judge can call a halt to the case on completion of the prosecution evidence if they are not satisfied that there is sufficient evidence to go before the jury, in which case the jury is asked to bring in a not-guilty verdict. For example, in a Crown Court hearing in Cardiff when two surgeons from Prince Philip Hospital Llanelli were charged with manslaughter following the removal of the wrong kidney, the pathologist giving evidence for the prosecution could not confirm that death was caused by the removal of the wrong kidney and thus the judge instructed the jury to bring forward a not-guilty verdict, since the causal link between an alleged act of gross negligence and the death had not been established by the prosecution. An NMC report[8] on 29 October 2003 stated that two nurses were convicted of manslaughter when an elderly patient died from septicaemia resulting from pressure sores while a resident in a nursing home, of which the nurses were managers. Their defence that it was the system, rather than themselves, that was to blame was rejected.

If the case proceeds, the defence calls its witnesses. At present, although the accused does not have to give evidence, the judge may in certain circumstances allow adverse inferences to be drawn by the jury.

After all the evidence has been given, the defence and prosecution conclude their cases in final speeches. The judge then sums up the case for the jury, and has the task of explaining to the jury all the relevant directions of law: the elements of the crime that the prosecution must prove the accused committed, the nature of the **burden of proof** that is on the prosecution. The judge also analyses the evidence which both sides have put before the jury.

The jurors then retire to decide their verdict and elect a foreman after they have retired. Initially, the jury is asked to return a unanimous verdict. If it is clear that they can never reach a unanimous verdict, then they can return to court and can be given instructions on returning a majority verdict which must be at least 10 to 2. The minimum period of jury discussion before a majority verdict is possible is 2 hours and 10 minutes, but in practice it may be a much longer time.

If the jury decides that the staff nurse is guilty, evidence of previous convictions (until this moment usually kept secret from the jury, but under the Criminal Justice Act 2003 evidence of bad character is admissible in certain circumstances) and her present social and economic circumstances will be given before sentencing. Sentencing will usually be adjourned for a pre-sentencing report from a probation officer. Box 2.7 sets out the powers of sentencing.

The staff nurse has the right to appeal against the finding of guilt on the grounds that the conviction is unsafe. She also has the right to appeal against the sentence imposed. The prosecution can appeal against sentencing by way of a reference by the Attorney General and it has the right to appeal on a point of law. Guidelines on sentencing are issued by the Sentencing Guidelines Council[9] and courts are required to follow relevant guidelines unless it is contrary to the interests of justice to do so.

> **Box 2.7 — Sentencing in the Crown Court**
>
> Absolute/conditional discharge
>
> Bindover
>
> Fine (and compensation)
>
> Community orders coupled with conditions such as unpaid work, supervision, attendance at a programme, residence and curfew which can be electronically monitored
>
> Suspended sentence with or without conditions, the maximum length of sentence is 2 years with a suspension of up to 2 years
>
> Restraining order
>
> Prison sentence
>
> Hospital order, Section 37 Mental Health Act 1983
>
> Hospital order and restriction order, Sections 37 and 41 Mental Health Act 1983
>
> For offences since October 2012 a victim's surcharge is also imposed
>
> The courts are required to take account of Sentencing Guidelines, unless it would be unjust to do so
>
> Credit is given for an early plea of guilty and the credit reduces with time.

Elements of a crime

In order to establish guilt, the prosecution must be able to show that each element of the crime charged is proved so that the jury is sure. Each crime thus has its ingredients that make up that particular offence. Examples are given of the elements of some crimes in Box 2.8.

> **Box 2.8 — Examples of the definition of certain crimes**
>
> 1. **Assault** (common law offence):
>
>   *actus reus:* an act that causes the victim to fear the immediate application of force against them
>
>   *mens rea:* an unlawful intention to cause the victim to apprehend the immediate application of force, or recklessness as to whether the victim might apprehend immediate force.
>
> 2. **Battery** (common law offence):
>
>   *actus reus:* an act that results in the application of force to the person of another
>
>   *mens rea:* an unlawful intention to apply force, or recklessness as to whether force might be applied.

3. Wounding or causing really serious harm, Section 18 Offences Against the Person Act 1861:

    actus reus: wound or cause any really serious harm to any person

    mens rea: unlawfully with intent to do really serious harm or an intent to resist or prevent lawful apprehension or detaining of any person.

4. Wounding or inflicting really serious harm, Section 20 Offences Against the Person Act 1861:

    actus reus: to wound or inflict any really serious harm on any other person, either with or without any weapon or instrument

    mens rea: unlawfully and maliciously (intentional or recklessly and without lawful justification).

5. Theft, Section 1(1) Theft Act 1968:

    actus reus: appropriate property that belongs to another

    mens rea: dishonest with the unlawful intention of permanently depriving the true owner of that property.

Mental and Physical Elements

There is a further breakdown of the elements that have to be established to prove that a crime has taken place, i.e. between the **actus reus** and the *mens rea*. The **mens rea**, or mental element, includes all those elements that relate to the mind of the accused. The *actus reus* is everything else. There are some crimes where there is no requirement to show a mental element. For example, the sale of medicine by a person who was not qualified and while unsupervised by a pharmacist and which was contrary to section 52 of the Medicines Act 1968 was held to be an absolute offence.[10] The law has now been changed to require a mental element to be proved.

If there were no requirement for the prosecution to establish a mental element in the crime of theft, Staff Nurse Jarvis could be successfully prosecuted for theft in circumstances where someone had accidentally dropped a bottle of tablets in the staff nurse's open bag and she had therefore taken them home inadvertently. In order to secure a conviction, whether the prosecution takes place in the magistrates' court or in the Crown Court, all the elements, mental and physical, must be shown to have existed at the time it was alleged that the crime was committed.

Several cases where nurses have been convicted of criminal offences are now discussed.

Case of Beverley Allitt

Following the deaths and injuries to children caused by the nurse Beverley Allitt, an independent inquiry was set up. (Its recommendations are considered in chapter 5.)

Case of Sister Salisbury

Sister Salisbury[11], a nurse of some 30 years' standing worked on a gastroenterology/general medical ward. She had the care of a number of terminally ill elderly patients. She was convicted of attempting to murder two of those patients by inappropriately administering diamorphine in a deliberate attempt to hasten the end of their natural life. Sister Salisbury argued that she gave the diamorphine lawfully, as prescribed and in the best interests of each patient.

On hearing evidence that Sister Salisbury had exaggerated the pain the patients were experiencing to get the doctor to prescribe diamorphine and to justify her administration of the drug, together with comments made to staff including a remark that a patient should be nursed lying flat on his back so his lungs would fill with fluid and he would die, the jury returned a verdict of guilty and she was sentenced to five years, imprisonment.

Sister Salisbury also lost her job and was struck off the nurses register by the NMC.

Case of Nurse Patel

Nurse Patel[12] was a registered nurse working in a nursing home reserved for elderly patients who were mentally ill. The victim was a patient who lacked capacity and on the day in question, Nurse Patel, who was in charge of the home, was told by a health care assistant that the patient was becoming ill because his breathing was shallow and his pulse was faint. Nurse Patel apparently panicked. Although she called for an ambulance, she did not perform cardiac pulmonary resuscitation despite being asked to do so by the ambulance clinical adviser on the telephone. The patient had died by the time the ambulance arrived.

Nurse Patel was charged and convicted of wilful neglect under the Mental Capacity Act 2005 section 44 for deliberately failing to carry out CPR even though it was clinically necessary, a requirement of the nursing home's policy and there was no 'do not attempt resuscitation' notice in place for the patient. The judge directed that neglect was a failure to do what was necessary for the proper care or treatment of a patient and that stress or panic was no defence to a charge of wilful neglect. Nurse Patel was sentenced to a 12-month community order and a requirement to do 100 hours of unpaid work.

Case of Lucy Letby

In 2023 Lucy Letby, a former neonatal nurse, was convicted of murdering seven infants and of the attempted murder of six others. She was found to have injected her victims with insulin or air and abused them with medical instruments. She was sentenced to a whole life term of imprisonment. The government has commissioned an independent statutory inquiry into the circumstances leading to the murders chaired by Lady Justice Thrilwall.

Offence of ill-treatment or wilful neglect

Section 44 of the Mental Capacity Act 2005 introduced a new offence of ill-treatment or wilful neglect of a person who lacks mental capacity (see chapter 18). Following the Francis Report on Mid Staffordshire NHS Trust a new statutory offence of ill-treatment or wilful neglect was introduced under section 20 of the Criminal justice and Courts Act 2015. (This is discussed in chapter 5.)

Failure to Call Medical Assistance

A husband was charged with manslaughter because he had failed to call medical assistance for his wife following a home birth when the baby was stillborn. The wife refused to allow him to call for help and she died. The judge directed the jury that because the wife was mentally competent and had refused assistance, the husband's duty of care to seek assistance was removed. He could not therefore be guilty of manslaughter.[13]

Case of Nurse Amaro

Nurse Amaro[14] admitted a charge of manslaughter by gross negligence following the death of a six-year-old boy with Down's syndrome who was admitted to hospital but died of sepsis the same day. Nurse Amaro admitted that she failed to monitor the boy properly because she failed to take regular readings of his temperature, respiratory rate, his pulse and his oxygen saturation levels. The judge found her monitoring of the boy's fluid balance as wholly inadequate and that his blood pressure was not recorded for the whole period he spent in the nurse's care.

Nurse Amaro was given a two-year suspended prison sentence and was later struck off the nurses register by the NMC.

Negligence as a crime

In accepting the recommendations of the Mid Staffordshire NHS Foundation Trust Inquiry[15]; the National Advisory Group on the Safety of Patients in England[16] and the review into Winterbourne View Hospital[17], the government has sought to restore public confidence in its management and supervision of the health service. It has done this, in part, by encouraging the prosecution of health professionals, resulting in matters that would have historically been dealt with by the professional regulator, employer or civil courts now coming before the criminal courts as well. This has resulted in an increase in the prosecution of nurses whose carelessness is linked to the death of a patient through a charge of gross negligence manslaughter.

Negligence is generally associated with the civil law. It is the law's way of imposing a standard of care on professionals such as district nurses and it provides redress by way of compensation for those harmed by another's careless act or omission. In cases where the negligent act of a nurse is linked to the death of a person in their care then a crime may have been committed and a charge of gross negligence manslaughter brought.

Development of the Crime of Gross Negligence Manslaughter

In *R v Bateman* [1925][18] the court decided that gross negligence occurs when someone shows such disregard for the life and safety of other persons as to constitute a crime worthy of punishment. That high initial threshold for prosecution was lowered in *R v Misra & Srivastava* [2004][19] where two doctors were found guilty of gross negligence when they failed to heed the warnings to call for senior assistance because a patient was seriously ill. The patient subsequently died of toxic shock. The judge held that,

> [A health professional] would be told that grossly negligent treatment of a patient which exposed him or her to the risk of death, and caused it, would constitute manslaughter.

The doctors each received a suspended jail term of 14 months and the NHS trust was subsequently fined £100,000 for failing to have proper systems in place to supervise their junior doctors. The court found that had these systems been in place the patient would not have died.

This was also the case in *R v Adomako* [1995][20] where the defendant, an anaesthetist, failed to notice for four minutes that an endotracheal tube had become disconnected during an operation. Although an alarm sounded, the tube was not checked until the patient suffered a cardiac arrest. An **expert witness** for the prosecution stated that a competent anaesthetist should have spotted the problem within 15 seconds. The House of Lords held that gross negligence would occur where a patient's death occurs as the result of a:

- health professional displaying an indifference to an obvious risk of injury to the patient;
- health professional being aware of the risk of injury to the patient but deciding to run the risk;
- health professional's attempt to avoid a known risk being so grossly negligent that it deserves to be punished; or
- health professional displaying inattention or a failure to avert a severe risk.

Based on the House of Lords ruling it can be seen that a failure to heed any risk of injury could be considered in a gross negligence manslaughter case with the jury then asked to decide whether the negligence was so careless as to be criminal.

Redefining the Threshold for Gross Negligence Manslaughter

The Court of Appeal has redefined the threshold for gross negligence manslaughter so as to limit prosecutions to situations where there is a serious and obvious risk of death at the time of the careless act or omission.[21] The requirement for there to be a risk of death raises the threshold from the risk of injury set out by the House of Lords in *R v Adomako* [1995].

In *R v Rose* [2017] the Court of Appeal overturned a conviction for gross negligence manslaughter against an optometrist who had conducted a routine eye test and examination on a boy aged seven and recorded no issues of concern. Five months after the examination, while at school, the boy was taken ill. He died in hospital the same day from acute hydrocephalus, a long-standing chronic problem, treatable up to the point of acute deterioration and death.

The optometrist accepted that her failure to examine the back of the eye without a good reason was a breach of her duty of care as it would have revealed swelling of the optic nerve. She was charged and convicted of gross negligence manslaughter but appealed, arguing that the incorrect elements of gross negligence manslaughter had been put to the jury.

The Court allowed the appeal and stressed that their judgment applied to all health professions including nurses. The Court held that in assessing either the foreseeability of risk or the grossness of the conduct in question, the court could not take into account information which would, could or should have been available to a careless health professional who had breached their duty of care. The charge of gross negligence manslaughter required a test of foreseeability, i.e. the risk was so serious and obvious that death was foreseeable.

The Court of Appeal also held that the implications for nurses and other professions if the threshold was any lower would be serious because they would be guilty of gross negligence manslaughter by reason of negligent omissions to carry out routine eye, blood and other tests which would have revealed fatal conditions notwithstanding that the circumstances were such that it was not reasonably foreseeable that a failure to carry out such tests would carry an obvious and serious risk of death. In reaching its decision, the court stressed that it did not condone the initial carelessness and negligence in the way that the eye examination was carried out and the failure to identify the defect, which ultimately led to the boy's death. That serious breach of duty was however a matter for the professional regulator. It did not constitute the crime of gross negligence manslaughter.

The requirement for there to be a serious and obvious risk of death at the time of the negligence so that death was reasonably foreseeable means that it is less likely that a nurse's carelessness will result in prosecution if the patient dies. It is likely that in practice a nurse who carelessly administers the incorrect medicine or carelessly omits to carry out tests, resulting in a later deterioration and death of the patient, would now be less likely to face prosecution for gross negligence manslaughter as, arguably, a serious and obvious risk of death is not reasonably foreseeable at the time the negligence occurred. However, where a nurse, for example, carelessly administers 250 milligrams of digoxin against a prescription of 250 micrograms, resulting in the patient's death from digoxin toxicity, then a prosecution is more likely as there is a reasonably foreseeable, serious and obvious risk of death.

Corporate Manslaughter and Corporate Homicide Act 2007

As well as the possibility of individual practitioners facing criminal charges, it is likely that the nurse's employing organisation would also face investigation under the provisions of the Corporate Manslaughter and Corporate Homicide Act 2007. The Act came into force in April 2008 and introduced a new statutory offence of corporate manslaughter in England, Wales and Northern Ireland. In Scotland, the offence is known as Corporate Homicide.

The 2007 Act focuses on whether the death of a patient was caused by failings in the way an organisation such as an NHS trust or health board was managed rather than the negligence of one individual. Those failings must be by senior management, defined as those whose role is decisive or influential. The management failure leading to the death must be serious enough to amount to a gross breach of the duty of care owed to the victim.

In deciding whether there has been a gross breach a jury will consider whether a trust failed to comply with health and safety legislation and the extent to which the evidence shows that there were attitudes, policies, systems or accepted practices within the organisation that were likely to have encouraged, or tolerated such failings. This was the first time that consideration of the 'corporate culture' has been enshrined in the law of the United Kingdom. Examples of a gross breach by senior managers could include a failure to ensure safe working practices, a lack of proper training and failing to maintain equipment or premises in a safe working condition.

Guidance to the courts says that a fine for an offence of corporate manslaughter will seldom be less that £500,000 and may be measured in millions of pounds, so it is essential that nurse managers ensure that their health and safety policies reflect current requirements and that their staff abide by these policies.

Administration of drug by epidural instead of intravenous injection

In 2003 a junior doctor in Nottingham pleaded guilty to the manslaughter of a patient suffering from leukaemia. Instead of administering the drug intravenously, he administered it epidurally and the patient died. The doctor was given a prison sentence. The National Patient Safety Agency is tasked with preventing the recurrence of such mistakes (see chapters 12 and 27).

Defences

The main defences to a criminal act are shown in Box 2.9. They are all given here for completeness, but not all of them are relevant to Staff Nurse Jarvis's case.

Box 2.9   Main defences to a criminal offence

1. Absence of any of the elements making up the offence: *actus reus* or *mens rea*
2. Infancy:
    below 10 years no crime (In Scotland the age is being raised from 8 to 12 years.)
3. Insanity:
    (a) unfit to plead and stand trial
    (b) not guilty by reason of insanity at the time of the crime
4. Diminished responsibility and loss of control (which reduce murder to manslaughter)
5. Mistake (Sometimes this is a statutory defence but usually only where the defendant has taken all reasonable steps. Normally the statute places the burden of proof on the defendant on a balance of probabilities.)
6. Necessity (now known as 'duress of circumstances')
7. Duress
8. Superior orders
9. Self-defence

Absence of Any of the Elements Making up the Offence

It will be apparent from what has been said thus far that if the accused can show that any of the required elements, either *actus reus* or *mens rea*, as defined in the Act of Parliament or the common law definition of the crime, are missing, then there should be an acquittal. Even though it is usually for the prosecution to show they exist rather than for the defence to prove their absence, it would clearly be an advantage for the defence to show their absence. Thus, for example, in the offence of theft, one of the elements is that the property that has been taken belonged to another.

If the defence can show that the property did not belong to anyone but had, in fact, been abandoned, then that would be a successful defence. A state of automatism by the defendant was accepted by the prosecution when it withdrew charges against a man who had strangled his wife while having a nightmare. Brian Thomas dreamt that intruders had broken into their camper van and he woke up to find his wife dead beside him. It was accepted that he was not in control of his actions at the time of the killing and the prosecution accepted the evidence of three psychiatrists that detention in a mental hospital would serve no useful purpose.[22]

Infancy

Children under 10 years are exempt from criminal responsibility and cannot be found guilty of a crime. The infant is known as *doli incapax*.

Minors over 10 years are presumed to be responsible for their actions but there are considerable procedural differences from the way in which an adult is proceeded against. The UK was criticised by the European Court of Human Rights for its handling of child criminals following the conviction of two boys for the killing of Jamie Bulger.[23] The Court held that Article 6 had been breached by the way the trial had been conducted. However, the court did not find that there was a breach of Article 3 (inhuman or degrading treatment). In March 2010 the Children's Commissioner called for the age of criminal responsibility to be raised from 10 to 12 years. Dr Maggie Atkinson pointed out that in some European countries the age of criminal responsibility was 14 years.[24] Her call was rejected by the Ministry of Justice. Scotland is raising the age of criminal responsibility from 8 years to 12 years. In England the defence of *doli incapax* for a child over 10 was abolished by the Crime and Disorder Act 1998 section 34 as interpreted by the House of Lords.[25]

The Supreme Court has held that under Articles 6 and 8 it was permissible for a child to testify in family proceedings, but the considerations of the advantages of the child giving evidence to determine the truth had to be balanced against the damage it might do to the child.[26] The Youth Justice and Criminal Evidence Act 1999 introduced a range of measures that can be used to facilitate the gathering and giving of evidence by vulnerable (which includes all those under 18) and intimidated witnesses. These are known as 'special measures' and include screens, the removal of wigs and gowns, live links, evidence given in private and video recorded interviews.[27]

Insanity

Insanity can be pleaded before or when the trial takes place so that the accused is held unable by reason of insanity to stand trial. Alternatively, it can be pleaded as a defence to the crime on the basis that at the time the crime was committed the accused was insane. The definition of insanity as a defence is based on the M'Naghten Rules, which were laid down in 1843. The basic propositions are:

> [E]very man is presumed to be sane and to possess a sufficient degree of reason to be responsible for his crimes, until the contrary be proved.
>
> [To] establish a defence on ground of insanity, it must be clearly proved that at the time of the committing of the act, the party accused was labouring under such a defect of reason, from disease of mind, as not to know the nature and quality of the act he was doing, or if he did know it, that he did not know he was doing what was wrong.

Since 1843 there have been many interpretations and refinements of this definition, but the substance has survived. The defence is available to any criminal charge. For example, a woman, who had an undiagnosed dementia at the time of the offence, turned her car into the path of a van and the collision forced the van into a woman and child on the pavement. The jury accepted that as a result of the dementia the driver did not know what she was doing and this was more than a momentary lapse of concentration. She was found not guilty of causing death by dangerous driving by reason of insanity. As a result of the special verdict, the judge imposed a 12 month supervision order on the driver (Woodcock 2022).

Diminished Responsibility and Loss of Control

These statutory defences provided by the Homicide Act 1957, as amended by the Coroners and Justice Act 2009, apply only to murder and have the effect of enabling the accused charged with murder to be found guilty of manslaughter on grounds of diminished responsibility or loss of control. (The former common law defence of provocation has been replaced by a new defence of loss of control.) The Law Commission published a consultation paper in 2006 which set out proposals for a new Homicide Act.[28] Some of its recommendations were included in the Coroners and Justice Act 2009. The Amendments to the Homicide Act 1957 by the Coroners and Justice Act 2009 are shown in Box 2.10.

Box 2.10 Amendments to the homicide act 1957

The Homicide Act 1957 is amended:

1. A person ('D') who kills or is a party to the killing of another is not to be convicted of murder if D was suffering from an abnormality of mental functioning which:
    (a) arose from a recognised medical condition;
    (b) substantially impaired D's ability to do one or more of the things mentioned in subsection (1A); and
    (c) provides an explanation for D's acts and omissions in doing or being a party to the killing.

1A. Those things are:
    (a) to understand the nature of D's conduct;
    (b) to form a rational judgement;
    (c) to exercise self-control.

1B. For the purposes of subsection (1)(c), an abnormality of mental functioning provides an explanation for D's conduct if it causes, or is a significant contributory factor in causing, D to carry out that conduct.

Loss of control

Section 54 of the Coroners and Justice Act 2009 provides a new partial defence to murder known as loss of control, which is shown in Box 2.11.

Box 2.11 — Loss of control Section 54 of the Coroners and Justice Act 2009

Section 54 Partial defence to murder: loss of control

1. Where a person ('D') kills or is a party to the killing of another ('V'), D is not to be convicted of murder if:

   (a) D's acts and omissions in doing or being a party to the killing resulted from D's loss of self-control;

   (b) the loss of self-control had a qualifying trigger; and

   (c) a person of D's sex and age, with a normal degree of tolerance and self-restraint and in the circumstances of D, might have reacted in the same or in a similar way to D.

2. For the purposes of subsection (1)(a), it does not matter whether or not the loss of control was sudden.

3. In subsection (1)(c) the reference to 'the circumstances of D' is a reference to all of D's circumstances other than those whose only relevance to D's conduct is that they bear on D's general capacity for tolerance or self-restraint.

4. Subsection (1) does not apply if, in doing or being a party to the killing, D acted in a considered desire for revenge.

5. On a charge of murder, if sufficient evidence is adduced to raise an issue with respect to the defence under subsection (1), the jury must assume that the defence is satisfied unless the prosecution proves beyond reasonable doubt that it is not.

6. For the purposes of subsection (5), sufficient evidence is adduced to raise an issue with respect to the defence if evidence is adduced on which, in the opinion of the trial judge, a jury, properly directed, could reasonably conclude that the defence might apply.

7. A person who, but for this section, would be liable to be convicted of murder is liable instead to be convicted of manslaughter.

8. The fact that one party to a killing is by virtue of this section not liable to be convicted of murder does not affect the question whether the killing amounted to murder in the case of any other party to it.

   The meaning of qualifying trigger is defined in section 55:

Section 55 Meaning of 'qualifying trigger'

1. This section applies for the purposes of section 54.

2. A loss of self-control had a qualifying trigger if subsection (3), (4) or (5) applies.

3. This subsection applies if D's loss of self-control was attributable to D's fear of serious violence from V against D or another identified person.

> 4. This subsection applies if D's loss of self-control was attributable to a thing or things done or said (or both) which:
>   **(a)** constituted circumstances of an extremely grave character; and
>   **(b)** caused D to have a justifiable sense of being seriously wronged.
> 5. This subsection applies if D's loss of self-control was attributable to a combination of the matters mentioned in subsections (3) and (4).
> 6. In determining whether a loss of self-control had a qualifying trigger:
>   **(a)** D's fear of serious violence is to be disregarded to the extent that it was caused by a thing which D incited to be done or said for the purpose of providing an excuse to use violence;
>   **(b)** a sense of being seriously wronged by a thing done or said is not justifiable if D incited the thing to be done or said for the purpose of providing an excuse to use violence;
>   **(c)** the fact that a thing done or said constituted sexual infidelity is to be disregarded.
> 7. In this section references to 'D' and 'V' are to be construed in accordance with section 54.

The Court of Appeal (Criminal Division) has held that on a charge of murder, where the defence of loss of self-control is raised, then whether the circumstances were extremely grave and whether the defendant's sense of being seriously wronged by them was justifiable required an objective assessment by the judge at the end of the evidence and by the jury.[29]

A man who caused fractures, when fighting two burglars of his premises, was acquitted of causing grievous bodily harm by the jury after 20 minutes' deliberation.[30]

Mistake

A defendant can argue self-defence if they honestly but mistakenly believed they were under attack. This can be an effective defence where it prevents the accused from being able to form the required mental element (i.e. *mens rea*) to be guilty of the offence charged. For example, a defendant to a charge of theft could argue that they honestly but mistakenly believed that they had permission to take the goods, i.e. mistake negatives dishonesty. Mistake of law is not sufficient, for knowledge that an act is a crime is not usually a necessary ingredient of the *mens rea*.

Necessity

There is no recognised principle that necessity is a valid defence to any crime.

Duress

This will be a valid defence where it can be established that the force or compulsion was such that the accused had no choice. There must be an immediate threat of death or serious harm. It is unlikely to be accepted as a defence to a charge of murder, but has been invoked in other lesser crimes.

Superior Orders

It is not a defence for the accused to argue that the crime was committed in obedience to the orders of a superior. However, it might be possible for a defendant to show that as a result of the orders they lacked the required mental element for the crime and that they were acting reasonably in all the circumstances. The issue of obeying orders as a defence in the civil courts is considered in chapter 4.

Self-defence

Reasonable force can be used to defend oneself or another person against an attack. However, greater force than is reasonable would result in the possibility of the defender being liable to prosecution for assault or, in the event of the assailant dying, murder or manslaughter. (This is considered further in chapter 12.)

Criminal injuries compensation

A scheme to compensate those who have suffered personal injuries as the result of criminal action has been in existence since 1964. A new scheme for compensation following injuries or death as a result of a crime was established on 1 April 1996 under the Criminal Injuries Compensation Act 1995, based on a statutory scale of awards known as the 'tariff'. Details of the scheme,[31] which was revised in 2008, and again in 2012[32] are available from the Criminal Injuries Compensation Authority (CICA) headquarters in Glasgow[33] and can be downloaded from the internet.[34]

The 2012 scheme excludes some injuries originally recognised as the subject of compensation, and payments for other injuries are reduced. Claims are processed by the CICA and claims officers, and adjudicators on a panel determine whether a claim can be met. Evidence is obtained from applicants, the police medical bodies and others such as witnesses to the incident. The CICA determines whether payments are to be made to victims of criminal acts. Those eligible (and these include the victims of crime as well as the dependants of homicide victims) must have reported the crime to the police as soon as possible. The application should be made within two years of the incident, but exceptions can be made to both these requirements. Payments are made against a tariff system up to a maximum of £500,000 (see Annex E of the scheme) and include the following items:

- medical expenses;
- mental health expenses;
- lost wages for disabled victims (but not for the first 28 full weeks of lost earnings or earning capacity);
- lost support for dependants of homicide victims;
- funerals;
- travel;
- rehabilitation for disabled victims;
- pain and suffering;
- bereavement; and
- loss of parental services.

Claims below £2500 are excluded from the new scheme. (Previously the minimum payment was £1000).

A crime must be established for compensation to be payable and a cyclist was stripped of his award of £500,000 for injuries he sustained when a dog chased him into the path of a car. The Court of Appeal held that he had not been the victim of a crime and was not entitled to the money.[35]

Conclusions

Significant changes have taken place in criminal law and procedure in recent years. The introduction of an offence of corporate manslaughter does not yet appear to have influenced the attitudes of senior management within the NHS, although the organisation can now be held to account for a death caused by gross negligence, and rules relating to health and safety of both staff and patients are likely to be strictly enforced. It is now more likely that the individual nurse will be involved in criminal law issues and should be aware that any successful prosecution of a registered practitioner will be notified to the NMC (see chapter 11).

Legal aid has been cut for criminal court hearings. Changes announced in September 2013 by the Justice Secretary Chris Grayling included removing legal aid in 11,000 cases brought by prisoners each year, a 30 per cent cut in the cost of long-running criminal cases; a staged 17.5 per cent cut in legal fees; and a new system for contracts for legal aid work, that came into force in 2015. However, these contracts will no longer be awarded to the lowest bidder (ridiculed as 'supermarket justice' by the barristers), with no cap on the number of firms to be awarded contracts.[36] In addition, a working party will look at how thousands of short hearings can be avoided and handled by email or video-link.

The Court of Appeal overruled the Crown Court which had held that because of a refusal by barristers to accept the lower level of fees paid in criminal cases the defendants could not be properly represented and therefore the cases adjourned or dismissed. The Court of Appeal decision has been criticised since it means that the prosecution with well-paid top barristers will be facing inexperienced junior barristers paid for out of the public defender service.[37]

Reflection questions

In the case of Staff Nurse Jarvis, trace the course that would be followed if:

(a) she were tried in a magistrates' court;
(b) she were tried in the Crown Court;
(c) she pleaded guilty in the magistrates' court; and
(d) she pleaded guilty in the Crown Court.

Further exercises

1. What do you consider are the advantages and disadvantages of trial before magistrates compared with a jury trial for an offence that is triable either way?

2. What evidence do you consider the prosecution would require in a case similar to that of Staff Nurse Jarvis and what evidence would the defence seek?
3. Visit your local magistrates' court and Crown Court and analyse the difference between the two in terms of formality, procedure and justice to the accused.
4. Ascertain whether there have been any prosecutions for corporate manslaughter or corporate homicide in the NHS and identify the implications of this offence for your own organisation.

References

[1] www.gov.uk/government/publications/pace-code-c-2017
[2] Police and Criminal Evidence Act 1984 (Codes of Practice) Revisions to Codes E and F Order 2010 SI 2010/1108
[3] www.cps.gov.uk
[4] Frances Gibb, Crime victims win right to appeal when prosecutors drop charges, *The Times*, 1 June 2013
[5] *R v Killick* [2011] EWCA Crim 1608
[6] www.legislation.gov.uk/uksi/2015/1490/contents/made
[7] https://www.justice.gov.uk/courts/procedure-rules/criminal/docs/criminal-procedure-amendment-rules-2018-guide.pdf
[8] www.nmc.org.uk
[9] www.sentencingcouncil.org.uk/publications/?type=publications&s=&cat=definitive-guideline&topic=&year=
[10] *Pharmaceutical Society of Great Britain v Logan* (1982) Crim LR 443
[11] *R v Salisbury* [2005] EWCA Crim 3107 (CA)
[12] *R v Patel* [2013] EWCA Crim 965
[13] *R v Smith* [1979] Crim LR 251
[14] www.nmc.org.uk/globalassets/sitedocuments/ftpoutcomes/2016/august/reasons-amaro-cccsh-36269-20160804.pdf
[15] House of Commons (2013) *Report of the Mid Staffordshire NHS Foundation Trust Public Inquiry Executive summary HC 947* retrieved from The Stationery Office website webarchive.nationalarchives.gov.uk/20150407084231/;www.midstaffspublicinquiry.com/report
[16] National Advisory Group on the Safety of Patients in England (2013) *A promise to learn – a commitment to act: Improving the safety of patients in England* London: Department of Health
[17] Department of Health (2012) *Transforming care: A national response to Winterbourne View Hospital Department of Health Review: Final Report* London: TSO
[18] *R v Bateman* [1925] Cr. App R. 8
[19] *R v Misra & Srivastava* [2004] EWCA Crim 2375
[20] *R v Adomako* [1995] 1 AC 171 (HL)
[21] *R v Rose* [2017] EWCA Crim 1168
[22] Simon de Bruxelles, Man with rare sleep illness who killed his wife of 40 years during nightmare is declared innocent, *The Times*, 21 November 2009
[23] *T v United Kingdom*; *V v United Kingdom* [2000] 2 All ER 1024 ECHR
[24] Rachel Sylvester et al., Children under 12 'can't be criminals', *The Times*, 13 March 2010
[25] *R v JTB* [2009] UKHL 20

26 *In re W (Children) (Family Proceedings: Evidence)*, The Times Law Report, 8 March 2010 Supreme Court
27 www.cps.gov.uk
28 Law Commission, A new Homicide Act for England and Wales, Consultation paper 177, 2006
29 *R* v *Dawes*, *R* v *Hatter*, and *R* v *Bowyer*, The Times Law Report, 25 July 2013 CA Crim
30 Oliver Moody, Gardener who fought burglars is cleared after 'ten months of hell', *The Times*, 24 January 2014
31 Criminal Injuries Compensation Scheme 2008, CICA Glasgow
32 Ibid.
33 Criminal Injuries Compensation Authority, Alexander Bain House, Atlantic Quay, 15 York Street, Glasgow G2 8JQ. Tel: 0300 003 3601
34 Ministry of Justice www.gov.uk
35 *Criminal Injuries Compensation Authority* v *First-Tier Tribunal*, The Times Law Report, 21 February 2014
36 Frances Gibb, Legal aid slashed for criminals and the rich, *The Times*, 5 September 2013
37 Phil Smith, Operation Cotton: the case with no barristers, *The Times*, 29 May 2014

Chapter 3

Liability in a Civil Court Case for Negligence

This chapter discusses

- Duty of care
- Standard of care
- Causation
- Liable for what?
- Harm

Introduction

Litigation to obtain compensation in the civil courts is one of the growth areas of recent years. In 2014 the NHS Litigation Authority stated[1] it had made provision for nearly £25.6 billion for future compensation payouts with clinical claims against the NHS being at a record high. Total negligence claims jumped 18 per cent to 11,945 which officials said was the result of new legal firms entering the market and cases being brought before the rules on no win, no fee were changed. Of the £1.2 billion paid out in 2013 almost a quarter (£259 million) was paid to claimants' solicitors. More recently, litigation costs have continued to rise. In 2022/23 almost £2.7 billion was paid by NHS Trusts and Health boards to settle claims made against GPs, hospitals and primary care settings. This represented an overall increase of 9.5% upon the 2021/22 figure, which stood at almost £2,5 billion. According to the National Patient Safety Incident Reports, there were 12,675 serious incidents per year in English NHS Trusts and 68,111 moderate incidents per year – serious and moderate incidents include acts and omissions in care that lead to an unexpected or avoidable death or injury causing a serious harm.[2,3] There is now a new approach to responding to patient safety incidents via the Patient Safety Incident Response Framework (PSIRF) which will examine why incidents happen, and associated contributing factors.

If harm has occurred to a patient, then the patient or their representatives can seek compensation. However, not all harm is compensatable. Accidents to patients are infinite: they include incidents where the patient falls out of bed, pressure sores develop, the wrong dose of medicine is given, it is given at the wrong time or at the wrong site by the wrong method or the expiry date is passed, the wrong limb is amputated, the treatment is given to the wrong patient, the patient dies as the result of a mistake. Some of these are the result of negligence and the victims may receive compensation. Not all accidents, however, will result in the payment of compensation to the patient or relatives. In some circumstances the defendant may pay a sum of money to the claimant without admitting liability. This is known as an **ex gratia** payment and may have the effect of resolving the issue and reducing the potential costs of further proceedings. For example, Camden and Islington Mental Health and Social Care Trust agreed to pay £400,000, without admitting liability, to a mental patient who leapt under an Underground train. The patient had walked out of the psychiatric department of the Whittington Hospital nine days before. The patient claimed that the trust failed to protect him from himself.[4] In a case where a woman aged 64 was told to suck ice cubes for a persistent cough and after being seen by five doctors over two years was found to be suffering from cancer and died, the husband accepted an undisclosed sum from the GP who originally treated her, but with no admission of liability.[5]

In contrast, liability was admitted by the Barking, Havering and Redbridge Hospital NHS Trust in 2013 when it was reported that a mother died after two trainee surgeons took out an ovary instead of her appendix.[6] In any subsequent court case the only issue would be over **quantum**, i.e. how much compensation was payable (if this could not be agreed between the parties) and not liability.

This chapter looks at the circumstances that must exist for compensation to be payable and the type of harm for which compensation will be paid. The personal liability of the nurse and the liability of her employer are considered in chapter 4. The calculation of compensation is considered in chapter 6.

In this section we are concerned with four basic questions:

1. What is meant by the term 'duty of care'; when does the nurse owe a duty of care; and to whom is it owed?
2. What is the appropriate standard of care and what criteria determine whether the nurse is in breach of that duty?
3. What is meant by 'reasonably foreseeably caused' and why and how must the claimant prove this in an action for negligence?
4. What type of harm do the courts recognise as capable of being compensated?

This chapter will answer these questions by providing examples where patients have been harmed. The next chapter will consider some specific problems of liability in relation to inexperienced staff, team responsibility, limits on resources and also the liability of the NHS trust.

Duty of care

Difficulties can arise as to whether a duty of care exists, especially outside the immediate employment situation. A duty of care is not owed universally and the claimant bringing the action has to show that a duty of care was owed to them personally.

The legal test of whether a duty of care exists was laid down in the case of *Donoghue* v *Stevenson*.[7] In this case, the manufacturer (Mr Stevenson) was held to owe a duty of care to the ultimate consumer, in this case Mrs Donoghue. The facts of this case were that a person who was bought a bottle of ginger beer discovered the decomposed remains of a snail when half the beer had been drunk and sued the manufacturer, arguing that the manufacturer owed a duty of care to the consumer. In the case, Lord Atkin stated that:

> **You must take reasonable care to avoid acts or omissions which you can reasonably foresee would be likely to injure your neighbour. Who then in law is my neighbour? The answer seems to be persons who are so closely and directly affected by my act that I ought reasonably to have them in contemplation as being so affected when I am directing my mind to the acts or omissions which are called in question.**

In other words, a duty of care can be said to exist if one can see that one's actions are reasonably likely to cause harm to another person.

It is important to acknowledge that Lord Atkin has made an essential point that it must be reasonable for a duty of care to be owed. For example, Nurse Jones is informed at handover to work on ward 3 instead of ward 2. Later on in the day, an incident happens on ward 2, and the patient's relative wishes to make a complaint against everyone working on ward 2. In these circumstances, it would be viewed as unreasonable for Nurse Jones to be included in the complaint as she spent the shift working on a different ward.

Duty of care was further defined in the case of *Caparo Industries* v *Dickman Plc* [1990] – in this case Lord Bridge made a fundamental point in that there must be a relationship between the parties owing a duty of care and the parties to which a duty is owed. It must also be fair, just and reasonable for a duty of care to be imposed upon a person or parties whose actions or omissions are under challenge. Proximity need not be geographical – a diabetes specialist nurse in the UK may forget to provide advice to a diabetic patient to avoid being barefooted on a beach during a holiday they are taking in Australia. During the holiday the patient, while barefooted, steps on broken glass, and due to peripheral neuropathy is unable to feel the glass penetrate their foot. While geographically the UK and Australia are thousands of miles apart, the nurse still owes a duty of care to provide correct advice to the patient, and the relationship between the nurse and the patient remains proximal, i.e. near.

In recent years, there have been several cases on whether a duty of care is owed to an individual by different public services: the ambulance service, social services, the police and the fire service. In one case, the Court of Appeal held that although the ambulance service owed no duty to the public at large to respond to a telephone call for help, once a 999 call had been accepted, it was arguable that the ambulance service did have an obligation to provide the service for a named individual at a specified address. Subsequently the Court of Appeal dismissed an appeal by the London Ambulance Authority that it should pay the victim £362,377. The facts of the case are shown in Case 3.1.

Case 3.1   *Kent* v *Griffiths and Others* [2000]

Ambulance slow to arrive[8]

A doctor called an ambulance for a woman who was asthmatic at 4.27 p.m. on 16 February 1991. The standards recommended were that the ambulance should come within 14 minutes. The husband phoned again at 4.39 p.m. and was told they would be there within 7 to 8 minutes. The doctor phoned at 4.55 p.m. and was told it would be a couple of minutes. The ambulance arrived at 5.05 p.m., 38 minutes after the first call. (A record prepared by a member of the crew indicated that it had arrived after 22 minutes.) During the journey, the claimant was given oxygen, but on the way suffered a respiratory arrest with tragic consequences, including serious memory impairment, change of personality and miscarriage. The judge found that the record of the ambulance's arrival had been falsified. The Court of Appeal refused to strike out the case as disclosing no reasonable **cause of action** for negligence, but held that the case should continue to trial.

The Court of Appeal held that a duty of care could be owed by the ambulance service, which was comparable to hospital services rather than to the police or fire services.

In the second appeal, the Court of Appeal held that the **acceptance** of the call in the present case established the duty of care. It was delay that caused the further injuries. If wrong information had not been given about the arrival of the ambulance, other means of transport could have been used.

In another case, in June 2014 a scientist who was brain damaged after waiting more than 100 minutes for an ambulance won compensation of £5 million. The ambulance service had given the call a high-risk register which required a police escort because of potential risks to the safety of staff.[9]

Does a Nurse have a Duty to Volunteer Help?

Practical Dilemma 3.1   Volunteering help

A nurse on her way to work passes a road accident. She sees that a man is still trapped in a vehicle. Does she have an obligation to stop and render first aid? If she does stop and help and something goes wrong, would she be liable?

Unless there is a pre-existing relationship between the parties (for example, if the nurse has caused the accident or if they are employed to assist people in such circumstances), the nurse has no duty in law to stop and render first aid. So if, for example, someone saw the nurse drive past and, knowing that they were a nurse, believed that the nurse could have saved the victim, and the nurse was consequently sued, the action would fail. The nurse's failure to help is not actionable. There is in law no duty to volunteer help. There must be a pre-existing duty. However, once the nurse undertakes the duty of care, the nurse is then bound to follow the standard of care that would be expected of a reasonable person. So, for example, imagine that the nurse moves the victim and causes spinal injury. If it can be shown that the nurse should have anticipated, and foreseen the dangers of moving a person when a spinal injury was possible, and if there were no immediate danger in leaving the man where he was, then the nurse could be sued for any further injuries she had caused him. As this event would have taken place outside of work, there would be no vicarious lability (where the employer takes the liability on behalf of the employee).

While there is no legal duty, the Nursing and Midwifery Council (NMC) has made it clear in paragraph 15 of The Code,[10] published in 2015 updated in 2018 to include Nursing Associates, that a nurse should:

Always offer help if an emergency arises in your practice setting or anywhere else.

It goes on to state in paragraph 15.1 that the nurse must:

only act in an emergency within the limits of your knowledge and competence.

The nurse who failed to volunteer help could therefore not be held legally liable in the civil courts for failing to act; they could, however, face professional conduct proceedings (see chapter 11). Where the nurse has volunteered help in such a situation, as previously stated, it is unlikely that the employer would accept any responsibility for the nurse's actions (i.e. would not be vicariously liable) and therefore the nurse would have to rely on personal insurance cover in the event of any action being brought against them. This cover, known as cover for Samaritan actions, is provided by some professional associations and such professional indemnity covered is recommended by the NMC. Professional indemnity cover is now required by all health professionals (see chapter 4). Lord Young's[11] review of health and safety laws recommends clarification of the laws relating to the liability of a volunteer because of fears that concern over liability is preventing people from volunteering help.

Clarify (through legislation if necessary) that people will not be held liable for any consequences due to well-intentioned voluntary acts on their part.

The Social Action, Responsibility and Heroism Act was passed by the UK Parliament in 2015. The Act protects volunteers, teachers and organisations from legal action if they act in an emergency or take reasonable steps in organising school trips (see chapter 12).

Practical Dilemma 3.2 A fall in the night

Mary Smith is in the postoperative ward following a gall bladder operation. She becomes very disturbed during the night and Staff Nurse Janice Parker hears a crash and rushes to the ward. She finds Mrs Smith on the floor.

How is the civil liability of the staff nurse determined? The questions to be answered are:

1. Does Staff Nurse Parker owe a duty of care to Mrs Smith?
2. Is she in breach of the duty of care?
3. Has her breach of care led to reasonably foreseeable harm?
4. Has the patient suffered compensatable harm?

To win compensation in a civil case, Mary Smith would have to show that the staff nurse failed to follow the approved accepted practice without good reason in carrying out her duty of care towards her and that, as a reasonably foreseeable result, she suffered harm.

Does a Duty of Care Arise?

A nurse, by virtue of the nurse/patient relationship, does owe a duty of care to her patients. Whether a duty of care exists will be decided by established legal principles. There is no doubt that, in these circumstances, the nurse does owe a duty of care to the patient. The duty of care in relation to independent contractors is considered in chapter 4. Once it is decided that a duty of care is owed, the next question is: has there been a breach of this duty? Before this can be answered, the nature of the standard of care owed must be established.

Standard of care

Approved Practice

Case 3.2 — Whitehouse v Jordan [1981]

Birth traumas[12]

Stuart Whitehouse was born on 7 January 1970 with severe brain damage. His mother alleged that the brain damage was caused because the doctor pulled too hard and too long with forceps, as a consequence of which the baby was severely disabled. The doctor denied the allegations.

The House of Lords stated that whether an error of judgement was negligence or not depended on the facts of the situation. The test to be applied to determine if there was negligence was the **Bolam Test** (from an earlier case in 1957).[13] In applying this test in this case, the House of Lords decided that Mr Jordan had not been negligent. The Bolam Test is as follows:

> **When you get a situation that involves the use of some special skill or competence, then the test as to whether there has been negligence or not is . . . the standard of the ordinary skilled man exercising and professing to have that special skill. If a surgeon failed to measure up to that in any respect ('clinical judgement' or otherwise), he had been negligent and should be so adjudged.**

In the last sentence, 'any other professional' can be substituted for 'surgeon'. Thus the negligence of a nurse is to be determined by the standard of the ordinary skilled nurse at the time that the events took place. Standards might have changed before any court case takes place. A doctor was not liable when the patient developed a later illness which the doctor could not have spotted at the time.[14]

Let us turn again to Practical Dilemma 3.2, of the patient falling out of bed, and see how the court would decide whether or not Staff Nurse Janice Parker was in breach of care in relation to the patient Mary Smith.

What would the ordinary skilled nurse be expected to do in those circumstances? Was it reasonably foreseeable that this patient was likely to be restless? If so, what additional precautions should have been taken? Was she in the right location and was she adequately supervised? Had the patient called earlier for help or a bedpan and did that request go unheard or unmet? In the actual court hearing, expert evidence would be given as to what would have been expected of a nurse in that context and the judge would decide what should be regarded as acceptable practice in that context.

Deviation from Approved Practice

It does not follow that simply to fail to follow the accepted practice is, in itself, evidence of negligence since there may well be very strong reasons why the usual properly accepted practice was not followed in a particular case. The following case illustrates this point.

Case 3.3   *Maynard* v *West Midlands* [1984]

Biopsy[15]

A consultant physician and a consultant surgeon, while recognising that the most likely diagnosis of the patient's illness was tuberculosis (TB), took the view that Hodgkin's disease, carcinoma and sarcoidosis were also possibilities. Because Hodgkin's disease is fatal unless remedial steps are taken in its early stages, they decided that, rather than wait several weeks for the result of a sputum test, the operation of mediastinoscopy should be performed to provide a biopsy. This involved some risk of damage to the left laryngeal recurrent nerve, even if correctly performed. The operation was carried out properly, but that damage did in fact occur. The biopsy proved negative and it was subsequently confirmed that the patient did have TB and not Hodgkin's disease. The patient brought an action against the health authority, claiming that the decision to perform the biopsy rather than wait for the result of the TB test had been negligent.

At the trial, a **distinguished** body of medical opinion was called approving of the action of the consultants in carrying out the operation, but the judge said that he preferred the evidence of an expert witness called for the claimant, who had stated that the case had almost certainly been one of TB from the outset and should have been so diagnosed and that it had been wrong and dangerous to undertake the operation. The trial judge gave judgment for the claimant. The defendants succeeded before the Court of Appeal and the claimant therefore appealed to the House of Lords. The House of Lords held that in the medical profession there was room for differences of opinion and practice, and that a court's preference for one body of opinion over another was no basis for a conclusion of negligence. Where it was alleged that a fully considered decision by two consultants in their own special field had been negligent, it was not sufficient to establish negligence for the claimant to show that there was a body of competent professional opinion that considered that the decision had been wrong if there was also a body of equally competent professional opinion that supported the decision as having been reasonable in the circumstances. The claimant therefore lost the appeal and the case.

While this decision might seem very hard for the patient, it is only fair to the professional staff where a decision has been made carefully and with great consideration and is supported by substantial professional opinion, even if not everyone would have followed the same practice. In applying this to nursing staff, it can be said that in most circumstances the nurse will be expected to follow the standards of practice laid down by the profession or the local policy of the employer, but there may be very exceptional circumstances where it is justifiable not to follow the accepted practice. In a more recent case, the Court of Appeal has suggested that, where there was more than one acceptable standard, competence should be gauged by the lowest of them.[16] The Bolam Test applied where there was a conscious choice of available courses made by a trained professional. It was inappropriate where the alleged neglect lay in an oversight.

Statute 3.1
Congenital Disabilities (Civil Liability) Act 1976 Section 1(5)

The defendant is not answerable to the child, for anything he did or omitted to do when responsible in a professional capacity for treating or advising the parent, if he took reasonable care having due regard to then received professional opinion applicable to the particular class of case; but that does not mean that he is answerable only because he departed from received opinion.

The wording of the Congenital Disabilities (Civil Liability) Act 1976 (which gives a right of action in cases of prenatal infliction of harm) puts the point very clearly.

The courts rely on expert evidence to decide on what is a reasonable standard of care and the House of Lords in the Bolitho case emphasised that such expert opinion must flow logically and reasonably from the specific circumstances:

> **The use of the adjectives 'responsible, reasonable and respectable' (in the Bolam case) all showed that the court had to be satisfied that the exponents of the body of opinion relied upon could demonstrate that such opinion had a logical basis.[17]**

It will be rare for a court to hold a school of medical opinion as irresponsible.[18]

Following the changes to the civil procedure as a result of the Woolf Reforms, parties to a civil action are required, if possible, to agree on experts who are to give evidence of the required standards and the extent to which what actually happened measured up to that standard.

The application of the Bolam Test was considered in the work of the laboratory screeners who read the slides for cervical cytology.[19] The High Court and Court of Appeal held that the Bolam Test did not apply where no professional judgement was required by the employee. The evidence of expert witnesses that the Standards of the Cervical Screening Programme, which required an absolute confidence test, had not been complied with was accepted by the judge. (The full facts of the case are given in chapter 22.) In a case which followed a skiing accident, the Court of Appeal held that the implementation of a duty of care never to allow skiing pupils to take risks beyond their capabilities depended on local standards.[20] An inquest in 2010 heard that a teenager suffering from meningococcal septicaemia died after she was moved to two incorrect wards rather than to intensive care. The coroner ruled that there was a lack of direction and urgency over her treatment which was characterised by seven errors. He was unable to say whether these failures had contributed to her death.

Policies, Protocol, Procedures, Guidelines, Benchmarks and their Effect

The questions arise: when must I follow a procedure and when should I not follow it? Is there any difference in law between a policy, a procedure and a guideline and their effect? In the main, guidance issued by an employer, by a professional association or by the registration body should as far as is reasonable be followed. However, there may be specific circumstances that make the following of a particular procedure inappropriate and therefore any reasonable practitioner would modify compliance with the procedure accordingly. Clearly, advice from others would be required to ascertain whether rigid compliance with the procedure would be justified. The courts require a reasonable standard to be followed, a standard that would be supported by competent professional opinion and practice. Where the practitioner decides that circumstances justify a modification of the usual procedure, it is essential that they record exactly why the usual practice was not followed.

Procedures, policies, protocols, benchmarks and guidelines do not have a recognised **hierarchy** in courts of law. The same principles would apply to them all. In general, they should be followed, if it would be reasonable to do so. If a policy or guideline is issued by an NHS trust or health board that is not acceptable in the light of professional practice, it should be challenged as soon as possible and a revised policy that does accord with reasonable standards of care issued. The significance of protocols has become more important as the work of the National Institute for Health and Care Excellence (NICE) has expanded (see chapter 5). Eventually, NICE guidelines are likely to be incorporated into the Bolam Test of reasonable practice, but it will be open for a health professional to argue that the guidelines were not appropriate in the particular circumstances of the patient for whom they were caring. In the case of *Early v Newham HA*,[21] the judge accepted that guidelines drafted locally by consultants on intubation could be seen as satisfying the Bolam Test. In a case in 2005[22] where a ventouse delivery was attempted at 9 cm of dilation and led to spastic tetraplegia and cerebral palsy in the baby, the court held that the clinician had failed to follow both the guidelines of the Royal College of Obstetricians and Gynaecologists and also the hospital's own guidelines, and held the defendant NHS trust liable.

The Bolam Test was applied in a case where a patient alleged that, had her general practitioner referred her for orthopaedic surgery the same day as she was seen by him, she would not have suffered from the severe side effects of the loss of function of her bowels and bladder. She failed since it was established that her GP's views were in accordance with the practice accepted as proper and there was no evidence that had there been a same-day referral, she would have had an operation immediately.[23] The Department of Health has updated the essence of care benchmarks which were first published in 2001 and following a consultation in 2009 were revised.[24] Twelve fundamental areas of patient care were identified and provide benchmarks for determining if the essential standards have been met. The areas include: bladder, bowel and continence care; care environment; communication; food and drink; prevention and management of pain; personal hygiene; prevention and management of pressure ulcers; promoting health and wellbeing; record keeping; respect and dignity; safety and self-care. The guide on how to employ the benchmarks shows how versatile they are for use in audit, education, checklists, and for use by the Care Quality Commission (CQC) and other regulators to ascertain compliance with recognised standards of care. Many professional bodies, including the Royal College of Nursing (RCN), have provided guidelines on clinical practice which could become absorbed within the Bolam Test of approved practice. For example, the RCN has published guidelines on the assessment and prevention of falls in older people,[25] venous leg ulcers,[26] irritable bowel syndrome,[27] pressure ulcer assessment and equipment,[28] recognition of acute pain in children,[29] management of violence in inpatient psychiatric services and emergency departments,[30] contingency management and delivery of critical care in a post anaesthesia care unit,[31] monitoring standards of care,[32] national standards and guidance in diabetes care,[33] and dementia.[34] They, and others, can be found on the RCN website.[35] (See also chapter 23 on the scope of professional practice and clinical guidelines.)

NICE published guidance on the use of intravenous drips in December 2013 pointing out that tens of thousands of patients were harmed every year because doctors and nurses made basic mistakes when using intravenous drips. The guidance emphasised that all doctors and nurses must be trained in how to use drips. They should also use new formulas to calculate what patients need, and the cost of this will be more than outweighed by savings from patients having fewer complications as a result.[36]

In 2014 NICE was given a new role to develop evidence-based guidelines which set out safe staffing levels for the NHS, focusing on nursing and midwifery staffing levels (see chapter 4). Further information on forthcoming NICE publications on staffing can be found on its website.[37]

Recent examples of possible negligence include:

> An inquest was told that a GP was visited four times by a 16-year-old girl with complaints of headaches and failed to diagnose a non-lethal brain tumour. He refused the mother's request to arrange an MRI scan.[38]
>
> An ambulance NHS trust was found liable for the negligence of paramedics who failed to take a proper history from the patient or to make a proper assessment of the symptoms and signs they did find, had insufficient training and knowledge of the potential consequences of her high blood pressure and had over reliance on ECGs. They did not advise the patient to attend hospital that day and she died five days later.[39]
>
> A liver surgeon was suspended after a review of 32 of his patients found that 10 later died and 8 of those deaths were avoidable.[40] He was reported to the GMC and the Cardiff and Vale University Health Board set up an emergency line for patients.
>
> A patient was found dead in the hospital fire exit.[41]
>
> A girl died when the paramedics went to the wrong RAF base.[42]
>
> A girl died from pneumonia after being sent home from an out-of-hours GP who gave her less than optimal treatment.[43]
>
> A girl died from an infection because a junior doctor with only four weeks in the post failed to spot a fatal infection. The junior doctor was left in charge of 130 patients overnight and the coroner stated that the medical records were a shambles.[44]
>
> The coroner recorded a narrative verdict in a case where a 64-year-old man died after apparently being ignored by staff who did not give him the necessary fluids for his kidney condition and were too busy to provide care at the Queens Medical Centre in Nottingham.[45]

In many of these cases, the inquest finding will be followed by either civil action to obtain compensation or an **offer** of an ex gratia payment by the hospital to settle the case.

The Court of Appeal refused to allow an appeal against the finding that there was no negligence by a GP who failed to refer a baby to hospital. Colic had been diagnosed. The baby was subsequently diagnosed with meningitis which left him with moderate learning difficulties, double incontinence and right hemiplegic cerebral palsy. It held that the experienced judge had come to a clear conclusion about the consultation with the GP and there was no material error in his approach or findings.[46]

The legal situation is thus as follows:

1. There is no breach of the standard of care if the professional has acted in accordance with the practice accepted as proper by a responsible body of professionals skilled in that particular art and this was appropriate in the circumstances of the case.

2. There is no breach of the standard of care if there is no acceptable body of opinion covering that situation, but what the professional did was considered reasonable in all the circumstances.

3. There is no breach of the standard of care if the professional did not follow the accepted practice, but their actions were reasonable in all the circumstances and would be supported by competent professional opinion.

Reasonable Foreseeability

Other criteria are considered in determining if the professional has been negligent. One of the basic principles of the law of negligence is that precautions can be taken only against reasonably known risks.

Case 3.4 *Roe v Ministry of Health* [1954]

Ampoules in phenol[47]

A local anaesthetic was given by injection in a hospital. The ampoule, which was stored in phenol to sterilise it, contained invisible cracks caused by some mishandling in the hospital, through which the phenol seeped into the ampoule. The injection caused paralysis.

The patient sued the anaesthetist and nurses and their employer. The patient, however, lost the case. The possibility of seepage through invisible cracks was not known at that time and precautions against an unforeseeable possibility are not required of the defendant. However, successful defence may, of course, mean that the next claimant has a greater chance of winning since such risks are now known. The standard of care thus increases.

The judge, Lord Denning, said in this case:

> It is so easy to be wise after the event and to condemn as negligence that which was only a misadventure. We ought always to be on our guard against it, especially in cases against hospitals and doctors. Medical science has conferred great benefits on mankind, but these benefits are attended by considerable risks. Every surgical operation is attended by risks. We cannot take the benefits without taking the risks. Every advance in technique is also attended by risks. Doctors like the rest of us have to learn by experience; and experience often teaches in a hard way. Something goes wrong and shows up a weakness, and then it is put right . . . We must not look at the 1947 accident with 1954 spectacles.

Exactly the same could be said of practice today and of nurses as well as doctors. There may be many occasions when one looks back and says, 'I would do things differently if I were to do it again', but that does not mean the professional has been negligent.

Keeping up to Date

When one looks at the many professional journals that exist, the question must arise as to what extent the professional can be expected to master all this knowledge. How up to date is one expected to be?

Case 3.5 *Crawford v Charing Cross Hospital* [1953]

A recent article[48]

A patient developed brachial palsy during a blood transfusion. An article had appeared in *The Lancet* six months previously describing this hazard.

The patient lost the case on the grounds that, provided the professional staff were following the accepted approved practice at that time, it could not be said that they were negligent in failing to apply or be aware of recent knowledge.

Articles in magazines and journals can be of very different status. Some are pure research articles, the lessons from which have not yet been absorbed into current accepted practice; others are controversial and their conclusions may never become part of recognised procedure. For example, if an article was from a tabloid paper, while it may have some merit, there is an onus on the nurse to seek more robust evidence before deciding a particular action. Other instructions, however, should have immediate effect. Thus, if a directive from the Medicines and Healthcare Products Regulatory Agency warned against prescribing a particular drug to a patient, to ignore that instruction might well be evidence of negligence. Nursing staff who had received comparable instructions from their profession or senior nurse management would be expected to be aware of these orders and to comply. The instructions would become part of the accepted practice.

Balancing the Risks

As the earlier quotation from Lord Denning points out, there are hazards in modern medicine, and much of professional discretion is concerned with balancing the risks of taking action A compared with action B or compared with taking no action at all.

Practical Dilemma 3.3 Meningitis

A patient was admitted with a provisional diagnosis of meningitis. She was immediately barrier nursed in a single room, even though that meant moving a very sick patient on to a four-bed ward. The patient who was moved died in the night. There was criticism from relatives that the patient should not have been moved and also a suggestion that the death was accelerated. Was the nurse at fault if, the next day, it was discovered that the suspected meningitis patient was only suffering from a non-fatal virus?

Provided the nurse used their professional judgement in making the decision to give the single room to that particular patient, with the knowledge available to them at that time, then there should be no finding of negligence. In fact, if meningitis had been confirmed, then the nurse may well have been negligent in not taking precautions to prevent any danger of staff or patients being infected. They have to use their judgement in determining the degree of risk to both patients.

Causation

The third element in the claimant's case against the NHS trust or the nurse is to establish that there is a causal link between the breach of the duty of care by the nurse and the harm suffered by the claimant. It is possible for the nurse to fail in their duty of care to the patient and for the patient to suffer harm, yet for the nurse or their employer not to be liable in civil law. This is because one of the essential elements that the claimant must establish in an action for negligence is that there is a causal link between the failure of the defendant to follow the approved practice and the harm suffered by the patient. The possibility that this harm could occur must be reasonably foreseeable and must also take place.

Factual Causation

Case 3.6 *Barnett v Chelsea HMC* **[1968]**

Causation[49]

A patient attended the casualty department after drinking tea that, unknown to him, had been contaminated with arsenic and that caused prolonged vomiting. The doctor did not examine him, but sent a message that he should see his own doctor. He died a few hours later.

The widow failed in her action because it was established that the patient would have died even if properly examined and treated. In this case, the pathological evidence on the progress of arsenic poisoning and the projected timetable of events had the patient been examined and admitted was of vital importance.

Similarly, the claimant lost where a doctor had been negligent in making a wrong diagnosis but nothing could have been done had the correct diagnosis been made.[50] In another case although there were breaches of care by doctors in the care of a patient following rectal surgery, the high court held that these breaches had not caused the death from compartment syndrome.[51]

In such circumstances, although a civil action fails there are likely to be professional and disciplinary proceedings by the professional body and the employer.

Barnett's case (Case 3.6) was an example of a lack of factual connection between the breach of duty of care and the harm suffered by the patient.

Another example of a case that has been before the House of Lords is the following.

Case 3.7 — Wilsher v Essex AHA [1988]

Blindness, but how caused?[52]

In the Wilsher case (considered in chapter 4 Case 4.3), the House of Lords decided that the case should be reheard by a new High Court judge on the issue of whether it was the defendant's negligence that had caused the harm to the child. In this case, it was agreed that there were several different factors that could have caused the child to become blind, and the negligence by the defendant was only one of these. The trial judge had failed to make a relevant finding of fact and could not presume that it was the defendant's negligence that had caused the harm.

Following the House of Lords' ruling, the parties came to a settlement and compensation was paid to the parents for the child.

In a case heard in 2008, the Court of Appeal held that weakness to the patient following the hospital's negligence in failing to resuscitate her properly after an operation combined with weakness caused by her pancreatitis led to her overall weakened state which resulted in her aspirating her vomit and suffering brain damage. It was not possible to determine the causative effects of each form of weakness, but the Ministry of Defence (in their role as managers of the Royal Haslar Hospital – the first hospital to which she was admitted) was held liable for the harm the patient suffered.[53]

In July 2009, the High Court held that Corby Borough Council was potentially liable for disabilities to young children whose mothers had been exposed to toxic materials when the former steelworks were reclaimed. The Council had argued that there was no link between the deformities and the removal of waste to a quarry.[54] The deformities included missing fingers, heart and eye defects and skin conditions.

Case 3.8 — Kay v Ayrshire and Arran Health Board [1987]

The cause of deafness[55]

A child suffering from meningitis was given 300,000 units of penicillin instead of 10,000 units. The mistake was discovered and remedial action taken. The health authority admitted liability and made an offer to the parents for the additional pain and suffering that the negligence caused the boy. However, the parents argued that the overdose had caused the boy to become deaf and they rejected the board's offer, claiming instead many thousands of pounds more because they held the health authority liable for the deafness.

The House of Lords decided that the parents had not made out the factual causation between the overdose and the deafness, and thus that the boy was not entitled to the larger amount. It is a well-known fact that meningitis itself can cause deafness.

Reasonably Foreseeable Consequence

In a civil case for negligence, the claimant also has to establish that the harm that occurred was a reasonably foreseeable consequence of breach of duty by the defendant.

Practical Dilemma 3.4 — Reasonable foreseeability

In breach of her duty of care, a nurse failed to dispose properly of contaminated dressings, which were left on a stainless steel trolley in the treatment area. By chance, two boys broke into the room looking for syringes and needles. When they heard footsteps approaching, they grabbed as much as they could from the trolley and ran off, taking a dressing with them. Subsequently, an outbreak of disease attributable to the dressing occurred in the neighbourhood. Was the nurse responsible in law for this?

The nurse was certainly at fault for not disposing correctly of the dressings. However, it could be argued that the subsequent events were not reasonably foreseeable and, in any event, the chain of causation between the nurse's action and the outbreak of the disease was broken by the action of the boys. This is sometimes known as a *novus actus interveniens* (i.e. a new act intervening).

Taking One's Claimant as One Finds Him

There is one important exception to the rule that the harm resulting from the breach of duty is reasonably foreseeable, known as the thin skull rule or 'you take your claimant as you find him'.

Practical Dilemma 3.5 — The thin skull rule

A nurse puts some drops in the wrong eye. They were meant to dilate the pupil in the other eye. They would not normally have caused any harm, but because of an existing defect in that eye the patient became blind.

The nurse in this case is clearly negligent. However, in the majority of patients her error would have caused no, or very little, harm. In this case, however, even though she could not have predicted the outcome, she would be liable for the harm that has occurred on the basis of the doctrine 'you take your claimant as you find him'.

Case 3.9 — *Smith v Leech Brain* [1961]

The thin skull rule[56]

An accident occurred at work when a labourer was splashed with a piece of molten metal and his lower lip was burnt. The burn was treated and the labourer thought nothing more about it. However, the place where the burn had been began to ulcerate and get larger. He consulted his general practitioner who sent him to hospital where cancer was diagnosed. Treatment by radium needles enabled the lip to heal and destroyed the primary growth. Subsequently, however, secondary growths were observed. He had six operations and died of cancer just over three years after the accident. His widow claimed compensation from the employers.

They admitted liability for the original accident, but denied that they were responsible for the man's death. Lord Parker in the Queen's Bench Division held that the test was not whether the defendants could reasonably have foreseen that a burn would cause cancer and that Mr Smith would die. The test was whether these defendants could reasonably foresee the type of injury that he suffered, namely the burn. The amount of damage suffered as a result of a burn depends on the characteristics and constitution of the victim. The widow therefore won her case.

In a case involving harm to a child who was playing about on a boat,[57] the House of Lords held that ingenuity of children in finding unexpected ways of doing mischief to themselves and others should not be underestimated. Reasonable foreseeability was not a fixed point on the scale of probability and the child won his case against the local authority as occupiers. (The case is discussed in chapter 12 Case 12.3.)

Loss of a Chance

Case 3.10   *Hotson v Berkshire AHA* [1987]

A lost chance[58]

A 13-year-old boy fell out of a tree and suffered a slipped femoral epiphysis. He attended the A&E department, but the doctor failed to carry out an X-ray of the hip. The boy suffered considerable pain and returned to hospital five days later, when the fracture was diagnosed. He developed avascular necrosis of the femoral head which medical evidence suggested occurred in 75 per cent of patients. Expert evidence for the claimant was that as a result of the delay in diagnosis he lost a 25 per cent chance of avoiding this complication. The judge awarded the boy £150 damages for the pain suffered by him for the five days, which he would have been spared by prompt diagnosis and treatment. In addition, the boy was awarded 25 per cent of the damages that would have been awarded had the entire injury been attributable to negligence (i.e. 25 per cent of £45,000), for the loss of the chance of recovery.

The House of Lords allowed the health authority's appeal, holding that the claimant had not established that the defendant's negligence had caused the avascular necrosis. The question of causation was to be determined on the balance of probabilities with the onus on the claimant. The cause of his injuries was the non-negligent falling out of the tree and that injury would on balance of probabilities have occurred anyway.

The loss of a chance argument by a claimant is particularly difficult in cases where there has been failure to diagnose a condition such as a malignancy. In such a case the patient may have died even had the correct diagnosis been made, but would attempt to argue that had the correct diagnosis been made, then he would have been in that category which would have obtained remission following the appropriate treatment. In order to obtain compensation when there has been negligence in diagnosis, the claimant may have to rely on the specific consequences of delayed diagnosis such as further protracted treatment, additional pain and suffering, or other harm, rather than being able to claim that he or she would have been cured.

The House of Lords, in a majority judgment (*Gregg* v *Scott*),[59] reaffirmed the use of the balance of probabilities test of causation in a 'lost chance' case and dismissed the claimant's appeal. The claimant alleged that negligent misdiagnosis of his tumour had caused a nine-month delay in the start of treatment. The trial judge held that this delay had reduced the claimant's chance of a cure from 42 per cent to 25 per cent. *Gregg* v *Scott* was applied in another case of failure to detect cancer, where the claimant partially succeeded in his claim. The GP admitted breach of her duty of care in failing to diagnose a malignant melanoma in 2006. A correct diagnosis was made seven months later by another doctor. The judge held that the tumour had already become ulcerated in 2006 and his chances of surviving a further 10 years were less than 50 per cent. The judge found that failure to diagnose the tumour in 2006 had caused his life expectancy to be reduced by three years[60]

Hotson was applied in a case where Cauda Equina Syndrome (CES) was not diagnosed but the court held that on the balance of probabilities the prospects of the claimant making a good recovery if surgery had been undertaken earlier were less than 50 per cent and his claim that earlier surgery might have resulted in some general improvement in his condition was entirely speculative and impressionistic.[61]

Liable for what?

A victim of the Ladbroke Grove rail crash who suffered depression which led to his killing someone, was unable to recover **damages** for the loss of his earnings after the manslaughter from the defendants who admitted liability for negligence up to the date of the manslaughter.[62] While his physical injuries were minor, the accident had a major psychological impact on him. He suffered post-traumatic stress disorder (see below) with a marked depressive component and a significant personality change. In August 2001, he stabbed a stranger to death. The Court of Appeal held that his claim was not founded on an illegal act. The manslaughter was not inextricably bound up with the claim for loss of earnings before and after the manslaughter, which resulted from the defendant's negligence. It was for the court to determine to what extent the manslaughter was the claimant's fault and therefore could be viewed as contributory negligence under the 1945 Act (see below).

However, the House of Lords allowed the defendant's appeal and held that the claimant could not recover damages for loss of earnings following his detention in prison and in mental hospital following the killing on the basis that a person cannot benefit from his own wrong (*ex turpi causa non oritur actio*). The defendants had accepted liability in negligence up to the date the claimant had committed the manslaughter.[63]

Harm

Not all forms of harm are compensatable by the civil courts. Grief itself is not a ground for a claim, although there is now a statutory right for compensation for bereavement where the death has resulted from negligence. This is considered in chapter 6 where the basis for the amount of compensation is discussed. The court recognises that harm that involves personal injury or death or loss or damage of property should be compensated if the other elements of negligence can be proved. However, the harm must be a reasonably foreseeable consequence of the breach of duty; it must not be too remote. This is a particularly difficult question when economic loss has occurred and the courts have limited the liability of the defendants to reasonably foreseeable economic loss. Similar difficulties arise over determining the liability for causing nervous shock, or post-traumatic stress as it is now termed.

Post-traumatic Stress

Case 3.11 *McLoughlin v O'Brian* [1982]

Post-traumatic stress syndrome (nervous shock)[64]

Mr Thomas McLoughlin and his three children, George (aged 17), Kathleen (aged 7) and Gillian (aged 3), were in a motorcar driven by George when it was in collision with a lorry. George was not at fault. Mrs McLoughlin, who was not in the vehicle, was told by a friend who was in the car behind (with Michael, another McLoughlin child, aged 11, who was a passenger) that George had probably died and that he was uncertain of the condition of the husband or the other children. She was driven to the hospital and saw Michael, who told her that Gillian was dead. She was taken down the corridor and, through a window, she saw Kathleen, crying with her face cut and begrimed with dirt and oil. She could hear George shouting and screaming. She was taken to her husband, who was sitting with his head in his hands. His shirt was hanging off him and he was covered in mud and oil. He saw his wife and started sobbing. She was then taken to see George. The whole of the left face and left side were covered. He appeared to recognise her and then lapsed into unconsciousness. Finally, she was taken to see Kathleen, who by now had been cleaned up. The child was too upset to speak and simply clung to her mother. As a result of this experience Mrs McLoughlin suffered from severe shock, organic depression and a change of personality. She was normally a person of reasonable fortitude.

Obviously, in a case like this, damages would be payable to the husband and the children for the harm that they had suffered, but in addition to that, compensation was claimed by Mrs McLoughlin for nervous shock. The defendants argued that she was too remote from the defendants' negligence: she was not herself a direct victim of the accident, neither was she a bystander witnessing what happened. The House of Lords decided that she was entitled to receive compensation since she was so closely related to those injured and the nervous shock that she suffered was close in both space and time.

Lord Wilberforce said:

> It is necessary to consider three elements inherent in any claim: the class of persons whose claims should be recognised; the proximity of such persons to the accident; and the means by which the shock is caused. As regards the class of persons the possible range is between the closest possible of family ties, of parent and child or husband and wife, and the ordinary bystander. Existing law recognises the claims of the first; it denies that of the second, either on the basis that such persons must be assumed to be possessed of fortitude sufficient to enable them to endure the calamities of modern life or that defendants cannot be expected to compensate the world at large.

Any persons wishing to claim compensation for nervous shock (now referred to as post-traumatic stress syndrome) would have to show that they were actually suffering from a mental illness and not simply grief, and that they were sufficiently closely related to the objects of the defendant's negligence and also in time and space.

The law has been further clarified by the House of Lords in the case of *Alcock* v *Chief Constable of the South Yorkshire Police*.[65] In this case, people who were present at or who watched the disaster at Hillsborough, where 96 people died (as a result of overcrowding in the stadium due to negligence by the police, which was determined by a second coroner's inquest held between April 2014 and April 2016), brought a claim in respect of post-traumatic stress syndrome. The House of Lords held that in order to establish a claim in respect of psychiatric illness resulting from shock it was necessary to show not only that such injury was reasonably foreseeable, but also that the relationship between the claimant and the defendant was sufficiently proximate. Proximity could include not only blood ties, but also ties of love and affection. The closeness would have to be proved in each individual case. The claimant would also have to show propinquity in time and space to the accident or its immediate aftermath. It was held that those claimants who viewed the disaster on television could not be said to be equivalent to being within sight and hearing of the event or its immediate aftermath.

In March 2014 the Association for Personal Injury lawyers pressed for the law to be reformed so that compensation for mental harm suffered by those who witness the death of a loved one is no longer based on the principles set down in the Alcock case but should be revised. The Alcock principles were held to be archaic, inflexible, unfair and needed to be changed as a matter of urgency.[66]

In *White and Others* v *Chief Constable of the South Yorkshire Police and Others*,[67] police officers sued for post-traumatic stress syndrome following the same disaster. The House of Lords decided that merely being an employee of the person/organisation responsible for the negligence did not automatically create sufficient proximity for the claimant to succeed in obtaining compensation for post-traumatic stress syndrome. The employee had to satisfy the usual rules of establishing proximity. To obtain compensation for psychiatric illness, a rescuer would have to show that he had objectively exposed himself to danger or reasonably believed that he was doing so. Rescuers were not entitled to claim compensation when they were not within the range of foreseeable physical injury and their psychiatric injury was caused by witnessing or participating in the aftermath of accidents that caused death or injury to others. The police therefore failed in their claim.

Both the McLoughlin and Alcock cases were referred to in a case in 1998,[68] where a mother failed in her case to obtain compensation for psychiatric illness following the abduction and death of her daughter by a mentally ill outpatient. The Court of Appeal held that the judge was correct to find that there was no proximity between the mother, the daughter and the Tees Health Authority. It was also relevant to consider how the offences could have been avoided even if sufficient proximity were established, having regard to the difficulty in identifying and protecting potential victims and to the limited effectiveness of the health authority's powers under the Mental Health Act 1983.[69]

The High Court[70] applied these House of Lords cases in a situation where a fire officer sued his son, claiming damages for psychiatric harm suffered as a result of attending the scene of an accident in which the son had suffered head injuries. The accident occurred as a result of the son driving a car negligently after drinking. The court held that a victim of self-inflicted injuries owed no duty of care to a secondary party who, after witnessing the event from which the injuries resulted or its aftermath, suffered psychiatric injury. In addition, in the circumstances of the case, to allow one family member to sue another would potentially result in an objectionable form of intra-family litigation.

An event may, in practice, cover a period of time, as the following case shows.

Case 3.12   *North Glamorgan NHS Trust* v *Walters* [2003]

Delayed transfer[71]

A 10-month-old boy was admitted to hospital suspected of suffering from hepatitis. The doctors failed to diagnose that this was acute and accepted that, had it been properly diagnosed and treated by means of a liver transplant, he may have lived. During the night he suffered a fit and the mother was told by the nurse that it was unlikely that he had suffered any brain damage. In fact, there had been a major epileptic seizure that led to a coma and irreparable brain damage. A scan was carried out and the mother was told incorrectly that it showed no brain damage. He was transferred to a London hospital where he was placed on a life support machine. A further scan showed that he had suffered severe brain damage and the parents agreed that it was in the boy's best interests for the life support to be turned off. He died in his mother's arms. She was subsequently told that had he been transferred earlier he would have had a far better chance of survival.

It was agreed that the mother was suffering from a pathological grief reaction, which was a result of witnessing, experiencing and participating in the events described. The judge found that the mother was a secondary victim and her psychiatric injury was caused by sight and sound of a horrifying event that had covered a period of time. The defendants appealed to the Court of Appeal on the grounds that the 36-hour period could not be regarded in law as one horrifying event, but the claimant's appreciation was not sudden. The Court of Appeal held that the 36-hour period could be viewed as a single horrifying event and the judge was correct to find that the claimant's appreciation of the events was sudden as opposed to an accumulation of gradual assaults on her mind.

A similar decision is seen in another Court of Appeal case[72] where the claimant suffered post-traumatic stress syndrome after her daughter was killed in a road accident when a car mounted the pavement. The claimant rushed to the scene of the accident, which was cordoned off, and she was prevented from crossing the tape. She was told that her daughter was dead and she screamed hysterically and collapsed to the ground. Subsequently, at the mortuary, while the worst of the injuries on the girl's lower part were covered by a blanket, the mother saw that the daughter's face and head were disfigured. She cradled the daughter, saying she was cold. She lost her case on the grounds that the judge could not accept that what happened in the mortuary could be said to be part of the aftermath. The shock from which she suffered was a result of what she had been told by the police. The Court of Appeal allowed the claimant's appeal, holding that the immediate aftermath extended from the moment of the accident until the moment that the claimant left the mortuary. The judge had artificially separated out the mortuary visit from what was an uninterrupted sequence of events.

A woman received more than £500,000 after paramedics arrived 17 minutes late to tend her dislocated knee. Her knee dislocated on a bus and she was trapped between two chairs. It took 50 minutes for the paramedics to arrive. The kneecap was manipulated back into place but she suffered immense psychological damages and she has been left house-bound.[73] In 2012 the High Court warned against the dangers of allowing claims for mental distress to creep into the forum of clinical negligence. In the case, parents failed in their claim for damages for psychiatric injury following the stillbirth of a child as a result of the hypercoiling of the umbilical cord. There had been negligence by the consultant in failing to advise a second meeting in relation to conception but this breach did not lead to the stillbirth.[74]

This topic of post-traumatic stress syndrome relates to the nurse in two ways. First, they may themselves be the victim of post-traumatic stress arising from another person's negligence, in which case they need to know whether they are likely to obtain compensation. Second, in their own work they should be aware of the dangers of causing stress shock in others and the possibility of claims for compensation arising out of this.

Conclusions

Claims in respect of clinical negligence are increasing in the NHS, and the nurse needs to be aware of the basic legal provisions which apply so that she can protect both the patient and herself. Following the Francis Report into the Mid Staffordshire NHS Trust scandal a duty of candour on organisations has been introduced together with a more effective complaints procedure. This duty of candour has been introduced into the The Code (NMC, 2015 updated 2018), adding a professional requirement for nurses to be open with mistakes made by them and other professionals. Being more open and transparent with patients and relatives will hopefully assist in earlier resolutions and foster a learning culture where staff can learn from mistakes made, to put in place steps to minimise future avoidable risks to patients. (See chapter 5 for the Francis Report and chapter 26 for complaints handling.) Identification and implementation of the appropriate standards is essential together with quality record keeping (see chapter 9) to ensure litigation is reduced.

Reflection questions

1. Consider the duty of care possibly owed by the nurse of an NHS trust and discuss whether and on what grounds you think a duty would be owed in the following circumstances:
   a. an informal psychiatric patient who wanders away from the hospital and damages cars in the vicinity of the hospital
   b. a patient detained under the Mental Health Act who does likewise
   c. a patient in the A&E department who, after an attempted suicide, insists on taking his own discharge and is shortly afterwards found dead on a railway line
   d. a doctor in a cinema who gives a person having a cardiac arrest the wrong treatment
   e. a community nurse who is caring for a neighbour, not on their list, and who accidentally leaves the door open. The neighbour is mugged and the house burgled.
2. If there has been a negligent act but no harm has occurred to the patient, what remedies are available (if any) for the patient to obtain compensation?

3. How would you determine the standard of care that should be adopted in carrying out the following procedures:

   a. lifting
   b. administering medication
   c. informing patients of their rights
   d. advising relatives on the procedures to be followed in dealing with death?

4. A man of 60 was told that he had terminal cancer and was unlikely to survive more than six months. He bought a car for a friend, had an expensive holiday and spent most of his savings. A year later he was informed that there had been a mistake in diagnosis and the growth was benign, and he could live to the usual age of life expectancy. He wishes to sue the trust for negligence. Analyse how such an action would proceed and what he would have to prove.

Further Exercises

1. Why do you consider that causation is an important element in an action for negligence? Would it be fairer to the claimant if causation did not need to be proved?
2. New Zealand and Finland have a system of no-fault liability for personal injury claims. What are the advantages and disadvantages of introducing such a scheme into the UK?

References

[1] NHS Litigation Annual Report for 2013 July 2014, www.gov.uk/government/publications/the-nhs-litigation-authority-report-and-accounts-2013-to-2014
[2] Blackwater Law (2018) Report into Serious Incidents at NHS Trusts and Health Boards in England and Wales. Braintree, Essex.
[3] www.npsa.nhs.uk/
[4] News item, *The Times*, 24 June 2009
[5] News item, Cancer victim was told to suck ice cubes by the GP, *The Times*, 3 August 2013
[6] Kat Lay, Mother died after doctors took out ovary instead of appendix, *The Times*, 11 June 2013
[7] *Donoghue* v *Stevenson* [1932] AC 562
[8] *Kent* v *Griffiths and Others*, The Times Law Report, 23 December 1998; The Times Law Report, 10 February 2000; [2000] 2 All ER 474
[9] Frances Gibb, Victim wins £5m after ambulance delay, *The Times*, 18 June 2014
[10] Nursing and Midwifery Council, The Code: standards for performance, conduct and ethics, NMC, 2015
[11] HM Government, Common Sense Common Safety 2010, Stationery Office; lordyoungreview@dwp.gsi.gov.uk
[12] *Whitehouse* v *Jordan* [1981] 1 All ER 267
[13] *Bolam* v *Friern Barnet HMC* [1957] 2 All ER 118
[14] *Ministry of Justice* v *Carter* [2010] EWCA Civ 694

15. *Maynard* v *West Midlands RHA* [1984] 1 WLR 634
16. *Michael Hyde and Associates Ltd* v *JD Williams and Co. Ltd*, The Times Law Report, 4 August 2000
17. *Bolitho* v *City and Hackney Health Authority* [1997] 3 WLR 115
18. *M* v *Blackpool Victoria Hospital NHS Trust* [2003] EWHC 1744
19. *Penney, Palmer and Cannon* v *East Kent Health Authority* [2000] Lloyd's Rep Med p. 41 CA
20. *Gouldbourn* v *Balkan Holidays Ltd.*, The Times Law Report, 3 May 2010
21. *Early* v *Newham HA* [1994] 5 Med LR 214
22. *Fotedar* v *St George's Healthcare NHS Trust* [2005] EWHC 1327 QBD
23. *Zarb* v *Odetoyinbo* [2006] EWHC 2880
24. Department of Health, Essence of Care, DH, TSO 2010
25. Royal College of Nursing 002772, RCN, London, November 2007
26. Royal College of Nursing 001214 October 2007; 003020 October 2007; 001204 October 2007; 001269 October 2007
27. Royal College of Nursing 003283 November 2008
28. Royal College of Nursing 002166 November 2007; 002444 November 2007
29. Royal College of Nursing 001597 November 2007; 003542 September 2009
30. Royal College of Nursing 003017 November 2007
31. Royal College of Nursing 003842 November 2010
32. Royal College of Nursing 2013
33. Ibid., 2013
34. Ibid., 2014
35. www.rcn.org.uk
36. Chris Smyth, Lives put at risk by nurses who can't use drips, *The Times*, 10 December 2013
37. www.nice.org.uk
38. Simon de Bruxelles, GP ignored tumour pain, *The Times*, 14 December 2013
39. *Taaffe* v *East of England Ambulance NHS Trust* [2012] EWHC 1335
40. News item, *The Times*, 11 December 2013
41. Rhys Blakely, Patient found dead in hospital fire exit, *The Times*, 11 October 2013
42. News item, *The Times*, 5 March 2014
43. David Sanderson, Dying student called mother after GP failed to give proper care, *The Times*, 8 January 2014
44. News item, *The Times*, 11 January 2014
45. News item, Hospital 'too busy' to treat dying man, *The Times*, 10 April 2014
46. *Doy (A child)* v *Gunn* [2013] EWCA Civ 547
47. *Roe* v *Minister of Health* [1954] 2 QB 66
48. *Crawford* v *Charing Cross Hospital*, The Times Law Report, 8 December 1953
49. *Barnett* v *Chelsea HMC* [1968] 1 All ER 1068
50. *Wright* v *Cambridge Medical Group* [2011] EWCA Civ 669
51. *Orwell* v *Salford Royal NHS Trust Foundation* [2013] EWHC 3245 QB
52. *Wilsher* v *Essex Area Health Authority* [1986] 3 All ER 801 CA; [1988] 1 All ER 871 HL
53. *Bailey* v *Minister of Defence* [2008] EWCA 883 Civ
54. *Cory Group Litigation Re* [2009] EWHC 1944 and 2109
55. *Kay* v *Ayrshire and Arran Health Board* [1987] 2 All ER 417
56. *Smith* v *Leech Brain & Co. Ltd* [1961] 3 All ER 1159 QBD
57. *Jolley* v *Sutton London Borough Council*, The Times Law Report, 24 May 2000; [2000] 1 WLR 1082
58. *Hotson* v *East Berks HA* [1987] AC 750
59. *Gregg* v *Scott* [2005] UKHL 2

60 *JD* v *Mather* [2012] EWHC 3063 QB.
61 *Hussain* v *Bradford Teaching Hospital NHS Foundation Trust* [2011] EWHC 2914
62 *Gray* v *Thames Trains Ltd and Another*, The Times Law Report, 9 July 2008 CA; [2008] EWCA Civ 713
63 *Gray* v *Thames Trains Ltd and Another*, The Times Law Report, 10 June 2009 HL; [2009] UKHL 33
64 *McLoughlin* v *O'Brian* [1982] 2 All ER 298
65 *Alcock* v *Chief Constable of the South Yorkshire Police* [1992] 2 AC 310 HL
66 www.apil.org.uk
67 *White and Others* v *Chief Constable of the South Yorkshire Police and Others* [1999] 1 All ER 1
68 *Palmer* v *Tees Health Authority and Another*, The Times Law Report, 1 June 1998; [1998] Lloyd's Rep Med 447 QBD
69 *Palmer* v *Tees HA* (2000) 2 LGLR 69 CA
70 *Greatorex* v *Greatorex and Another* (Pope, Pr 20 Defendant) [2000] 4 All ER 769
71 *North Glamorgan NHS Trust* v *Walters*, Lloyd's Rep Med 2 [2003] 49 CA
72 *Giullietta Galli-Atkinson* v *Sudhaker Seghal* Lloyd's Rep Med 6 [2003] 285
73 News item, *The Times*, 21 February 2014
74. *Less* v *Hussein* [2012] EWHC 3513 QB

Chapter 4

Specific Problem Areas in Civil Liability

Personal Liability of the Nurse, Vicarious Liability of the Employer and Managerial Issues

This chapter discusses

- Negligence in communication
- Inexperience
- Team liability and apportionment of responsibility
- Taking instructions: refusal to obey
- Nurse as manager
- Pressure on the manager
- Vicarious liability of employer
- In the course of employment
- Liability for negligence of volunteers
- Duty of care and liability for independent contractors
- Direct liability of employer
- Indemnity from the employee at fault
- Pressure from inadequate resources
- Public Interest Disclosure Act 1998 and whistleblowing

Introduction

In this chapter, we explore some of the particular difficulties that can arise in determining the liability of a professional in some specific situations, beginning with liability for negligence in communicating. In addition, we consider the problems that can arise from inadequate resources;

the nurse as a manager; and the liability of the employer. (The scope of professional practice and the role of the clinical nurse specialist and consultant nurse are considered in chapter 23.)

Negligence in communication

It is possible to be negligent in failing to communicate with the appropriate person at the correct time and in the proper way.

Case 4.1 Coles v Reading HMC [1963]

Crushed fingers[1]

Mr Coles suffered a crush injury to his finger. He went to the cottage hospital where the nurse cleaned the wound of dust and dirt and told him to go to a proper hospital where he would have an anti-tetanus injection. But neither she nor anyone else impressed on him the purpose and importance of the visit and so he did not go. He later saw his general practitioner who believed that he had had the injection and so he did not give him one. He subsequently died of tetanus.

In this case, there was negligence by all those professional staff (including the nurse) who had failed to communicate adequately with other professionals and with the patient. Failure to communicate, if it falls short of the required professional standard, can be regarded as negligence and is actionable if it causes reasonably foreseeable harm to the patient.

Failure to communicate rarely causes such devastating harm as in this tetanus case, but there are other well-known examples where it is vital that the patient receives certain information and it cannot be assumed that the patient is aware of the dangers. For example, in head injury cases there may be no detectable sign of head injury when the patient is seen in the emergency department. However, it is essential that the patient be warned to return if certain symptoms appear. Comparable instructions must be given after plastering and in many other situations. In such circumstances, it is advisable for a strict procedure to be implemented to ensure that the correct information is given both by word of mouth and in writing. If there is likely to be any dispute as to whether the information was given and/or where there are considerable dangers if the patient is not informed, it is possible to ask the patient to acknowledge in writing their receipt of that information. This procedure has the added advantage of making the patient aware of the importance of the information or instructions. A report of the National Patient Safety Agency in 2010[2] into delayed diagnoses of cancer revealed appalling faults in communication between GP, hospitals and diagnostic departments such as radiology and pathology. For example, a chest X-ray suggesting lung cancer taken on 1 November 2007 and reported on 23 days later was not delivered until 1 February 2008. In 2023 the Patients Association found that 55% of people had experienced poor communication from the NHS in the previous five years, and that 1 in 10 of the respondents said their care had been affected because of poor communication.

Negligence in instructing others is considered in further detail in chapter 17, which deals with the law and the nurse educator. Liability for a negligent misstatement was found when a local authority recommended a registered childminder to a mother despite an earlier case of non-accidental injury by the minder.[3]

Inexperience

Does a newly qualified nurse have to follow the same standard of care as an experienced nurse?

In practical terms, it is, of course, impossible to expect the same standard of care from the inexperienced nurse as from the experienced senior nurse. However, in law that is what the patient is entitled to expect. You cannot say in defence to a patient, 'The reason that you were given the wrong drug is that nurse X administered it and they have only just qualified.' The patient is entitled to receive the accepted standard of care whoever provides it. It is, however, essential that staff work within their field of competence and that work requiring greater experience is performed by those with the appropriate skills or that those lacking in experience have adequate supervision to ensure the task is safely undertaken. This point is discussed in the Wilsher case (see Case 4.3).

Case 4.2 *Nettleship v Weston* [1971]

A learner driver[4]

Mr Nettleship was teaching Mrs Weston to drive in her husband's car. On the third lesson, he was helping her by moving the gear lever, applying the handbrake and occasionally helping with the steering. In the course of the lesson, they made a slow left-hand turn after stopping at a halt sign. However, Mrs Weston did not straighten up the wheel and panicked. Mr Nettleship got hold of the handbrake with one hand and tried to get hold of the steering wheel with the other. The car hit a lamp standard. Mr Nettleship broke his kneecap. He claimed compensation and succeeded before the Court of Appeal.

The crucial question in the case was: since Mrs Weston was not a qualified driver, was the standard of care that she owed to the instructor lower than would otherwise have been the case? The court decided not. They preferred to have one standard of driving, not a variable standard depending on the characteristics of the individual driver. 'The certainties of a general standard are preferable to the vagaries of a fluctuating standard' (Lord Justice Megaw).

This might seem irrelevant to the standard of the nurse but Lord Justice Megaw, in discussing the issue, used the example of the young surgeon:

> Suppose that to the knowledge of the patient, a young surgeon, whom the patient has chosen to operate on him, has only just qualified. If the operation goes wrong because of the surgeon's inexperience, is there a defence on the basis that the standard of care and skill was lower than the standard of a competent and experienced surgeon? In cases such as the present it is preferable that there should be a reasonably certain and reasonably ascertainable standard of care, even if on occasion that may appear to work hardly against an inexperienced driver.

Mr Nettleship obtained his compensation, subject to a reduction for contributory negligence.

Practical Dilemma 4.1 No experience

Ruth Evans is recently qualified and is a staff nurse at Roger Park Hospital. She is asked to work initially on the orthopaedic ward until a vacancy occurs on the children's ward, which is her chosen specialty. The orthopaedic consultant suggests that Fred Timms, who has recently been taken off traction, could start some mobility exercises. Ruth, following this advice, approaches Fred's bed with a nursing auxiliary and with a pair of crutches. She suggests that Fred should manoeuvre himself to the side of the bed and gently put his sound leg on the floor. Then, when he feels steady enough, he should take the crutches and start to walk. Fred shifts to the side of the bed, puts his sound leg on the floor, but, as he stands up holding on to the crutches, they slide away from him and he falls heavily to the ground. Subsequently, X-rays reveal a further fracture of the injured leg and a fresh fracture in the other leg. Where does Ruth stand as far as liability is concerned? Is the fact that she has only just commenced on the orthopaedic ward and has never specialised in it a good defence for her personally against any potential court action that Fred might bring?

It is quite likely that if this case were investigated it would be established that there was a recognised procedure for mobilisation of orthopaedic patients, which would most likely involve the physiotherapist, and that Ruth had failed to follow this and probably was not even aware of its existence. This would be no defence against Fred. If he can establish the four elements of negligence – (a) a duty of care was owed to him, (b) Ruth was in breach of that duty by failing to follow the accepted approved practice and that (c) as a reasonably foreseeable consequence, he has (d) been caused harm – then he would succeed in his action. Ruth would be held to be negligent. Fred is, however, more likely to sue the NHS trust as Ruth's employer on the grounds that it is vicariously liable for her negligence (see below) and is also directly liable for failing to ensure a system of supervision of inexperienced staff. Other staff may also be held negligent. For example, who should have ensured that Ruth had the requisite training, that she was made aware of ward procedures and that she had adequate support? Someone else should have ensured that she was aware of the role of the physiotherapist.

In practice, of course, the experience of individual staff varies greatly and even where staff have had the same experience and training, their level of skill and manual dexterity may also vary greatly. However, the patient should be assured that the recognised approved standard of care will be given. Occasionally, a patient may require a higher standard.

For example, Mr Links may have held himself up as a specialist in a complex ear operation that is not often performed because of its particular hazards and difficulties. A GP might refer a patient to Mr Links because of his particular skill. If Mr Links then fails to perform the operation carefully and the patient suffers harm, it is no defence for Mr Links to claim that he knows he did not perform it correctly, but no other ear surgeon could have done it. He has held himself up as having that particular skill. Of course, it would have to be shown that he had failed to perform the operation with the required level of care and skill. The fact that things go wrong does not in itself mean that there has been negligence.

Team liability and apportionment of responsibility

Team Liability

If harm is caused by another member of the team, is the nurse responsible?

Work in the health service is, above all, team-oriented. Very few tasks are performed entirely on one's own. In the community, particular tasks are often allocated not purely on a professional basis, but on a key worker basis, which enables one person to take responsibility for a wide range of tasks.

Practical Dilemma 4.2 The team

Jane is a third-year student who, together with other members of staff on the ward, is caring for orthopaedic patients. The nursing process is in operation. One day Jane is asked to work in the plaster unit where it is her task to bind the plaster bandage around the patients' limbs. One of the patients, a young boy called Sam, has a broken wrist and Jane is told to strap it up. She bandages the wrist and then calls the sister to look at it. The sister glances at it, but does not touch it and the boy's mother is asked to bring him back in three weeks' time. No instructions are given about checking the tightness of the bandage or moving the hand. Three weeks later the boy returns with his mother and it is noticed that the bandage has been put on too tightly and it appears that permanent damage has been done to the boy's hand. What is Jane's responsibility?

Jane is, of course, the person who actually bandaged his wrist. Whether the trust is vicariously responsible for her actions will depend on any memorandum of agreement between her university and the NHS trust/Health Board offering clinical placements. Jane's personal liability will depend on such questions as: Had Jane been trained to plaster? Was such a task entirely within her competence? Should she have refused to undertake an activity for which she was not competent? Was her level of expertise such that the ward manager should have checked her work? If, for example, it should have been quite clear that Jane was too inexperienced to undertake the task without supervision, the fact that she asked the ward manager to check over the work might be sufficient to relieve her of personal responsibility. The failure to communicate to the parent the need to check on the plaster is also a breach of duty, and liability will depend on who had the responsibility of ensuring that this was done. As has been noted in the first section of this chapter, failure to communicate can itself be grounds for an allegation of negligence.

The team may be a group of nurses working together – it might be a multidisciplinary group (sometimes referred to as the team around the patient to recognise patients as being an integral part of the decision making in relation to their own care). In the following case, the team was made up of doctors and nurses working under one consultant.

Case 4.3 Wilsher v Essex AHA [1986]

No team liability[5]

A premature baby was placed in a special care baby unit staffed by a medical team consisting of two consultants, a senior registrar, several junior doctors and trained nurses. A junior doctor, while monitoring the oxygen intake, inadvertently put the catheter in a vein rather than in an artery. He asked the senior registrar to check what he had done. The registrar failed to see the mistake and several hours later made exactly the same mistake himself. As a result, the catheter failed to monitor the oxygen correctly and it was alleged that the child suffered from an incurable condition of the retina resulting in near blindness.

At the trial, the judge awarded £116,199 to the child. The health authority appealed to the Court of Appeal on the grounds that: (1) there had been no breach of duty of care owed to the child because the standard of care required of doctors in the unit was only that reasonably required of doctors having the same formal qualifications and practical experience as the doctors in the unit; and (2) the child had failed to show that the health authority's actions had caused or contributed to his condition since excess oxygen was merely one of several different factors, any one of which could have caused or contributed to the eye condition from which the child suffered. (This last point is known as causation and is discussed in chapter 3.)

On the point of the standard of care, the Court of Appeal held that there was no concept of team negligence, in the sense that each individual team member was required to observe standards demanded of the unit as a whole, because it could not be right, for example, to expose a student nurse to an action for negligence for her failure to possess the experience of a consultant. The standard of care required was that of the ordinary skilled person exercising and professing to have that special skill, but that standard was to be determined in the context of the particular posts in the unit rather than according to the general rank or status of the people filling the posts, since the duty ought to be tailored to the acts which the doctor had elected to perform rather than to the doctor himself. It followed that inexperience was no defence to an action for negligence. One judge, however, stated that an inexperienced doctor who was called on to exercise a specialist skill and who made a mistake nevertheless satisfied the necessary standard of care if he had sought the advice and help of his superior when necessary. The court in this case applied the same standard as the court in the Whitehouse and Jordan case (see chapter 3 Case 3.2), i.e. the Bolam Test. The judges held that the junior doctor had not been negligent and had upheld the relevant standard of care by consulting his superior. His superior had, however, been negligent in failing to notice that the catheter had been mistakenly inserted in a vein rather than an artery and, accordingly, the health authority was vicariously liable for the registrar's negligence.

An additional finding was that there was no reason why, in certain circumstances, a health authority could not be directly liable to a claimant if it failed to provide sufficient or properly qualified and competent medical staff for the unit. The House of Lords subsequently ordered a new trial on the issue of causation and the parties then settled the case (see chapter 3).

Apportioning Responsibility

Although there is no concept of team negligence in law, each person is individually responsible for his/her negligence; it does not follow that there are no occasions of multiple liability, i.e. in a given situation several different professionals might be individually responsible for their own individual negligence. An example of this is given in chapter 27 on the prescribing of medicines.[6] Under the Civil Liability (Contribution) Act 1978, if there are several defendants, a successful claimant can recover damages from any one of the defendants. That defendant may then sue the other defendants to recover a sum that represents their responsibility for the harm which has occurred.

Taking instructions: refusal to obey

General Principles

When we look at the scope of professional practice (see chapter 23), we will consider the possibility that the nurse might have to refuse to undertake a task where, for example, she was not trained to perform it or where she had insufficient time to undertake it safely. In this section, we look at the wider field of obeying orders.

Practical Dilemma 4.3   Orders are orders

A registrar decides that Margaret Brown should be prescribed a new drug that has only just been released on to the market and writes her up for it. The staff nurse on that ward is not familiar with the drug and says that they would like to check it with the pharmacist before they administer it. The doctor is furious with this insolence and says that if he has written it up then the nurse should administer it without questioning his competence. The nurse says that they need some understanding of the drug before they administer the medicine to the patient. The doctor insists the nurse gives it. Where does the nurse stand?

This is a simplified version of situations that often confront nurses. This particular example raises the issue of what the nurse's responsibility is in relation to the administration of drugs, but examples could be given from other fields such as obeying the order 'not for resuscitation', not passing certain information on to a patient, etc.

It is impossible to give an answer that would apply to every situation. In an emergency, for example, certain risks have to be taken which would not be appropriate in non-urgent circumstances. In Practical Dilemma 4.3, the nurse would be quite correct in obtaining further information about the drug in question. When a nurse administers a drug, they must be sure that they are administering the right drug, at the right time, in the right place, at the right dosage, in the right way, to the right patient. The nurse should not administer a drug of which they have no or little knowledge without taking all reasonable steps to ascertain that it is appropriate for that particular patient. If in this situation the nurse were to go ahead and administer the drug on the orders of the doctor and the patient were to die or suffer harm as a result, the nurse could be held to be negligent in any civil action (for which the employers would be held vicariously liable) since the nurse failed to follow the reasonable standards of care expected of a nurse. The nurse could also face professional disciplinary proceedings before the Fitness to Practise Committee (FtPC) of the NMC and disciplinary proceedings before their own line manager because the nurse had failed to use all care and skill in carrying out their contract of employment. If the patient died, the nurse might have to appear in the coroner's court and there might also be criminal proceedings brought against both the nurse and the doctor. See The Code[7] (NMC, 2015), which states that:

> **You put the interests of people using or needing nursing or midwifery services first. You make their care and safety your main concern and make sure their dignity is preserved and their needs are recognised, assessed and responded to . . . (you must) work in partnership with people to make sure you deliver care effectively.**

In all these courts and hearings, saying, 'I was only carrying out orders' will not be sufficient defence on its own. In the civil courts, the fitness to practise proceedings of the NMC and the employer's disciplinary proceedings, the nurse would have to show that what they did was reasonable, having regard to the approved accepted practice to be expected from any qualified nurse. In the criminal courts, the nurse would have to show that their acts or omissions did not constitute the ingredients of the particular charge and/or that the nurse lacked the required mental state (see chapter 2).

Obeying Orders in an Emergency

In certain circumstances, time does not permit the usual practice to be followed, but the risks taken must be balanced against the risk of the patient dying.

Practical Dilemma 4.4 — Emergency

A patient has been brought into the A&E department with severe bleeding. A blood sample is taken for cross-matching and he is immediately put on an intravenous infusion of plasma. The doctor places the cannula in the patient's arm for the intravenous infusion and asks the nurse to set up a saline solution for administration straight away. Staff Nurse Bryant takes the bag that the doctor is holding out to her and attaches it to the IV line. She does not check the bag. The patient's condition worsens and he eventually dies. It is then discovered that the doctor inadvertently gave the nurse a bag containing a substance other than saline. What is the nurse's liability?

It is clear that a quick check of the label on the bag would not have delayed the patient's treatment and could have been done by the nurse without any difficulty. It is most likely that the nurse would be found personally negligent in these circumstances (although the employer would have to pay compensation because of its **vicarious liability** for the nurse's negligence) and any defence of 'but that was the bag the doctor gave me' would be unlikely to succeed. There could be other circumstances where emergency life-saving measures are required and the nurse would be unable to make the same checks. Very rarely, however, would the defence of 'obeying orders' succeed, since as a professionally qualified person the nurse would be expected to act responsibly and carefully and to ensure that her own personal actions are safe.

Nurses sometimes complain that the misgivings they express to doctors are ignored. What do they do then? Obviously, it depends on the circumstances. Where the misgivings concern treatment that could be harmful to the patient and if one doctor ignored the nurse's concern, then the nurse should express their misgivings to their own line manager and, if necessary, the advice of a more senior doctor should be sought. Much depends on the approach made by the nurse and the nature of the relationship and understanding that exists between the nurse and the doctor. Undoubtedly, encouragement of a team approach to patient care could prevent many unnecessary confrontations of this kind. It should, of course, be stressed that a nurse should not disobey the instructions of a doctor lightly; they should have compelling reasons from the patient's point of view. The nurse should ensure that they keep detailed records indicating the reasons for their actions and that the nurse manager is brought in at the earliest opportunity. If it should happen that the nurse's attitude was unreasonable then the nurse would, of course, face disciplinary action and, if the patient has been harmed as a result of the nurse's action, civil proceedings and **professional misconduct** proceedings may be sought. (See the discussion of whistleblowing later in this chapter.)

In a case heard by the Court of Appeal in 1942[8], Lord Goddard said:

> If a doctor in a moment of carelessness, perhaps by the use of a wrong symbol in a prescription, ordered a dose which to an experienced ward sister was obviously incorrect and dangerous, I think it might well be held to be negligence if she administered it without obtaining confirmation from the doctor or higher authority. In the stress of an operation, however, I should suppose that the first thing required of a nurse would be an unhesitating obedience to the orders of the surgeon.

Since 1942, as the recognition of the nurse's personal professional accountability has strengthened, the number of occasions on which a nurse would be expected to obey orders without question has clearly diminished.

Nurse as manager

Delegation and Supervision

As the role of the nurse develops (see chapter 23), more and more work that is currently undertaken by registered staff will have to be delegated to nursing associates and healthcare support workers under the supervision of the registered nurse. Delegation may take place to other trained staff, learners and nursing assistants and also volunteers. On some occasions, these volunteers may be very unwilling helpers as, for example, where youth training schemes include an attachment to a hospital. If such persons are assigned to work on a ward or department and the nurse manager is responsible for them, then they would have to ensure that their training and the tasks delegated to them are appropriate and that adequate supervision is provided. (This topic is further considered in chapter 23.)

As a manager, the nurse would be responsible for ensuring that the resources were effectively used and were sufficient for treating patients according to the approved standard of care. If harm is caused by inadequate resources and it is established that the manager failed to take the appropriate measures to prevent unreasonable risks arising, then the manager may well be liable. Delegation to support workers and the recommendations of the Francis Inquiry on the training and registration of support workers are considered in chapter 23.

Pressure on the manager

Practical Dilemma 4.5 | Manager's nightmare

Unit Manager Janice Clarke is on duty and is informed by the staff in the surgical ward that, although they are on intake and have three empty beds, owing to illness and the failure to fill vacancies they are so far below their establishment that the situation is dangerous and the present staff cannot cope with any more patients.

Obviously, the unit manager would ensure that the facts are correct and that the nurses on that ward are using their time appropriately and not undertaking tasks that could safely be left, in order to give priority to the work that is most important. Having assured herself that the situation is critical, she would then look internally at other wards and decide whether staff could be transferred. She might also have to consider bringing in bank or agency nurses. If necessary, she would consider the situation on a district basis, which might mean that she would have to discuss the possibility of another hospital taking over the intake at the present. Ultimately, she might have to bring in other districts or at least refer the problems to a more senior manager. The decision might be made that waiting list admissions are cancelled for the time being. Clearly, at all stages in this decision the evidence of the individual ward staff on the dangers and hazards is vital for informed decisions to be made. Like the ward sister or staff nurse, the nursing officer herself should keep records of the reasons behind the actions she has taken since this information may well be relevant to a court or fitness to practise hearing. (Whistleblowing is considered below.)

Practical Dilemma 4.6 On holiday

Anita Patel is a ward manager of an acute surgical ward of 30 patients. While she is on holiday, a patient is given a pre-medication prior to the form of consent for his operation being signed. The mistake is discovered and because it was felt that there was no doubt that the patient wanted to have the operation he was still asked to sign the form. He was then taken to theatre. Subsequently, he disputed the extent of his operation, as he had understood that the operation was only exploratory, but he received radical surgery including the provision of a colostomy. He argued that had he known that this was a possibility he would not have agreed to have the operation and he could not remember signing any form of consent. The circumstances of his signature were then discovered. Since the ward manager was on holiday at the time, is there any possibility of her being liable?

It would be cheering for ward managers if the question could be answered with a definite 'no'. However, this is not possible. A manager has a continuing responsibility to ensure that procedures and policies are designed and implemented to prevent any likelihood of harm to the patient. A vital question to be answered would be: had a procedure been established to ensure that the nursing staff checked that the consent form had been signed before administration of pre-medication? It would be the ward manager's responsibility to ensure that those procedures that come under the responsibility of the nursing staff are carried out competently and diligently, even when she is not there. In this example, the doctor would be liable for failing to obtain consent. In addition, as far as the immediate responsibility is concerned, the manager in charge of the ward at the time would also share liability for the events, but if, for example, it were established that there was no clear system for ensuring a correct procedure in relation to the checking of consent forms prior to the pre-medication being given, then the ward manager who should have implemented and supervised such a procedure would share some responsibility for the events. It is likely, too, that evidence of similar events in the past would be used to show the deficiencies in overall ward management in this particular context. In these circumstances, the ward manager's liability is not vicarious (see next section), i.e. it does not concern taking responsibility for the fault of others. It is directly her own personal liability for failing in her management role. If, of course, it can be shown that a sound practice had been implemented and was not followed on that occasion owing to the negligence of the staff on duty at that time, then there is less likelihood that the ward manager would be held liable.

Her failings in her responsibilities as manager could result in her having to give evidence in the civil courts, if her employer were to be sued for its vicarious liability for her negligence and, in addition, it could result in her facing a hearing for professional misconduct before the Fitness to Practise Committee of the NMC. The definition of unfitness to practise by reason of conduct unworthy of a nurse, which may justify removal from the Register, is sufficiently wide to cover mismanagement by a nurse. Nurse managers may appear before the FtPC to answer the charge of misconduct in failing to take responsibility for the situation and having shown a failure in management. A nurse manager who was aware that a nurse was on drugs or under the influence of drink at work and who failed to take appropriate action would be in breach of the NMC Code of Practice and could face a fitness to practise hearing.

The Francis Report of the Mid Staffs Inquiry[9] made the following recommendation in relation to ward nurse managers:

> **Recommendation 195:** Ward nurse managers should operate in a supervisory capacity, and not be office-bound or expected to double up except in emergencies as part of the nursing provision on the ward. They should know about the care plans relating to every patient on his or her ward. They should make themselves visible to patients and staff alike, and be available to discuss concerns with all, including relatives. Critically, they should work alongside staff as a role model and mentor, developing clinical competencies and leadership skills within the team. As a corollary, they would monitor performance and deliver training and/or feedback as appropriate, including a robust annual appraisal.

Vicarious liability of employer

Vicarious Liability

The NHS trust, health board or employer has two forms of liability in negligence: one is known as direct liability, i.e. the trust/health board itself is at fault; the other is known as vicarious liability or indirect liability, i.e. the trust is responsible for the faults of others, mainly its employees. In this first section, we look at the vicarious liability of the employer, which could be an NHS trust, health board, a clinical commissioning group, a private hospital, a company or even a GP who employs their own staff.

Practical Dilemma 4.7 — Assault on behalf of the employer

Kate was a staff nurse in casualty where, at weekends, there tended to be a problem with drunks. The hospital was close to the town centre and to several pubs and, not infrequently, people needing some assistance were accompanied by friends who were incoherent and abusive. One evening Kate was very busy and therefore extremely annoyed to find some very obstreperous men accompanying another man who had a cut head. She asked them to leave him and wait outside. They refused to go. She said she would have to summon the police if they did not leave quietly. One particularly aggressive visitor moved towards the treatment trolley and Kate, fearing that he would knock it over, raised her arm to prevent him. He was taken by surprise at her actions and fell heavily to the ground, catching his head on the side of the trolley. Kate has subsequently learnt that he intends to sue her and her employer.

In a personal action against her for assault, Kate would have to prove that she took reasonable action in self-defence or in protecting her employer's property or in evicting on behalf of the occupier a trespasser who refused to go. In such cases, it is more likely that the claimant would sue the NHS trust or health board responsible for the wrongs of its employees. The claimant does not have to choose whether to sue the employer or the employee. He can sue both. The obvious advantage of suing the employer is that funds will be available to pay him should he win the case. To win against the employer, he has to establish the following:

1. Kate was negligent or was liable for a civil wrong (see chapter 3).
2. Kate was an employee.
3. Kate was acting in the course of her employment (see below).

There is no problem with the second element in this case. Kate was an employee, but there may be cases where this is not so clear; for example, if Kate were an agency nurse it might not always be obvious whether Kate is considered to be an employee of the authority to which she is sent or whether she continues to be an employee of the agency.

In practice, the first element could cause some considerable difficulty. Much would depend on the circumstances of the assault: whether she had lost her temper, the level of provocation she was subjected to, etc. Let us assume, for the purpose of this discussion, that it was established as a matter of fact that Kate had acted unlawfully and that personal action against her would therefore succeed.

In the course of employment

In the Employer's Interests

The third element now needs to be considered. Was the nurse acting in the course of her employment when she assaulted the visitor? The test used to answer this question is as follows: what was she employed to do and when she carried out that act was she acting for the benefit of her employer? In this case, she was clearly not employed as a bouncer, but she was trying to prevent a trolley from being upset by an obstreperous visitor (or even trespasser). This could certainly be seen as being in the interests of the employer's business. Even if there were a clear policy that nursing staff should not attempt to deal with aggressive visitors on their own, this should not necessarily prevent the act from being in the course of employment. The performance of a prohibited act does not on its own mean that the employee has ceased to be acting in the course of employment. All the facts have to be considered. If it can be shown that all three elements were present (i.e. Kate was liable for a civil wrong, was an employee and was acting in the course of employment), the NHS trust or health board could be held vicariously liable for the harm caused by the nurse.

There have been difficulties in establishing whether an act is in the course of employment, and Box 4.1 sets out the criteria which have been used by the courts to decide if an act is in the course of employment.

Box 4.1

The term may cover:

1. Acts authorised by employer.
2. Acts not authorised by employer, but
   (a) performed for the purpose of the employer's business;
   (b) prohibited acts, but the prohibition does not take the conduct outside the sphere of employment[10];
   (c) acts incidental to the employment, undertaken for the employee's benefit while the employee is working on the employer's business (e.g. smoking on duty)[11];
   (d) acts for the protection of the employer's property and business[12]; or
   (e) dishonest or fraudulent acts of the employee, if the employer is under a duty to the person suffering the loss[13]

Outside the Job Description

Practical Dilemma 4.8   Helping others

Chibuzo Barrett was a staff nurse on a medical ward and was concerned that the kitchen had not sent up the diets. He telephoned for them and was told that he would have to wait since there were no porters available. Rather than wait, he decided to fetch them himself He went to the kitchen, passing the notice saying: 'No admission, kitchen staff only.' He went across to the diet bay and as he did so he knocked into a cook who was removing a pan of gravy from the stove. The gravy splashed over the cook and also over Chibuzo. What remedies do the cook and Chibuzo have in this situation and is the employer vicariously liable for Ann's negligence?

    The cook could, of course, sue Chibuzo personally. Chibuzo owed a duty of care to the cook and, by his carelessness, he caused reasonably foreseeable harm to the cook. However, is the employer vicariously liable for Chibuzo's actions? There is no doubt that he is an employee. There is also no doubt that he was negligent in knocking into the cook. However, is the third element satisfied, i.e. was he acting in the course of employment when he went to the kitchens and when he knocked into the cook? He was employed as a nurse, not as a kitchen porter, but he was acting in the care of the patients (his employer's business) when he went to the kitchens. Even if there were a clear prohibition on non-kitchen staff entering the kitchens, this would not in itself remove the act from the course of employment. The crucial point would be whether he was acting on the employer's business when he entered the kitchen and the answer to that in this case is yes. It would be very different if he entered the kitchen to have a chat on non-hospital business with a friend of his who worked there.

    It is not, of course, uncommon for staff in the health service to step outside the strict confines of their job descriptions. If the employer is aware of this and turns a blind eye to it, then it could be said that the employer condones it and accepts that the employee's duties have been expanded to include the additional tasks. In such cases, if the employee acts negligently while carrying out these duties, it could be argued that he or she is acting within the course of his or her employment. In addition, particularly during times of industrial action, employers specifically authorise staff to cover for the strikers or those working to rule. In such cases, the employees are acting in the course of their employment: they have the express authorisation of the employer.

Activities Incidental to the Work

Practical Dilemma 4.9   Smoking on duty

There was a clear and enforced policy at Roger Park Hospital that there was no smoking anywhere. One of the nurses ignored these instructions and regularly smoked with the patients in the ward area. On one such occasion, he accidentally dropped the cigarette and burned a patient's foot. The patient threatened to sue the NHS trust. Was the nurse acting in the course of employment?

> **Case 4.4**   *Century Insurance Co. Ltd v Northern Ireland Road Transport Board* [1942]
>
> ## Lighting up[14]
>
> A tanker driver ignored his instructions not to light matches when loading or unloading his vehicle and, as a result, the tanker, a vehicle belonging to the garage and several nearby houses were destroyed.

The answer is probably yes, based on the above case.

In this case, the court held that even though the act of lighting a cigarette is for the employee's own comfort and even though it is prohibited, the act could not be separated from the circumstances of his employment. The driver was held to be negligent in the course of performing his authorised work and the employers (and therefore their insurers) were liable.

In our example of the smoking nurse, it is highly likely that he will face disciplinary proceedings and possibly even dismissal, yet he may still be held to be acting in the course of employment and therefore the employer is liable for any harm which his negligence has caused.

In Case 4.5 the House of Lords held that school owners were vicariously liable for acts of sexual abuse committed by the school warden against pupils – the abusive acts were sufficiently connected with his work as to be in the course of employment.

> **Case 4.5**   *Lister v Hesley Hall* [2001]
>
> ## Sexual abuse by warden[15]
>
> The board of governors were sued by the victims of abuse by the warden at Hesley Hall, a children's home, because of its vicarious liability for his actions. The Home denied liability on the grounds that the abuse was not committed in the course of his employment. The House of Lords held that it was vicariously liable for the acts of the warden in abusing the claimants: the Home had undertaken the care of the children and entrusted the performance of that duty to the warden and there was therefore sufficiently close connection between his employment and the acts committed by him.
>
> The House of Lords stated that the approach which was best when determining whether a wrongful act was to be deemed to be done by the employee in the course of his employment was to concentrate on the relative closeness of the connection between the nature of the employment and the particular wrongdoing. The defendant undertook to care for the claimants through the services of a warden, so there was a very close connection between the torts of the warden and the defendant. The torts were also committed at a time and place when the warden was busy caring for the claimants. The warden was carrying out his duties though in an unauthorised and improper mode.

The Lister case was followed by the Court of Appeal when an archdiocese of the Catholic Church was held vicariously liable for the abuse of a boy by a priest. It was held that sufficient connection existed between what a priest with special responsibility for youth work was employed to do and his sexual abuse of a non-Catholic boy to hold the Church vicariously liable for his abuse.[16]

The House of Lords held that an employer could be vicariously liable for harassment by an employee which was contrary to the Protection from Harassment Act 1997[17] (see chapter 12). In *Weir* v *Chief Constable of Merseyside Police*,[18] a policeman was helping his girlfriend to move house when he assaulted a man who was rummaging through his girlfriend's possessions. He was held to be acting in the course of employment because he had identified himself to the victim as a policeman and told him he was taking him to the police station. In contrast, in *N* v *Chief Constable of Merseyside Police*[19], a policeman who raped a woman and made a video film of the assault was held not to be acting in the course of employment even though he was in his uniform and displayed his warrant card. In *Gravil* v *Redruth Rugby Football Club*,[20] the Court of Appeal held that the club was vicariously liable for a player who punched an opponent, causing serious injuries. The punch was thrown in the course of the game and could be fairly regarded as a reasonably incidental risk to the playing of rugby.

What if a Nurse is Off Duty?

There can be no easy answer. It depends entirely on what the nurse is doing and in what way they have been negligent. In one case, the Court of Appeal allowed an appeal with costs against the decision of the Professional Conduct Committee (PCC), who found that a nurse was guilty of misconduct when she refused to answer a heart patient's call for help because she was having her tea break. The decision was based on the fact that it had not been established that the nurse knew it was an emergency. However, this case was before the PCC and different principles might apply in a civil case.

In one case, for example, some employees in their employer's van left the authorised route and went to a café to have a snack. On the way back, they had an accident and the court held that they were not acting in the course of employment.[21] It might have been different had they deviated from their route to collect goods for the employer.

Non-employees

It will be recalled that, in order to establish vicarious liability, it must be established that the negligent person is an employee of the defendant. Box 4.2 shows some of the criteria used by the courts to decide if an individual is an employee. Case 4.6 illustrates this principle.

The Court of Appeal held that the boy was not an employee of the authority, that he was doing those duties as part of his education and that the authority was therefore not vicariously liable.

Box 4.2

1. The employee agrees that in consideration of a wage or other remuneration he will provide his own work and skill in performance of some service for the employer.
2. He agrees, expressly or impliedly, that in the performance of that service he will be subject to the other's control in a sufficient degree to make that other the employer.
3. The other provisions of the contract are consistent with its being a contract of service. 'Control in itself is not always conclusive', *Ready-Mixed Concrete (South-East) Ltd* v *Ministry of Pensions and National Insurance* [1968] 1 All ER 433.

> **Case 4.6**   *Watkins v Birmingham City Council* [1975]
>
> ## Classroom chaos[22]
>
> A deputy headmistress was injured when she fell over a tricycle that had been negligently placed near a classroom door by a ten-year-old boy in the course of carrying out his assigned task of distributing milk in the classrooms. There was a strict rule that tricycles were not to be removed from their safe position in the middle of the assembly hall.

In a case in 1999[23], the Court of Appeal held that it was necessary for a contract of employment to contain an obligation on the part of the employee to provide services personally. A contract that allowed services to be provided by another person was a **contract for services** and not a **contract of service**.

Liability for negligence of volunteers

What about volunteers? Do the same principles apply? Is the NHS trust liable for the negligent acts of the volunteer? If we follow the basic principles of vicarious liability, it could be argued that since the volunteer is not an employee, then the NHS trust should not be liable. However, the philosophy that underlies the concept of vicarious liability is one of public policy, i.e. the person or organisation that has set in motion a particular activity that has caused harm should bear the loss rather than an innocent victim. In addition, one of the essential elements in the principle of vicarious liability is that the master is in control of the servant's activity. Whether or not an NHS trust would be liable to a third person for the negligence of a volunteer would, of course, depend on the circumstances of the volunteer's negligence. It may be that the NHS trust or its staff are themselves at fault in failing to provide adequate training or supervision, or have delegated an entirely inappropriate task to the volunteer.

Duty of care and liability for independent contractors

> **Practical Dilemma 4.10**   Agency liability
>
> Mary Downs is employed by a nursing agency and is often sent to work in NHS hospitals that call on the agency for additional staff to cover any crises. While she is assisting on the ITU, she fails to notice that one of the monitoring machines has ceased to function and she then discovers that the patient has died. The relatives wish to bring a complaint or even take the NHS trust or the agency to court.

In a case like this, there may well be direct responsibility of the NHS trust for failing to provide a machine that had an effective alarm system or had been satisfactorily maintained. If there is also negligence on the part of the agency nurse, does it make any difference that she is not an employee of the NHS trust, but is employed by the agency? Could the NHS trust still be liable for her negligence? The answer would depend to a considerable extent on the agreement between the NHS trust and the agency on the terms of employment of their staff. In the unlikely event that this has not been predetermined, the control test would be applied. The general or permanent employer has to shift the presumption of responsibility for the negligence of the employee on to the hirer. He can do this by showing that the control of the employee has passed to the hirer. In a health service context, this should be relatively easy since an agency staff nurse sent to help out at an NHS hospital would automatically become part of the ward/department, would be under the control of the ward sister or departmental head and would be subject to their supervision. In most cases, unless there is a clear agreement to the contrary, the NHS trust would probably be vicariously liable for the negligence of the agency staff.

In a significant decision with wide implications, the Supreme Court ruled in October 2013 that a school had a duty of care to a pupil who was severely brain damaged during a swimming lesson run by an independent swimming instructor in a council-run pool in Essex.[24] It was alleged that the swimming instructor's negligence had caused the injuries. The Supreme Court ruled that the school had a non-delegable duty of care towards its pupils – not merely to take reasonable care of them but also to provide that reasonable care is taken of them by third parties, even while outside the premises of the school. It stated that 'the duty extends beyond being careful, to procuring the careful performance of work delegated to others'. Five defining features justified departure from the established principle of the delegation of the duty of care:

1. The claimant is a child or vulnerable person.
2. There is a pre-existing duty owed by the defendant to the claimant with a positive obligation to protect the claimant from harm.
3. The claimant has no control over the defendant's performance of that obligation.
4. The defendant has delegated some part of its function to a third party.
5. The third party has been negligent.

This ruling has significant implications for both health and local authorities as they delegate services to be performed by outside organisations. Having established this principle, the victim now has to establish that there was negligence which led to her brain injuries in order to obtain the £3 million compensation.

In 1947 the House of Lords[25] held that any written agreement between the parties was not conclusive and the actual facts of the case were more significant: the firm which paid the employee and hired out a crane was vicariously liable for personal injury caused by the crane operator. In *Hawley* v *Luminar Leisure Ltd* a night club was held vicariously liable for injuries caused by a door steward, even though he was employed by another company with whom the night club contracted.[26] The issue of which of several organisations is vicariously liable for harm caused by negligence is likely to arise more frequently as diverse arrangements between the public and private sector operate in the NHS following the Health and Social Care Act 2012 (see chapters 5 and 12).

Direct liability of employer

The Secretary of State has a statutory duty (i.e. one laid down by Act of Parliament) under the NHS Act 1977 (now re-enacted in the National Health Service Act 2006 as amended by the

Health and Social Care Act 2012) to provide medical services throughout England, and to direct the appropriate health service bodies to exercise these functions on his behalf. It has been argued that if any employee or independent contractor or agency person is negligent, then there is a breach of duty under the Act and the NHS trust is primarily liable, without having to establish all the elements of vicarious liability. This was the opinion of Lord Denning in the case now described.

Case 4.7 Cassidy v Ministry of Health [1939]

A hand operation[27]

The patient lost the use of his left hand and had severe pain and suffering as a result of negligent treatment following an operation on his hand. The evidence showed a *prima facie* case of negligence on the part of the persons in whose care the plaintiff was, although it was not clear whether this was to be imputed to Dr Fahrni, the full-time assistant medical officer, to the house surgeon or to one of the nurses.

The Court of Appeal held that the hospital authority was liable. Lord Denning said:

> **Whenever (hospital authorities) accept a patient for treatment, they must use reasonable care and skill to cure him of his ailment. The hospital authorities cannot, of course, do it by themselves. They have no ears to listen through the stethoscope, and no hands to hold the knife. They must do it by the staff which they employ, and, if their staff are negligent in giving the treatment, they are just as liable for that negligence as is anyone else who employs others to do his duties for him . . . I decline to enter into the question whether any of the surgeons were employed only under a contract for services, as distinct from a contract of service. The evidence is meagre enough in all conscience on that point, but the liability of the hospital authorities should not, and does not, depend on nice considerations of that sort. The plaintiff knew nothing of the terms on which they employed their staff. All he knew was that he was treated in the hospital by people whom the hospital authorities appointed, and the hospital authorities must be answerable for the way in which he was treated.**

This suggests that the NHS trust cannot delegate its duty by providing competent trained staff. It will always be primarily responsible for any negligence to the patients whether the negligent person is an employee, a volunteer, an independent contractor or an agency employee.

A case on this point is that of *Wilsher* v *Essex Area Health Authority*[28], discussed earlier. In this case, it was held that there was no reason why, in certain circumstances, a health authority could not be directly liable to a plaintiff (claimant) if it failed to provide sufficient or properly qualified and competent medical staff for the unit. In a case where the Ministry of Defence ceased to arrange direct care for British forces in Germany, their families entered into an arrangement whereby an English NHS trust procured services in Germany and a baby was subsequently brain damaged. The High Court held that there was no negligence by the NHS trust and there was no appeal against that finding. The Court of Appeal held that the Ministry of Defence was not liable.[29] It considered that there was no non-delegable duty which made the Ministry liable for acts of negligence by the provider. This must be contrasted with the recent judgment of the Supreme Court which held that an education authority was liable for injuries to a pupil in a swimming pool even though the swimming lessons had been contracted out to an independent contractor.[30]

It must be pointed out, however, that even where it is possible to hold the NHS trust directly liable for the harm caused to the patient under the principle set out by Lord Denning, those individuals who were negligent could still face an action for their personal liability. In addition, if the NHS trust pays out compensation as a result of an employee's negligence, it would be possible for it to seek an indemnity from the negligent person. At present, this indemnity is rarely sought.

Indemnity from the employee at fault

This indemnity arises as a result of an implied term in the contract of employment, that the employee will indemnify the employer as a result of any losses caused by a breach of contract by the employee. In these circumstances, this would be a breach of the term 'to use all reasonable care and skill'.

Case 4.8 Lister v Romford Ice and Cold Storage Co. Ltd [1957]

Family trouble[31]

Lister was employed as a lorry driver who worked with his father. He negligently ran down his father while backing the lorry in a yard. The father recovered damages from the employers on the grounds of their vicarious liability for the negligence of their employee. The employers' insurers then brought an action against the son for damages for breach of an implied term in his contract of employment that he would exercise reasonable care and skill in his driving. The son in his defence claimed that he was entitled to the benefit of any insurance that his employer either had or should have taken out. Therefore, they could not claim an indemnity from him.

The House of Lords held by a majority decision that they could claim an indemnity from the employee and they refused to imply a term in the contract of employment that the employer would not seek to claim an indemnity from the negligent employee.

Case 4.9 Jones v Manchester Corporation [1952]

Anaesthetic[32]

The widow of a patient who died as a result of negligent hospital treatment sued for damages. The hospital board claimed an indemnity from Dr Wilkes, an inexperienced physician, who had administered the fatal anaesthetic under the instructions of Dr Sejrup, a house surgeon.

The Court of Appeal rejected this claim for an indemnity partly because the hospital itself was at fault.

Claims brought against NHS organisations are handled by the NHS Litigation Authority (NHSLA). Trusts have joined in a clinical negligence scheme (CNST) whereby resources are pooled and claims over a certain amount are met from the pool. (This is discussed further in chapter 6.)

Professional Indemnity Insurance Cover

A new clause 9 was included in the amended NMC's Code of Professional Conduct in 2004, and the 2008 edition is as follows:

> The NMC recommends that a registered nurse, midwife or specialist community public health nurse, in advising, treating and caring for patients/clients, has professional indemnity insurance. This is in the interests of clients, patients and registrants in the event of claims of professional negligence.
>
> Although employers have vicarious liability for the negligent acts and/or omissions of their employees, such cover does not normally extend to activities undertaken outside the registrant's employment. Independent practice would not be covered by vicarious liability. It is the individual registrant's responsibility to establish their insurance status and take appropriate action.
>
> In situations where an employer does not have vicarious liability, the NMC recommends that registrants obtain adequate professional indemnity insurance. If unable to secure professional indemnity insurance, a registrant will need to demonstrate that all their clients/patients are fully informed of this fact and the implications this might have in the event of a claim for professional negligence.

This compromise is not now possible as a result of the European Directive on cross-border healthcare.

The Health Care and Associated Professions (Indeminity Arrangements) Order 2014[33]

This order was passed in 2013, and came into effect on the 1st August 2015. The order made it a statutory requirement to 'have in force in relation to him an indemnity arrangement which provides appropriate cover for practicing as such'.

Appropriate cover is in relation to ensuring appropriate cover is in place against liabilities that may occur during the nurses' practice. In most cases this cover will be provided by the nurses' employer. If not, the nurse needs to pay personal indemnity insurance themselves.[34]

For employees who are covered by the employer's vicarious liability, the need for personal public indemnity cover will only become necessary if they work outside the course of employment and therefore the employer does not accept vicarious liability – for example, if they undertake Good Samaritan acts. Professional associations often provide cover for such actions by their members. However, the Order has clear implications for all those who undertake private practice. They now require personal public indemnity cover for their private work. Independent midwives who have found that professional indemnity cover is too costly can no longer practice without such cover. The impact of this has been spelt out by Richard Griffith.[35]

The NMC requires all its registrants to sign a self-declaration when registering and renewing, stating that they have (or will have prior to commencing any practice) appropriate indemnity arrangements. Legislation requiring registrants to have professional indemnity insurance cover came into force on 17 July 2014.

Pressure from inadequate resources

Unfortunately, harm to the patient can occur because of shortage of staff, inadequate equipment and unsafe premises. This section deals with the liability of those concerned. The Code[36] (NMC, 2015) sets out clearly the practitioner's duty in relation to managing risk and the environment of care:

Manage Risk

- You must act without delay if you believe there is a risk to patient safety or public protection.
- Raise and, if necessary, escalate any concerns you may have about patient or public safety, or the level of care people are receiving in your workplace or any other healthcare setting, and use the channels available to you in line with our guidance and your local working practices.
- You must inform someone in authority if you experience problems that prevent you working within this Code or other national standards, taking prompt action to tackle the causes of concern if you can.

General Principles

> **Practical Dilemma 4.11   Resources**
>
> Pauline Cross is working on a busy medical ward with only two staff. The patients are severely confused and can do little for themselves. As she is transferring a patient from a wheelchair into bed, the patient falls to the floor and breaks her hip bone. Is Pauline likely to be held responsible in law for the patient's injuries?

It could be argued that this incident took place because there was inadequate staffing. However, there are many factors to be considered. Were they so short-staffed that even when priorities were set it would have been impossible for another member of the staff to help Pauline? Had the staff been trained in manual handling and was a risk assessment carried out? Was such an incident reasonably foreseeable such that additional precautions should have been taken or was it an inevitable accident? If the conclusion is that the accident was avoidable and another nurse should have been assigned to assist Pauline, then this will not automatically relieve Pauline of responsibility, especially if she were in charge of the ward. The question arises whether it would not have been possible to have transferred the patient to bed later when more help would have been available. Alternatively, could the tasks that were occupying the other nurses have been given a lower priority?

Even if all the questions could be answered negatively, i.e. they were so short-staffed that they could not take the necessary foreseeable precautions to ensure the patient was put to bed safely, Pauline may still be responsible. If she was in charge of the ward, had she warned her senior nurse management of the staffing difficulties and suggested remedial action such as discharging patients to other wards or home or suggesting the use of agency nurses if nurses could not be transferred from other wards? Failure to take such action where her management role requires it would mean that Pauline would have to share some measure of responsibility for the occurrence.

Employer's Responsibility

If a patient is harmed because of an accident that would not have occurred had reasonable resources been available, then the patient would have a valid action to recover compensation in the civil courts. It is no defence to say to a patient, 'We are sorry we amputated the wrong leg, but

Wednesday is our busiest day and we had a lot of staff off with flu.' A patient is entitled to the approved standard of care. Even in an emergency situation, staff would be expected to take additional precautions to prevent further harm arising on the basis of a clear order of priorities. In such circumstances, the patient would be able to sue the NHS trust for its vicarious liability for the negligence of the staff. However, it is probable, too, that an action of direct liability also might succeed against the trust because harm was caused to the patient as a result of inadequate resources. If there has been a failure to provide a reasonable standard according to the Bolam Test, it does not matter what the cause was: staffing shortages, lack of equipment, or inexperience, there will either be direct liability of the organisation or vicarious liability for the negligence of its staff.[37] The claimant must, of course, be able to show that there is a causal link between the failure to maintain the reasonable standard of care and the harm which has occurred.[38]

Case 4.10   *McCormack v Redpath Brown* [1961]

Inadequate resources (1)[39]

A doctor working in the Emergency Department through pressure of work, made only a brief examination and treated a major head injury on the assumption that it was a minor one.

Both he and the health authority were held liable. The judge held that pressure of work was no defence to the patient's claim.

Case 4.11   *Deacon v McVicar and Another* [1984]

Inadequate resources (2)[40]

Several allegations were made by a patient that she was not treated with proper professional care and skill during the delivery of her first child. A Shirodkar suture had been fitted at an earlier stage because of an incompetent cervix. It was important that the suture should be removed promptly once labour had commenced; otherwise there was a danger that the cervix could be damaged. The patient claimed that the staff had failed to act speedily and as a consequence her cervix was damaged. The defendants claimed that the ward was very busy that night and the patient received appropriate care.

At the defendants' request, the judge directed that the notes of the other patients should be made available to show what was going on in the labour ward that evening. He did so with reluctance because he did not wish a breach of the duty of confidentiality owed to the patients and the defendants had not pleaded any special emergency that prevented speedier attention to the patient. These patients were referred to by code names. Their notes were exhaustively examined in the course of the evidence. 'In summary they showed that the doctors were busy and that the patient bringing the action was not the only patient who presented problems. But they did not show there was anything to prevent the doctors performing a vaginal examination or removing the suture sooner than they did.'

One of the criticisms was that the doctors had failed to give the patient sufficient priority. The doctor in his defence said that on a busy labour ward the doctors do not sit down and work out a list of priorities. The judge, however, had to decide if the patient had been kept waiting too long. He said: 'I appreciate that one must not be too critical of what goes on in a busy ward but it is difficult to understand why the patient did not have a vaginal examination until two hours after admission. Other ladies were admitted at about the same time as she was and whose cases were of no greater urgency had their examinations far sooner.'

Commenting on the statement of one of the experts for the defence who had said, 'I think the time scale is within the pattern of what occurs in a busy ward', the judge said:

> **That may well be, but it does not resolve the question whether this particular patient was given proper care . . . I do not pinpoint any particular moment when a particular doctor did something wrong. It was rather a case where there was a lack of sufficient sense of urgency on all sides. In these circumstances I hold that the second defendants (Leicester Health Authority) did not treat the patient with proper professional care and skill.**

The patient was awarded £1500.

Several important points emerge from this case:

1. The assessment of priorities can be carried out negligently or not at all and can itself form the basis of a claim for compensation.
2. To ascertain the workload and other demands, it is possible with the approval of the judge for the records of other patients to be made available. It is essential that comprehensive records are always kept.

Coping Under Pressure

One question often asked by nursing staff in relation to shortage of resources is, 'What happens if we are dangerously short of staff and yet we cope? What is the situation then?' This is a frequent situation. Yet if no person suffers harm as a result of the inadequate levels, then there can be no action for negligence, since harm must be established. However, it would be part of the duties of the nurse, both in her professional duties and as a manager, to ensure that senior levels are notified of any dangers or hazards so that harm does not eventually occur. An inadequate number of trained staff in proportion to the demands of patients could lead to inexperienced people administering drugs, using specialised equipment or assisting doctors in complex treatments, and patients could therefore suffer overdoses or other forms of harm. In extreme situations, where it is impossible to obtain sufficient numbers of staff to run a service safely or to run a service with the correct skill mix, then the provision of that service may have to be transferred to other providers.

Legal Requirements on Staffing

Another question that is raised is: 'What are the legal staffing levels or of what legal significance is a particular staffing ratio that has been recommended by different researchers?' Minimum staffing levels or ratios are unlikely to be laid down by Act of Parliament or by the courts. (Note, however, guidance by NICE in 2014 discussed below). Under the principles relating to liability in negligence, sufficient resources must be provided to ensure that the patients being cared for are provided with the approved accepted standard of care, i.e. the Bolam Test. All circumstances must be taken into account in determining whether this has been provided in respect of a given patient who has suffered harm. Obviously, evidence could be given of the extent to which the staffing levels had fallen below the levels considered by experts in the field to be the minimum consistent with good practice, but this is evidence, not law.

One of the recommendations from the Francis Inquiry on Mid Staffordshire Hospital related to the need to prioritise nurse staffing levels. It was, however, pointed out in a letter to *The Times* that 'there is a danger that mandated staffing levels will be perceived as an optimum staffing level, when in our experience, the number of staff required may differ according to patient need and may be in excess of the mandated level'. The correspondent recommended the use of the Safer Nursing Care Tool to determine optimal nurse staffing levels for inpatient wards.[41]

In May 2014 NICE stated that it planned to develop guidance on staffing levels for doctors following guidance it had given for nurse staffing. Numbers of nurses must be set and monitored on a shift-by-shift basis. Death rates rose if each nurse was looking after more than eight patients. In July 2014 NICE suggested the following red alerts/flags to indicate that wards were short-staffed:

- patients not receiving medication when they should;
- delays of more than 30 minutes in providing pain relief;
- patients not asked about their pain levels;
- patients not helped to use the lavatory;
- food or other items out of reach;
- patients left uncomfortable and at risk of pressure sores; and
- only one registered nurse on duty on a shift.

Guidance was issued on calculating the number of nurses required on each shift in relation to the needs of patients and activities to be performed. The deputy CEO of NICE estimated that an extra 5 per cent of current nursing costs would be required to implement the guidance.[42] Further information on NICE publications on staffing guidance can be found on its website.[43]

However, in Wales the Nurse Staffing Levels (Wales) Act was passed in 2016; which places a legal duty upon a Local Health Board or NHS trust in Wales to calculate and take steps to maintain nurse staffing levels. The Act came into force on 6 April 2018. A similar Act was passed in Scotland in 2019 (The Health and Care (Staffing) (Scotland) Act 2019), and this Act came into force on the 1st April 2024. Legislating for safe staffing levels in the devolved nations will no doubt increase the debate for similar legislation to be passed in England.

Failures by Management

What does a nurse do if she has drawn the attention of management to a situation that she considers dangerous and nothing is done about it? Whatever the situation, whether it is concerned with inadequate resources or incompetent staff, the nurse should not give up if she feels her concern about a dangerous situation is being ignored. She has a duty to ensure that the patients are cared for appropriately. She should therefore put her concerns in writing with evidence of hazards that have occurred. Her report would need to be a detailed account that is meaningful to management of the levels of staffing and the needs of the patients. If nothing is done, she should then be prepared to refer the matter to a higher level of management. Eventually, if she is still concerned that the dangers are being ignored, she should take the matter to her NHS trust or the NMC and utilise the procedure set up under the Public Interest Disclosure Act 1998. This is preferable to bringing the local or national press into a field that should be sorted out internally.

Public interest disclosure act 1998 and whistleblowing

Nurses are required under the The Code (see above) to identify any risks or problems that have arisen and the steps taken to deal with them. The Code also added a duty to be candid (truthful), about all aspects of care and treatment, including when any mistakes or harm have taken place. Practitioners whose fitness to practise is doubted must also be reported to line managers, and/or the NMC, or their respective regulatory body (for example the General Medical Council for doctors).[44] Many nurses have feared victimisation (see report on Rodney Ledward, chapter 5). To allay such fears and prevent victimisation, the NHS Management Executive issued Guidelines for Staff on Relations with the Public and the Media (1993). This emphasised that under no circumstances are employees who express their views about health service issues in accordance with this guidance to be penalised in any way for doing so (paragraph 6). Each NHS employer has a duty to establish a procedure for employees to raise concerns. Statutory provision was made in the Public Interest Disclosure Act 1998 to ensure that a procedure is set up to ensure that staff who raise justifiable concerns are protected from victimisation. Justifiable concerns are shown in Box 4.3.[45] The charity Protect provides a helpline and information service for the promotion and protection of responsible whistleblowing.[46] A claim by an employee of the North Glamorgan NHS Trust that he had been unfairly dismissed because he had made allegations of fraud against other employees was allowed to proceed on the grounds that in a fact-sensitive situation such as a whistleblowing claim a full hearing was necessary to resolve the dispute.[47]

The Employment Rights Act 1996 provides protection for workers who suffer a detriment or are dismissed as a result of blowing the whistle by making a qualified **disclosure** in accordance with sections 43C to 43H (as amended by the Enterprise and Regulatory Reform Act 2013). Qualifying disclosure has the meaning given in section 43B of the Act. Section 43F provides that a qualifying disclosure will be protected if it is made to a prescribed person and relates to matters in respect of which that person is protected. Amendments made by the Enterprise and Regulatory Reform Act 2013 include the provision that disclosures (after 25 June 2013) are not protected unless the worker reasonably believes that the disclosure is in the public interest. The tribunal is given the power to reduce the compensation where the disclosure is not made in good faith. In addition a worker is protected if they are subjected to detriment by co-worker or agent of employer. (See Section 19 Enterprise and Regulatory Reform Act 2013.)

The Schedule of the 1999 Public Interest Disclosure (Prescribed Persons) Order[48] sets out the list of prescribed persons and the matters in respect of which they are prescribed for the purposes of section 43F. The list has subsequently been amended in 2003, 2009, 2010 and 2013 to include the General Social Care Council, the Health and Safety Executive, local authorities responsible for enforcing health and safety legislation, the Information Commissioner and the Pensions Regulator. The worker must reasonably believe that the relevant failure is within the concern of that person and the information is substantially true.

The protected disclosures in Box 4.3 are extensive and would cover most of the situations in which a registered practitioner would have a professional duty to inform an appropriate person or authority under the Code of Professional Conduct.

> **Box 4.3** **Protected disclosures under the public interest disclosure act 1998**
>
> 1. That a criminal offence has been, is being or is likely to be committed.
> 2. That a person has failed, is failing or is likely to fail to comply with any legal obligation to which he is subject.
> 3. That a miscarriage of justice has occurred, is occurring or is likely to occur.
> 4. That the health or safety of any individual has been, is being or is likely to be endangered.
> 5. That the environment has been, is being or is likely to be damaged.
> 6. That information tending to show any matter falling within any of the above paragraphs has been, is being or is likely to be deliberately concealed.

Under the Act, as amended, the disclosure is only protected if certain conditions are satisfied. If bad faith is found to exist, damages can be reduced by up to 25 per cent. Disclosure is also protected if it is made in the course of obtaining legal advice; or if the employer is a body any of whose members are appointed by a minister of the Crown, then the disclosure can be made to a minister of the Crown. This would cover disclosures by employees working within the NHS. The employee must believe the disclosure to be in the public interest. Disclosures to prescribed persons are protected if made in good faith to a person prescribed by the Secretary of State. Other disclosures are protected if the conditions set out in Box 4.4 are satisfied.

> **Box 4.4** **Conditions for other protected disclosures**
>
> 1. The worker reasonably believes that the information disclosed, and any allegations contained in it, are substantially true.
> 2. The disclosure is made in the public interest (added by section 17 of the Enterprise and Regulatory Reform Act 2013).
> 3. The worker does not make the disclosure for personal gain.
> 4. Any of the conditions in subsection 2 is met (see below).
> 5. In all the circumstances of the case, it is reasonable for the worker to make the disclosure.

The subsection 2 conditions referred to in Box 4.4 include the reasonable belief that the employee would be subjected to detriment by their employer if they make the disclosure. Factors determining the reasonableness of the disclosure include the identity of the person to whom it is made; the seriousness of the failure; whether it is continuing or likely to occur in future; whether the disclosure is made in breach of a duty of confidentiality; previous disclosures to the employer or to another person prescribed by the Secretary of State; and compliance with any procedure specified for making disclosures.

Disclosures Relating to Exceptionally Serious Failures

Special provisions apply to a disclosure of an exceptionally serious failure. Such a disclosure is protected if the employee makes the disclosure in good faith, reasonably believing the allegations to be true, not making the disclosure for personal gain and in all the circumstances it is reasonable to make the disclosure and to that particular person.

Gagging of an Employee

The Act states that any provision in an agreement is void in so far as it purports to preclude an employee from making a protected disclosure. Thus, if a trust attempts to introduce a term into a contract of employment that prevents an employee making a disclosure that comes under the protection of the Act, that term is void.

Before the Public Interest Disclosure Act, a student nurse reported a Rampton Hospital nurse for ill-treating and assaulting patients.[49] The abuser was subsequently convicted in the criminal courts and struck off the UKCC Register. The student nurse, however, suffered considerable abuse after blowing the whistle. Such victimisation should now lead to compensation for the person raising the concern. Under section 19 of the Enterprise and Regulatory Reform Act a worker (W) has the right not to be subjected to any detriment by any act, or any deliberate failure to act, done (a) by another worker of W's employer in the course of that other worker's employment, or (b) by an agent of W's employer with the employer's authority, on the ground that W has made a protected disclosure. Where a worker is subjected to such detriment then that is treated as also done by the worker's employer. It is immaterial whether the thing is done with the knowledge or approval of the worker's employer. However, it is a defence for the employer to show that the employer took all reasonable steps to prevent the other worker so acting. This fills the gap highlighted in the case of *NHS Manchester* v *Fecitt and others*.[50]

In 2013 the employment charity Public Concern at Work[51] set up a commission to look into whistleblowing. It recommended that a statutory code of practice should be created which can be taken into account when courts and tribunals are considering whistleblowing cases.

A consultant cardiologist Raj Mattu won a landmark tribunal ruling for unfair dismissal against Walsgrave Hospital in Coventry in the longest-running and most expensive whistleblowing case in NHS history. He first blew the whistle in 1998 about concerns on patient safety. The tribunal judgment was given in April 2014 and held that he suffered a detriment as a whistleblower and was found to have been unfairly dismissed. He claimed that he had been harassed by senior management when he drew attention to the need for reforms. His whistleblowing attempts were dismissed by Sir David Nicholson as an employment matter in 2010. Dr Mattu subsequently met with the new head of the NHS Simon Stevens, who has called for a new culture of openness in the NHS.[52] Documents released under the Freedom of Information Act revealed that officials from various national health bodies joined meetings to discuss the case without Dr Mattu's knowledge. He initially claimed £6.5 million in damages, however the trust awarded him with £1.2 million in damages.

The following case is reported by Public Concern at Work.

Case 4.12   *Kay v Northumberland Healthcare NHS Trust* [2001]

A protected disclosure bid[53]

Kay managed a ward for the elderly. Kay internally raised concerns about bed shortage but was told there were no resources. The problem worsened and some elderly patients were moved to a gynaecological ward. Kay wrote a satirical open letter to the Prime Minister for his local paper. With the trust's agreement, Kay was photographed for the local press. When the letter was published, the trust gave a final written warning for totally unprofessional and unacceptable conduct. Kay won the case as the disclosure was protected because (a) disclosure under 43G of the 1998 Act was balanced with Article 10 and freedom of expression in the European Convention on Human Rights, (b) Kay did not know of the trust's whistleblowing policy, (c) there was no reasonable expectation of action following earlier concerns, and (d) it was a serious public concern.

Margaret Haywood, a registered nurse, was struck off the Register by the NMC as a consequence of her breach of confidentiality in participating in a TV programme which highlighted abuse of elderly residents in a care home. She appealed to the High Court against the decision. A joint NMC and RCN statement was made in December 2009 as follows:

> **The NMC and the Royal College of Nursing (RCN) are pleased to announce a settlement in the case of nurse Margaret Haywood.**
> **This was an extremely difficult and complex case in which the NMC panel had to balance Ms Haywood's duty to protect patient confidentiality with her duty to raise concerns about poor standards of care.**
> **The NMC and RCN put forward terms of settlement for the Court's consideration and the Court approved those terms which led to the replacement of the striking off order with a 12 month caution.**

Subsequently, Kathy George, the thenChief Executive and Registrar, NMC said:

> **Raising concerns about poor standards of care is a difficult and brave step for any nurse or midwife to take and is vitally important in driving improvements in patient care. One of the lessons of Margaret Haywood's case is that nurses and midwives need clearer information about how to appropriately raise and escalate concerns in a way that is safe for patients and in a way that will not bring them into conflict with their code of conduct.**

The RCN on its website (61) has a raising concerns toolkit. The toolkit gives guidance to all practitioners on how they should raise concerns about a patient's care. It explains the process of raising concerns, offers information about legislation and indicates where staff can get confidential support and advice.[54]

In the NHS an associate Emergency Department specialist who had reported clinical failings by a colleague was ostracised by senior management, refused access to important meetings and offered a £96,000 pay-off with a gagging clause which she turned down.[55] Enquiries using the Freedom of Information Act found that 71 NHS trusts admitted reaching settlements with doctors over the past decade. Forty admitted making pay-offs totalling £3 million.

In 2014 the Supreme Court held on the preliminary issue of the definition of a worker for the purposes of bringing a whistleblowing case that a partner was eligible to bring a case. The action was then remitted to the employment tribunal to determine whether the applicant had been the victim of discrimination on the grounds of sex and whistleblowing.[56]

Kennedy Report

The Kennedy Report,[57] following the inquiry into children's heart surgery at Bristol Royal Infirmary, recommended that there should be openness and honesty in the NHS and a partnership between patients and professionals. It set out the principles which should be recognised within NHS management.

In considering the topic of 'respect and honesty', the Report recommended that:

Patients in their journey through the healthcare system are entitled to be treated with respect and honesty and to be involved, wherever possible, in decisions about their care.

To achieve this aim the Report makes recommendations on achieving a partnership between healthcare professionals and the patient, whereby the patient and the professional meet as equals with different expertise. Patients must be kept informed about their treatment and care. Communications must be improved, including the use of tape-recording facilities to enable patients, should they so wish, to make a tape-recording of a discussion with a healthcare professional when a diagnosis, course of treatment or prognosis is being discussed. Support services should be provided for patients, including counselling and a professional bereavement service. Voluntary organisations that provide care and support for patients should, where they meet the appropriate standards, receive state funding to contribute their services. Consent to treatment should be seen as a process and not simply the signing of a form. Feedback from patients should be encouraged. There should be a duty of candour, to tell a patient if adverse events have occurred, and patients should receive an acknowledgement, an explanation and an apology. Complaints should be dealt with swiftly and thoroughly, keeping the patient informed, and the present system of compensation should be reviewed.

The Department of Health announced its response to the Report in 2002 and both the full response and an executive summary are available from the Department of Health website.[58]

Subsequently many of the recommendations in the Kennedy Report on Bristol have been repeated in the Francis Report on Mid Staffordshire Hospital (see chapter 5). A duty of candour was one of the recommendations put forward by the Francis Inquiry and section 81 of the Care Act 2014 enables regulations to be drawn up to place such a duty on health service organisations (see chapter 5).

Kay Sheldon, a whistleblower on the board of the Care Quality Commission (CQC), was threatened with losing her post following the failure of the CQC adequately to inspect baby deaths at Morecambe Bay NHS Trust.[59] Subsequently, Health Secretary Jeremy Hunt stated that he had approved a CQC recommendation that she be reappointed to the Board when her five-year term expired.[60]

Amanda Pollard, an inspector for the CQC, brought an action for constructive dismissal claiming that she was vilified, bullied, ridiculed and ostracized when she tried to blow the whistle on the organisation. The employment tribunal found that her resignation, some 14 months after the Public Inquiry, was not protected by the whistleblowing law.

Two whistleblowers in South Devon, Penny Gates and Clare Sardari, won a tribunal ruling that they suffered by making whistleblowing allegations, but an allegation of unfair dismissal was dismissed. They alleged that the Chief Executive was guilty of nepotism by hiring her daughter's boyfriend for a role for which he had little experience. The tribunal ruled that South Devon Healthcare NHS Foundation Trust made a dishonest attempt to suppress the findings of an internal investigation.[61]

In evidence given to the Commons Health Select Committee in March 2013 Sir David Nicholson, Chief Executive of the NHS, denied that he had tried to silence whistleblowers and pledged that no one in the NHS would be asked to sign gagging clauses banning them from talking about patient safety.[62] Great Ormond Street Hospital was accused of changing the report it submitted to the Baby P inquiry as part of a cover-up. It denied this, saying that the 2007 report was amended on legal advice. The Secretary of State for Health Jeremy Hunt asked the hospital for a response to the allegations.[63]

Criticism was made by the Public Accounts Committee in January 2014 of the fact that public sector bodies may have handed whistleblowers generous payoffs to keep quiet in a series of 'shocking' cover-ups.[64] It recommends that the Cabinet Office should require public sector organisations to secure its agreement for all special severance payments. (See also chapter 5 and the Stafford Report.)

In June 2014 the Secretary of State for Health announced an independent review into whistleblowing in the NHS to be led by Sir Robert Francis QC who chaired the Mid Staffs Inquiry, to ensure that where NHS whistleblowers are mistreated there are appropriate remedies for staff and accountability for those mistreating them. On 7 August 2014 he urged doctors and nurses to tell him what is going wrong and pledged to prise open an NHS 'closed ranks culture' that harms patient care. The review completed its work in November 2014. The main recommendations from this review included:

- NHS workers can raise concerns in the public interest with confidence that they will not suffer detriment as a result.
- Appropriate action is taken when concerns are raised by NHS workers.
- Where NHS whistleblowers are mistreated, those mistreating them will be held to account.

Conclusions

This chapter has covered a wide range of topics relating to the role of the nurse in communicating, delegating, managing and dealing with inadequate resources. It has also considered the direct and vicarious liability of the employer. Nurses and employers, however, work within the wider scope of the NHS and it is the structure and management of the NHS to which we now turn.

Reflection questions

1. There can be liability for failure to communicate. Apply this principle to your particular post and consider how and to what extent communication with the patient could be improved.
2. Consider any work you undertake as a member of a team and assess the extent to which it is clear where the boundaries of individual responsibility lie.
3. There are times when it is essential that a nurse follows the instructions of a doctor and others when it is imperative that he/she check that the instructions are appropriate. What distinguishing features would decide whether an order falls in the first category or in the second?
4. What is the difference between direct and vicarious liability?
5. In what way do you think that the liability of the NHS trust for the safety of the volunteer differs from its liability for the safety of staff (see, in addition, chapter 12)?
6. An employee can be liable for the negligent actions of another person if the employee should not have delegated a task to them or, having correctly delegated it, has failed to provide the appropriate level of supervision. Apply this principle to the role of the nurse manager in relation to junior registered staff, learners, volunteers and untrained assistants.

Further exercises

1. Obtain a copy of your NHS trust's policy on the use of volunteers and study in particular those parts that relate to liability for the negligence of volunteers.
2. Obtain a copy of your employer's policy on raising concerns and familiarise yourself with its contents. Do you understand how the procedure would work in practice?
3. Obtain a copy of the Mid Staffs Inquiry Report and consider the extent to which your department could implement any of its recommendations that are not yet in place.

References

[1] *Coles* v *Reading HMC* (1963) 107 SJ 115
[2] National Patient Safety Agency, Delayed Diagnosis of Cancer: thematic review, NPSA 2010
[3] *Harrison* v *Surrey County Council and Others*, The Times Law Report, 27 January 1994
[4] *Nettleship* v *Weston* [1971] 3 All ER 581
[5] *Wilsher* v *Essex Area Health Authority* [1986] 3 All ER 801 CA; [1988] 1 All ER 871 HL
[6] *Dwyer* v *Roderick*, 20 June 1984 QBD
[7] Nursing and Midwifery Council, The Code: standards for performance, conduct and ethics, NMC, 2015
[8] *Gold* v *Essex County Council* [1942] 2 All ER 237
[9] Report of the Mid Staffordshire NHS Foundation Trust Public Inquiry HC 947, February 2013, Stationery Office; www.midstaffspublicinquiry.com
[10] *Rose* v *Plenty* [1976] 1 All ER 97
[11] *Century Insurance Co. Ltd* v *Northern Ireland Road Transport Board* [1942] 1 All ER 491
[12] *Poland* v *Parr and Sons CA* [1926] All ER 177
[13] *Lloyd* v *Grace Smith & Co.* [1912] AC 716; *Morris* v *C.W. Martin & Sons Ltd* [1965] 2 All ER 725
[14] *Century Insurance Co. Ltd* v *Northern Ireland Road Transport Board* [1942] 1 All ER 491
[15] *Lister & Others* v *Hesley Hall Ltd* [2001] UKHL 22; [2002] 1 AC 215; The Times Law Report, 10 May 2001; [2001] 2 WLR 1311
[16] *MAGA* v *Trustees of the Birmingham Archdiocese of the Roman Catholic Church* [2010] EWCA 256
[17] *Majrowski* v *Guy's and St Thomas's NHS Trust* [2006] UKHL 34; [2007] 1AC 224; [2005] ICR 977
[18] *Weir* v *Chief Constable of Merseyside Police* [2003] EWCA Civ 111 CA
[19] *N* v *Chief Constable of Merseyside Police* [2006] EWHC 3041 QB
[20] *Gravil* v *Redruth Rugby Football Club* [2008] EWCA Civ 689
[21] *Hilton* v *Thomas Burton* (Rhodes) Ltd [1961] 1 WLR 705
[22] *Watkins* v *Birmingham City Council,* The Times Law Report, 1 August 1975
[23] *Express and Echo Publications Ltd* v *Taunton*, The Times Law Report, 7 April 1999; [1999] EWCA Civ 949
[24] *Woodland* v *Essex County Council* [2013] UKSC 66
[25] *Mersey Docks and Harbour Board* v *Coggins and Griffith (Liverpool) Ltd* [1947] AC 1 HL
[26] *Hawley* v *Luminar Leisure Ltd* [2006] EWCA Civ 18
[27] *Cassidy* v *Ministry of Health* [1939] 2 KB 14
[28] *Wilsher* v *Essex Area Health Authority* [1986] 3 All ER 801 CA
[29] *A* v *Ministry of Defence* [2004] EWCA 641
[30] *Woodland* v *Essex County Council* [2013] UKSC 66
[31] *Lister* v *Romford Ice and Cold Storage Co. Ltd* [1957] 1 All ER 125 HL

32 *Jones* v *Manchester Corporation* [1952] 2 All ER 125 CA
33 EU Directive 2011/24/EU Patient Rights in Cross-Border Healthcare
34 www.nhs.uk
35 Richard Griffith, Impact of the cross-border health-care directive on independent midwives, *British Journal of Midwifery*, 21(8):601–2, August 2013
36 Nursing and Midwifery Council, Code of Professional Conduct: standards for conduct, performance and ethics, NMC, 2008
37 *Ball* v *Wirral Health Authority* [2003] WLR 117
38 *Aisha Qureshi* v *Royal Brompton and Harefield NHS Trust* [2006] EWHC 298 QB
39 *McCormack* v *Redpath Brown*, *The Times*, 24 March 1961
40 *Deacon* v *McVicar and Another*, 7 January 1984, QBD
41 Dalya Wittenberg, The Shelford Group Chief Nurses Letter to editor, *The Times*, 21 November 2013
42 Chris Smyth, Patients 'must demand faster pain relief', *The Times*, 15 July 2014
43 www.nice.org.uk
44 UKCC, Reporting Unfitness to Practise – Information for Employers and Managers, UKCC, August 1996
45 Royal College of Nursing, Raising Concerns, Raising Standards 003532, RCN London, May 2009
46 www.pcaw.org.uk/case-studies; 020 3117 2520
47 *Ezsias* v *North Glamorgan NHS Trust* [2007] EWCA Civ 330
48 Public Interest Disclosure (Prescribed Persons) Order (SI 1549)
49 News item, *Nursing Times*, 96(23):48, June 2000
50 *NHS Manchester* v *Fecitt and others* [2011] EWCA 1190
51 www.pcaw.org.uk
52 Moody Oliver, Doctor to tell NHS chief of war against him, *The Times*, 24 April 2014
53 *Kay* v *Northumberland Healthcare NHS Trust 2001*, available on the Public Concern at Work website: www.pcaw.org.uk/case-studies
54 The Royal College of Nursing, Raising Concerns Toolkit at https://www.rcn.org.uk/employment-and-pay/raising-concerns/Raising-concerns-toolkit#introduction Accessed, April 2024
55 Steve Boggan, 'It was like a bad gangster movie – they were trying to blackmail me', *The Times*, 28 August 2010
56 *Bates van Winkelhof* v *Clyde and Co LLP* [2014] UKSC 32, The Times Law Report, 4 June 2014
57 Bristol Royal Infirmary Inquiry (Kennedy Report), Learning from Bristol: the report of the public inquiry into children's heart surgery at the Bristol Royal Infirmary 1984–1995 (chaired by Professor Ian Kennedy), Command Paper Cm 5207, July 2001
58 Department of Health's Response to the Report of the Public Inquiry into children's heart surgery at the Bristol Royal Infirmary 1984–1995, DH, January 2002, Cm 5363; www.gov.uk/government/uploads/learningfromBristol or webarchive www.bristol-inquiry.org.uk
59 Sarah-Kate Templeton, Minister tried to gag NHS whistleblower, *Sunday Times*, 23 June 2013
60 News item, NHS Whistleblower to keep job on CQC Board, *The Times*, 3 July 2013
61 News item, BBC News, 30 January 2014, www.bbc.co.uk
62 Chris Smyth, Under fire NHS chief denies trying to gag whistleblowers, *The Times*, 6 March 2013
63 Sarah-Kate Templeton, Baby P hospital ordered to look into cover-up, *Sunday Times*, 30 June 2013
64 House of Commons Public Accounts Committee 36th Report: Confidentiality Clauses and Special Severance Payments, January 2014

Chapter 5

Statutory Functions and Management of the NHS

This chapter discusses

- National Health Service
- White Paper *Equity and Excellence: Liberating the NHS*
- Enforcement of statutory duties
- NHS England (the National Health Service Commissioning Board)
- Clinical commissioning groups
- The mandate
- NHS foundation trusts
- NHS Improvement (formerly Monitor)
- Clinical governance
- Duty of quality
- Care Quality Commission
- National Institute for Health and Care Excellence (NICE)
- NHS 111 and walk-in clinics
- NHS inquiries
- Mid Staffordshire
- NHS Foundation Trust Inquiry
- The NHS Constitution
- NHS and the private sector

Introduction

This chapter considers the statutory background to the NHS and the functions of the Secretary of State. It looks at the present organisations which run the NHS following the Health and Social Care Act 2012 and considers the duty of quality, the Care Quality Commission and the National Institute for Health and Care Excellence. Issues of resource management and the Public Interest

Disclosure Act 1998 are considered in relation to whistleblowing in chapter 4. The role of NHS professionals is considered in chapter 11. The administrative structure of the NHS in the four constituent countries of the UK is increasingly moving in different directions as can be seen from the analysis by Nicholas Timmins.[1] This chapter will focus on the changes which have taken place in England and readers are referred to the websites of the three assemblies for further details of health services in each country.

National Health Service

The National Health Service (NHS) was set up on 5 July 1948 as a result of the National Health Service Act 1946. It was based on the principle that services should be provided free at the point of delivery unless there was clear statutory authorisation for any charges. Charges for prescriptions were the first to be introduced. The duty to provide services was placed on the Secretary of State who delegated these functions to regional hospital boards, hospital management committees and other statutory organisations. Family practitioner services were administered by the executive councils, later superseded by the family practitioner committees. A major reorganisation of healthcare provision took place in 1973 and the statutory duties were re-enacted in the National Health Service Act 1977. Health Service legislation has since been consolidated in the National Health Service Act 2006 with the NHS Consequential Amendments Act 2006 and separate legislation for Wales and in the legislation of 2008 and 2012.

White Paper Equity and Excellence: Liberating the NHS

The White Paper *Equity and Excellence: Liberating the NHS* was published by the coalition government in July 2010 on reforming the NHS.[2] It laid the foundation for a radical reorganisation of the NHS, abolishing strategic health authorities and primary care trusts and making all NHS trusts into foundation trusts. The executive summary of the White Paper can be found on the website of this book. Its themes were:

- Putting patients and public first;
- Improving healthcare outcomes;
- Autonomy, accountability and democratic legitimacy;
- Cutting bureaucracy and improving efficiency; and
- Making it happen.

Addressing the White Paper's recommendations, Monitor, now part of NHS Improvement,[3] has become an economic regulator with three key functions: to promote competition; to regulate prices; and to support continuity of services. The Care Quality Commission (CQC) has received enhanced powers to be an effective quality inspectorate across both health and social care. The majority of NHS funds have passed to GP practices to commission services for patients. Local authorities have been given control over local health improvement budgets. The role of the Department of Health and Social Care has been reduced and NHS England promotes equality and tackles inequalities in access to healthcare. NHS England allocates resources according to the needs of local areas, and leads specialised commissioning. The key roles of the Department of Health and Social care are:

- Setting a formal mandate for NHS England;
- Holding NHS England to account;
- Arbitration;
- The legislative and policy framework; and
- Accounting annually to Parliament.

Healthwatch has been established nationally and locally, based on local involvement networks to champion the needs of the public and patients at every level. The focus now is on giving patients and the public more choice and involvement. Providers should respond to their needs. The internal market was not reintroduced but the concept of 'contestability' was envisaged.

Contestability means that there is the threat of competition, rather than there actually being competition. If the threat of competition exists, then providers in the market will respond as if they are in competition and act accordingly. This means that the benefits of competition can be achieved even in the absence of competition.[4]

Health and Social Care Act 2012

The Health and Social Care Act 2012 put the changes into law.

The duties placed on the Secretary of State are shown in Statute Box 5.1, which outlines how the 2006 Act was amended by the 2012 Act.

Statute 5.1

Duties of the Secretary of State under the National Health Service Act 2006 as amended by 2012 Act

Secretary of State's duty as to health service

Section 1(1)

1. The Secretary of State must continue the promotion in England of a comprehensive health service designed to secure improvement:
   (a) in the physical and mental health of the people in England; and
   (b) in the prevention, diagnosis and treatment of illness.
2. For that purpose, the Secretary of State must exercise the functions conferred by this Act so as to secure that services are provided in accordance with this Act.
3. The Secretary of State retains ministerial responsibility to Parliament for the provision of the health service in England.
4. The services provided as part of the health service in England must be free of charge except in so far as the making and recovery of charges is expressly provided for by or under any enactment, whenever passed.

1A Duty as to improvement in quality of services

1. The Secretary of State must exercise the functions of the Secretary of State in relation to the health service with a view to securing continuous improvement in the quality of services provided to individuals for or in connection with—
   (a) the prevention, diagnosis or treatment of illness, or
   (b) the protection or improvement of public health.
2. In discharging the duty under subsection (1) the Secretary of State must, in particular, act with a view to securing continuous improvement in the outcomes that are achieved from the provision of the services.
3. The outcomes relevant for the purposes of subsection (2) include, in particular, outcomes which show—
   (a) the effectiveness of the services,
   (b) the safety of the services, and
   (c) the quality of the experience undergone by patients.
4. In discharging the duty under subsection (1), the Secretary of State must have regard to the quality standards prepared by NICE under section 234 of the Health and Social Care Act 2012.

1B Duty as to the NHS Constitution
In exercising functions in relation to the health service, the Secretary of State must have regard to the NHS Constitution.

1C Duty as to reducing inequalities
In exercising functions in relation to the health service, the Secretary of State must have regard to the need to reduce inequalities between the people of England with respect to the benefits that they can obtain from the health service.

1D Duty as to promoting autonomy

1. In exercising functions in relation to the health service, the Secretary of State must have regard to the desirability of securing, so far as consistent with the interests of the health service—
   (a) that any other person exercising functions in relation to the health service or providing services for its purposes is free to exercise those functions or provide those services in the manner that it considers most appropriate, and
   (b) that unnecessary burdens are not imposed on any such person.
2. If, in the case of any exercise of functions, the Secretary of State considers that there is a conflict between the matters mentioned in subsection (1) and the discharge by the Secretary of State of the duties under section 1, the Secretary of State must give priority to the duties under that section.

1E Duty as to research
In exercising functions in relation to the health service, the Secretary of State must promote—
   (a) research on matters relevant to the health service, and
   (b) the use in the health service of evidence obtained from research.

1F Duty as to education and training

1. The Secretary of State must exercise the functions of the Secretary of State under any relevant enactment so as to secure that there is an effective system for the planning and delivery of education and training to persons who are employed, or who are considering becoming employed, in an activity which involves or is connected with the provision of services as part of the health service in England.
2. Any arrangements made with a person under this Act for the provision of services as part of that health service must include arrangements for securing that the person co-operates with the Secretary of State in the discharge of the duty under subsection (1) (or, where a Special Health Authority is discharging that duty by virtue of a direction under section 7, with the Special Health Authority).
3. In subsection (1), 'relevant enactment' means—
    (a) section 63 of the Health Services and Public Health Act 1968,
    (b) this Act,
    (c) the Health and Social Care Act 2008,
    (d) the Health Act 2009, and
    (e) the Health and Social Care Act 2012.

1G Secretary of State's duty as to reporting on and reviewing treatment of providers

1. The Secretary of State must, within one year of the passing of the Health and Social Care Act 2012, lay a report before Parliament on the treatment of NHS health care providers as respects any matter, including taxation, which might affect their ability to provide health care services for the purposes of the NHS or the reward available to them for doing so.
2. The report must include recommendations as to how any differences in the treatment of NHS health care providers identified in the report could be addressed.
3. The Secretary of State must keep under review the treatment of NHS health care providers as respects any such matter as is mentioned in subsection (1).
4. In this section—
    (a) 'NHS health care providers' means persons providing or intending to provide health care services for the purposes of the NHS, and
    (b) health care services for the purposes of the NHS' has the same meaning as in Part 3 of the Health and Social Care Act 2012.

Secretary of State's general power as to services

Section 2(1)

The Secretary of State may:

(a) provide such services as he considers appropriate for the purpose of discharging any duty imposed on him by this Act; and
(b) do any other thing which is calculated to facilitate, or is conducive or incidental to, the discharge of such a duty.

> **Section 2(2)**
>
> Subsection (1) does not affect:
>
> (a) the Secretary of State's powers apart from this section,
>
> (b) Chapter 1 of Part 7 [of this Act] (pharmaceutical services).
>
> **3B Secretary of State's power to require Board to commission services**
>
> 1. Regulations may require the Board to arrange, to such extent as it considers necessary to meet all reasonable requirements, for the provision as part of the health service of—
>
>   (a) dental services of a prescribed description;
>
>   (b) services or facilities for members of the armed forces or their families;
>
>   (c) services or facilities for persons who are detained in a prison or in other accommodation of a prescribed description;
>
>   (d) such other services or facilities as may be prescribed.
>
> 2. A service or facility may be prescribed under subsection (1)(d) only if the Secretary of State considers that it would be appropriate for the Board (rather than clinical commissioning groups) to arrange for its provision as part of the health service.
>
> 3. In deciding whether it would be so appropriate, the Secretary of State must have regard to—
>
>   (a) the number of individuals who require the provision of the service or facility;
>
>   (b) the cost of providing the service or facility;
>
>   (c) the number of persons able to provide the service or facility;
>
>   (d) the financial implications for clinical commissioning groups if they were required to arrange for the provision of the service or facility.

Other services which the Secretary of State has a duty to provide are set out in Schedule 1 of the NHS Act 2006 and include the medical inspection of pupils, contraceptive services, provision of vehicles for disabled persons, microbiological services and research activities.

Part 4 of the 2006 Act covers primary medical services; Part 5 the provision of dental services; Part 6 ophthalmic services; and Part 7 pharmaceutical services as amended by the Health and Social Care Act 2012.

The 2012 Act also saw the introduction of Healthwatch England and local Healthwatch organisations (see chapter 26).

The Health and Social Care Information Centre was set up under section 252 of the Health and Social Care Act 2012.

Enforcement of statutory duties

Failure to provide reasonable services continues to be a political issue and Section 1(3) of the 2006 Act (as amended by the 2012 Act) states that 'the Secretary of State retains ministerial responsibility to Parliament for the provision of the health service in England'. However, there have been several cases where patients who have waited a considerable time for operations or for other treatments have brought legal action to enforce the provision for them of health services. By and large, the courts have taken the view that it is not for the court to become involved in issues relating to resource allocation, unless there are clear failures in public duty (see Case 5.1). However, a decision of the Court of Appeal in 2004 held that the NHS should pay for a patient to have treatment abroad, if the patient had waited a significantly long time for NHS treatment.[5] (The case is considered later in this chapter on page 100.) Where a patient is kept waiting for treatment, there is an interesting distinction in the following three situations.

1. Where the treatment has commenced, it must be carried out according to the accepted approved standard. If a negligent act occurs that causes harm to the patient, then this is actionable by the patient (see chapters 3, 4 and 6).

2. Where treatment has not commenced and the patient has to wait on a waiting list, then even though the patient's condition might deteriorate this is not actionable provided the health service body has carried out its provision of health services rationally and determined priorities between patients appropriately. It may, of course, be the subject of a complaint since the provider has failed to comply with the standards set by the Department of Health, but these standards do not have any legal effect unless they are already incorporated in an Act of Parliament or a decided case or unless they infringe the European Convention on Human Rights. The Secretary of State has a duty under section 1A of the 2006 Act to secure continuous improvement in the quality of services and must have regard to the quality standards prepared by NICE under section 234 of the Health and Social Care Act 2012. However, it would appear that breach of this duty would give rise to a complaint rather than court action.

3. As a result of the *Watts* case,[6] where it is held that the patient has waited an unreasonable length of time for treatment, the NHS may be obliged to pay for treatment provided abroad.

Case 5.1   R v *Secretary of State for Health* [1979]

Inadequate resources[7]

Orthopaedic patients at a hospital in Birmingham, who had waited for treatment for periods longer than was medically advisable, brought an action against the Secretary of State, the regional health authority and the area health authority. They were seeking a declaration that the defendants were in breach of their duty under Section 1 of the National Health Service Act 1977 to continue to promote a comprehensive health service designed to secure improvement in health and the prevention of illness, and under Section 3 to provide accommodation, facilities and services for those purposes.

The judge held that it was not the function of the court to direct Parliament as to what funds to make available to the health service and how to allocate them. The Secretary of State's duty under Section 3 to provide services 'to such extent as he considers necessary', gave him discretion as to the disposition of financial resources. The court could interfere only if the Secretary of State acted so as to frustrate the policy of the Act or as no reasonable minister could have acted. No such breach had been shown in the present case. The court could not grant **mandamus** or a declaration against area or regional authorities since specific remedies against them were available by Section 85 and Part V of the 1977 Act. Nor, if a breach were proved, did the Act admit of relief by way of damages. The application was therefore dismissed.

The reasoning behind the above ruling was confirmed in the following case.

Case 5.2 *In re Walker Application* [1987]

Postponed operation[8]

Mrs Walker's baby son required a heart operation and was on the waiting list. A date was fixed for the operation to be performed, but it was postponed by the Birmingham Health Authority. She applied to the court for a judicial review of the decision of the health authority. The High Court judge refused her application. She appealed to the Court of Appeal which upheld the earlier decision.

The health authority had accepted that the regional district health authorities could be subject to judicial review where there was reason to believe that they might be in breach of their public duties. There would always be individuals who believed that treatment was not provided quickly enough, but the financial resources were finite and always would be. The court held that it was not for the court to substitute its own judgment for that of those responsible for the allocation of resources. It would interfere only if there had been a failure to allocate funds in a way that was reasonable or where there had been breaches of public duties. Mrs Walker's application was refused.

Case 5.3 *R v Cambridge HA* [1995]

Bone marrow transplant postponed operation[9]

A 10-year-old girl was suffering from acute myeloid leukaemia and required a further session of chemotherapy and a second bone marrow transplant to survive. It was estimated that the chance of success was between 10 per cent and 20 per cent. Costs of the drug and transplant were estimated as £15,000 and £60,000, respectively. The health authority refused to resource this and the father challenged its decision. The High Court upheld his application for judicial review. The health authority appealed to the Court of Appeal and the case was heard that same day. The Court of Appeal held that the four criticisms made by the trial judge of the health authority's decision were not acceptable. The court should confine itself to the lawfulness of the decision. It held that it was not in the best interests of the child to undergo further treatment and that resources had to be taken into account.

While the general principle that the courts will not intervene in resourcing issues of the NHS appears to continue to be accepted by the courts, there have been several cases where health authorities have been held liable for failure to provide services and in one case it was ruled that in certain circumstances the NHS should pay for treatment overseas.

In one case,[10] the health authority decided that it would not enable beta interferon to be prescribed for patients in its catchment area, since it was not yet proven to be clinically effective for the treatment of multiple sclerosis. A sufferer from multiple sclerosis challenged this refusal of the health authority and succeeded on the grounds that the health authority had failed to follow the guidance issued by the Department of Health.[11] A declaration was granted that the policy adopted by the health authority was unlawful and an order of mandamus was made requiring the defendants to formulate and implement a policy that took full and proper account of national policy as stated in the circular. In a later case the Court of Appeal held that the policy of a primary care trust on the availability of Herceptin for breast cancer was irrational since there were no clinical or personal considerations which led to one patient being preferred over another. It asked the primary care trust (PCT) to formulate a lawful policy upon which to base decisions in particular cases, including that of Mrs Rogers, in the future.[12] On 18 July 2007 the High Court ruled that, although the PCT policy on the drug Avastin was entirely rational and sensible, the PCT had made a flawed and irrational decision when it refused to fund Avastin for cancer treatment for a specific patient, Ms Otley.[13] As a consequence the PCT agreed to fund five cycles of treatment for her, the treatment being reviewed after those treatments and a CT scan. The guidance issued by NICE on drugs for Alzheimer's was also challenged in a case in 2007.[14]

Another case concerned three transsexuals who wished to undergo gender reassignment.[15] The health authority refused to fund such treatment on the grounds that it had been assigned a low priority in its lists of procedures considered to be clinically ineffective in terms of health gain. Under this policy, gender reassignment surgery was listed among others as a procedure for which no treatment, apart from that provided by the authority's general psychiatric and psychology services, would be commissioned, save in the event of overriding clinical need or exceptional circumstances. The transsexuals sought judicial review of the health authority's refusal and the judge granted an order quashing the authority's decision and the policy on which it was based. The health authority then took the case to the Court of Appeal, but lost its appeal.

The Court of Appeal held that:

1. While the precise allocation and weighting of priorities is a matter for the judgment of the authority and not for the court, it is vital for an authority:
   (a) to accurately assess the nature and seriousness of each type of illness;
   (b) to determine the effectiveness of various forms of treatment for it; and
   (c) to give proper effect to that assessment and that determination in the formulation and individual application of its policy.

2. The authority's policy was flawed in two respects:
   (a) it did not treat transsexualism as an illness, but as an attitude of mind which did not warrant medical treatment;
   (b) the ostensible provision that it made for exceptions in individual cases and its manner of considering them amounted to the operation of a 'blanket policy' against funding treatment for the condition because it did not believe in such treatment.

3. The authority were not genuinely applying the policy to the individual exceptions.

4. Article 3 and Article 8 of the European Convention on Human Rights (see Chapter 1) did not give a right to free healthcare and did not apply to this situation, where the challenge is to a health authority's allocation of finite funds. Neither were the patients victims of discrimination on the grounds of sex.

It is inevitable that there will always be a gap between the demands that are made for healthcare and the resources to meet those demands. Decisions will therefore have to be made on priorities and who is refused treatment. New developments in technology, such as the identification of the human genome and the treatment possibilities for identified genetic diseases, are just one example of increasing pressures. The Human Rights Act 1998 has seldom been successfully relied upon in disputes over access to services. As we examine later in this chapter, NICE is tasked with determining priorities and quality standards. There is evidence that, in the current time of financial pressures, many elective or cosmetic treatments are ceasing to be provided on the NHS.[16] However, since the statutory duty on the clinical commissioning group (see Statute Box 5.4) is to 'arrange for the provision of the following to such extent as it considers necessary to meet the reasonable requirements of the persons for whom it has responsibility'; it is unlikely that any court action to enforce provision (for example of removal of tattoos, surgery to prevent snoring, hair transplantation) would succeed. In a poll commissioned by the NHS Confederation which reported in March 2014, half of the politicians surveyed in Britain think a free NHS could be consigned to history unless challenges are tackled to ensure that it meets future patient needs. The Chief Executive of the NHS Confederation expressed concern about how the NHS could make provision of services for an ageing population and an increase in long-term health conditions. See also the interim report of the King's Fund discussed below.[17]

Another case where the claimant challenged a failure to provide services was that of Mr Condliff who alleged that failure to provide bariatric surgery for his obesity was a breach of his Article 8 rights. He failed: the court held that there had to be a balancing act between individual needs and the community as a whole and that the Trust had acted reasonably.[18] Where a health service body has been negligent in the performance of its duties, then a civil claim for compensation may be brought. (This is considered in chapters 3, 4 and 6.) Where a death has occurred as a result of gross negligence by the organisation then proceedings under the Corporate Manslaughter and Homicide Act in 2007 may be brought (see chapter 2).

Distinction between Statutory Duties and Guidance from the Department of Health and Social Care

In fulfilling its statutory duties, the government issues circulars providing guidance to NHS organisations on how they should function. These are available from the Department of Health (DHSC) website.[19]

While in general the advice in these circulars is not the law as such, there is a clear responsibility on organisations to follow the recommendations. The failure by a health authority to follow DH guidelines on the prescribing of beta interferon led to a successful action being brought by a patient suffering from multiple sclerosis[20]. In a contrasting case,[21] a court held that government circular 1998/158, which limited the powers of GPs to prescribe Viagra, was unlawful as by preventing the issue of a prescription, where the GP considered it to be justified, the clinical judgment of the GP was usurped. As a consequence, regulations were then issued by the Secretary of State which placed restrictions on the prescription of Viagra on the grounds of cost to the NHS. Pfizer's challenge to the legality of these regulations failed. (The restrictions were removed on 1 August 2014 when the price of Viagra fell by 93 per cent as generic versions of the drug became available.)

NHS England (the National Health Service Commissioning Board)

The Health and Social Care Act 2012 established the NHS Commissioning Board which is now known as NHS England.

Regulations[22] provide for a range of matters relating to the functions of NHS England, which is subject to the same duty under Section 1(1) as the Secretary of State except for public health functions (see chapter 25). In discharging that duty NHS England has the functions set out in Statute Box 5.2.

Statute 5.2

Section 1H of the 2006 Act as Amended by Section 9(1) of the 2012 Act

NHS Commissioning Board (now NHS England)

1H The National Health Service Commissioning Board and its general functions

1. There is to be a body corporate known as the National Health Service Commissioning Board ('the Board').
2. The Board is subject to the duty under section 1(1) concurrently with the Secretary of State except in relation to the part of the health service that is provided in pursuance of the public health functions of the Secretary of State or local authorities.
3. For the purpose of discharging that duty, the Board—
   (a) has the function of arranging for the provision of services for the purposes of the health service in England in accordance with this Act, and
   (b) must exercise the functions conferred on it by this Act in relation to clinical commissioning groups so as to secure that services are provided for those purposes in accordance with this Act.

Schedule A1 of the 2012 Act makes further provision about NHS England.

NHS England was established as an arm's length independent body. Its initial function was to authorise clinical commissioning groups (CCGs) and it took up its full functions on 1 April 2013. From this date NHS England has taken on many of the current functions of primary care trusts with regard to the commissioning of primary care health services, as well as some nationally based functions previously undertaken by the Department of Health.

NHS England Aims

1. to end unjustifiable variations in services and a reduction of health inequalities;
2. to secure better outcomes for patients as primary care clinicians are empowered to focus on delivering high quality, clinically effective, evidence-based services;
3. to achieve greater efficiencies in the delivery of primary care health services through the introduction of standardised frameworks and operating procedures.

NHS England is required to meet the objectives set out in the mandate (see below) which is to be published each year by the Secretary of State (section 13A and 13B of the 2006 Act as amended by section 23 of the Health and Social Care Act 2012). The functions of NHS England include those specified in the 2012 Act which are shown in Statute Box 5.3.

Statute 5.3
Specified functions of NHS England

13C. Duty to promote NHS Constitution
  (a) act with a view to securing that health services are provided in a way which promotes the NHS Constitution, and
  (b) promote awareness of the NHS Constitution among patients, staff and members of the public.

13D. The Board must exercise its functions effectively, efficiently and economically.

13E. The Board must exercise its functions with a view to securing continuous improvement in the quality of services provided to individuals for or in connection with—
  (a) the prevention, diagnosis or treatment of illness, or
  (b) the protection or improvement of public health

  In particular, the Board must act with a view to securing continuous improvement in the outcomes that are achieved from the provision of the services, in particular—
  (a) the effectiveness of the services,
  (b) the safety of the services, and
  (c) the quality of the experience undergone by patients.

It must have regard to (a) any document published by the Secretary of State relating to this duty and (b) the quality standards prepared by NICE under section 234 of the Health and Social Care Act 2012.

13F. Duty as to promoting autonomy
13G. Duty as to reducing inequalities
13H. Duty to promote involvement of each patient
13I. Duty as to patient choice
13J. Duty to obtain appropriate advice
13K. Duty to promote innovation
13L. Duty in respect of research
13M. Duty as to promoting education and training
13N. Duty as to promoting integration of those services
13O. Duty to have regard to impact on services in certain areas
13P. Duty as respects variation in provision of health services
13Q. Public involvement and consultation by the Board
13R. Information on safety of services provided by the health service
13S. Guidance in relation to processing of information
13T. Business plan
13U. Annual report
13V. Establishment of pooled funds
13W. Board's power to generate income etc.
13X. Power to make grants etc.
13Y. Incidental powers
13Z. Exercise of functions and interpretation.

Further rules relating to the functions of NHS England and the clinical commissioning groups are set out in Regulations.[23] Further regulations require NHS England and clinical commissioning groups to ensure good practice when procuring healthcare services for the purposes of the NHS, to protect patients' rights to make choices and to prevent anti-competitive behaviour. The regulations also provide scope for complaints to, and enforcement by Monitor as an alternative to challenging decisions in the courts.[24]

Clinical commissioning groups

The Health and Social Care Act 2012 abolished strategic health authorities and placed the responsibility for the commissioning of health services upon corporate bodies known as clinical commissioning groups (CCGs). Each clinical commissioning group has the function of arranging for the provision of services for the purposes of the health service in England in accordance with the Health and Social Care Act 2012 (which amended section 3 of the NHS Act 2006).

The statutory duties placed upon CCGs are set out in Statute Box 5.4.

Statute 5.4
Statutory Duties of Clinical Commissioning Groups

Duties of clinical commissioning groups as to commissioning certain health services (S. 13 of 2012 Act amending S. 3 of 2006 Act)

3(1) A clinical commissioning group must arrange for the provision of the following to such extent as it considers necessary to meet the reasonable requirements of the persons for whom it has responsibility.
  (a) Hospital accommodation;
  (b) Other accommodation for the purpose of any service provided under this Act;
  (c) Medical, dental, nursing and ambulance services;
  (d) Such other facilities for the care of pregnant women, women who are breast feeding and young children as the group considers are appropriate as part of the health service;
  (e) Such other services or facilities for the prevention of illness, the care of persons suffering from illness and the after-care of persons who have suffered from illness as the group considers are appropriate as part of the health service;
  (f) Such other services as are required for the diagnosis and treatment of illness.

(1A) For the purposes of this section, a clinical commissioning group has responsibility for—
  (a) persons who are provided with primary medical services by a member of the group, and
  (b) persons who usually reside in the group's area and are not provided with primary medical services by a member of any clinical commissioning group.

(1B) Regulations may provide that for the purposes of this section a clinical commissioning group also has responsibility (whether generally or in relation to a prescribed service or facility) for persons who—

(a) were provided with primary medical services by a person who is or was a member of the group, or

(b) have a prescribed connection with the group's area

(1C) The power conferred by subsection (1B)(b) must be exercised so as to provide that, in relation to the provision of services or facilities for emergency care, a clinical commissioning group has responsibility for every person present in its area.

(1D) Regulations may provide that subsection (1A) does not apply—

(a) in relation to persons of a prescribed description (which may include a description framed by reference to the primary medical services with which the persons are provided);

(b) in prescribed circumstances.

(1E) The duty in subsection (1) does not apply in relation to a service or facility if the Board has a duty to arrange for its provision.

(1F) In exercising its functions under this section and section 3A, a clinical commissioning group must act consistently with—

(a) the discharge by the Secretary of State and the Board of their duty under section 1(1) (duty to promote a comprehensive health service), and

(b) the objectives and requirements for the time being specified in the mandate published under section 13A. [See Statute Box 5.5]

3(2) For the purposes of the duty in subsection (1) services provided under—

(a) section 83(2) (primary medical services), section 99(2) (primary dental services) or section 115(4) (primary ophthalmic services) or,

(b) a general medical services contract, a general dental services contract or a general ophthalmic services contract must be regarded as provided by the Secretary of State.

3(3) This section does not affect Chapter 1 of Part 7 (pharmaceutical services).

(3A) Power of clinical commissioning groups to commission certain health services

1. Each clinical commissioning group may arrange for the provision of such services or facilities as it considers appropriate for the purposes of the health service that relate to securing improvement—

   (a) in the physical and mental health of the persons for whom it has responsibility, or

   (b) in the prevention, diagnosis and treatment of illness in those persons.

2. A clinical commissioning group may not arrange for the provision of a service or facility under subsection (1) if the Board has a duty to arrange for its provision by virtue of section 3B or 4.

3. Subsections (1A), (1B) and (1D) of section 3 apply for the purposes of this section as they apply for the purposes of that section.

The general duties of clinical commissioning groups are set out in section 26 of the Health and Social Care Act 2012, which adds sections 14P to 14Z24 to the 2006 Act. These duties include the following:

14P	Duty to promote the NHS Constitution
14Q	Duty to exercise its functions effectively, efficiently and economically
14R	Duty as to improvement in quality of services
14S	Duty in relation to quality of primary medical services
14T	Duties as to reducing inequalities
14U	Duty to promote involvement of each patient
14V	Duty as to patient choice
14W	Duty to obtain appropriate advice
14X	Duty to promote innovation
14Y	Duty in respect of research
14Z	Duty as to promoting education and training
14Z1	Duty as to promoting integration
14Z2	Public involvement and consultation by clinical commissioning groups
14Z3	Arrangements by clinical commissioning groups in respect of the exercise of functions
14Z4	Joint exercise of functions with Local Health Boards
14Z5	Raising additional income
14Z6	Power to make grants
14Z7	Responsibility for payments to providers
14Z8	Guidance on commissioning by the Board
14Z9	Exercise of functions by the Board
14Z10	Power of Board to provide assistance or support
14Z11	Commissioning plan
14Z12	Revision of commissioning plans
14Z13	Consultation about commissioning plans
14Z14	Opinion of Health and Wellbeing Boards on commissioning plans
14Z15	Reports by clinical commissioning groups
14Z16	Performance assessment of clinical commissioning groups
14Z17	Circumstances in which powers in sections 14Z18 and 14Z19 apply
14Z18	Power to require documents and information, etc.
14Z19	Power to require explanation
14Z20	Use of information
14Z21	Power to give directions, dissolve clinical commissioning groups, etc.
14Z22	Procedural requirements in connection with certain powers
14Z23	Permitted disclosures of information.

The financial arrangements for clinical commissioning groups are covered by section 27 of the 2012 Act, which inserts sections 23G to 23K into the 2006 Act.

Further information on clinical commissioning groups and their location can be found on the NHS website.[25] The reorganisation of health services and in particular the establishment of CCGs was intended to give General Practitioners a greater voice in the commissioning of local health services. However, concerns about the availability of services and the pressure on A&E departments (see chapter 20) have led to concerns about GP services. There are also concerns about revised payment methods. In the contracts agreed in 2004, GP practices received a minimum practice income guarantee (MPIG) which protected the smaller practices from falls in funding. However, current plans to phase out the MPIG by 2021 may lead to the closure of many smaller practices.[26]

Both NHS England and the clinical commissioning groups have a statutory responsibility (the former under 13N and the latter under 14Z1 of the amended 2006 Act) to promote integration with social services. This is comparable to the duty under section 3 of the Care Act 2014 which requires local authorities to ensure the integration of care and support provision with health provision and health-related provision in carrying out its functions.

The mandate

Under Section 13A of the amended NHS Act 2006 before the start of each financial year, the Secretary of State must publish and lay before Parliament a document to be known as 'the mandate'. In this the Secretary of State must specify the points set out in Statute Box 5.5.

Statute 5.5
Section 13A of the NHS Act 2006

The mandate contents to be specified by Secretary of State

(a) the objectives that the Secretary of State considers the NHS Commissioning Board should seek to achieve in the exercise of its functions during that financial year and such subsequent financial years as the Secretary of State considers appropriate, and

(b) any requirements that the Secretary of State considers it necessary to impose on the Board for the purpose of ensuring that it achieves those objectives.

The Secretary of State must also specify in the mandate the amounts that the Secretary of State has decided to specify in relation to the limits on capital and revenue resource use. Also specified may be the ways in which the Secretary of State proposes to assess the Board's performance in relation to the first financial year to which the mandate relates.

The NHS Commissioning Board has the responsibility of seeking to achieve the objectives specified in the mandate, and complying with any specified requirements.

In preparing the mandate the Secretary of State must consult the NHS Commissioning Board, the Healthwatch Committee England of the Care Quality Commission and any other appropriate persons.

Regulations[27] impose requirements on the NHS England and CCGs in order to ensure good practice in relation to the procurement of healthcare services for purposes of the NHS, to ensure the protection of patients' rights to make choices regarding their NHS treatment and to prevent anti-competitive behaviour by commissioners with regard to such services.

NHS foundation trusts

NHS trusts were established by the NHS and Community Care Act 1990 which saw the introduction of the internal market in the NHS. NHS trusts were established to provide services under a non-legally enforceable contract or agreement with the health authorities. In addition, group fundholding practices of GPs were established which were allocated the funds to purchase services for the patients on their lists from the providers. Foundation trusts were set up in 2004 following the Health and Social Care (Community Health and Standards) Act. The statutory provisions were consolidated in the National Health Service Act 2006 sections 30–65 and Schedules 7, 8, 9 and 10. The transition from the status of NHS trusts to foundation trusts was overseen by an independent regulator (Monitor) which had the power to licence the trusts as foundation trusts. Section 179 of the Health and Social Care Act 2012 abolishes NHS trusts, with transition provisions, and from 2014 all NHS trusts are expected to be foundation trusts.

NHS Improvement (formerly Monitor)

A body corporate known as the Independent Regulator of NHS Foundation Trusts (then called Monitor, now NHS Improvement)[28] was set up under Section 31 of the 2006 Act with additional provisions relating to membership, tenure of office, general and specific powers, finance and reports set out in Schedule 8. It has a duty to exercise its functions in a manner consistent with the performance by the Secretary of State of the duties under Sections 1, 3 and 258 of the NHS Act 2006 (duty as to health service and services generally and as to university clinical teaching and research).

There are set criteria for the licensing of a healthcare service for the purposes of Part 3 of the Health and Social Care Act 2012.[29] A Schedule to the Order sets out criterion 1 in relation to registration with the Care Quality Commission and criterion 2 in relation to provider fitness.

The Health and Social Care Act 2012 and Monitor

Sections 61 to 71 and Schedule 8 of the 2012 Act set out provisions relating to Monitor. Under section 61 Monitor, the body corporate known as the Independent Regulator of NHS Foundation Trusts, is to continue to exist, and is to be known as Monitor. Schedule 8 (which makes further provision about Monitor) has effect.

Section 62 sets out the general duties and is shown in Statute Box 5.6.

Statute 5.6
Section 62 of the Health and Social Care Act 2012

General Duties of Monitor

1. The main duty of Monitor in exercising its functions is to protect and promote the interests of people who use health care services by promoting provision of healthcare services which—
   (a) is economic, efficient and effective, and
   (b) maintains or improves the quality of the services.
2. In carrying out its main duty, Monitor must have regard to the likely future demand for healthcare services.
3. Monitor must exercise its functions with a view to preventing anti-competitive behaviour in the provision of healthcare services for the purposes of the NHS which is against the interests of people who use such services.
4. Monitor must exercise its functions with a view to enabling healthcare services provided for the purposes of the NHS to be provided in an integrated way where it considers that this would—
   (a) improve the quality of those services (including the outcomes that are achieved from their provision) or the efficiency of their provision,
   (b) reduce inequalities between persons with respect to their ability to access those services, or
   (c) reduce inequalities between persons with respect to the outcomes achieved for them by the provision of those services.
5. Monitor must exercise its functions with a view to enabling the provision of healthcare services provided for the purposes of the NHS to be integrated with the provision of health-related services or social care services where it considers that this would—
   (a) improve the quality of those healthcare services (including the outcomes that are achieved from their provision) or the efficiency of their provision,
   (b) reduce inequalities between persons with respect to their ability to access those healthcare services, or
   (c) reduce inequalities between persons with respect to the outcomes achieved for them by the provision of those healthcare services.
6. Monitor must, in carrying out its duties under subsections (4) and (5), have regard to the way in which—
   (a) the National Health Service Commissioning Board carries out its duties under section 13N of the National Health Service Act 2006, and
   (b) clinical commissioning groups carry out their duties under section 14Z1 of that Act.

> 7. Monitor must secure that people who use healthcare services, and other members of the public, are involved to an appropriate degree in decisions that Monitor makes about the exercise of its functions (other than decisions it makes about the exercise of its functions in a particular case).
> 8. Monitor must obtain advice appropriate for enabling it effectively to discharge its functions from persons who (taken together) have a broad range of professional expertise in—
>   (a) the prevention, diagnosis or treatment of illness (within the meaning of the National Health Service Act 2006), and
>   (b) the protection or improvement of public health.
> 9. Monitor must exercise its functions in a manner consistent with the performance by the Secretary of State of the duty under section 1(1) of the National Health Service Act 2006 (promotion of comprehensive health service).
> 10. Monitor must not exercise its functions for the purpose of causing a variation in the proportion of healthcare services provided for the purposes of the NHS that is provided by persons of a particular description if that description is by reference to—
>   (a) whether the persons in question are in the public or (as the case may be) private sector, or
>   (b) some other aspect of their status.

Under section 63 the Secretary of State is empowered to give guidance to Monitor for the purpose of assisting Monitor to comply with its duty under section 62(9).

Section 64 gives supplementary guidance on the meaning of anti-competitive behaviour, healthcare and the NHS.

Regulations can be made under section 65 to extend Monitor's scope to cover adult social care services which are defined to include all forms of personal care and other practical assistance provided for individuals who, by reason of age, illness, disability, pregnancy, childbirth, dependence on alcohol or drugs, or any other similar circumstances, are in need of such care or other assistance, but (b) does not include anything provided by an establishment or agency for which Her Majesty's Chief Inspector of Education, Children's Services and Skills is the registration authority under section 5 of the Care Standards Act 2000.

Section 66 sets out the matters to which Monitor must have regard to in exercise of functions and these are shown in Statute Box 5.7.

Statute 5.7

Section 66 of the Health and Social Care Act 2012

Matters to which Monitor must have regard

1. In exercising its functions, Monitor must have regard, in particular, to the need to maintain the safety of people who use healthcare services.

2. Monitor must, in exercising its functions, also have regard to the following matters in so far as they are consistent with the matter referred to in subsection (1)—

   (a) the desirability of securing continuous improvement in the quality of healthcare services provided for the purposes of the NHS and in the efficiency of their provision,

   (b) the need for commissioners of healthcare services for the purposes of the NHS to ensure that the provision of access to the services for those purposes operates fairly,

   (c) the need for commissioners of healthcare services for the purposes of the NHS to ensure that people who require healthcare services for those purposes are provided with access to them,

   (d) the need for commissioners of healthcare services for the purposes of the NHS to make the best use of resources when doing so,

   (e) the desirability of persons who provide healthcare services for the purposes of the NHS cooperating with each other in order to improve the quality of healthcare services provided for those purposes,

   (f) the need to promote research into matters relevant to the NHS by persons who provide healthcare services for the purposes of the NHS,

   (g) the need for high standards in the education and training of healthcare professionals who provide health care services for the purposes of the NHS, and

   (h) where the Secretary of State publishes a document for the purposes of section 13E of the National Health Service Act 2006 (improvement of quality of services), any guidance published by the Secretary of State on the parts of that document which the Secretary of State considers to be particularly relevant to Monitor's exercise of its functions.

Section 67 is concerned with the conflicts between functions, and the role of Monitor to ensure that the conflict is resolved in the manner it considers best. The section prioritises the different duties Monitor has.

Under Section 68 Monitor has a duty to review regulatory burdens and in reviewing the exercise of its functions must secure that it does not impose burdens which it considers to be unnecessary nor maintain burdens which it considers to have become unnecessary. It must publish a statement relating to what it proposes to do.

Where Monitor is intending to do something which could have a significant impact on service providers, then, under section 69, it must carry out an impact assessment.

Section 70 relates to information which can be used by Monitor and the duty of Monitor to provide the Secretary of State with such information as he may specify.

Section 71 makes provision for a situation where the Secretary of State considers that Monitor is failing to perform its functions.

From 1 April 2016 NHS Improvement became the operational name for an organisation that brought together:

- Monitor
- NHS Trust Development Authority

- Patient Safety
- Advance Change Team
- Intensive Support Teams

NHS Improvement's role is to oversee foundation trusts and NHS trusts, as well as independent providers that provide NHS-funded care. It offers support the providers need to give patients consistently safe, high quality, compassionate care within local health systems that are financially sustainable. It can hold providers to account and, where necessary, intervene to ensure patient safety and financial sustainability.

Licensing

Sections 81 to 110 of the Health and Social Care Act 2012 make provisions relating to the licensing of health service providers, their **conditions** and their enforcement. Under section 81 it is a requirement that all health service providers are licensed. Any person who provides a healthcare service for the purposes of the NHS must hold a licence under the 2012 Act and regulations may make provision for determining, in relation to a service provided by two or more persons acting in different capacities, which of those persons is to be regarded as the person who provides the service.

Under section 86 Monitor has the responsibility of setting the criteria for obtaining a license. In February 2013 Monitor published the NHS Provider licence setting out conditions for providers of NHS services valid from April 2013. Further information for independent providers of NHS trusts was circulated in 2014. The licensing documents are available on the NHS Improvement website.

National Health Service Trust Development Authority

The National Health Service Trust Development Authority (NHSTDA), which is now also part of NHS Improvement, was established under section 28 of the NHS Act 2006 regulations for membership and procedure set out in National Health Service Trust Development Authority Regulations.[30] Further regulations set out the establishment and constitution.[31] Functions specified under section 28 of the 2006 Act are to exercise such of the Secretary of State's functions in connection with the performance management and development of NHS trusts in England and the making of certain public appointments to NHS bodies in England and such other functions as the Secretary of State may direct. The NHSTDA is responsible for overseeing the performance management and governance of NHS trusts, including clinical quality.

NHS Trust Development Authority (Establishment and Constitution) Order 2012 is amended by a later order[32] to provide for the transfer of property and liabilities from the Secretary of State to the Authority plus the transfer of staff from the Secretary of State for Health, strategic health authorities, primary care trust and the National Institute for Improvement and Innovation to the Authority. Further information, including its NHS foundation trust quality reports requirements, can be found on its website.[33]

Community and Primary Care Services

The NHS and Community Care Act 1990 changed the basis of community care, implementing the recommendations of the Griffiths Report.[34] Instead of places in nursing homes and residential care homes being funded on a means-tested basis by social security, funds were given to the local authority social services departments to become the purchasers of places, on a means-tested basis, for those residents in its catchment area who required nursing or residential care (see chapter 23 for community provisions).

Care Trusts

The NHS Plan[35] envisaged that care trusts would be established to commission and provide social services as well as community healthcare (see chapter 23). Further provisions to regulate care trusts are contained in the Health and Social Care Act 2001 Part 3 re-enacted in section 77 of the NHS Act 2006 as amended by section 200 of the Health and Social Care Act 2012. Care trusts enable social services as well as health services to be provided by the same trust. Section 77 enables an organisation to be designated as a care trust. Regulations relating to care trusts were enacted in 2012 replacing those of 2001.[36] A list of all NHS care trusts can be found on the nhs.uk website.[37]

Clinical governance

One of the most significant changes envisaged by the government in its 1997 White Paper was the concept of clinical governance. It was defined as:

A framework through which NHS organisations are accountable for continuously improving the quality of their services.[38]

The idea of clinical governance is simple. In the past, the trust board and its chief executive have been responsible for the financial probity of the organisation; there has been no statutory responsibility of the trust for the overall quality of the organisation. Under the concept of clinical governance, the board and its chief executive are responsible for the quality of clinical services provided by the organisation. In theory, this could mean that a board is removed or a chief executive dismissed if a baby suffers brain damage at birth or a mother dies in childbirth as a result of negligence.

Duty of quality

The concept of clinical governance was based on the statutory duty of quality under section 18 of the Health Act 1999 which has now been replaced by section 45 of the Health and Social Care (Community Health and Standards) Act 2003, which places on each NHS body the duty to put and keep in place arrangements for the purpose of monitoring and improving the quality of healthcare provided by and for that body.

Section 45 of the Health and Social Care Act 2008 (replacing section 46 of the Health and Social Care (Community Health and Standards) Act 2003 is shown in Statute Box 5.8.

> ## Statute 5.8
> ### Section 45 of the Health and Social Care Act 2008
>
> **Standards set by Secretary of State**
>
> 1. The Secretary of State may prepare and publish statements of standards in relation to the provision of NHS care.
> 2. The Secretary of State must keep the standards under review and may publish amended statements whenever the Secretary of State considers it appropriate.
> 3. The Secretary of State may direct a person—
>   (a) to prepare a draft statement of standards for the purposes of subsection (1), submit it to the Secretary of State for approval and publish it in the form approved or modified by the Secretary of State;
>   (b) to keep standards under review for the purposes of subsection (2) and, whenever the person considers it appropriate, submit a draft amended statement to the Secretary of State for approval and publish it in the form approved or modified by the Secretary of State.
> 4. The Secretary of State must consult such persons as the Secretary of State considers appropriate—
>   (a) before publishing a statement under subsection (1) or approving a statement under subsection (3)(a);
>   (b) before publishing under subsection (2), or approving under subsection (3)(b), any amended statement which in the opinion of the Secretary of State effects a substantial change in the standards.

The role of Healthwatch and local Healthwatch in standard setting is discussed in chapter 26. Standard setting and monitoring have become an even more significant part of the practitioner's professional responsibilities. (Standards in relation to the law are discussed in chapter 3 on the law of negligence.)

The Care Quality Commission (CQC) will have regard to the adherence to these standards in its inspections, inquiries and investigations. Under section 46(4) of the Health and Social Care Act 2008 the Secretary of State can devise or approve the indicators of quality which are to be used by the CQC, and under subsection 46(5) the Secretary of State can direct the CQC to devise these indicators for his approval.

Under section 234 of the Health and Social Care Act 2012 NHS England can direct NICE to prepare statements of standards (known as quality standard) in relation to the provision of:

(a) NHS services,
(b) public health services, or
(c) social care in England.

NICE quality standards can be accessed on its website.

The Care Quality Commission

In 2009 the Care Quality Commission took over the responsibilities of three commissions: the Healthcare Commission (i.e. the Commission for Health Audit and Inspection – formerly the Commission for Health Improvement (CHI)); the Commission for Social Care Inspection; and the Mental Health Act Commission.[39] CQC was intended to be a stronger force in the raising and implementation of standards across the NHS than its predecessor.

Its main functions, objectives and matters to which it had to have regard under the Health and Social Care Act 2008 are listed in Statute Box 5.9. Regulations were enacted setting out its duties of registration.[40] Additional duties as the replacement body of the Mental Health Act Commission were later added.[41] Since April 2010 all NHS trusts have been registered with the CQC, some conditional on action being taken to meet concerns about safety and quality of care.

Statute 5.9
Sections 2, 3, 4 and 5 of the Health and Social Care Act 2008

Care Quality Commission

S.2 Main functions

1. Registration functions under chapter 2.
2. Review and investigation functions under chapter 3.
3. Functions under the Mental Health Act 1983.

S.3 The Commission's objectives

1. The main objective of the Commission in performing its functions is to protect and promote the health, safety and welfare of people who use health and social care services.
2. The Commission is to perform its functions for the general purpose of encouraging—
   (a) the improvement of health and social care services,
   (b) the provision of health and social care services in a way that focuses on the needs and experiences of people who use those services, and
   (c) the efficient and effective use of resources in the provision of health and social care services.
3. In this chapter, 'health and social care services' means the services to which the Commission's functions relate.

S.4 Matters to which the Commission must have regard

1. In performing its functions the Commission must have regard to—
   (a) views expressed by or on behalf of members of the public about health and social care services,
   (b) experiences of people who use health and social care services and their families and friends,

(c) views expressed by local involvement networks about the provision of health and social care services in their areas,

(d) the need to protect and promote the rights of people who use health and social care services (including, in particular, the rights of children, of persons detained under the Mental Health Act 1983, of persons who are deprived of their liberty in accordance with the Mental Capacity Act 2005 (c. 9), and of other vulnerable adults),

(e) the need to ensure that action by the Commission in relation to health and social care services is proportionate to the risks against which it would afford safeguards and is targeted only where it is needed,

(f) any developments in approaches to regulatory action, and

(g) best practice among persons performing functions comparable to those of the Commission (including the principles under which regulatory action should be transparent, accountable and consistent).

2. In performing its functions the Commission must also have regard to such aspects of government policy as the Secretary of State may direct.

3. In subsection (1)(c), 'local involvement network' has the meaning given by section 222(2) of the Local Government and Public Involvement in Health Act 2007 (c. 28).

S.5 Statement on user involvement

1. The Commission must publish a statement describing how it proposes to—

    (a) promote awareness among service users and carers of its functions,

    (b) promote and engage in discussion with service users and carers about the provision of health and social care services and about the way in which the Commission exercises its functions,

    (c) ensure that proper regard is had to the views expressed by service users and carers, and

    (d) arrange for any of its functions to be exercised by, or with the assistance of service users and carers.

2. The Commission may from time to time revise the statement and must publish any revised statement.

3. Before publishing the statement (or revised statement) the Commission must consult such persons as it considers appropriate.

4. In this section—

    (a) 'service users' means people who use health or social care services, and

    (b) 'carers' means people who care for service users as relatives.

Care Quality Commission (Membership) Regulations 2008 amended by the CQC membership Amendment Regulations in 2013 (SI 2157) to increase the maximum number of members from 12 to 14. Other amendments were made by SI 2011/2547 and 2012/1186; the latter substituted references to the National Patient Safety Agency by the NHS Commissioning Board Authority, increased numbers of members to no more than 12 (subsequently 14) and removed the bar on the Secretary of State appointing CQC employees as members.

It can be seen that the CQC's main statutory duty is to protect and promote the health, safety and welfare of those who use health and adult social care services in England. To meet that duty the CQC has the power to formulate policies and standards that health and adult social care services have to comply with including:

- Registration of health services to ensure that required standards of safety and quality are being met.
- Monitoring of health providers to check that they are meeting essential standards of safety and quality.
- Using enforcement powers to take speedy and effective action where services are not to the required standard.
- Carrying out periodic reviews of services to assess how well those providing and arranging services are performing.
- Offering advice and making recommendations to help improve services.

(Care Quality Commission 2009)

Registration with the CQC

Under the Health and Social Care Act 2008 all providers of health and services, including NHS trusts providing nursing services, have to register with the CQC if they undertake regulated activities as defined in the Health and Social Care Act 2008 (Regulated Activities) Regulations 2014. The range of regulated activities subject to registration include hospital and community nursing services undertaken by NHS trusts.

The 2014 regulations were introduced following the Francis Report into the care of patients at the Mid Staffordshire Hospital (House of Commons 2013). They came into force in April 2015.

All service providers must submit evidence, including evidence from people who use the services, confirming that each standard and outcome imposed for the regulated activity is complied with. These include person-centred care, dignity and respect, consent, meeting nutritional and hydration needs, safeguarding and providing safe care and treatment. Where a service provider does not meet the required standards it must be declared and an action plan submitted with the reasons for non-compliance and how they will be achieved.

The fundamental standards set in law a clear baseline below which care must not fall and the CQC can take enforcement action against providers that do not meet these standards. Some of these standards have offences attached, and the CQC can bring prosecutions if these are breached and the breach causes avoidable harm or risk of such harm.

Safe Care and Treatment

One fundamental standard that has an offence attached for breach is the requirement to provide safe care and treatment under the Health and Social Care Act 2008 (Regulated Activities) Regulations 2014, regulation 12.

The regulation places a duty on NHS Trusts to ensure that care and treatment is provided in a safe way for service users.

To comply with regulation 12 the NHS trust must ensure that they:

- assess the risks to the health and safety of service users of receiving the care or treatment;
- do all that is reasonably practicable to mitigate any such risks;

- ensure that persons providing care or treatment to service users have the qualifications, competence, skills and experience to do so safely;
- ensure that the premises used by the service provider are safe to use for their intended purpose and are used in a safe way;
- ensure that the equipment used by the service provider for providing care or treatment to a service user is safe for such use and is used in a safe way;
- ensure that there is sufficient equipment and medicine to ensure the safety of service users and to meet their needs;
- manage medicines safely and properly;
- assess the risk of, and prevent, detect and control the spread of, infections; and
- ensure that timely care planning takes place to ensure the health, safety and welfare of service users during transfers of care.

(Health and Social Care Act 2008 (Regulated Activities) Regulations 2014, regulation 12 (2))

It is an offence for an NHS trust to breach regulation 12 where that breach results in avoidable harm to a service user, a risk of avoidable harm occurring or a loss of money or property due to theft or misuse (Health and Social Care Act 2008 (Regulated Activities) Regulations 2014, regulation 22).

CQC's First Prosecution for Failing to Provide Safe Care and Treatment

The CQC brought their first prosecution against an NHS foundation trust in England under regulation 12 of the 2014 regulated activities regulations following an incident at an inpatient mental health unit.

Since 2010, patients detained under the Mental Health Act 1983 had climbed onto the roof of the unit from a courtyard in an attempt to abscond from detention on no fewer than seven separate occasions. The CQC argued that the trust had failed to act to prevent access to the roof by patients even after one patient fell sustaining serious life changing neck injuries in 2015. When a further three patients gained access to the roof, with one sustaining an injury, the CQC prosecuted the NHS foundation trust after that incident.

Guidance from the CQC on compliance with the Health and Social Care Act 2008 (Regulated Activities) Regulations 2014, regulation 12(2) requires care providers and their staff, including nurses, to:

- assess and manage risk to health and safety of service users;
- ensure the safety of premises by making adjustments to the premises, staff practice and equipment to protect service users;
- ensure staff, such as nurses, have training on the safe operation of premises that includes incident reporting and emergency and contingency planning;
- ensure health and safety concerns are included in service users care and treatment plans; and
- report, escalate, act on and disseminate health and safety concerns that might affect service users.

(Care Quality Commission 2015)

The NHS trust admitted that it had failed to meet this fundamental standard and as a result avoidable harm was caused to service users in their care and other service users were put at risk of further avoidable harm, and so pleaded guilty to the offence (Care Quality Commission 2017). The case highlights the need for nurses to have a good working knowledge of the requirements of the Health and Social Care Act 2008 (Regulated Activities) Regulations 2014 so that they act to ensure that their employing trust discharges their obligations.

The other enforcement powers of the CQC include the power to impose, vary or remove conditions, of cancelling registration or issuing a warning notice, issuing a penalty notice in lieu of prosecution and suspending registration.

The CQC also works with various bodies to enforce the standards. It has a reciprocal statutory duty with NHS Improvement to cooperate together, and memoranda of understanding with the professional regulators including the NMC to exchange information relating to the fitness to practice of a nurse.

The Care Act 2014 section 89 inserts new provisions into the Health and Social Care Act 2008 to require the non-executives to appoint a Chief Inspector of Hospitals, a Chief Inspector of Adult Social Care, and a Chief Inspector of General Practice. Section 90 of the Care Act 2014 makes amendments to the Health and Social Care Act 2008 to ensure the independence of the Care Quality Commission by removing the Secretary of State's power in various functions such as making regulations as to procedure for representations before report publication or the need for the approval of the Secretary of State in conducting studies as to economy, efficiency, the frequency of inspections, etc.

Regulations drawn up under section 20 of the Health and Social Care Act 2008 which enable the CQC to set standards for regulated organisations across a range of areas are amended by section 95 of the Care Act 2014 to enable provision to be made for a specified person to set the standards for management and training in regulated activities. Section 46 of the Health and Social Care Act 2008 imposed a duty on the CQC to conduct reviews and performance assessments of the carrying on by prescribed registered service providers of specified regulated activities and publish reports of these assessments. Regulations in 2014 prescribe the registered service providers and regulated activities for those purposes.[42]

The CQC has carried out a survey of 69,000 NHS inpatients which revealed some major concerns, including the fact that 45 per cent of patients responding were not told about the side effects of their medication.[43] In October 2010 the CQC stated that almost 1000 care homes in England were not being properly run by a qualified manager and faced closure.[44] A rehab clinic, the Causeway Retreat, was fined £8000 and had to pay costs of £30,000 for failure to register with the CQC.[45]

The CQC has also carried out an inquiry into the health organisation's involvement in the case of Baby P, showing that communication between the different health bodies was systematically poor (see chapter 13).[46] It also reviewed a mental health unit in Devon where six elderly patients died and found nursing failures and poor staff supervision.[47]

The CQC has reported Colchester Hospital University NHS Trust to the police following disclosure that staff were 'pressured, bullied and harassed' to change the data on cancer waiting times to make it look as though targets had not been missed.[48] The Chief Inspector of Hospitals recommended that the trust be put into special measures. The medical director of NHS England had alerted the CQC to a whistleblower's allegations about the hospital. Monitor also launched an investigation to establish whether other patients did not receive treatment in accordance with national standards.

The results of the CQC inpatient survey for 2017 showed gradual improvement since 2009 in a number of areas including:

- the quality of communication between themselves and medical professionals (doctors and nurses),
- the quality of information about operations or procedures,

- privacy when discussing their condition,
- quality of food, and
- cleanliness of their room or ward.

However, the results also indicated that responses to some questions were less positive or have not improved, including patients' perceptions of:

- noise at night from other patients,
- emotional support from staff during their hospital stay,
- information on new medications prescribed while in hospital, and
- the quality of preparation and information for leaving hospital.

Certain groups of patients consistently report poorer experiences of their time in hospital, including:

- patients with mental health conditions,
- younger patients (aged 16–35 years), and
- patients with Alzheimer's or dementia.

In 2017 the CQC reported that the majority of care that people receive is good, and there were providers and services that delivered outstanding care including 6 per cent of NHS acute hospital and mental health core services, and 4 per cent of GP practices. However, some 3 per cent of NHS acute hospital core services, 2 per cent of GP practices and 1 per cent of adult social care and NHS mental health core services were rated as inadequate, with a further 37 per cent of NHS acute core services, 24 per cent of NHS mental health core services and 6 per cent of GP practices being rated as requiring improvement.[49]

The Care Act 2014 section 92 creates an offence for a care provider to supply or provide false or misleading information unless it can prove that it took all reasonable steps and exercised all due diligence.

National Institute for Health and Care Excellence (NICE)

The National Institute for Clinical Excellence (NICE) (subsequently renamed National Institute for Health and Care Excellence) was established on 1 April 1999 to promote clinical excellence and cost-effectiveness.[50] Subsequently it was abolished (section 248 of the Health and Social Care Act 2012) and re-established on a new statutory basis under Sections 232–249 and Schedule 16 of the Health and Social Care Act 2012. Regulations relating to its constitution and functions were subsequently enacted.[51]

The statutory provisions are shown in Statute Box 5.10.

Statute 5.10
Sections 232–234 of the Health and Social Care Act 2012

Statutory provisions on the National Institute for Health and Care Excellence (NICE)

Section 232

1. There is to be a body corporate known as the National Institute for Health and Care Excellence (referred to in this Part as 'NICE').
2. Schedule 16 (which makes further provision about NICE) has effect.

233 General duties

1. In exercising its functions NICE must have regard to—
   (a) the broad balance between the benefits and costs of the provision of health services or of social care in England,
   (b) the degree of need of persons for health services or social care in England, and
   (c) the desirability of promoting innovation in the provision of health services or of social care in England.
2. NICE must exercise its functions effectively, efficiently and economically.
3. In this Part—

   'health services' means services which must or may be provided as part of the health service in England;
   'social care' includes all forms of personal care and other practical assistance provided for individuals who, by reason of age, illness, disability, pregnancy, childbirth, dependence on alcohol or drugs, or any other similar circumstances, are in need of such care or other assistance.

234 Quality standards

1. The relevant commissioner may direct NICE to prepare statements of standards in relation to the provision of—
   (a) NHS services,
   (b) public health services, or
   (c) social care in England.
2. In this Part such a statement is referred to as a 'quality standard'.
3. In preparing a quality standard NICE must consult the public and, for that purpose, may publish drafts of the standard.
4. NICE must keep a quality standard under review and may revise it as it considers appropriate.
5. A quality standard (and any revised standard)—
   (a) has no effect unless it is endorsed by the relevant commissioner, and
   (b) must not be published by NICE unless the relevant commissioner so requires.

6. The relevant commissioner may require NICE—
   (a) to publish the standard (or revised standard) or to disseminate it to persons specified by the relevant commissioner, and
   (b) to do so in the manner specified by the relevant commissioner.
7. NICE must—
   (a) establish a procedure for the preparation of quality standards, and
   (b) consult such persons as it considers appropriate in establishing that procedure.
8. Subsection (9) applies in a case where the Secretary of State and the Board each has power under this section to give NICE a direction to prepare a quality standard in relation to the same matter or connected matters.
9. In such a case—
   (a) the Secretary of State and the Board may issue a joint direction under subsection (1), and
   (b) if they do so, NICE must prepare a joint quality standard in respect of the matter or matters concerned.
10. In this section 'the relevant commissioner'—
    (a) in relation to a quality standard in relation to the provision of NHS services, means the Board, and
    (b) in relation to a quality standard in relation to the provision of public health services or of social care in England, means the Secretary of State, and a reference to the relevant commissioner in relation to a joint quality standard is a reference to both the Secretary of State and the Board.
11. In this Part—
    NHS services' means services the provision of which is arranged by the Board or a clinical commissioning group under the National Health Service Act 2006 (including pursuant to arrangements made under section 7A of the National Health Service Act 2006) or section 117 of the Mental Health Act 1983 (after-care); 'public health services' means services provided pursuant to the functions of—
    (a) the Secretary of State under section 2A or 2B of, or paragraph 7C, 8 or 12 of Schedule 1 to, that Act, or
    (b) a local authority under section 2B or 111 of, or paragraphs 1 to 7B or 13 of Schedule 1 to, that Act.

Section 235 covers the supply of quality standards to other persons such as devolved authorities. Section 236 requires NICE to give advice or guidance to the Secretary of State or NHS England on any quality matter referred to it by the Secretary of State or (as the case may be) NHS England. Under section 237, regulations may confer functions on NICE in relation to the giving of advice or guidance, provision of information or making of recommendations about any matter concerning or connected with the provision of:

(a) NHS services,
(b) public health services, or
(c) social care in England.

However, the regulations cannot permit a direction to be given about the substance of advice, guidance or recommendations of NICE. Section 238 enables the regulations to stipulate provisions on appeals against NICE recommendations. Section 239 enables the regulations to confer functions on NICE in relation to providing or facilitating the provision for training in connection with the provision of NHS services, public health services or social care in England. Section 240 enables the regulations to cover advisory services by NICE.

Under section 241, NHS England may direct NICE to exercise any of its functions in relation to the preparation of the guidance required to be published under section 14Z8 of the National Health Service Act 2006 (the 'commissioning guidance'). A direction under subsection (1) may direct NICE to exercise the functions in such manner and within such period as may be specified in the direction.

Under section 241(3) NICE must, if requested to do so:

(a) provide NHS England with information or advice on such matters connected to its functions in respect of the commissioning guidance as may be specified in the request, and

(b) disseminate the commissioning guidance to such persons and in such manner as may be specified in the request.

Regulations (under section 242) may make provision requiring NICE to publish a document (known as 'the charter') explaining the functions of NICE and how NICE intends to exercise them.

Section 245 makes provision for the situation if NICE is failing to discharge its functions.

In April 2014 NICE announced that it was not recommending Kadclya (a drug for breast cancer estimated to extend life by an average of six months) for NHS use because it was too expensive at £90,000 per patient. NICE was attempting to negotiate with Roche over the price.[52] Individual patients could apply to the government's Cancer Drugs Fund (CDF). Kadclya was out of CDF funding and into routine NHS funding in 2017 following a deal between the manufacturer and NHS England that allowed NICE to recommend its use.[53]

The fact that NICE has recommended certain treatments does not automatically mean that patients can insist on them. For example, NICE recommended that three courses of IVF treatment should be available to infertile couples. However, as a result of financial pressures the Mid Essex Clinical Commissioning Group decided to restrict IVF treatments to HIV-positive men and to cancer patients. The CCG said that after consultation local GPs agreed that other types of care should take priority over fertility services in any spending decisions.[54] In another example NICE has approved the prostrate drug enzalutamide for men after chemotherapy has been exhausted but NHS England is refusing to fund it for those men who had already tried abiraterone.[55] NICE has come under criticism for its recommendations that statins should be taken by more than 4 million additional persons who would benefit from cholesterol lowering drugs. Critics fear that GPs will be unable to cope with the additional demands.[56]

NHS 111 and walk-in clinics

NHS Direct, which enabled patients to seek advice on health problems, both by telephone and online, was replaced in England in 2014 by a new NHS 111 service. NHS 111 provides a free-to-call service but it is not an emergency number. The website[57] states that it can be used: if medical help is needed but it is not a 999 emergency; if you think you may need to get to A&E; you don't know who to call or you do not have a GP; if you need health information or reassurance about what to do next. The NHS 111 service is staffed by trained advisers supported by experienced nurses and paramedics.

Walk-in centres (WICs) are managed by clinical commissioning groups. A registered nurse is usually in charge of each WIC and patients do not usually need an appointment. Most centres are

The National Quality Board

The National Quality Board was re-established by NHS England as a forum where key NHS oversight organisations come together to share intelligence, agree action and monitor overall quality assurance in the NHS in England. The board is composed of senior clinicians and representatives from NHS England, the CQC, NHS Improvement, Department of Health and Social Care, Health Education England, Public Health England, NICE and NHS Digital.

NHS inquiries

Airedale Inquiry Report

In 2010 the report of an inquiry into events at Airedale Foundation NHS Trust Hospital was published.[58] Anne Grigg-Booth, a night nurse, was accused of killing three patients by illegally administering opiates.

Winterbourne View Hospital Report

An undercover operation by BBC *Panorama* revealed cruel, callous and degrading abuse of residents at this private hospital and led to the imprisonment of six care workers and five others were found guilty. The government published a full response in December 2012 and set out a programme of action including tighter inspections and regulation by the Care Quality Commission.

Beverly Allitt

Beverly Allitt, a state-enrolled nurse, was convicted of murdering four children, of attempting to murder three others and of causing grievous bodily harm to six more. She was sentenced to life imprisonment on every count. An independent inquiry,[59] chaired by Sir Cecil Clothier, made significant and substantial recommendations on the selection procedures for nurses, including the prohibition of employment of those with a personality disorder, and that there should be formal health screening; that post-mortem reports should be sent by the coroner to doctors involved in the patient's care; that there should be a review of paediatric pathology services; that there should be a review of sickness information being referred to occupational health and of the criteria for management referrals to occupational health; that there should be untoward incident reports if there is a failure of an alarm on monitoring equipment; and that reports of serious untoward incidents should be made in writing to district and regional health authorities. The Department of Health drew the attention of NHS managers to the report's recommendations.[60] The report accepted that no measures can afford complete protection against a determined miscreant and emphasised that:

> Our principal recommendation is that the Grantham disaster should serve to heighten awareness in all those caring for children of the possibility of malevolent intervention as a cause of unexplained clinical events.

A High Court judge ruled on 6 December 2007 that Beverly Allitt must serve a minimum of 30 years in custody and will therefore be over 60 years old before she is eligible for release.

Shipman Inquiry

It was apparent from the prosecution of a GP, Dr Shipman, for the murder of 15 patients, that the principal recommendation of the Allitt Inquiry applies as much to the care of adults as to children. An inquiry was set up after his conviction and several reports have been published: the first[61] identified the patients for whose deaths he was probably responsible (possibly over 200); the second[62] reviewed a police investigation into early police enquiries; and the third[63] made fundamental recommendations on the reform of the present system of death certification and the office and function of the coroner (see chapter 28). The fourth Shipman report, which was published in July 2004,[64] considered the regulation of controlled drugs in the community (see chapter 27). The fifth report of this inquiry was published in December 2004[65] and was concerned with the complaints against and the regulation of doctors. The sixth, and final, Shipman report considered how many patients Shipman killed during his career as a junior doctor at Pontefract General Infirmary and in his time at Hyde.[66] Shipman committed suicide in Wakefield prison on 13 January 2004.

Dr Rodney Ledward

Rodney Ledward was struck off the medical register after being found guilty of bungling 13 gynaecological operations. He died in 2000. An inquiry found that there had been a climate of fear and intimidation preventing nurses and junior doctors from telling tales in case they lost their jobs. It condemned NHS consultants for allowing him to carry on working for years and made recommendations that each trust should develop a list of untoward clinical events which should trigger an incident report. It also made recommendations relating to the function of each Royal College and clinical governance principles should apply to private practice as well as the NHS.[67] It was subsequently reported[68] that 59 women were suing the Kent and Medway Health Authority and East Kent Hospitals NHS Trust for damages. They alleged that they were raped or sexually assaulted by Rodney Ledward when they were in his care in the early 1980s.

Gosport War Memorial Hospital Inquiry

The Gosport Independent Panel,[69] set up to address concerns raised by families about the care and deaths of patients in Gosport War Memorial Hospital, delivered its report in June 2018. The panel found that in some 456 cases there was evidence that opioids were used without clinical indication, resulting in the shortening of the lives of those people as a result of the pattern of prescribing and administering those drugs.

Nurses use controlled drugs, including opioids, for their contribution to the care of patients, especially those in intractable pain or receiving palliative care. Such care often requires the dose to be increased in response to greater pain and suffering by the patient.

The report of the Gosport Independent Panel can be found on its website.[70]

Reports of other inquiries which can be downloaded from the Department of Health website include the inquiry into Clifford Ayling (a GP from Kent who was convicted of indecently assaulting women patients); Richard Neale (a gynaecologist who was struck off the GMC register for poor standards in a number of cases); and the Kerr/Haslam Inquiry (two psychiatrists in Yorkshire about whom several patients raised concerns).

Mid Staffordshire NHS foundation trust inquiry

The report of Robert Francis QC of the independent inquiry into the failures of the trust to provide basic patient care between 2005 and 2009, published in February 2010, stated that the deaths of 400 people were attributable to major failings in the quality of care. It recommended that Monitor should be asked to deauthorise Mid Staffs as a foundation trust. The response of the government to the report, published the same day, emphasised the need to learn lessons from the failure and a further inquiry under Robert Francis was set up to look at why the commissioning, regulatory and supervisory bodies did not detect the failures earlier. The GMC and NMC were asked to review the evidence and report on whether any action was necessary. Action by the NMC against individual registered nurses involved in the Mid Staffs scandal was taken.[71] The Staffordshire Inquiry chaired by Robert Francis QC was followed by the setting up of a public inquiry. The NHS Medical Director led a working group to look at hospital standardised mortality rates and develop a single clearer measure for the NHS and for patients. The government also called for greater openness and transparency among foundation trusts, with a strong presumption that, where appropriate, trust boards should meet in public and governors should have access to papers.

The report of the Francis Inquiry[72] was published on 6 February 2013. It made 290 recommendations to change the culture of the NHS to avoid a repeat of the tragedy. The report can be downloaded.[73] Robert Francis, in a letter to the Secretary of State for Health published with the executive summary of the report, described the essential aims of the report and these are shown in Box 5.1.

Box 5.1 Essential aims of the Francis Report on Mid Staffordshire NHS foundation trust

(a) Foster a common culture shared by all in the service of putting the patient first.

(b) Develop a set of fundamental standards, easily understood and accepted by patients, the public and healthcare staff, the breach of which should not be tolerated.

(c) Provide professionally endorsed and evidence-based means of compliance with these fundamental standards, which can be understood and adopted by the staff who have to provide the service.

(d) Ensure openness, transparency and candour throughout the system about matters of concern.

(e) Ensure that the relentless focus of the healthcare regulator is on policing compliance with these standards.

(f) Make all those who provide care for patients – individuals and organisations – properly accountable for what they do to ensure that the public is protected from those not fit to provide such a service.

(g) Provide for a proper degree of accountability for senior managers and leaders to place all with responsibility for protecting the interests of patients on a level playing field.

(h) Enhance the recruitment, education, training and support of all the key contributors to the provision of healthcare, but in particular those in nursing and leadership positions, to integrate the essential shared values of the common culture into everything they do.

(i) Develop and share ever improving means of measuring and understanding the performance of individual professionals, teams, units and provider organisations for the patients, the public and all other stakeholders in the system.

Some of the key recommendations to secure the achievement of the aims shown in Box 5.1 included:

- Changing the culture of the NHS, for which three characteristics are required: openness, transparency and candour.
- A statutory obligation should be imposed on healthcare providers, registered medical and nursing practitioners to observe the duty of candour.
- There should be a statutory obligation on directors of healthcare organisations to be truthful in any information given to a regulator or commissioner.
- There should be a criminal offence for any registered doctor, nurse or allied health professional or director of a registered or authorised organisation to obstruct the performance of these duties or dishonestly or recklessly make an untruthful statement to a regulator.
- Enforcement of the statutory duties should be by the Care Quality Commission.
- Increased focus on a culture of compassion and caring in nurse recruitment, training and education.
- Registration system to be introduced for healthcare support workers.
- NHS Constitution should be the first reference point for all NHS patients and staff and the common values of the service should be enshrined and effectively communicated by the NHS Constitution which should set out the system's values and the rights, obligations and expectations of patients.
- A simpler system of regulation.
- Non-compliance with a fundamental standard leading to death or serious harm of a patient should be capable of being prosecuted as a criminal offence, unless the provider or individual concerned can show that it was not reasonably practical to avoid this.
- Complaints relating to possible breaches of fundamental standards and serious complaints, should be accessible to the CQC, relevant commissioners, health scrutiny committees, communities and Local Healthwatch. Recommendations of the Patient's Association on complaints handling should be implemented. Any expression of concern by a patient should be treated as a complaint unless the patient's permission is refused.

Many of the recommendations from the Francis Public Inquiry were enacted in Part 2 of the Care Act 2014 on Care Standards. Sections 81–95 create a duty of candour; impose licence conditions on NHS foundation trusts; provide for the appointment of a trust special administrator; increase the independence of the CQC; and create an offence of a care provider providing false or misleading information.

Offence of Ill-Treatment or Wilful Neglect

The Government accepted in the autumn of 2013 a recommendation of the National Advisory Group on the Safety of Patients in England (2013) that called for a new statutory criminal offence of ill-treatment or wilful neglect of patients to be created covering all patients regardless of age or decision-making capacity.

This call to criminalise ill-treatment and wilful neglect for all patient groups echoed the view of the official inquiry into Mid Staffordshire NHS Trust, that more criminal sanctions should be available to prosecute poor care (Mason 2013).[74]

The numbers of prosecutions for ill-treatment and wilful neglect by nurses and other care workers has risen considerably since the Francis Report in England (House of Commons 2013) and the Andrews Report in Wales (Andrews and Butler 2014)[75] highlighted episodes of poor care resulting in the death of vulnerable patients.

Police investigations arising from the Andrews Report saw three nursing staff pleading guilty to wilful neglect with two others denying the charges and awaiting trial. At the conclusion of the investigation the police made clear that many more staff at the Abertawe Bro Morgannwg Health Board would have faced prosecution, as the evidence suggested the poor care they gave patients amounted to ill-treatment or wilful neglect, but the patients had decision-making capacity (McCarthy 2015).[76]

The police's limited ability to charge nurses who they believed had ill-treated or wilfully neglected their patients was due to the limits placed on them by the law as it applied at that time. There were three offences available but they only applied to specific classes of patient:

- The Mental health Act 1983, section 127 made it an offence to ill-treat or wilfully neglect a patient receiving treatment in a hospital for a mental disorder.
- The Children and Young Persons Act 1933, section 1 made it an offence to ill-treat or neglect a person under 16.
- The Mental Capacity Act 2005, section 44 made it an offence to ill-treat or wilfully neglect a person who lacked decision-making capacity.

The Revised Criminal Offence

Parliament has now removed the limits on when a prosecution for ill-treatment and wilful neglect can occur and introduced a new law covering all patients. Although health care is a devolved issue for the governments of England and Wales the law has been introduced through a criminal justice statute, which is not devolved, and so it applied in England and Wales.

The Criminal Justice and Courts Act 2015, section 20 now makes it an offence for a care worker to ill-treat or wilfully neglect a person in their care. A care worker is defined as anyone who is paid to provide health or social care and so includes nurses. The requirement for a care worker to be paid was included to ensure that relatives, volunteers and other informal carers would not be subject to prosecution under the Act.

The wording of the 2015 Act also makes it clear that in the case of healthcare the offence applies to those who ill-treat or wilfully neglect adults and children but for social care the offence only applies if the victim is an adult (Criminal Justice and Courts Act 2015, section 20(3)).

Healthcare is defined by the 2015 Act as including, but is not limited to, health care relating to physical health, mental health, public health, and procedures that are similar to forms of medical or surgical care but are not provided in connection with a medical condition. This comprehensive definition is designed to ensure that patients undergoing public health measures such as smoking cessation and those receiving cosmetic procedures are protected by the Act. A nurse guilty of either offence can now face a maximum sentence of up to five years in prison.

Care Provider Offence

The Criminal Justice and Courts Act 2015, section 21 creates an offence that applies to care providers, including organisations that arrange for the provision of healthcare to adults or children. This would include hospital and community trusts, health boards, GP practices and clinical commissioning groups.

A care provider commits an offence where

- a care worker ill-treats or wilfully neglects an individual,
- the care provider's activities are managed or organised in a way that amounts to a gross breach of their duty of care, and
- in the absence of the breach the ill-treatment or wilful neglect would not have occurred or would have been less likely to occur.

(Criminal Justice and Courts Act 2015, section 21 (1))

To be guilty of an offence a care provider would have to be in gross breach of their duty of care to the patient, i.e. the organisation will have had to have fallen far below the standard normally expected of it in the discharge of its duty of care. The wording of the offence means that it will be much easier for the police and Crown Prosecution Service to bring charges against individual nurses than their employing hospitals, community services or GP practices.

Ill-Treatment and Wilful Neglect

The specifics of the offences are not statutorily defined under the Criminal Justice and Courts Act 2015. The police and Crown prosecutors rely on the specific circumstances of the case and on cases previously decided by the Courts.

Ill-Treatment

Ill-treatment is given its ordinary English meaning and so includes any behaviour that a court would reasonably consider to be abusive. In *R v Strong* [2014] a care worker pleaded guilty to ill-treatment when she participated in bullying, harassing and assaulting vulnerable older people with dementia.

A support worker was convicted of ill-treatment after she pushed a cleansing wipe into a vulnerable patient's mouth and poured water over another patient (Barnett 2015).[77]

Wilful Neglect

Neglect occurs where a nurse fails to do what they would be expected to do in the care and treatment of a person in their care. This has been held to include falsifying records, failing to give medication and failing to provide CPR (2013).[78]

To be convicted the neglect must be wilful. In *R v Patel* [2013] a nurse refused to perform cardiac pulmonary resuscitation (CPR) when instructed to do so. A post-mortem revealed that the patient had been suffering from pneumonia which caused respiratory arrest, which in turn caused a cardiac arrest. CPR would have been unlikely to have saved the patient.

The Court of Appeal nevertheless held that the nurse had been properly convicted of wilful neglect and reiterated that neglect occurs where a nurse fails to do that which ought to be done in the treatment of a patient. For the neglect to be wilful it must be shown that the nurse knew it was necessary to administer treatment but deliberately decided not to do so because they could not face it.

R v Patel [2013] highlights that the offence of wilful neglect is not based on outcome or harm. It is enough for the prosecution to show that a nurse failed to do what they should have done and failed to do it deliberately to make out the offence.

Accidents and Errors

In its response to its consultation on the new offences the Department of Health (2014) stressed the offences are not meant to

- penalise genuine accidents or errors,
- hinder the free exercise of clinical judgement, or
- hinder organisations from making considered decisions on selection criteria for particular treatments.

This suggests that there would need to be a significant or serious breach of the standards of care for the offence to be committed but the decision on prosecution is not the Department of Health's to make – it will be for the police and Crown prosecutors to decide.

The Government Response to the House of Commons Health Committee Third Report of Session 2013–4 *After Francis: Making a difference* CM 8755 was published in November 2013. A statutory duty of candour is included in the Care Act, not on individuals but on the providers and will be included as a new registration requirement for health and social care providers registered with the Care Quality Commission. Section 81 of the Care Act 2014 provides for a duty of candour. It inserts into section 20 of the Health and Social Care Act 2008 (regulation of regulated activities), a new (5A) which states that regulations under this section must make provision as to the provision of information in a case where an incident of a specified description affecting a person's safety occurs in the course of the person being provided with a service. The NMC has included a duty of candour in its revised Code.

The recommendation in the Francis Report that healthcare support workers should receive training and supervision is considered in chapter 23.

The NHS Constitution

Professor Lord Darzi was appointed by the government to undertake a review of the NHS, with four main objectives: to put clinical decisions at the centre of the NHS; to improve patient care, particularly for those with long-term and life-threatening conditions; to make care more accessible and convenient; and to establish a vision for the next decade based less on central direction and more on patient control. An interim report was published, followed on 9 May 2008 by a review, Leading Local Change, and the final report, High Quality of Care for All, on the future of the NHS was published in 2008.[79] This made many radical recommendations, including enhancing the enforcement powers of the CQC. The Darzi Report also included in a draft format, an NHS Constitution[80] which can be seen on the website of this book in its finalised format. The Constitution sets out the seven key principles which guide the NHS; the rights and responsibilities of patients, the rights and responsibilities of staff and the values underpinning the NHS. It thus attempts to consolidate all the existing legal rights of patients, staff and public in one document and to set down some pledges such as:

> **The NHS will strive to provide all staff with personal development, access to appropriate training for their jobs, and line management support to succeed. (pledge)**

The NHS Constitution is accompanied by a statement of accountability. All organisations providing NHS services will be obliged by law to take account of the Constitution and its principles and values in their decisions and actions.

The Darzi review has been subject to many criticisms, including the absence of a timeframe and clear additional resources for its implementation. However, the Darzi review did set out a strategy which can be used by health professionals to develop their own services according to established values and clear standards. For example, it was planned that about 15 million clients with long-term conditions will have individual care plans.

Statutory provisions for the recommendations in the Darzi review were contained in the Health Act 2009. Under section 2 of the Act it is a requirement of specified NHS organisations to have regard to the NHS Constitution in performing their functions. Section 3 of the Health and Social Care Act 2012 inserts into the NHS Act 2006 the requirement that 'in exercising functions in relation to the health service, the Secretary of State must have regard to the NHS Constitution' (see Statute Box 5.1). Similarly in section 23 of the Health and Social Care Act 2012 the NHS Commissioning Board (NHS England) must, in the exercise of its functions:

(a) act with a view to securing that health services are provided in a way which promotes the NHS Constitution, and
(b) promote awareness of the NHS Constitution among patients, staff and members of the public (see Statute Box 5.3).

Section 26 places a similar duty upon the clinical commissioning groups.

An NHS Handbook providing guidance on the NHS Constitution was also drawn up and under the 2009 Act the Secretary of State must ensure that the Handbook continues to be available to patients, staff and members of the public and at least once in any period of three years the Secretary of State must carry out a review of the Handbook. The first review was completed in July 2012 and updated in October 2015 and again in 2017.

A summary of the Seven Principles of the NHS as revised in 2015 is shown in Box 5.2.[81]

Box 5.2 Principles of the NHS Constitution

1. The NHS provides a comprehensive service, available to all.
2. Access to NHS services is based on clinical need, not an individual's ability to pay.
3. The NHS aspires to the highest standards of excellence and professionalism.
4. The patient will be at the heart of everything the NHS does.
5. The NHS works across organisational boundaries.
6. The NHS is committed to providing best value for taxpayers' money.
7. The NHS is accountable to the public, communities and patients that it serves.

NHS and the private sector

In a development which can be seen as a sign of future changes it was announced that Hinchingbrooke Hospital in Cambridgeshire was to be run by a private company.[82] The hospital had an annual turnover of £92 million and debts of £40 million. All prospective NHS bidders had pulled out of the tender process, leaving only private companies bidding. The contract required the maternity and emergency services to be kept open, the NHS staff to retain their employment and the hospital assets to continue to be owned by the NHS. The first private company to take over an NHS hospital was Circle Health, to which Hinchingbrooke Hospital was franchised out in November 2010, but the experiment ended in failure when Circle announced they intended to withdraw from the contract just three years into their 10-year franchise.[83]

NHS Charges

A basic principle of the NHS when established was that it should be free at the point of use. However, charges for prescriptions (with exemptions) were soon levied and subsequently other charges have been raised but each must be based on specific legislation. Charges following treatment after a road accident were initiated in 1999 and have been amended in subsequent years. The NHS Injury Cost Recovery scheme recovers costs from insurers where personal injury compensation is paid. The cost increases each year to take account of hospital and community services inflation. In 2017 the charges stood at £678 for outpatient appointments, £883 per day for inpatient care and treatment to a cap of £49,824 and £205 per ambulance journey.[84] Since the spring of 2015, patients from outside the EU seeking treatment in Britain are charged 150 per cent more of the cost of their care in an attempt to deter 'health tourism', saving the NHS an estimated £500 million per year.

An independent commission set up by the King's Fund and chaired by Kate Barker stated that NHS charges such as for GP appointments, A&E and other services and taxes on pensioners need to be considered to fix the fracture between the health service and councils, which condemns the elderly to confusing and chaotic care. The report recommended that means-tested social care run by councils should be unified in a single, ring-fenced budget. It noted that it is unfair that people with some conditions such as cancer have their treatment fully paid by the NHS but those with others such as dementia or Parkinson's often have to pay many costs themselves.[85]

Conclusions

This chapter has considered the statutory duties placed on the Secretary of State and the organisations that have been introduced in recent years to ensure that accountability and high standards of care are provided in the NHS. It is perhaps too soon to evaluate the implications of the Health and Social Care Act 2012 and the new institutions established under that Act. However, the impact of the Mid Staffordshire scandal and the subsequent Francis Report are still reverberating around the NHS in England. The NHS is facing the most significant funding problems in its entire history and there are calls for major changes in how the organisation should be financed and how the long-term problems of an aging population and increasing numbers suffering from chronic diseases together with the challenges of meeting the opportunities arising from new technologies such as genetic screening are to be managed. In 2014 Unite estimated that 70 per cent of NHS contracts had been awarded to private companies over the previous two years and the number of contracts for tender was up by 30 per cent. Unite questioned the impact of these developments on patient care and service quality.

Reflection questions

1. Assess the likely contribution of NICE, CQC and the statutory duty of quality to the standards of care within your own sphere of professional practice.
2. Discuss the national scheme for the reporting of adverse healthcare incidents. How does it operate within your particular field of work? (See also chapter 12.)
3. Consider the effects of the Health and Social Care Act 2012. What impact have they had upon your work and how has its implementation improved standards of care within the NHS?

Further exercises

1. Consider the present organisation of primary health and social care services as a result of the Health and Social Care Act 2012 and Care Act 2014. To what extent do you think that patient care has improved?
2. Analyse the NHS Constitution (see the website of this book) and consider specifically the effects that it could have in the area in which you work. To what extent do you consider that it affects your own working practices?

References

[1] Nicholas Timmins, The four UK health systems, The King's Fund, London, 2013
[2] Department of Health, Equity and Excellence: Liberating the NHS, White Paper Cm 7881, 2010
[3] gov.uk/government/organisations/monitor/about
[4] Department of Health, Equity and Excellence: Liberating the NHS: Analytical strategy
[5] *R (Watts)* v *Bedford Primary Care Trust and Another*, The Times Law Report, 3 October 2003; [2004] EWCA Civ 166; (C372/04) [2006] ECJ
[6] Ibid *R* v *Secretary of State for Social Services ex parte Hincks and Others*, Solicitors' Journal, 29 June 1979, 436
[7] Ibid *R* v *Secretary of State for Social Services ex parte Hincks and Others*, Solicitors' Journal, 29 June 1979, 436
[8] *R* v *Central Birmingham HA ex p Walker* (1987) 3 BMLR 32
[9] *R* v *Cambridge Health Authority ex parte B (A Minor)* (1995) 23 BMLR 1 CA; [1995] 2 All ER 129
[10] *R* v *North Derbyshire Health Authority* [1997] 8 Med LR 327
[11] NHS Executive Letter, EL (95)97
[12] *R (on the application of Rogers)* v *Swindon NHS Primary Care Trust and Another* [2006] EWCA Civ 392
[13] *R (on the application of Otley)* v *Barking and Dagenham NHS Primary Care Trust* [2007] EWHC 1927
[14] *Eisai Ltd v National Institute for Health and Clinical Excellence (Alzheimer's Society and Shire Pharmaceuticals Ltd Interested parties)* [2007] EWHC 1941

[15] *North West Lancashire Health Authority* v *A, D and G* [1999] Lloyd's Rep Med; (1999) 2 CCL Rep 419; [2000] 1 WLR 977
[16] Sam Lister, 'Traffic light' rationing in NHS trusts forces more to go private, *The Times*, 13 November 2010
[17] King's Fund, A new settlement for health and social care: interim report April 2014; www.kingsfund.org.uk
[18] R (*on the application of Condliff*) v *North Staffordshire Primary Care Trust* [2011] EWCA 910
[19] www.gov.uk
[20] *R* v *North Derbyshire Health Authority* [1997] 8 Med LR 327
[21] *R* v *Secretary of State for Health ex p Pfizer Ltd* [1999] 3 CMLR 875; Lloyd's Rep Med 289
[22] The National Health Service and Public Health (Functions and Miscellaneous Provisions) Regulations 2013 SI 2013/261
[23] Ibid
[24] National Health Service (Procurement, Patient Choice and Competition) Regulations 2013 SI 2013/257; and No 2 SI 2013/497
[25] www.nhs.uk
[26] Charlie Cooper, GPs appeal to patients for help to stop funding cuts, *The Independent,* 29 May 2014
[27] National Health Service (Procurement, Patient Choice and Competition) Regulations 2013 SI 2013/257
[28] https://improvement.nhs.uk
[29] National Health Service (Approval of Licensing Criteria) Order 2013 No 2960
[30] National Health Service Trust Development Authority Regulations 2012 SI 2012/922
[31] National Health Service Trust Development Authority (Establishment and Constitution) Order 2012 SI 2012/901
[32] Ibid., 2013 SI 2013/260
[33] https://improvement.nhs.uk/improvement-hub
[34] Sir Roy Griffiths, Community Care: agenda for action, HMSO, 1988; followed by Command Paper 849, Caring for People: community care in the next decade and beyond, HMSO, November 1989
[35] Department of Health, The NHS Plan: a plan for investment, a plan for reform, Cm 4818-1, Stationery Office, London, July 2000
[36] The NHS Bodies and Local Authorities (Partnership Arrangements, Care Trusts, Public Health and Local Healthwatch) Regulations 2012 SI 2012/3094
[37] www.nhs.uk/servicedirectories/pages/nhstrustlisting.aspx
[38] Department of Health, A First Class Service: quality in the new NHS, DH, 1998
[39] Care Quality Commission (Membership) Regulations 2008 SI 2008/2252
[40] Care Quality Commission (Registration) Regulations 2009 SI 2009/3112
[41] Care Quality Commission (Additional Function) Regulations 2009 SI 2009/410
[42] Care Quality Commission (Reviews and Performance Assessments) Regulations 2014 SI 2014/1788
[43] Care Quality Commission, Supporting briefing note: issues highlighted by the 2009 survey of patients in NHS hospitals in England, CQC, 2010
[44] David Rose, Care homes with no qualified manager face closure, The Times, 8 October 2010
[45] News item, The Times, 20 November 2010
[46] Care Quality Commission, Review of the involvement and action taken by health bodies in relation to the care of Baby P, CQC, 2009
[47] Care Quality Commission, Investigation into the mental health care for older people provided by the Devon Partnership NHS Trust, CQC, 2010

[48] Chris Smyth, Hospital lied to authorities over waiting times for cancer care, The Times, 6 November 2013
[49] www.cqc.org.uk/publications/major-report/state-care
[50] National Institute for Clinical Excellence (Establishment and Constitution) Regulations SI 1999/220; amendments SI 2002/1759 and 2002/1760
[51] National Institute for Health and Care Excellence (Constitution and Functions) and the Health and Social Care Information Centre (Functions) Regulations 2013 SI 2013/259
[52] Chris Smyth, Anger as latest breast cancer treatment is blocked, The Times, 8 August 2014
[53] www.nice.org.uk/news/article/kadcyla-new-deal-for-breast-cancer-patients-given-green-light-in-final-draft-guidance
[54] Chris Smyth, IVF restricted to cancer patients and HIV men, The Times, 23 July 2014
[55] News item, The Times, 23 July 2014
[56] Chris Smyth, Rush for statins 'will clog up GPs with worried well', The Times, 19 July 2014
[57] www. nhs.uk
[58] K Thirwell, E Kinsella, A Mullen, The Airedale Inquiry Report to the Yorkshire and Humber Strategic Health Authority, 2010
[59] Clothier Report, The Allitt Inquiry: an independent inquiry relating to deaths and injuries on the children's ward at Grantham and Kesteven General Hospital during the period February to April 1991, HMSO, London, 1994
[60] Alan Glasper, The Care Quality Commission: criteria for assessing NHS trusts, British Journal of Nursing, 19(5):280–1, 2010
[61] Shipman Inquiry First Report: Death Disguised, 19 July 2002; webarchive.nationalarchives.gov.uk
[62] Shipman Inquiry Second Report: The Police Investigation of March 1998, 14 July 2003
[63] Shipman Inquiry Third Report: Death and Cremation Certification, 14 July 2003
[64] Shipman Inquiry Fourth Report: The Regulation of Controlled Drugs in the Community, Cm 6249, 15 July 2004, The Stationery Office
[65] Shipman Inquiry Fifth Report: Safeguarding Patients: Lessons from the Past – Proposals for the Future, Command Paper Cm 6394, December 2004, Stationery Office
[66] Shipman Inquiry Sixth Report: Shipman: The Final Report, January 2005, Stationery Office
[67] Jean Ritchie, Inquiry into quality and practice within the NHS arising from the actions of Rodney Ledward, DH, 2000
[68] News item, The Times, 4 November 2003
[69] Gosport Independent Panel (2018) Gosport War Memorial Hospital, Report of the Gosport Independent Panel; retrieved from www.gosportpanel.independent.gov.uk
[70] www.gosportpanel.independent.gov.uk
[71] David Rose, Nurses face disciplinary action over NHS scandal, The Times, 19 June 2010
[72] Report of the Mid Staffordshire NHS Foundation Trust Public Inquiry, HC 947 February 2013, Stationery Office; www.midstaffspublicinquiry.com
[73] www.midstaffsublicinquiry.com
[74] R. Mason (2013) NHS staff could be prosecuted for wilful neglect or manslaughter, says Francis retrieved from The Telegraph, 12 February www.telegraph.co.uk/news/politics/9865105/NHS-staff-could-be-prosecuted-for-wilful-neglect-or-manslaughter-says-Francis.html
[75] J. Andrews and M. Butler (2014) Trusted to Care An independent Review of the Princess of Wales Hospital and Neath Port Talbot Hospital at Abertawe Bro Morgannwg University Health Board Stirling: University of Stirling

[76] J. McCarthy (2015) Police: more staff failing in duty, *Wales on Sunday*, 8 March
[77] Barnett (2015) Cruel hospital worker stuffed wet wipe into dementia sufferer's mouth to stop her screams *Daily Express*
[78] Griffith R. (2013) *Extending the scope of wilful neglect will result in paternalistic nursing care*. Br J Nurs; 22(20):1190–1.
[79] Department of Health, High Quality of Care for All, Cm 7432, 2008, DH, London
[80] Available on the DH website with supporting documents; www.dh.gov.uk
[81] National Health Service (Revision of NHS Constitution Principles) Regulations 2013 SI 2013/317
[82] Sam Lister, NHS hospital to be run by private company, *The Times*, 18 February 2010
[83] www.parliament.uk/business/committees/committees-a-z/commons-select/public-accounts-committee/news/report-circle-withdrawal-from-hinchingbrooke-hospital
[84] https://assets.publishing.service.gov.uk/government/uploads/system/uploads/attachment_data/file/655585/ICR_guidance_2017_2018.pdf
[85] King's Fund, A new settlement for health and social care: interim report, April 2014; www.kingsfund.org.uk

Chapter 6

Progress of a Civil Claim: Defences and Compensation

This chapter discusses

- Civil proceedings
- Compensation in civil proceedings for negligence
- Defences to a civil action
- Clinical Negligence Scheme for Trusts (CNST) and the NHS Litigation Authority (NHSLA)
- NHS Redress Act 2006
- Reforms to civil litigation

Introduction

This chapter considers the likely course that any civil case against a nurse and/or NHS trust might follow, the ways in which compensation in the civil courts is assessed and the defences that may be available. It takes into account the major reforms in civil procedure which came into effect in April 1999, following the Report on Access to Justice by Lord Woolf[1] and the more recent changes.

Civil proceedings

Two Issues

In any civil case there are two separate issues:

1. Is the defendant liable?
2. How much compensation is payable?

It is sometimes possible that one of these issues has been agreed, e.g. the defendant accepts liability, but disagrees with the amount of compensation (known as quantum) claimed by the victim, or that the amount of compensation that would be payable is agreed, but the defendant refuses to accept liability for that sum. Sometimes both issues are disputed. Evidence will therefore be required on both issues. The elements to establish liability and the kinds of harm for which compensation is payable are discussed in chapter 3. In some cases a defendant may be prepared to pay compensation without admitting liability. This is known as an *ex gratia* payment and is considered below.

A nurse is first likely to be asked by management to provide a statement on the events. Care should be taken in the completion of this and guidelines are given in chapter 9. If the victim has sought advice and has decided to commence an action, the next stages are set out below. The High Court hears claims exceeding £50,000. Claims below that amount are heard in the county court and follow different tracks. Claims up to £10,000 are dealt with in the small claims branch. Claims between £10,000 and £25,000 are heard in the fast track branch and those between £25,000 and £50,000 are heard in the multi-track branch of the county court (see chapter 1 for civil courts).

Mediation

One of the results of the Woolf reforms in civil justice is that the parties are encouraged to resolve the dispute before going to court using mediation or other forms of resolution, such as **alternative dispute resolution**. Often such processes can be linked with the complaints procedure (see chapter 26) to avoid litigation. In mediation, an independent mediator attempts to assist the parties to reach an agreement to resolve the dispute. Unlike arbitration, the parties are under no compulsion to accept any ruling by the independent person. Changes to legal aid recommended by the Justice Secretary announced in November 2010 included the removal of legal aid for most clinical negligence claims and also the encouragement for mediation to resolve issues. Legal aid changes were implemented from 1 April 2013.

Case Management

The overriding principle enshrined in the Civil Procedure Rules[2] (see Box 6.1) is that all cases should be dealt with justly. The court must seek to give effect to this overriding principle when it exercises any powers under the rules and when it interprets any rule. The parties also have a duty to help the court to further this overriding objective. The court, in furthering this principle of dealing with cases justly, must actively manage the cases. Active management includes:

1. Encouraging the parties to cooperate with each other in the conduct of the proceedings.
2. Identifying the issues at an early stage.
3. Deciding promptly which issues need full investigation and trial and accordingly disposing summarily of the others.
4. Deciding the order in which the issues are to be resolved.
5. Encouraging the parties to use an alternative dispute resolution procedure if the court considers that appropriate, and facilitating the use of such procedure.
6. Helping the parties to settle the whole or part of the case.
7. Fixing timetables or otherwise controlling the progress of the case.
8. Considering whether the likely benefits of taking a particular step justify the cost of taking it.

9. Dealing with as many aspects of the case as it can on the same occasion.
10. Dealing with the case without the parties needing to attend court.
11. Making use of technology.
12. Giving directions to ensure that the trial of a case proceeds quickly and efficiently.

> ### Box 6.1 The Civil Procedure Rules
>
> The Civil Procedure Rules are a procedural code with the overriding objective of enabling the court to deal with cases justly. They are available online.[3]
>
> Dealing with a case justly includes, so far as is practicable:
>
> 1. Ensuring that the parties are on an equal footing.
> 2. Saving expense.
> 3. Dealing with the case in ways which are proportionate:
>   (a) to the amount of money involved;
>   (b) to the importance of the case;
>   (c) to the complexity of the issues; and
>   (d) to the financial position of each party.
> 4. Ensuring that it is dealt with expeditiously and fairly.
> 5. Allotting to it an appropriate share of the court's resources, while taking into account the need to allot resources to other cases.

A prime mechanism for judicially-led case management is the introduction of three tracks:

1. Small claims track
2. Fast track
3. Multi-track.

The court allocates each case to one of these three tracks on the basis of information provided by the claimant on the statement of the case. If it does not have enough information to allocate the claim then it will make an order requiring one or more parties to provide further information within 14 days.

Small Claims Track (CPR Part 27)

This provides a procedure for straightforward claims that do not exceed £10,000, without the need for substantial pre-hearing preparation and the formalities of a traditional trial and where costs are kept low.

Fast Track (CPR Part 28)

Factors deciding whether a case is allocated to the fast track include: the limits likely to be placed on disclosure; the extent to which expert evidence may be necessary; and whether the trial will last longer than a day. Case management directions will be given at the allocation stage or at the listing stage.

Multi-Track (CPR Part 29)

Other cases may be allocated to be dealt with on a multi-track basis and dealt with at a civil trial centre.

Pre-Action Protocol

Lord Woolf found that one of the major sources of increased costs and delay in clinical negligence litigation is at the pre-litigation stage and he therefore recommended the development and introduction of a **pre-action protocol**. A draft protocol was drawn up in 1997 by the Clinical Disputes Forum and was formally launched on 23 July 1998.[4] The protocol sets a standard of good practice with emphasis on better handling of potential disputes and more effective and efficient management of information and investigation. It also sets out the steps to be followed where litigation is in prospect.

Summary Judgment or Other Early Termination

Part of the court's duty of active case management is the summary disposal of issues that do not need full investigation and trial. The court can strike out a statement of case or give a **summary judgment** where either claimant or defendant has no reasonable prospect of success.

Disclosure and Inspection of Documents

A party discloses a document by stating that the document exists or has existed. Rules relating to the disclosure and inspection of documents are to be found in Part 31 of the Civil Procedure Rules. There are rules relating to standard disclosure that list the documents that are to be disclosed. These include:

1. the documents on which the party relies;
2. the documents that adversely affect his own case or another party's case or support another party's case;
3. the documents that he is required to disclose by a relevant practice direction.

A party is required to make a reasonable search for any relevant documents. Some documents are obtainable before a case begins under the Supreme Court Act 1981 section 33. The nurse may well not be aware of this activity unless they are being personally sued or unless good communication ensures that they are kept in the picture. In *Harris* v *Newcastle HA* [1989] 2 All ER 273, the court allowed pre-trial disclosure of records relating to events 26 years before, even though the health authority intended to plead that the case was out of time. The emphasis now is on full disclosure by each party to ensure that the case can be dealt with as promptly as possible.

Claim Form is Issued

This marks the beginning of the case. There are important time limits (discussed below) within which the claim form (originally known as a writ) is issued. The claim form indicates that action is now being commenced. It is preceded by what is known as a letter before action, i.e. a warning by the claimant (usually the claimant's solicitor) that if there is no acceptance of the claim, then the legal action will commence. The claim form usually names the NHS trust as the defendant, but it is possible for an individual employee to be named as a party and more than one defendant can be named.

Service of Claim Form (CPR Part 7)

This must be sent to the defendant within four months of its issue. (In the past there was a requirement for personal service, i.e. the claim form had to be handed to the defendant personally. Now, however, the claim form is sent to a known address or sent by fax or electronic methods under Rule 7.5.) The defendant must then respond by filing a defence or an admission or filing an acknowledgement of service. If the defendant fails to respond, the claimant may be able to obtain judgment in default.

The drafting of the documents or statements of case (these were once known as pleadings) is arranged by the respective parties' solicitors, who often instruct counsel (i.e. barristers). A litigant may, however, represent themselves personally. Strict time limits are laid down for the service and response to the documents. Under the Woolf reforms, the documents exchanged between the parties should be simpler and be verified by the parties. If there are uncertainties, the court can require the parties to clarify any matter in dispute.

Pre-trial Review

Eventually, there will be an assessment of the situation by the parties, together with a registrar or judge, account taken of the number of witnesses to attend, exchange of any experts' medical reports and, finally, the case will be set down for hearing.

Payment into Court

Rules about offers to settle and **payments into court** are set out in Parts 36 and 37 of the Civil Procedure Rules. In some cases where there is dispute over the amount of compensation, but liability is accepted, the defendant will probably be advised to pay a sum in settlement of the case into court. If the claimant accepts this payment in, then the defendant will be liable for the claimant's costs up to that point. The court will be notified that there has been a settlement of the case. A payment in may also be made where the defendant does not accept liability, but they are not confident of winning the case and rather than risk losing and having to pay the costs of both sides they offer a sum in full and final settlement.

If the claimant decides that the payment in is not acceptable, the case will continue. In these circumstances, the judge is not told that there has been a payment in. He or she will not therefore be influenced by that in determining the case and deciding what compensation to award. If they award less than the payment in or if they decide there is no liability by the defendant, then the claimant will have to pay both the defendant's costs from the time of the payment in as well as their own, since, of course, had the claimant accepted that sum deemed reasonable in comparison with the judge's award, there would have been no time-consuming and costly court hearing. These costs may well exceed the amount of the award. The judge has a discretion over whether to award the defendant the costs in these circumstances. An example of a refusal to accept a reasonable offer and becoming liable for the costs of a defendant is a case brought by a tourism student who sued his college for not warning him of leeches on a barefoot walk through a jungle. He was awarded £4795,[5] however the college's insurers covered the cost of defending the case. The student was left £11,000 out of pocket, with Judge William Gaskell QC only awarding 40 per cent of his costs for the student failing to seriously negotiate a settlement.[6]

The hearing

Claimant's Case

Examination in chief

This is when questions are put to the witness by the party that has called him or her to give evidence.

The claimant has the burden of establishing to the satisfaction of the judge, on a **balance of probabilities**, that there has been negligence or some other alleged civil wrong. The claimant will therefore be asked to give evidence first.

His or her witnesses will be sworn in, in turn, and will then give evidence under examination of the claimant's legal representative. This has, in the past, usually been a barrister (counsel), instructed by the solicitor; however, increasingly solicitors are taking on an advocacy role. Sometimes the claimant appears personally. This initial questioning is known as **examination in chief**. The witness cannot be asked leading questions when being examined in chief. Counsel will have before them the proof of the witness statements to the solicitor and will take him or her through this to bring their evidence to the court.

Expert evidence

Expert evidence from witnesses may be required on the nature of the standard of care that should have been provided or on the amount of compensation payable. The new Civil Procedure Rules have led to major changes in the giving of expert evidence and these are discussed in chapter 9.

Cross-examination

Counsel for the defence is then able to question the witness, i.e. cross-examine. Here the task is to discredit the evidence by showing that it is irrelevant, unreliable or for some other reason is of no weight against the defendant. Alternatively, the witness can be used to support the case of the other side. Leading questions are allowed when the witness is under cross-examination. The judge will, however, intervene to protect the witness from harassment. (See chapter 9 on giving evidence in court.) At this stage, the judge may wish to question the witness to clarify points on which he or she is not certain.

Re-examination

Finally, the side calling that witness has the chance of repairing any damage that the cross-examination has inflicted, but the re-examination is confined to points that have arisen during cross-examination or under questioning by the judge. All the claimant's witnesses give evidence in this way.

When the case for the claimant has ended, the judge has the opportunity of ending the case at this point and of finding against the claimant on the grounds that he or she has not established a *prima facie* case and therefore the defence is not required to give evidence. The judge cannot, of course, decide at this point against the defendant because the defence has not as yet given evidence.

Defendant's Case

If the case proceeds, the defence must put forward its witnesses who are examined in chief, cross-examined and then re-examined as previously described. If it is alleged that the nurse has been negligent, they will be called as a witness for the defence. Several years may have elapsed since the events and their recall may be limited or even nil. The nurse is able to refresh their memory by referring to contemporaneous records and therefore they should refer to the case notes. In this situation, the nurse will appreciate the value of detailed, accurate, clear information on those events. Counsel who examines the nurse in chief will have a copy of statements they have previously given. The nurse should ensure that they had help in making this statement and prior to the court hearing they should be instructed on the procedure to be followed and some of the pitfalls they may encounter. Most of those who have appeared in court describe the event as particularly harrowing, and preparation is essential. (Giving evidence in court is discussed further in chapter 9.)

Judge's Summing Up

After summaries by counsel, the judge then has the task of making his or her judgment. This may be reserved, i.e. the parties are notified that they will be informed of the outcome, or it might be given immediately. The judge will determine both liability and damages (whichever are in dispute). The party having to pay costs will usually depend on the outcome, i.e. the loser pays the costs of both sides. There is no jury in a civil case (except in defamation cases, if the judge directs).

Res IPSA Loquitur

In certain cases, inferences can be made from the facts about the existence of negligence.[7] If the claimant can establish that it is a *res ipsa loquitur* situation ('the matter speaks for itself'), then the defendant can be asked to show how the incident occurred without negligence on their part. The claimant would have to show the following factors to raise a presumption of *res ipsa loquitur*:

1. What has occurred would not normally occur if reasonable care were taken.
2. The events were under the control or management of the defendant.
3. The defendant has not offered any reasonable explanation for what occurred.

The most obvious example is leaving a swab inside a patient or amputating the wrong limb. The doctrine was applied when a patient went into hospital with two stiff fingers and was discharged with four stiff fingers: he was entitled to receive an explanation from the hospital as to how this could have happened without negligence on its part.[8] This procedure gives the claimant a technical advantage that is very necessary when he is ignorant of the actual events that caused harm. If the defendant fails to give a reasonable explanation of the events, the court can draw the inference that there was negligence. In a case brought against Tesco by a woman who slipped on some yoghurt that had been spilt on the floor, the doctrine was applied and Tesco found liable.[9] In medical negligence cases the effect of *res ipsa loquitur* is to enable the claimant to force the defendant to respond at peril of having a finding of negligence made against them.[10]

A surgeon who had been found negligent in carrying out a gall bladder operation appealed on the grounds that the judge should not have disapplied the *res ipsa loquitur* principle failed in his appeal. The Court of Appeal held that the judge had correctly addressed the issue as to whether negligence had been proved in the circumstances. The award of £92,391 damages was not unreasonable.[11]

Compensation in civil proceedings for negligence

Nurses sometimes meet patients who are hesitant to undertake all the necessary physiotherapy and other rehabilitative work lest the compensation (known as quantum) will be reduced because they are seen to have made a full recovery. However, the powers of the court to make provisional awards or award interim amounts of compensation should make it easier for a claimant to focus on rehabilitation. There is also a duty on a claimant to mitigate or reduce their loss. In medical cases the test will be whether in all the circumstances and the medical advice given the claimant acted reasonably (for example, in refusing surgery).[12] The chance of a recommended remedial operation failing to rectify the claimant's condition has to be taken into account in determining compensation payable. In 2009 the NHS Litigation Authority applied to set aside an award in the case of *Michael Spence* v *Angela Naveda and Barking, Havering and Redbridge University Hospitals NHS Trust* of over £3 million paid to the claimant on the grounds that video evidence showed that he had not suffered such serious injuries as he claimed. A new figure of £300,500, of which the NHS trust was liable for £141,250, was agreed.[13]

An attempt to recover money already paid out was made by Bedford Hospital NHS Trust which had failed to detect fetal spina bifida. It had paid an interim sum of £705,000 with the final moneys due when the boy was 10, but he died aged 6 in 2011. The trust claimed back £330,000 paid for his care. The mother had bought a four-bedroomed house adapted to his needs, which solicitors advised her to sell in order to repay the trust.[14]

A patient whose cancer was not diagnosed received £300,000 in an out-of-court settlement after losing his tongue and vocal cords. He went to his GP with a lump in his throat and suggested it may be cancerous since he worked with chemicals, but cancer was not diagnosed until the following year.[15]

A £2.8 million lump sum plus £383,000 a year until the victim was 19 when it would rise to £424,000 a year was paid by Great Ormond Street Hospital for Children to Maisha Najeeb whose brain was injected by glue. She was being treated for a brain condition where arteries and veins had been disentangled. There was no system in place to distinguish between two syringes: one with glue to block off bleeding blood vessels, and one with a harmless dye to monitor the flow of blood around the brain and head. As a result of the error, glue was wrongly injected into the artery causing catastrophic and permanent brain damage. She needed 24-hour care.[16]

How do you quantify compensation for a person who is wrongly told that they have a terminal illness? Denise Clark, aged 34, was told that she had terminal cancer, arranged her funeral and was then told the diagnosis was wrong. NHS Grampian is reported to have settled her case for a large five-figure sum.[17]

Practical Dilemma 6.1 — Leslie's Leg

Leslie was travelling on his motorbike when a car started to overtake him. Unfortunately, a lorry was coming in the opposite direction and the vehicle pulled in to the side, knocking Leslie off. Leslie was admitted to the orthopaedic ward from A&E. He suffered a serious compound fracture. The prognosis was that he was unlikely to make a complete recovery and could anticipate further problems with the leg, a slight limp and a vulnerability to arthritis later on. He had been advised not to expect to return to his existing job (a PE instructor) for at least nine months. How will his likely compensation be calculated?

Ian Knauer was awarded £642,972, the bulk of it for lost services, following the death of his wife as a result of exposure to asbestos while employed at HM Prison Guys Marsh Dorset. The Ministry had admitted liability but disputed the amount of compensation.[18]

Special Damages

Leslie will first be entitled to receive special damages. These are amounts to cover specific losses that have already been suffered and where the amount can therefore be accurately stated. For example, the loss and damage to his motorbike, damage to his clothing, loss of wages up to the present day. Interest is allowed on the items.

General Damages

The headings under which such damages are calculated are shown in Box 6.2.

Box 6.2 Types of damages

1. Special damages: expenses and losses to the date of judgment.
2. General damages:
    a. *non-pecuniary loss:*
        pain and suffering
        loss of amenity
    b. *pecuniary loss:*
        loss of earnings
        loss of earning capacity
        cost of future care and expenses
        interest.

Non-pecuniary loss (i.e. non-financial loss)

1. *Pain and suffering*: this is to cover the pain from the injury itself, as well as from any consequential medical treatment and worry about the effects of the injury on the patient's lifestyle. It could also include damages for the mental suffering resulting from the fact that the person's life has been shortened. (Administration of Justice Act 1982 section 1(1)(a) introduced this form of compensation since there is no longer any compensation for the actual shortening of life itself. This used to be known as 'loss of expectation of life' and was abolished by this Act.)
2. *Loss of amenity*: Leslie will be able to recover additional compensation if it is established that his activities will be restricted because of the injuries to his leg. Clearly, if his leg had to be amputated, then he would recover an additional sum for that loss.

These non-pecuniary losses are notoriously difficult to calculate. How can money ever be an adequate compensation for blindness or loss of the ability to have children or to enjoy normal activities? The answer is that it cannot. However, since there is no other form of compensation, the non-pecuniary loss has to be converted into pecuniary form. Judges follow precedents in calculating the awards. They examine decisions in preceding cases, taking into account any relevant differences between the present case and the earlier cases and allowing for inflation. A judge's award is subject to appeal.

Pecuniary loss

1. *Loss of earnings*: Leslie's loss of future earnings would be calculated by determining his net annual loss multiplied by a figure to cover the number of years the disability will last. The figure takes into account the fact that the compensation will be paid out all at once rather than each week or month over the next few years. (Structured payments are now being introduced.)
2. *Loss of earning capacity*: because of his injury Leslie may never be able to work as a PE instructor again. Alternatively, he may retain his job initially, but with the risk that if he loses it he might never get similar paid work again because of his disability. He is entitled to be compensated for this risk.
3. *Expenses*: Leslie would also be entitled to recover reasonable expenses in getting to and from hospital, medical and similar expenses (e.g. physiotherapy) and, in some circumstances, domestic help. This may also include the costs of hospice care.[19]
4. *Interest*: interest is payable on the pecuniary loss already suffered and on the non-pecuniary loss.
5. *Deductions*: deductions are made in respect of the value of certain social security benefits, which are paid to the compensation recovery unit.

Interim payments can be made by the court under the Rules of the Supreme Court. The claimant can apply for an interim payment at any time after the claim form has been served on the defendant. Thus, where the defendant has admitted liability, but disputes the amount of damages payable, the court could make an order for an interim payment to be made. Because of the uncertainty of prognosis, there is the power for an order of provisional damages for personal injuries to be made if there is a chance that at some time in the future the injured person will, as a result of the act or omission, develop some serious disease or suffer some serious deterioration in his physical or mental condition (Supreme Court Act 1981 section 32A). Provisional damages in relation to exposure to asbestos were awarded in one case.[20] Where large settlements are to be paid, parties often agree a structured settlement whereby an annuity is purchased with part of the lump sum, thus providing an income to the claimant for life.

> **Case 6.1** S (a child) v Royal Bournemouth and Christchurch Hospital NHS Trust [2012]

Brain damage at birth[21]

The boy was aged 14 at the date of the child settlement approval hearing. He had sustained severe brain injury during delivery resulting in his being diagnosed with severe four-limb athetoid cerebral palsy. His multiple difficulties led to his being highly dependent on others for his care needs. In particular he was unable to walk or stand independently, unable to care for his own hygiene and could not feed himself. He would never be able to achieve independence or undertake gainful employment. He was predicted to live for a further 40 years.

Past losses:	including sums for gratuitous care, accommodation, and aids and appliances	£273,227
Future losses:	Loss of earnings	£437,797
	Physiotherapy	£67,000
	Occupational therapy	£40,440
	Speech therapy	£150,000
	Assistive technology	£200,000
	Holiday expenses	£133,045
General damages for pain suffering and loss of amenity:		£230,000
Total damages on capitalised basis:		£7,102,012
Periodical payments:		£60,318 for two years
		£77,618 for three years
		£180,000 p.a. for life

Periodical payments based on a whole life multiplier of 25.42.

In December 2003 £5.75 million in agreed damages was awarded to Matthew King, then aged 8, who had been starved of oxygen at birth and suffered from cerebral palsy. South Kent Hospitals NHS Trust admitted liability for his injuries, but the valuation of his claim had been deferred so that his needs could be assessed.[22] In January 2004 Oliver Davies, then 8 years old, received £3.4 million damages for oxygen starvation at birth which led to acute cerebral palsy. Oxford Radcliffe Hospitals NHS Trust admitted liability. There had been an inexcusable delay in arranging an emergency delivery.[23]

Where there has been a failure to diagnose a terminal condition such as cancer, damages can be awarded for the loss of a chance of successful treatment being given, but it may be difficult for the claimant to establish, on a balance of probabilities, that it was more probable than not that the outcome would have been materially different had the diagnosis been made earlier[24] (see chapter 3 and causation).

Calculating Amount of Compensation

The House of Lords ruled that in awarding compensation, victims should not be expected to speculate on the stock market and therefore lower levels of return based on index-linked government securities can be used as the basis of calculation. The effect of this ruling was to increase the capital amount awarded to victims. In the case itself, James Thomas, a cerebral palsy victim as a result of negligence at birth, was awarded £1,285,000 by the High Court judge, but this was reduced by the Court of Appeal by £300,000 on the basis that the capital could be invested in higher return (but more risky) equities. The House of Lords restored the original amount.[25] Subsequently the Lord Chancellor issued a statement[26] which recognised that the use of index-linked government stock as the basis for calculation was appropriate, even though the Court of Protection invested client funds partly in equities. Courts were able to adopt a different rate if there were exceptional circumstances under section 1(2) of the Damages Act 1996.

The Law Commission recommended changes to the present system relating to the quantifying of damages for personal injury[27] in 1996 and suggested, among other recommendations, that the NHS should be able to recover the costs arising from the treatment of road traffic and other accident victims. It is estimated that this would bring in £120 million to the NHS. A later report by the Law Commission[28] in 1999 recommended that compensation for non-pecuniary loss (e.g. pain, suffering and loss of amenity) should be increased and this could be implemented through the courts' decisions on damages. The Court of Appeal gave judgment in March 2000[29] and decided that a modest increase was required to bring some awards up to a figure that was fair, reasonable and just. It recommended that damages for claims above £10,000 should be raised by a maximum of about 35 per cent with increases tapering downwards. The Court of Appeal acknowledged that the life expectancy for many seriously injured claimants has increased and they can now survive for many years. In 2012 the Court of Appeal announced an increase in general damages by 10 per cent in accordance with the recommendations of the Jackson final report on civil litigation costs.[30] The Court of Appeal has the responsibility of monitoring and where appropriate altering the guideline rates for general damages in personal injury cases. The continuity of future periodic payments as a result of the possible failure of the NHS foundation was questioned in one case. The judge held that the continuity was reasonably secured because arrangements had been agreed whereby the NHS Litigation Authority was the source of the payments and was therefore legally responsible for the payments.[31]

The principles of determining the compensation payable when a child is born following a failed sterilisation or a failure to advise a woman that the foetus is suffering from disabilities (and therefore the possibility of a termination not being discussed) are considered in chapter 14.

Defences to a civil action

A considerable number of claims that are brought against NHS trusts and health authorities are dropped before they reach a final outcome, and many of those that survive to the end are unsuccessful. They may fail because on investigation there are no grounds for negligence or some of the other defences succeed. This section looks at the defences open to a nurse or her employer in civil actions for negligence.

Denial of Facts

It often happens that, when things go wrong, it is one person's word against another. The patient might complain that the nurse has been negligent, but the nurse might be able to show that the events were not as the patient describes. Many court cases are simply disputes over facts. Where only two people are involved, with no other witnesses and no other circumstantial evidence, if such a case comes before the courts, the judge will have to decide, on the basis of the evidence in court and the way the parties stand up to cross-examination, which account of the events is acceptable. Records of what took place can be of considerable significance in determining the outcome of the hearing.

In civil cases, the burden is on the claimant to establish, on a balance of probabilities, that the defendant has been negligent.

A Missing Element

Even where the facts are not disputed, it might still be possible for an action for negligence to be defended on the grounds that one of the essential elements is missing. To succeed in a negligence case it is necessary for the claimant to establish that a duty of care was owed by the defendant, that the defendant was in breach of this duty and that this breach caused reasonably foreseeable harm to the claimant (see chapter 3). If one of these elements has not been established on a balance of probabilities, then the defendant will win the case.

Contributory Negligence

Practical Dilemma 6.2 — Walking aids

Fred, who has recently had an operation for a fractured leg, has been receiving help from the physiotherapist in walking with crutches. Fred asks a Health Care Assistant, who has only just come on to the ward, for help in going to the toilet. She is not aware that Fred has been told not to try to walk yet unless he is accompanied by a qualified person. She assists him out of bed and on to the crutches. As she does so, the crutches slip from under Fred and he falls to the ground, sustaining another fracture.

In this situation, the Health Care Assistant or the ward management are clearly at fault in allowing Fred out of bed in these circumstances. However, Fred is also at fault. He should have followed the advice provided. Fred's responsibility for the harm that has occurred depends to a large extent on his level of understanding, how clear the advice provided to him was and how reasonable it was to expect him to have waited for experienced help in using the crutches. If he were to sue the NHS trust and its staff, they may well defend themselves on the grounds that he was partly at fault in not taking care of himself. This defence is known as a defence of contributory negligence. The defendant is saying to the claimant: 'You failed to take care of yourself and that has led to or increased the harm that you have suffered.' If the judge is satisfied that the defendant has succeeded in this defence, he or she is able to reduce the compensation by the extent to which they consider the claimant's fault has contributed to the harm. The wording of section 1 of the Law Reform (Contributory Negligence) Act 1945 is shown in the following Statute Box 6.1.

Statute 6.1
Law Reform (Contributory Negligence) Act 1945 Section 1

1. **Apportionment of liability in case of contributory negligence**

1. Where any person suffers damage as the result partly of his own fault and partly of any other person or persons a claim in respect of that damage shall not be defeated by reason of the fault of the person suffering the damage, but the damages recoverable in respect thereof shall be reduced to such an extent as the court thinks just and equitable having regard to the claimant's share in responsibility for the damage.

The trial judge decided that failure to wear a seatbelt was not contributory negligence. The defendant appealed to the Court of Appeal and won his appeal. Lord Denning emphasised that where the damage to the claimant would not have been reduced by failure to wear the seatbelt, then there should be no reduction of compensation, but where, as here, the injuries would have been reduced by wearing a seatbelt, there should be a reduction of compensation. In Mr Froom's case, the injuries to the head and chest would have been prevented by wearing a seatbelt. His finger would have been broken anyway and therefore there was no reduction on that account. The overall deduction of compensation for Mr Froom's contributory negligence was held to be 20 per cent. (This case was heard before the wearing of front seatbelts was compulsory.)

Case 6.2 *Froom* v *Butcher* [1975]

No seatbelt[32]

Mr Froom was driving his car carefully at a speed of 30–35 mph with his wife sitting beside him and his daughter in the back seat. The front seats were fitted with seatbelts, but neither Mr nor Mrs Froom was wearing one. Unfortunately, Mr Froom's car was struck head-on by a car travelling at speed in the opposite direction and on the wrong side of the road as it had pulled out to overtake a line of traffic.

Reductions of compensation on grounds of contributory negligence can vary from 95 per cent to 5 per cent. When it is larger, then there is held to be no liability on the part of the defendant; when it is smaller it is considered to be too insignificant to count. To succeed, the defendant has to establish that the claimant failed to take reasonable care of themselves and that this failure contributed to the harm they suffered, or increased it. In the case of *Badger* v *The Home Office*[33] the deceased was employed by the defendants as a boiler maker and it was established that he had been exposed to asbestos. However, he was also a smoker and that had contributed to his death by lung cancer. The compensation awarded to his widow was reduced by 20 per cent because a reasonably prudent man would have stopped smoking.

Contributory Negligence and Children

Lord Denning has said:

> A very young child cannot be guilty of contributory negligence. An older child may be; but it depends on the circumstances. A judge should only find a child guilty of contributory negligence if he or she is of such an age as reasonably to be expected to take precautions for his or her own safety: and then he or she is only to be found guilty if blame should be attached to him or her.

In the same case, Lord Justice Salmon said:

> The question as to whether the plaintiff can be said to have been guilty of contributory negligence depends on whether any ordinary child of 13½ years could be expected to have done any more than this child did. I say 'any ordinary child'. I do not mean a paragon of prudence; nor do I mean a scatter-brain child; but the ordinary girl of 13½ [the age of the child in that case].[34]

Willing Assumption of Risk (Volenti non fit Injuria)

Sometimes, where there is a known risk, the possibility of this taking place is accepted and the defendant is not liable. The most obvious example is dangerous sports where both players and spectators are at some risk. If that risk occurs, it is assumed that there will be no court action, but that the risk has been willingly accepted (known as **volenti non fit injuria**). For example, in a rugby match it is possible that a player may be seriously injured, even though no rules have been broken and there is no criminal act. This is a risk of the game and is accepted by the players. If, of course, the rules have been broken and thus resulted in injuries, then the injured player may well have an action for assault.

In the health service context, the agreement by the patient that treatment can proceed counts not only as consent to what would otherwise constitute a trespass to the person, but it is also an acceptance of the possibility that those hazards that are an inextricable risk of that particular treatment could occur. Consent, however, does not imply consent to the risk that the professional will be negligent (see chapter 7 on consent).

Practical Dilemma 6.3   Blood donor

Rachel had been giving blood for many years. She was summoned on one occasion to the session. As the needle was inserted and the cannula put in place, she felt an appalling pain. She shrieked and the needle was quickly withdrawn and a new painless site was found. After the session, Rachel found that it was very difficult to move her hand, arm and fingers. She was examined by a doctor who sent her for tests and eventually she was told that a very rare damage to the nerve had occurred. However, she was assured that with physiotherapy she would soon recover full function. Unfortunately, this did not prove to be true. She was eventually forced to take early retirement on the grounds of ill health and did not recover full arm or hand movement. She sought advice about suing the doctor and was given an expert's report that such a rare event could occur without any negligence on the part of the doctor, so that there was no point in suing either the doctor or the blood transfusion authority. However, Rachel argued that if she had known of the risk she would not have agreed to give blood unless she had been given an assurance that in the event of the risk taking place she would have received compensation.

As the law stands at present, unless Rachel can show negligence (either in carrying out the treatment or in failure to warn her of the risk of harm) by the professional staff or the employer, she would be unable to recover compensation in court. We do not have a system of no-fault liability. As a volunteer, she can be assumed to have accepted the possibility of those risks occurring, although she may well be able to show that there was a breach of the duty owed to her as a volunteer if certain risks were not pointed out to her. The Pearson Report on compensation for personal injuries recommended that there should be an acceptance of no-fault liability for volunteers in medical research. These recommendations have not been implemented in law (although pharmaceutical companies offer compensation on a no-fault liability basis to those who take part in drug trials (see chapter 27)) and it could be argued that if the recommendations are ever implemented they should be extended to cover such situations as donation of blood. In such situations, many NHS trusts would make an *ex gratia* payment, i.e. a payment without any acceptance or implication of liability on its part.

To establish a defence of willing assumption of risk, the defendant has to show that the claimant knew of the risk, willingly consented to run it and waived any right to sue for compensation. If it is successfully pleaded, it operates as a total defence.

Sometimes employers have tried to rely on this defence when sued by an employee for injuries at work. For example, it has been said that back injuries are an occupational hazard for nurses; all psychiatric nurses accept the risk of physical violence; central sterile supply department (CSSD) assistants are likely to suffer from 'sharp' injuries as an occupational hazard. However, it is quite clear that where there is a failure of the employer in his duty to care for the employee's safety, then the defence of willing assumption of risk will not prevail. (See chapter 12 on health and safety law.)

Exemption from Liability

NHS trust premises are a blaze of exemption notices: 'no responsibility is taken for cars parked in this area'; 'the "X" NHS trust accepts no liability for patients' property'. How effective are these notices if the NHS trust or its employees are negligent? Can a patient be persuaded to sign a form saying that they will not hold the 'X' NHS trust liable in any respect? Sometimes an NHS trust responds to a complaint by asking for a declaration that if the complaint is to be pursued and an investigation conducted, then the NHS trust requires an assurance that there will be no civil action. Can such a declaration be held against the person who signed? The answer to these questions is to a considerable extent given by reference to the Unfair Contract Terms Act 1977. This Act prevents anyone in the course of any business activity (and this covers professional, local and public authority activity) from exempting themselves from negligence if that negligence gives rise to personal injury or death. Any agreement, notice or clause to that effect is void (see Statute Box 6.2 below).

Statute 6.2
Sections from the Unfair Contract Terms Act 1977

1. Scope of Part I

1. For the purposes of this part of this Act, 'negligence' means the breach—

    (a) of any obligation, arising from the express or implied terms of a contract, to take reasonable care or exercise skill in the performance of the contract

    (b) of any common law duty to take reasonable care or exercise reasonable skill (but not stricter duty)

    (c) of the common duty of care imposed by the Occupiers' Liability Act 1957 or the Occupiers' Liability Act (Northern Ireland) 1957.

2. This part of this Act is subject to Part III; and in relation to contracts, the operation of Sections 2 to 4 and 7 is subject to the exceptions made by Schedule 1.

3. In the case of both contract and tort, Sections 2 to 7 apply (except where the contrary is stated in Section 6(4)) only to business liability, that is liability for breach of obligations or duties arising—
   (a) from things done or to be done by a person in the course of a business (whether his own business or another's), or
   (b) from the occupation of premises used for business purposes of the occupier; and references to liability are to be read accordingly. (Addendum added by Occupiers' Liability Act 1984 on liability of an occupier of premises for recreational or educational purposes not a business liability unless granting the person access falls within the business purposes of the occupier.)

4. In relation to any breach of duty or obligation, it is immaterial for any purpose of this part of this Act whether the breach was inadvertent or intentional, or whether liability for it arises directly or vicariously.

2. Negligence liability

1. A person cannot by reference to any contract term or to a notice given to persons generally or to particular persons exclude or restrict his liability for death or personal injury resulting from negligence.

2. In the case of other loss or damage, a person cannot so exclude or restrict his liability for negligence except insofar as the term or notice satisfies the requirement of reasonableness.

3. Where a contract term or notice purports to exclude or restrict liability for negligence a person's agreement to or awareness of it is not of itself to be taken as indicating his voluntary acceptance of any risk.

11. The 'reasonableness' test

1. In relation to a notice (not being a notice having contractual effect), the requirement of reasonableness under this Act is that it should be fair and reasonable to allow reliance on it, having regard to all the circumstances obtaining when the liability arose or (but for the notice) would have arisen.

2. Where by reference to a contract term or notice a person seeks to restrict liability to a specified sum of money, and the question arises (under this or any other Act) whether the term or notice satisfies the requirement of reasonableness, regard shall be had in particular (but **without prejudice** to subsection (2) above in the case of contract terms) to—
   (a) the resources which he could expect to be available to him for the purpose of meeting the liability should it arise, and
   (b) how far it was open to him to cover himself by insurance.

3. It is for those claiming that a contract term or notice satisfies the requirements of reasonableness to show that it does.

14. Interpretation of Part I

In this part of this Act: 'business' includes a profession and the activities of any government department or local or public authority.

> ### Practical Dilemma 6.4 — No liability
>
> A surgeon said: 'I am prepared to carry out upon you a very risky operation and I want you to sign that you will exempt me from all blame if anything goes wrong.' The patient, in his desire to have the operation, signed the form, but, unfortunately, the surgeon made a very careless error that no competent surgeon would have made, leaving the patient severely disabled.

Is the patient bound by that form? The answer is no. The Unfair Contract Terms Act prevents the surgeon relying on that form as a defence against the patient. He cannot exclude or restrict his liability for death or personal injury resulting from his negligence. The same principles do not apply to loss of or damage to property. Under the Unfair Contract Terms Act 1977, an exemption for damage to or loss of property is valid if it is reasonable (see Statute Box 6.2). (For further discussion on this, see chapter 24.)

Limitation of Time

Most civil court actions must be brought within a certain length of time. The time limit for actions concerning personal injury and death is three years from the cause of action arising or the date of the knowledge of the cause of action arising. The issue of the claim form marks the beginning of the court action and it is the time that elapses from the cause arising to the day the claim form is issued that is critical.

Knowledge of the harm

If a patient did not realise that they were suffering from the effects of someone's negligence in that time, then the time limit does not apply until they have that knowledge. It used to be law that if the claimant was out of time for whatever reason then they were barred from proceeding with the case. The injustice of this rule is very easy to see from cases involving such long-term diseases as pneumoconiosis, asbestosis and similar conditions. The law was therefore amended so that the period did not start to run until the claimant had knowledge of the facts shown in Statute Box 6.3.

> # Statute 6.3
> ## Limitation Act 1980 Section 14
>
> **Definition of knowledge**
> (a) that the injury in question was significant
> (b) that the injury was attributable in whole or in part to the act or omission which is alleged to constitute negligence
> (c) the identity of the defendant, and
> (d) the identity of any other defendant.

> The term 'significant' is further defined as where 'the person whose date of knowledge is in question would reasonably have considered it sufficiently serious to justify instituting proceeding against a defendant who did not dispute liability'. (A subsection 1A to section 14 is added by the Consumer Protection Act 1987 to cover the date of knowledge for the purposes of that Act.)

The potential claimant cannot, however, simply turn a blind eye to knowledge that any reasonable person would acquire from the facts around him. If, however, he had no knowledge of the facts, then he is not barred from proceeding.

In a significant decision the House of Lords[35] ruled in January 2008 that claims could be brought by the victims of rape and sexual assault outside the time limit, if the judge ruled that the personal characteristics of the claimant might have prevented him or her acting as a reasonable person. Three of the cases were remitted to High Court for reconsideration in the light of the House of Lords ruling. It overruled its previous decision in the case of *Stubbings* v *Webb*[36] and allowed time-barred appeals in cases which involved a rape victim, whose rapist had subsequently won the lottery, and several victims of sexual assault by council employees in council run schools or residential homes. The consequence of the decision is that many thousands of victims of indecent assault may pursue claims against councils and churches. The High Court also held that claims by former servicemen for radiation injury resulting from nuclear tests in the 1950s could go ahead and were not to be struck out on grounds that they were time-barred or had no reasonable prospect of success.[37] The Court of Appeal held that all the cases but one were statute-barred ([2010] EWCA Civ 1317). The Supreme Court in 2012[38] dismissed the appeals by a 4 to 3 majority. The Supreme Court was divided on how knowledge should be determined. The majority took the view that a reasonable belief of the possibility that injuries were the result of fault was what was required; the minority held that a claimant's knowledge, not belief, was the relevant issue and that by definition knowledge must be based on fact. The majority also held that the use of the judge's discretion under section 33 to permit the case to continue would not be appropriate.

Practical Dilemma 6.5 — Delay

Claire French was admitted for an appendicectomy. The operation was performed successfully and she was discharged. From time to time, however, she complained of violent stomach pain for which she took very strong painkillers. Some six years after the first operation, she was admitted to hospital in intense agony and no painkiller could relieve it. The consultant was reluctant to operate since he could not identify any possible cause for which surgery was the solution. However, a laparoscopy was performed and it was then discovered that a swab had been left behind in the previous operation. The consultant was completely open with Claire about his findings and assured her that from now on she should not get any pain. She felt that she should be compensated for the fact that she had already suffered much pain and had had to endure the risks, pain and suffering of a second operation. Is she entitled to compensation?

As a result of the changes by the Limitation Act 1980, she would not be barred on the grounds of exceeding the time limit, which would run from the time she was informed of the cause of her suffering. The House of Lords has eased the time limit of those suing for rape or sexual assault.[39]

Judge's Discretion to Extend Time Limit

In addition, under section 33 of the Limitation Act 1980 the judge has the discretion to allow a case to proceed that would otherwise be outside the time limit where it would be equitable to allow the claimant to continue. A judge refused to extend the time limit in the following case.

Case 6.3 *Fenech v E. London and City Health Authority* [2000]

No extension of time[40]

On 5 July 1960 the claimant gave birth to her first child. Afterwards, the doctor suturing her episiotomy informed her that the needle that he had been using had broken. In fact, a two-inch piece of the needle had been left inside the wound. The claimant experienced pain in the area of the episiotomy, but was too embarrassed to discuss her symptoms with her general practitioner. She gave birth to five more children. In 1983, she came under the care of a female gynaecologist and underwent a number of negative investigations and operations over a period of 11 years. The fragment of the needle was identified on a hip X-ray when she was being reviewed by orthopaedic surgeons in 1991, but it was not until a repeat X-ray in 1994 that she was informed of the needle's presence. She issued proceedings in January 1997 and the issue of limitation was tried as a preliminary point. At the county court, her claim was held to be statute-barred: although she had not attained actual knowledge until 1994, she had had constructive knowledge 'long before 1994'. She appealed to the Court of Appeal on the grounds that the judge had erred in refusing to take into account her embarrassment when considering when she ought reasonably to have sought medical advice and the defendant could not prove that such earlier advice would have led to an earlier detection of the needle fragment.

The Court of Appeal dismissed the appeal on the grounds that she should have sought medical advice earlier; she failed to give the gynaecologist sufficient information about her symptoms and, while the 1991 X-ray had revealed the fragment of the needle, its significance and relationship to her gynaecological problems were not realised by the orthopaedic specialists who were reviewing her for a hip replacement.

In contrast, in the case of *Amanda Godfrey* v *Gloucester Royal Infirmary NHS Trust*,[41] in which the claimant argued that while she had been told following an ultrasound scan that her baby (who was born in 1995) had severe abnormalities, she did not have sufficient information to make a decision about a termination until she read the medical report in 2001, the judge did not accept this argument but was still prepared to exercise his discretion under section 33 of the Limitation Act 1980 and held that it was equitable to allow the case to proceed. In the case[42] of a boy born with cerebral palsy, the Court of Appeal held that he was expected to bring a claim of negligence within three years of his actual knowledge or such knowledge as he might reasonably be expected to acquire to mount a claim against the defendant responsible for causing the injury. Applying this test, the claimant had **constructive knowledge** of the facts by 1998 and the claim (which was brought in 2006) was statute-barred but the Court exercised its discretion under section 33 and allowed the claim to proceed on equitable grounds.

Extension of the Time Limit on Other Grounds

Where minors under 18 years of age have suffered personal injury, there is no time barrier to bringing an action until they reach the age of 18 years, at which time the time limit comes into operation. (See chapter 13 on children.) The same principle applies to those of unsound mind whose disorder prevents them from bringing an action within the appropriate time limits. The time limits do not commence until the disorder ceases, which in most cases will be at death.

Legal Aid and Conditional Fees

One of the recent changes in civil justice is the withdrawal of legal aid in personal injury claims. The introduction of **conditional fee systems** into civil litigation, sometimes referred to as 'no win, no fee', enables an agreement to be drawn up between solicitor and client, whereby the former would act on behalf of the latter in civil proceedings and only claim a fee if the outcome is satisfactory to the client. Regulations[43] that came into force in June 2003 enabled clients to enter into simpler, more transparent conditional fee agreements (CFAs) with the solicitors and enable solicitors to guarantee to clients that they would get all the damages awarded. In some cases, especially those involving clinical negligence, it may be necessary for the client to purchase insurance cover for possible witnesses and other costs. The Conditional Fee Regulations 2000 and 2003 were revoked in November 2005[44] with the aim of simplifying CFAs and making them more transparent and easier to use for both solicitors and their clients. Further information on CFAs is available from the Bar Council website.[45]

From April 2013 the attractions of no win, no fee have been reduced by changes which mean that claimants can no longer recover the extra fees that they must pay their lawyers or their legal insurance premiums from the losing side.[46] Commercial third party funding schemes have begun whereby they agree to fund a case if the claimant's solicitor provides a convincing argument that it will ultimately succeed. The fee comes out of recovered damages.[47] The fees which lawyers can charge for personal injury cases have also been reduced from May 2013. Fees for minor injuries in road accidents have been cut from £1200 to £500. Referral fees paid between lawyers, insurers, claims firms, garages and others when cases are passed on are banned.[48]

Insurers are also seeking MRI scans on claimants who are seeking compensation for alleged whiplash injuries.[49]

Section 44 of the Legal Aid, Sentencing and Punishment of Offenders Act 2012 amended the Act 1990 so that a success fee payable under a CFA may no longer be recovered by a lawyer from a losing party but is subject to additional conditions.[50] The Conditional Fee Agreements Order 2013/689 makes provision as to how the success fee should be calculated: in a claim for personal injuries the success fee is limited to a maximum of 25 per cent of damages awarded for pain, suffering and loss of amenity and pecuniary loss. The Damages-Based Agreements (DBA) Regulations[51] set conditions for them to be enforceable under the Courts and Legal Services Act 1990. A cap of 25 per cent for a DBA is set in a claim for personal injuries.

The Financial Services (Banking Reform) Act 2013 places claims management complaints in the jurisdiction of the Legal Ombudsman who has the power to force companies to pay compensation or provide another form of redress. The result is that those bombarded by ambulance chasers could receive compensation through the Legal Ombudsman. The Claims Management Regulation Unit (at the Ministry of Justice) will be able to fine companies which use information provided by unsolicited calls and texts or who provide poor quality services. Referral fees paid to middlemen are banned. The Legal Ombudsman[52] reported in January 2014 that nearly £1 million in compensation was ordered to be paid to clients because of disputes over no win, no fee agreements.[53]

A special out-of-court scheme to settle compensation for those with asbestos-related disease has been set up. The Mesothelioma Act 2014 creates a package of support – funded by insurance firms – to pay in excess of 800 eligible people from 2014, and 300 every year after that until 2024. Further information is available on the government website[54] and from the Asbestos Victims Support Group Forum.[55] (See chapter 25.)

Clinical Negligence Scheme for Trusts (CNST) and the NHS Litigation Authority (NHSLA)

The CNST was established in 1996[56] to administer trusts and other NHS bodies that take part in a voluntary scheme whereby compensation is met from a pooling system. The payment into the pool depends on an assessment of the risk presented by that particular trust and amounts over a specified minimum will be met from the pool. The CNST visits organisations that belong to or wish to belong to the scheme to assess their risk: they examine, in particular, the standard of risk assessment and management in the organisation, and the standards of record keeping. In the light of their assessment, premiums payable into the scheme are assessed. Over 95 per cent of NHS trusts are members of CNST. Liabilities prior to April 1995 are covered by the Existing Liabilities Scheme (ELS), which is centrally funded.

The NHS Litigation Authority (NHSLA) was a special health authority, i.e. a statutory body, set up in 1995 to oversee the CNST in the handling of claims. The NHSLA used an approved list of solicitors to handle litigation. In one case,[57] when the parties disputed the details for the setting up of a structured settlement, the claimant gave notice that they would ask the judge to summon the NHSLA's chief executive to explain why the defendants were attempting to charge the claimant for setting up the structured settlement. The defendants then reached agreement with the claimant. The NHSLA was subject to an annual performance review. A key function for the NHSLA was to contribute to the incentives for reducing the number of negligent or preventable incidents. It aimed to achieve this through an extensive risk management programme. It designed a set of risk management standards for each type of healthcare organisation, incorporating organisational, clinical, and health and safety risks. They covered: NHSLA Acute, PCT and Independent Sector Standards; NHSLA Mental Health and Learning Disability Standards; and NHSLA Ambulance Standards. Since April 2017 the NHSLA has been renamed NHS Resolution. The above-mentioned work of the NHSLA continues under NHS Resolution. According to the NHS Resolution website, its strategy to 2022 includes:

> a move to an organisation which is more focused than before on prevention, learning and early intervention to address the rising costs of harm in the NHS. This means an earlier involvement, where we are well placed to respond sooner when something goes wrong, as well as identifying opportunities for prevention.
>
> From 2022 to 2025 its strategy was updated and is focused on four priorities:-
>
> > Priority 1: Deliver fair resolution, and trying to keep patients and healthcare staff out of formal processes to minimise distress and costs.
> > Priority 2: Share data and insights as a catalyst for improvement.
> > Priority 3: Collaborate to improve maternity outcomes by bringing together key parties to decide what further improvements can be made to improve maternity safety.
> > Priority 4: Invest in our people and systems to transform our business.

In addition, the CNST has devised a set of standards for maternity services. These standards can be accessed on the NHSLA webpage,[58] which can be accessed via the NHS Resolution website.[59]

Amendments to the Clinical Negligence Scheme for Trusts were enacted through regulations in 2014.[60] These update the definition of relevant function relating it to how services are now commissioned and covers the activities of bodies exercising other functions in relation to the health service and other powers to generate income.

NHS Redress Act 2006

The National Audit Office reported in May 2001 that almost £4 billion would be required to meet the costs of known and anticipated claims in the NHS.[61] In the light of this report, the DH announced in July 2001 that it was setting up a committee under the chairmanship of the Chief Medical Officer of Health to consider a new scheme for compensation for clinical negligence and published a consultation paper.[62] This was followed, on 30 June 2003, by a further consultation document, 'Making Amends',[63] which provided a comprehensive account of the background to the present situation. It looked at the present system of medical negligence litigation and its costs. It analysed public attitudes and concerns and the earlier reviews of the negligence system by the Pearson Commission,[64] the Woolf Report on Access to Justice[65] and the National Audit Office Report in 2001.[66] It considered recent action taken to reform civil court procedures, claims handling by the NHS Litigation Authority and the use of alternative dispute resolution. It analysed systems of no-fault liability in Denmark, Finland, France, New Zealand, Norway and Sweden and discussed no-fault liability as an option along with continued reform of the present tort process, a tariff-based national tribunal or a composite option drawing on all three. The scheme eventually recommended in 'Making Amends' was a composite package of reform drawing on the best elements of these three options. It included suggestions for the care and compensation for severely neurologically impaired babies; for the NHS redress scheme to be part of the system for handling complaints; for the retention of right to pursue litigation through the courts and changes to the existing scheme for civil proceedings; and for a duty of candour to be placed on healthcare professionals and managers to inform patients where they become aware of a possible negligent action or omission.

The NHS Redress Act which was eventually agreed was a very much less radical scheme than that proposed in the consultation paper. It gave power to the Secretary of State to establish a scheme for the purpose of enabling redress to be provided without recourse to civil proceedings. The NHS (Clinical Negligence Scheme) Regulations 1996 SI were the principal regulations and have been amended most recently by an SI in 2013[67] which added a number of additional bodies to be eligible to take part in the scheme including NICE, the Health and Social Care Information Centre, local authorities which provide or arrange for the provision of NHS services plus other changes.

On 1 April 2011 in Wales regulations were implemented to deal with complaints against the NHS providers. There is a redress scheme for the resolution of low-value clinical negligence claims (those under £25,000). Further details can be found on the Welsh Government website.[68]

On 18 March 2009, in response to a written question, a statement was made by Lord Darzi to the effect that the government's priority was to put in place across the health and social care in the country general foundations of redress, in its wider sense, by placing the patient at the heart of any complaints system and move to a more robust sensitive complaints procedure. In other words, the government's priority was the NHS Constitution and the rights and pledges outlined in that, rather than the implementation of the NHS redress scheme, which has not yet been enacted in England and at the time of writing in 2024 is still not being used.

Reforms to civil litigation

In 2010 the Final Report of Lord Jackson's review on civil litigation costs was published and has resulted in many of the changes to the conditional fee system outlined above being implemented.[69] The Review considered that the consequences of its recommendations were that:

- Most personal injury claimants will recover more damages than they do at present, although some will recover less;
- Claimants will have a financial interest in the level of costs which are being incurred on their behalf;
- Claimant solicitors will still be able to make a reasonable profit;
- Costs payable to claimant solicitors by liability insurers will be significantly reduced; and
- Costs will also become more proportionate, because defendants will no longer have to pay success fees and after-the-event insurance premiums.

Conclusions

Unfortunately, little progress seems to have been made in the reform of the current system for obtaining compensation for clinical negligence. Earlier criticisms of the handling of clinical negligence cases from the Public Accounts Committee[70] and the Health Service Committee of the House of Commons with the possible introduction of no-fault compensation being introduced[71] have not been acted upon. The NHS redress scheme, which does not contain the radical proposals set out in 'Making Amends', has not at the time of writing been implemented in England though it has been in Wales and there is ongoing concern that in the vast bills for clinical negligence more money is going to lawyers than to claimants.[72] The Jackson Report has not met with unqualified support from lawyers,[73,74] but the Young Report recommended its speedy implementation (see chapter 12). Obtaining legal aid in civil cases has become more difficult and there is more regulation of no win, no fee schemes. For those who have suffered harm as a result of negligence by health and social care providers obtaining compensation is becoming more and more difficult. It may be that the statutory duty of candour by organisations may assist potential litigants (see chapter 5).

Reflection questions

1. Look at the aspects of case management as set out and consider the extent to which this should ensure that cases are dealt with faster and more justly to the parties.
2. What is meant by *res ipsa loquitur*? In what situations in healthcare do you think it could apply?
3. What is the difference between pecuniary loss and non-pecuniary loss as a result of a civil wrong? How is compensation for the latter calculated?
4. What is meant by contributory negligence? What are the principles on which the judge works in deciding the level of deduction of compensation? (See Statute Box 6.1.)
5. Are there any tasks that you perform that are likely to cause harm to you? Do you consider the principle of *volenti non fit injuria* applies to any of them and, if so, why?

Further exercises

1. Examine the notices in your hospital that disclaim any responsibility for loss or damage. Consider any ways in which they might not be completely effective in the light of the Unfair Contract Terms Act 1977.
2. What action do you consider could be taken to reduce the level and therefore the cost of litigation within the NHS?
3. Obtain a copy of your local complaints scheme and consider the extent to which its implementation could reduce civil action being brought within the NHS.

References

[1] Lord Woolf, Access to Justice. Full details of the Civil Procedure Rules are available on the website at www.justice.gov.uk/courts/procedure-rules/civil
[2] Ian Grainger and Michael Fealy, *Introduction to the New Civil Procedure Rules*, Cavendish Publications Ltd, London, 1999
[3] www.justice.gov.uk/courts/procedure-rules/civil
[4] NHS Executive, Handling Clinical Negligence Claims, HSC 1998/183
[5] News item, *The Times*, 29 November 2007
[6] Robin Turner, £11,000 blow for victorious jungle bite claimant, *Wales Online*, 5 June 2008
[7] *Roe* v *Minister of Health* [1954] 2 QB 66
[8] *Cassidy* v *Ministry of Health* [1951] 2 KB 343
[9] *Cassidy* v *Ministry of Health* [1951] 2 KB 343
[10] *Ratcliffe* v *Plymouth and Torbay HA* [1998] PIQR P170
[11] *Thomas* v *Curley* [2013] EWCA Civ 117
[12] *Selvanayagam* v *University of West Indies* [1983] 1 All ER 824
[13] https://resolution.nhs.uk/

[14] News item, *The Times*, 16 May 2013
[15] News item, *The Times*, 30 August 2010
[16] News item, Girl who had brain injected with glue wins payout, *The Times*, 28 January 2014
[17] News item, *The Times*, 25 July 2014
[18] *Knauer* v *Ministry of Justice* [2014] EWHC 2553
[19] *Drake and Another* v *Foster Wheeler Ltd*, The Times Law Report, 20 September 2010
[20] *Hurditch* v *Sheffield HA* [1989] 2 All ER 869
[21] *S (a child)* v *Royal Bournemouth and Christchurch Hospital NHS Trust* October 2012 (taken from Quantum of Damages, Vol. 3, Kemp and Kemp, Sweet & Maxwell, B1-014)
[22] News item, £5.75m for palsy boy, *The Times*, 20 December 2003
[23] News item, Hospital payout, *The Times*, 20 January 2004
[24] *Gregg* v *Scott* [2003] Lloyd's Rep Med 3
[25] *Wells* v *Wells* [1999] 1 AC 345
[26] Lord Chancellor Statement, 27 July 2001; Kemp and Kemp, *The Quantum of Damages*, Vol. 2, 36090/2, 2007 edition
[27] Law Commission, Damages for Personal Injury: medical, nursing and other expenses, Stationery Office, London, 1996
[28] Law Commission Report No. 257, Personal Injury Compensation for Non-pecuniary Loss, 19 April 1999
[29] *Heil* v *Rankin* [2000] 2 WLR 1173, The Times Law Report, 24 March 2000
[30] *Simmons* v *Castle* [2012] EWCA Civ 1039
[31] *YM (A child)* v *Gloucestershire Hospitals NHS Foundation Trust*; *Kanu* v *King's College Hospital NHS Trust* [2006] EWHC 820; [2006] PIQR P27
[32] *Froom* v *Butcher* [1975] 3 All ER 520
[33] *Badger* v *Ministry of Defence* [2005] EWHC 2941 QBD
[34] *Gough* v *Thorne* [1966] 3 All ER 398 CA
[35] *A* v *Hoare; X and Another* v *Wandsworth LBC; C* v *Middlesborough Council; H* v *Suffolk CC; Young* v *Catholic Care (Diocese of Leeds) and Another*, The Times Law Report, 31 January 2008
[36] *Stubbings* v *Webb* [1993] AC 498
[37] *AB and others* v *Ministry of Defence*, The Times Law Report, 10 June 2009; [2010] EWCA Civ 1317
[38] *AB and others* v *Ministry of Defence* [2012] UKSC 9
[39] *A* v *Hoare* (and other cases) [2008] UKHL 6
[40] *Alice Maud Fenech* v *East London and City Health Authority* [2000] Lloyd's Rep Med p. 35 CA
[41] *Amanda Godfrey* v *Gloucester Royal Infirmary NHS Trust* [2003] Lloyd's Rep Med 8
[42] *Whiston* v *London Strategic Health Authority*, The Times Law Report, 4 May 2010; [2010] EWCA 195
[43] Conditional Fee Agreements (Miscellaneous Amendments) Regulations 2003
[44] Conditional Fee Agreements (Revocation) Regulations 2005 SI 2005/2305
[45] www.barcouncil.org.uk
[46] Legal Aid Sentencing and Punishment of Offenders Act 2012
[47] Jonathan Ames, Another litigation industry is born?, *The Times*, 20 June 2013
[48] Frances Gibb, Lawyers' fees for accident claims slashed in attempt to drive down insurers' costs, *The Times*, 2 May 2013
[49] Miles Costello, Insurers want MRI scans to curb whiplash claims, *The Times*, 15 July 2013
[50] Section 58(4A) and (4B) of the Courts and Legal Services Act 1990
[51] Damages-Based Agreements Regulations 2013/609

52 www.legalombudsman.org.uk
53 Frances Gibb, No win, no fee clients saddled with huge bills, *The Times*, 6 January 2014
54 www.gov.uk
55 www.asbestosforum.org.uk
56 National Health Service (Clinical Negligence Scheme) Regulations XI 1996/251; amendment regulations SI 2002/1073
57 *Inman v Cambridge Health Authority*, January 1998 (taken from Quantum of Damages, Vol. 2, Kemp and Kemp, Sweet & Maxwell, 1998 edn)
58 National Health Service Litigation Authority, *Clinical Negligence Scheme for Trusts: Maternity Clinical Risk Management Standards*, Version 1, 2013/14; www.nhsla.com/Safety/Documents/CNST%20Maternity%20Standards%202013-14.pdf
59 www.resolution.nhs.uk/about
60 National Health Service (Clinical Negligence Scheme) (Amendment) Regulations 2014 SI 2014/933
61 National Audit Office, *Handling Clinical Negligence Claims in England*, Report of the Comptroller and Auditor General, HC 403 Session 2000–2001, 3 May 2001
62 Department of Health press release 2001/0313, New Clinical Compensation Scheme for the NHS, 20 July 2001
63 Department of Health, Making Amends: a consultation paper setting out proposals for reforming the approach to clinical negligence in the NHS, CMO, June 2003
64 Pearson Report, Royal Commission on Civil Liability and Compensation for Personal Injury, Cmnd 7054, HMSO, London, 1978
65 Lord Woolf, Final Report: Access to Justice, HMSO, London, July 1996
66 National Audit Office, Handling Clinical Negligence Claims in England, Report of the Comptroller and Auditor General, HC 403 Session 2000–2001, 3 May 2001
67 NHS (Clinical Negligence Scheme) Regulations 2013 SI 2013/497
68 https://gov.wales
69 Lord Jackson, Review of Civil Litigation Costs: Final Report, Stationery Office, London, 2010
70 Committee of Public Accounts HC 619-1 (1998–99) Hansard
71 Health Select Committee HC 549 (1998–99) Hansard, October 1999
72 Sam Lister, Lawyers take half of NHS damages claim, *The Times*, 18 December 2009
73 See Law Society website: www.lawsociety.org.uk
74 Alex Wade, Fewer than 10 per cent of my clients would be able to sue if Jackson is implemented, *The Times*, 25 March 2010

Chapter 7

Consent to Treatment and Informing the Patient

This chapter discusses

- Basic principles
- Requirements of a valid consent
- How should consent be given?
- Right to refuse treatment
- Taking one's own discharge
- Definition of mental capacity under the Mental Capacity Act 2005
- Hunger strikes
- Amputation of healthy limbs
- Defences to an action for trespass to the person
- Mental Capacity Act 2005
- Mental Health Act 1983
- Giving information to a patient prior to consent being obtained
- Non-therapeutic procedures
- Giving information to the terminally ill patient
- Notifying the patient of negligence by a colleague
- No decision about me, without me

Introduction

This chapter covers the principles relating to consent to treatment and giving information to the patient.

Basic principles

Any adult, mentally competent person has the right in law to consent to any touching of his person. If he is touched without consent or other lawful justification, then the person has the right of action in the civil courts of suing for **trespass to the person – battery** where the person is actually touched, **assault** where they fear that they will be touched. The fact that consent has been given will normally prevent a successful action for trespass. However, it may not prevent an action for negligence arising on the ground that there was a breach of the duty of care to inform the patient. This chapter explores both these aspects of consent and looks at the information that must be legally given to the patient and other questions that arise on informing the patient. Reference should be made to chapter 13 on consent in relation to children and young persons – those under 18 years; to chapter 19 on consent in relation to the mentally disordered; to chapter 18 on consent in relation to the elderly; and to chapter 16 in relation to those with learning disabilities. The situation relating to AIDS and HIV is considered in chapter 25 and to operations in chapter 15.

Requirements of a valid consent

To be valid, consent must be given voluntarily by a mentally competent person without any duress or fraud. In the case of *Freeman* v *Home Office*,[1] a prisoner challenged the legality of his being injected with drugs for his personality disorder on the basis that he had not given his consent and that being given medicine by a doctor in a custodial situation precluded consent being voluntarily given. The Court of Appeal refused to accept this proposition and agreed with the High Court judge that: 'Where, in a prison setting, a doctor has the power to influence a prisoner's situation and prospects, a court must be alive to the risk that what may appear, on the face of it, to be real consent is not in fact so.' There is a presumption that the patient is mentally competent, now enshrined in statutory form in section 1(2) of the Mental Capacity Act 2005. However, this can be rebutted on a balance of probabilities (s. 2(4) of the Mental Capacity Act 2005) if there is evidence to the contrary. The criteria to be used in assessing competence are set by sections 2 and 3 of the Mental Capacity Act 2005 and are shown in Statute Box 7.1. Where a person falsely claims to be a doctor and gave a woman a breast examination, she had not consented to the treatment.[2]

How should consent be given?

Figure 7.1 illustrates the different forms of giving consent. As far as the law is concerned, there is no specific requirement that consent for treatment should be given in any particular way. They are all equally valid. However, they vary considerably in their value as evidence in proving that consent was given. Consent in writing is by far the best form of evidence and is therefore the preferred method of obtaining the consent of the patient when any procedure involving some risk is contemplated. The Department of Health updated its guidance on consent to examination and treatment in 2001 and produced two publications: a reference guide to the principles on

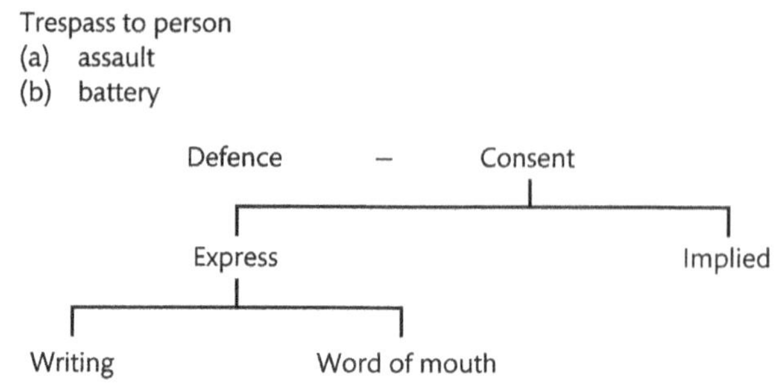

Figure 7.1

Various forms of consent to a trespass to the person

```
Trespass to person
(a) assault
(b) battery

       Defence  —  Consent
                ┌─────┴─────┐
              Express      Implied
          ┌─────┴─────┐
       Writing    Word of mouth
```

consent to examination and treatment[3] and a good practice in consent implementation guide.[4] Subsequently the Department of Health amended the reference guide[5] and indicated the changes necessary to the forms of consent in the light of the Mental Capacity Act and recent court decisions.[6] The forms recommended for use by the Department of Health in the implementation guide are considered below.

In certain circumstances the fact that consent has been given does not prevent a criminal offence occurring. In the case of R v Brown sadomasochists were prosecuted for an offence of causing actual bodily harm under the Offences Against the Person Act 1861 and the defence that they were consenting to the activities was not accepted.[7] In another case the House of Lords held that an irrational fear preventing the free exercise of choice by B was sufficient to make criminal A's sexual touching of B, who was unable to refuse through a mental disorder. Inability to communicate any choice made was not limited to physical inability.[8] In an unreported case[9] a deputy manager at a care home was sentenced to 3 months for assault when he attempted to carry out manual evacuation of faeces on a resident, when he was not qualified to carry out the procedure. Consent by the resident was not an effective defence.

Consent in Writing

The forms of consent to examination and treatment that are contained in the Department of Health guidance[10] require the health professional providing the treatment (and this can include a nurse practitioner or midwife) to discuss with the patient the benefits of the treatment and also any serious or frequently occurring risks associated with it and also identify any additional procedures which may be necessary, including the possibility of a blood transfusion or other specified procedure.

Consent is not simply a signature on a form: it is the result of a process of communication between patient and professional that may result in the patient signing a form, which is evidence that the patient agrees to the proposed treatment. Significant recommendations were made in the Kennedy Report[11] following the inquiry into paediatric heart surgery at Bristol Royal Infirmary on greater openness and honesty between health professionals and the patient. The recommendations on consent included those shown in Box 7.1 (numbers refer to recommendations in the Report).

If a nurse were to become aware that the patient who has put their signature to a consent form has very little idea of what the patient has given consent to, then the nurse should ensure that the health professional concerned gives more information to the patient about what is proposed. Where does the nurse stand if they are aware that the patient has signed a form without realising what is involved?

> **Box 7.1** **Recommendations on consent in kennedy report**
>
> 1. In a patient-centred healthcare service patients must be involved, wherever possible, in decisions about their treatment and care.
> 5. Information should be tailored to the needs, circumstances and wishes of the individual.
> 23. We note and endorse the recent statement on consent produced by the DH reference guide to consent for examination and treatment (DH 2001). It should inform the practice of all healthcare professionals in the NHS and be introduced into practice in all trusts.
> 24. The process of informing the patient, and obtaining consent to a course of treatment, should be regarded as a process and not a one-off event consisting of obtaining a patient's signature on a form.
> 25. The process of consent should apply not only to surgical procedures but also to all clinical procedures and examinations that involve any form of touching. This must not mean more forms: it means more communication.
> 26. As part of the process of obtaining consent, except when they have indicated otherwise, patients should be given sufficient information about what is to take place, the risks, uncertainties, and possible negative consequences of the proposed treatment, about any alternatives and about the likely outcome, to enable them to make a choice about how to proceed.

Practical dilemma 7.1   Ignorance is bliss

Susan Wnek had signed the form to consent to an operation for the investigation of a lump in her breast. She was very distressed to be undergoing surgery and ever since she had come into hospital had been able to understand and take in very little of what was said to her. The doctor had explained that a biopsy would be carried out and if that were positive further surgery would be undertaken. It was apparent to Staff Nurse Rachel Bryant that Susan had very little awareness that a radical mastectomy could be performed.

Where does Staff Nurse Bryant stand in relation to the proposed operation? The staff nurse has a legal duty to the patient and if she knows that the patient did not understand what she signed or failed to take in the information given by the doctor, she should arrange for the doctor to return and give the patient more information. From the court's point of view, the fact that the patient has signed the form and expressly agreed to a named procedure or course of treatment and that she understands that 'any procedure in addition to those described on this form will only be carried out if it is necessary to save my life or to prevent serious harm to my health' would be very strong evidence to defend any action for trespass to the person.

There is a possibility, however, of a successful action in negligence if the patient has not been given relevant information (see below). There is a clear duty on any health practitioner to take reasonable care that a patient receives the appropriate information before any consent form is signed and treatment proceeds. The nurse should, as far as possible, take appropriate steps to inform the relevant health practitioner if she discovers that this duty has not been carried out.

Consent by Word of Mouth

Many of the less risky treatments are carried out without any formal signature of the patient. Consent by word of mouth is valid, but it may be far more difficult to establish in court, since it might be one person's word against another. Many of the day-to-day treatments and tests are, however, carried out on this basis.

Case 7.1 *Davis v Barking, Havering and Brentwood HA* [1993]

Consent to anaesthesia[12]

The claimant signed a consent form giving consent to a general anaesthetic. She was subsequently given a caudal block and, unfortunately, suffered some harm as a result. She claimed that she had not given consent to this block, which therefore amounted to a trespass to her person, i.e. battery. The High Court judge held that separate consent was not required for each part of the treatment.

The Department of Health recommends that consent in writing be obtained for any significant procedure such as a surgical operation or when the patient participates in a research project or a video recording (even if only minor procedures are involved).[13]

Implied Consent

It is sometimes said that the fact that a patient comes into hospital means that he or she is giving their consent to anything that the consultant deems appropriate. That, however, is not supported in law. There are many choices of available treatment and when care is provided there must be evidence that the patient has agreed to that particular course. Similarly, it is said that when an unconscious patient is treated in the A&E department, he implies consent to being treated. This, however, is likewise not so. An unconscious patient implies nothing. The professionals care for him in the absence of consent as part of their duty to care for the patient out of necessity in an emergency[14] and could defend any subsequent action for trespass to the person on that basis. They would now be acting under the statutory duty provided by the Mental Capacity Act 2005 to act in the best interests of a mentally incapacitated person.

Implied consent is better reserved for situations where non-verbal communication by the patient makes it clear that he is giving consent. Nurses are familiar with the signs: the patient rolls up his sleeve for an injection; the patient opens his mouth as the nurse waves the thermometer in the air. Such actions indicate to the nurse that the patient agrees to the treatment/care proceeding. No words are spoken, there is no signature, but it is clear that the patient is in agreement. In a Massachusetts case of 1891, a passenger on a ship who held out her hand to be vaccinated lost her action for battery.[15]

The weakness of implied consent is, however, that it is not always clear that the patient is agreeing to what the nurse intends to do. Thus the patient who rolls up their sleeve for blood pressure to be taken would get a nasty shock when the nurse gives him an injection, yet that is how the nurse has interpreted his non-verbal actions. To avoid such misunderstandings, it is preferable if the nurse tells the patient what they wish to do and obtains a spoken consent from the patient. (The problems in giving day-to-day care to the confused elderly are considered in chapter 18.)

Once a mentally competent patient has given a valid consent to treatment, then he/she cannot succeed in an action for trespass to the person,[16] but if it is claimed insufficient information on the risks of the treatment was given to them they would have to bring an action in negligence alleging a breach of the duty of care in failing to provide sufficient information (see pages 169–3).

Right to refuse treatment

It is a basic principle of law in this country that an adult, mentally competent person has the right to refuse treatment and take his own discharge contrary to medical advice. The Court of Appeal has emphasised that provided the patient has the necessary mental capacity, which is assessed in relation to the decision to be made, then he or she can refuse to give consent for a good reason, a bad reason or no reason at all. This was the principle set out in the case of *Re MB* shown in Case 7.2.

Case 7.2   *Re MB* [1997]

Consent to a caesarean section[17]

A pregnant woman suffered from needle phobia as a result of which she was unable to agree to have an injection that would precede a Caesarean section. The High Court judge held that her needle phobia rendered her mentally incapacitated to take the decision not to have a Caesarean operation. The Court of Appeal confirmed that decision, but emphasised that had she been competent, she could have refused the operation. The Court of Appeal in *Re MB* laid down the steps and rules that should be followed when a health professional is faced with a patient who appears to be mentally incompetent.

The ruling in *Re MB* was followed by the Court of Appeal in a case brought against St George's Hospital,[18] while in a more recent case a judge declared that a Caesarean and all necessary procedures could be performed on a woman detained under Section 5(2) of the Mental Health Act 1983.[19]

Mental Capacity of the Patient

The fact that mentally capacitated adult patients can refuse life-saving treatment can be upsetting for staff, as the following case shows.

> ### Case 7.3 Re C (An Adult: Refusal of Medical Treatment) [1994]
>
> ## The patient's autonomy[20]
>
> The patient was a 68-year-old man who suffered from paranoid schizophrenia and was detained at Broadmoor Hospital. He developed gangrene in one foot and doctors believed an amputation to be a life-saving necessity. He refused to give consent and sought an **injunction** restraining the hospital from carrying out an amputation without his express written consent. He succeeded on the grounds that the evidence failed to establish that he lacked sufficient understanding of the nature, purpose and effects of the proposed treatment. Instead, the evidence showed that he:
>
> 1. had understood and retained the relevant treatment information
> 2. believed it, and
> 3. had arrived at a clear choice.

The sole issue in this case was whether the patient had the mental capacity to give a valid refusal. It should be noted that the presence of a mental disorder does not automatically mean that a person is incapable of making a valid decision in relation to treatment. *Re C* should be contrasted with a case[21] where a patient refused a blood transfusion which was required because she self-harmed. She described her blood as being evil and it was held that this was evidence of mental disorder which made her incapable of using and weighing the relevant information.

In a more recent case with similar facts to those in Case 7.3 the Court of Protection ruled that doctors must respect the wishes of a patient with schizophrenia who refused to undergo a potentially life-saving amputation of her leg. JB had a gangrenous foot after an ulcer became infected. Judge Jackson ruled that her mental illness had not robbed her of the power to make rational decisions. 'The freedom to choose for oneself is part of what it means to be human'[22] (see also the case of *Nottinghamshire Healthcare NHS Trust* v *RC* where the patient was detained under the Mental Health Act 1983) (see chapter 19).

In contrast, a compulsory Caesarean was authorised on a woman with autistic spectrum disorder and borderline learning disabilities who lacked the requisite mental capacity.[23] (The case is discussed in chapter 16.)

In *Re MB*[24] the Court of Appeal laid down a test for the competence of the patient which was applied in the case of Miss B, where a woman who had been paralysed refused to be placed on a ventilator and when that refusal was ignored applied to the court for the ventilator to be switched off. The facts are shown in the following case.

The main issue in the case was the mental competence of Miss B. If she were held to be mentally competent, she could refuse to have life-saving treatment for a good reason, a bad reason or no reason at all. She was interviewed by two psychiatrists who gave evidence to the court that she was mentally competent. The judge therefore held that she was entitled to refuse to be ventilated. The judge, Dame Elizabeth Butler-Sloss, President of the Family Division, held that Miss B possessed the requisite mental capacity to make decisions regarding her treatment and thus the administration of artificial respiration by the trust against her wishes amounted to an

Case 7.4   Ms B [2002]

Refusal to be ventilated[25]

Miss B suffered a ruptured blood vessel in her neck which damaged her spinal cord. As a consequence she was paralysed from the neck down and was on a ventilator. She was of sound mind and knew that there was no cure for her condition. She asked for the ventilator to be switched off. Her doctors wished her to try out some special rehabilitation to improve the standard of her care and felt that an intensive care ward was not a suitable location for such a decision to be made. They were reluctant to perform such an action as switching off the ventilator without the court's approval. Miss B applied to court for a declaration to be made that the ventilator could be switched off.

---

unlawful trespass. Dame Elizabeth Butler-Sloss restated the principles which had been laid down by the Court of Appeal in the case of St George's Healthcare Trust:

- There was a presumption that a patient had the mental capacity to make decisions whether to consent to or refuse medical or surgical treatment offered.

- If mental capacity was not an issue and the patient, having been given the relevant information and offered the available option, chose to refuse that treatment, that decision had to be respected by the doctors, considerations of what the best interests of the patient would involve were irrelevant.

- Concern or doubts about the patient's mental capacity should be resolved as soon as possible by the doctors within the hospital or other normal medical procedures.

- Meanwhile, the patient must be cared for in accordance with the judgement of the doctors as to the patient's best interests.

- It was most important that those considering the issue should not confuse the question of mental capacity with the nature of the decision made by the patient, however grave the consequences. Since the view of the patient might reflect a difference in values rather than an absence of competence, the assessment of capacity should be approached with that in mind and doctors should not allow an emotional reaction to or strong disagreement with the patient's decision to cloud their judgement in answering the primary question of capacity.

- Where disagreement still existed about competence, it was of the utmost importance that the patient be fully informed, involved and engaged in the process, which could involve obtaining independent outside help, of resolving the disagreement since the patient's involvement could be crucial to a good outcome.

- If the hospital were faced with a dilemma that doctors did not know how to resolve, this must be recognised and further steps taken as a matter of priority. Those in charge must not allow a situation of deadlock or drift to occur.

- If there was no disagreement about competence, but the doctors were for any reason unable to carry out the patient's wishes, it was their duty to find other doctors who would do so.

- If all appropriate steps to seek independent assistance from medical experts outside the hospital had failed, the hospital should not hesitate to make an application to the High Court or seek the advice of the Official Solicitor.

- The treating clinicians and the hospital should always have in mind that a seriously physically disabled patient who was mentally competent had the same right to personal autonomy and to make decisions as any other person with mental capacity.

It was reported on 29 April 2002 that Miss B had died peacefully in her sleep after the ventilator had been switched off.

The patient therefore has a right to refuse treatment, but it must be clear that he has the requisite mental capacity. The case of *Re C* (Case 7.3) clearly brings out the clash between the patient's autonomy and the professional duty of care. Clearly, it would be essential for those in charge of the patient to take all reasonable precautions to ensure that the patient has appropriate counselling and all the necessary information and help in facing the future, but if this fails, it is the competent patient's right to refuse. Similarly, an adult Jehovah's Witness is able to refuse a blood transfusion. It was reported that a young mother who was a Jehovah's Witness died on 25 October 2007 after giving birth to twins because she refused a life-saving blood transfusion.[26] Different principles apply in relation to children and these are discussed in chapter 13.

The Court of Appeal in the case of *Re T* (see Case 7.5) emphasised the importance of ensuring that, when a patient refuses treatment, the patient has the mental capacity to make a valid decision and has not been subjected to the undue influences of another.

Case 7.5   *Re T* [1992]

Refusal of blood transfusion[27]

A young pregnant woman was injured in a car accident and told the staff nurse that she did not want a blood transfusion. Her mother was a Jehovah's Witness. At the time, it was unlikely to be necessary. However, subsequently she went into labour and a Caesarean was necessary. She told medical staff that she would not want a transfusion and had signed a form to that effect. She was not told that it might be necessary to save her life. After the operation, she required blood as a life-saving measure and her father and co-habitee applied to court. The judge authorised the administration of blood on the ground that the evidence showed that she was not in a fit condition to make a valid decision: pain or exhaustion can lead to lack of capacity.

For a case on refusal of treatment by a 16-year-old, see *In Re W* (see chapter 13 Case 13.1).

The common law principles relating to the presumption of capacity in the person over 16 years and the definition of capacity and best interests have now been placed on a statutory basis by the Mental Capacity Act 2005 (see pages 165–9).

Taking one's own discharge

It follows from what has been said so far that the adult, mentally competent patient is able to take his own discharge. However, this principle may, in practice, cause concern for staff, as Practical Dilemma 7.2 illustrates.

Practical dilemma 7.2 Self-discharge

Don Pritchard was admitted from the A&E department with a suspected head injury. Before X-rays had been taken, he insisted on leaving the hospital, contrary to medical advice. The nursing staff knew that he was still very confused and it seemed likely that his aggression was a result of a brain injury.

This is a difficult situation because it could be argued here that, as a result of the brain injury, the patient was not mentally competent and therefore his decision to discharge himself was an irrational one. If the patient is mentally incapacitated and there is clear danger to the patient's life if he is allowed to leave, it could be argued that these are circumstances in which the staff would be justified in acting in an emergency to save the patient's life. If this does not apply, then the patient has the right to go. An assessment should be carried out of his mental competence. If he is deemed mentally competent, he cannot be compelled to stay, unless he presents a danger to other people. If possible, he should be persuaded to sign a form that he took his own discharge contrary to medical advice. However, it is not always possible to get this signature and therefore it is necessary to ensure that another member of staff can act as a witness to what occurred. In either case, it is essential that full records be made of the circumstances leading to the patient's discharge and the efforts made to persuade him to stay. If harm eventually befalls the patient as a result of his taking his own discharge contrary to medical advice, if there is evidence that the staff did all they could to persuade him to stay and if there was clear evidence that the patient was mentally competent, there is unlikely to be a successful action for negligence against the staff.

Definition of mental capacity under the Mental Capacity Act 2005

The definition of mental capacity under Sections 2 and 3 of the Mental Capacity Act (MCA) is shown in Statute Box 7.1.

Statute 7.1
Sections 2 and 3 of the Mental Capacity Act 2005

Section 2 People who lack capacity

1. For the purposes of this Act, a person lacks capacity in relation to a matter if at the material time he is unable to make a decision for himself in relation to the matter because of an impairment of, or a disturbance in the functioning of, the mind or brain.
2. It does not matter whether the impairment or disturbance is permanent or temporary.

3. A lack of capacity cannot be established merely by reference to:
   (a) a person's age or appearance, or
   (b) a condition of his, or an aspect of his behaviour, which might lead others to make unjustified assumptions about his capacity.
4. In proceedings under this Act or any other enactment, any question whether a person lacks capacity within the meaning of this Act must be decided on the balance of probabilities.
5. No power which a person ('D') may exercise under this Act:
   (a) in relation to a person who lacks capacity, or
   (b) where D reasonably thinks that a person lacks capacity, is exercisable in relation to a person under 16.
6. Subsection (5) is subject to section 18(3).

Section 3 Inability to make decisions

1. For the purposes of section 2, a person is unable to make a decision for himself if he is unable:
   (a) to understand the information relevant to the decision,
   (b) to retain that information,
   (c) to use or weigh that information as part of the process of making the decision, or
   (d) to communicate his decision (whether by talking, using sign language or any other means).
2. A person is not to be regarded as unable to understand the information relevant to a decision if he is able to understand an explanation of it given to him in a way that is appropriate to his circumstances (using simple language, visual aids or any other means).
3. The fact that a person is able to retain the information relevant to a decision for a short period only does not prevent him from being regarded as able to make the decision.
4. The information relevant to a decision includes information about the reasonably foreseeable consequences of:
   (a) deciding one way or another, or
   (b) failing to make the decision.

From Statute Box 7.1 it will be noted that there are two stages for the definition of mental capacity. The first is: is the person suffering from an impairment of, or a disturbance in, the functioning of the mind or brain? The second is: is the effect of the impairment or disturbance an inability to make a decision?

In the case of *RT* v *LT & Anor*[28] the Court of Protection had to decide if a young woman aged 23 lacked the capacity to make decisions: (1) about where she should live; and (2) what contact she should have with members of her family. The judge held that she lacked the requisite mental capacity because of her inability to use or weigh that information as part of the process of making the decision (s. 3(1)(c)).

On 26 May 2010 the Court of Protection gave permission to an NHS trust to sedate a cancer patient (PS) with a phobia of hospitals and needles, and to perform a hysterectomy considered necessary to save her life, treatment which was necessary in her best interests. PS, who was represented by the Official Solicitor, had a significant impairment in intellectual functioning as a consequence of a learning disability which meant that she lacked the requisite mental capacity to give or refuse consent under the Mental Capacity Act 2005.[29] It was recognised that some force may be necessary to sedate her, convey her to hospital and care for her in the period of postoperative recovery. The judge did not consider it necessary to invoke the Deprivation of Liberty Safeguards (DoLS) under Schedule 1 of the MCA (see chapter 16).

The Supreme Court ruled on the definition of mental capacity in March 2014 in a case following a road accident. The defendant motor cyclist had knocked down the claimant who was crossing the road. An initial agreement had been reached whereby the claimant received £12,500 with costs. That was a gross undervaluation of the claim which was assessed as £2 million by the claimant's advisers and about £800,000 by the defendant. The Supreme Court held that the claimant lacked the capacity to commence and conduct proceedings. She should have had a litigation friend from the outset and the settlement should have been approved by the court under rule 21(10)(1) of the civil procedure rules. The consent order was set aside and the case was to go to trial.[30]

In the case of *A Local Authority* v *SY*, (where S had mild learning disabilities and entered into a sham marriage with T and unsuccessfully used the marriage to prevent deportation) the Court of Protection stated that while it was usual for an assessment of capacity to be undertaken by a medical practitioner or a psychiatrist an appropriately qualified social worker was eminently suited to undertake such assessments. It granted the declarations sought by the local authority (LA): that S lacked the capacity to litigate, to make decisions about her residence, contact and care or to enter into a contract of marriage; that it was both lawful and in S's best interests for her to reside at a placement identified by the LA, to receive a care package in accordance with her assessed needs and for her contact with others to be regulated by the local authority. The Court of Appeal also declared that the marriage ceremony was a non-marriage and stated that it would not tolerate the exploitation of young and vulnerable adults.[31]

The Court of Appeal emphasised that the statutory test for capacity was decision specific, rather than being 'person' or 'act' specific, when allowing an appeal in part against a decision by the Court of Protection. The judge held that W did not have sufficient mental capacity to decide whether to live with her husband on his release from prison. The judge had found that she had the capacity to marry but he failed to explain how and why her mental impairment did not rob her of capacity in other aspects of her life, yet caused an inability for her to decide to live with her husband. He had not given the explanations required by section 2(1) and his decision had to be set aside.[32]

Hunger strikes

In an old case,[33] a suffragette went on hunger strike and was force-fed in prison. She lost her claim for trespass to the person. The court held that the prison doctor was justified in feeding her on the grounds that it was the duty of the officials to preserve the health and lives of prisoners. However, in a case in 1995,[34] a prisoner went on hunger strike and the application was made to court to decide whether it was lawful for his doctors and nurses to abstain from force-feeding him. The judge held that there were four grounds for intervening against the prisoner's right of self-determination:

1. The interest that the state holds in preserving life.
2. The interest of the state in preventing suicide.

3. Maintaining the integrity of the medical profession.
4. The protection of the rights of innocent third parties.

He concluded that these did not overrule the right of self-determination of a mentally competent person and the prisoner could be permitted to starve himself to death, provided that he has the legal capacity. The European Court of Human Rights held in a case in 2007 brought against Moldova that a prisoner's forced feeding with no medical justification was a breach of his Article 3 rights.[35]

In a more recent case in 2013 (*A NHS Trust v Dr A*)[36] an Iranian doctor who was detained under section 3 of the Mental Health Act was on hunger strike and the NHS trust sought a declaration that he lacked capacity and that he could be given artificial nutrition and hydration. The judge held that he would not make an order under the Mental Health legislation nor under the Mental Capacity Act but under the inherent jurisdiction of the court to act in the best interests of Dr A and declared that it would be lawful for Dr A to be provided with artificial nutrition and hydration and to use reasonable force and restraint for that purpose even though there would be deprivation of liberty. It was subsequently reported that as a result of the feeding, Dr A's mental state improved and he recovered his capacity and returned to Iran.

In a case in 2000,[37] the Moors murderer Ian Brady, who was in Ashworth Special Hospital, applied to court to be allowed to starve himself to death. The court held that he did not have the mental competence to make that decision. The decision to commence force-feeding was in all respects lawful, rational and fair. Brady was incapacitated by his mental illness. The failed attempts by the Ashworth Special Hospital Authority to discover who had leaked information about Brady to a journalist are considered in chapter 8. Brady applied in 2013 to a Mental Health Review Tribunal to be transferred to prison. The tribunal did not accede to his request and he remained detained in hospital until his death in May 2017.[38] (The case is considered in chapter 19.)

Amputation of healthy limbs

Media attention has been given to the condition of body dysmorphic disorder, where the patient wishes to have his healthy limbs removed. A surgeon in Falkirk and District Royal Infirmary, in a private operation, removed one lower limb from each of two patients who suffered from this disorder.[39] The hospital has subsequently banned such operations. In the absence of any doctor prepared to amputate, patients are known to have shot their limbs off or committed suicide. The General Medical Council has offered ethical guidance and the Medical Defence Union has emphasised that the utmost caution should be taken by doctors considering such an operation. They must be certain that the operation is right and that the patient has had full counselling as to the consequences. Everything must be carefully documented.[40] The House of Lords has held that consent is not a defence to an offence of grievous bodily harm.[41]

Defences to an action for trespass to the person

Consent is the main form of defence to an action for trespass to the person. However, it is not the only one and Box 7.2 shows the other defences.

Box 7.2 Defences to an action for trespass to the person

1. Consent
2. Acting under a statutory power, e.g. Mental Capacity Act (see below), Mental Health Act 1983 (see chapter 19)
3. Making a lawful arrest
4. Parental powers (see chapter 13)

Patients Lacking Mental Capacity

This issue is considered below under the defence of statutory powers and also in chapter 19 in relation to mentally disordered persons. Where a patient lacks the capacity to give consent then treatment without consent may be given under statutory powers. Detention and compulsory treatment for mental disorder may be justified under the Mental Health Act 1983 (as amended by the 2007 Act) (see chapter 19). Alternatively, care and treatment can be given under the Mental Capacity Act 2005. Powers under this Act could be used not only if temporary restraint is justified in the interests of the patient but also if it is necessary to detain patients in hospitals or care homes when the use of the Mental Health Act powers is not required. This loss of liberty is possible under the Deprivation of Liberty Safeguards (Bournewood), which are explained below and considered in detail in chapter 16. In this chapter we look at the provisions of the Mental Capacity Act 2005 and the care and treatment of those adults who are incapable of giving the requisite consent.

Unconscious patients

It was mentioned earlier that the doctors and nurses in their duty of care for the patient may take life-saving action. This was originally on the basis of their common law powers (recognised in the *Re F* case)[42] to act out of necessity in the best interests of a mentally incapacitated adult, but is now on the basis of the statutory powers in the Mental Capacity Act 2005. The Act requires actions to be taken in the best interests of a person who lacks mental capacity and this requires ascertaining from relatives and friends information about the personal beliefs and views and feelings of the patient. Where serious medical treatment decisions are to be made on behalf of a person who lacks mental capacity, then in the absence of a relative or informal carer or person

Case 7.6 *Malette* v *Shulman* [1991]

Do not give me blood[43]

In a Canadian case, an unconscious patient was given a life-saving blood transfusion in spite of the fact that she was carrying a card refusing such treatment. She was awarded C$20,000. The doctor had ignored her written request not to give her blood and this constituted a trespass to her person.

who can be consulted on the person's best interests, an independent mental capacity advocate must be appointed to report on the patient's best interests (see below). This topic of lack of mental capacity is also considered in relation to the care of the elderly in chapter 18 and of those with learning disabilities in chapter 16. The legal situation relating to a patient in a persistent vegetative state is considered in chapter 28.

In this case, the card setting out the wishes of the patient acted as a living will or advance directive. These are now placed on a statutory footing under the Mental Capacity Act 2005 (see chapter 28).

Mental Capacity Act 2005

Where a practitioner takes measures to save the life of an unconscious patient, that is not a situation of implied consent, but a situation of necessity which is now covered by the Mental Capacity Act 2005. In such circumstances, the Mental Capacity Act 2005 recognises the duty of a professional to take action in the best interests of the patient following the accepted standard of care of the reasonable professional. The House of Lords had established the principle of acting out of necessity in the case of *Re F*,[44] which concerned the sterilisation of a woman who suffered from severe learning disabilities and who was incapable of giving consent. However, the principle of acting out of necessity where an adult was incapable of giving consent also applied to day-to-day care. In the case of a girl of 18 with an intellectual age of between 5 and 8, the Court of Appeal held that the court had the power under its inherent jurisdiction and in the best interests of that person to hear the issues involving her future and to grant the necessary declarations.[45] The House of Lords (in the Bournewood[46] case) also held that the common law powers can be used to detain a mentally incapable adult if that is in the person's best interests but this was overruled by the European Court of Human Rights[47].

Recommendations were made by Law Commission No. 231[48] for a statutory duty to replace this common law power, with specific requirements depending on the seriousness of the treatment to be undertaken. Following further consultation by the Lord Chancellor,[49] the government published its proposals for decision making on behalf of mentally incapacitated adults[50] and this was followed by a draft Bill.[51] The Bill was subject to scrutiny by a Joint Committee of Parliament[52] and revised in the light of its recommendations. The Mental Capacity Act 2005 came into force partly on 1 April 2007 and on 1 October 2007. The Act will be considered under the following headings:

Principles

Definition of mental capacity

Best interests

Code of Practice

Independent mental capacity advocate

Lasting powers of attorney

Court of Protection, deputies and the Office of Public Guardian

The Deprivation of Liberty Safeguards (Bournewood)

(In chapter 28 will be found a discussion of the statutory provisions for advance decisions. The Mental Capacity Act 2005 protections provided in relation to research on those lacking capacity can be found in chapter 17.)

Principles of the Mental Capacity Act 2005

The basic principles set out in section 1 of the Act are shown in Statute Box 7.2.

Statute 7.2
Principles set down in Section 1 of the Mental Capacity Act 2005

1. The following principles apply for the purposes of this Act.
2. A person must be assumed to have capacity unless it is established that he lacks capacity.
3. A person is not to be treated as unable to make a decision unless all practicable steps to help him to do so have been taken without success.
4. A person is not to be treated as unable to make a decision merely because he makes an unwise decision.
5. An act done, or decision made, under this Act for or on behalf of a person who lacks capacity must be done, or made, in his best interests.
6. Before the act is done, or the decision is made, regard must be had to whether the purpose for which it is needed can be as effectively achieved in a way that is less restrictive of the person's rights and freedom of action.

Definition of Mental Capacity

Sections 2 and 3 provide a statutory definition of mental capacity (see Statute Box 7.1). The definition is decision-specific, i.e. a person may have the capacity to make a decision on one matter but not on another. For example, a person with learning disabilities may be able to decide on the food to eat and clothes to wear, but not whether to have an operation for an appendectomy. In the case of *PH* v *Local Authority*[53] the Court of Protection held that PH, a 49-year-old man suffering from Huntington's disease, did not have the capacity to make decisions about his care and treatment and also about his future care and residence. The second declaration was to remain in force for six months. A final declaration was not to be made until all practical steps to assist him in acquiring the necessary capacity had been taken.

In contrast in the case of SB[54] the Court of Protection judge decided that a 37-year-old woman with bipolar disorder did have the mental capacity to make her own decisions and this included her wish to have a termination. The judge stated that:

> It seems to be, therefore, that even if aspects of the decision making are influenced by paranoid thoughts in relation to her husband and her mother, she is nevertheless able to describe, and genuinely holds, a range of rational reasons for her decision. When I say rational, I do not necessarily say they are good reasons, nor do I indicate whether I agree with her decision, for section 1(4) of the Act expressly provides that someone is not to be treated as unable to make a decision simply because it is an unwise decision.

(Holman J)

Best Interests

The Mental Capacity Act sets out the steps which must be taken in determining what are the best interests of the patient. They are shown in Statute Box 7.3.

Statute 7.3
Best interests

Section 4 of the Mental Capacity Act

1. In determining for the purposes of this Act what is in a person's best interests, the person making the determination must not make it merely on the basis of:
   (a) the person's age or appearance, or
   (b) a condition of his, or an aspect of his behaviour, which might lead others to make unjustified assumptions about what might be in his best interests.

2. The person making the determination must consider all the relevant circumstances and, in particular, take the following steps.

3. He must consider:
   (a) whether it is likely that the person will at some time have capacity in relation to the matter in question, and
   (b) if it appears likely that he will, when that is likely to be.

4. He must, so far as reasonably practicable, permit and encourage the person to participate, or to improve his ability to participate, as fully as possible in any act done for him and any decision affecting him.

5. Where the determination relates to life-sustaining treatment he must not, in considering whether the treatment is in the best interests of the person concerned, be motivated by a desire to bring about his death.

6. He must consider, so far as is reasonably ascertainable:
   (a) the person's past and present wishes and feelings (and, in particular, any relevant written statement made by him when he had capacity),
   (b) the beliefs and values that would be likely to influence his decision if he had capacity, and
   (c) the other factors that he would be likely to consider if he were able to do so.

7. He must take into account, if it is practicable and appropriate to consult them, the views of:
   (a) anyone named by the person as someone to be consulted on the matter in question or on matters of that kind,
   (b) anyone engaged in caring for the person or interested in his welfare,
   (c) any donee of a lasting power of attorney granted by the person, and
   (d) any deputy appointed for the person by the court, as to what would be in the person's best interests and, in particular, as to the matters mentioned in subsection (6).

> 8. The duties imposed by subsections (1) to (7) also apply in relation to the exercise of any powers which:
>   (a) are exercisable under a lasting power of attorney, or
>   (b) are exercisable by a person under this Act where he reasonably believes that another person lacks capacity.
> 9. In the case of an act done, or a decision made, by a person other than the court, there is sufficient compliance with this section if (having complied with the requirements of subsections (1) to (7)) he reasonably believes that what he does or decides is in the best interests of the person concerned.
> 10. 'Life-sustaining treatment' means treatment which in the view of a person providing health care for the person concerned is necessary to sustain life.
> 11. 'Relevant circumstances' are those:
>   (a) of which the person making the determination is aware, and
>   (b) which it would be reasonable to regard as relevant.

The implication of the statutory steps which must be taken in determining what are a person's best interests is a modified best interest test. For example, if a person, who was once a firm believer in the sin of any surgical intervention, lost the mental capacity to make their decisions, then their earlier views on non-surgical intervention would be taken into account in determining what was in their best interests.

In 2013 the Supreme Court held that in deciding whether medical treatment should be withheld from a person lacking the requisite mental capacity the focus had to be on whether it would be in the patient's best interests to give the treatment, rather than on whether it would be in his best interests to withhold it. The Supreme Court held that the Court of Appeal had been in error in using an objective approach to decide what the patient would think rather than the subjective test used by the trial judge.[55] The patient was a guitarist who had been treated for cancer of the colon but then suffered a serious infection. He lost the capacity to make his own decisions and the Trust sought a declaration that it would be in his best interests to have certain painful and deeply physical treatments withheld from him in the event of clinical deterioration. His family accepted that he would never return to full health but believed that he gained pleasure from his present life and would want it to continue. The judge held that it would not be appropriate to make the declarations sought. The Court of Appeal reversed the decision on the ground that futility was to be judged by the level of improvement the treatment would bring to the general health of the patient and recovery meant that the patient would recover to the extent that imminent death was averted. The patient died but the family wished the Supreme Court to hear the appeal.

Code of Practice

The Department for Constitutional Affairs (now absorbed in the Ministry of Justice) prepared guidance on the Mental Capacity Act in the form of a Code of Practice. There is a statutory duty for those professionals involved in the care of those lacking mental capacity to have regard to the Code of Practice (s. 42(4)). It can be accessed via the internet.[56] While not statutorily bound by the Code of Practice, informal carers and others caring for those lacking the requisite mental capacity should find it of assistance both in determining whether a person lacks capacity and also in deciding what are the person's best interests.

Independent Mental Capacity Advocate

Where serious medical treatment is proposed or accommodation arrangements are being made then, in the absence of an informal carer, relative or friend who can be consulted on behalf of a person lacking the capacity to make his or her own decisions, an independent mental capacity advocate (IMCA) must be appointed to report on the best interests of the patient. A report is given of one of the first situations where an IMCA was appointed where a patient had lost consciousness and had no meaningful brain activity and no next of kin had been traced.[57] The IMCA reported on the patient's best interests and the treating clinicians decided that antibiotics would not be administered for an infection and the patient passed away.

Lasting Power of Attorney

The Mental Capacity Act enables a person, when competent, to set up a lasting power of attorney (LPA) by which the donee of the power can make decisions on their behalf. Unlike the earlier enduring power of attorney, which could only relate to the delegation of decisions relating to property and affairs, the LPA can be set up for both property and affairs and also for decisions relating to personal welfare. There are different LPA forms for property and finance and for personal welfare. From 1 October 2007 enduring powers of attorney can no longer be set up, but those which are already in existence can continue to be used. There is one major difference between the two kinds of delegation. Although the donee under an LPA relating to property and affairs can exercise those powers while the donor still has the mental capacity to make their own decisions (for example, the donor might appoint an attorney to sell his house for him while he is abroad), the donee under an LPA relating to personal welfare decisions can only make decisions for the donor if the donor lacks the requisite mental capacity. Practical Dilemma 7.3 illustrates the effect of the appointment of an LPA for a patient in hospital. Further details and the forms to be completed can be obtained from the government website.[58]

Practical dilemma 7.3 — Lasting power of attorney

Meryl, the ward sister of a medical ward, was informed that a patient, Agnes, recently admitted with a severe chest infection and who appeared unable to make her own decisions, had set up an LPA giving the power to make personal welfare decisions to her daughter, Nicky. Meryl was concerned about whether Nicky could refuse antibiotics and resuscitation on Agnes's behalf if it were to be a life-saving necessity.

Nicky should be asked to show Meryl the LPA which Agnes has drawn up so that the specific instructions were made known to the ward team. Life-sustaining treatment, which was in her best interests, could only be refused on Agnes's behalf if she had specifically included that in the LPA, which had been appropriately drawn up, witnessed and registered. The LPA would only come into effect if Agnes lacked the capacity to make her own decisions.

Court of Protection, Deputies and the Office of Public Guardian

Another significant innovation of the Mental Capacity Act 2005 was the establishment of a new Court of Protection with the jurisdiction to make decisions relating to personal welfare as well as property and finance. (The predecessor Court of Protection could only cover issues relating to property and affairs.) The court can either make one-off decisions (with or without a court hearing) or appoint deputies with powers to make specific decisions on behalf of those lacking the requisite mental capacity who were over 16 years. Property decisions could be made on behalf of those under 16 years, if the mental capacity was likely to extend after they became 16 years. For example, if a young boy was badly brain-damaged in a road accident at 12 years old and received compensation from the driver responsible, decisions relating to the property and finances could be made by the Court of Protection while he was still under 16 years, because he was unlikely to recover his mental capacity. It might decide to appoint a deputy to make decisions relating to his finances. The Mental Capacity Act also made provision for an Office of Public Guardian. This keeps registers of deputies and LPAs and keeps a watching brief of their functioning. Complaints about the donee under an LPA who appeared not to be acting in the best interests of the donor could be made to the Office of Public Guardian which might decide to appoint a Visitor (General or Specific) to investigate the situation. The Court of Protection has opened its hearings to the public with reporting restrictions, and reports of cases can be accessed on its website. Further discussion of the Court of Protection and its role in property matters can be found in chapter 24 and from the Court of Protection website.[59] See also the website of 39 Essex Chambers.[60]

The Deprivation of Liberty Safeguards (Bournewood)

The European Court of Human Rights ruled that there was a breach of Article 5.4 of the European Convention on Human Rights where a person with learning disabilities, and incapable of consenting to the admission, was detained in a hospital without being placed under the Mental Health Act 1983.[61] The facts of the case are given in chapter 16 (Case 16.3). As a consequence of the case the UK government had to ensure that legislation was introduced to safeguard those who were incapable of giving consent to admission to hospitals and care homes but needed to be kept there for their safety, in a situation where the powers of detention under the Mental Health Act 1983 were inappropriate. Following extensive consultation the Department of Health decided in favour of amending the Mental Capacity Act 2005 to safeguard the rights of those kept in hospitals and care homes and ensure that there was no violation of Article 5. (See chapter 16 for further details of the Bournewood safeguards.) A Supreme Court decision on the right of those with severe disabilities to enjoy the protection of the Deprivation of Liberty Safeguards[62] is discussed in chapter 16 (Case 16.4).

Mental Health Act 1983

Justification for acting without the consent of a patient may also be provided by the Mental Health Act 1983 (as amended by the Mental Health Act 2007) and this is considered in chapter 19.

Giving information to a patient prior to consent being obtained

As has been mentioned, there are two main actions in relation to consent:

1. An action for trespass to the person.
2. An action in negligence for a breach of the duty of care to inform the patient.

We now turn to the action for negligence. The courts have made it clear that if a competent patient has given a willing consent for a procedure, then an action for trespass to the person cannot proceed. If the patient alleges that they were not given significant information about possible side effects, then the action will be one of negligence. This raises the question of how much information must be given to the patient. The leading case on this question is Case 7.7 presented here.

Case 7.7 *Sidaway v Bethlem Royal Hospital Governors* [1985]

Failing to inform[63]

Amy Sidaway suffered from persistent pain in her neck and shoulder and was advised by a surgeon to have an operation on her spinal column to relieve the pain. The surgeon warned her of the possibility of disturbing a nerve root and the possible consequences of doing so, but did not mention the possibility of damage to the spinal cord, even though he would be operating within 3 millimetres of it. The risk of damage to the spinal cord was very small (less than 1 per cent), but if the risk materialised, the resulting injury could range from mild to very severe. Amy consented to the operation, which was performed with due care and skill. However, in the course of the operation, she suffered an injury to her spinal cord that resulted in her being severely disabled. She sued the surgeon and the hospital governors, alleging that the surgeon had been in breach of a duty owed to her to warn her of all possible risks inherent in the operation, with the result that she had not been in a position to give an informed consent to the operation. Amy lost the case before the trial judge and her appeal to the Court of Appeal. She then appealed to the House of Lords.

The House of Lords held that her appeal should fail. Three of the judges held that the test of liability in respect of a doctor's duty to warn his patient of risks inherent in treatment recommended by him was the same as the test applicable to diagnosis of treatment, i.e. the doctor was required to act in accordance with a practice accepted as proper by a responsible body of medical opinion. This is known as the 'Bolam Test' (see page 50). Since the surgeon's non-disclosure of risk of damage to the plaintiff's spinal cord accorded with a practice accepted as proper by a responsible body of neurosurgical opinion, the defendants were not liable to the plaintiff.

The other two judges (Lord Scarman and Lord Templeman) were also of the opinion that Amy's appeal must fail since she had not proved on the evidence that the surgeon (who had died since the operation) had been in breach of duty by failing to warn her of the risks. Lord Scarman, while finding against her, alone of all the judges held that a patient had a right to give informed consent and he followed an American case,[64] where the 'prudent patient' test was applied to decide on the information a patient should be given prior to any consent, i.e. 'What would a reasonable prudent patient think significant if in the situation of this patient?' Lord Scarman concluded that:

> English law must recognise a duty of the doctor to warn his patient of risk inherent in the treatment which he is proposing, and especially so if the treatment be surgery. The critical limitation is that the duty is confined to material risk. The test of materiality is whether in the circumstances of the particular case the court is satisfied that a reasonable person in the patient's position would be likely to attach significance to the risk. Even if the risk be material, the doctor will not be liable if on a reasonable assessment of his patient's condition he takes the view that a warning would be detrimental to his patient's health.

Comment on the Sidaway Case

While the case was concerned with treatment by a doctor, the same principles would apply to treatment by any other professional. Although the judges turned down Amy's appeal, their reasons for doing so were extremely varied. The majority applied the Bolam Test of the accepted approved professional practice.

Even Lord Scarman, who used the 'prudent patient' test, still agreed that there may well be exceptions where the doctor is entitled to use 'therapeutic privilege' in deciding what to tell or what not to tell the patient prior to any procedure. This exception means that in the end the professional must follow the accepted approved practice in so far as it is applicable to the particular needs of that specific patient. However since the Montgomery ruling in 2015 (see later on in this chapter), Lord Scarman's 'prudent patient' test has been adopted by the courts.

The Sidaway case was cited and followed in the case of *Blyth* v *Bloomsbury Health Authority*.

Case 7.8 *Blyth* v *Bloomsbury HA* [1987]

Depo-provera[65]

In this case, a patient had been given an injection of Depo-Provera and claimed that she had suffered harm as a result of it and that knowledge that was possessed by hospital researchers about some of the side effects of the drug was not made known to her at the time that she was prescribed it. The Court of Appeal applied the Bolam Test and the Sidaway case to the facts and decided that there was no negligence by the doctors who cared for her in the information they gave to her. They emphasised that the extent of the duty to give information is to be judged in the light of the state of medical knowledge at the time and one must avoid the danger of being wise after the event. In addition, they refused to interpret the Sidaway judgments as implying that where the patient asked specific rather than just general questions this meant that the doctor is under an obligation to tell the patient all he knows about the subject.

> The amount of information to be given must depend on all the circumstances, and as a general proposition it is governed by what is called the Bolam Test.
>
> *(Lord Justice Neill)*

Another important point is that in subsequent cases (see below), the courts have held that the professional's duty is not divisible. Diagnosis, treatment, carrying out that treatment and informing the patient are all part of the doctor's duty of care and cannot be separated into different boxes. Informing the patient of risks is as much a part of the clinical judgement of the doctor as all his other tasks.

The general proposition therefore is that a person giving information to the patient must follow the reasonable standard of approved practice, i.e. the Bolam Test. However, in one case, a judge held that what was purported to be the approved practice was not acceptable.

Case 7.9 *Smith v Tunbridge Wells HA* [1994]

Failure to warn[66]

Evidence given by experts to the court suggested that a body of experienced competent surgeons would not have warned the patient of a risk of impotence from the operation. The judge disagreed with this and held that the failure to warn of the risk of impotence was neither reasonable nor responsible and the surgeon was therefore in breach of his duty to warn the patient.

In the following case, the court had to decide whether the doctors had followed the reasonable standard of care when they gave advice that the baby should not be induced.

Case 7.10 *Pearce v United Bristol Healthcare NHS Trust* [1998]

Clinical opinion[67]

Mrs Pearce was expecting her sixth child. The expected date of delivery was 13 November 1991, but it had still not arrived on 27 November. She begged the consultant to give her an induced labour or a Caesarean section. He suggested that she should have a normal birth and let nature take its course. He pointed out that it would be very risky to induce the birth and she would take longer to recover from a Caesarean. He did not tell her that there was an increased risk of a stillbirth as a result of the delay in delivery between 13 and 27 November. She accepted his advice. The baby died *in utero* some time between 2 and 3 December.

The trial judge dismissed the claim. The Court of Appeal dismissed the appeal. It applied the reasoning in the Sidaway case and held that this was a case 'where it would not be proper for the courts to interfere with the clinical opinion of the expert medical man responsible for treating Mrs Pearce'.

Subsequently the House of Lords had to decide if the patient has to prove that they would not have had the treatment had they known of the serious risks of harm.

Case 7.11   *Chester v Afshar* [2002]

Warning the patient of risks[68]

The patient suffered from severe back pain and gave consent to an operation for the removal of three intravertebral discs. The neurosurgeon failed to give a warning to her about the slight risk of post-operative paralysis, which the patient suffered following the operation. The trial judge held that the doctor was not negligent in his conduct of the operation, but was negligent in failing to warn her of the slight risk of paralysis which she suffered. He also held that, had she been aware of the risk, she would have sought advice on alternatives to surgery and the operation would not have taken place when it did, if at all. He therefore held that there was a sufficient causal link between the defendant's failure to warn and the damage sustained by the claimant and that link was not broken by the possibility that the claimant might have consented to surgery in the future. He gave judgment for damages to be assessed. The defendant appealed to the Court of Appeal which dismissed the appeal. The defendant then appealed to the House of Lords which by a majority verdict dismissed his appeal.[69]

The House of Lords held that the claimant had shown that had she been notified of the risk, which in fact occurred, she would have had to think further about undergoing the surgery and therefore she had established a causal link between the breach and the injury she had sustained and the defendant was liable in damages. Lord Hope's reasoning is shown in Box 7.3.

Box 7.3   *Chester v Afshar* (Lord Hope)

I start with the proposition that the law which imposed the duty to warn on the doctor has at its heart the right of the patient to make an informed choice as to whether, and if so when and by whom, to be operated on. Patients may have, and are entitled to have, different views about these matters. All sorts of factors may be at work here – the patient's hopes and fears and personal circumstances, the nature of the condition that has to be treated and, above all, the patient's own views about whether the risk is worth running for the benefits that may come if the operation is to be carried out. For some the choice may be easy – simply to agree to or to decline the operation. But for many the choice will be a difficult one, requiring time to think, to take advice and to weigh up the alternatives. The duty is owed as much to the patient who, if warned, would find the decision difficult as to the patient who would find it simple and could give a clear answer to the doctor one way or the other immediately.

To leave the patient who would find the decision difficult without a remedy, as the normal approach to causation would indicate, would render the duty useless in the cases where it may be needed most. This would discriminate against those who cannot honestly say they would have declined the operation once and for all if they had been warned. I would find that result unacceptable. The function of the law is to enable rights to be

> vindicated and to provide remedies when duties have been breached. Unless this is done the duty is a hollow one, stripped of all practical force and devoid of all content. It will have lost its ability to protect the patient and thus to fulfil the only purpose which brought it into existence. On policy grounds therefore I would hold that the test of causation is satisfied in this case. The injury was intimately involved with the duty to warn. The duty was owed by the doctor who performed the surgery that Miss Chester consented to. It was the product of the very risk that she should have been warned about when she gave her consent. So I would hold that it can be regarded as having been caused, in the legal sense, by the breach of that duty.

The outcome of *Chester* v *Afshar*, therefore, was that the appeal by the surgeon failed and the patient won the case.

The Supreme Court judgment made in the case of *Montgomery* v *Lanarkshire* [2015], reaffirmed the principles laid out in Chester; percentages of risk were dispensed with, and the Bolam principles no longer applied to information giving with regard toward patients with capacity. Rather:

> **The doctor is . . . under a duty to take reasonable care to ensure that the patient is aware of any material risks involved in any recommended treatment, and of any reasonable alternative or variant treatments. The test of materiality is whether, in the circumstances, of the particular case, a reasonable person in the patient's position would be likely to attach significance to the risk, or the doctor is or should reasonably be aware that the particular patient would be likely to attach significance to it.**[70]

Non-therapeutic procedures

It was suggested in a case in 1987 (see Case 7.12) that the principles set out in the Sidaway case did not apply where non-therapeutic care was being provided but this was not accepted by the Court of Appeal.

Case 7.12 *Gold v Haringey Health Authority* [1987]

Risk of sterilisation failing[71]

The claimant had two children and when she became pregnant with her third child agreed with her husband that they would have no further children after that pregnancy. She was seen by a consultant who suggested sterilisation following the birth of the child, but made no mention of the possibility of her husband having a vasectomy. Neither did he give her any warning of the risk of the sterilisation failing. The sterilisation operation was performed the day after the birth, but she subsequently became pregnant with her fourth child. She brought an action against the health authority alleging that there was negligence in failing to warn her of the risk of the operation failing and that the statement to her that the operation was irreversible amounted to a negligent misrepresentation.

The trial judge held that there was a distinction in the information that should be given in a non-therapeutic context compared with a decision on therapeutic treatment and that a sterilisation operation was non-therapeutic. He awarded her damages of £19,000. On appeal, the Court of Appeal held that the principles set out in the Sidaway case should apply in both contexts and it did not accept the validity of a distinction between therapeutic and non-therapeutic:

> The [Bolam] principle does not depend on the context in which any act is performed or any advice given. It depends on a man professing skill or competence in a field beyond that possessed by the man on the Clapham omnibus. If the giving of contraceptive advice required no special skill, then I could see an argument that the Bolam Test should not apply. But that was not, and could not have been suggested. The fact (if it be a fact) that giving contraceptive advice involves a different sort of skill and competence from carrying out a surgical operation does not mean that the Bolam Test ceases to be applicable. It is clear from Lord Diplock's speech in Sidaway that a doctor's duty of care in relation to diagnosis, treatment and advice, whether the doctor be a specialist or general practitioner, is not to be dissected into its component parts. To dissect a doctor's advice into that given in a therapeutic context and that given in a contraceptive context would be to go against the whole thrust of [the decision in Sidaway].

The judge should have accepted the body of responsible medical opinion on the standard that should have been followed in giving her information.

Giving information to the terminally ill patient

In research reported by the Marie Curie Palliative Care Institute in Liverpool and the Royal College of Physicians,[72] it was found that only 45 per cent of patients know that they are in 'the dying phase', compared with 80 per cent of their carers. The failure to inform patients was also evidenced in a report by the Royal College of Physicians in May 2014 which is considered in chapter 28.[73]

If a patient is terminally ill, should the nurse tell the patient contrary to medical advice? What is the position if the relatives do not wish the patient to be told?

Practical dilemma 7.4   Silence or lies?

Paul George has been operated on for 'ulcers'. Unknown to him, the surgeons actually found an inoperable tumour with wide spreading of the malignancy throughout the body. It is estimated that death is likely to occur in a few months. The consultant, who is normally in favour of a very open approach to patients, believes that Paul, who is 54, would not be able to cope with this news yet and he discusses this with Paul's wife, who agrees. The nursing staff are advised accordingly.

This kind of situation is in substance not unfamiliar to nursing staff and is repeated in different guises on many occasions. Unfortunately, however, it is the nursing staff who are most frequently with the patients and who are most likely to be asked: 'I don't have cancer, do I nurse?' or 'When am I likely to get out of here?' or 'Is it worth my while booking for this holiday next year?' and other direct or indirect questions designed to obtain a little more information for the patient as to where he stands. The questions that then arise in the nurse's mind are: Where does the patient stand in law? Does the patient have a legal enforceable right to obtain this information? What is the nurse's position in regard to the patient, the doctor and the relative?

Patient's Rights

As has been seen in the discussion thus far, there is a duty on professional staff when advising certain forms of treatment to ensure that the patient is notified of any material risks of substantial side effects. However, this duty on the professional used to be qualified by the power to withhold information in the rare cases where it was deemed to be in the patient's interest not to know. This was known as therapeutic privilege, and in previous years informing the patient that they are terminally ill may well have come under this heading. Thus, if, in the opinion of the doctor, it would be harmful to tell a patient such disturbing news, then the doctor could withhold such information on the grounds that they are acting in the patient's best interest.

Since the ruling from Montgomery the law is now less clear. A doctor may not withhold information about risks because he believes the patient would refuse consent if he were aware of them. There must be other reasons to justify withholding this information, and with the case of Montgomery the test to be used is the prudent patient test rather than the prudent doctor test – that being, as Lord Scarman referred to in Sidaway, would a reasonable patient agree with positional stance of the doctor/healthcare professional? If under the circumstances the prudent patient test showed that the patient has a right to be informed, the healthcare professional has no right to withhold information merely because they view it to be in the best interests of the patient. In the past paternalistic practice was accepted. In the twenty-first century, this practice is being challenged, often in the courts. With this in mind, the nurse needs to be very mindful of patient autonomy and its strengthening because of the Montgomery ruling. When examining consent issues and the withholding of information, it is no longer permissible for healthcare professionals (HCPs), including the nurse to utilise the Bolam principles (Bolam 1957) to justify their actions (where the actions of the HCP are judged to be of a sufficient standard (or not) by other HCPs), but instead it is for the prudent patient to determine. In other words if the ordinary patient would expect all material risks to be disclosed to them in relation to a proposed treatment, this is the minimum standard expected of the HCP; anything less can result in the HCP being held negligent for their actions (or omissions). Nurses need to remind colleagues of patient autonomy if a colleague is not involving the patient in their care, or not listening to the patient.

The consultant or general practitioner has clinical responsibility for the patient. If in the doctor's opinion the patient would be harmed by any disclosure and he has exercised his judgement on this in accordance with the approved professional practice, then that decision must be accepted and implemented by the rest of the team of professionals. The nurses might disagree with the decision and, of course, they may well have the opportunity of persuading the doctor to change his mind, based on their own personal knowledge of the patient, his needs and his own understanding. Ultimately, however, they would be obliged to defer to the clinical decision of the doctor. Any nurse who flagrantly went against the doctor's view on this might well face disciplinary proceedings. What is clear at the present is that in the absence of any absolute statutory provision for accessing information, patients do not have a clear right to obtain this information. It may be that future cases based on the Articles of the European Convention on Human Rights may hold that keeping significant information from patients is a breach of Article 3 or Article 8 (see website of this book).

The court has yet to deal directly with the question as to whether the patient has a right to be told and whether the doctor has a duty to tell when the patient is in a terminal condition. It is quite likely that if this is put before the courts, the court will apply the Bolam Test and leave it to the approved professional practice in relation to that particular patient. (The issue of obeying instructions is considered in chapter 4.)

Relatives' Rights

It is not uncommon for relatives, on hearing of a particularly upsetting diagnosis, to ask for the patient not to be informed of it 'because he could not cope with that yet'. Often, perhaps, it is not the patient's inability to deal with the information, but the relatives' inability to cope with the patient's knowledge of it. The conspiracy of silence thus begins. As far as the law is concerned, unless the patient is mentally incompetent, this should not arise. The patient is entitled to have information about him kept confidential (see chapter 8). It is a breach of this duty to the patient when the relative is told first. It is always open to the patient to say to the doctor, 'I would rather that my wife was not told about my diagnosis yet.' That is his right. Yet, when terminal illness or chronic sickness are concerned, the rules of confidentiality are broken and the relative is often informed first. Obviously, there are exceptions to this duty of confidentiality when the patient is too ill to be told and decisions have to be made that therefore involve the relative. However, that should be the exception.

Let us return to the situation of Paul George (Practical Dilemma 7.4). If the nurse has received clear instructions that Paul should not be told that he is terminally ill, the nurse should not act contrary to these instructions. Neither, however, should she lie to Paul. If Paul makes it clear that he is seeking more information, the nurse should arrange for Paul to speak with the doctor concerned and express to the doctor her own views of Paul's needs. Ultimately, the wife has no right to insist that information is withheld from Paul. Obviously, because of her knowledge of Paul, she should be involved in any discussions on the correct approach.

Notifying the patient of negligence by a colleague

If a colleague has been negligent or even acts criminally, should the nurse inform the patient? This is not a hypothetical question, as the cases of Beverly Allitt, Dr Shipman and the Francis Inquiry[74] into Mid Staffordshire NHS Trust (see chapters 2 and 5) show, and it sometimes happens that a nurse is aware that a mistake has been made and that neither patient nor relatives have been made aware of this, although they may realise that all has not gone according to plan. What is the nurse to do in these circumstances? Do they have a duty to inform the patient?

The nurse should take every action that they reasonably can to ensure that the patient is fully informed. Reference must also be made to the Code of Professional Conduct (2015) and the practitioner's duty to ensure that any untoward occurrences are brought to the attention of the appropriate officer. Under the 'preserve safety' heading (section 14) of the Code (2015), there is a requirement for registered nurses to 'be open and candid with all service users about aspects of care and treatment, including when any mistakes or harm have taken place'.

Where the nurse is herself at fault the NMC has made it clear that, where a practitioner has honestly admitted an error, she should be treated differently from a practitioner who has attempted to cover up a mistake.[75] NHS trusts and health authorities are required to establish procedures to implement the Public Interest Disclosure Act 1998, known as the whistleblower's charter. Guidance is given in HSC 1999/198 by the Department of Health on the implementation of this Act. Its aim is to protect any employee who brings a protected disclosure (e.g. a criminal offence, health and safety danger, failure to fulfil legal duty) to the attention of the appropriate person in the organisation from any victimisation. (This legislation is further discussed in chapter 4.) The Kennedy Report on Bristol paediatric heart surgery[76] recommended that there should be openness and honesty with patients. The Francis Report recommended that there should be a duty of candour on the individual but the government has instead opted for a duty of candour to be placed on the organisation and section 81 of the Care Act 2014 enables the appropriate regulations to be made (see chapter 5). The National Patient Safety Agency's effectiveness depends on health professionals being prepared to admit when hazards exist or where accidents have occurred. The Action for Victims of Medical Accidents is campaigning for a duty of candour to be included as one of the standards required for registration with the Care Quality Commission (CQC). They call it 'Robbie's Law', after Robbie Powell whose family fought for justice against cover-up and alleged fraud (Robbie Powell died in 1990 of Addison's disease which was not diagnosed, but suspected. The medical records were found to have been falsified. Subsequently the parents accepted an out-of-court settlement with the health authority, and have called for a public inquiry into his death and the post-death cover-up.) Barrister Nicholas David Jones conducted an inquiry which reported in February 2012 and the report was presented to the Welsh Assembly in July 2012 heavily redacted. Jonathan Evans MP, who has supported the Powell family, has called for greater openness in disclosing the reasons why failures occur and for a duty of candour to be recognised.

The CQC stated on its website that the 'CQC has been working closely with the Department of Health and the National Patient Safety Agency (NPSA) to address concerns about outstanding safety alerts. On 1 April [2010], CQC implemented a new regulatory scheme and now uses information about safety alerts to monitor standards in the NHS.'[77] The CQC's own problems with its own failures are considered in chapter 5. (See also chapter 12 and the reporting of safety alerts.)

No decision about me, without me

The White Paper *Equity and Excellence: Liberating the NHS* set out the government's vision of an NHS that puts patients and the public first, where 'no decision about me, without me' was the norm. It made proposals on giving everyone more say over their care and treatment with more opportunity to make informed choices, as a means of securing better care and better outcomes. The Department of Health (DH) issued two consultations: the first, *Greater choice and control* (2010) sought views on the choices people wanted to make and led to the introduction of choice in the providers of community services. The second (2012) was on how to make patient choice a reality in primary care, before diagnosis at referral and after diagnosis. The government published its response to the results of the latter consultation in December 2012.[78] It noted that the Health and Social Care Act 2012 made clear the duties on the NHS Commissioning Board and the clinical commissioning groups to promote the involvement of patients and carers in decisions about their care and treatment, and to enable patient choice. In addition the Care Act 2014 focused on the personalisation of care, with people, not institutions, in control. It also created a right to a care and support plan, which should be prepared in consultation with the person and carer. It also created a new entitlement to a personal budget (see chapter 22). A pledge was to be introduced into the NHS Constitution to involve patients in care planning discussions and to offer them a written record of what is agreed, if they want one. The NHS Commissioning Board will be held to account for delivering this. As part of the implementation strategy, the Department of Health's Choice Framework for NHS-funded care and treatment in England will set out the choices that people can expect to be offered, which will raise awareness of these choices, including where people have legal rights to make choices, as well as screening. The NHS Choice Framework can be found on the DH website and on gov.uk. The Department of Health also intended to establish regulations that would include requirements to safeguard patients' rights to exercise choice, and Monitor would oversee the regulations.

Conclusions

The government's strategy for the past two years has been to involve patients in the decisions relating to their care and to ensure that they have the necessary information. This has been bolstered by statutory duties placed on the NHS Commissioning Board, on the clinical commissioning groups, NHS Improvement and in the NHS Choice Framework and in revisions to the NHS Constitution. However, it is not clear that this explicit recognition of patients' rights provides any greater protection than the existing laws in relation to trespass to the person and the duty of care to inform. The new statutory provisions are likely to be enforced through the NHS complaints procedures and these have been notorious failures in ensuring that complaints are dealt with effectively and efficiently. (See chapter 26.)

The implementation of the Mental Capacity Act 2005 and the establishment of the new Court of Protection with its extended remit to cover personal welfare has had a radical impact on decision making on behalf of the mentally incapacitated. There should now be clear policies in place in each health and social care organisation. The consent forms used by health service organisations should have been amended to take account of the new legislation. Increasingly, too, it is likely that more relatives will have lasting powers of attorney in relation to decisions on personal welfare and more advance decisions will be created. (Advance decisions are considered in chapter 28.)

Reflection questions

1. What is meant by implied consent to treatment? Consider examples of implied consent from your own practice.
2. Consider the implications of the Mental Capacity Act for your particular specialty.
3. What is the difference between the 'Bolam Test' and the 'prudent patient' test so far as consent to treatment is concerned?

Further exercises

1. Refer to the specialist subject areas in Part II of this book and consider the principles that apply to consent by children under 16, consent by young persons of 16

and 17, consent by a person with learning disabilities and by a mentally disordered person and on behalf of an unconscious patient.
2. Consider the first Schedule to the Human Rights Act 1998 (see website of this book) and consider any other rights in relation to healthcare that you consider should be included.

References

[1] *Freeman* v *Home Office* [1984] 1 All ER 1036
[2] *R* v *Tabassum* [2000] 2 Cr App Rep 328
[3] Department of Health, Reference guide to consent for examination or treatment, DH, 2001; www.dh.gov.uk/consent
[4] Department of Health, Good practice in consent implementation guide, DH, November 2001, amendments 2009
[5] Department of Health, Reference guide to consent for examination or treatment, DH, 2nd edition 2009; www.gov.uk
[6] Department of Health, Information to assist in amending consent forms, DH, 2009
[7] *R* v *Brown and Others*, House of Lords, The Times Law Report, 12 March 1993
[8] *R* v *Cooper*, The Times Law Report, 7 August 2009
[9] *R* v *Williams*, 24 November 2004, Llanelli Magistrates unreported
[10] Department of Health, Reference guide to consent for examination or treatment, DH, 2nd edition 2009
[11] Bristol Royal Infirmary Inquiry (Kennedy Report), Learning from Bristol: the report of the public inquiry into children's heart surgery at the Bristol Royal Infirmary 1984–1995, Command paper Cm 5207, Stationery Office, London, 2001
[12] *Davis* v *Barking*, *Havering* and *Brentwood HA* [1993] 4 Med LR 85
[13] Department of Health, Reference guide to consent for examination or treatment, DH, 2nd edition 2009 (Paragraph 35); www.gov.uk
[14] *F* v *West Berkshire Health Authority* [1989] 2 All ER 545; [1990] 2 AC 1
[15] *O'Brien* v *Cunard Steamship Co.* (1891) 28 NE 266
[16] *Chatterton* v *Gerson* [1981] 1 All ER 257
[17] *Re MB (An Adult: medical treatment)* [1997] 2 FLR 426
[18] *St George's Healthcare NHS Trust* v *S* [1998] 3 All ER 673
[19] *Great Western Hospitals NHS Foundation Trust* v *AA and others* [2014] EWHC (Fam)
[20] *Re C (An Adult: refusal of medical treatment)* [1994] 1 All ER 819; (1993) 15 BMLR 77
[21] *NHS Trust* v *Ms T* [2004] EWHC 1279
[22] *Heart of England NHS Foundation Trust* v *JB* [2014] EWHC 342
[23] *The Mental Health Trust* and *Anor* v *DD and Anor* [2014] EWCOP 11
[24] *Re MB (An Adult: medical treatment)* [1997] 2 FLR 426
[25] *Re B (Consent to treatment: capacity)*, The Times Law Report, 26 March 2002; [2002] 2 All ER 449
[26] Jehovah's Witness mother dies after refusing blood transfusion after giving birth to twins, *Daily Mail*, 5 November 2007; ww.dailymail.co.uk/news/article-491791/Jehovahs-Witness-mother-dies-refusing-blood-transfusion-giving-birth-twins.html
[27] *In re T (An Adult: refusal of medical treatment)* [1992] 4 All ER 649
[28] *RT* v *LT & Anor* [2010] EWHC 1910 (Fam)
[29] *DH NHS Foundation Trust* v *PS* [2010] EWHC 1217
[30] *Dunhill* v *Burgin*, The Times Law Report, 28 March 2014 SC; [2014] UKSC 18
[31] *A Local Authority* v *SY* [2013] EWHC 3485

[32] *York City Council v C* [2013] EWCA 478
[33] *Leigh v Gladstone* (1909) 26 TLR 139
[34] *Secretary of State for the Home Department v Robb* [1995] 1 All ER 677
[35] *CIORAP v Moldova* [2007] ECHR 502
[36] *A NHS Trust v Dr A* [2013] EWHC 2442 (COP)
[37] *R v Collins, ex p Brady* (2001) 58 BMLR 173; [2000] Lloyd's Med Rep 355
[38] *Re Ian Brady* [2013] MHLO 89 (FTT)
[39] Gillian Harris, Surgeon happy he removed healthy limbs, *The Times*, 1 February 2000
[40] For further discussion of this topic, see Dimond, B., *Legal Aspects of Consent*, Quay Publications, Dinton, 2nd edition 2009
[41] *R v Brown and Others*, The Times Law Report, 12 March 1993 HL
[42] *F v West Berkshire Health Authority* [1989] 2 All ER 545
[43] *Malette v Shulman* [1991] 2 Med LR 162
[44] *F v West Berkshire Health Authority* [1989] 2 All ER 545
[45] *In re F (An adult: court's jurisdiction)*, The Times Law Report, 25 July 2000; [2000] 2 FLR 512
[46] *R v Bournewood Community and Mental Health NHS Trust ex parte L* [1999] AC 458
[47] *HL v United Kingdom* [2004] ECHR 720 Application No. 45508/99 5 October 2004; The Times Law Report, 19 October 2004
[48] Law Commission, *Mental Incapacity*, HMSO, London, 1995
[49] Lord Chancellor, Who Decides? Lord Chancellor's Office, Stationery Office, London, 1997
[50] Lord Chancellor, Making Decisions, Lord Chancellor's Office, Stationery Office, London, 1999
[51] Department of Health, Reference guide to consent for examination or treatment, DH, 2001; www.gov.uk
[52] House of Lords and House of Commons, Joint Committee on the Draft Mental Incapacity Bill Session 2002–3, HL paper 189-1; HC 1083-1
[53] *PH v Local Authority* [2011] EWHC 1704
[54] *SB (a patient, Capacity to consent to termination) Re* [2013] EWHC 1417
[55] *Aintree University Hospitals NHS Foundation Trust v James* [2013] UKSC 67
[56] www.gov.uk/government/publications/mental-capacity-act-code-of-practice
[57] Robert Tobin, Pioneering use of Independent Mental Capacity Advocate, *Clinical Risk*, 13(5):199, September 2007
[58] www.gov.uk/lasting-power-of-attorney
[59] www.gov.uk/court-of-protection
[60] www.39essex.com/court_of_protection/browse
[61] *HL v United Kingdom* [2004] ECHR 720 Application No 45508/99 5 October 2004; The Times Law Report, 19 October 2004
[62] *P (by his litigation friend the Official Solicitor) v Cheshire West and Cheshire Council and Anor* [2014] UKSC 19
[63] *Sidaway v Bethlem Royal Hospital Governors and Others* [1985] 1 All ER 643
[64] *Canterbury v Spence* [1972] 464 F 2d 772
[65] *Blyth v Bloomsbury Health Authority*, The Times Law Report, 11 February 1987; [1993] 4 Med LR 151
[66] *Smith v Tunbridge Wells Health Authority* [1994] 5 Med LR 334
[67] *Pearce v United Bristol Healthcare NHS Trust* (1998) 48 BMLR 118 CA
[68] *Chester v Afshar*, The Times Law Report, 13 June 2002; [2002] 3 All ER 552 CA
[69] *Chester v Afshar*, The Times Law Report, 19 October 2004 HL; [2004] UKHL 41; [2004] 3 WLR 927
[70] *Montgomery v Lanarkshire Health Board* [2015] UKSC 11

[71] *Gold* v *Haringey Health Authority* [1987] 2 All ER 888
[72] Rosemary Bennett, Patients 'not told they are dying', *The Times*, 5 December 2007
[73] Royal College of Physicians, Significant variation in standards of care for people dying in hospital, Press Release 14 May 2014
[74] Report of the Mid Staffordshire NHS Foundation Trust Public Inquiry, HC 947 February 2013, Stationery Office; www.midstaffspublicinquiry.com
[75] Nursing and Midwifery Council, Standards for medicines management, NMC, 2007
[76] Bristol Royal Infirmary Inquiry (Kennedy Report), Learning from Bristol: the report of the public inquiry into children's heart surgery at the Bristol Royal Infirmary 1984–1995, Command paper Cm 5207, The Stationery Office, London, 2001
[77] www.cqc.org.uk
[78] Department of Health, Liberating the NHS: No decision about me, without me, Government Response, December 2012

Chapter 8

Data Protection: Confidentiality and Access

This chapter discusses

- General Data Protection Regulation (including Data Protection Act 2018)
- Duty of confidentiality
- Caldicott Guardians
- Freedom of Information Act 2000
- DNA databases
- Access to Medical Reports Act 1988

Introduction

Two main laws regulate privacy and access to information: the General Data Protection Regulation that establishes principles for the control over and access to personal information, and the Freedom of Information Act 2000 which enables individuals to obtain, subject to major exceptions, information held by public bodies. This chapter explains these provisions in the light of the duty of confidentiality binding upon health professionals and the patient's right to access their health records.

General Data Protection Regulation (including Data Protection Act 2018)

The General Data Protection Regulation (UK GDPR) is European Union law that came into force in all member states, including the United Kingdom, on 25 May 2018. The UK GDPR will be supplemented by the Data Protection Act 2018 and together they replace the Data Protection Act 1998.

The UK GDPR sets out the law relating to the protection of personal data and brings data protection into line with other human rights and fundamental freedoms. The regulation applies to personal data that is either processed automatically or which forms part of or is intended to form part of a filing system, such as patient records. The UK GDPR unifies all EU member states' approaches to data regulation, ensuring all data protection laws are applied identically in every country within the EU. It gives greater rights to and protects EU citizens from organisations using their data irresponsibly and puts them in charge of what information is shared, and where and how it is shared.

Information Commissioner

The Information Commissioner's Office (ICO) will remain the overall policing authority in respect of these regulations in the United Kingdom. The ICO was established as an independent authority to uphold information rights in the public interest, and promote openness by public bodies and data privacy for individuals. Both the UK GDPR and Freedom of Information Act 2000 fall within the jurisdiction of the Information Commissioner (IC), together with the Environmental Information Regulations and the Privacy and Electronic Communications Regulations. Good practice notes, codes of practice and technical guidance notes on all this legislation are available on the IC's website.[1]

The ICO has legal powers to ensure that organisations comply with the legal requirements, and details of cases where these powers of enforcement have been used are available on the ICO website. An application for judicial review by the Secretary of State of an information tribunal decision which had quashed a ministerial certificate claiming exemption from providing subject access on grounds of national security failed. The High Court held that the IC had the power to check whether an exemption was properly claimed.[2] The powers of the IC were strengthened by the UK GDPR (see Breach of the UK GDPR below). Fines are part of the ICO's overall regulatory toolkit, which includes the power to serve an enforcement notice and the power to prosecute those involved in the unlawful breaches of the UK GDPR.[3]

Personal Data

The UK GDPR, article 4, defines data as any information relating to an identified or identifiable natural person known as the data subject.

Identifiable means the person can be identified either directly or indirectly by:

- name
- ID number
- location data
- online identifier
- one or more factors specific to the natural person's
  - physical,
  - psychological,
  - genetic,
  - mental,
  - cultural, or
  - societal identity.

The UK GDPR also defines special categories of personal data to which further requirements apply before processing is lawful. In general the processing of personal data is prohibited if it reveals the:

- racial or ethnic origin,
- political opinions,
- religious or philosophical beliefs,
- trade union membership,
- genetic data,
- biometric data for the purpose of uniquely identifying a natural person,
- data concerning health, or
- data concerning a natural person's sex life or sexual orientation.

Processing

Under the UK GDPR, processing means any operation or set of operations performed on personal data, whether or not by automated means, such as collection, recording, organisation, structuring, storage, adaptation or alteration, retrieval, consultation, use, disclosure by transmission, dissemination or otherwise making available, alignment or combination, restriction, erasure or destruction.

Obtaining, recording, sharing and storing of patient information – whether on paper or electronically – by nurses are everyday examples of data processing. Much of that data will be related to the health of the person, their religion, ethnic origin and in some cases the sexual orientation and sex life of the person so will fall into the special category of personal data.

UK GDPR principles

The UK GDPR, article 5, sets out principles relating to personal data. It requires that personal data shall be:

(a) processed lawfully, fairly and in a transparent manner;
(b) collected for specified, explicit and legitimate purposes;
(c) adequate, relevant and limited to what is necessary;
(d) accurate and, where necessary, up to date;
(e) stored for no longer than is necessary; and
(f) processed in a manner that ensures integrity and confidentiality.

Accountability

NHS Trusts, Health Boards and GP practices, as data controllers, are responsible for and must be able to demonstrate that they are complying with the principles of UK GDPR. As public bodies, NHS organisations are now required to appoint a data protection officer whose role is to ensure that a record is kept of what data is collected, what it is used for and the lawful reason for processing. This record must be available to the ICO. Where there is a breach of the UK GDPR, NHS organisations have a duty to report that breach to the ICO.

In some cases, NHS organisations will have to undertake Data Protection Impact Assessments where they undertake high-risk processing activities such as large-scale processing of sensitive data or large-scale automated profiling using sensitive data.

Where NHS organisations contract with other organisations to process data, they must ensure that they stipulate what processing can be undertaken, ensure that contractors are subject to a duty of confidence and ensure that appropriate security measures are in place to protect against a data breach. NHS organisations also have an obligation to assist contractors with Data Protection Impact Assessments, data subject access requests, upholding the rights of data subjects, submitting to audits, providing information and ensuring any breach of the regulation is reported to the ICO. At the end of the contract, data must be deleted or returned to the NHS organisation who initiated the contract.

Transparency

The transparency requirement of the UK GDPR, article 12, requires that NHS organisations have a duty to tell patients, as data subjects, why data is being collected in a concise, transparent, intelligible and easily accessible form, using clear and plain language, with particular provision made for any information addressed specifically to a child.

Nurses must ensure that any assessment forms, emails, questionnaires, surveys or other record they send to patients or ask patients to complete now have a privacy notice that complies with the requirements of the UK GDPR, article 13, by providing the following information:

About the organisation:

- Organisation and its contact details
- Details of representative if relevant
- Contact details of Data Protection Officer (DPO)

Purpose of collecting data:

- What data will be used for, including whether it will be used to make automated decisions
- The legal basis for using the data, including any legitimate interests relied on
- What categories of people will receive or have access to the data

Other information:

- Whether data will be sent or stored abroad and on what basis
- How long will it be stored
- Whether provision of data is required and consequences of not doing so

Rights:

- To withdraw consent for processing (where consent is used as the basis of processing)
- Of access, notification of erasure, restriction, objection and portability
- Right to lodge a complaint to ICO.

Lawful processing (UK GDPR articles 6 and 9)

The UK GDPR requires a lawful reason for the processing of personal data. Those lawful reasons are set out in the UK GDPR, article 6 and require that at least one of the following reasons apply:

(a) Data subject has given consent to the processing
(b) Processing is necessary under a contract to which the data subject is a party
(c) Processing is necessary for compliance with a legal obligation
(d) Processing is necessary in the public interest or exercise of official authority

(e) Processing is necessary for legitimate interests – this does not apply to public bodies such as statutory organisations and publicly funded contractors.

NHS Trusts, Health Boards and GP practices cannot therefore use the legitimate interests clause under article 6 as a lawful reason for processing personal data. They will have to rely on one or more of the other lawful reasons to justify the processing of information.

In many cases the data NHS organisations and their nurses process will be special category personal data relating to a person's health. The UK GDPR defines health data as:

personal data relating to the person's physical or mental health including the provision of health services that reveal information about the person's health status.

Special categories of personal data can be processed where:

- the data subject gives explicit consent,
- processing is necessary for employment law or trade union purposes,
- processing is necessary to protect the vital interests of a data subject who lacks capacity to give consent,
- processing is necessary for the functions of a legitimate association such as a church or other not-for-profit body,
- processing is necessary for legal proceedings and claims, or
- processing is necessary in the public interest.

For health purposes the UK GDPR, article 9(2)(h), allows the processing of special categories of personal data where it is necessary for:

- preventive or occupational medicine,
- the assessment of the working capacity of the employee,
- medical diagnosis,
- the provision of health or social care or treatment, or
- the management of health or social care systems and services.

Consent

The UK GDPR requires organisations that process personal data establish and publish the lawful basis that they are relying on for processing personal data. Consent and explicit consent are options for lawful processing of personal data and special categories of personal data under the UK GDPR but other lawful reasons are available to NHS organisations and in most cases consent is not the most efficient way to process data in the NHS.

Under article 4 of the UK GDPR consent must be:

- given by a statement or by a clear affirmative action, and
- freely given, specific, informed and unambiguous.

The UK GDPR, article 7, holds that consent is not regarded as freely given if the data subject has no genuine or free choice or is unable to refuse or withdraw consent without detriment. The article also holds that consent will not provide a valid legal ground where there is a clear imbalance between the data subject and the controller and in particular where the controller is a public authority.

As NHS organisations are public bodies it is unlikely that consent provides a lawful basis for processing personal data under the UK GDPR, article 6.

For the processing of health data as a special category of personal data, Article 9 of the UK GDPR requires that explicit consent is obtained from the patient. The ICO argues that explicit consent has to be expressly confirmed and recorded in writing, in a very clear and specific statement. This is likely to be impractical and even detrimental to a patient if it causes delay in the sharing of information.

Using consent as the lawful basis for processing personal data would also require NHS organisations to:

- facilitate withdrawal of consent – it must be as easy to withdraw as to give
- demonstrate that consent has been obtained
- ensure the availability of:
  - the right to erasure (where the subject withdraws consent and there is no overriding legitimate grounds to continue processing the data), and
  - the right to data portability.

Lawful basis for processing data in the NHS

Under the UK GDPR, articles 6 and 9, NHS organisations are able to rely on clauses for the lawful processing of personal and special category data other than consent. As a publicly funded health body the NHS and its organisations can rely on article 6(1)(e) for direct care and administration purposes as it allows processing that is 'necessary for the performance of a task carried out in the public interest or in the exercise of official authority'.

Where the direct care or administration concerns a special category of personal data, such as health data, then the NHS can rely on article 9(2)(h) that allows the processing of data for health purposes including 'medical diagnosis, the provision of health or social care or treatment or the management of health or social care systems'.

UK GDPR and the nurse's duty of confidence

The nurse's legal and professional duties of confidence to patients will not be affected by the UK GDPR unless their employing organisation uses consent as the basis for processing personal data. As this will not normally be the case, for the reasons set out above, the nurse will continue to be required to discharge their obligations under the duties of confidence by respecting patient confidences unless one of the exceptions to the duty applies.

Article 9(3) of the UK GDPR makes clear that the processing of data for health or social care purposes must be done by or under the responsibility of a professional under a professional obligation of secrecy under domestic law or rules established by national competent bodies (European Parliament and of the Council 2016). The nursing regulator is a national competent body for the purpose of the UK GDPR and the Nursing & Midwifery Council (NMC) Code (Nursing and Midwifery Council 2018) establishes a professional duty of secrecy through standard 5, that requires nurses to respect people's right to privacy and confidentiality.

Data Subject Rights

The UK GDPR, chapter III, sets out a range of rights for data subjects that NHS bodies as data controllers must respect and comply with:

- **Right to be informed:** This reflects the transparency principle and requires information, usually in the form of clear and concise privacy notices, to be provided to patients.

- **Right to access data held:** Patients continue to have the right to access data held about them. The time limit is now one month and there is no longer any fee for providing the information requested.
- **Right to rectification:** Data controllers, including NHS bodies, have to ensure that information is accurate. Patients have the right to require rectification of inaccurate personal data. NHS bodies must reply to the request for rectification within one calendar month.
- **Right to erasure:** The right to be forgotten is available for circumstances such as where the basis for lawful processing is consent and the subject withdraws consent, and there is no other legal ground for processing; the data subject objects and there are no overriding legitimate grounds (see below); the personal data have been collected in relation to information society services (commercial websites such as eBay); or the personal data are no longer necessary for the purposes for which they were collected.

  The right is not available in cases where the conditions relied upon for processing are for the performance of a task carried out in the public interest or for reasons of public interest in the area of public health in accordance with Art. 9(2)(h) or (i).
- **Right to restriction of processing:** Data subjects have the right to require data controllers to restrict processing where the accuracy is contested by the data subject; processing is unlawful, and the subject opposes erasure; the data controller no longer needs the data, but the subject requires it to be kept for legal claims; or the data subject has objected, pending verification of legitimate grounds.
- **Right to data portability:** Data subjects have the right to receive personal data about them in a commonly used and machine-readable format but only where the processing is based on consent and the processing is automated.
- **Right to object to processing:** In health and social care this would apply where the lawful basis for processing was the performance of a task in the public interest or exercise of official authority. Where a patient objects, an NHS organisation must not continue to process data unless it can demonstrate compelling legitimate grounds for the processing which override the interests, rights and freedoms of the individual or for the establishment, exercise or defence of legal claims. The right to object does not apply where the data processing is for statistical or research purposes.
- **Right to object to processing for direct marketing:** This is absolute and the processor would need to stop processing.
- **Right not to be subject to decision based on automated processing, including profiling:** Data subjects have the right not to be subject to a decision based solely on automated processing, including profiling, which produces legal effects concerning them, or similarly significantly affects them.

In addition to these rights the UK GDPR, article 25, stresses the need for NHS organisations to ensure that there are measures in place to minimise the risk to data subjects' rights in the design and operation of their data processing activities. Only personal data that is necessary for each specific purpose should be processed under the concept of data minimisation. NHS organisations should also consider pseudonymisation to achieve this where possible. The UK GDPR, article 4, defines this as:

> the processing of personal data in such a manner that the personal data can no longer be attributed to a specific data subject without the use of additional information, provided that such additional information is kept separately and is subject to technical and organisational measures to ensure that the personal data are not attributed to an identified or identifiable natural person.

Breach of the UK GDPR

If a breach of security leads to data being destroyed, lost, altered, unauthorised disclosure or access to personal data then the NHS body must report the breach to the ICO within 72 hours of discovery unless the breach is unlikely to result in risk to rights and freedoms of persons.

The breach must also be reported to data subjects if it is likely to result in a high risk to rights and freedoms of persons. There is no time limit on when this must be done, but the UK GDPR requires it to be carried out without undue delay.

Increased penalties have been introduced for any breach of the UK GDPR.

A fine of up to 10 million euros can be levied by the information commissioner for:

- Failure to maintain records of processing activities;
- Failure to report breach; or
- Failure to implement appropriate technical and organisational measures.

A more severe fine of up to 4 per cent of global annual turnover or 20 million euros (whichever is greater) can be levied for:

- A breach of basic principles for processing;
- A breach of data subjects' rights; or
- A breach of obligations regarding international transfers.

Human Rights

The UK GDPR must be read in conjunction with the Human Rights Act 1998 (see chapter 1), since Article 8 recognises an individual's right to private and family life (see website of this book). The Freedom of Information Act 2000 gives a right of access to information held by public authorities, but this is subject to many exceptions, including personal information where the UK GDPR applies (Freedom of Information Act 2000, section 40). The courts have issued injunctions to grant people lifetime anonymity. Thus, where two young boys had been convicted of killing James Bulger, a toddler, there was a fear for their safety (and therefore their Article 2 rights were at stake) if their new identities were disclosed, and an injunction was ordered forbidding disclosure of their identities;[4] a woman who had been convicted of manslaughter for killing two young children when she was 11 years old succeeded in obtaining an injunction to protect the privacy of herself and her daughter. There was no real fear of danger to her life (and therefore Article 2 rights), but her right to private and family life under Article 8 was threatened.[5] The Supreme Court held that the automatic release of a person's convictions, cautions and warnings regardless of the length of time that had elapsed, when that person was required to obtain an enhanced criminal record certificate for the purposes of obtaining employment which involved working with children or other vulnerable persons was incompatible with their Article 8 right to respect for their private life.[6] The European Court of Human Rights held that journalists were entitled to protection under Article 10 (freedom of expression) and were not required to disclose the source of their information.[7] The public interest in the protection of journalists' sources was sufficient to outweigh any threat of damage through future dissemination of a company's confidential information. In a case in 2010 the Court of Appeal held that confidentiality of commercial information could be seen as a possession and under the Human Rights Act private and public interests had to be balanced in the interests of proportionality.[8] The dispute about the use of super-injunctions, where the very existence of the application for an injunction cannot be mentioned, is still unresolved despite the Master of the Rolls Lord Neuberger's report in May 2011.

In May 2014 the Supreme Court held that courts had an inherent jurisdiction under the common law and statutory power to depart from the principle of open justice and interfere with the right of freedom of expression by prohibiting the publication of names and other details in court proceedings if that was necessary in the interests of justice or for the protection of an individual. The BBC were prevented from identifying an immigrant who had committed sexual offences and feared for his safety if his identity was known when deported.[9]

In 2014 the European Court of Justice[10] held that Google, as an internet search engine, had a legal duty to remove search results that are 'inadequate, irrelevant or no longer relevant, or excessive', i.e. there is a *right to be forgotten*. This right has now been included in the UK GDPR as one of several rights given to data subjects.

Duty of confidentiality

The patient is entitled to confidentiality of the information about them. There is therefore a duty on every nurse and indeed every employee to ensure confidentiality of information. The duty arises:

1. From the duty of care in negligence (discussed in chapter 3).
2. From the implied duties under the contract of employment (see chapter 10).
3. From the duty to keep information that has been passed on in confidence, confidential, even when there is no pre-existing relationship or legally enforceable contract between the parties (a duty based on equity and only recently recognised by the courts and discussed in the case of *Stephens* v *Avery and Others*).[11]
4. From requirements by professional registration bodies as part of the professional conduct, such as the Nursing and Midwifery Council.

In the case of Naomi Campbell, the House of Lords in a majority decision held that even though she had brought into the public domain the fact that she was being treated for drug addition, certain information could still be kept confidential, including the time, form and place of the drug therapy, and she was therefore entitled to damages against the Mirror Group Newspapers (MGN) for that breach of confidence.[12] In this respect her right to privacy succeeded against the right to freedom of expression under Article 10. Article 8 rights were also upheld in a case brought by Max Mosley against the *News of the World* which published accounts of his alleged sadomasochistic sex sessions. The judge decided that there was no evidence of Nazi behaviour and his private rights under Article 8 should be upheld. There was no public interest which justified a breach of Article 8.[13] The European Court of Human Rights held that secret interception by the Ministry of Defence of the external communications of Liberty were not dealt with adequately under the Interception of Communications Act 1985 with sufficient clarity to give individuals protection and there was therefore a breach of Article 8 rights.[14]

A complaint was made about a consultant psychiatrist who read notes and discussed patients while on public transport. She admitted the confidentiality breaches, apologised and promised not to repeat the conduct. She was referred to a disciplinary panel but argued that the 'fair blame' procedure should be implemented. The Court of Appeal held that the case manager had been entitled to regard a breach in a public place as a potentially serious offence and was justified in referring the case to a disciplinary hearing.[15]

Under the duties implied in the contract of employment, the employee has a responsibility to the employer to keep information acquired from work confidential (see chapter 10). For the nurse, too, that duty is also spelled out by The Code: Professional standards of practice and behaviour for nurses and midwives[16] (see Box 8.1). (See Box 8.2 on page 190 for exceptions to the duty of confidentiality.)

> **Box 8.1 The code: Professional standards of practice and behaviour for nurses and midwives**
>
> ## Respect people's right to privacy and confidentiality
>
> As a nurse or midwife, you owe a duty of confidentiality to all those who are receiving care. This includes making sure that they are informed about their care and that information about them is shared appropriately.
>
> To achieve this, you must:
>
> - respect a person's right to privacy in all aspects of their care
> - make sure that people are informed about how and why information is used and shared by those who will be providing care
> - respect that a person's right to privacy and confidentiality continues after they have died
> - share necessary information with other healthcare professionals and agencies only when the interests of patient safety and public protection override the need for confidentiality, and
> - share with people, their families and their carers, as far as the law allows, the information they want or need to know about their health, care and ongoing treatment sensitively and in a way they can understand.

While this code is not enforceable in a court of law, it reflects what the law upholds and is used by the NMC and its committees as a guideline in determining whether the nurse is guilty of professional misconduct and therefore whether their fitness to practise is impaired. Difficulties arise not in understanding the duty of confidentiality, but in knowing when the exceptions arise and in what circumstances breaking the duty is permissible. The NMC has produced an advice sheet providing guidance on confidentiality and the circumstances in which disclosure is justified.[17]

In a case brought by Ashworth Hospital against MGN, the judge made an order requiring the newspaper group to disclose to the hospital the identity of the source of their information about a convicted murderer who was a patient at Ashworth. The Court of Appeal upheld this judgment, holding that the protection of patient information was of vital concern to the NHS.[18] MGN disclosed that the clinical notes had been received from a freelance investigative journalist, Mr Ackroyd. He then refused to identify his sources within the hospital. The hospital then sought an order requiring him to disclose the source of the notes. Mr Ackroyd stated that although he had been paid £1250 from the *Daily Mirror*, his sources at the hospital had not received any payment and were not motivated by financial gain, but to reveal publicly the way in which Ian Brady had been treated.

The Court of Appeal held that the protection of journalistic sources was one of the basic conditions of press freedom and the hospital had to establish an overriding public interest amounting to a pressing social need to which the need to keep press sources confidential should give way. The current case was different from the original MGN case, since as a journalist he was entitled to present different evidential material from a different perspective. The passage of time since the original case meant that there was no cloud of suspicion that was still blighting activity at the hospital and there had been no breach of confidentiality.[19] On 27 July 2007 the House of Lords refused leave to appeal against the Court of Appeal decision. Robin Ackroyd was thus not forced to disclose the source of his information.

The High Court has also recognised that in exceptional circumstances the court has the jurisdiction to extend the protection of confidentiality of information even to the extent of imposing restrictions on the press where a failure to do so would probably lead to serious physical injury or the death of the person seeking that confidentiality. Thus it granted an injunction to prohibit the publication of the details of the boys who killed James Bulger.[20]

In 2003 the DH issued an NHS Confidentiality Code of Practice.[21] This supersedes the earlier advice on the protection and use of patient information issued in 1996 and is quoted in new guidance from NHS England in a Confidentiality Policy.

In 2013 NHS England published a Confidentiality Policy, the purpose of which was to lay down principles that must be observed by all who work within NHS England and have access to person-identifiable information or confidential information. A summary of Dos and Don'ts is set out in Appendix A. Appendix B sets out the legal framework and the Caldicott principles.

National Data Opt-out

The national data opt-out was introduced on 25 May 2018, providing a facility for individuals to opt-out from the use of their data for research or planning purposes. NHS Digital takes the lead on implementation of the national data opt-out. Individual person preferences are being collected from 25 May 2018 and by 2020 all health and care organisations are required to have applied these preferences in all research and planning situations in which confidential patient information is used. NHS Digital will apply these preferences with immediate effect.

The national data opt-out will replace the previous 'type 2' opt-out, which required NHS Digital to refrain from sharing a patient's confidential patient information for purposes beyond their direct care. Any person with an existing type 2 opt-out will have it automatically converted to a national data opt-out from 25 May 2018.

The national data opt-out choice can be viewed or changed at any time by using the online service at www.nhs.uk/your-nhs-data-matters.

NHS Digital also provides guidance on the national data opt-out to nurses on their website.[22]

Exceptions to the Duty of Confidentiality

In chapter 5 of the Review of Information Governance carried out by Dame Fiona Caldicott in 2012[23] (see page 203) four legal bases for processing personal confidential data are identified. They are: the consent of the patient, statutory provisions, court order and in the public interest. These have been expanded for the purpose of this chapter and are shown in Box 8.2.

Box 8.2 Exceptions to the duty of confidentiality

1. Consent of a patient.
2. Interests of patient.
3. Court orders:
    subpoena
    civil procedure rules.
4. Statutory duty to disclose:
    Road Traffic Act 1988 (as amended)
    Prevention of Terrorism (Temporary Provisions) Act 1988
    Public Health Acts
    Misuse of Drugs Acts
    Health and Social Care Act 2008.
5. Public interest.
6. Police.
7. UK GDPR and Data Protection Act 2018 provisions.

Consent of the patient

The duty is owed to the patient and it is therefore in the power of the mentally capacitated patient to authorise disclosures to be made. Thus announcements to the press, notification of relatives and spouses and provision of information to a solicitor or to an insurance company are all legitimate disclosures with the consent of the patient. If the patient is unconscious and an adult, the consent of the relatives is often used to justify disclosure on behalf of the patient, but there may well be little justification for this in law, unless the patient has appointed that relative as his agent and given him that authority. The Court of Appeal held that no confidentiality arose in relation to a decision made by the Law Society on the outcome of a complaint made about a solicitor.[24] Similarly, if a patient wished to give details about a complaint he had made about his healthcare, subject to the laws of defamation, he would be legally able to do so. In contrast, if anyone else published details of the complaint without the patient's consent, this would be a breach of confidentiality.

Practical Dilemma 8.1 Spouse's confidence

Annabel was involved in a serious road accident and admitted to hospital. While on the orthopaedic ward, a telephone request came in asking for information on her progress. The nurse taking the call asked who the caller was. The answer was 'her husband'. The nurse then gave the caller full details of Annabel's progress. She then told Annabel that her husband had phoned, asking for information about her; the nurse was surprised at Annabel's fury. It appeared that she had recently separated from him, she had not notified him of where she was now living and did not want any communication with him because of his violence.

The difficulties of the nurse's position in a situation like this are easily understood. In 99 out of 100 cases, Annabel would be delighted to receive a message of concern and interest. However, it is the 100th case that causes concern and procedures have to be established to prevent any unauthorised information being disclosed. Annabel is entitled to withhold information of her condition from her relatives and friends. In some cases, even an acknowledgement that a patient is on a particular ward, e.g. psychiatric or gynaecology (abortion), might be an unwarranted disclosure. In Practical Dilemma 8.1, the nurse was at fault in not checking with Annabel first and it is now standard practice not to disclose information over the phone unless checks on the caller have been made and the patient is agreeable to the information being given.

There can often be a problem in caring for elderly patients where the patient has made a special request to the nurses that the relatives should not be told about their condition. However, it can give rise to additional problems for staff. 'Where do I stand if I do not contact the relatives regarding the condition of the elderly patient because the elderly patient has asked me not to do so?' is a not infrequent question. Applying the principles discussed here, the patient does have the right to refuse to allow this information to be passed on. However, if the relatives are to care for the patient eventually, there may well be information that they need to know for the patient's own safety and thus disclosure is justified in the interests of the patient (see below).

Disclosure refused by the patient

In the following case the patient refused to permit disclosure of her records to her employer.

Case 8.1 *Nicholson v Halton General Hospital NHS Trust* [1999]

Waiver of patient's right to confidentiality[25]

The claimant issued proceedings against her employer, alleging that she had sustained radial tunnel syndrome in her right wrist as a result of his negligence in requiring her to perform repetitive movements at work. She had undergone a remedial operation and the employer wished to have details of the reasons for the operation and the nature of the condition. She refused to give permission for the employer's legal and medical advisers to discuss the operation with her consultant. The employer sought an 'unless' order from the court, that unless she provided the necessary consent, the proceedings would be stayed. Her consultant also stated that he would not become involved unless instructed by the court. The judge refused the 'unless' order.

The Court of Appeal upheld the appeal and granted the 'unless' order. It stated that the court could not order a claimant to waive her right of confidentiality, but could stay proceedings until the claimant waived the right of confidentiality. Information requested from a claimant in a case of this kind should be confined to that which was relevant to the issues between the parties and a claimant could not restrict the information requested to a written rather than an oral form.

Disclosure to the press

Exactly the same principles apply when the press are asking for information about a patient. If the patient consents, the information can be given. If the patient refuses, then no information should be given and this includes a condition check, where the press phone up to find out the latest condition of the patient. Where the patient is unconscious, confidentiality should be respected.

Disclosure in the interests of the patient

Disclosure between professionals caring for the patient is justified on the basis that if information obtained by the doctor and relevant to the care of the patient is not passed on to the appropriate professional, then the patient might suffer. An obvious example is the patient's history of allergy to certain medication: if the pharmacist and the nurse were not told of a known allergy or allowed to see the records, they would be unable to ensure that the patient was given appropriate medication. Traditionally, nurses have not usually had difficulties over access to the patient's records. Other professional groups have encountered difficulties: occupational therapists, physiotherapists, social workers and other groups have sometimes been refused access to the patient's records on the grounds that it is unnecessary and also a breach of confidentiality. This is a difficult problem. On the one hand, the wider the range of people who have access to the medical records of the patient, the more difficult it is to maintain the duty of confidentiality. On the other hand, there are many situations where a professional caring for the patient, in ignorance of certain facts known to the doctor, could do the patient considerable harm.

The problem becomes even more complex when we consider the question of how much confidential information should be given to a volunteer who is taking the patient out. For example, if the volunteer is taking a patient with learning disabilities out for the day, it might be vital in the interests of the safety of the patient to advise the volunteer that the patient is epileptic and to ensure that the volunteer would know how to cope should the patient have a fit. Contrariwise, the fact that the patient had an abortion five years ago would be irrelevant and thus would be a disclosure that would not be justified in the interests of the patient.

In conclusion, it could be said that disclosure of confidential information to others is justified if it is necessary in the interests of the health and/or safety of the patient or the professional. Those to whom this information is disclosed would themselves be subject to the same duty of confidentiality. AIDS/HIV has raised many significant problems in this field and these are discussed further in chapter 25. The UK GDPR does not change the nurse's duty of confidence or their ability to share clinical information about a patient with others professionally involved in the care of that patient unless the NHS body is relying on consent as the lawful reason for processing personal data. Although the implied consent on which such disclosures are based would not meet UK GDPR requirements, the data processing of such information is lawful under the UK GDPR, article 9, for the provision and management of health and social care. The right to access records in the interests of the patient does not cover 'snooping'. A nurse faced fitness proceedings before the Conduct and Competence Committee because she abused her position by checking the medical records of a patient who was having an affair with her husband, a GP. She looked at the woman's computer records 230 times in two years. She was allowed to stay on the Register because her misconduct was during a sustained period of personal stress and was unlikely to recur.[26]

Court orders

Subpoena

This is an order made by the court, which must be obeyed under threat of punishment for contempt of court.

The court has the power to **subpoena** any relevant evidence or witnesses in a case in the interests of justice. The court can also place conditions on an order for disclosure, as in the case of *A Health Authority* v *X*.[27] In this case, the health authority received information about a child protection case from the local authority from which it considered that there had been possible medical malpractice. The health authority sought an order for production of certain case papers, which the judge allowed and ordered the respondent doctor to produce the medical records. The judge placed certain conditions on the order to ensure the confidentiality of the documents and to prevent disclosure to third parties without the permission of the court. The health authority appealed against these conditions, but the Court of Appeal held the judge had been correct to exercise his discretion to impose conditions on the orders for disclosure.

There are only two exceptions to the power of the court to order disclosure and these are known as being privileged from disclosure.

Privilege on grounds of public interest (sometimes known as public interest immunity). An example of public interest protected from an order for disclosure is national security. It would usually be claimed by a minister of the Crown when a certificate is signed to the effect that disclosure of a particular document or information would be contrary to the public interest. Following the Scott Inquiry into the Matrix Churchill case, it was recommended that **privilege** on the grounds of the public interest should not be claimed when prosecution of a criminal offence was being brought. The House of Lords laid down guidelines for claiming privilege on grounds of public interest in a case in 2004.[28] It stated that withholding information (as an exception to the golden rule of disclosure) may be justified but it always had to be the minimum necessary to protect the public interest in question and could never imperil the overall fairness of the trial. Further clarification of the issue can be found on the Serious Fraud Office website.[29]

Legal professional privilege This second exception to the power of the court to order disclosure covers communications between client and legal adviser where litigation is envisaged or is taking place. In the interests of total disclosure between client and lawyer, and in the advancement of justice, these communications are free from an order of discovery or disclosure. Difficulties have arisen over the disclosure of statements taken from witnesses to an accident that might be used later in any court proceedings. Are such statements protected from disclosure on the grounds of legal professional privilege?

In the case of *Waugh* v *British Railway Board*,[30] it was held that where a document comes into being after an accident and where there are two purposes for its use (e.g. management purposes to ensure that the accident does not happen again and legal purposes to defend any potential action), then if the dominant purpose is for management purposes, the document is not privileged from disclosure under the rules of professional legal privilege. This ruling by the House of Lords was upheld in the following case.

Case 8.2   *Lee v SW Thames RHA* [1985]

Disclosure[31]

Marlon Lee, a young boy, was severely scalded and was initially treated in a hospital run by one health authority, then subsequently transferred to a burns hospital run by another district authority. Shortly afterwards, he developed breathing problems and was transferred to the first hospital by the ambulance that came under the South West Thames Regional Health Authority. He suffered brain damage, which was considered to be due to lack of oxygen. The mother asked for disclosure of the ambulance report produced by the regional health authority for the first hospital, but was refused it. Her application to the court for disclosure failed on the basis that the report was prepared in contemplation of litigation and to assist the legal advisers and disclosure could not be ordered even though it had been initiated as a result of the request by the first hospital authority, not by the authority responsible for the ambulance service.

This case shows the disadvantages faced by potential litigants since the health authority or NHS trust is, of course, both custodian of the records and a potential defendant, and can use its first function to enable it to have immediate access to all the relevant records.

The test to decide whether communication between a solicitor and his client was privileged from disclosure was to consider whether it was made confidentially for the purposes of legal advice, constructing such purposes broadly.[32] A person could agree to a partial waiver of the right to legal professional privilege without having to lose the right entirely.[33] Section 42 of the Freedom of Information Act recognises the exception of legal professional privilege and an Awareness Guidance note is available from the Information Commissioner's website.[34] The court held in March 2008 that the mention of a document in a written statement did not constitute an automatic waiver of legal professional privilege so as to entitle the other party to inspect it.[35] The House of Lords held in March 2009 that covert surveillance of communications between clients and their lawyers was permitted under the Regulation of Investigatory Powers Act 2000 and was not protected by legal professional privilege notwithstanding any statutory rights of persons in custody to consult their lawyers in private.[36]

Apart from these exceptions, the judge has the power to order the production of any evidence relevant to the case. There is no recognition of the privilege of confidential medical information, neither do the courts recognise the secrecy of the confessional. In the case of *Deacon* v *McVicar*[37] (see Case 4.11, page 93), the judge ordered the production of the records of other maternity patients.

Health visitors are more likely than any other group of nurses to be summoned by subpoena to appear in court. They had adopted a procedure whereby they would normally require service of a subpoena before giving evidence in court. In this way, they were able to make it clear to their clients that they had no option but to attend court and were obliged to disclose confidential information. The Children Act 1989 has led to health visitors giving evidence in the interest of the child without waiting for a subpoena.

Disclosure in personal injury cases

Disclosure can be made of relevant records under the Supreme Court Act 1981, sections 33 and 34: section 33 enables disclosure to be made between parties to a case before litigation commences; section 34 enables an order for disclosure to be made against a third party. In addition, as a result of pressure from the Health Service Commissioner and also from judges in several cases where there has been evidence of unnecessary delay in the production of medical records, NHS trusts nowadays rarely wait to be issued with an order for disclosure, but are more likely to produce the relevant documents when the solicitor requests them. Access by the claimant can be sought under the statutory provisions of the data protection legislation. In addition, the Woolf reforms in civil justice have led to earlier disclosure of relevant information as part of the pre-action protocol (see chapter 6).

Disclosure before trial

In addition to the rules under the Supreme Court Act 1981, the rules of the High Court enable an order for relevant information to be made once the claim form has been issued and the case commenced. This order for the production of documents is part of the exchange of information that takes place between the parties before the hearing takes place in the court. The aim is to ensure that the parties understand the main points in dispute and are not surprised when the oral hearing takes place. The days in court should thus be kept to a minimum and should take place only when there really is an outstanding issue between the parties. As a consequence of the changes to the civil law procedure following Lord Woolf's report on access to justice, the emphasis is on openness between the partners and early disclosure between them of all relevant information, including the reports of experts. Under the new system of case management by the courts introduced under the new Civil Procedure Rules, directions have been given to facilitate the exchange of information and the progress of the case (see chapter 6).

In exceptional circumstances, the court could order disclosure to a person who was neither a party to the case nor a lawyer. Thus, in the case over the alleged harm caused by the drug Opren, the Court of Appeal allowed disclosure to the medical and scientific journalist and writer who was assisting the many claimants in their case against Eli Lilly.[38]

Although not a court, the Health Service Ombudsman has the power to order the production of documents, including personal health records and the attendance and examination of witnesses.

Statutory duty to disclose

Whatever the views of the patient, there are certain circumstances in which disclosure of otherwise confidential information must be made by law. The following are the main provisions:

1. *Road Traffic Act 1988 Section 170 as amended by the Traffic Act 1991*: this requires any person to give information to the police relating to a road traffic accident involving personal injuries. A doctor was prosecuted under its predecessor for failing to disclose the relevant information and was fined £5.[39] His claim that he should not be required to give information that would be a breach of the patient's confidence was not accepted either by the trial judge or by the divisional court (see also chapter 20). In a case in 1999,[40] it was held that there was a statutory duty to report a road accident, even when the driver was not actually driving at the time.

2. *Prevention of Terrorism (Temporary Provisions) Act 1988, Section 11 (Continuous Order SI 1993/747)*: this makes it an offence for any person having information, which he believes may be of material assistance in preventing terrorism or apprehending terrorists, to fail without reasonable cause to give that information to the police. This therefore places a burden on staff, for example in A&E departments, to disclose the existence of wounds that may have resulted from terrorist acts.

3. *Public Health (Control of Disease) Act 1984*: as amended in 2010 requires a medical practitioner attending a patient who appears to be suffering from a notifiable disease to notify the medical officer of the district of the name and whereabouts of the patient and the disease. Notifiable diseases include cholera, plague, smallpox and typhus (see chapter 25).

4. *Abortion Act 1967*: requires doctors to inform the Chief Medical Officer of the DH of detailed information relating to the termination of pregnancy (see chapter 14).

5. *Drugs*: The Misuse of Drugs (Supply to Addicts) Regulations 1997 have abolished the requirement for a doctor to notify the Home Office of any patient who appears to be drug-dependent, but a doctor is expected to notify the local drug misuse database (see chapter 27).

6. *Health and Social Care Act 2008*: The Care Quality Commission has powers of inspection, entry and to require documents and information. Sections 76–79 cover its use and disclosure of confidential information. The NHS Act 2006 gives powers to the NHS Counter Fraud Service to require the production of documents to prevent, detect and prosecute fraud in the NHS.

Public interest

Unfortunately, many of the difficulties relating to the exceptions to the duty of confidentiality come under the broad heading of 'public interest' where there is little guidance from the courts.

> **Practical Dilemma 8.2**   **An epileptic lorry driver**
>
> Bill, a long-distance lorry driver, is diagnosed as having epilepsy, which is not yet under control through medication. The doctor has advised him to notify his employers and cease driving until the epilepsy is under control. Bill does not wish to do this since he has just been interviewed for the job of coach driver on the continent and he has been hoping for this chance for years. April, a nurse in the neurology ward, recognises Bill as her neighbour and is horrified when she hears from Bill's wife that Bill has been given the job of driving a coachload of schoolchildren to France. She knows several children who will be on that trip.

Many would argue that in these circumstances a breach of the duty of confidentiality owed to Bill is justified on grounds of the public interest. Obviously, there are advantages in Bill's being persuaded of the dangers of driving on the trip, but if he fails to disclose this and continues with his plans, then many would justify the doctor making the disclosure. If the doctor is adamant that he will not breach that confidence, does the nurse have any right to do so? The General Medical Council states specifically that it would defend any practitioner who disclosed confidential information in such circumstances. However, it is for each specific practitioner to decide personally if the particular circumstances justify disclosure in the public interest. There is no statutory definition of the public interest. Failure to notify the Vehicle Licensing Authority that a particular driver was not medically fit to drive could even be seen as a breach of a duty of care towards those persons who may be harmed as a result of that person driving. The success of such a hypothetical case would depend on establishing the following:

1. The doctor (or the nurse or other professional) owed a duty of care to the person who was eventually injured.
2. There was a breach of this duty in that the relevant information was not passed to the appropriate authority.
3. The personal injuries or death were a reasonably foreseeable result of that failure and were caused by that failure.

Until such a case is heard, or a law is enacted, a firm decision cannot be made, but some guidance is provided by the Tarasoff case heard in America and considered in Case 8.3. In addition, it should be pointed out that any person who drives a vehicle contrary to medical advice would themselves be committing a criminal offence.

> **Case 8.3**   *Tarasoff Case* [USA 1976]

Confidentiality and psychotherapy[41]

A psychologist in California was told by a patient that he intended to kill a girl. The psychologist informed the campus police, who detained the man, but soon after released him. They did not inform the girl's parents of the danger to her. The patient subsequently killed the girl. The parents sued the university for breach of its duty of care to the girl in failing to warn them. They succeeded in a majority verdict. The court held that the therapist owes a legal duty of care not only to his patient, but also to his patient's would-be victim. This duty of care is subject to scrutiny by judge and jury.

A **dissenting judge**, Judge Clark, was concerned that the very practice of psychiatry vitally depended on the reputation in the community that the psychiatrist would not tell. He considered that assurance of confidentiality was important to ensure patients were not deterred from seeking treatment; to ensure that they made a full disclosure to the doctor and to ensure that the patient maintains his trust in his doctor, which is vital for successful treatment. The NMC recognises that the public interest may be a justification for disclosing confidential information. Box 8.3 shows the NMC advice on disclosure without the consent of the patient.

In a more recent case concerning a psychiatrist, it was reported that a psychiatrist treating a paedophile had broken confidentiality by telling the police her concerns about his intentions. As a consequence of this information the paedophile was arrested, his house searched and he was sentenced to a community order. He was already on the sex register. The psychiatrist's actions in putting the duty under the Children Act before her duty of confidentiality to her client was commended by the NSPCC.[42]

Box 8.3 What is disclosure without consent? NMC guidance

- The term 'public interest' describes the exceptional circumstances that justify overruling the right of an individual to confidentiality in order to serve a broader social concern.
- Under common law, staff are permitted to disclose personal information to prevent and support detection, investigation and punishment of serious crime and/or to prevent abuse or serious harm to others. Each case must be judged on its merits.
- Examples could include disclosing information in relation to crimes against the person, e.g. rape, child abuse, murder, kidnapping, or as a result of injuries sustained from knife or gunshot wounds.
- These decisions are complex and must take account of both the public interest in ensuring confidentiality against the public interest in disclosure. Disclosures should be proportionate and limited to relevant details.
- Nurses and midwives should be aware that it may be necessary to justify disclosures to the courts or to the NMC and must keep a clear record of the decision-making process and advice sought. Courts tend to require disclosure in the public interest where the information concerns misconduct, illegality and gross immorality.

(NMC Regulation in practice topics: confidentiality. Paragraphing by author)

Reference should be made to chapter 4 and the discussion on whistleblowing. A registered nurse may face allegations of breach of confidentiality if she raises concerns about patient care outside the organisation. See the Haywood case and the new guidance published by the NMC on raising concerns discussed in chapter 4.

The Court of Appeal has given guidance on the public duty of confidence in the following case.

Case 8.4 W v Egdell [1989] Disclosure in the Public Interest[43]

W, a psychiatric patient, brought an action against an independent psychiatrist, the health authority, the mental health review tribunal and the Secretary of State for breach of confidentiality. The psychiatrist had sent a copy of his report on W's mental condition to the hospital on grounds of public interest on the basis of W's particular circumstances. The High Court judge held that no distinction should be drawn between a psychiatrist who was independent and one employed by the health authority. The report did not come under the heading of legal professional privilege (see page 193). The judge relied on the General Medical Council's Advice on Standards of Professional Conduct and Medical Ethics and refused an injunction against the use or disclosure of the report and dismissed his claims for damage.

The Court of Appeal dismissed W's appeal and held that the balance came down in favour of the public interest in the disclosure of the report and against the public interest in the duty of confidentiality owed to the patient. Unlike the trial judge, the Court of Appeal considered the General Medical Council's rules as inappropriately relied on by the judge, since Dr Egdell did not have clinical responsibility for W. The Court of Appeal quoted Article 8(2) of the European Convention on Human Rights which permits intervention by a public authority in the duty of professional secrecy in the interests of public safety and the prevention of crime (see website of this book). The same considerations justified Dr Egdell's actions.

Practical Dilemma 8.3 Occupational health

Brenda works as a nurse in the occupational health department and is horrified to discover that a paediatric nurse, Karen, has an unusual bacterial infection which makes it very dangerous for her to work in the unit, particularly with the premature babies. However, she knows that Karen has exhausted all her sick pay allowance from the authority and would be dependent on DSS benefits. She is bringing up two children on her own and would have great difficulty managing without her NHS pay. Karen herself is not ill: she appears to be a carrier rather than a sufferer of this particular germ and is anxious to continue to work and does not want her nursing officer to be notified.

An occupational health department is sometimes caught in the clash between its duty to keep information acquired from its clients/patients confidential and the interest of the employer in being aware of that information, especially where there is danger to the health or safety of other employees as a result of the person's medical condition. (The cases of *X v Y*[44] and *H (A Healthcare Worker) v Associated Newspapers Ltd*[45] and disclosure in relation to HIV/AIDS are considered separately in chapter 25.) Exactly the same principles apply as in the situation described above, with the additional dimension of the employer's duty to other employees in the workplace. There is a clear duty owed by the employer to his employees under an implied term in the contract of employment (see chapter 10), whereas the duty owed in the law of negligence in the situation of the epileptic lorry driver described in Practical Dilemma 8.2 is not at all clear.

In Brenda's case, there is clear justification for advising Karen that the information cannot be withheld. The dangers to the patients and to other staff are such that she cannot continue to work until she is free of the germ. Karen may have the right to claim the statutory right of payment on the grounds of medical suspension (see chapter 10). This breach of confidentiality can be justified by reference to a preceding agreement, namely the contract of employment and the implied terms in it (see chapter 10). Some authorities may well have an express term in their contract of employment authorising the occupational health department to notify the employer of any condition that would be dangerous to patients or other employees. Guidance is given by the RCN on confidentiality and the occupational health nurse.[46]

The Clothier Report following the conviction of Beverley Allitt[47] made recommendations for occupational health departments. It recommended that they should be involved in the selection of prospective employees and should monitor ongoing health problems of employees, alerting the employers when there were any serious risks to others. (See chapter 12 for a discussion on the National Patient Safety Agency and chapter 4 for whistleblowing.) The recommendations of the Clothier Report were reinforced by the report of an inquiry chaired by Richard Bullock following the case of Amanda Jenkinson, a Nottinghamshire nurse who was imprisoned for harming a patient. Similar recommendations were made to occupational health departments on risks from employees.

Disclosure to a registration body

In some cases, disclosure to a state registration body may be justified in the public interest, as the following case shows.

Case 8.5 *Re L* [2000]

Disclosure to a registration body in the public interest[48]

In care proceedings about a pre-school child, expert psychiatric evidence concluded that the mother was suffering from a severe personality disorder. The mother was a paediatric nurse and the three doctors involved in the case were agreed that there would be concern for any child in the mother's care. The court went on to consider whether the matter should be reported to the UKCC for the protection of any children who might be put at risk by contact with the mother in her professional capacity. The court decided that the court's judgment, the expert medical reports, and the minutes of the experts' two meetings should be given to the UKCC. The court had to decide on the balance of the rights of the mother and the child against the public interest in demanding protection from nurses who were, or who were potentially, unfit to practise.

Disclosures to the police

There are very few occasions on which the citizen is obliged as a duty by Act of Parliament to provide the police with information. The main statutes requiring disclosure are cited above. Many quandaries arise outside those areas and concern the powers of the police to require a professional to disclose confidential information during police investigations. Another difficulty is the position where, by chance, particularly through work in the community, the professional obtains evidence that a crime has been committed or is being committed: for example, stolen goods are seen in a client's home; there is evidence of drug abuse; there is evidence that a child is being physically or mentally ill-treated or sexually abused; there is evidence that a patient has had an illegal abortion; there has been an attempt to conceal the birth of a stillborn child; a wife has suffered a severe battering by the husband.

The police powers are contained in the Police and Criminal Evidence Act 1984. Medical records and human tissue or tissue fluid that has been taken for the purposes of diagnosis or medical treatment and which a person holds in confidence are subject to special procedures (see below).

Statute 8.1
Sections 9, 12 and 14 from the Police and Criminal Evidence Act 1984

Section 9. A constable may obtain access to excluded material or special procedure material by making an application under Schedule 1.

Section 11. Excluded material means:

(a) personal records which a person has acquired or created in course of any trade, business, profession . . . and which he holds in confidence

(b) human tissue or tissue fluid which has been taken for the purposes of diagnosis or medical treatment and which a person holds in confidence

(c) . . .

Section 12. Personal records means documentary or records concerning an individual (whether living or dead) who can be identified from them and relating:

(a) to his physical or mental health

(b) to spiritual counselling or assistance given or to be given to him

(c) to counselling or assistance given or to be given to him, for the purposes of his personal welfare, by any voluntary organisation or by any individual who:

   (i) by reason of his office or occupation has responsibilities for his personal welfare; or

   (ii) by reason of an order of a court has responsibilities for his supervision.

Section 14. Special procedure material means material other than items subject to legal privilege and excluded material in the possession of a person who:

(a) acquired or created it in course of any trade, business, profession or other occupation or for the purpose of any paid or unpaid office

(b) and holds it subject
   (i) to an express or implied undertaking to hold it in confidence or
   (ii) to a restriction or obligation such as is mentioned in S.11(2)(b).

A circuit judge can make an order that the person who appears to be in possession of the specified material should produce it to a constable for him to take it away or give a constable access to it, not later than the end of the period of seven days from the date of the order. The judge must be satisfied that specific access conditions are fulfilled before making the order.

Disclosure where a criminal offence is believed to have taken place

Practical Dilemma 8.4   Rape?

The police arrive at the A&E department one night enquiring about the possibility of a young man in his twenties having been admitted with severe lacerations to his face and neck. About two hours earlier, a girl of 15 had been found in a serious condition having suffered an attack. She had tried to defend herself by hitting the assailant in the face with a mirror. There was blood on the mirror and she believed she had cut him severely. The police arrive in the department and ask the duty nurse if they can go through the admissions during the last two hours.

The information required by the police is related to the medical records and thus comes under the special procedure. The police can make an application to a circuit judge for an order for the production of special procedure material. He will do so only if he is satisfied that certain conditions are present. However, these are the ultimate powers. It is unlikely that the police would be obliged to go to this length against an NHS trust. If it is known that the police can ultimately seek an order for disclosure, then the NHS trust policy is likely to be one of cooperation with them. In a case such as the rape case above, the nurse would be advised to call the medical officer in charge of the A&E department who would identify any patients who come within a fairly detailed description of the likely assailant. Giving the police the admission book would be beyond this duty.

In a case in 1993,[49] an order for disclosure to the police of the social security records giving dates of admission and discharge to the hospital was held not to come within the provisions of Schedule 1 of the Police and Criminal Evidence Act 1984.

Department of health advice

The Department of Health in its NHS Confidentiality Code of Practice[50] (see page 188) considers disclosure to the police and states:

> In the absence of a requirement to disclose there must be either explicit patient consent or a robust public interest justification. What is or [is not] in the public interest is ultimately decided by the courts.
>
> Where disclosure is justified it should be limited to the minimum necessary to meet the need and patients should be informed of the disclosure unless it would defeat the purpose of the investigation, allow a potential criminal to escape or put staff or others at risk.

The Department of Health quotes the definition of serious crime used by the GMC, i.e. 'a crime that puts someone at risk of death or serious harm and would usually be crimes against the person, such as abuse of children'.[51]

Practical Dilemma 8.5 — Let me know!

The police are investigating a burglary in which the householder came back early and surprised the burglar, who fell from a first-floor window, but still managed to escape. The police have enquired at the various A&E departments in the vicinity. At one hospital, they heard of an admission following a road accident where a man said he fell from a motorcycle when it crashed against a tree. There were no witnesses. They believe that the injuries are comparable to those the burglar might have sustained. Since the patient is not yet fit for interrogation as he has just come from the operating theatre, the police ask the ward sister:

1. to let them know when he can be questioned, and
2. not to let him go until the police arrive.

What is the ward sister's position? Must she obey this order?

Notifying the police of the patient's fitness for questioning: There is no clear legal right for the police to insist that this is done. For example, if the ward sister decides that her duty is to the patient, not to the police, and thus fails to notify the police, could she then be prosecuted for obstructing the police in the execution of their duty? The answer is probably not, unless it can be shown that they had express legal powers to demand the information from her. In practice, of course, staff often rely on the help of the police when they have aggressive visitors, or even aggressive patients, and are therefore prepared to reciprocate. What we are concerned with here is the legal duty on the ward sister to provide this information and it is unlikely that this power exists.

Keeping the patient until the police arrive: The citizen does have wide powers of arrest, although they are, of course, more limited than police powers. The sister would have no statutory power of keeping the patient (which would, in fact, be arresting him) until the arrival of the police unless either she knows that an **arrestable offence** has been committed and the patient is guilty of this or she has reasonable grounds for suspecting that he is guilty. In the circumstances described above, it would not appear likely that the ward sister has those grounds since, as far as she knows, the patient could well have fallen from his motorcycle. She would therefore be on very weak ground if she refused to allow him to take his own discharge other than on the basis that she was acting out of her duty of care to save his life. In this situation, the police would have to provide a policeman to wait until such time as the patient could be questioned or taken to the police station under arrest.

Reporting crime to the police

Practical Dilemma 8.6 — Discovery in the community

Jane, a health visitor, goes to enquire at a house where there is a young child of 18 months, since she has not seen her in the clinic and the child is due for several vaccinations and tests. While in the house, she notices the following: small burn marks on the child who looks very undernourished; four brand new video recorders in the corner of the room; and a pipe from the gas supply which bypasses the meter. One might question her imagination over the last item, but if this is in fact what she spotted, does she have any duty in respect of them?

---

1. *Non-accidental injury*: Jane's duty is to the child, so there can be no doubt that if she has reasonable grounds for suspecting that there is any abuse, then she must take the appropriate action to safeguard the child. There is a clear procedure for action if such a situation exists and Jane would have the responsibility to set it in motion. Even if Jane were a district nurse and visiting the mother rather than the child, she would still have a duty to ensure that the appropriate care was taken. (See chapter 13 for child protection procedures.)

2. *Suspected stolen goods*: there is no duty on Jane to act as police informer in such circumstances. If, of course, the goods were subsequently found to be stolen and Jane were summoned to court as a witness, she would have to give evidence of what she had seen. What, however, if the goods were NHS trust property? Does she have a duty to inform her employer that goods are being stolen? The answer depends on whether a term can be implied into the contract of employment that any employee must inform the employer of any thefts from the workplace. It would appear to make business sense of the contract of employment if such a duty could be seen to be implied. (See chapter 10 on implying terms into a contract of employment.)

3. *Gas*: it could be argued that the system for bypassing the meter is simply another case of stolen goods and theft. However, there are additional problems here, since there is a considerable public danger risking fire or an explosion. It could therefore be argued that Jane did have a public duty to notify the police, since her client and others could be in considerable danger.

Reporting suspected child abuse to the police

The Director of Public Prosecutions called for the creation of a statutory duty for teachers, social workers and doctors to report allegations of child sexual abuse to the police. He pointed out that Australia, the US and Canada have mandatory reporting systems. The response from the Department of Education was that mandatory reporting was not the answer to protecting children.[52] However, in July 2014 the Prime Minister said that mandatory reporting was under consideration (see chapter 13).

Disclosure by the police to employers and the NMC

Where a registered practitioner is charged or convicted of an offence, the police would ensure that both the employers and the NMC or other registration body are informed.

Case 8.6 *Woolgar v Chief Constable of Sussex Police* [1999]

Disclosure to the UKCC[53]

Junia Woolgar, a registered nurse and matron of a nursing home, was arrested and interviewed by the police following the death of a patient in her care. The police concluded the investigation without bringing any charges and they referred the matter to the UKCC, which asked for further information. It was the practice of the police to seek the consent of those who had given statements. Ms W refused to give consent and sought an injunction to restrain the police from disclosing to the UKCC the contents of an interview they had taped. She appealed against the High Court judge's refusal to grant the injunction. The Court of Appeal held that the police were entitled to release the information to a regulatory body, if they were reasonably persuaded that it was relevant to an inquiry being conducted by the regulatory body. She lost her appeal.

Rebecca Leighton, a nurse who had been cleared of poisoning patients, sued the police force on the grounds that they gave the public access to her private Facebook account and leaked her name to the media. She sought compensation in a claim for aggravated damages for breach of confidence, misuse of private information, negligence and breach of a statutory duty and her legal costs.[54] In June 2014 it was reported that she had received a £53,000 payout from the police.

Disclosure to parents

Information can be given to parents about their child's health if it is in the best interests of the child, and if a competent child has consented to the information being given. A mentally competent young person under 16 years has the right to request the withholding of information from the parents. This principle, established in the Gillick case, was upheld in the Axon case. In the Axon case,[55] a mother of teenage daughters applied for judicial review of DH guidelines on advice and treatment of young people under 16 years on contraception, sexual and reproductive health which was based on the Gillick judgment. She claimed that she should have been told that her daughter had given consent to an abortion. The High Court dismissed her application, upholding the guidance laid down by Lord Fraser in the Gillick case (see chapters 13 and 14).

Disclosure of information relating to a mentally incapacitated adult

In a case in 2002[56] the Court of Appeal recognised the duty of confidentiality owed to the mentally incapacitated adult, but in the circumstances, and taking account of the limited information required by his mother, allowed disclosure of information to her. She had applied in her capacity as nearest relative under the Mental Health Act 1983 for access to his medical records. Disclosure of information about those adults lacking mental capacity (who are outside the provisions of the Mental Health Act 1983) would now come under the Mental Capacity Act 2005 and the jurisdiction of the Court of Protection.

Disclosure on an anonymous basis

The laws of confidentiality usually apply to the disclosure of information when the identity of the patient is made known. However, the Department of Health challenged a data-collecting company that was using information provided by GPs and pharmacists about prescribing habits.[57] The company believed the information would be useful to drug companies and would provide useful data for those interested in monitoring prescribing patterns. Even though the information would be anonymous, the Department of Health challenged the use of this information as a breach of the guidelines put forward by the Department of Health[58] in 1996. It succeeded before the High Court but the Court of Appeal[59] reversed this decision. It held that GPs and pharmacists providing prescription information that did not identify the patient was not a breach of confidence. Anonymous data did not involve a risk to the patient's privacy, even if, with effort, the patient could be identified.

Disclosure and Article 8 rights

In another case, a health authority sought to obtain disclosure of patient records to consider the compliance of a medical practice with the terms of service of the practitioners. Two patients had not given consent to the disclosure and therefore the GPs involved, not wishing to risk a breach of confidence by disclosing the information, applied to the court for a ruling as to whether they were entitled to make the disclosure. The court considered earlier cases heard by the European Court of Human Rights on medical data and Article 8[60] and ordered the disclosure of the records but on condition that the confidentiality of the personal information should be maintained and the patients' anonymity preserved as far as possible. The court also ordered that the data could not be disclosed more widely than was necessary to deal with the problem.[61]

A claim for privacy protected by Article 8 failed when a judge ordered *The Times* to disclose the name of a blogger who had sought an injunction to stop *The Times* revealing his name.[62] In contrast, the Court of Appeal upheld a claim by a member of the Campaign against the Arms Trade that being photographed and details of his identity obtained by police were a breach of his Article 8 rights. The court held that breach of privacy required compelling justification such as terrorism or serious criminal activity rather than low level crime.[63]

Caldicott Guardians

Concern about the need to improve the way in which the NHS managed patient confidentiality led to the appointment of a committee chaired by Dame Fiona Caldicott. It reported in December 1997 and included in its recommendations the need to raise awareness of confidentiality requirements, and specifically recommended the establishment of a network of Caldicott Guardians of patient information throughout the NHS. Subsequently, a steering group was set up to oversee the implementation of the report's recommendations. A circular issued in 1999[64] gave advice on the appointment of the Guardians, the programme of work for the first year for improving the way each organisation handles confidential patient information and identified the resources, training and other support for the Guardians.

Caldicott Review on Information Governance in Health and Social Care 2013

Dame Fiona Caldicott was appointed in 2012 to review the balance between protecting patient information and its sharing, to improve patient care. (The full terms of reference can be found in Appendix 2 of the report.) The review was published in April 2013[65] and it is available on the government website.[66]

The principles set out in the original Caldicott Report of 1997 were revised and are as follows:

1. Justify the purpose
2. [Do not] use personal confidential data unless it is absolutely necessary
3. Use the minimum necessary personal confidential data
4. Access to personal confidential data should be on a strict need-to-know basis
5. Everyone with access to personal confidential data should be aware of their responsibilities
6. Comply with the law
7. The duty to share information can be as important as the duty to protect patient confidentiality.

The review made 26 recommendations all of which were accepted by the government which published its response in September 2013[67] and in its final chapter drew up a table of commitments to be fulfilled by itself and identified organisations. The Department of Health stated that the duty to share information can be as important as the duty to protect patient confidentiality.[68] The review found that the culture in the health service had unfortunately become one of anxiety, some say fear (over data protection laws). Health workers were scared to share data with other health professionals. It also found that some patients had been denied access to their own records because NHS bosses were so scared of fines for breaching data protection laws. The Department of Health subsequently appointed Dame Fiona Caldicott as chair of an independent panel to oversee and scrutinise implementation of the review's recommendations and to provide advice on information governance issues.

Guardians

Each health body was required to appoint a Caldicott Guardian by the 31 March 1999. Ideally, the Guardian would be at board level, be a senior health professional and have responsibility for promoting clinical governance within the organisation. A manual for Caldicott Guardians published in November 2006 and updated in 2010 can be downloaded from the DHSC website.[69]

The UK Caldicott Guardian Council is the national body for Caldicott Guardians and has produced an online manual for Calidcott Guardians to assist them in discharging their duties.

Freedom of Information Act 2000

The Act gives a general right of access to information held by public authorities, but this right is subject to significant exceptions. The main exemptions from the duty are set out in Part 2 of the Act. Some of the exemptions are subject to a public interest test and these are shown in Box 8.4. Others are absolute exemptions and these are shown in Box 8.5. In addition to these exemptions, under section 14 a request that is vexatious or that the public authority has already complied with does not have to be complied with. For the exemptions listed in Box 8.4, a public interest test applies. This means that a public authority must consider whether the public interest in withholding the exempt information outweighs the public interest in releasing it. The majority of exemptions fall into this category. For those exemptions listed in Box 8.5, there is no requirement for the public authority to consider the public interest.

Box 8.4 — Exempt information where the public interest test applies

Information intended for future publication
National security
Defence
International relations
Relations within the UK
The economy
Investigations and proceedings conducted by public authorities
Law enforcement
Audit functions
Formulation of government policy
Prejudice to effective conduct of public affairs
Communication with Her Majesty, etc. and honours
Health and safety
Environmental information
Personal information
Legal professional privilege
Commercial interests

Box 8.5 — Absolute exemptions from the Act

Information accessible to the applicant by other means
Information supplied by or relating to bodies dealing with security matters
Court records
Parliamentary privilege
Prejudice to effective conduct of public affairs
Personal information where the applicant is the subject of the information
Information provided in confidence
Prohibitions on disclosure where a disclosure is prohibited by an enactment or would constitute contempt of court

Data Protection and Freedom of Information Legislation

From Box 8.5 it will be noted that personal information where the applicant is the subject of the information is absolutely exempt from the Freedom of Information Act. Section 40 states that:

> [A]ny information to which a request for information relates is exempt information if it constitutes personal data of which the applicant is the data subject.

If a data subject wants access to personal information, then the route for that application is the UK GDPR and in general the Freedom of Information Act 2000 tries to prevent an overlap between the two laws.

In a dispute between Health and Care Professions Council (HCPC) and the Information Commissioner, the Tribunal[70] held that the ICO was entitled to see information which the HCPC had refused to disclose to an applicant under the Freedom of Information Act. Sue Lee had applied for information relating to her complaint about a registrant which had been turned down. The HCPC refused her request and she then applied to the ICO under section 50 of the Freedom of Information Act. The ICO issued an information notice requesting sight of the information which the HCPC had refused to disclose. HCPC appealed the Information Notice under section 57(2) of the Freedom of Information Act. The Tribunal upheld the Information Notice and dismissed the appeal. The HCPC had argued that it had a duty of confidentiality to its registrants, that its procedures in protecting the public would be jeopardised by such disclosure. However, the Tribunal was of the view that the HCPC would be able to revise its procedures to ensure that those providing information were accurately forewarned that the HCPC's dealing with this information would be subject to its duties under the Freedom of Information Act and the now the UK GDPR. If registrants enquired further they could be provided with a number of reassurances. Failures by a public body to provide information to an applicant under the Freedom of Information Act relying on the grounds of legal professional privilege have been challenged before the Information Tribunal. The applicant succeeded in one case where the application under the Freedom of Information Act was for information related to the withdrawal of treatment from the applicant, and the policy under which the treatment was withheld. The Tribunal held that the trust was in breach of its obligations.[71] In contrast, in another case a widow whose husband had died following a fall from a hospital bed was given a report of the trust's inquiry but she was refused the witness statements. The Commissioner upheld the trust's decision that they were exempt from the Freedom of Information Act under sections 31 and 36, and her appeal to the Tribunal failed.[72] Ann Clywd has complained that a Welsh Health Board illegally gave confidential information relating to her husband, a patient, to a Welsh Assembly member under the Freedom of Information Act. She stated that this information was not covered by the Act and the information was passed on because of political motives as a result of her complaints about her husband's ill-treatment. She has called for an Inquiry[73] which was rejected by the Welsh Assembly government. The rejection of most of her complaints by the University Hospital of Wales was ridiculed by Camilla Cavendish.[74]

In a landmark decision the Supreme Court held in March 2014 that while the Charity Commission did not have to disclose information to *The Times* about a charity involving the MP George Galloway and Iraq under the Freedom of Information Act or under the European Convention on Human Rights, there was at common law a right in the public interest for the information to be disclosed. 'There was a common law presumption in favour of openness.'[75] The Charity Commission stated that it would assess future requests for disclosure of information in the light of the Supreme Court judgment. In its leader, *The Times* said that 'the consequences of this Supreme Court ruling cannot be overstated . . . This newspaper believes that it is both politically healthy and ethically correct that the conduct of any public body be scrutinized closely, confidently and consistently.'[76] The implications for the NHS and its dealings with the public in the light of the Francis Inquiry are obvious (see chapter 5).

The Court of Appeal has held that where a person claims information under the Freedom of Information Act he is entitled to stipulate which software format should be used when the information was provided to him.[77]

The mother of a girl who had died in hospital appealed against the decision of the Information Commissioner to refuse her access to her daughter's records.[78] The trust was unwilling to release the records without the consent of the daughter's husband as her next of kin. The hospital had admitted liability for the daughter's death and had reached a settlement with the husband involving payment of substantial compensation. The mother contended that the records did not fall within the exception for confidential information under the Freedom of Information Act 2000 section 41. The judge refused the application on the following grounds:

1. The public interest ensuring that patients retained trust in confidentiality of information they gave to doctors outweighed, by some way, the countervailing public interest in disclosure of a deceased's medical records.

2. If disclosure would be contrary to an individual's reasonable expectation of maintaining the confidentiality of his or her private information, then the absence of detriment in the sense contemplated by the mother was not a necessary ingredient of the **cause of action**.

3. The duty of confidence was capable of surviving the death of the confider.

4. The trust would be in breach of confidence owed to the daughter if it disclosed her medical records other than under the terms of the Act, and the breach would be actionable by the daughter's personal representatives. Her records were exempt information under section 41 and should not be disclosed.

5. The rights of the next-of-kin had to prevail where the rights and wishes of family members differed.

A journal sought disclosure of letters written by the Prince of Wales to the government and succeeded before the Upper Tribunal which held that the communications should be disclosed. Subsequently the Attorney General used a ministerial veto to prevent the public seeing the documents. The Court of Appeal ruled that he had no good reason to overrule the decision of the Upper Tribunal and his certificate should be quashed.[79]

Codes of practice

Codes of practice giving practical guidance to public authorities on the discharge of their duties under the Act have been issued by the Lord Chancellor as required under section 45 of the Act[80] (referred to as the Section 45 Code of Practice). In December 2003 a model action plan for preparation for the implementation of the Freedom of Information Act 2000 was published.[81] While this model action plan is not compulsory, it was intended as a tool to disseminate ideas and best practice and to assist public authorities in creating a structured path towards full implementation of the Act in 2005. Freedom of Information Act Awareness Guidance leaflets are available from the Information Commissioner's website.[82]

Records of deceased persons

The only surviving provisions of the Access to Health Records Act 1990 are those relating to the records of deceased persons. Under section 3(1)(f) of the Access to Health Records Act 1990 where a person has died, the patient's personal representative and any person who may have a claim arising out of the patient's death may apply for access to the deceased patient's health records. Where such an application is made, access shall not be given if the record includes a note, made at the patient's request, that they did not wish access to be given on such an application. Nor will access be given by the record holder to any part of the record, if they are of the opinion that it would disclose information which was not relevant to any claim which may arise out of the patient's death.

Every NHS contract of employment or contract with an external contractor must contain a confidentiality clause that extends to both living and deceased patients.

Standard 5.3 of the NMC Code requires that nurses also have a professional duty to respect the right to privacy and confidentiality of patients even after they have died.

A life insurance company may seek information to decide whether to make a payment under a life assurance policy and require doctors to give information about the cause of death. Doctors could release information in accordance with the Access to Health Records Act 1990.

Access at common law

The Court of Appeal held in the case of Martin[83] that there is no absolute right to access personal health records.

DNA databases

In a case before the European Court of Human Rights concerning the National DNA database, two men from Sheffield, Michael Marper and S, sought the destruction of their DNA samples. They had been arrested in 2001 and had their fingerprints and DNA samples taken. They were not convicted of any crime and argued that the samples should have been destroyed. Their case was rejected by the British courts and in February 2008 the ECHR gave permission for the case to proceed.[84] The ECHR subsequently held that storage of DNA profiles of suspects who were not convicted was a breach of Article 8 and constituted a disproportionate interference with the applicants' right to privacy.[85] The ECHR considered that the blanket and indiscriminate nature of the powers given to the police could not be regarded as necessary in a democratic society. As a consequence of this judgment more than 1.6 million DNA and fingerprint samples must be destroyed from police databases.[86] The Information Tribunal held that police were breaking rules on the holding of personal details and that they should remove information about minor crimes from their records because storing it breached data protection laws.[87] However, this decision was overruled by the Court of Appeal.[88] It held that it was for the data controller to determine the purposes for which data were processed and it was a registered purpose to hold information so that it could be supplied to others in legitimate need such as the courts and Crown Prosecution Service. Liberty has asked the Health Secretary to investigate the holding of secret databases of DNA from newborns by the NHS where the appropriate consent has not been obtained.[89] The annual report for the National DNA Database Strategy Board for 2012/13 is available on the government website.[90] It reports on the progress of the removal of the DNA data of 1.7 million innocent persons and children from the National Database in accordance with the Protection of Freedoms Act 2012 which came into force on 31 October 2013.

A requirement that a man formerly convicted of manslaughter should attend a police station and provide a non-intimate DNA sample was held to be a proportionate and justified interference with his Article 8 rights. Amendments had been made to the Police and Criminal Evidence

Act 1984 to provide a scheme for the taking and retention of samples which complied with Article 8.[91]

In May 2013 the Supreme Court held that fingerprints which had been taken by an electronic device which had not been approved as required by statute were admissible in evidence at the suspect's trial. It was a well-established rule of English law that (apart from confessions to which special considerations applied) any evidence which is relevant is admissible even if it has been obtained illegally.[92]

Genetic data and biometric data are now defined as special personal data and its processing is unlawful unless one of the exemptions under the UK GDPR article 9 applies.[93]

Access to Medical Reports Act 1988

This Act came into force on 1 January 1989. It gives an individual a right of access to any medical report relating to him that has been supplied by a medical practitioner for employment purposes or insurance purposes. Before any such medical report can be supplied, the individual must be notified that it is being requested and the individual must give his consent to that request. The medical practitioner must not supply the report unless he has the consent of the individual. He is also required to give the individual the opportunity of access to it and to be allowed to correct any errors. These provisions apply unless 21 days have elapsed since the practitioner notified him of his intention to provide a report. The medical report must be retained by the medical practitioner for at least six months from the date on which it was supplied.

There is an exemption from individual access where the medical practitioner is of the opinion that disclosure would be likely to cause serious harm to the physical or mental health of the individual or would indicate the intentions of the practitioner in respect of the individual or where the identity of another person would be made known (unless that person has consented to the disclosure or is a health professional involved in the individual's care).

Concern was expressed by the Information Commissioner that insurers were regularly accessing the full medical records of patients contrary to data protection rules and an investigation has been initiated.

Conclusions

The NHS Confidentiality Code of Practice is of considerable guidance to healthcare staff in deciding whether the disclosure of confidential information is justified. However, the fact that many of the underpinning laws are based on common law, rather than statute, does make for difficulties. For example, whether a disclosure is justified as being in the public interest is determined by case law. The individual nurse practitioner still has to use her professional judgement in determining whether disclosure is justified, and she is personally and professionally accountable for her decision. The UK GDPR has tightened up access to and disclosure of personal information, putting more pressure on the decisions of the individual practitioner. Nurses should ensure that they make use of the existence of the Caldicott Guardian in their organisations to advise on issues relating to confidentiality and to assist in protecting the interests of the patient. If necessary, the protection of the Public Interest Disclosure Act 1998 could be sought if concerns on confidentiality need to be made known at a senior level within the organisation (see chapter 4 and whistleblowing). The Human Rights Act, in enabling persons to bring actions against public authorities that have failed to uphold a person's right to respect for private and family life, as set out in Article 8, has led to more litigation on grounds that confidentiality has not been respected.

The protection of patient confidentiality and the rights of access to information on health records thus continue to be a legal battleground. There are fears that the developing computerised system for patient records will provide inadequate protection for patient confidentiality. The Information Commissioner in his dual role as enforcement officer for both UK GDPR and Freedom of Information legislation has a major role to play in ensuring that patient confidentiality is respected, but legitimate claims to access information held by public authorities is granted. Regular updating can be obtained via the Information Commissioner's website.[94] Serious losses of data by the Child Support Agency, the Driving Standards Agency, the Ministry of Works and Pensions and the Ministry of Defence in 2007 and 2008 have raised further concerns about the security of NHS information and strengthened the opposition of many doctors to the NHS electronic patient record systems. The Information Commissioner now has powers to fine up to 20 million euros, and custodial sentences are being considered for the most serious breaches of the data protection laws. The second Caldicott review emphasised that appropriate sharing of patient information can be as important as protecting confidentiality.

Reflection questions

1. Prepare guidelines for a new employee on the duty of confidentiality.
2. Do you consider that there is a breach of confidentiality if a nurse returns home and tells her husband that they are treating a patient with AIDS on the ward? She does not mention the patient's name.
3. Consider the exception to the duty of confidentiality entitled 'public interest' and consider examples from your own experience that may come under that heading. What justifications could you give for and against disclosure?
4. Do you consider that the patient should have an absolute right of access in law to health records? Justify your answer.
5. Hospitals are often seen as the most difficult institutions in which to keep personal matters secret. What action do you think could be taken to enforce the duty of confidentiality in practice?

Further exercises

1. Identify who the Caldicott Guardian is in your organisation and establish the role that they play in maintaining standards of confidentiality.

References

On the protection of natural persons with regard to the processing of personal data and on the free movement of such data (United Kingdom General Data Protection Regulation) 2016 (2016/679)

Nursing and Midwifery Council (2018) *The Code: Professional standards of practice and behaviour for nurses and midwives* London: NMC

[1] www.ico.org.uk
[2] *R (on the application of the Secretary of State for the Home Department)* v *Information Tribunal (Information Commissioner, interested party)* [2006] EWHC 2958 Admin; [2007] 2 All ER 703
[3] www.ico.org.uk
[4] *Venables* v *News Group Newspapers Ltd* [2001] Fam 430
[5] *X (A woman formerly known as Mary Bell)* v *SO* [2003] EWHC 1101; [2003] 2 FCR 686
[6] *R (T)* v *Chief Constable of Greater Manchester Police and others*, The Times Law Report, 23 June 2014
[7] *Financial Times Ltd and others* v *United Kingdom* (Application O 821/03), The Times Law Report, 16 December 2009
[8] *R (Veolia ES Nottinghamshire Ltd* v *Nottinghamshire County Council)*, The Times Law Report, 9 November 2010
[9] *A* v *British Broadcasting Corporation*, The Times Law Report, 15 May 2014
[10] *Google Spain SL, Google In* v *Agencia Espanola de Protection Datos, Mario Costeja Gonzalez* Case C-131/12, 13 May 2014 ECJ
[11] *Stephens* v *Avery and Others* [1988] 2 All ER 477
[12] *Campbell* v *MGN Ltd* [2004] UKHL 22; [2004] 2 AC 457 HL
[13] *Mosley* v *News Group Newspapers* [2008] EWHC 1777
[14] *Liberty and others* v *United Kingdom*, The Times Law Report, 11 July 2008
[15] *Chhabra* v *West London Mental Health NHS Trust* [2013] EWCA Civ 11
[16] Nursing and Midwifery Council, The Code: Professional standards of practice and behaviour for nurses and midwives, NMC, London, 2015
[17] Nursing and Midwifery Council, Advice sheet on confidentiality, NMC, London, 2009
[18] *Ashworth Hospital Authority* v *MGN Ltd* [2001] 1 All ER 991
[19] *Mersey Care NHS Trust* v *Ackroyd* [2007] EWCA 101
[20] *Venables and Another* v *News Group Newspapers Ltd and Others* [2001] 1 All ER 430 FD
[21] Department of Health, NHS Confidentiality Code of Practice, DH, 2003, available on www.gov.uk/government/publications/confidentiality-nhs-code-of-practice (superseding HSG (96) 18 LASSL (96)5)
[22] https://digital.nhs.uk/services/national-data-opt-out-programme/guidance-for-health-and-care-staff
[23] Fiona Caldicott, The Information Governance Review: To share or not to share, Department of Health, March 2013
[24] *Napier and Another* v *Pressdram Ltd*, The Times Law Report, 2 June 2009
[25] *Nicholson* v *Halton General Hospital NHS Trust, Current Law*, 46, November 1999
[26] News item, Snooping nurse, *The Times*, 21 September 2010
[27] *A Health Authority* v *X, The Independent*, 17 January; [2002] 2 All ER 780 CA
[28] *R* v *H; R* v *C*, The Times Law Report, 6 February 2004; [2004] 2 WLR 335
[29] www.sfo.gov.uk
[30] *Waugh* v *British Railway Board* [1980] AC 521
[31] *Lee* v *South West Thames Regional Health Authority* [1985] 2 All ER 385
[32] *Balabel and Another* v *Air India*, The Times Law Report, 19 March 1988
[33] *Fulham Leisure Holdings Ltd* v *Nicholson Graham and Jones (a firm)* [2006] EWHC 158 Ch; [2006] 2 All ER 599
[34] Information Commissioner, Freedom of Information Act Awareness Guidance No. 4, 2004, updated 2006
[35] *Expandable Ltd and others* v *Rubin*, The Times Law Report, 10 March 2008

36 *McE v Prison Services of Northern Ireland and Another; C and A v Chief Constable of the Police Service of Northern Ireland; M v Same*, The Times Law Report, 12 March 2009
37 *Deacon v McVicar and Another*, 7 January 1984 QBD
38 *Davies v Eli Lilly and Co.* [1987] 1 All ER 801
39 *Hunter v Mann* [1974] 1 QB 767
40 *Cawthorne v Director of Public Prosecutions*, The Times Law Report, 31 August 1999
41 *Tarasoff v Regents of the University of California* 17 Cal 3d 425 (1976) (USA)
42 Simon de Bruxelles, Psychiatrist breaks confidence to help snare paedophile, *The Times*, 23 July 2013
43 *W v Egdell* [1989] 1 All ER 1089 HC; [1990] 1 All ER 835 CA
44 *X v Y and Another* [1988] 2 All ER 648
45 *H (A Healthcare Worker) v Associated Newspapers Ltd; H (A Healthcare Worker) v N (A Health Authority)* [2002] Civ 195; [2002] Lloyd's Rep Med 210 CA
46 80 Royal College of Nursing, Confidentiality: RCN, guidance for occupational health nurses, No. 002 043 October 2003, RCN
47 Clothier Report, The Allitt Inquiry: an independent inquiry relating to deaths and injuries on the children's ward at Grantham and Kesteven General Hospital during the period February to April 1991, HMSO, London, 1994
48 *Re L (Care Proceedings: disclosure to third parties)* [2000] 1 FLR 913
49 *R v Cardiff Crown Court ex parte Kellam*, The Times Law Report, 3 May 1993
50 Department of Health, NHS Confidentiality Code of Practice, DH, 2003, available on www.gov.uk/government/publications/confidentiality-nhs-code-of-practice (superseding HSG (96)18 LASSL (96)5)
51 GMC guidance, Confidentiality: protecting and providing information, GMC, London, 2004
52 Fiona Hamilton, Reporting child sex abuse 'must be made compulsory', *The Times*, 4 November 2013
53 *Woolgar v Chief Constable of Sussex Police and Another* [1999] 3 All ER 604 CA
54 William Chester and David Brown, Nurse cleared of poisoning patients sues police force, *The Times*, 3 June 2013
55 *R (on the application of Axon) v Secretary of State* [2006] EWHC 37 Admin; [2006] 2 WLR 1130
56 *R (on the application of S) v Plymouth City Council* [2002] EWCA Civ 388
57 *R v Department of Health ex p Source Informatics Ltd* [1999] Lloyd's Rep Med 264; [1999] 4 All ER 185
58 Department of Health HSG (1996) 18, Protection and Use of Patient Information, DH circular, March 1996 (superseded by Department of Health, NHS Confidentiality Code of Practice, DH, 2003, available on www.gov.uk/government/publications/confidentiality-nhs-code-of-practice)
59 *R v Department of Health ex p Source Informatics Ltd* [2000] TLR 17, [2000] 1 All ER 786 CA
60 *Z v Finland* [1998] 25 EHRR 371 and *MS v Sweden* [1999] 28 EHRR 91
61 *A Health Authority v X* [2001] 2 FLR 673 Fam Div; [2002] EWCA Civ 2014 CA
62 *The Author of A Blog v Times Newspapers Ltd* [2009] EWHC 1358
63 *R (Wood) v Commissioner of Police of the Metropolis*, The Times Law Report, 1 June 2009
64 NHS Executive, HSC 1999/012, Caldicott Guardians, 31 January 1999
65 Fiona Caldicott, The Information Governance Review: To share or not to share, Department of Health, March 2013
66 www.gov.uk
67 Department of Health, Information: To share or not to share. Government response to the Caldicott Review, DH, 2013

68 Chris Smyth, Staff must share patients' data, says Hunt, *The Times*, 13 September 2013
69 Department of Health www.gov.uk
70 *Health Professions Council* v *Information Commissioner* [2008] UKIT EA/2007/0116 14 March 2008
71 *Brigden* v *Information Commissioner* [2007] UKIT EA/2006/0034 (5 April 2007)
72 *Galloway* v *IC* [2009] UKIT EA/2008/0116 (20 March 2009)
73 The Health and Social Care Information Centre (HSCIC), Guide to confidentiality in health and social care, September 2013
74 Camilla Cavendish, Help us, Doctor. We're frightened of being ill in Cover-up General, *The Sunday Times*, 27 April 2014
75 *Kennedy* v *Charity Commission* [2014] UKSC 20
76 *Leader The Times*, 27 March 2014
77 *Innes* v *Information Commissioner and Another*, The Times Law Report, 8 August 2014
78 *Bluck* v *Information Commissioner* (2007) 98 B.M.L.R. 1
79 *R (Evans)* v *Attorney General and Information Commissioner* [2014] EWCA 254
80 Lord Chancellor, Code of Practice on the Discharge of Public Authorities' Functions under Part 1 of the Freedom of Information Act 2000; Lord Chancellor, Code of Practice on the Management of Records (Section 46 Code of Practice)
81 www.dca.gov.uk/foi/map/modactplan.htm
82 www.ico.org.uk
83 *R* v *Mid Glamorgan Family Health Services Authority, ex p. Martin* [1995] 1 All ER 356
84 *Marper* v *UK* [2007] EHCR 110; Application nos 30562/04 and 30566/04
85 *S and Marper* v *UK* (Application Nos 30562/04 and 30566/04) ECHR [2008], The Times Law Report, 8 December 2008 [2008] ECHR 1581
86 Richard Ford, Police are ordered to destroy all DNA samples taken from innocent people, *The Times*, 5 December 2008, page 16
87 Richard Ford, Ruling could wipe out criminal records, *The Times*, 22 July 2008, page 5
88 *Chief Constable of Humberside Police and others* v *Information Commissioner, Secretary of State for the Home Department intervening,* The Times Law Report, 22 October 2009
89 Marie Woolf, NHS uses babies' blood for secret database, *The Sunday Times*, 23 May 2010
90 www.gov.uk
91 *R (On the application of R)* v *A Chief Constable* [2013] EWHC 2864 Admin
92 *Public Prosecution Service of Northern Ireland* v *Elliott and another*, The Times Law Report, 18 June 2013
93 https://UK GDPR-info.eu/art-9-UK GDPR/
94 www.ico.org.uk

Chapter 9

Record Keeping, Statements and Evidence in Court

This chapter discusses

- Record keeping
- Statements
- Evidence in court
- Defamation
- Internet

Introduction

Good standards of record keeping are an essential part of professional practice and the duty of care owed to the patient. This chapter provides guidance on record keeping and advice on statement and report writing and giving evidence in court.

Record keeping

General Principles

The NMC considers record keeping a crucial aspect of a nurse's professional duty. Failing to meet the standard for record keeping remains an instance that can lead to one's name being removed from the professional register.

Standard 10 of the Code[1] imposes a duty on nurses to keep clear and accurate records relevant to their practice. The Code makes clear that the standard applies to all records relevant to a nurse's practice and not just patient records. To achieve the standard, nurses must be able to show that they:

- complete all records at the time or as soon as possible after an event, recording if the notes are written some time after the event;
- identify any risks or problems that have arisen and the steps taken to deal with them, so that colleagues who use the records have all the information they need;

- complete all records accurately and without any falsification, taking immediate and appropriate action if they become aware that someone has not kept to these requirements;
- attribute any entries they make in any paper or electronic records to themselves, making sure they are clearly written, dated and timed, and do not include unnecessary abbreviations, jargon or speculation;
- take all steps to make sure that all records are kept securely; and
- collect, treat and store all data and research findings appropriately.

Failure, therefore, to maintain reasonable standards of record keeping could be evidence of unprofessional behaviour and subject to fitness to practice proceedings.

Guidance on record keeping is also provided by NHS Digital.[2] The Audit Commission made recommendations to improve the standard of record keeping in hospitals in 1995.[3] It reviewed the situation in 1999 and concluded that, although progress had been made, there was still scope for further improvements.[4] The Clinical Negligence Scheme for Trusts monitors standards of record keeping and risk management by NHS organisations as part of its work in setting levels for membership of the NHS pool for sharing liability for compensation claims (see chapter 6). The standards set by the NHS Resolution include in their criteria principles relating to documentation. For example, criterion 8 for the governance standard relates to health records management. This states that chief executives and senior managers of all NHS organisations are personally accountable for records management within their organisation. Records are now kept of the many assessments which have to be carried out, including risk assessment, manual handling assessment, tissue viability assessment, social care, nutrition, and many others.

Increasingly, the records include a care pathway tracked out for that particular patient and nurses would be expected to identify the progress of the patient along that pathway.

CQC fundamental standards

Regulation 17(2)(c) of the Health and Social Care Act 2008 (Regulated Activities) Regulations 2014 requires that NHS care providers maintain securely an accurate, complete and contemporaneous record in respect of each service user, including a record of the care and treatment provided to the service user and of decisions taken in relation to the care and treatment provided.

Box 9.1 sets out the Care Quality Commission (CQC) requirements for meeting that regulation.

Box 9.1 CQC requirements for records that are fit for purpose

Records relating to the care and treatment of each person using the service must be kept and be fit for purpose. Fit for purpose means they must:

- be complete, legible, indelible, accurate and up to date, with no undue delays in adding and filing information, as far as is reasonable. This includes results of diagnostic tests, correspondence and changes to care plans following medical advice.
- include an accurate record of all decisions taken in relation to care and treatment and make reference to discussions with people who use the service, their carers and those lawfully acting on their behalf. This includes consent records and advance decisions to

refuse treatment. Consent records include when consent changes, why the person changed consent and alternatives offered.
- be accessible to authorised people as necessary in order to deliver people's care and treatment in a way that meets their needs and keeps them safe. This applies both internally and externally to other organisations.
- be created, amended, stored and destroyed in line with current legislation and nationally recognised guidance.
- be kept secure at all times and only accessed, amended, or securely destroyed by authorised people.

Both paper and electronic records can be held securely providing they meet the requirements of the General Data Protection Regulation (UK GDPR) and Data Protection Act 2018.

Decisions made on behalf of a person who lacks capacity must be recorded and provide evidence that these have been taken in line with the requirements of the Mental Capacity Act 2005 or, where relevant, the Mental Health Act 1983, and their associated Codes of Practice.

Information in all formats must be managed in line with current legislation and guidance.

Systems and processes must support the confidentiality of people using the service and not contravene the UK GDPR and Data Protection Act 2018.

Common errors noted in record keeping

These are listed in Box 9.2 and are the most common errors in record keeping.

Box 9.2 Common errors in record keeping

Times omitted

Illegible handwriting

Lack of entry in the record when an abortive call has been made

Abbreviations were ambiguous

Record of phone call (e.g. to social services) that omitted the name of the recipient (e.g. social worker)

Use of correction fluid and covering up of errors

No signature

Absence of information about the child

Inaccuracies, especially of the date

Omission of date of medical check-up and hearing test and records for immunisation

Delay in completing the record; sometimes more than 24 hours elapsed before the records were completed

Record completed by someone who did not make visit

Inaccuracies of name, date of birth and address

Unprofessional terminology, e.g. 'dull as a doorstep'

Meaningless phrases, e.g. 'lovely child'

> Opinion mixed up with facts
>
> Reliance on information from neighbours without identifying the source
>
> Subjective not objective comments, e.g. 'normal development'

The errors shown in Box 9.2 are not of course exhaustive and each practitioner could add others they have noticed to the list. However high a standard of record keeping is maintained, this is of little value if the records are not read. An inquest heard in 2010 that a diabetic patient died in hospital because the nurses had failed to read the records and to ensure that she received her insulin.[5] The CQC criticised Manchester Royal Infirmary in its inspection in December 2013 because notes were illegible which meant that records were incomplete and increased the chance of patients failing to get the treatment they needed. In its report the Manchester Children's Hospital was told that 'we found that many entries in the medical notes were illegible'. In a news item in May 2014 it was reported that the wrong notes were used for a patient with the same name. An arm operation was carried out based on the records of another patient with the same name at Westmorland General Hospital Cumbria.[6]

Clarity

Records should be meaningful, clear accounts of the patient's care. 'Had a good day', which is one of the most unhelpful statements, should not feature in the records. Why did she have a good day? Had her appetite returned? Had she spent most of the time sleeping? Alternatively, had she spent most of the day awake? Had she been of minimal trouble to the nursing staff? Had she in contrast been lively and interacted with the nursing staff? All these situations, many of them incompatible, are within the meaning of those words.

Comprehensiveness

Some nurses might see this paperwork as a distraction from the real task of nursing, i.e. caring for the patient. However, records are an integral part of nursing care. Failure to record an important item, e.g. administration of a drug, may mislead other professionals, such as those on a later nursing shift, and the patient could consequently be given an overdose. Accurate, comprehensive information relating to the care and the condition of the patient is a vital part of the professional role of the nurse. In addition, the information could be used for many other purposes of which the nurse may not be aware at the time.

Use of abbreviations

Standard 10 of the Code (NMC, 2015) makes it clear that good record keeping includes ensuring that you:

> **attribute any entries you make in any paper or electronic records to yourself, making sure they are clearly written, dated and timed, and do not include unnecessary abbreviations, jargon or speculation**

This is a move away from the NMC's earlier advice that abbreviations should not be used. There are of course dangers in the use of abbreviations:

1. PID: **p**elvic **i**nflammatory **d**isease or **p**rolapsed **i**ntervertebral **d**isc?
2. pt: **p**atien**t**, **p**hysiotherapis**t** or **p**art **t**ime?

3. CP: **c**erebral **p**alsy or **c**hartered **p**hysiotherapist?
4. MS: **m**ultiple **s**clerosis or **m**itral **s**tenosis?
5. NFR: **n**ot **f**or **r**esuscitation or **n**europhysiological **f**acilitation of **r**espiration?
6. NAD: **n**othing **a**bnormal **d**iscovered or **n**ot **a d**rop!

Nurses must ensure that all colleagues and service users have a clear understanding of entries within their records. The general rule is that abbreviations should not be used in clinical records. Some abbreviations, such as where the full term is lengthy, may be used only after the term is written in full for the first time, with the abbreviation placed in brackets immediately following, e.g. Methicillin-Resistant Staphylococcus Aureus (MRSA). The abbreviation should be for that specific entry only and a term generally recognised within the National Health Service. This also applies to the use of symbols and signs and other hieroglyphics.

Who should sign or write the records?

Any individual, and this would include unregistered staff or learners who have first-hand knowledge of any events regarding the care of the patient, should write up the relevant record and initial or sign it. Countersigning might be required by trained staff in certain circumstances and the procedure for this would be laid down locally. Any member of staff, registered or not, could be summoned to court to give evidence of what took place.

What about errors and mistakes?

If it is necessary to change what has been written, it is good practice for a line to be put through the incorrect statement with brackets being used to set out the extent of the error and the correct statement made underneath rather than heavily scoring out the incorrect sentence or using correction fluid. These and other such deletions should not be used on records. It should always be clear what was originally written and any corrections should be signed and dated. If the records are then used in evidence, it should be clear what was originally written and why it was changed. It must be emphasised that these records are not proof of the truth of what they contain, but the writer of the records could be summoned to court to give direct evidence as to their accuracy and reliability.

Use in court

What constitutes a legal document?

There is sometimes confusion over what is a legal document. For example, are nursing care plans legal documents? The answer is that any document requested by the court becomes a legal document. The court could subpoena the disclosure of care pathway records or the nursing process documents, medical records, X-rays, pathology laboratory reports, social workers' records, any document in fact that may be relevant to the case. If they are missing, the writer of the records could be cross-examined as to the circumstances of their disappearance.

While the main purpose of record keeping is the care of the patient, considerable reliance will be placed on the records in any court hearing. Any weaknesses in record keeping will hamper the professional when it comes to giving evidence in court and will render them vulnerable in cross-examination, especially when there has been a considerable delay between the events recorded and the court hearing.

On some occasions, records may be looked at in a matter unconnected with the treatment of that particular patient. For example, in the case of *Deacon* v *McVicar*[7] (see chapter 4 Case 4.11), there was a dispute as to the priority that a particular patient should have been given and the judge ordered the records of the other patients on the ward at the time to be disclosed in order to assess whether or not they would have been making demands on medical and nursing time at a particular point in time.

The preceding chapter considers the rules relating to the disclosure of medical records in cases of personal injury litigation, and the powers of the court to order the discovery of any relevant documents, with only privileged records being exempt from disclosure. Health records are not proof of the truth of the facts stated in them, but the maker of the record must be called to give evidence as to the truth of what is contained in them. There are exceptions under civil evidence legislation that permit the records to be used in evidence without the presence of the maker (where, for example, the maker is dead or overseas), but due warning of the intent to use the records in evidence must be given to the other side.

Maintaining high standards of record keeping

The pressures of work and the lack of adequate time for record keeping make it extremely difficult to ensure that standards of record keeping are kept high. Constant vigilance is required. Clinical governance requires each NHS organisation to have a clear system of setting and maintaining high standards of record keeping on a multidisciplinary basis.

Computerised Records

The 1997 White Paper on the NHS[8] envisaged a vast investment in information technology within the NHS that would ultimately link GP surgeries and hospitals to an NHS-wide information network. Despite an investment of many billions of pounds neither the time scale nor the full implementation of the strategy has been achieved.

The Department of Health pledged guarantees in May 2005 relating to patients' control over access to their health records.[9] The Care Record Guarantee, drawn up by the Care Record Development Board, included the commitments that access to records by NHS staff will be strictly limited to those having a need to know to provide effective treatment to a patient; patients will be able to block off parts of their record to stop it being shared with anyone in the NHS, except in an emergency, and individuals will be able to stop their information being seen by anyone outside the organisation which created it.

The Information Governance Toolkit can be obtained from the website of the Health and Social Care Information Centre, which took over the functions of NHS Connecting for Health.[10]

In April 2007 the House of Commons Public Accounts Committee concluded that the 'NHS IT project was the biggest in the world and it is turning into the biggest disaster'. In 2010 it was running four years late and the budget had grown from £2.3 billion to £12.7 billion. Increasingly, there were concerns about patient consent to the inclusion of records on a national database and the fact that the pack sent to 12 million persons did not contain an opt-out form. In 2014 it was reported that the failed £11.4 billion plan to digitise medical records in the NHS had led to an arbitration decision that the NHS should pay Fujitsu £400 million in addition to the £250 million already paid.[11] The Public Administration Select Committee were due to open an investigation. In 2013 the Department of Health issued a press release which challenged the NHS to go paperless by 2018.[12] The Information Governance Review (led by Fiona Caldicott) supported plans for patients to have online access to their GP records by 2015 and recommended sharing information across hospitals, social care and public health. Jeremy Hunt, the Secretary of State for Health, stated that patients should have compatible digital records so their health information can follow them around the health and social care system. The Professional Records Standards Body (PRSB)[13] has been established to provide structure and contents standards for health and social care records so that the information can be recorded for the purposes of direct care and reused for management, policy and research purposes, maximising the benefits of information technology. The establishment of the PRSB was supported by NHS Digital.

NHS Digital

NHS Digital is the national information and technology partner to the national health and the social care system. Its responsibilities were set out in the Health and Social Care Act 2012 and are considered in chapter 8. NHS Digital created the Summary Care Record (SCR), which is an electronic record of important patient information that is created from GP records. The SCR can be seen and used by health and care staff in other areas who are involved in the care of the person. People can ask to view or add information to their SCR by visiting their GP. Further information on the SCR can be obtained from the NHS Digital website.[14]

While computerisation will resolve some of the problems arising from manually held records, such as illegible spelling, the principles of good record keeping in terms of the content, clarity and accuracy of the information put on to the computer will still apply. Data protection requirements on security and access to the data are enforced through the criminal law (see chapter 8).

The law relating to DNA databases is considered in chapter 8.

Statements

Figure 9.1 illustrates some of the many occasions on which staff may be required to produce a statement. The statements produced on different occasions have very different purposes and effects. For example, where a statement is taken by the police, it can be used as formal evidence in criminal proceedings and the person who made the statement can be questioned on it. Where it has been made under caution, it can be used in evidence against an accused. In civil

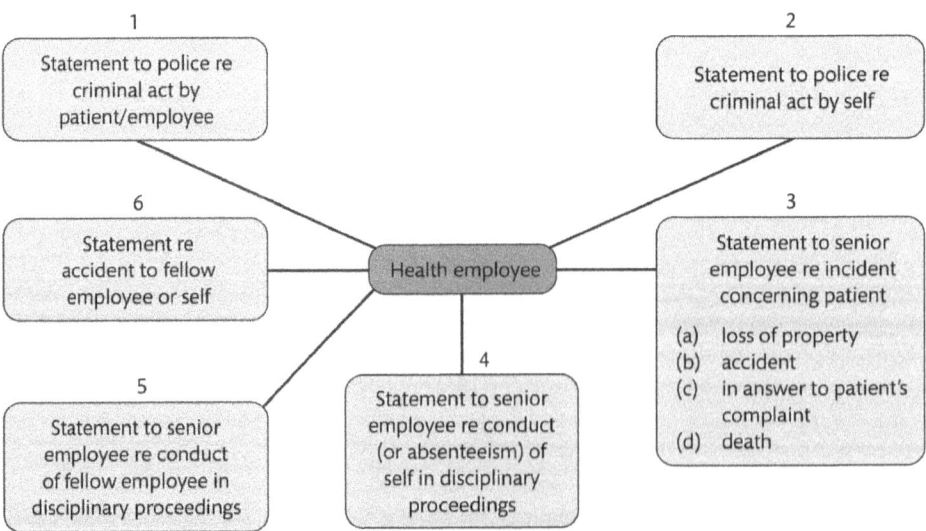

Figure 9.1
Occasions when a statement might be requested

1 and 2 criminal proceedings; 3(a–c) and 6 civil proceedings; 4 and 5 tribunal proceedings; 3(d) coroner's proceedings.

proceedings, the statement is not regarded as formal evidence, although the civil court now has the power to order disclosure of witnesses' statements.

The purpose of this section is to explore the principles of statement making and highlight some of the dangers.

Does a Nurse have to Make a Statement?

The one occasion on which a nurse can refuse to make a statement is if it criminally implicates them. No one can be forced to answer a question if the effect of the answer is to incriminate them. There is a right to remain silent when questioned by the police about an alleged offence and also if a defendant is in a criminal court, but failure to reply or remaining silent can result in an adverse conclusion being drawn about this failure in an address to the jury.

There are considerable advantages in setting out exactly what took place as a record, although help and guidance are clearly essential. In general, a statement is required, not for self-defence, but as evidence of the events to which the nurse was a witness. There have been examples where hospital staff have refused to participate in an inquiry set up by the health authority. For example, in the Shewin case, where a patient went into hospital for a gall bladder operation and suffered irreversible brain damage, the doctors initially refused to take part in the health authority inquiry. They eventually did so and were exonerated.[15]

In general, it could be argued that provided a member of staff is given appropriate guidance in making a statement, then the statement should be a valuable reminder at a later date of the details of what took place. It would seem to be reasonable to imply a term into the contract of employment that a National Health Service employee, in the course of his or her employment, would cooperate with the police and the coroner's court and would give a statement and information relevant to civil claims. It could also be argued that the employee should have assistance from senior managers or from the employer's solicitors in preparing a statement.

Standard 23 of the Code (NMC, 2015) places a duty on nurses to cooperate with all investigations and audits even where they are against the nurse.

What is the Status of a Statement as Evidence in Court?

In criminal proceedings

Where the statement forms part of a police investigation and a caution has been given as to its effect, it could be used in evidence against the person who gave it, especially where the account they are now giving is entirely different from the statement.

Where the statement has been given by a person who is a witness to the events, then the statement, if it was made contemporaneously with the events described, can be used as an aid to memory. It must be emphasised that the statement is not in itself proof of the truth of the events therein described. Any number of lies or exaggerations can be recorded in a statement. However, except for certain exceptions, the person who made the statement would be expected to give evidence in court and could be cross-examined on the statement, from which the court could deduce the weight to be attached to the statement. Documentary evidence is permissible under the Criminal Justice Act 1988 sections 23–28 (as amended by the Criminal Justice Act 2003).

In civil proceedings

The statement can be used by its maker to refresh their memory. The court now has access to the statement; it can order disclosure of the witness statements. Written documents can be entered as evidence under the provisions of the Civil Evidence Act 1968. Further details relating to statements and documents can be found in the Civil Procedure Rules, which are available online.[16]

Can the Court always Insist on the Statement being Produced?

In chapter 8, the occasions on which documents are regarded as privileged were discussed. Where the statement, document, letter, etc. has come into existence as a result of and for the purposes of proposed or existing litigation, they are covered by professional legal privilege and the courts cannot enforce disclosure.

Should a Nurse make a Statement?

A distinction must again be made between the criminal and the civil courts. Where the police are investigating a crime and seeking information from witnesses, then it could be an offence to refuse to cooperate with them. There is, however, no duty to incriminate oneself. Recent legal advice to the NMC suggests that registered nurses are not under a duty to provide a statement to the police if it would incriminate them.[17]

In potential civil cases, there is no duty to make a statement, except possibly under the contract of employment.

However, if one considers the time it takes for a case to come to court – in the civil courts sometimes as long as five or six years – it is highly unlikely that anyone would have a detailed recollection of the facts when they finally come under cross-examination or are giving evidence in chief. A detailed comprehensive statement of the events, drawn up at the time of the incident or events, is essential to refresh one's memory. In addition, a detailed, sensibly prepared statement may eliminate the chance of a nurse being called as a witness and thus save a needless attendance in court.

What Points should be followed in Making a Statement?

Purpose

Before a statement is made, it is always advisable for its maker to have an idea of the purposes for which it is being made. Is it going to the coroner's office? Is it for internal information only? Is it to be used in a criminal prosecution? The purpose will affect the detail, style and content of the statement. The maker should therefore find out from the person who has asked for the statement who will read it and to what varied purposes it will be put. If there is any danger that the maker would incriminate themselves, they should ask for legal advice before making the statement. It is not necessary to wait for a request before writing a statement about a certain occurrence. In some situations, it may be wise for a witness or participant to write down a brief account of the events immediately.

Guidance

Even in circumstances where there is no question of self-incrimination, it is always advisable to seek advice in making the statement. An objective reader can see gaps, ambiguities and confusion in a statement and give much valuable assistance.

Who should provide the guidance?

Normally, a senior nurse manager or the solicitor to the employer should provide this assistance. There will be occasions, however, where advice from a union officer is sought. In disciplinary proceedings, this depends on how far the proceedings have been taken. It would, for example, be contrary to the guidelines for good practice for management to refuse to allow an employee to receive the advice of the union representative prior to any formal disciplinary action being taken (see chapter 10).

The essential elements in a statement are shown in Box 9.3.

Box 9.3 — Essential elements of a statement

1. Date and time of incident
2. Full name of maker, position, grade and location
3. Full name of any person involved, e.g. patient, visitor, other staff
4. Date and time the statement was made
5. A full and detailed description of the events that occurred
6. Signature
7. Any supporting statement or document attached

Principles to be Followed

Box 9.4 sets out the nine principles to be followed in preparing a statement.

Box 9.4 — Principles to be followed in preparing a statement

1. Accuracy
2. Factual
3. Avoid hearsay
4. Conciseness
5. Relevance
6. Clarity
7. Legibility
8. Overall impact
9. Keep copy

Accuracy

It is essential that the statement should set out clearly the facts that took place. There should be no exaggeration or minimisation. The statement should be read through carefully to ensure that there are no inconsistencies, mistakes or other faults. There should be access to the relevant records so that the statement maker does not rely on memory in preparing the statement. If the record keeping has been of a high standard, this will facilitate the writing of the statement.

Keeping to the facts

The maker should, if at all possible, avoid value judgements and should keep to the facts. For example, a health visitor might have formed the opinion that one of her clients was lazy. If this is relevant to the statement, it is of far more value if she were to write down a description of the facts that led her to that opinion than to make value judgements. Thus 'there were 12 dirty milk bottles on the living room floor and piles of papers on every seat, etc.' is more useful than expressing an opinion that may or may not be acceptable and is not on its own very meaningful. The facts on which those opinions are based are more useful. There are occasions where it is necessary to express opinions, especially where they led one to act in a particular way. Even here, however, it is still necessary to record the facts that led to those opinions. For example: 'Because I felt she was a danger to herself I put the bed rails up.' This statement needs to be amplified to expand on what has caused the nurse to believe that the patient was a danger to herself. For example, had she fallen out of bed? Had she tried to leave the ward? Was she in a confused state and, if so, how did she show it?

Where it is possible to check facts before making the statement, this should be done. For example, a statement that a patient had a high temperature should be checked against the patient's record; similarly, a description that the patient had been written up for a particular form of medication should be checked against the drug card. Sometimes it is helpful to draw a sketch of the ward layout or where the patient was found or where there is a need to identify the exact location, but only if the plan is a help rather than a further source of confusion.

Avoidance of hearsay

Hearsay is the recording or repetition of what someone else has seen or heard. If possible, it is best to avoid this as the person making the statement is only repeating what someone else has said and cannot give first-hand evidence of what was heard or seen. Imagine a situation where a nurse hears a fall in the night and runs into the ward to find a patient on the floor. It is better for her statement to cover what she herself saw and heard rather than to repeat what another employee heard and saw. This other person should be asked to provide a statement of what she witnessed at first hand. Where the only witness to the events may have been another patient, it may be possible to obtain a statement from that patient, but that does depend on his physical and mental condition.

Conciseness

The statement must not ramble. It must be to the point in a logical sequence. Padding, waffle and meaningless generalisations should all be avoided. However, essential detail should not be sacrificed on the altar of brevity. The amount of detail required will, of course, depend on the facts described.

Relevance

It is a useful exercise to question oneself on the events to establish what detail a stranger to the situation would require. This questioning would have to take place in the context of the purpose for which the statement is required. In some circumstances, it may be important to describe the colour, material and style of the patient's clothes – in other circumstances, this may be entirely irrelevant. If there is any doubt as to what is relevant or not, one should err on the side of inclusion. What is in can always be omitted on the grounds of relevance at a later stage; what is left out is left out for good, because such details would soon be forgotten if not recorded.

Clarity

It is essential that the maker should read through the statement to ensure that it is clear and meaningful. If there are any doubts as to what is meant, it should be rewritten until one is sure that it is an exact clear record of what happened. Substitutes for any misleading or ambiguous words or phrases should be found. The use of clichés should be avoided. Abbreviations should be used only after the full terms are set out in full, with the abbreviation set out in brackets after the words. They should not be used for any other meaning. The level of technical language used should relate to the likely readership. In some circumstances, it will be necessary to explain technical procedures in full. In others, there will be no need. Emphasis should be on simplicity rather than complexity. The writer should make sure that he or she understands the statement.

Legibility

If the statement is handwritten, it should be legible. If it is typed at a later date, then the typed copy must be checked for errors.

Overall impact

The statement should be read through and its overall impact assessed. Does it give sufficient detail? Is it clear exactly what happened? Is it accurate? Is there any further information that should be included? Is it internally consistent? Have any facts been checked?

Any necessary changes should be made and the maker should not sign the statement unless they are entirely satisfied with it. The maker must be satisfied with every aspect of the statement. The maker must not allow themselves to be browbeaten into including information that is not within their knowledge or that they know is not entirely accurate. Personal accountability must be accepted for the statement. Putting a signature to a statement implies that the maker is satisfied that it is accurate in every detail and they take personal responsibility for it. A copy should always be kept. The confidentiality of the statement should be protected in accordance with the principles considered in chapter 8.

Practical Dilemma 9.1 Statement writing

Consider any incident which has occurred in recent days and draft a statement including all the points made in Box 9.3 and 9.4.

If possible ask your tutor or mentor to read through your draft and comment on it. Imagine that the events become subject to a court hearing in 10 years' time. What questions could be asked and to what extent does the statement provide the answers?

Evidence in court

Reference should be made to chapters 2 and 6 for procedures followed in criminal and civil courts, respectively.

Fears of Giving Evidence in Court

There are few health professionals who relish the possibility of being required to give evidence in court. Preparation and guidance in facing the ordeal are essential, whether it is a criminal court, coroner's court, civil court, conduct and competence committee hearing or employment tribunal. Of equal importance, however, are comprehensive, clear and accurate records. Box 9.5 sets out some of the fears expressed by nurses.

Box 9.5 Fears over a court appearance

Fear of the unknown

Hearing the client call one a liar

Publicity

Waiting and the build-up in tension that can arise

Remembering the detail of what took place

Fear of being made to look a fool

Being unable to express oneself concisely

Contradicting oneself

Omissions in one's statement on which one could be cross-examined

Being made to feel guilty

Downright rudeness and offensiveness of the others in court, especially the barristers

Tension and nerves

Being turned into the betrayer of the client

Waste of time

Being cross-examined by the client when he is not represented but is conducting his case personally

Failure to understand the legal jargon, procedure and gestures

Manipulation under cross-examination and being forced to change one's evidence.

Preparation for a Court Appearance

Experience in giving evidence in court will undoubtedly clear some of the anxieties illustrated in Box 9.5. Many can be solved by a private visit to a court hearing (they are all open to the public except for the few cases, such as children's and matrimonial proceedings, which are heard in private), and going on one's own or in a group without any personal involvement gives a sense of the procedure and language used and provides a chance of familiarising oneself with the process.

Witnesses are of two kinds: a witness of fact and an expert witness. The witness of fact is required to describe what they saw and did and give direct evidence of the facts in dispute. Their opinion is not usually required. An expert witness, by way of contrast, provides evidence of opinion of professional practice and approved standards of care or of causation or the appropriate level of compensation. The expert will be chosen because of their personal standing within a particular specialty.

Witness of fact

If a nurse were asked to attend court as a **witness of fact**, a solicitor would normally assist in explaining the procedure and in preparing the nurse for giving evidence. Considerable expertise can often be built up within a department and the lessons learnt passed from one to another. Confidence in the records that have been kept and the statements made should ensure that nerves are kept under control. The nurse should know the contents of the original records and where the entries appear so that there is no fumbling through the original records in the course of giving evidence.

Advice on court procedure and giving evidence in court is available from the county courts or High Court and also from the website at the Ministry of Justice.[18] Forms and guidance are also available from His Majesty's Courts Service.[19] Failure to respond to a witness summons can lead to the person being in contempt of court and a fine of up to £1000. A witness could apply to have the summons withdrawn.

Expert witness

The Civil Procedure Rules Part 35, which can also be accessed via the internet, set down detailed rules relating to the role of the **expert witness** and the contents of the expert's report. Rule 35.3 on expert witnesses states:

1. It is the duty of experts to help the court on matters within their expertise.
2. This duty overrides any obligation to the person from whom experts have received instructions or by whom they are paid.

Practical issues such as 'What do I call the judge?' often worry potential witnesses.

- A High Court judge is called 'My Lord' or 'My Lady'
- A circuit judge is called 'Your Honour'
- A district judge is called 'Sir' or 'Madam'.

Expert evidence has come into focus recently following the discrediting of evidence given in the trial of mothers accused of causing the deaths of their babies. Dr Meadows, a paediatrician, gave evidence for the prosecution in the trial of C for the murder of her two sons and she was convicted. Her second appeal to the Court of Appeal against the conviction succeeded on the grounds that the verdicts were unsafe because of material non-disclosure by the Crown's pathologist. A complaint was made to the General Medical Council (GMC) about the evidence of Dr Meadows, which the Court of Appeal had indicated was also probably unsafe. The GMC concluded that he was guilty of serious professional misconduct and ordered his name to be struck off the register. Meadows appealed against this striking off to the High Court, which found for him on the grounds that an expert witness should be immune from subsequent legal proceedings. The GMC appealed to the Court of Appeal, which held that immunity from suit did not apply to disciplinary, regulatory or fitness to practise proceedings. However, Meadows's mistake had not amounted to serious professional misconduct. He had not intended to mislead the trial court and he had honestly believed in the validity of his evidence when he gave it.[20]

Cross-examination

As far as the cross-examination is concerned, it should be remembered that following a few guidelines should limit the damage to one's evidence in chief.

> Go prepared to the court hearing with the relevant records and documentation.
> Read through the contemporaneous notes beforehand.
> Go through the evidence with a senior nurse manager.

In court, be honest; do not exaggerate; do not be drawn into saying something that is not true; do not rush the answers; take time to think.

Be aware of the 'Catch 22'-type question:

> Q. You are a nurse?
>
> A. Yes.
>
> Q. You are therefore observant?

How do you answer this? If you say, 'Yes', the next questions could be:

> Q. How fast was the car going?
>
> A. Er . . . I'm not sure.
>
> Q. But I thought you said you were observant?

If you say, 'No', the next question could be:

> Q. Then your observations in this case are entirely useless?
>
> A. Er . . .

If you answer the original question, 'Sometimes, it depends on what I am observing', it is likely to lead to a question or comment such as, 'Then we cannot rely on your evidence in this case'.

Such tactics are unlikely to have any effect on the judge's view, but they can sometimes influence the jury's thinking. (It must be remembered, however, that there is usually no jury in the civil court and the nurse's involvement in a jury trial in the Crown Court is likely to be rare.) What is more likely, however, is that the tactics used unnerve the person being cross-examined and cause difficulties for the future. The witness feels discredited. One way of avoiding the Catch 22 question is to expand on the answer so that one is answering fully and accurately.

> Q. You are therefore observant?
>
> A. My training has taught me to observe a patient's condition.

It is important under such pressure to avoid becoming angry or upset.

It is likewise important to avoid commenting on the relevance of the question. 'Do I have to answer that question, my Lord?' is fine on a TV drama, but unnecessarily dramatic in court. In most circumstances, one can rely on one's own lawyer or the judge to protect one from unnecessary harassment.

It must be remembered that in cross-examination there are two purposes. One is to discredit the witness's potentially hostile evidence against a client by showing the witness to be unreliable, dishonest, exaggerated, given to imagination, inconsistent (either internally, i.e. within their own evidence, or externally, i.e. in contrast to what another witness has said or what other evidence shows), unclear, confused, suffering from amnesia or (and this may be the most effective) irrelevant.

The other purpose of cross-examination is to build up the strength of the side undertaking the cross-examination. Thus, the witness being cross-examined can be used to bolster the good character and reputation of the defendant. 'What were his good qualities?' 'Was she a good mother?' 'Did you see her show any kindness to the child?' 'Did you like her?' is another Catch 22 question since once again to answer negatively implies that the witness being cross-examined is prejudiced; to answer affirmatively shows that the client has likeable qualities.

It is important in this context for the professionals to remember that in cases where they are giving evidence as witnesses as a result of their professional work, they are not on a particular side. They are called to give evidence of facts that they themselves witnessed. Their reputation does not hang on getting a particular outcome in a negligence case or in a non-accidental injury case. Where the client is personally cross-examining the professional, there should be no sense of betrayal since the professional would have been subpoenaed to attend court and is not there voluntarily.

Defamation

One concern of anyone asked to provide a statement or give evidence is that he or she could face an action for defamation. The main principles of such an action will be discussed very briefly here. The Defamation Act 2013 has introduced some significant changes to the law. A statement is not defamatory unless its publication has caused or is likely to cause serious harm to the reputation of the claimant. Where an organisation which trades for profit is the claimant, then harm to its reputation is not serious harm, unless it caused or is likely to cause serious financial loss.

The Defamation Act 2013 provides the following defences to an action for defamation:

Truth: the defendant can show that the imputation conveyed by the statement complained of is substantially true.

Honest opinion: the following conditions must be met:

1. the statement complained of was a statement of opinion;
2. the statement complained of indicated, whether in general or specific terms, the basis of the opinion;
3. an honest person could have held the opinion on the basis of
    (a) any fact which existed at the time the statement was complained of was published;
    (b) anything asserted to a fact in a privileged statement (see below) published before the statement complained of.

The defence of honest opinion is defeated if the claimant shows that the defendant did not hold the opinion.

Publication of a matter in the public interest: the defendant must also reasonably believe that publishing the statement complained of was in the public interest.

Operators of websites: it is a defence for the operator to show that it was not the operator who posted the statement on the website. This defence, however, can be defeated if:

(a) it was not possible for the claimant to identify the person who posted the statement,
(b) the claimant gave the operator notice of complaint in relation to the statement, and
(c) the operator failed to respond to the notice of complaint.

Regulations provide further details of this defence.

Peer-reviewed statement in a scientific or academic journal: subject to specified conditions including that there has been an independent review of the article. This makes statutory provision for the defence recognised by the Court of Appeal in the case of Dr Singh (see chapter 17).[21]

Reports Protected by Privilege

Another significant change is that trial is to be without a jury unless the court directs.

The court has the power to order the defendant to publish a summary of the judgment when giving judgment for the claimant.

While Article 10 of the European Convention on Human Rights recognises the right of freedom of expression, this is qualified by the need to protect the reputation or rights of others. This is examined in the discussion of the case of Dr Simon Singh, a science writer who successfully defended an action for libel brought against him by the British Chiropractic Association (BCA) (see chapter 17).[22]

Practical Dilemma 9.2   **Providing references**

A ward sister is asked to provide a reference for a staff nurse who has been working on her ward. The staff nurse came under suspicion of theft shortly before this request and the ward sister felt that she would not be honest or accurate if she omitted this fact. The staff nurse failed to get the job she was applying for and subsequently learnt of the contents of the reference. In the meantime, a cleaner was charged and found guilty of the theft. The staff nurse is threatening to sue the ward sister for defamation. Would she succeed?

There is no doubt that to say someone is guilty of theft would be a defamatory statement if it were untrue and had caused or was likely to cause serious harm. However, writing a reference would probably be regarded as an occasion of qualified privilege. If the ward sister wrote the reference without any improper motive, she should have a good defence in an action for defamation. If, however, she made that statement for some other purpose, then the privilege is destroyed by malice. What if she merely stated that the nurse was under suspicion for theft, which would be true? If the words conveyed the impression that there were grounds for considering the nurse to be guilty of theft, then they could be regarded as defamatory and therefore actionable, unless protected by qualified privilege.

Liability for References

Any person asked to provide a reference owes a duty of care to both the subject of the reference and also to the recipient of the reference. In the case of *Hedley Byrne* v *Heller*,[23] the House of Lords[24] held that a duty of care was owed where a person gave advice that he knew would be relied on by the person seeking that advice. If the person suffered harm as a result of reliance on advice that was given negligently, then an action for compensation could be brought against the person who gave the advice. An employer who suffered harm from relying on a reference, which had been given negligently, could sue for compensation. Alternatively, if the reference contained inaccuracies and had been prepared negligently, the subject of the reference could sue the person providing the reference for harm, including financial loss, arising from the breach of the duty of care owed to him or her. To win the case the employee would have to show that the reference was misleading and led the recipient to act to the disadvantage of the subject of the reference and as a consequence he or she has suffered harm.[25] The Court of Appeal has held that an employer has a duty to undertake a reasonable inquiry into the factual basis of statements in a reference in order to discharge its duty to provide an accurate and fair reference.[26] The Information Commissioner's Office (ICO) has published an Employment Practices Code which is available on the ICO website.[27] The Court of Appeal has held that writing a bad reference for a former employee could, under the Equality Act 2010 (see chapter 10), be seen as victimisation of the person even after the employee had left work. An employee failed in his claim against his employers for providing him with an unsatisfactory reference. The High Court held that the employers were protected by qualified privilege and there was no malice shown by the employer.[28]

Internet and social media

The openness and the wide, rapid dissemination of information through the internet and social media have raised concerns about their recreational use by nurses who often fail to realise how widely-linked groups of online contacts are and how quickly information is spread through social media.

When using social networks nurses have to consider whether their remarks or photographs are in keeping with their duty of confidence.

The NMC[29] has issued advice to nurses on the standards expected of them when using social networks. It makes clear that the Code (NMC, 2015) applies to the use of social networking sites and other forms of online communication and nurses must 'uphold the reputation of your profession at all times'. Conduct online is judged in the same way and to the same standard as conduct in a nurse's work and private life. Fitness to practice will be impaired if a nurse acts inappropriately online including where they:

- share confidential information online
- post inappropriate comments about colleagues or patients
- use social networking sites to bully or intimidate colleagues
- pursue personal relationships with patients
- distribute sexually explicit material, or
- use social networking sites in any way which is unlawful.[30]

The NMC recommend that nurses exercise caution when interacting online and in particular to ensure they:

- keep their personal and professional life separate as far as possible;
- uphold the reputation of their profession even where they have not identified themselves as a nurse;
- protect privacy by adjusting privacy settings online;
- must not use social networks to build or pursue relationships with patients;
- must not accept a friendship request from a current or former patient;
- must not discuss work-related issues online even where anonymised;

- must never post pictures of patients online;
- must never use their mobile phone camera in the workplace;
- do not use social networks for raising and escalating concerns or whistleblowing;
- must treat everything online as public, permanent and shared; and
- follow workplace policy for staff and students on the use of social networking sites.[31]

Conclusions

Litigation and complaints within the NHS have continued to increase, so it is inevitable that greater and greater emphasis is placed on records and record keeping in the context of the nurse giving evidence and the nurse is increasingly likely to have to appear in court. However, it must not be forgotten that the most important aspect of record keeping is the fulfilment of the duty of care to the patient and ensuring that others who care for the patient are fully informed through the records of the action that has been taken or that still needs to be done. If the standard of record keeping meets the needs for patient care, then the records will be of sufficient quality to protect the practitioner should they have to defend their practice in any forum or court of law. Regular audit and monitoring are essential for standards to be set and maintained. If records are maintained at a high standard, then the making of statements and giving evidence in court are greatly facilitated. The NHS strategy for electronic patient records has had immense problems in keeping to its timetable, but eventually it should lead to a significant improvement in standards of documentation within the NHS. Constant audit and monitoring will continue to be essential.

Reflection questions

1. What errors have you noticed in record keeping? In what ways do you consider that standards of record keeping could be raised?
2. Consider the implications of electronic patient recording systems for your speciality and analyse its benefits for patient care.
3. Prepare a statement concerning an incident that has recently occurred. Read it through and consider if there are any errors.
4. What is meant by hearsay? Give several examples of it.

Further exercises

1. Arrange a visit to court. Write up the points that any potential witness should be aware of in relation to the procedure, formality and language used. If you have the chance to visit more than one court (e.g. Crown or magistrates' or county or High Court), draw up a list of the differences between them.
2. What most concerns you about the possibility of giving evidence in court? Prepare a list of your concerns, then consider ways of meeting some of these anxieties.

References

[1] Nursing and Midwifery Council (2015) The Code: Professional standards of practice and behaviour for nurses and midwives
[2] https://digital.nhs.uk/data-and-information/looking-after-information/data-security-and-information-governance
[3] Audit Commission, Setting the Records Straight: a study of hospital medical records, Audit Commission, Abingdon, 1995
[4] Audit Commission, Update Setting the Records Straight, Audit Commission, Abingdon, 1999
[5] News item, Diabetic patient died after nurses failed to give insulin, *The Times*, 7 September 2010
[6] News item, *The Times*, 28 May 2014
[7] *Deacon v McVicar and Another*, 7 January 1984 QBD
[8] Department of Health, White Paper on the NHS, The New NHS – modern, dependable, The Stationery Office, London, 1997
[9] Department of Health, Clear rules set for patients' electronic records, May 2005
[10] www.hscic.gov.uk
[11] Jill Sherman, NHS fiasco to cost taxpayer millions, *The Times*, 1 August 2014
[12] Department of Health, NHS challenged to go paperless by 2013, Press Release 2013
[13] www.theprsb.org.uk
[14] https://digital.nhs.uk/services/summary-care-records-scr
[15] *BMJ*, 1979, 1232
[16] www.justice.gov.uk/civil/procrules_fin/menus/rules.htm
[17] Chris Smyth, Nurses told they don't have to co-operate with police, *The Times*, 25 January 2014
[18] Ministry of Justice www.gov.uk
[19] www.hmcourts-service.gov.uk
[20] *Meadows v General Medical Council* [2006] EWCA Civ 1390, [2007] 1 All ER 1
[21] *British Chiropractic Association v Singh* CA, The Times Law Report, 23 April 2010
[22] Ibid.
[23] *Hedley Byrne v Heller* [1963] 2 All ER 575 HL
[24] *Spring v Guardian Assurance Co. Plc and Others*, The Times Law Report, 8 July 1994; [1995] 2 AC 296
[25] *Bartholomew v London Borough of Hackney* [1999] IRLR 448
[26] *Cox v Sun Alliance* [2001] EWCA Civ 649; [2001] IRLR 448 CA
[27] https://ico.org.uk/media/for-organisations/documents/1064/the_employment_practices_code.pdf
[28] *Thour v Royal Free Hampstead NHS Trust* [2012] EWHC 1473
[29] www.nmc.org.uk/globalassets/sitedocuments/nmc-publications/social-media-guidance.pdf
[30] Nursing and Midwifery Council (2011) Social Networking Sites
[31] Griffith, R. and Tengnah, C., District nurses' use of social networking sites: caution required, *British Journal of Community Nursing*, 16(9):455–7, 2011

Chapter 10
The Nurse and Employment Law

This chapter discusses

- Human rights
- Contract of employment
- Statutory provisions covering employment
- Unfair dismissal
- Trade union rights
- Public and private employees
- Discrimination: The Equality and Human Rights Commission
- Equality Act 2010

Introduction

The complexities of employment law can be bewildering, yet the nurse needs to know the way through the maze for two basic reasons: on the one hand, the nurse is an employee and therefore should be acquainted with the rights of an employee; on the other hand, the nurse may be or become a manager in which case they will need to be able to advise staff on their rights and also to understand the relevant employment law covering the nurse's role as manager. The areas discussed in this chapter are set out above. No attempt is made to give the full detail of all the employment statutes but instead the basic principles are set out together with the statutory framework. References are provided so that more detailed information can be obtained.

The legal relationship of employee/employer is composed of many terms drawn from a variety of sources. These are shown in Figure 10.1. First we look at human rights and then how the contract of employment comes into existence.

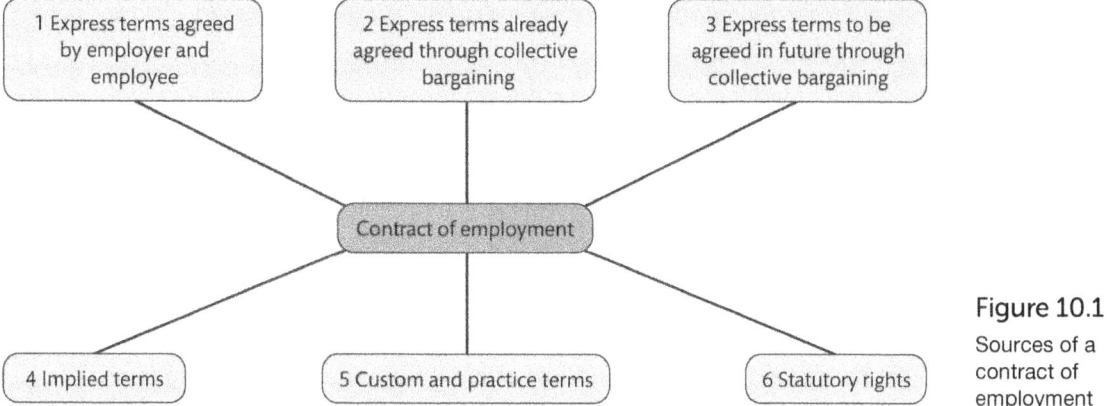

Figure 10.1
Sources of a contract of employment

Human rights

Since October 2000 the European Convention on Human Rights has been directly enforceable in the UK courts. (See the website of this book for Schedule 1 to the Human Rights Act 1998.) Employees in the NHS are entitled to have their rights as set out in the Schedule respected by their employers. Of particular significance to the employment situation are:

- Article 3 and the right not to be subjected to inhuman or degrading treatment or punishment
- Article 6, which gives a person a right to have their civil rights and obligations determined in a fair and public hearing within a reasonable time by an independent and impartial tribunal
- Article 8, which gives a person a right to personal and family life, home and correspondence (subject to specified qualifications) and has implications for any monitoring by the employer of emails, telephone conversations and video surveillance
- Article 9 and the right to freedom of thought, conscience and religion (subject to specified qualifications)
- Article 10 and the right to freedom of expression (subject to specified qualifications)
- Article 11 and the right to freedom of peaceful assembly and to freedom of association with others, including the right to form and to join trade unions for the protection of his interests
- Article 14 and the right not to be discriminated against in the exercise of other rights (examples are given of forms of discrimination, but these are not intended to be exhaustive).

A claim before the European Court of Human Rights under Article 8 succeeded when a transsexual complained that the refusal by the Department of Social Security to pay her a state pension on reaching her sixtieth birthday violated her right to respect for her private life under the Charter Article 8.[1]

If a court considers that any existing legislation is incompatible with the European Convention on Human Rights, it can make a declaration of incompatibility, so that Parliament can decide what action to remove the incompatibility is necessary. A court cannot overrule statutory provisions (see chapter 1). The Equality and Human Rights Commission replaced the Commissions covering equal opportunities, disability rights and race equality on 1 October 2007, and its website[2] is a useful source of information about human rights and discrimination. Please note the Commission only has effect in England, Scotland and Wales. The Information Commissioner's website covers human rights and the duties of an employer in relation to data protection and freedom of information[3] (see chapter 8).

Contract of employment

Formation of Contract

Stages leading to formation of a contract of employment

When a nurse accepts the **offer** of a post, a contract then comes into existence and the nurse will be bound by its terms, unless the terms are interpreted by a court as unreasonable. In this sense the contract is an abstract concept; there may be nothing in writing but the relationship of the parties is radically altered by that agreement.

In any negotiation leading up to a contract of employment many documents may be circulated: an advertisement, an application form, perhaps a job description and often an interview. All these stages are known as an '**invitation to treat**'. Neither party is bound by them and can usually pull out of the negotiations at any stage. Thus an employer is not bound to appoint after advertising a post. Similarly, someone who has sent in an application form can withdraw at any stage from the field prior to **acceptance** of an offer. A contract only comes into being once an offer has been accepted. The offer is usually made by the employer. This could be in writing (for example, after holding interviews the applicants could be sent away without knowing the results and be told that they will be notified) or it could be at the actual interview when the applicants wait until the successful one is summoned and offered the post. Good practice however is for the interviewer to take a candidate's contact details, and let the candidate know that they will be informed later in the day or the next day, the outcome of the interview. Sometimes, this might be a conditional offer: it might, for example, be an offer dependent on a satisfactory medical examination or references, or the selection panel might not have the power to offer the post but can only recommend to the authority that X be appointed. The candidate should be absolutely clear as to the nature of the offer since if it were subject to approval by a higher authority, which did not agree to that appointment or indeed to any appointment, the candidate would have no remedy if they have undergone expenses or even terminated their existing job believing that they had a contract. If the candidate accepts an unconditional offer then and there, they are bound by that contract.

Practical Dilemma 10.1 — Better prospects

A ward manager applies for, is offered and accepts a post in a neighbouring NHS trust. The manager then sees a senior nurse manager post advertised in their own trust, applies and is accepted before they have commenced work in the new post. What is their position in law?

Technically, the ward manager is in breach of contract with the neighbouring NHS trust. They are bound by the contract they have agreed with that trust. In practice, the trust is unlikely to take action against the ward manager; certainly the publicity that would arise would do little to enhance the reputation of that trust and the courts are unlikely to order the ward manager to commence work with the new trust, preferring to compensate by an order for damages to be paid rather than make what is known as an order for specific performance of the contract. The amount payable would be minimal, simply the loss incurred by the trust as a result of the ward manager's breach of contract. The cost of taking the breach to court would probably outweigh the losses they would have incurred via the advertising and the subsequent re-advertising of the post.

Failure to Declare a Particular Medical Condition or Criminal Record

Pre-employment checks

It is for the prospective employer to ascertain the good and bad about any prospective employee. There is no obligation on the candidate to present their inadequacies. However, if the applicant is questioned about medical history or criminal record and lies or fails to disclose relevant information and if this information is later discovered after the applicant has been offered the post and accepted, then the employer is entitled to terminate the contract on the grounds of the misrepresentation provided that they would not have offered the post had they known of the facts. In addition, making a false statement can also be a criminal offence, and a declaration to this effect can be found within most application forms.

The Rehabilitation of Offenders Act 1974 protects those who have a past criminal record from being compelled to disclose it. The rehabilitation periods were changed in 2012.[4] Former prisoners sentenced to six months or less will have to admit their criminal history on job application forms for only two years from the end of their sentence instead of the current seven years from the date of conviction. A person sentenced to up to four years in jail will have to declare their conviction for seven years after the end of their sentence compared with the current provision of disclosure for the rest of their lives. However, this Act does not apply to most health service posts and thus the applicant would have to disclose a criminal record when asked. Where the appointment involves working with children or vulnerable adults, then the employer would be required to check that the person's name is not contained on lists of those considered unsuitable for such work. The Disclosure and Barring Service (which was formed from the merger of the Independent Safeguarding Authority (ISA) with the Criminal Records Bureau on 1 December 2012) should be contacted to ensure that the individual is not on its list.

In 2020 the law has been amended so even with enhanced DBS checks, any spent convictions even when an individual has more than one conviction will not be automatically disclosed, and youth cautions, reprimands and warnings will also not be automatically disclosed. However, any convictions or cautions that are not suitable for being filtered (not needing to be declared) will still be disclosed via an enhanced DBS. Such offences include assault on a child, murder and manslaughter, wounding a person with intent to do grievously bodily harm, and making false statements in an application leading to registration.

> **Practical Dilemma 10.2**   **Undisclosed epilepsy**
>
> An applicant for a post of Health Care Assistant is not asked and fails to disclose that they suffer from epilepsy. This is discovered subsequently when the employee has a fit at work. The employers send the Health Care Assistant a letter dismissing them from their post. What are the legal rights of the Health Care Assistant?

The employers can either give the Health Care Assistant the requisite notice or they could dismiss the employee instantly on the grounds that they are not capable of performing the job safely. However, this is subject to the laws on disability discrimination as re-enacted in the Equality Act 2010, which is considered below. If the applicant had lied about their health, this would be taken into account in determining whether a dismissal would be fair. See also the definition of good health by the NMC, albeit the NMC will only apply to registered nurses and nursing associates (discussed in chapter 17).

Are Terms Agreed at an Interview Binding?

It sometimes happens that at an interview an applicant is given certain assurances about the conditions of work: shifts, hours, days off, holiday dates, location of the workplace, etc. These terms can be made **conditions** of the contract. Thus an applicant who had already booked a holiday can obtain an agreement that one of the terms of the contract is that these dates can be retained. Failure to keep to this agreement would constitute a breach of contract by the employer. However, it is a question of fact as to whether the discussion leads to an agreed term or is merely a working arrangement that can be changed by the employer at a later date. In order to safeguard their position, the nurse, in accepting the post in writing, could confirm that certain terms have been agreed as part of the contract. A job description is not regarded in law as setting out terms of the contract. The list of duties contained therein can be changed unilaterally by the employer (within the overall contractual title) and the job description will usually end with a final requirement of 'and any other reasonable instructions of the employer'. This is perfectly lawful since it is an implied obligation on the part of the employee to obey the reasonable instructions of the employer.

Content of Contract

Figure 10.1 (see the introduction to this chapter) shows sources of the various terms that comprise a contract of employment.

Express terms agreed between employer and applicant

These would include the starting date, the grade and title of post, the point on the salary scale at which the employee would start and many others. It is a matter of interpretation as to how many of the details in the advertisement become terms of the contract.

Express terms already agreed for the post

The bulk of the terms and conditions of posts in the National Health Service were nationally agreed and contained in the Whitley Council Agreements and the health service bodies were bound by these. The Agreements comprised the General Council Conditions, and conditions relating to particular staff groups are negotiated by the NHS Staff Council. The employee's contract should make it clear that it is subject to nationally negotiated conditions. They should be available for inspection by any employee or applicant. NHS trusts also have the power to negotiate some terms locally. Agenda for Change is a nationally agreed pay framework which applies to all NHS staff, except for doctors, dentists and very senior managers. Pay recommendations are made by the NHS Pay Review Body (NHSPRB), and if accepted by Parliament are implemented on a national level. However, devolution allows the respective legislative bodies in Scotland, Wales and Northern Ireland to determine the rates of pay for NHS staff working in one of those countries. In the past few years, there has been varying levels of strike action across the four UK countries, although in Scotland strike action was limited due to the Scottish Government negotiating a pay deal with nurses that to date (2024) is more generous than in other parts of the UK. Please note that if taking strike action is technically a breach of contract, although as long as the union has undertaken a proper ballot of members with sufficient notice provided, there is less likelihood of dismissal, although the employer does have the right to withhold pay for hours/days not worked.

Statutory terms

Additional terms are added by Act of Parliament which are binding on the employer.

Implied terms

Additional terms are also implied in a contract of employment which place obligations on the employer or employee. Past court rulings by judges have decided whether certain specific terms should be implied and also what tests should be used to decide if a particular term is implied.

Box 10.1 sets out implied terms placing obligations on the employer. Box 10.2 sets out implied terms placing obligations on the employee.

Box 10.1 Implied terms binding on the employer

1. A duty to take reasonable care for the health and safety of the employee
2. A duty to pay and to provide work
3. A duty to treat the employee with consideration and support them
4. A duty to deal promptly and properly with grievances

Box 10.2 Implied terms binding on the employee

1. A duty to obey the reasonable orders of the employer
2. A duty to act with reasonable care and skill
3. A duty not to compete with the employer's enterprise
4. A duty to keep secrets and confidential information

> **Practical Dilemma 10.3** — **Implied terms**
>
> An emergency arises in Y Hospital following a multiple pile-up on the nearby motorway. A call is put out to those off duty in the nurses' home, which is onsite, that help is urgently required. Sarah, a staff nurse who has just come off duty after an eight-hour shift, is asked to return. She refuses, saying she is too tired. She has actually arranged to go out with her boyfriend. Her absence is noted and she is subsequently disciplined. She argued that her off duty was her own time and she had no obligations to the employer during it. Also she was far too tired to be of any assistance and in fact would have been positively dangerous to the patients. The employers, in contrast, might argue that there is an implied term in the contract that even when the employee is off duty, she can still be summoned to assist in an emergency.

The outcome of a case such as Practical Dilemma 10.3 will hinge on whether such a term should be implied and also whether a nurse is correct in refusing to help when she is tired and therefore a potential hazard to the patient. A paramedic who refused to take a woman to hospital for an emergency Caesarean section because he was on his break was sacked by his employers and was struck off by the HPC.[5] However, it is worth noting that being on a break while in the course of your shift will be viewed differently to summoning a nurse who is off duty. There may well be an ethical, and even a professional duty a nurse should adhere to; however, to compel someone outside their hours of work to come back into work might be deemed unreasonable by the courts.

There is no decided case on the situation in Practical Dilemma 10.3. The NMC set out an express duty to provide care in or outside the work setting in an emergency in its Code of Professional Conduct published in 2004,[6] but this was not repeated in the 2008 or 2015 edition (see chapter 3 and duty of care).

What about Sarah's fitness to work? It is true that an employee who is unfit to work and is likely to be a danger to fellow employees and patients should stay away. However, in an emergency situation, risks might have to be taken and the risk of potential harm to the patient balanced against the value of that additional pair of hands. It would be a question of fact as to where the balance lay.

Terms resulting from custom and practice

This overworked phrase has been used by trade unionists to give contractual force to certain work practices and privileges that were not original terms of the contract. However, the judicial meaning is much narrower and is confined to special trades and works where the nature of the work has led to special terms being implied. To be legally recognised by the courts, a custom must be 'reasonable, certain and notorious'.

Can an Employee see or have a Copy of her Contract?

A statutory right is given to employees to receive a written statement of particulars of employment. Previously, NHS employees, as Crown employees, were excluded from these provisions. However, under section 60 of the NHS and Community Care Act 1990, health service bodies lost the status of being Crown bodies and all NHS employees now have this statutory right.

Employers are required within two months of the commencement of employment, and as soon as possible after any change in the contract, to give written particulars of the terms set out in Box 10.3. This statement is not the contract itself, but provides *prima facie* evidence of the contractual terms. While the written statement can refer to another document or manual for sickness, sick pay or pensions and the length of notice, all other particulars must be specifically included in the single written statement of employment particulars. Further information on employment contracts can be found on the government website.[7]

Box 10.3 Written statement of employment particulars

Name of employer and employee

Date when employment (and the period of continuous employment) began

Remuneration and the intervals at which it is to be paid

Hours of work

Holiday entitlement

Notice entitlement

Job title or brief job description

Period of employment, or date of ending fixed term, if post not permanent

Place of work or locations if more than one, and the employer's address

Details of collective agreements affecting employment

Additional detail if employee is expected to work abroad

How to complain about a grievance or disciplinary/dismissal decision

Where information about disciplinary and dismissal procedures, grievance procedures, pensions and pension schemes and sick pay and procedures can be found

Changing the Contract

Practical Dilemma 10.4 Job title

Marcus was appointed on the basis that he worked on the surgical ward at Roger Park Hospital. After two years, he was asked to work on the medical wards at Green Down Hospital. He was unwilling either to change his specialty or to move from the present hospital. Could Marcus refuse to move?

The answer depends on whether the location and the specialty are terms of the contract. If they were, then it would be a breach of contract for the employer to change the contract unilaterally. This is because one of the basic principles of contract law is that one party cannot change the terms without the agreement of the other party to the contract (unless there is specific contractual agreement for this, as in the terms and conditions of senior civil servants). Thus, if these issues are seen to be contractual conditions, then the nurse is entitled to retain them. However, care must be taken in insisting on legal rights since it may be that a redundancy situation exists in which case a nurse who refused unreasonably to accept suitable alternative work would lose both his job and the right to obtain compensation. In addition, if someone has been unfairly dismissed, he has a duty to mitigate the loss.

Often, however, the location and ward are not contractual terms, but simply a working arrangement, in which case they can be reasonably altered by the employer without the consent or the right of refusal of the employee. How does one know if the issue in dispute is a contractual term or not? This would depend on the nature of the agreement between them, on the letter (if any) offering the post and on other evidence of the understanding between the parties as to the nature of the contract. Contracts cannot usually be changed unilaterally. Where, however, the employee seeks to obtain promotion or change their post they may be asked to accept new contractual provisions which may not be based on NHS terms and conditions of service.

Breach of Contract

By employee

The employee, as has been seen, has an implied duty to take reasonable care and skill in their work and to obey the reasonable orders of the employer. If the employee is in breach of these terms, they can be disciplined. In extreme cases, the employee's actions may justify summary dismissal by the employer. Other sanctions by the employer include suspension, demotion, warnings, etc.

By employer

The duty to abide by the contractual agreement is reciprocal and the employee is therefore entitled to expect that they will be treated with consideration and that there will be no unilateral change of contract conditions. If it is apparent that the employer is in fundamental breach of contract, then the employee may be able to consider himself constructively dismissed. The recent change in the law whereby breach of health and safety regulations can no longer be the basis for an action for compensation may lead to an increase in claims for the failure of the employer to respect the duty to take reasonable care of the employee's health and safety (see chapter 12).

Statutory provisions covering employment

The Protection of Children Act 1999, the Protection of Vulnerable Adults scheme and the Sexual Offenders Act 1997 enabled employers to establish if there are grounds for not employing prospective employees. Consequently there were three separate lists of persons who were barred from working with children or vulnerable adults. The lists operated under different legislation with different criteria and procedures. Following a public consultation[8] undertaken in the light of the Bichard Inquiry[9] (which was set up following the murders of Holly Wells and Jessica Chapman), the Safeguarding Vulnerable Groups Act 2006 was passed to provide the legislative framework for a revised vetting and barring scheme for people who work with children and vulnerable adults. It aimed at minimising the risk of harm to children and vulnerable adults by barring unsuitable individuals not just on the basis of referrals but also at the earliest possible opportunity as part of a centralised vetting process that all those working with children and vulnerable adults must go through. Subsequently the Disclosure and Barring Service (DBS) has been established.

Sexual Offenders Act 1997 and 2003

The Sexual Offenders Act 1997 was passed to ensure that once a sex offender had served their sentence and was about to be released, they would still be subject to some form of supervision to protect persons against the risk of their reoffending. Part I of the Act requires the notification of information to the police by persons who have committed certain sexual offences.

The Sexual Offenders Act has now been replaced by the Sex Offences Act. This Act required relevant offenders to notify certain personal information to the police. New 2004 regulations[10] set out travel notification requirements which were further amended in 2012.[11]

Protection of Children Act 1999

This legislation had four purposes.

1. It made statutory the Department of Health's Consultancy Service Index list and it required childcare organisations to refer the names of individuals considered unsuitable to work with children for inclusion on the list.
2. It provided rights of appeal against inclusion.
3. It required regulated childcare organisations to check the names of anyone they propose to employ in posts involving regular contact with children with the list and not to employ them if listed.
4. It amended Part V of the Police Act 1997 to allow the Criminal Records Bureau (now the Disclosure and Barring Service, DBS) to act as a central access point for criminal records information, the Children's Barred List[12] and the Department of Health list. In other words, the DBS process would act as a one-stop shop in the carrying out of checks.

The effect of the legislation was that organisations working with children, such as local authorities and health trusts, had a statutory duty from 2 October 2000 to vet prospective employees, paid or unpaid, for work involving contact with children.

Protection of Vulnerable Adults

Provision was made in the Care Standards Act 2000 for a scheme to protect vulnerable adults. The protection of vulnerable adults (POVA) scheme enabled a list to be kept of anyone who has harmed or placed at risk of harm a vulnerable adult in their care, and providers of care are not able to offer employment to such individuals. Those on the list who sought employment in care positions would be committing a criminal offence. Checks against the POVA list were requested as part of disclosures from the Criminal Records Bureau.[13] Care workers who had challenged their provisional placement on the POVA list as being contrary to their Article 6 and 8 rights won their case in the High Court, which held that the provisions of the Care Standards Act 2000 in relation to provisional listings were not compatible with their human rights.[14] The Court of Appeal held that those who worked with vulnerable adults should be given the opportunity to make representations before being placed on the POVA list. That would prevent section 82(4)(b) of the Care Standards Act being incompatible with Article 6 of the European Convention on Human Rights. The POVA list whilst still in common usage has now been renamed the Children's and Adults' Barred Lists and is managed by the Independent Safeguarding Authority.

Safeguarding Vulnerable Groups Act 2006

This Act set up a new scheme for barring those unsuitable for work with children and vulnerable adults. Vulnerable adult is defined in section 59 and includes many categories of adults, such as those in residential care, those receiving healthcare or a welfare service of any description and those who require assistance in the conduct of their affairs. Regulations which came into force in October 2009[15] amplify the definition of a welfare service by stating that it includes the provision of support, assistance or advice by any person, the purpose of which is to develop an individual's capacity to live independently in accommodation, or sustain their capacity to do so. The regulations also prescribe the circumstances in which driving children and adults can become a regulated activity.

The Supreme Court held that the absence of an individual review of the notification requirements on a sex offender who had been placed under lifelong notification duties constituted a disproportionate interference with Article 8 rights.[16]

Protection of vulnerable adults: no secrets

No Secrets guidance[17] was issued in 2000 for the protection of the elderly and vulnerable adults against abuse. In 2008–9 an extensive consultation exercise was carried out with both professionals and service users, and in January 2010 the government published its response in a written ministerial statement. This stated that the following action would be taken:

- an inter-departmental ministerial group (IDMG) would be set up to determine policy and work priorities; provide a strategic and coordination role and provide public and parliamentary advocacy;
- Safeguarding Adult Boards would be put on a statutory footing by legislation;
- a programme of work with representative agencies and stakeholders would be launched to support effective policy and practice in safeguarding vulnerable adults.

Disclosure and Barring Service

The Protection of Freedoms Act 2012 section 87(1) established the Disclosure and Barring Service (DBS) with the transfer of functions from Independent Safeguarding Authority.[18] The functions of the Secretary of State performed by the Criminal Records Bureau are also transferred to the DBS, which can be accessed on the government website.[19] The DBS processes requests for criminal records checks; decides whether it is appropriate for a person to be placed on or removed from a barred list and places or removes people from the DBS children's barred list and adults' barred list for England, Wales and Northern Ireland. It has published a code of practice for recipients of DBS certificates. Part 5 of the Protection of Freedoms Act 2012 defines the scope of the regulated activities in relation to children and vulnerable adults and sets out the information required for the purposes of making barring decisions; the review of barring decisions; information about barring decisions and the duty to check on whether a person is barred. Sections 21 to 27 of the Safeguarding Vulnerable Groups Act 2006 covering controlled activity and monitoring are repealed. Regulations implement the changes.[20] Access to the Disclosure and Barring Service is through the government website.[21]

In England and Wales, the Child Sex Offender Disclosure Scheme (known as Sarah's Law – resulting from the campaign by Sara Payne whose daughter Sarah was murdered by a convicted paedophile in 2000) enables parents to inquire about any person who has access to their children and has led to 4,754 applications since the launch of the scheme in 2011 with the disclosure of more than 700 paedophiles to parents.[22] In Scotland a similar scheme exists entitled Keeping Children Safe, while in Northern Ireland, Child Protection Disclosure Arrangements was launched via the Justice Act (Northern Ireland) 2015, and acts in a similar way to Sarah's Law in England and Wales.

The Supreme Court has ruled that the automatic release of a person's convictions, cautions and warnings regardless of the length of time that had elapsed, when that person was required to obtain an enhanced criminal record certificate for the purposes of obtaining employment which involved working with children or other vulnerable persons, was incompatible with their Article 8 right to respect for their private life.[23]

Statutory Rights for Employees

Certain Acts of Parliament provide additional rights to employees.[24] The most significant Acts are the Employment Rights Act 1996, Employment Relations Act 1999, Employment Act 2002, Employment Relations Act 2004, Employment Act 2008, the Equality Act 2010, Enterprise and Regulatory Reform Act 2013 and the Children and Families Act 2014. Table 10.1 sets out some of the statutory rights and the minimum time of **continuous service** that the employee must have in order to claim these rights. They include medical suspension payments, guaranteed pay, rights for the pregnant employee, time off work provisions, rights in relation to trade unions and many others. In addition, after 2 October 2000, those employees working for a public organisation or an organisation that exercises functions of a public nature may have grounds for claiming a breach of their human rights if the employer does not respect the rights set out in the European Convention on Human Rights.

Table 10.1 Statutory rights

Right	Period of continuous employment
Flexible working	26 weeks
Not to be dismissed because of medical suspension	4 weeks
Written statement of terms and conditions of employment	4 weeks
Written reasons for dismissal	1 year (2 for those employed after 6.04.12)
Not to be unfairly dismissed	2 years
Maternity rights	
1. Paid time off work to receive antenatal care	No minimum period
2. Right to return to work after pregnancy	No minimum period
3. Not to be unfairly dismissed on grounds of pregnancy	No minimum period
Redundancy pay	2 years
Not to be dismissed because of trade union activities	No minimum period
Time off for trade union duties, trade union activities and public duties	No minimum period

Some of the main employment rights are shown in Box 10.4.

> **Box 10.4 Statutory rights**
>
> 1. Employment particulars
> 2. Protection of wages
> 3. Guaranteed payments
> 4. Sunday working for shop and betting workers
> 5. Protection from suffering detriment in employment
> 6. Time off work
> 7. Suspension from work
> 8. Maternity rights
> 9. Termination of employment
> 10. Unfair dismissal rights
> 11. Redundancy payments, etc.
> 12. Insolvency of employers
> 13. Whistleblowing
> 14. Part-time workers' rights
> 15. Notice of dismissal
> 16. Itemised pay slip
> 17. Right not to be discriminated against
> 18. Holiday and holiday pay

Rights of the pregnant employee

The employment rights set out in Box 10.4 have been strengthened by the implementation of the European Pregnant Workers Directive and recent implementation of rights for parents and those with dependants. No continuous service is required to obtain these rights. The rights include:

1. The right not to be dismissed on grounds of their sex, pregnancy or maternity leave.
2. The right to receive 26 weeks' ordinary maternity leave and 26 weeks' additional maternity leave. Pregnant women who meet qualifying conditions may receive up to 39 weeks' Statutory Maternity Pay (those not entitled may receive 39 weeks' Maternity Allowance).
3. The right to return to work after confinement.
4. The right to attend antenatal classes.
5. The right to be offered suitable alternative work or be paid during suspension from work on maternity grounds.
6. The right to have their health and safety protected when they are pregnant, have recently given birth or are breastfeeding (see chapter 12).

Further details on all these rights are to be found on the government website[25] and also the ACAS website.[26] The Citizen's Advice Bureau also has useful information on employment rights[27] as well as the Northern Ireland government website NIDirect.[28]

In addition to the statutory rights, NHS conditions covering the same field often exist. The employee usually has the right to choose whichever benefits are more favourable to them. The RCN has provided guidance for nursing, midwifery staff and students.[29]

Right not to be unfairly dismissed on grounds of pregnancy

Practical Dilemma 10.5   Morning sickness

Barbara is two months pregnant and suffering very badly from morning sickness and hypertension. Her absence from the ward is causing considerable difficulties and she is not popular with the other staff. She has worked with the authority for three years. It has been agreed that she should be dismissed because of the continual absences. What are her rights?

She is pregnant, a full-time employee for three years and is therefore able to claim the right of not being unfairly dismissed on the grounds of pregnancy. The authority might argue that her pregnancy is making it impossible for her to do her job adequately, there is no suitable alternative work and therefore they are justified in dismissing her. This is, however, no longer an acceptable defence to an application for unfair dismissal on grounds of pregnancy and the employee would probably succeed in her application. No continuous service is required. Furthermore, the employee is entitled to receive pay during a time of suspension from work on maternity grounds, if suspension results from a health ground specified by statute (i.e. pregnancy, birth or breastfeeding) or to be offered suitable alternative work. If suitable alternative work is not available, the employee can claim pay during the time of suspension from work. Claims in relation to dismissal on grounds of pregnancy can also be brought under the Equality Act under which there is no upper limit to the amount of compensation. (In 2010 a banker who was not allowed to return to work after her maternity leave was awarded £1.5 million for sex discrimination and unfair dismissal.)[30]

Maternity right to return to work

In *Halfpenny* v *IGE Medical System Ltd* 1999,[31] a woman who had left work to have a child exercised her statutory right to return to work after her maternity leave by giving the appropriate notice. She then sought to delay her return to work on grounds of sickness. The employers allowed a first extension, but then notified her that her job was no longer available. At an industrial tribunal she lost her application for unfair dismissal, wrongful dismissal and unlawful sex discrimination, and her appeal before the employment appeal tribunal was also unsuccessful. Her appeal to the Court of Appeal, however, succeeded on the grounds that the exercise of her statutory right to return to work was made complete and effective by the giving of the appropriate notice at the appropriate time. The employers were guilty of unfair dismissal, wrongful dismissal and unlawful sex discrimination.

The European Court of Justice held that a woman who gave up work or looking for work because of the physical constraints of the late stages of pregnancy and the aftermath of childbirth retained the status of worker within the meaning of Article 45 of the Treaty on the Functioning of the European Union, provided she returned to work or found another job within a reasonable period after the birth of the child.[32]

Dismissal of maternity leave replacement

A case that came before the European Court in Luxembourg concerned an employee who was appointed to the post to provide maternity cover for an employee during maternity leave.[33] However, she became pregnant and was dismissed. The court ruled that it was an unfair dismissal on the grounds of pregnancy. Its decision was therefore that EEC Directive 76/207 precluded dismissal of an employee who had been recruited for an unlimited term with a view initially to replacing another employee during maternity leave and could not do so because, shortly after her recruitment, she was herself found to be pregnant. Subsequently, the Sex Discrimination Act 1975 was amended in 2005 and again in 2008 to clarify the protection provided to the pregnant employee. The provisions are now re-enacted in the Equality Act 2010. The Protection from Redundancy (Pregnancy and Family Leave) Act 2023, further strengthens the law, and any pregnant employees, and those returning from maternity and adoption leave have special protection from redundancy, and this includes employees with shared parental leave.

Antenatal visits

There is a statutory right to attend antenatal examinations with paid leave. For the first visit, there is no requirement to show the certificate for the expected date of confinement or the appointment card, but for subsequent visits the employer can insist on seeing both. The right is not absolute, however. It depends on the reasonableness of the request and it may be reasonable to refuse such time off if an employee can reasonably make arrangements for an appointment outside normal working hours. There is no statutory right for the father to have paid leave to accompany his wife on antenatal visits, but the government is encouraging employers to adopt a flexible approach and has published a fathers-to-be and antenatal[34] appointments good practice guide. Under the Children and Families Act 2014 fathers have a right to unpaid leave to attend up to two antenatal appointments.

In a case reported on 18 March 2014 the European Court ruled that a woman, who had made arrangements with a surrogate to have a child for her, was not entitled to receive maternity benefits.[35] Changes introduced by the Children and Families Act 2014 make it easier for intended parents in a surrogacy arrangement to access adoption leave and pay, and shared parental leave and pay.

Parental leave for caring for a child (including adopted child)[36]

A right was given by the Employment Relations Act 1999 to enable either parent to be absent from work for the purpose of caring for a child or making arrangements for the child's welfare.[37] Following an EU directive, amendment regulations were passed which enable a qualifying employee's entitlement to parental leave to be increased from 13 weeks to 18 weeks.[38] Under the Children and Families Act 2014 all parents of children under 18 are able to take up to 18 weeks of unpaid parental leave per parent per child.

Emergency leave can be taken to deal with an emergency involving a dependant. There is not a set amount of time and there is no right to paid time off, but some employers might be prepared to give paid time off. An emergency includes illness, injury, assault, having a baby, disruption of care arrangements, if a child is involved in an incident during school time.

Statutory maternity leave and pay

Statutory maternity leave of 52 weeks is made up of 26 ordinary maternity leave for the first 26 weeks and additional maternity leave for the last 26 weeks. The earliest date it can commence is 11 weeks before the expected week of the childbirth or the day after the birth if the baby is early. It will automatically start if the employee is off work for a pregnancy-related illness in the 4 weeks before the week that the baby is due. Statutory maternity pay (SMP) is paid for up to 39 weeks; 90 per cent of average weekly earnings (before tax) for the first 6 weeks, then £145.18 or 90 per cent of average weekly earnings (whichever is the lower) for the next 33 weeks. To be eligible for leave, employees must be an employee, give the employer the correct notice, earn on average at least £116 a week, give proof of the pregnancy and have worked for the employer continuously for 26 weeks up to the qualifying week – the fifteenth week before the expected week of childbirth. An employee cannot get SMP if they go into police custody during the maternity pay period. Further details of the statutory maternity pay scheme are available.[39]

Maternity allowance

This is payable to those employees who do not qualify for statutory maternity pay. The higher amount is payable for 39 weeks for employees who are not eligible for SMP, for the self-employed and those who have recently stopped working. Employees must have worked for at least 26 weeks in the 66 weeks before the week the baby is due and have earned at least £30 a week over any 13 week period. Allowance at present (April 2024) is £184.03 (full rate) a week for up to 39 weeks.

Maternity allowance at the lower level is paid for 14 weeks if for at least 26 weeks in the 66 weeks before the baby is due the person is married or in a civil partnership, is not employed or self-employed, worked with a spouse or a partner in a business and is not paid. The person must not be eligible for statutory maternity pay or the higher amount of maternity allowance. The amount payable is £27 a week for up to 14 weeks.

Paternity leave and pay

Statutory paternity pay (SPP) is payable by employers to eligible employees to take paid leave to care for his baby or support the mother following birth. He can take either one week's or two consecutive weeks' paternity leave and during this time he may be entitled to SPP. The baby's mother and father are able to share leave between them and alternate, discontinuous periods of time off can be taken by both parents with the employer and employee agreeing the pattern of leave. The mother could transfer all her leave to the father except for the two weeks' compulsory leave she must take. The maximum entitlement is 52 weeks to be shared between them. Further details are available on the government website.[40]

Time-off provisions

Paid or unpaid time off (depending on the benefit) is also a statutory right and can be seen in Box 10.5. Again, there are comparable NHS rights and the employee is entitled to choose whichever is more advantageous.

Box 10.5 — Time-off provisions

Time off for:

1. Trade union duties (officer): reasonable paid time off to carry out duties in connection with industrial relations and for training relevant to carrying out those duties (as a learning representative) (reasonable defined in ACAS Code of Practice No. 3)
2. Trade union activities (member): reasonable unpaid time off during working hours to take part in TU activities (see ACAS Code of Practice No. 3)
3. Public duties – local authority member, school governor, JP: reasonable unpaid time off (take into account time off given in relation to 1 or 2 above and other public duties)
4. To seek job in redundancy situation: reasonable paid time off to seek work or seek retraining
5. Jury service: unpaid time off
6. Health and safety representative: reasonable paid time off to perform function and train for it
7. Time off for dependants

In Practical Dilemma 10.6, Mary took the case to an industrial tribunal and won since it was held that rearranging a timetable was not giving time off. However, Mary was still receiving her full pay and the time-off provisions were only for unpaid time off. (The school could have reduced her workload, reduced her salary accordingly and then employed a locum to teach in Mary's place with the money saved. Mary might have preferred the existing arrangements!)

Practical Dilemma 10.6 — Rearranging a timetable

Mary Briggs was a nurse lecturer. She was also very involved in local government and had recently been elected as leader of the opposition on the county council. She was appointed to several subcommittees. She applied for time off to attend the meetings. The principal was extremely helpful and rearranged her timetable so that she would not have to teach in the afternoons when the council meetings took place. Mary complained that her workload had not decreased and she now found that she was having to spend several evenings doing work that normally she would have done during her free periods, which had now been lost.

Time off for dependants[41]

From 15 December 1999, reasonable time off is permitted where it is reasonable for an employee to deal with an emergency involving a dependent. This includes when a dependant is ill, gives birth or is injured; dies; where there is unexpected disruption of arrangements for the care of the dependant; or an incident at school. The employee must notify the employer of the reason for their absence as soon as is reasonably practicable and how long they are likely to be off. Dependants include a spouse, a child, a parent, a person who lives in the same household as the employee (other than a tenant or lodger) and includes any person who reasonably relies on the employee for assistance when ill or injured. An employer's refusal to give time off for dependants could be followed by an application by the employee to an employment tribunal.

Flexible working

Section 47 of the Employment Act 2002 introduced a statutory right from April 2003 for an employee to request a variation in her contract, known as making a statutory application. Only employees who have worked continuously for the same employer for 26 weeks are eligible to make a statutory application and only one a year can be made. The employer has a statutory duty to consider the request but can refuse the request if a refusal is justified. Clear procedures for dealing with requests by employees for changes in their contracts are essential. From 30 June 2014 all employees with 26 weeks' continuous service are able to apply for flexible working, thus removing the previous restriction of those with children under 17 years or those with caring responsibilities. The statutory process and all its deadlines are removed and new regulations replaced the 2002 regulations for applications after 30 June 2014.[42] Employers are required to consider the request in a reasonable manner and within a reasonable time and can legitimately refuse if a refusal is justified. A code of practice to assist employers on flexible working came into force on 30 June 2014.[43] The Employment Rights (Flexible Working) Act 2023 allows employees to request flexible working arrangements right from day one of employment. Employees mist also provide a good reason for denial and must respond to any requests within two months (previously it was three months). Employees can also make two requests for flexible working within a twelve-month period (previously it was only one month). Under the Carer's Leave Act 2023, an employee also has the right to one week of carer's leave in addition to any annual leave entitlement. However, this one week is unpaid leave. The Employer cannot refuse carer's leave but can ask for a postponement if the request is for a critical working period (for example a winter crisis situation at the local health board/trust or dealing with a pandemic).

Statutory Sick Pay Scheme

Most NHS employees are entitled to six months' full pay and six months' half-pay, after a determined length of service, while absent on grounds of sickness. The employer is able to recover some of this from the statutory sick pay (SSP) scheme. Details of the operation of the scheme are available from the government website. All employers can offset any contractual liability to pay sick pay against their payments under SSP.

Redundancy

The NHS has its own redundancy scheme set out in the general conditions of service. It broadly follows the statutory scheme from the point of view of consultation when redundancies are envisaged. However, the NHS has a much wider definition of suitable alternative work. The Information and Consultation with Employees Regulations[44] came into force in April 2005 and require consultation with and information to be given by employers where there are decisions likely to affect future employment.[45] Initially this applied to organisations where there are more than 150 employees. From 2008 the regulations apply to organisations of 50 or more employees. Employees could also seek personal information about themselves from the employer under the General Data Protection Regulations 2016 and general information under the Freedom of Information Act 2000 (see chapter 8).

Working Time Directive (WTD)

A Directive had been adopted by the member states of the European Union on 23 November 1996, but implementation in the UK was delayed until 1 October 1998, when the Working

Time Regulations[46] came into force.[47] Although the UK is no longer a member of the European Union, the Working Time Regulations remain in force under UK law.

Main principles

The fundamental provision is that a worker's working time, including overtime, should not exceed an average of 48 hours for each 7 days over a specified period of 17 weeks. Regulations also specify provisions for rest breaks and annual leave. Night work should not normally exceed an average of 8 hours for each 24 hours. The employer has a duty to ensure that no night worker, whose work involves special hazards or heavy physical or mental strain, works for more than 8 hours in any 24-hour period. Before assigning a worker to night work, the employer has to ensure that the worker has the opportunity of a free health assessment before they take up the assignment. There should be a weekly rest period of not less than 24 hours in each 7-day period: alternatively, two rest periods each of not less than 24 hours in each 14-day period or one rest period of not less than 48 hours in each 14-day period.

Employers are required to keep records relating to the hours of work, which can be inspected by enforcement agencies. The Health and Safety Executive and local authority environmental health officers are responsible for enforcing the working time limits. Individual employees can, if internal appeals mechanisms fail, apply to the employment tribunal for alleged infringements of their statutory rights. The application must be made within 3 months of the infringement and the Advisory, Conciliation and Arbitration Service (ACAS) will provide conciliation services. The European Court of Justice has held the UK requirement of 13 weeks' work before being eligible to have annual leave illegal.[48] In a later case, the European Court of Justice held that UK guidelines on the WTD were incompatible with the Directive, in that the guidelines did not make clear that employers had to ensure that workers actually did take a rest break according to the regulations.[49] Although the European Court of Justice no longer has jurisdiction over the UK, any deviance from the regulation can still be brought before the UK courts for a ruling.

Working longer than 48 hours a week

Individual employees can, if they wish, agree to work more than the average of 48 hours a week. However, this must be an individual decision. It cannot be negotiated as part of the collective agreement and it must be agreed in writing by the employee. The employee should not be placed under pressure to agree to a longer time. The employee can end the agreement by giving notice to the employer, as specified in the agreement, or, if no notice time is specified, then seven days' notice must be given. The employer is required to keep records of this agreement and the term of notice and the number of hours worked since the agreement came into effect.

National Minimum Wage (NMW) Act 1998

From 1 April 1999, employers have been obliged to pay a minimum wage to employees, with those aged between 18 and 20 years receiving a lower figure. Employees can appeal to an employment tribunal without any continuous service requirement if they are dismissed because they qualify for the NMW or because they have attempted to enforce the NMW right.[50] The Court of Appeal has held that a restaurant cannot use tips to achieve the minimum wage level.[51] The House of Lords held that non-payment of holiday pay is an unlawful deduction from wages;

employees who were entitled to statutory holiday pay were also entitled to claim its non-payment as an unlawful deduction from wages.[52] The current national minimum wage (as at April 2024) is £11.44 per hour for adults over the age of 21, and £8.60 per hour for those aged between 18 and 20 years. Care workers won a significant victory when a firm was successfully prosecuted by HM Revenue and Customs for refusing to pay staff for the time it takes them to travel between appointments. HMRC claimed the practice breached minimum wage legislation. The firm concerned has to pay staff £600,000 in arrears.[53] In another case an employee successfully appealed to the Employment Appeal Tribunal (EAT) claiming that her employer had failed to pay her the national minimum wage for sleepovers and the time she spent travelling between clients' homes. The EAT held that the sleepovers were part of time work, irrespective of the level of activity and that time spent travelling was working time.[54]

Part-time Employees

On 1 July 2000 regulations came into force to prevent part-time workers being treated less favourably than full-time workers,[55] implementing the EU Part-Time Work Directive.[56] Paragraph 5 of the UK regulations gives the part-time worker:

> [T]he right not to be treated by his employer less favourably than the employer treats a comparable full-time worker as regards the terms of his contract, or by being subjected to any other detriment by any act, or deliberate failure to act of his employer.

The right applies only if the treatment is on the grounds that the worker is a part-time worker and the treatment is not justified on objective grounds. The part-time worker has to compare himself with full-time workers working for the same employer. The right also applies to workers who become part-time or, having been full-time, return part-time after absence, to be treated not less favourably than they were before going part-time. It does not give an employee the right to insist on having part-time work.

The regulations (paragraph 6) also entitle a worker, who considers that he has been treated in a manner that infringes this right, to request from his employer a written statement giving particulars of the reasons for the treatment. The worker must be provided with a statement within 21 days of his request. Failure to provide a statement at all or only in an evasive or equivocal way will enable the tribunal to draw any inference that it considers just and equitable to draw, including an inference that the employer has infringed the right in question. The regulations also protect the part-time worker from unfair dismissal and give a right not to be subjected to any detriment (paragraph 7).

Any worker who considers that his rights have been infringed can present a complaint to an employment tribunal within three months of the day of less favourable treatment or detriment taking place. This is subject to the right of the tribunal to consider out-of-time cases, if in all the circumstances it is just and equitable to do so.

The European Union issued a Directive[57] giving new rights for temporary workers, including workers hired through agencies. After twelve weeks in a given job, an agency worker will be entitled to equal treatment (at least the basic working and employment conditions that would apply to the worker concerned if s/he had been recruited directly by that undertaking to occupy the same job). Regulations implementing this Directive were passed in 2010 and came into force on 1 October 2011. This is referred to as the Agency Workers Regulations 2010 and is a part of UK domestic legislation that has not been affected by the UK's withdrawal from the European Union in 2020.

Dismissal and Professional Conduct and Competence

Where a registered practitioner has been dismissed by his or her employer this will be reported to the NMC and the investigating committee or other practice committees may look into the situation with a view to deciding whether the practitioner is fit to practise (see chapter 11). Other disciplinary action may or may not be reported to the NMC depending on the extent to which the fitness to practise of the practitioner is impaired. The NMC is concerned to ensure that employers take greater responsibility over the competence of their registered practitioners to practise and that issues relating to contractual matters are dealt with by employers rather than being referred to the NMC. It has issued guidance to employers on their responsibilities in relation to professional registration.[58] (This replaces the earlier publications on reporting unfitness to practise and lack of competence.) The National Audit Office[59] considered the management of suspensions of clinical staff in NHS hospital and ambulance trusts in England and suggested significant reforms, highlighting concerns about the length of suspensions of clinical staff on full pay and the fairness, openness and transparency of existing procedures.One of the new powers introduced in 2002 for the NMC was to permit a registrant to remain on the Register subject to specified conditions (see chapter 11). This would require monitoring of the practitioner however it allows the registrant to continue working as a registrant as long as they adhere to the conditions provided.

Surveillance by Employers

The European Court of Human Rights, in the case brought before it by Alison Halford, held that her rights of privacy had been invaded when her employers, the Merseyside Police Authority, intercepted the private telephone calls she made from the office. The court held, however, that provided that the employer warned the employees that their calls could be tapped, there would be no breach of the right to privacy as guaranteed by the European Convention.[60] Article 8 of the Convention recognises the right to respect for private and family life, home and correspondence (see chapter 1). The Information Commissioner's Office has published, as part of its Employment Practices Data Protection Code, a code of practice relating to the monitoring of employees' emails by employers.[61] The Regulation of Investigatory Powers Act 2000[62] and the Telecommunications (Lawful Business Practices) (Interception of Communications) Regulations 2000[63] enable emails to be monitored without consent in specified circumstances such as the prevention or detection of crime or the investigation of unauthorised use of the system. The employer must have taken reasonable steps to inform users of the monitoring or have reasonable grounds to believe that employees are aware that this may happen. There are considerable advantages for employers to have a code of practice covering all aspects of surveillance and ensure that it is regularly updated, that employees are aware of its existence and that consent to the monitoring is a term of the contracts of employment. The Information Commissioner's office has published the Employment Practices Code, Part 3 of which includes a section on monitoring at work.[64]

Unfair dismissal

General Principles

One of the most important of the statutory rights is the right not to be unfairly dismissed. Every employee has a right by virtue of his contract, statute or the common law to receive notice unless the employee is themselves in breach of contract and is summarily dismissed. Thus, without a concept of unfair dismissal, a nursing officer who has worked for 20 years with that employer could lawfully be given her requisite notice under the contract with no particular reasons for the notice being specified and be lawfully dismissed. This would be contractually acceptable, but highly unjust. The right not to be unfairly dismissed protects employees who meet certain conditions against this unjust treatment. There is also a right not to suffer a detriment or dismissal in health and safety cases. It is unfair to dismiss an employee in circumstances arising out of health and safety matters, e.g. carrying out health and safety activities at the request of the employer, being a safety representative or a member of a safety committee, bringing the employer's attention to harmful circumstances, refusing to work in dangerous conditions or taking appropriate steps to protect themselves or others from damage.

There is now a continuous service requirement of two years for unfair dismissal unless the application is based on the specific grounds shown in Table 10.1.

The Public Interest Disclosure Act 1998 extends these provisions and protects an employee from victimisation where the employee has made a protective disclosure in accordance with the provisions of this Act and its subsequent amendments (see chapter 4).

An employee must apply to ACAS and seek conciliation. Individuals wanting to bring a tribunal claim must inform ACAS first. Claims are no longer made direct to the tribunal. If conciliation is unsuccessful, the individual can continue with a tribunal claim. If employers lose a claim, tribunals will have the power to fine them, with a minimum of £100 in addition to the award made to the claimant and fee reimbursement.

The conditions that the employee must satisfy to bring an action for unfair dismissal are set out in Box 10.6. If these conditions are met, the employee can then, within three months of the dismissal, apply to the employment tribunal for an unfair dismissal hearing. The three-month time limit can be extended if the tribunal considers that it was not reasonably practicable for the employee to comply with it. Reforms introduced under the Enterprise and Regulatory Reform Act 2013 (ERRA) include capping the compensation payable – payouts to be limited to up to one year's pay or £74,200, whichever is the lower; and fees to be introduced to restrict spurious cases. Claimants have to pay fees of between £390 and £1200 if the case goes to a tribunal. The time limit for bringing an unfair dismissal application is extended (by the 2013 Act section 8 and Schedule 2) to allow time for conciliation.

Figures suggest that the fees to bring an application to the employment tribunal have led to an 80 per cent reduction in the number of applications. The Chair of the Industrial Law Society wrote to *The Times* deploring the consequential injustices for many employees who could no longer afford to bring action for breach of their statutory rights. He called on the government to review the effects of the fees urgently.[65] However to date (April 2024) no changes have been made.

Box 10.6 Conditions for bringing an unfair dismissal action

1. Two years' continuous service with that employer (except for example in cases of trade union activity or discrimination and dismissal on grounds of pregnancy or childbirth or health and safety (see Table 10.1)
2. Eligibility under the legislation
3. Being below retirement age
4. Dismissal (i.e. termination by employer, expiry of fixed-term contract or constructive dismissal)

Unfair Dismissal and Record Keeping

Case 10.1 *Barchester Healthcare Ltd v Tayeh [2013]*

False entry in records[66]

Tayeh was a registered nurse employed in a care home run by the defendant. In disciplinary proceedings she admitted making a false entry on a patient's drip-feed record and failing to make proper observations in respect of a patient who had fallen, and was summarily dismissed for gross misconduct. She succeeded before the employment tribunal which held that the falsification of records did not amount to serious misconduct, she had not been promptly suspended after the incident, and the employer had not taken into account mitigation available to her in relation to the fall, and the dismissal was therefore unfair. The employers appealed to the Employment Appeal Tribunal (EAT), which upheld the appeal holding that the dismissal was fair and that the employers had been entitled to dismiss Tayeh for gross misconduct. Tayeh appealed to the Court of Appeal which upheld the decision of the EAT. The falsification of written records was a serious matter capable of meriting dismissal.

Unfair Dismissal and Length of Continuous Service and Compensation

From 6 April 2012 the qualifying period for bringing unfair dismissal claims was increased from one year's continuous service to two years' continuous service. The compensation comprises a basic award based on a maximum week's pay (£700) multiplied by the number of years of continuous service (depending on age) (with a maximum of 20 years), and a compensatory award designed to compensate the employee for the financial results of losing his or her job. In April 2018 the ceiling was £115,115. This ceiling does not apply to awards under sex discrimination, equal pay and whistleblowing victimisation claims. Furthermore, an additional award can be made under section 117 of the Employment Rights Act 1996 (ERA) where the employer refuses a tribunal order to reinstate or re-engage the employee. The additional award is limited to between 26 and 52 weeks' pay with a ceiling on the maximum week's pay which can be used in the calculation. The ceiling is raised each year. Further information is available from the government website.[67] The Court of Appeal reviewed the compensation payable to a nanny who had been unfairly dismissed while off sick and held that if she had not been dismissed she would have been paid statutory sick pay, so that was the measure of her loss. The Court of Appeal accepted that it was good employment practice for an employer who has dismissed an employee without notice to make a payment in lieu of notice which should not be subject to any deduction for sums earned elsewhere.[68]

The Court of Appeal held that costs could be awarded against an unreasonable claimant by an employment tribunal.[69]

Constructive Dismissal

Practical Dilemma 10.7   Dangerous conditions

Kay was a directorate manager in charge of the acute wards of Roger Park Hospital. She had warned the senior managers that the situation was dangerous since, owing to an acute shortage of nurses which coincided with a vigorous attempt to reduce the waiting lists, with extra beds being put up on all the wards, there was a danger that accidents could happen. No notice was taken of her warnings and, in fact, more patients were admitted. She advised the consultants that nurses would not be able to carry out certain tasks normally undertaken by doctors and that the junior doctors would be expected to add the drugs to intravenous transfusions. Her senior nurse manager was advised by the consultants that this was unacceptable and Kay was asked to withdraw that instruction and notify the nurses that they must continue to undertake such tasks. She pointed out that they did not have the time to do these. She was warned that she would face disciplinary proceedings if she continued to defy the managers. She said she would prefer to leave than endanger the lives of patients and stated that the managers were in breach of contract in failing to support her attempt to maintain professional standards. She left and subsequently brought an action for unfair dismissal.

Assuming that Kay qualifies as far as the conditions set out in Box 10.6 are concerned, she needs to establish as a preliminary point that she was dismissed and did not resign. The employers are likely to argue that they did not dismiss her, that she left work of her own free will and that she is therefore ineligible to bring an unfair dismissal action.

The question is: Have the managers acted in such a way that she is entitled to see the contract as at an end? It will be remembered that one of the implied terms in a contract of employment is that the employer will act reasonably towards the employee and support him/her. It could be argued here that in failing to support Kay's endeavours in this situation, the employers are in fundamental breach of contract. If this can be established, then Kay can argue that there is a constructive dismissal, she is entitled to bring her action before the tribunal and it is then for the managers to establish that the dismissal was fair. By the same token, the employers will be arguing that Kay was not dismissed, that she had failed to do all she could to work with them and that she had defied reasonable orders from them. Kay should also refer to the Public Interest Disclosure Act 1998 to show that her concerns about health and safety come under the disclosures protected by that Act and that she followed the procedure required by the Act (see chapter 4 on whistleblowing). Ultimately, the outcome will depend on the evidence from both sides: Kay would have to show evidence, both documentary and through witnesses, of earlier attempts to persuade management that the situation was dangerous and that the managers were acting in fundamental breach of contract. An example of constructive dismissal is the case of a professor who complained that degrees were being cheapened and a complete mockery was being made of the examination process. Professor Buckland protested when exam papers were marked a third time and higher marks awarded and subsequently won his case for unfair dismissal. In 2008 the employment tribunal decided that there had been a fundamental breach of the implied term of trust and confidence in his employment contract and he had been constructively dismissed. Bournemouth University won its appeal to the employment appeal tribunal but the Court of Appeal restored the original ruling, holding that the university had undermined his position. If damages could not be agreed between the parties then the employment tribunal would be asked to assess them.[70]

Case 10.2 Atkin v Enfield Group HMC [1975]

Fair dismissal[71]

The Court of Appeal heard a case where a senior nurse had been dismissed for failure to wear the appropriate uniform. They held that the dismissal was fair.

Procedure in an Application for Unfair Dismissal

The employee is normally expected to exhaust the internal appeal machinery set up by their employer before an application to an employment tribunal is heard. But owing to time limits (an application for unfair dismissal should be brought within three months of the date of dismissal, if reasonably practicable, which now takes into account mediation through ACAS), the employee should instigate the application in any case and ask for an adjournment pending the outcome of the internal appeal. In this way, they will not be out of time. The application must first be made to the Advisory, Conciliation and Arbitration Service (ACAS) who will attempt to resolve the dispute.[72] ACAS has published a Code of Practice on the disciplinary and grievance procedures in employment. This was last updated in March 2015.[73] Employers must comply with the Code, which requires that disciplinary rules and procedures are clearly set out and accessible to the employees. Failure by any employer to follow the ACAS guidelines will not make the employer liable to proceedings in itself, but evidence of this failure could be used against the employer in evidence before an employment tribunal. Since September 2000 employees have had a statutory right to be accompanied at any disciplinary or grievance hearing. Failure by the employer to permit the employee to be accompanied or to postpone (for up to five days) a hearing to enable the person to attend can lead to up to two weeks' compensation payable to the employee. Employees seeking to bring applications before an employment tribunal can brief a barrister direct without having to hire a solicitor first. New regulations for employment tribunals came into force in July 2013 which simplified the procedure.[74]

Automatically Unfair Dismissals

Some dismissals are automatically unfair and whether the employer acted reasonably or not is irrelevant. These have been expanded recently and include dismissals connected with:

pregnancy or childbirth;
parental leave and time off for dependants;
jury service;
health and safety;

exercise of a right under the Working Time Regulations;
making a protected disclosure;
performing a function of an employee representative;
assertion of a statutory right;
membership or non-membership of a trade union;
taking of protected industrial action;
acting in connection with an employee's rights under the Part-time Workers (Prevention of Less Favourable Treatment) Regulations 2000;
Fixed-term Employees (Prevention of Less Favourable Treatment) Regulations 2002;
an application for flexible working;
the Tax Credits Act 2002;
the Information and Consultation of Employees Regulations 2004;
a request not to retire;
discrimination – relating to age, disability, gender reassignment, marriage and civil partnership, pregnancy and maternity, race, religion or belief, sex and sexual orientation; and
failure by the employer to comply with the relevant statutory disciplinary and dismissal procedures.

Hearing

If the employee is able to show that she satisfies the conditions set out in Box 10.6, the burden will be on the employer to show that the dismissal was based on a statutory reason. These are set out in Box 10.7. The tribunal must then decide if the employer has acted reasonably in treating this reason as sufficient to justify dismissal. The criteria that have been considered by the tribunals in determining the reasonableness of employers' actions are set out in Box 10.8. Every circumstance must be taken into account, and the fact that the tribunal might not have acted in the way in which the particular employer acted is not relevant. The crucial question is: Was *that* employer acting reasonably? One important point is whether the disciplinary Code of Practice and the guidelines prepared by ACAS were followed.

Box 10.7 Statutory reasons to dismiss

1. Capability or qualifications
2. Conduct
3. Some other substantial reason
4. Redundancy
5. Statutory prohibition
6. Lockout or participation in strike or industrial action
7. National security

> **Box 10.8 Criteria for the reasonableness of the employer**
>
> 1. Code of practice
> 2. Nature of employment situation, e.g. size and resources of organisation, type of work
> 3. Consistency of employer
> 4. Timing of dismissal
> 5. Length of service of employee
> 6. In cases of dishonesty and other misconduct:
>   - the employer must show that he genuinely believes the employee to be guilty of the misconduct in question
>   - he must have reasonable grounds on which to establish that belief
>   - he must have carried out such investigation into the matter as was reasonable in all the circumstances (see *British Home Stores* v *Birchell* 1978 IRLR 379)
> 7. Principles of natural justice

Outcome

If the employee's application for unfair dismissal is upheld, the following remedies are available to the tribunal:

1. Reinstatement/re-engagement.
2. Compensation – basic award; compensatory award; special award.

In assessing compensation, the tribunal will take into account any fault on the part of the employee. In a case in 2004,[75] the House of Lords held that compensation for injury to feelings and other non-economic loss could not be awarded in unfair dismissal cases.

Trade union rights

It is impossible in a work of this nature to be other than superficial in relation to the status and powers of trade unions. (Reference should be made to the Further Reading section for special books in this field.) Box 10.9 illustrates some of the present rights of the independent trade union. Information on the rights of trade union representatives to have paid time off for training and for carrying out their duties is available on the government website.[76] The members, however, only have the right of reasonable unpaid time off work for union activities. Employees have the right not to be dismissed for being, or refusing to be, union members or for taking part in union activities.[77]

> **Box 10.9** **Trade union rights and the role of safety representatives**
>
> 1. A union is independent if it is not under the domination or control of an employer and not liable to interference by an employer. Its independence can be certified by the certification officer and his certificate is conclusive evidence that the union is independent.
> 2. Independence is an essential feature if the union is to enjoy the following statutory rights:
>   - to take part in trade union activities
>   - to be given information and be consulted over 'transfers of undertaking'
>   - to gain information for collective bargaining
>   - to secure consultation over redundancies
>   - to insist on time off for trade union duties and activities
>   - to appoint health/safety representatives
> 3. A trade union is fully liable for any of its acts that constitute a tort (civil wrong) *except* where it acts in contemplation or furtherance of a trade dispute. The meaning of these words has been narrowed since 1980 so that, in general, secondary action (e.g. where employees of A go on strike to support the employees of B) is not covered and therefore the union would be liable for the damage that results from the unlawful action
> 4. Safety representatives are appointed by a recognised trade union from among the employees. Names are to be notified to the employer in writing. They represent employees in consultation with the employer under section 2(4) and (6) of the Health and Safety at Work Act 1974. Functions are set out in Regulation 4 of statutory instrument 1977 No. 500:
>   - Investigate potential hazards and dangerous occurrences at workplace and examine cause of accidents at work
>   - Investigate complaints of employees relating to health, safety or welfare at work
>   - Make representations to employer under (a) and (b)
>   - Make representations to employer on general matters affecting health, safety or welfare
>   - Carry out inspections under Regulations 5, 6 and 7
>   - Represent employees in consultation with Health and Safety Inspectorate
>   - Receive information from inspectors under section 28(8)
>   - Attend meetings of safety committees
>
> 'No function given to a safety representative by this paragraph shall be construed as imposing any duty on him.'

The trade union officers do not have any management rights: they have no power as part of their function as union officials to give orders to the employees. Obviously, they might advise their members to follow a particular course, but it is up to the members' own judgement whether they follow the advice or not. The Employment Act 1988 gave additional protection to the employee: he has the right not to be denied access to the courts by union rules; the right not to be unjustifiably disciplined by a union; the right to complain to an employment tribunal and obtain compensation if this latter right is infringed.

Public and private employees

Those nurses who work as employees in the private sector enjoy much the same rights as those who work in the NHS. There are, however, some major differences. If the nurse is only one of a few employees, then she may not enjoy all those statutory rights enjoyed by those working for employers of large concerns. This also applies to those NHS nurses who work for single-handed general practitioners or group practices.

In addition, they may not be subject to NHS conditions of service. In this case, there will be other provisions relating to holidays, pay, sick pay, pensions, time off, etc., which will either have been laid down in advance or which will have to be agreed with the employer. The nurse should make sure that she is aware of these provisions before she accepts the post.

Discrimination: The Equality and Human Rights Commission

The Equality and Human Rights Commission (EHRC) was established on 1 October 2007 under the Equality Act 2006, replacing the Equal Opportunities Commission, the Disabilities Rights Commission and the Commission for Racial Equality. It also assumed responsibility for promoting equality and combating unlawful discrimination in three new areas: sexual orientation, religion or belief and age. It also has responsibility for the promotion of human rights. The Commission has a general duty under section 3 to exercise its functions with a view to encouraging and supporting the development of a society in which:

(a) people's ability to achieve their potential is not limited by prejudice or discrimination;

(b) there is respect for and protection of each individual's human rights;

(c) there is respect for the dignity and worth of each individual;

(d) each individual has an equal opportunity to participate in society; and

(e) there is mutual respect between groups based on understanding and valuing of diversity and on shared respect for equality and human rights.

More specific duties relate to equality and diversity (section 8), human rights (section 9), groups (section 10), monitoring the law (section 11) and monitoring progress (section 12). It has powers to publish or disseminate ideas or information, undertake research, provide education or training, give advice or guidance, and issue codes of practice. It also has the power to carry out an investigation, to apply to court for an injunction against a person who it believes to be committing an unlawful act, to bring proceedings in its own name and to give legal assistance to an individual who alleges that he is a victim of behaviour contrary to the equality enactments. The following sections consider the basic provisions in law against discrimination, and further information can be obtained from the EHRC website.[78] In November 2011 the EHRC published the report of an inquiry into older people and human rights in home care. It uncovered areas of real concern in the treatment of some older people and significant shortcomings in the way that care is commissioned by local authorities. The report is available on its website. In May 2014 it called for clear national and local guidance on the Do Not Resuscitate Notices.

Equality Act 2010

The Equality Act 2010, which was passed through Parliament before the general election in 2010, had the purpose of harmonising discrimination law and of strengthening the law to support progress on equality. It places duties in relation to discrimination on to a new statutory footing. The major legislative enactments of the past 40 years were repealed (Equal Pay Act 1970; Sex Discrimination Act 1975; Race Relations Act 1976 and the Sex Discrimination Act 1986). Nine key characteristics were recognised as requiring protection from discrimination. In time case law on the 2010 Act will develop, but where the 2010 Act simply repeats the earlier legislation, the case law before 2010 will still be relevant.

Key Characteristics which are Protected

The Equality Act recognises nine characteristics for protection against discrimination:

age

disability

gender reassignment

marriage and civil partnership

pregnancy and maternity care

race

religion or belief

sex

sexual orientation.

Six of these characteristics are further defined below.

Disability

A person has a disability if he or she has a physical or mental impairment, and the impairment has a substantial and long-term adverse effect on his or her ability to carry out normal day-to-day activities. In the case of *J v DLA Piper*,[79] the employment appeal tribunal overruled the employment tribunal and held that depression could be a disability under the Disability Discrimination Act 2005. The House of Lords has held that in determining whether a person was disabled under the Northern Ireland Disability Discrimination Act 1975 by reason of having an impairment which, although capable of being controlled by measures taken to treat it, would be likely to have substantial adverse effects but for those measures, the word 'likely' did not mean 'probably' but 'could well happen'. The employee whose propensity to develop vocal nodules was controlled by a strict management regime based on avoiding raising her voice, was a disabled person for the purposes of the Act. The employers who placed her in a noisier work environment in spite of her claim that it would require her to speak louder and jeopardise her voice management regime, had to answer her claim that they had failed to make reasonable adjustments for her disability.[80] The Ministry of Justice accepted that there was a breach of the Equality Act 2010 when there was a failure to provide a disabled prisoner with a wheelchair-accessible toilet and bath.[81] An action is being brought before the European Court of Justice to determine whether EU law bans discrimination on grounds of obesity. A childminder, weighing more than 25 stone, in Denmark was sacked because he was no longer able to perform his duties. He needed the help of a colleague to tie a child's shoelace. A preliminary ruling by the advocate general on 17 July 2014 stated that obesity could be seen as a disability; however, the European Court of Justice did not stipulate a general principle against discrimination due to obesity nevertheless did acknowledge that severe obesity could fall under a disability. Therefore, it would be actionable via the Equality Act.

The limitations of the powers of the court were shown in the Supreme Court decision that a disabled air traveller could not obtain damages from the airliner because the terms of the Montreal Convention unifying rules for international carriage by air adopted by the EU excluded an award of damages.[82]

Gender reassignment

A person has the protected characteristic of gender reassignment if the person is proposing to undergo, is undergoing or has undergone a process (or part of a process) for the purpose of reassigning the person's sex by changing physiological or other attributes of sex.

Race

Race is defined to include (a) colour; (b) nationality; (c) ethnic or national origins.

The Supreme Court held in 2009 that the admissions policy of a Jewish school which, in the event of oversubscription, gave priority to children of matrilineal descent was discriminatory on the ground of ethnic origin and was thus racial discrimination.[83]

The employment appeal tribunal held that there had been discrimination on grounds of race and ethnic origin when a North Sudanese was refused promotion because she would have been exposed to safety risks when visiting Sudan and Eastern Chad. The employment appeal tribunal held that Amnesty International's defence that the appointment would have breached the Health and Safety at Work Act discriminated against her on the grounds of her race and ethnic origin.[84]

The Supreme Court refused to allow an employer to raise the fact that the employee was an illegal immigrant in an action brought by the employee for racial discrimination. The Court of Appeal had set aside the tribunal decision, holding that the illegality of the contract of employment formed a material part of the complaint and that to uphold it would be to condone the illegality. The Supreme Court held that to apply the defence of illegality would be an affront to the public policy of protecting the victims of human trafficking. The claimant had been employed as a home help after the defendant had helped her obtain false identity papers and worked illegally in the UK. She had been subjected to serious physical, emotional and verbal abuse and been unfairly dismissed.[85]

Religion

Religion means any religion and a reference to religion includes a reference to a lack of religion; belief means any religious or philosophical belief and a reference to belief includes a reference to a lack of belief. The employment appeal tribunal held that belief based on science was covered by the religion and belief regulations and was entitled to protection under equal treatment legislation.[86] In this case the claimant had a philosophical belief that mankind was heading towards catastrophic climate change and that he had a moral duty to lead a life in a manner that mitigated that catastrophe for the benefit of future generations and to persuade others to do the same.

The Court of Appeal[87] held that it was not indirect discrimination for an employer's dress code to prevent a staff member from wearing a cross as a visible neck adornment when her Christian religion did not require adherents to wear a public display of their faith. She took her case to the ECHR which ruled that British Airways had breached her human rights: her right to freedom of thought, conscience and religion. The government was ordered to pay her £26,600 in damages and costs. However, the ECHR[88] ruled that three other Christians were not discriminated against: an NHS nurse who had been banned from wearing a cross on health and safety grounds; a marriage counsellor and a registrar who refused to deal with same-sex couples on religious grounds.

Dispute over prohibitions on religious conventions such as the wearing of veils have emerged. For example, in September 2013 a judge ruled that a Muslim woman could wear a veil in court, but must remove it when giving evidence. The Lord Chief Justice subsequently announced in November 2013 that guidance is to be issued on the wearing of veils in court following a consultation. A Private Members' Bill, the Face Coverings (Prohibition) Bill, which would have prohibited face coverings in public, failed to complete its passage through Parliament in 2013–14 and therefore made no further progress. In July 2014, however, the ECHR ruled that the French ban on burkas in a public place was not a breach of human rights. The court held that promoting respect for the conditions in which people live together in public places was legitimate.

In other developments the Supreme Court held that the Church of Scientology was a religion for the purposes of marriage law and the conduct of weddings.[89] While the Marriage (Same Sex Couples) Act 2013 makes amendments to the Equality Act 2010 to provide that it is not unlawful discrimination for a religious organisation or individual to refuse to marry a same-sex couple in a religious ceremony.

Sex

In relation to a protected characteristic of sex, a reference to a person who has a particular protected characteristic is a reference to a man or to a woman. A nurse won her case against the Ministry of Defence (MoD) when an employment tribunal found that the MoD discriminated against women when recruiting to senior military roles filled by doctors and nurses.[90]

Sexual orientation

Sexual orientation means a person's sexual orientation towards (a) persons of the same sex, (b) persons of the opposite sex, or (c) persons of either sex. The Supreme Court held that guest house owners who turned away a gay couple were guilty of discrimination under the Equality Act.[91]

The ECHR held that a divorced partner living with a same-sex partner was discriminated against because her child support contributions were higher than they would have been had she been living in a heterosexual relationship.[92] In another case the House of Lords found in favour of a transsexual whose application to be a constable had been turned down because she could not perform full searching duties.[93]

Nature of the Protection

The Act protects those with the key characteristics from direct discrimination, indirect discrimination, harassment and victimisation. The Act prohibits conduct which amounts to direct and indirect discrimination, harassment and victimisation in the providing of a service, disposing or managing premises, work or employment services and the other areas shown in Statute 10.1, which provides an overview of the Act.

Statute 10.1

Equality Act 2010

An overview

Providing a service

Part 3 (+ Schedules 2 and 3) Makes it unlawful to discriminate against, harass or victimise a person when **providing a service** (which includes the provision of goods or facilities) or when exercising a public function

Disposing or managing premises

Part 4 (+ Schedules 4 and 5) Makes it unlawful to discriminate against, harass or victimise a person when **disposing** of (for example, by selling or letting) **or managing premises**

Work or employment services

Part 5 (+ Schedules 6, 7, 8 and 9) Makes it unlawful to discriminate against, harass or victimise **a person at work or in employment services**. Also contains provisions relating to equal pay between men and women; pregnancy and maternity pay; provisions making it unlawful for an employment contract to prevent an employee disclosing his or her pay; and a power to require private sector employers to publish gender pay gap (the size of the difference between men and women's pay expressed as a percentage) information about differences in pay between men and women. It also contains provision restricting the circumstances in which potential employees can be asked questions about disability or health

Education bodies

Part 6 (+ Schedules 10, 11, 12, 13 and 14) Makes it unlawful for **education bodies** to discriminate against, harass or victimise a school pupil or student or applicant for a place

Associations

Part 7 (+ Schedules 15 and 16) Makes it unlawful for associations (for example, private clubs and political organisations) to discriminate against, harass or victimise members, associates or guests and contains a power to require political parties to publish information about the diversity of their candidates

Other forms of conduct

Part 8 Prohibits **other forms of conduct**, including discriminating against or harassing of an ex-employee or ex-pupil, for example: instructing a third party to discriminate against another; or helping someone discriminate against another. Also determines the liability of employers and principals in relation to the conduct of their employees or agents

Enforcement of the Act's provisions

Part 9 (+ Schedule 17) Deals with **enforcement of the Act's provisions**, through the civil courts (in relation to services and public functions; premises; education; and associations) and the employment tribunals (in relation to work and related areas, and equal pay)

Terms in contracts

Part 10 Makes **terms in contracts**, collective agreements or rules of undertakings unenforceable or void if they result in unlawful discrimination, harassment or victimisation

General duty on public authorities

Part 11 (+ Schedules 18 and 19) Establishes **a general duty on public authorities to have due regard, when** carrying out their functions, to the need: to eliminate unlawful discrimination, harassment or victimisation; to advance equality of opportunity; and to foster good relations. Also contains provisions which enable an employer or service provider or other organisation to take positive action to overcome or minimise a disadvantage arising from people possessing particular protected characteristics

Taxis, other private hire vehicles, public service vehicles

Part 12 (+ Schedule 20) **Requires taxis, other private hire vehicles, public service vehicles** (such as buses and rail vehicles) to be accessible to disabled people and to allow them to travel in reasonable comfort

Reasonable adjustments to premises

Part 13 (+ Schedule 21) Deals with consent to **make reasonable adjustments to premises and improvements to let dwelling houses**

Exceptions

Part 14 (+ Schedules 22 and 23) Establishes **exceptions** to the prohibitions in the earlier parts of the Act in relation to a range of conduct, including action required by an enactment; protection of women; educational appointments; national security; the provision of benefits by charities and sporting competitions

Family property

Part 15 Repeals or replaces rules of family property law which discriminated between husbands and wives

Power for a Minister of the Crown

Part 16 (+ Schedules 24, 25, 26, 27 and 28) Contains a power for a Minister of the Crown to harmonise certain provisions in the Act with changes required to comply with EU obligations. It contains general provisions on application to the Crown, subordinate legislation, interpretation, commencement and extent. It also contains amendments to the Civil Partnership Act 2004 to allow civil partnership registrations to take place on religious premises that are approved for that purpose

---

Section 15 provides that a person (A) discriminates against a disabled person (B) if:

(a) (A) treats (B) unfavourably because of something arising in consequence of (B)'s disability; and

(b) (A) cannot show that the treatment is a proportionate means of achieving a legitimate aim.

This does not apply if (A) shows that (A) did not know, and could not reasonably have been expected to know, that (B) had the disability.

Section 16 covers gender reassignment discrimination in cases of absence from work. A person (A) discriminates against a transsexual person (B) if, in relation to an absence of (B)'s that is because of gender reassignment, (A) treats (B) less favourably than (A) would treat (B) if:

(a) (B)'s absence was because of sickness or injury; or
(b) (B)'s absence was for some other reason,
(c) and it is not reasonable for (B) to be treated less favourably.

A person's absence is because of gender reassignment if it is because the person is proposing to undergo, is undergoing or has undergone the process (or part of the process) mentioned in section 7(1).

Under section 17 pregnancy and maternity discrimination in non-work cases are protected characteristics in relation to:

(a) Part 3 (services and public functions);
(b) Part 4 (premises);
(c) Part 6 (education);
(d) Part 7 (associations).

Discrimination can arise if a person (A) discriminates against a woman if (A) treats her unfavourably because of a pregnancy of hers or, in the period of 26 weeks beginning with the day on which she gives birth, (A) treats her unfavourably because she has given birth (including, in particular, a reference to treating her unfavourably because she is breastfeeding). Giving birth includes giving birth to a stillborn child (i.e. after 24 weeks' gestation).

Under section 18 pregnancy and maternity discrimination in employment, a person (A) discriminates against a woman if, in the protected period in relation to a pregnancy of hers, (A) treats her unfavourably:

(a) because of the pregnancy, or
(b) because of illness suffered by her as a result of it.

Person (A) also discriminates against a woman if he treats her unfavourably because she is on compulsory maternity leave, or because she is exercising or seeking to exercise, or has exercised or sought to exercise, the right to ordinary or additional maternity leave.

Direct Discrimination

Section 13 defines direct discrimination as where a person (A) discriminates against another (B) if, because of a protected characteristic, (A) treats (B) less favourably than (A) treats or would treat others. The European Court of Justice (ECJ) held in January 2008 that direct discrimination existed when a woman with a disabled son claimed that she was discriminated against at work because of her child. The ECJ held that there was direct discrimination where a person suffered discrimination and/or harassment because he or she is associated with a disabled person. It was described as a landmark case, which could bring new rights for the 6 million carers in the UK.[94]

Combined Discrimination

Section 14 provides protection when there is combined discrimination, i.e. dual characteristics. A person (A) discriminates against another (B) if, because of a combination of two relevant protected characteristics, (A) treats (B) less favourably than (A) treats or would treat a person who does not share either of those characteristics. For example, an employer may treat a Muslim woman differently than he would treat a Christian woman or a Muslim man. The protection applies to the key characteristics except for civil partnership and marriage and pregnancy and maternity care.

Indirect Discrimination

The Equality Act 2010 defines as indirect discrimination where a person (A) applies to another (B) a provision, criterion or practice which is discriminatory in relation to a relevant protected characteristic of (B)'s. A provision, criterion or practice is discriminatory in relation to a relevant protected characteristic of (B)'s if:

(a) (A) applies, or would apply, it to persons with whom (B) does not share the characteristic;

(b) it puts, or would put, persons with whom (B) shares the characteristic at a particular disadvantage when compared with persons with whom (B) does not share it;

(c) it puts, or would put, (B) at that disadvantage; and

(d) (A) cannot show it to be a proportionate means of achieving a legitimate aim.

The relevant protected characteristics are: age; disability; gender reassignment; marriage and civil partnership; race; religion or belief; sex and sexual orientation (i.e. pregnancy and maternity are not included).

Duty to make Adjustments for Disabled Persons

Section 20 of the Act specifies three requirements in making adjustments for a disabled person. The first requirement is a requirement, where a provision, criterion or practice of (A)'s puts a disabled person at a substantial disadvantage in relation to a relevant matter in comparison with persons who are not disabled, to take such steps as it is reasonable to have to take to avoid the disadvantage.

The second requirement is a requirement, where a physical feature puts a disabled person at a substantial disadvantage in relation to a relevant matter in comparison with persons who are not disabled, to take such steps as it is reasonable to have to take to avoid the disadvantage.

The third requirement is a requirement, where a disabled person would, but for the provision of an auxiliary aid, be put at a substantial disadvantage in relation to a relevant matter in comparison with persons who are not disabled, to take such steps as it is reasonable to have to take to provide the auxiliary aid.

A person who has a duty to make reasonable adjustments is not entitled to require a disabled person, in relation to whom (A) is required to comply with the duty, to pay to any extent (A)'s costs of complying with the duty. The Equality and Human Rights Commission welcomed the decision of the Supreme Court in the case[95] where disabled persons lacking mental capacity were held to be entitled to have the same protections of their liberty as the non-disabled. Lady Hale stated that a gilded cage is still a cage. (The case is considered in chapter 16.)

Harassment

The Act defines harassment as where (A) engages in (a) unwanted conduct related to a relevant protected characteristic, and (b) the conduct has the purpose or effect of:

1. (a) violating (B)'s dignity, or
    (b) creating an intimidating, hostile, degrading, humiliating or offensive environment for (B).
2. (A) also harasses (B) if:
    (a) (A) engages in unwanted conduct of a sexual nature, and
    (b) the conduct has the purpose or effect referred to in subsection (1)(b).
3. (A) also harasses (B) if:
    (a) (A) or another person engages in unwanted conduct of a sexual nature or that is related to gender reassignment or sex,
    (b) the conduct has the purpose or effect referred to in subsection (1)(b), and
    (c) because of (B)'s rejection of or submission to the conduct, (A) treats (B) less favourably than (A) would treat (B) if (B) had not rejected or submitted to the conduct.

In deciding whether conduct has the effect referred to in subsection (1)(b), each of the following must be taken into account:

4. (a) the perception of (B),
    (b) the other circumstances of the case,
    (c) whether it is reasonable for the conduct to have that effect.

The relevant protected characteristics for harassment are: age; disability; gender reassignment; race; religion or belief; sex and sexual orientation (i.e. civil partnership and marriage and pregnancy and maternity are excluded).

The Protection from Harassment Act 1997 provides additional protection and remedies against harassment and has wider coverage. (The 1997 Act is not restricted to the nine characteristics, there is a six-year limitation period rather than three months under the 2010 Act and there is no employer's defence that it took all reasonable steps to avoid it (see chapter 12).)

Victimisation

1. A person (A) victimises another person (B) if (A) subjects (B) to a detriment because:
    (a) (B) does a protected act, or
    (b) believes that (B) has done, or may do, a protected act.
2. Each of the following is a protected act:
    (a) bringing proceedings under this Act;
    (b) giving evidence or information in connection with proceedings under this Act;
    (c) doing any other thing for the purposes of or in connection with this Act;
    (d) making an allegation (whether or not express) that (A) or another person has contravened this Act.
3. Giving false evidence or information, or making a false allegation, is not a protected act if the evidence or information is given, or the allegation is made, in bad faith.
4. This section applies only where the person subjected to a detriment is an individual.
5. The reference to contravening this Act includes a reference to committing a breach of an equality clause or rule.

The Court of Appeal held that a former employee could claim that he had been victimised when the former employer wrote a bad reference because he had initiated employment tribunal proceedings.[96] The court interpreted the Equality Act 2010 to give effect to the UK's obligations under European Union law which aimed to proscribe post-employment victimisation.

Positive Action

Section 158 applies where a person (P) reasonably thinks that:

1. persons who share a protected characteristic suffer a disadvantage connected to the characteristic;
2. persons who share a protected characteristic have needs that are different from the needs of persons who do not share it; and
3. participation in an activity by persons who share a protected characteristic is disproportionately low, then positive action may be permissible under section 158. Person (P) is not prohibited by the Equality Act from taking any action which is a proportionate means of achieving the aim of:
    (a) enabling or encouraging persons who share the protected characteristic to overcome or minimise that disadvantage;
    (b) meeting those needs; or
    (c) enabling or encouraging persons who share the protected characteristic to participate in that activity (section 158(2)).

    Exclusions to this can be made by regulations.

(This section does not apply to selection and recruitment, which is covered by section 159, nor to selection of candidates which is covered by section 104.)

Positive action in relation to recruitment and promotion

Under section 159(1) positive action is permissible in relation to recruitment and promotion if a person (P) reasonably thinks that:

(a) persons who share a protected characteristic suffer a disadvantage connected to the characteristic; or
(b) participation in an activity by persons who share a protected characteristic is disproportionately low.

However, positive action is not permissible if the person without the protected characteristic is better qualified. The positive action must be a proportionate means of achieving the specified aim.

Under section 159(2) Part 5 (work) does not prohibit (P) from taking action within subsection (3) with the aim of enabling or encouraging persons who share the protected characteristic to:

(a) overcome or minimise that disadvantage; or
(b) participate in that activity.

Section 159(3) stipulates that action is treating a person (A) more favourably in connection with recruitment or promotion than another person (B) because (A) has the protected characteristic but (B) does not.

But under section 159(4), subsection (2) applies only if:

(a) (A) is as qualified as (B) to be recruited or promoted;

(b) (P) does not have a policy of treating persons who share the protected characteristic more favourably in connection with recruitment or promotion than persons who do not share it; and

(c) taking the action in question is a proportionate means of achieving the aim referred to in subsection (2).

Public Sector Equality Duty

Specific duties are imposed on public authorities (as defined in Schedule 19) under Section 149 of the Act. The first duty of eliminating discrimination, harassment, victimisation or any other prohibited conduct applies to the nine characteristics listed above. The other two duties, advancing equality of opportunity and fostering good relations, apply to all those characteristics except civil partnership and marriage.

Statute 10.2
Public Sector Equality Duty

Section 149 of the Equality Act 2010

1. A Public authority must, in the exercise of its functions, have due regard to the need to:
   (a) eliminate discrimination, harassment, victimisation and any other conduct that is prohibited by or under this Act;
   (b) advance equality of opportunity between persons who share a relevant protected characteristic and persons who do not share it;
   (c) foster good relations between persons who share a relevant protected characteristic and persons who do not share it.

2. A person who is not a public authority but who exercises public functions must, in the exercise of those functions, have due regard to the matters mentioned above.

3. Having due regard to the need to advance equality of opportunity between persons who share a relevant protected characteristic and persons who do not share it involves having due regard, in particular, to the need to:
   (a) remove or minimise disadvantages suffered by persons who share a relevant protected characteristic that are connected to that characteristic;
   (b) take steps to meet the needs of persons who share a relevant protected characteristic that are different from the needs of persons who do not share it;
   (c) encourage persons who share a relevant protected characteristic to participate in public life or in any other activity in which participation by such persons is disproportionately low.

4. The steps involved in meeting the needs of disabled persons that are different from the needs of persons who are not disabled include, in particular, steps to take account of disabled persons' disabilities.

> 5. Having due regard to the need to foster good relations between persons who share a relevant protected characteristic and persons who do not share it involves having due regard, in particular, to the need to:
>   (a) tackle prejudice, and
>   (b) promote understanding.
> 6. Compliance with the duties in this section may involve treating some persons more favourably than others; but that is not to be taken as permitting conduct that would otherwise be prohibited by or under this Act.

The Mental Health (Discrimination) Act 2013 repealed section 141 of the Mental Health Act 1983 which disqualified MPs and members of devolved bodies on grounds of mental illness and any rule of common law which disqualifies a person from membership of the House of Commons on grounds of mental illness and also changed the rules in relation to jurors and company directors.

A claimant who was visually impaired successfully sought judicial review of a local authority's failure to fulfil its public equality duty when it failed to follow national guidance in relation to the design and specification of tactile paving. The High Court held that there was no justification for departing from national guidance.[97]

Discrimination in the NHS

A plan called 'Tackling Racial Harassment' in the NHS was launched in February 1999 by the then Health Minister Alan Milburn. He described it as 'the most concerted drive the NHS has ever seen on the issue'. The plan envisaged that by April 2000 every NHS employer would need to be in a position to tackle racial harassment whether committed by staff or by patients. NHS England has stated that it will work to ensure that advancing equality and diversity is central to how it conducts its business as an organisation. There is, however, evidence that racism is endemic in the NHS. A former NHS manager was awarded £1 million in a racial discrimination case against Central Manchester University NHS Foundation Trust in January 2012.[98]

Male midwives

Originally midwifery was one of the exemptions to the Sex Discrimination Act 1975 and the employment and training of men as midwives was restricted. However, under Order 1983 SI No. 1202 the exemptions were brought to an end. The health authorities were notified that when implementing these legislative changes they must make appropriate arrangements to ensure that:

(a) women have the freedom of choice to be attended by a female midwife;
(b) where male midwives are employed, provision is made for them to be chaperoned as necessary.

Subsequently it was held that the requirement that a male nurse be chaperoned which did not apply to female nurses was unlawful direct discrimination.[99]

Conclusions

It is inevitable that there are constant changes to the law relating to employment, human rights and equality. It is hoped that the Equality Act 2010 – in replacing previous legislation and with the Equality and Human Rights Commission monitoring the implementation of the law and taking legal action where appropriate – will ensure that the law is clearer and more easily enforceable. The duty placed upon public bodies to eliminate discrimination, harassment, victimisation and any other prohibited conduct has unfortunately not yet ensured that the NHS has been able to rid itself of the reputation for being a racist organisation.

Reflection questions

1. If you have a letter that purports to be your contract of appointment, compare it with the particulars set out in Box 10.3.
2. Take any statutory right and contrast it with the comparable rights given in your contract of employment by national NHS conditions. Which right would be of most benefit to the employee?
3. A manager is both an employee and the representative of the employer. In what way, if any, is there likely to be a conflict between these two roles?
4. If you were preparing to interview prospective employees, what questions do you consider would be unlawful under the Equality Act 2010?

Further exercises

1. Obtain a copy of your employer's disciplinary procedure and apply the procedure to any of the situations of alleged negligence by a nurse set out in this book.
2. Visit an employment tribunal and prepare a brief guide for a potential applicant on the procedure and formalities.

References

[1] *Grant v United Kingdom* [2003] (32570/03) 44 EHRR 1
[2] www.equalityhumanrights.com
[3] www.ico.org.uk
[4] Legal Aid, Sentencing and Punishment of Offenders Act 2012 sections 139–141
[5] News item, *The Times*, 3 September 2010
[6] Nursing and Midwifery Council, Code of Professional Conduct: standards for performance, conduct and ethics, NMC, 2004
[7] www.gov.uk

8 Department for Education and Science, Making Safeguarding Everybody's Business: a post-Bichard vetting scheme, 1485–2005DOC-EN; www.dfes.gov.uk/consultations
9 www.dera.ioe.ac.uk/6394/1/report
10 SI 2004/1220
11 Sexual Offences Act 2003 (Notification Requirements) (England and Wales) Regulations 2012 SI 2012/1876
12 List 99 is a list held by the Department for Children, Schools and Families of those considered unsuitable to work with children. It has always been a statutory list
13 www.gov.uk/publications/safeguarding-policy-protecting-vulnerable-adults
14 *R (on the application of Wright and others)* v *Secretary of State for Health and Another* [2006] EWHC 2888; [2007] 1 All ER 825; The Times Law Report, 16 November 2007 CA
15 The Safeguarding Vulnerable Groups Act 2006 (Miscellaneous Provisions) Regulations 2009 SI 2009/1548
16 *R (F)* v *Secretary of State for Justice; R (Thompson)* v *Secretary of State for the Home Department*, The Times Law Report, 22 April 2010
17 Department of Health and Home Office, No Secrets: guidance on developing and implementing multi-agency policies and procedures to protect vulnerable adults from abuse, DH and Home Office, London, 2000
18 Protection of Freedoms Act 2012 (Disclosure and Barring Service Transfer of Functions) Order 2012 SI 2012/3006
19 www.gov.uk
20 SIs 2012/2113 and 2112 amend the regulations Safeguarding Vulnerable Groups Act 2006 (Barred List Prescribed Information) Regulations 2008 SI 2008/16
21 www.gov.uk
22 Rosemary Bennett, Sarah's Law unmasks 700 paedophiles, *The Times*, 23 December 2013
23 *R (T)* v *Chief Constable of Greater Manchester Police and others*, The Times Law Report, 23 June 2014
24 Further details of statutory rights are available from the Department for Business, Innovation and Skills, www.legislation.gov.uk
25 www.gov.uk
26 www.acas.org.uk
27 www.adviceguide.org.uk
28 www.nidirect.gov.uk
29 Royal College of Nursing, Your Rights and Safety: an A–Z guide, Order No. 001771, RCN, July 2002
30 News item, *The Times*, 20 November 2010
31 *Halfpenny* v *IGE Medical System Ltd* [1999] 1 FLR 944 CA
32 *Saint Prix* v *Secretary of State for Work and Pensions* (Case C-507/12), The Times Law Report, 26 June 2014. The Protection from Redundancy (Pregnancy and Family Leave) Act 2023
33 *Webb* v *EMO Air Cargo (UK)*, The Times Law Report, 15 July 1994; [1995] IRLR 645, HL
34 www.gov.uk/news/new-rights-for-fathers-and-partners-to-attend-antenatal-appointments
35 *CD* v *ST* [2014] EUECJ 167/12
36 Paragraphs 76–80 Part I Schedule 4 of Employment Relations Act 1999
37 Maternity and Parental Leave Regulations 1999 SI 1999/3312
38 The Parental Leave (EU Directive) Regulations 2013 SI 2013/283
39 www.gov.uk/maternity-pay-leave/overview/
40 www.gov.uk
41 Part II Schedule 4 Employment Relations Act 1999
42 The Flexible Working Regulations 2014 SI 2014/1398

[43] Code of Practice (Handling in a reasonable manner requests to work flexibly) Order 2014 SI 2014/1665. The Employment Rights (Flexible Working) Act 2023. Carer's Leave Act 2023
[44] Information and Consultation with Employees Regulations 2004 SI 2004/3426
[45] www.bis.gov.uk; DTI guidance 2006
[46] Working Time Regulations 1998 SI 1998/1833
[47] NHS Executive, Working Time Regulations: implementation in the NHS, HSC 1988/204; DTI, A Guide to the Working Time Regulations, URN 1998/894
[48] *R v S of S for Trade and Industry*, The Times Law Report, 28 June 2001
[49] *Commission of the European Communities* v *UK* (C484/04) [2006] IRLR 888 ECJ
[50] Further information is available on 0845 8450 360
[51] *Commissioners for Revenue and Customs* v *Annabel's (Berkeley Square) Ltd and others,* The Times Law Report, 13 May 2009
[52] *Ainsworth and others* v *Inland Revenue Commissioners* HL, The Times Law Report, 15 June 2009
[53] Rosemary Bennett, Care staff win £600,000 pay for travel time, *The Times*, 6 June 2014
[54] *Whittlestone* v *BJP Home Supplies Ltd* [2014] ICR 275
[55] The Part-time Workers (Prevention of Less Favourable Treatment) Regulations 2000 SI 2000/1551
[56] Directive 97/81/EC, Part-time Work Directive as extended to the UK by Directive 98/23/EC
[57] Directive 2008/104/EC
[58] Nursing and Midwifery Council, Advice and information for employers of nurses and midwives, NMC, London, March 2010
[59] Report by the Comptroller and Auditor General on Management of Suspensions of Clinical Staff in NHS Hospitals and Ambulance Trusts in England, HC 1143, 6 November 2003
[60] *Halford* v *United Kingdom* (1997) 24 EHRR 523; [1997] IRLR 471; [1998] Crim LR 753
[61] www.ico.gov.uk
[62] Regulations of Investigatory Powers (Interception of Communications: Code of Practice) Order 2002, SI 2002/1693
[63] Telecommunications (Lawful Business Practices) (Interception of Communications) Regulations 2000, SI 2000/2699
[64] www.ico.org.uk
[65] Caspar Glyn QC, Letter to the Editor, *The Times*, 3 April 2014
[66] *Barchester Healthcare Ltd* v *Tayeh* [2013] EWCA Civ 29
[67] www.gov.uk
[68] *Burley* v *Langley* [2006] EWCA Civ 1778; [2007] 2 All ER 462
[69] *Sud* v *Ealing Borough Council*, Times Law Report, 23 October 2013 CA
[70] *Buckland* v *Bournemouth University Higher Education Corporation* [2010] EWCA Civ 121
[71] *Atkin* v *Enfield Group Hospital Management Committee* [1975] IRLR 217
[72] Employment Tribunals Act 1996 (Application of Conciliation Provisions) Order 2014 SI 2014/431
[73] www.acas.org.uk
[74] The Employment Tribunals (Constitution and Rules of Procedure) Regulations 2013 SI 2013/1237
[75] *Dunnachie* v *Kingston upon Hull County Council* [2004] IRLR 727
[76] www.gov.uk/browse/employing-people/trade-unions
[77] See DTI booklet PL871 for details of union membership and non-membership rights
[78] www.equalityhumanrights.com

[79] *J v DLA Piper UK LLP* [2010] UKEAT 0263_09_1506
[80] *Boyle* v *SCA Packaging Ltd*, Equality and Human Rights Commission Intervening, The Times Law Report, 6 July 2009 HL
[81] News item, *The Times*, 9 November 2010
[82] *Scott* v *Thomas Cook Tour Operators*, The Times Law Report, 13 March 2014
[83] *R (E)* v *Governing body of JFS and another*, United Synagogue and Others intervening, The Times Law Report, 17 December 2009
[84] *Amnesty International* v *Ahmed*, The Times Law Report, 6 October 2009
[85] *Hounga* v *Allen (Anti-Slavery intervening)*, The Times Law Report, 6 August 2014
[86] *Grainger plc* v *Nicholson*, The Times Law Report, 11 November 2009
[87] *Eweida* v *British Airways plc*, The Times Law Report, 18 February 2010; [2010] EWCA Civ 80
[88] *Eweida and others* v *United Kingdom* [2013] ECHR 37
[89] *Hodkin and Anor, R (on the application of)* v *Registrar General of Births, Deaths and Marriages* [2013] UKSC 77
[90] Martin Barrow, Nurse wins sexism case against MoD, *The Times*, 26 June 2013
[91] *Bull and Anor* v *Hall and Anor* [2013] UKSC 73
[92] *JM* v *United Kingdom*, Application No. 37060/06, The Times Law Report, 11 October 2010
[93] *A* v *West Yorkshire Police* [2004] UKHL 21
[94] *S. Coleman* v *Attridge* [2008] ECJ Case C-303/06, 31 January 2008; [2008] ICR 1128
[95] *P (by his litigation friend the Official Solicitor)* v *Cheshire West and Cheshire Council and Anor* [2014] UKSC 19
[96] *Jessemey* v *Rowstock Ltd and Another*, The Times Law Report, 15 April 2014
[97] *R (on the application of Ali)* v *Newham LBC* [2012] EWHC 2970
[98] *Central Manchester University Hospitals NHS Foundation Trust* v *Browne* [2011] UKEAT 0294
[99] *Moyhing* v *Barts and London NHS Trust* [2006] IRLR 860

Chapter 11

The Nurse as a Registered Professional

This chapter discusses

- Background to the establishment of the Nursing and Midwifery Council
- Nursing and Midwifery Council
- Registration and removal
- Professional standards and codes of practice
- Education and training
- Post-registration revalidation and continuing professional development (CPD)
- Fitness to Practise Annual Report 2016/17
- Professional Standards Authority for Health and Social Care (formerly the Council for Healthcare Regulatory Excellence (CHRE))
- Nursing associates

Introduction

It will be recalled from chapter 1 that there were four fields of accountability to be faced by the nurse: the civil and criminal courts; the disciplinary proceedings of the employer; and the Fitness to Practise Committee (FtPC) of the Nursing and Midwifery Council (NMC). This chapter considers the procedure for a hearing before the FtPC and the other practice committees. First, however, the constitution of the NMC will be considered. Significant changes came into force in April 2002, when the United Kingdom Central Council for Nursing, Midwifery and Health Visiting was replaced by the NMC and in 2004 new procedures for Fitness to Practise were introduced.[1]

Background to the establishment of the nursing and midwifery council

The Nurses, Midwives and Health Visitors Act 1979 had set up the previous framework for the United Kingdom Central Council, the national boards and the professional register, and

Statutory Instruments passed in the exercise of powers conferred by the principal Act provided the detail. At the request of the Department of Health, a review of the statutory regulation of nurses, midwives and health visitors was undertaken by JM Consulting. It reported in 1999[2] and made significant recommendations for a major reorganisation of the work, functions and organisation of the statutory regulation machinery. Its main recommendations were accepted by the government and the necessary legislative beginning was made in the Health Act 1999. In August 2000, the government issued a consultation paper[3] giving three months for feedback. The amending regulations were passed by order under section 60 of the Health Act 1999, with a new Nursing and Midwifery Council replacing the UKCC and the four national boards, maintaining a professional register with some 640,000 entries. Contrary to initial suggestions, health visitors continued to have separate registration and representation within the new Council, but were absorbed into a new part of the register named **specialist community public health nurses**.

New procedures for Fitness to Practise came into force in 2017.[4] They can be downloaded from the NMC website or obtained from the legislation website.[5]

The Health Act 1999 Schedule 3 paragraph 8 defines four fundamental functions of the new Council, which cannot be transferred by order to another body. These are:

1. keeping the register of members admitted to practise
2. determining the standards of education and training for admission to practise
3. giving guidance about standards of conduct and performance
4. administering procedures (including making rules) relating to misconduct, unfitness to practise and similar matters.

The Nursing and Midwifery Order 2001[6] provided detailed rules on the constitution of the Council and its functions.

Following extensive consultation by the NMC, new rules were enacted in Statutory Instruments, which can be downloaded from the NMC or legislation websites.

Nursing and midwifery council

The constitution of the NMC is given in Box 11.1 and its functions can be seen in Box 11.2. The Nursing and Midwifery Order requires the NMC to have specific statutory committees and these can be seen in Box 11.3.

Box 11.1 Constitution of the NMC (schedule 1 of the nursing and midwifery order 2001 as amended[7])

The Nursing and Midwifery Council shall consist of:

(a) 7 members who are appointed by the Privy Council (registrant members); and

(b) 7 members who are appointed by the Privy Council (lay members).

At least one member shall be elected from each of the national constituencies for each part of the register.

> **Box 11.2**   **Functions of the NMC[8]**
>
> ## The nursing and midwifery council and its committees
>
> Article 3:
>
> 3(2) The principal functions of the Council shall be to establish from time to time standards of education, training, conduct and performance for nurses and midwives and to ensure the maintenance of those standards.
>
> 3(3) The Council shall have such other functions as are conferred on it by the Order or as may be provided by the Privy Council by order.
>
> 3(4) The main objective of the Council in exercising its functions shall be to safeguard the health and well-being of persons using or needing the services of registrants.
>
> 3(5) In exercising its functions, the Council shall:
>
> (a) have proper regard for:
>
>   (i) the interests of persons using or needing the services of registrants in the United Kingdom, and
>
>   (ii) any differing interests of different categories of registrants;
>
> (b) cooperate, in so far as is appropriate and reasonably practicable, with public bodies or other persons concerned with:
>
>   (i) the employment (whether or not under a contract of service) of registrants,
>
>   (ii) the education or training of nurses, midwives or other health care professionals,
>
>   (iii) the regulation of, or the coordination of the regulation of, other health or social care professionals,
>
>   (iv) the regulation of health services, and
>
>   (v) the provision, supervision or management of health services.
>
> 3(5A) In carrying out its duty to cooperate under paragraph (5)(b), the Council shall have regard to any differing considerations relating to practising as a nurse or midwife which apply in England, Scotland, Wales or Northern Ireland [and the Isle of Man and the Channel Islands].

A new Article 6A[9] enables the Registrar, on advice from the Secretary of State that an emergency has or is occurring, to annotate in the Register against the name of a registrant to indicate that the registrant is qualified to order drugs, medicines and appliances in a specified capacity, notwithstanding that the registrant is not so qualified. The Registrar must consider that the registrant is a fit, proper and suitably experienced person to order drugs, medicines and appliances in that capacity with regard to the emergency. Once the emergency is over, the annotation must be removed.

Box 11.3 Statutory committees of the NMC

There shall be four committees of the Council, to be known as:

1. the Investigating Committee
2. the Conduct and Competence Committee (now referred to as the Fitness to Practise Committee)
3. the Health Committee (since removed)
4. the Midwifery Committee (since removed)

These were referred to as the statutory committees.

The Investigating Committee, the Conduct and Competence Committee and the Health Committee were also referred to as the 'practice committees'.

Registration and removal

Council has the duty of preparing and maintaining a register of qualified nurses, midwives and health visitors and setting out rules in relation to the entry on to, removal from, and restoration to the Register. These rules are set out in Part III of the Nursing and Midwifery Order 2001.

False Representation

Practical dilemma 11.1 False qualifications

Brenda had always wanted to be a nurse, but lacked the educational background. When she left school, she worked as a Health Care Assistant for many years and was given much responsibility. She then left the district when her husband moved jobs. She applied for the job of a night nurse in a private nursing home. At the interview, she was asked where she trained and she gave false information about her background. Because of her great experience, they were very impressed with her and failed to take up her references. After she had worked there for two years, a former colleague from her previous hospital came to visit a relative in the home and was surprised to discover that Brenda was referred to as 'sister'. The colleague made some enquiries and realised that Brenda was being treated as a registered nurse when in fact she was not one. She felt that it was her duty to point this out to the owners of the home because of the possibility that a patient could suffer harm. When the owners discovered the truth, Brenda was dismissed on the spot.

In a situation like this, as well as a loss of job, Brenda could face a criminal charge of falsely representing that she was on the Register or falsely representing that she possessed qualifications in nursing, midwifery or health visiting. These are offences under Article 44 of the Nursing and Midwifery Order 2001. The matter would not be one for the NMC since she is not registered, but would be a matter for the criminal courts. An offence is committed if a person falsely represents themselves as registered or uses a title set out in the Register indicative of different qualifications and different kinds of education or training, to which they are not entitled, or falsely represents themselves as possessing qualifications in nursing or midwifery. In October 2003 it was reported that a person who had worked as a GP nurse for 15 years was convicted after pleading guilty to deception at the Crown Court and was given a nine-month suspended sentence. The deception came to light when she used false documents to gain a job as clinical coordinator.[10]

In such a case the Council would be required to provide evidence of the fact that she was not on the Register and not entitled. Of course, if she was on the Register for one purpose, e.g. a general nurse, it would be an offence for her to pretend that she was a midwife. This would then be a matter that could be heard before the Fitness to Practise Committee (formerly the Conduct and Competence Committee (CCC)) as well as the criminal court, since, as she is already registered, the Committee could decide if she should remain on the Register or if any other action should be taken against her. In a separate case, a registered nurse who was training as a midwife was found to be unfit to practise because of her misconduct as a student midwife.[11]

The Statutory Instrument also sets out rules relating to registration, renewal of registration and readmission, lapse of registration and approved qualifications and EEA qualifications. Part IV of the order covers education and training, the appointment of visitors, information to be given by institutions, refusal or withdrawal of approval of courses, qualifications and institutions and post-registration training.

Removal from the Register

Under Article 21 of the Nursing and Midwifery Order 2001, the Council is required to establish and keep under review the standards of conduct, performance and ethics expected of registrants and prospective registrants and give them such guidance on these matters as it sees fit and to establish and keep under review effective arrangements to protect the public from persons whose fitness to practise is impaired.

The circumstances in which a person can be removed from the Register are:

1. Her fitness to practise is impaired by reason of:
   - misconduct
   - lack of competence
   - a conviction or caution in the UK for a criminal offence, or a conviction elsewhere for an offence which, if committed in England or Wales, would constitute a criminal offence
   - her physical or mental health
   - a determination by a body in the UK responsible under any enactment for the regulation of a health or social care profession to the effect that her fitness to practise is impaired or a determination by a licensing body elsewhere to the same effect, or barring by the Independent Safeguarding Authority (ISA) (now the Disclosure and Barring Service).

2. An entry in the Register relating to her has been fraudulently procured or incorrectly made.

Suspension from the Register

This power was introduced in 1993 and can be exercised where the Fitness to Practise Committee find an allegation well founded, and so serious as to warrant suspension from the Register, namely on misconduct and/or public interest grounds. Usually suspension is related to a serious episode within a short timeframe of the nurse's practice, rather than a series of events, which if serious would be more likely to warrant removal from the Register. The suspension must be for a specified period, which shall not exceed one year.

Interim Order

An interim order (IO) hearing can be held if the screening team following its risk assessment identify particular risk factors. An interim order can then be made if it is considered necessary to protect the public, is in the public interest or in the registrant's interest (see Box 11.6). The Fitness to Practise Committee or Investigating Committee can also decide to hold an interim orders hearing at any time. Since 1 April 2014, when an IO is imposed the NMC will no longer publish on its website the full determination but only the period of the order and the panel outcome. The Court of Appeal has held that an interim hearing to determine whether a registrant should be suspended or placed under conditions did not have to hear the substantive evidence of the registrant since fairness would necessitate the complainant being called and the hearing would thus become a trial before a tribunal. It ruled that the NMC guidance on interim hearings was fair and there was no breach of Articles 6 or 8 of the Human Rights Convention.[12]

Removal on Grounds of Fitness to Practise

Practical dilemma 11.2　Missing ampoule

Janice Lane was a ward manager on a busy surgical ward. One day she was preparing the midday medications on her own and while preparing a morphine injection for a patient dropped the ampoule, which broke. Ashamed of what had happened, she locked up the cupboard and pretended that it had not happened instead of following the correct procedure and writing the loss in the correct book and getting a witness. Subsequently, the loss of the ampoule was noticed by the following shift, and a search and an inquiry commenced which revealed nothing. The police were brought in and eventually Janice confessed.

Case examiners and practice committees

Case examiners can be appointed under Article 23. At least two case examiners (one lay person and one registrant selected with regard to the professional field of the person concerned) must consider the allegation and establish whether, in their opinion, power is given under the order to deal with it if it proves to be well founded. If in their opinion there is such power then the case examiners can refer the matter together with a report of the result of their consideration to such practice committee as they see fit. If they consider there is no such power then they can close the case, provided, if there are two screeners, the lay person agrees and, if there are more than two case examiners, the majority agrees.

The constitution of the practice committees is shown in Box 11.4 and the standards for members of practice committees are set out in Box 11.5.

Box 11.4 — Constitution of the practice committees

Membership of a practice committee shall comprise a chairperson, a registrant member and a lay member who shall be appointed by the Council. However, all three are independent of the NMC – in other words, the members are self-employed, and not employees of the NMC, to ensure independent judgement is made.

These members are appointed by Council in accordance with paragraph 18 of Schedule 1 of the order.[13]

The quorum of a practice committee shall be three and shall include at least one registrant and one lay member. The chairperson can be a lay member or a registrant member.

Box 11.5 — Standards for members of a practice committee

1. A member of a practice committee shall:
   - prepare for any meeting of the committee by reading the agenda and any papers issued by the committee of the Council which are relevant to any subject to be considered at that meeting, and
   - if he or she will not be attending a meeting of the committee, take all reasonable steps to give advance warning of their absence to the council.

2. A member of a practice committee shall undertake education and training provided or organised by the Council from time to time so that they are properly informed about their responsibilities and in particular shall receive training in:
   - the functions of the Council and the role of the committee and its place in the work of the Council—
     (i) the effective conduct of proceedings by the committee and
     (ii) the discharge by the committee of its functions under Part V of the Order (Fitness to Practise), including the principles of natural justice, human rights and Community law.

Investigating committee

The Investigating Committee has the function of assessing the risk of any allegation referred to it by Council or by the case examiners. The Investigating Committee does not 'test' the evidence, but instead evaluates whether the evidence provided forms a prima facie case. In other words, is there evidence of the alleged wrongdoing? After a referral, the Investigating Committee shall:

(a) decide that there is no current risk to the public or to the public interest, therefore the nurse can continue to practice without any restriction placed upon their registration.

(b) That there this is real and significant risk to the public if the nurse was to practice without restriction. In these circumstances the Investigating Committee can make an interim order. For risks that can be managed via conditions, a nurse will need to follow the conditions prescribed but will remain on the register and can continue to practice as a nurse. For risks that cannot be managed via conditions (very serious departures from the Code, or serious criminal allegations) the Investigating Committee can impose an interim suspension order.

(c) The Investigating Committee cannot remove a nurse from the register, as this can only happen at the substantive stage (the Fitness to Practice Committee).

(d) An interim order can last up to 18 months and needs to be reviewed at least every six months. Any extension to the interim order must be agreed by the High Court in England and Wales.

If the allegation relates to an entry on the Register being fraudulently procured or incorrectly made, then the Investigating Committee can, if it is satisfied that the allegation is correct, make an order that the Registrar remove or amend the entry and it must notify the person concerned of her right to appeal under Article 38, but this order can be reviewed if new evidence comes to light (Article 26(7) and (12)).

The Investigating Committee also has the power to make an interim order at the same time or at any time before referring a case to a Fitness to Practise Committee.

If the Investigating Committee concludes that there is no case to answer or that the relevant entry was not fraudulently procured or incorrectly made, it must make a declaration to that effect, with reasons.

Since 2017 case examiners have the power to give advice, issue a warning and recommend undertakings in less serious cases, which the registrant can choose to accept or not accept. If it is not accepted, the case examiners will refer the matter to a Fitness to Practise Committee for a full hearing. Undertakings are utilised if a nurse agrees to address areas of their practice which cause a current clinical risk to patients, and the undertaking is published against the nurse or midwife's entry on the Register. Warnings are only used if the nurse or midwife shows insight, remediation and there is no current risk to patients. Warnings are also published again the entry of the nurse or midwife for a period of 12 months. Advice is considered as private guidance and is not published against the name of the registrant.

Fitness to practise committee

It may be that, after scrutiny of the evidence in Janice's case (Practical Dilemma 11.2), the Case Examiners decide that the case should be referred first to the Investigating Committee and eventually to the Fitness to Practise Committee (the substantive stage).

The FtPC has the function of advising the Council on:

1. the performance of the Council's functions in relation to standards of conduct, performance and ethics expected of registrants and prospective registrants;
2. requirements as to good character and good health to be met by registrants and prospective registrants;
3. the protection of the public from people whose fitness to practise is impaired and to consider:
   - any allegations referred to it by the Council, Case Examiners, the Investigating Committee, and
   - any application for restoration referred to it by the Registrar.

Rules to be followed in Fitness to Practise hearings were set out in a Statutory Instrument,[14] which can be downloaded from the NMC or legislation websites.

The Rules cover the following topics in relation to the Fitness to Practise Committee:
Action upon referral of an allegation
    Meetings and hearings
        Notice of hearing
        Procedure of the FtPC
        Notice of decision

The hearing

The Rules also lay down the procedure which should be followed at a hearing covering preliminary meetings, public and private hearings, representation and entitlement to be heard, absence of the practitioner, witnesses, vulnerable witnesses, and the order of proceedings at the initial hearing, a review or restoration hearing or at an interim orders hearing and the notes and transcript of the proceedings. The details can be seen in the Statutory Instruments which are available from the NMC and legislation websites. In the case of *McDaid* v *NMC*[15] one of the grounds for the midwife's appeal against being struck off the Register was that the panel should not have proceeded with the case in her absence. No satisfactory explanation of her failure to attend was given. The judge found against her on that point but ruled that the panel's decision should be quashed and another panel should hear the case because she succeeded on one ground (that a letter from the Trust's head of employment stated that it was up to her to write to a complainant which was contrary to the trust's assertion that she had made inappropriate contact with a complainant). Details of the case are discussed by Andrew Symon.[16]

In the case of Becky Read, an independent midwife working with the Albany Group Practice, 63 charges against her were dismissed when the NMC failed to offer evidence to the court.[17]

Two nurses were struck off following the Mid Staffordshire Inquiry: Sharon Turner who had said that she didn't give a flying f*** about patients, falsified A&E waiting time records, bullied a colleague and called Asian doctors names; and Tracey White who changed A&E data to make it look as though waiting targets had been met, abused a woman who had had an abortion and called an elderly patient a naughty little monkey.[18] The panel found that their actions constituted misconduct and their fitness to practise was impaired. Earlier in 2013 the NMC decided that Helen Moss, the director of nursing at the hospital between 2006 and 2009, had no case to answer.

In another case a nurse whose job was to accompany sick patients home from abroad was removed from the Register after it was found that he wrongly gave patients a clean bill of health to fly and unnecessarily delayed the flights of others by creating false records.[19]

Further information on hearings can be found on the NMC website.

The NMC consulted on whether the criminal standard of proof (beyond reasonable doubt) used in practice committees should be replaced by the civil standard of proof (on a balance of probabilities) (see chapter 1) and concluded in the light of the response that the criminal standard should be kept, but that rules relating to civil procedures should be followed (see NMC website). However, the Health and Social Care Act 2008 Section 112 added a new section 60A to the Health Act 1999:

> **60A Standard of proof in fitness to practise proceedings**
> 1. **The standard of proof applicable to any proceedings to which this subsection applies is that applicable to civil proceedings.**
> 2. **Subsection (1) applies to any proceedings before—**
>   (a) the Office of the Health Professions Adjudicator, or
>   (b) a committee of a regulatory body, a regulatory body itself or any officer of a regulatory body, which relate to a person's fitness to practise a profession to which Section 60(2) applies.
> 3. **In subsection (2) 'regulatory body' means the body (or main body) responsible for the regulation of a profession to which Section 60(2) applies.**

This section cannot be amended by an order in council (s. 112(4)).

The civil standard of proof came into force for new proceedings on 3 November 2008.[20] An NMC briefing note for legal assessors in 2008 sets out the House of Lords' judgments in two cases where it was emphasised that the civil standard of proof was a balance of probabilities and did not alter according to the gravity of the allegations. The civil standard of proof is simply that it was more likely than not that the proposition is true. Usually the panel have to decide it was 51 per cent more likely that the nurse did or did not commit the mischief in the case. If the balance is 50 per cent, and 50 per cent of the panel cannot find the charge proven, then the charge will fall as benefit is given to the defendant (the registered nurse).

There are essentially two distinct stages to a hearing: the first is to determine whether the facts which have been alleged are proved and whether these facts mean that the registrant is guilty of misconduct and if their fitness to practise is impaired. The second stage is the determination of what action should be taken by the practice committee. Rule 24 was amended by SI 2007/893 changing the procedure to be followed from the initial hearing.

The outcome

Once there has been a decision that misconduct has been proven against the nurse and that their fitness to practise is currently impaired, the Committee then has to decide what sanction to adopt. There are several choices as outlined in Box 11.6.

Box 11.6 — Outcomes available to the fitness to practise committee

1. Take no further action
2. Caution the practitioner and make an order directing the Registrar to annotate the Register accordingly for a specified period which shall not be for less than 1 year and not more than 5 years (a caution order)
3. Impose conditions with which the person must comply for a specified period which shall not exceed 3 years (a conditions of practice order)
4. Suspension for a specified period from the Register (not exceeding 1 year): on expiry of this time, the person shall be restored to the Register (a suspension order)
5. Strike off the Register
6. Interim orders: Article 31 enables an order to be made to suspend the person's registration or imposing conditions with which the person must comply for a period not exceeding 18 months, if it is necessary for the protection of members of the public or otherwise in the public interest, or is in the interests of the person concerned At the FtPC stage interim orders are normally used to cover the appeal period, in case the nurse or midwife wishes to appeal sanctions imposed against their practice.

The professional screeners, and the courts can refer a case back to the FtPC. Under Article 30 any practice committee has power to vary the orders that it has made or refer the matter to another committee.

In all cases the respondent must be notified by recorded delivery of the decision of the FtPC.

Criminal misconduct

If the charge relates to criminal misconduct, then slightly different rules apply. Evidence as to a conviction on a criminal charge can be put before the FtPC and the respondent can adduce evidence to prove beyond reasonable doubt that they are not the person referred to in the certificate of conviction or that the offence referred to in the certificate of conviction was not that of which they were convicted (this prevents a second trial on the actual charge that was before the criminal courts).

The FtPC will determine whether any conviction has been proved and after that the validity of the conviction will not be questioned. Proof of a conviction alone will not in itself be considered to be evidence of impairment of fitness to practise. However, proof of the conviction is evidence of the commission of the offence. It then has to be decided whether that offence constitutes impairment of fitness to practise.

In the case of Balamoody against the UKCC,[21] the court held that the terms of the professional conduct rules covered all criminal convictions regardless of either the seriousness of the offence or whether it was committed in the course of nursing. While a criminal conviction did not of itself constitute misconduct, some offences would almost certainly amount to misconduct and therefore, where a professional had failed to adhere to important statutory requirements while discharging functions of a senior and supervisory nature, resulting in a criminal conviction, the relevant professional body and the court would be forced to regard that person's actions as a cause for serious concern. In Practical Dilemma 11.2, if Janice were convicted of a criminal offence and the FtPC were satisfied that the certificate of conviction applied to Janice, they would have to determine if her actions showed that she was unfit to practise and determine the action to be taken. Even if no criminal proceedings were brought, the Investigation Committee of the NMC would initiate proceedings to determine if there was a case to answer following the procedure set out in Rule 4 of the Statutory Instrument (SI).

Practical dilemma 11.3 | Breach of the peace

A district nurse was very angry to discover that a traffic warden was standing by her car as she returned from visiting a patient. She pointed out her nurse's sticker and explained that she was visiting only for a few minutes to give an injection. The traffic warden was unimpressed by her pleading and took no notice of what she was saying. The nurse became very heated and an argument broke out during which the traffic warden said: 'You nurses are all the same. You all think the law does not apply to you.' The nurse lost her temper and pushed the warden. She was subsequently charged with conduct likely to cause a breach of the peace. She was found guilty and fined. She eventually found herself facing FtPC proceedings.

A case such as that in Practical Dilemma 11.3 would be conducted under the procedure to be followed where a conviction is alleged. Rule 31 of the SI states that where a registrant has been convicted of a criminal offence a copy of the certificate of conviction shall be conclusive proof of the conviction and the findings of fact upon which the conviction is based shall be admissible as proof of those facts. The only evidence which may be adduced by the registrant in rebuttal of the conviction is evidence that she is not the person referred to in the certificate. If the district nurse in Practical Dilemma 11.3 fails to put forward such evidence, then the FtPC would hold that the conviction had been proved, and decide if this was evidence of impairment of fitness to practise. It is then open to the nurse to submit that the charges are not in themselves proof of unfitness to practise.

In the case of *Isaghehi* v *NMC*[22] where the NMC struck off a psychiatric nurse who had been convicted and imprisoned for dangerous driving, the High Court decided that the striking off was disproportionately high and that a year's suspension from the Register was the appropriate sanction.

In contrast Shackleford, a registered nurse, appealed to the High Court against his being struck off, alleging that the panel had come to the wrong decision about his impairment and the sanction was wrong. He had been given a community order after being convicted of assault on his pregnant partner. The High Court judge stated that this was unacceptable conduct for the profession of nursing. The profession must maintain high standards of personal behaviour. His appeal was dismissed.[23]

Removal on Grounds of Health

At any time, the case examiners, when investigating a case of alleged unfitness to practise or a complaint against a nurse, can refer the case to the Fitness to Practise Committee of the NMC.

The FtPC is constituted to determine whether or not:

1. a practitioner will be removed from the Register or part of it;
2. a person who has been removed from the Register or part of it may be restored;
3. a practitioner's registration shall be suspended; and
4. the suspension of a person's registration shall be terminated.

The rules relating to membership of a practice committee and a panel are shown in Box 11.7.

Box 11.7 Rules relating to membership of a practice committee and a panel

The members of each practice committee shall include registered professionals and other members, of whom at least one shall be a registered nursing or midwifery practitioner.
The number of registered members on a practice committee may, but need not, exceed the number of other members on the committee and shall not in any case exceed that number by more than one.
The chairperson of the committee shall be either a lay or registrant member.
No one shall be a member of more than one practice committee and shall not be both a Case Examiner and a member of a practice committee.
The constitution of a panel hearing the matter is:

- At least one registered nurse or midwifery member.
- At least one member of the panel must be a lay member and not a registered nursing practitioner.
- Non-Council members may be members of the panel.
- The number of registrants on the panel may exceed the number of lay members but not by more than one.
- No person who is a member of Council or a committee may take part in proceedings of a practice committee while the subject of any allegations or investigations about their fitness to practise.

Case examiners

Allegations may be referred to Case Examiners in accordance with the Nursing and Midwifery Order or rules made under it (Article 23 applies). No person may be a Case Examiner if they are:

- a member of a practice committee,
- a legal, medical or registrant assessor, or
- employed by the Council.

Detailed rules relating to the appointment and function of Case Examiners are laid down in Article 24.

Procedure

Information, in writing and received by the Registrar, which raises any question of the practitioner's fitness to practise being seriously impaired by reason of their physical or mental condition shall be submitted to the professional case examiners. Anyone wishing to lay information before the Registrar may make a statutory declaration.

1. If the professional case examiners decide there is no reasonable evidence to support the allegations, they shall direct the Registrar to inform the complainant and, if they consider it necessary or desirable, the practitioner. The professional case examiners may obtain the opinion of a selected medical examiner on the information and evidence that they have received.

2. If they feel that the matter should proceed further, they shall direct the Registrar to write to the practitioner by recorded delivery:

    - notifying the registrant that information has been received that appears to raise a question as to whether their fitness to practise has become seriously impaired by reason of their physical or mental condition and indicating the symptomatic behaviour that gives rise to that question
    - if a health case, inviting the practitioner to agree within 14 days to submit to examination at the Council's expense by two medical examiners to be chosen by the professional case examiners and to agree that such examiners should furnish reports to the Registrar on the practitioner's fitness to practise
    - informing the practitioner that it is open to them to nominate other medical practitioners to examine the registrant at their own expense and to report to the Registrar on the practitioner's fitness to practise
    - inviting the practitioner to submit to the Registrar any observations or other evidence that they may wish to offer as to their own fitness to practise.

    If the two medical practitioners are not able to agree, a third can be appointed at the Council's expense. The professional case examiners can make their own enquiries before giving any of the above directions.

Action following reports received from the medical examiners

1. If the medical examiners are unanimously agreed that the registrant is not fit to practise, then the Registrar shall refer the information, together with the medical examiners' reports, to the

Fitness to Practise Committee. The solicitor may be directed to take all necessary steps for verifying the evidence to be submitted to the FtPC and for obtaining any necessary documents and the attendance of witnesses.

2. If there is considered to be insufficient evidence of illness, the practitioner and the complainant shall be informed.

If the registrant refuses to submit to such an examination or nominate their own medical examiner, the professional case examiners shall decide whether or not to refer the information received to the Fitness to Practise Committee, indicating the reason why no medical report is available.

Notice of referral

The procedure relating to the notice of a hearing is set down in Rule 11. The notice must be sent at least 28 days before the date of the hearing.

Restoration to the Register

This is governed by Article 33: unless new evidence has come to light that enables a practice committee to review its order under Article 30(7), no application for restoration to the Register may be made:

- before the end of the period of five years beginning with the date on which the order for striking off took effect, or
- in any period of twelve months in which an application for restoration to the Register has already been made by the person who had been struck off.

The Registrar shall refer the application for restoration to the committee that made the striking-off order or, where a previous application has been made, to the committee that last gave a decision on an application for restoration.

The Committee shall give the applicant an opportunity to appear before it and to argue their case in accordance with rules made by the Council.

The Committee may not grant an application for restoration unless it is satisfied that the applicant not only satisfies the educational requirements and that they are capable of safe and effective practice as a nurse or midwife but, having regard to the circumstances of the striking-off order, is also a fit and proper person to practise the relevant profession. The Committee can, in granting the application for restoration, make it subject to the applicant satisfying such requirements as to additional education or training and experience as the Council has specified under its rules relating to return to work after an absence (Article 19(3)). When making an order for restoration to the Register, the Committee shall direct the Registrar to register the applicant in the relevant part, subject to payment of the prescribed fee and may also make a conditions of practice order with respect to the applicant.

Amendments have been made to the 2001 rules[24] so that Rule 14 which enables a registrant to apply for voluntary removal from the registrar, must now include in the declaration details of any matters which the registrant is aware of which may give rise, or have given rise, to a fitness to practise allegation. The Registrar must seek the advice of a Practice Committee if the application for voluntary removal is received at a time when the registrant is subject to fitness to practise allegations. The Registrar must also obtain comments from the maker of the allegations. The amendments also change Rule 15 to set out the matters which the Registrar must take into account where a registrant's registration has lapsed and the registrant has applied for readmission to the Registrar.

The proceedings of the FtPC are subject to review by the High Court. For example, in *Slater* v *United Kingdom Central Council for Nursing, Midwifery and Health Visitors*,[25] the Queen's Bench Division quashed the decision of the Professional Conduct Committee (PCC) in removing Mr Stephen Slater's name from the Register of nurses and remitted the case to a freshly constituted Committee for a rehearing on the grounds that the practitioner's case had not been fully considered by the Committee and an injustice might therefore have been done. In a later case, *Hefferon* v *Committee of the UKCC, Current Law*, May 1988, 221, the High Court quashed the decisions of the Committee on the grounds that there had been a breach of natural justice. With the establishment of the Council for the Regulation of Healthcare Professions, then known as the Council for Healthcare Regulatory Excellence and now known as the Professional Standards Authority for Health and Social Care (see page xxx), it is possible for a complainant to apply to the Council if they are aggrieved at a decision made by a health registration body, including the NMC.

Professional standards and codes of practice

The functions of the NMC set out in Box 11.2 include that of establishing and improving standards of training and professional practice and also providing, in such manner as it thinks fit, advice for nurses, midwives and health visitors on standards of professional conduct. In fulfilment of this duty, the NMC has made several revisions to the Code of Professional Conduct and Guidance on different aspects of professional practice. The NMC has established a Library of Standards Project to review the NMC's approach to the development and dissemination of standards for NMC approved programmes of education and training leading to entry on the professional Register. *Standards to Support Learning and Assessment in Practice*[26] was published by the NMC in 2006 and revised in 2008. In 2018 the NMC published new standards for pre-registration nurse and midwifery training (see below). The standards can all be found on the NMC website.[27]

Education and training

The statutory duty to establish and improve standards of training falls on the NMC. A team of professional officers works with members through specialist committees, including the Educational Policy Advisory Committee, the Midwifery Committee and a committee on research. The NMC published standards of proficiency for pre-registration nursing and midwifery education in March 2004 which were updated in 2010.[28] Revised pre-registration standards for midwifery education were published in February 2009. In January 2010 the NMC published consultation standards for pre-registration nursing education which came into force in 2011.[29] These include standards for education and also standards for competence and replace those published in 2004. The NMC has also provided guidance on the recognition of Accreditation of Prior (Experiential) Learning (AP(E)L) in the approval and monitoring of NMC approved programmes.[30]

In May 2018 the NMC published new standards for pre-registered nurse training entitled *Future nurse: Standards of proficiency for registered nurses*. There are various proficiencies that a student nurse will need to demonstrate in order to apply for registration with the NMC.

The proficiencies are spread across seven platforms:

1. Being an accountable professional;
2. Promoting health and preventing ill health;
3. Assessing needs and planning care;
4. Providing and evaluating care;
5. Leading and managing nursing care and working in teams;
6. Improving safety and quality of care; and
7. Coordinating care.[31]

Approved education institutions are responsible for ensuring that the quality of their programmes complies with the Standards and proficiencies.

The NMC, the Health Care Professions Council and the Department of Health work in partnership with the NHS higher education providers and other stakeholders to develop quality assurance arrangements for professional healthcare education. Five elements have been identified as forming a quality assurance framework:

- major review;
- ongoing quality monitoring;
- approval and re-approval processes;
- benchmarks and quality standards; and
- evidence on which conclusions and judgements are based.

The new quality assurance framework and the appointment of Mott McDonald was announced by the NMC in June 2013.[32] Further information on the NMC Quality Assurance Framework for Nursing, Midwifery and Specialist Community Public Health Nursing is available on the NMC website where reports of the monitoring of individual institutions can be found.

Post-registration revalidation and continuing professional development (CPD)

From 2015 new procedures for revalidation were introduced, building on existing processes and systems. Registrants renew their registration every three years, declaring that they have practiced for 450 hours over that time, that they have undertaken continual professional development and that they are of good health and character. They must also declare any police charges, cautions or convictions. From 2014 registrants must also declare that they hold an appropriate level of professional indemnity insurance. Since 2016 they also need to confirm that they have sought and received third party feedback and third party confirmation. The NMC code has been revised to ensure that it will support revalidation. Revisions have taken into account recommendations from the Francis Report[33] and Compassion in Practice.[34]

As part of revalidation, nurses also have to complete 35 hours of continuing professional development (CPD), including 20 hours of participatory learning. Nurses also have to gather five pieces of practice-related feedback. The nurse will need to undertake five written reflective accounts and have a reflective discussion with another registrant (normally a line manager).

In 2017, section 60 changes to the Nursing and Midwifery Order 2001 (the Order) allowed case examiners to issue undertakings, warning and advice; created a single FtPC panel by amalgamating the Conduct and Competence Committee with the Health Committee; removed the requirement for an interim order review every three months, although the registrant can still request an early review; removed a review of a substantial order, although the registrant can still request an early review; and finally there is no longer a requirement that the registrant has their hearing in the country where the registrant lives. In the future it would be possible for a nurse living in Newcastle to have their case heard in Edinburgh, rather than having to travel to London. The full Annual Report and the reports relating to the business plan, statistics and financial report can be downloaded from the NMC website. The NMC has provided guidance for employers on the role of the NMC and when and how to make referrals to the NMC in relation to fitness to practise of a nurse or midwife.[35]

A Fitness to Practise Case

An example of a case heard by the CCC (now the FtPC) was that of Jane Hirst. A conditions of practice order had been imposed on her registration on 3 April 2013. This was reviewed in April 2014 in her absence since she failed to attend in spite of having notice of the hearing. The charges which were found proved in April 2013 were that she had:

1. slept on duty;
2. allowed a healthcare assistant to sleep on duty and/or failed to adequately supervise her; and
3. failed to ensure that the care needs of the residents were met, by failing to ensure that some residents had been turned every two hours from 20.00 to prevent pressure sores from developing, and failed to adequately care for some residents' continence needs.

The panel accepted that this type of misconduct was remediable but her failure to attend meant that the panel was unable to explore with her any steps she might have taken to remedy her behaviour or to explore any insight she may have into her failures. She had shown no remorse, insight or remediation. The panel considered all the options available to it (allowing the order to lapse; a caution order; a further conditions of practice order; a period of suspension and striking off). It concluded that a four-month suspension with immediate effect was the most appropriate action to take to protect the public, to address the issue of public interest and to uphold the standards of the profession. The four-month time limit would give the registrant sufficient time to re-engage with the NMC proceedings.

In another fitness to practise case a nurse who forgot to give a blood transfusion to a patient overnight was suspended for nine months.[36]

The Court of Appeal held that the timeline of 28 days (set in Article 29(10) of the 2001 Order) to appeal against an order for removal from the Register was absolute and the appellants had left it too late.[37]

Professional Standards Authority for Health and Social Care (PSA) (formerly the Council for Healthcare Regulatory Excellence (CHRE))

The Council for the Regulation of Health Care Professionals (CRHCP)[38] was set up under the NHS Reform and Healthcare Professions Act 2002 in the wake of the Kennedy Report into children's heart surgery at Bristol Royal Infirmary.[39] Its remit covered nine regulatory bodies, including the NMC. A White Paper was published in February 2007 on the future of health professional regulation,[40] which envisaged major changes for the CRHCP, including a smaller and more board-like Council with all members being appointed and the national regulators no longer nominating their presidents to the Council. These changes were effected by the Health and Social Care Act 2008 and the Council's name was changed to the Council for Healthcare Regulatory Excellence. In 2010 a review of arm's-length bodies[41] recommended that the CHRE should cease to be an executive non-departmental public body and instead should be self-funded with fees paid by the regulatory bodies. In addition, its remit should be extended to set standards and to quality assure other voluntary registers and professional bodies.

These changes were made in 2013.[42] The name of the CHRE was changed to the Professional Standards Authority for Health and Social Care, with the remit of protecting users of healthcare, users of social care in England and users of social work services in England.[43] The NHS Reform and Health Care Professions Act 2002 was amended to include the power of the Secretary of State to request the Authority for advice on any matter connected with the social work profession, or social care workers in England. The Authority can provide advice and auditing services to a regulatory body. The PSA is accountable to Parliament and provides an annual report which is available on its website.[44] It describes its functions as regulating the statutory bodies and 'we assess their performance, conduct audits, scrutinize their decisions and report to Parliament. We also set standards for organisations holding voluntary registers for health and social care occupations and accredit those that meet them.' It has the power to refer to the High Court cases which have been heard by the regulatory body including those cases where there has been an acquittal.[45]

In 2008 the CHRE published a report on the NMC[46] pointing out serious weaknesses in the NMC's governance and culture, in the conduct of its Council and in its ability to protect the interests of the public through the operation of fitness to practise processes. The NMC took appropriate action. In 2013 the House of Commons Select Committee on Health reported on an accountability hearing with the Nursing and Midwifery Council and published the latter's response as an appendix.[47] The NMC accepted the recommendations for change and improvement and noted that significant changes had already taken place. It concluded that, 'We are determined to continue to improve delivery of our core functions and build confidence in our work and look forward to providing confirmation of further progress at our next hearing.'

In June 2018 the Professional Standards Authority (in its annual review for 2016–17) reported that the NMC had continued to achieve improvements across each of its regulatory functions.

Public Involvement

One of the main features of the new registration system was that public involvement should increase. Under Article 3(5) of the 2001 Order[48] as amended in 2008[49] in carrying out its functions the NMC has a duty to cooperate, in so far as is appropriate and reasonably practicable, with public bodies or other persons concerned with—

    (i)   the employment (whether or not under a contract of service) of registrants,

    (ii)   the education or training of nurses, midwives or other healthcare professionals,

    (iii) the regulation of, or the coordination of the regulation of, other health or social care professionals,

(iv) the regulation of health services, and

(v) the provision, supervision or management of health services.

(5A) In carrying out its duty to cooperate under paragraph (5)(b), the Council shall have regard to any differing considerations relating to practising as a nurse or midwife which apply in England, Scotland, Wales or Northern Ireland.

The NMC predecessor, the UKCC, issued in October 2000 a strategy for public involvement[50] which identified the current public involvement in the work of the UKCC. The NMC has continued to ensure good communications with the general public and its website is accessible not only to registered practitioners and health service employers, but also to the general public.

Nursing associates

Since 2015 the NMC has also validated nursing associate programmes with selected higher education institutions. The first nursing associate students are due to register in January 2019. They will be join a new nursing associate part of the Register; however they will not be registered nurses. Nursing associates will be able to perform a wide range of nursing skills including medicines administration. Nursing associate is at present an England only role, and to date there are no plans to introduce the role in, Scotland or Northern Ireland.[51] However in Wales there are plans to introduce nursing associates by 2026/2027. The NMC Code 2015 has recently been updated in 2018 to include the nursing associate role.

Conclusions

There is no doubt that the Professional Standards Authority for Health and Social Care (replacing the Council for Healthcare Regulatory Excellence) in its focused remit and constitution should exercise a significant role in regulatory standards, not only through its powers to refer individual decisions to the High Court but also through its overall review of the performance of the different regulatory bodies. The critical report of the CHRE in 2008 of the NMC has led to significant changes. The CHRE identified the need to reduce the backlog of conduct and competence cases and the NMC planned to reduce the waiting time to six months by 2010. Legislation implementing fundamental changes to the registration provisions of all healthcare professionals following the White Paper *Trust, Assurance and Safety*[52] was enacted in the Health and Social Care Act 2008 and subsequently in the Health and Social Care Act 2012.

The importance of professional regulation of health professions and also of the unregistered health care assistants was emphasised in the recommendations of the Francis Report on Stafford Hospital which is considered in chapter 5. To date (2018) Healthcare Assistants are not regulated by any professional body.

The Law Commission in 2014 recommended a single clear and consistent legal framework for all health and social care professionals in a new UK-wide single statute. New powers and duties would be set with the main objective of protecting the public. The report includes a draft bill which would enact the reforms.[53]

Reflection questions

1. How would you define fitness to practise by a nurse? Would any of the following count as evidence of unfitness to practise by your definition?

    (a) a nurse has an illegitimate child
    (b) a nurse is convicted of shoplifting
    (c) a nurse is found guilty of a breach of the peace after being involved in an argument with a traffic warden
    (d) a nurse is fined for speeding
    (e) a nurse borrows money from a junior member of staff on her ward
    (f) a nurse is discovered to be drunk when off duty, but still in her uniform.

2. Since the decision as to whether there is misconduct or not and therefore whether there is impairment of fitness to practise depends on the detailed circumstances, what additional information would you need to answer question 1 and how would that information affect your answer?

Further exercises

1. The FtPC sits in different parts of the country and is open to the public and members of the profession. Next time it meets in your vicinity, try to attend and write up the hearing from the point of view of the formality, the procedure followed, justice to the nurse defendant and justice to the general public.
2. In what ways does a hearing before the FtPC differ from a hearing before a civil court? To what extent do you consider that the hearing and its procedure comply with Article 6 of the European Convention on Human Rights? (See the website of this book.)
3. What do you consider should be the time limit before a nurse who has been struck off can apply to be restored to the Register?
4. To what extent do you consider that the Professional Standards Authority for Health and Social Care influences and affects the professional status of the nurse or midwifery practitioner?

References

[1] The Nursing and Midwifery Council (Fitness to Practise) Rules 2004, SI 2004/1761
[2] J.M. Consulting Ltd, The Regulation of Nurses, Midwives and Health Visitors: report on a review of the Nurses, Midwives and Health Visitors Act 1997, J.M. Consulting Ltd, February 1999
[3] NHS Executive, Modernising Regulation: the new Nursing and Midwifery Council: a consultation document, DH, August 2000

[4] www.nmc.org.uk/concerns-nurses-midwives/fitness-to-practise-a-new-approach
[5] www.legislation.gov.uk
[6] Nursing and Midwifery Order 2001, SI 2002/253
[7] The Nursing and Midwifery Council (Constitution) Order 2008 SI 2008/2553
[8] Nursing and Midwifery Order 2001 SI 2002/253, as amended by the Nursing and Midwifery (Amendment Order) SI 2008/1485
[9] Inserted by the Nursing and Midwifery (Amendment Order) SI 2008/1485 Schedule 1 paragraph 2
[10] News item, Bogus nurse, *The Times*, 10 October 2003
[11] Andrew Symon, Legal challenges to the NMC's Fitness to Practise decisions, *British Journal of Midwifery*, 18(6):390–1, June 2010
[12] *Perry v Nursing and Midwifery Council* [2013] EWCA Civ 145
[13] Nursing and Midwifery Order 2001, SI 2002/253
[14] The Nursing and Midwifery Council (Fitness to Practise) Rules 2004, SI 2004/1761
[15] *McDaid v NMC* [2013] EWHC 586
[16] Andrew Symon, The Nursing and Midwifery Council faces more legal challenges, *British Journal of Midwifery*, 21(6):449–450, June 2013
[17] Martin Barrow, Midwife is cleared after three-year 'witch-hunt', *The Times*, 3 July 2013
[18] Chris Smyth, Nurses are first to be struck off after Mid Staffs scandal, *The Times*, 26 July 2013
[19] David Brown, Nurse who risked patients' lives as he enjoyed jet-set lifestyle struck off, *The Times*, 4 September 2013
[20] Health and Social Care Act 2008 (Commencement Order No. 3) SI 2008/2717
[21] *Balamoody v UKCC*, *Independent*, 15 June 1998
[22] *Isaghehi v NMC* [2014] EWHC 127
[23] *Shackleford v NMC* [2014] EWHC 1112
[24] SI 2004/1767 and by SI 2012/2754
[25] *Slater v United Kingdom Central Council for Nursing, Midwifery and Health Visitors*, The Times Law Report, 10 June 1987
[26] Nursing and Midwifery Council, Standards to Support Learning and Assessment in Practice, NMC, 2006, revised 2008
[27] www.nmc.org.uk
[28] Nursing and Midwifery Council, Standards for Proficiency for Pre-registration Nursing Education, NMC, 2010
[29] Nursing and Midwifery Council, Standards for Pre-registration Nursing Education: draft for consultation, NMC, January 2010
[30] Nursing and Midwifery Council, Accreditation of Prior (Experiential) Learning (AP(E)L) Fact sheet 1/2004, NMC, 2010
[31] Nursing and Midwifery Council, Future nurse: Standards of proficiency for registered nurses, NMC, May 2018
[32] www.nmc.org.uk
[33] Francis Report of the Mid Staffordshire NHS Foundation Trust Public Inquiry 2013
[34] Department of Health, Compassion in Practice: Nursing, midwifery and care staff, our vision and strategy, NHS Commissioning Board, 2012
[35] Nursing and Midwifery Council, Advice and information for employers of nurses and midwives, NMC, 2010
[36] News item, *The Times*, 20 June 2009
[37] *Adesina v Nursing and Midwifery Council; Baines v Nursing and Midwifery Council* [2013] EWCA Civ 818
[38] Section 25 National Health Service Reform and Health Care Professions Act 2002

[39] Bristol Royal Infirmary Inquiry (Kennedy Report), Learning from Bristol: the report of the public inquiry into children's heart surgery at the Bristol Royal Infirmary 1984–1995, Command Paper Cm 5207, July 2001, www.gov.uk/government/uploads/learningfromBristol or webarchive www.bristol-inquiry.org.uk
[40] White Paper, Trust, Assurance and Safety: the regulation of health professionals in the 21st century, 2007
[41] Department of Health 2010, Liberating the NHS: report of the arm's length bodies, London, Crown, 2010
[42] Sections 222 to 229 Health and Social Care Act 2012
[43] Health and Social Care Act 2012 (Consequential amendments – the Professional Standards Authority for Health and Social Care) Order SI 2012/2672
[44] www.professionalstandards.org.uk
[45] *Ruscillo v Council for the Regulation of Health Care Professionals & Anor; Council for the Regulation of Health Care Professionals v NMC and Truscott* [2004] EWCA Civ 1356
[46] Council for Healthcare Regulatory Excellence, Special report to the Minister of State for Health Services on the Nursing and Midwifery Council, CHRE, 2008
[47] Health Committee Fifth report: 2013 accountability hearing with Nursing and Midwifery Council Report HC 699
[48] Nursing and Midwifery Order 2001 SI 2002/253
[49] Nursing and Midwifery (Amendment Order) SI 2008/1485
[50] UKCC, Strategy for Public Involvement, 2000
[51] www.nmc.org.uk/standards/nursing-associates
[52] White Paper, Trust, Assurance and Safety: the regulation of health professionals in the 21st century, 2007
[53] Law Commission, Regulation of Health Care Professionals and Regulation of Social Care Professionals in England 2014, www.lawcom.gov.uk

Chapter 12
Health and Safety and the Nurse

This chapter discusses

- Statutory provisions
- Corporate manslaughter and corporate homicide
- Common law duties: employer's duty
- Remedies available to an injured employee
- Special areas

Introduction

This chapter covers the basic principles of law relating to health and safety at work, taking examples from nursing practice. It covers both the statutes (Acts of Parliament and Statutory Instruments) and the common law (decided cases or judge-made law) that set out the legal requirements on health and safety. Statute law and common law work in parallel and cover similar duties (although statute law is more specific).

Statutory provisions

Health and Safety at Work Act 1974 (HASWA)

General principles

The Health and Safety at Work Act 1974 is enforced through the criminal courts by the Health and Safety Inspectorate, on behalf of the Health and Safety Executive, which has the power to prosecute for offences under the Act and under the regulations, also powers of inspection, and which can issue enforcement or prohibition notices.

The employer has two parallel duties – one under the civil law and enforced through the civil courts, the other under the criminal law and enforced through the criminal courts. The Health and Safety at Work Act is an Act that is enforceable through the criminal courts and places on both employer and employee considerable duties in relation to health and safety. Originally some regulations made under the Health and Safety at Work Act 1974 (such as the manual handling regulations) could also be used as the basis for a claim for compensation in the civil courts. However, under section 69 of the Enterprise and Regulatory Reform Act 2013 breach of the Health and Safety regulations is not actionable in the civil courts except to the extent that the regulations specify. It follows that negligence by the employer and not a simple breach of the regulations must be proved by the employee to obtain compensation in the civil courts. Statute Box 12.1 sets out the general duties under section 2 of the Act. Statute Box 12.2 sets out the duties of the individual employee. A glance will show how comprehensive they are.

A freedom of information request to the NHS litigation authority (now NHS Resolution) in 2012 revealed that some £20 million a year is paid to staff as compensation for health and safety failures that result in accidents at work. The sum included £3980 paid to a nurse who slipped on a piece of potato left on a ward floor.[1]

Statute 12.1

Section 2 of the Health and Safety at Work Act 1974: Duty of Employer

General duties of employers to their employees

1. It shall be the duty of every employer to ensure, so far as is reasonably practicable, the health, safety and welfare at work of all his employees.
2. Without prejudice to the generality of an employer's duty under the preceding subsection, the matters to which that duty extends include in particular:
    (a) the provision and maintenance of plant and systems of work that are, so far as is reasonably practicable, safe and without risks to health;
    (b) arrangements for ensuring, so far as is reasonably practicable, safety and absence of risks to health in connection with the use, handling, storage and transport of articles and substances;
    (c) the provision of such information, instruction, training and supervision as is necessary to ensure, so far as is reasonably practicable, the health and safety at work of his employees;
    (d) so far as is reasonably practicable as regards any place of work under the employer's control, the maintenance of it in a condition that is safe and without risks to health and the provision and maintenance of means of access to and egress from it that are safe and without such risks; and
    (e) the provision and maintenance of a working environment for his employees that is, so far as is reasonably practicable, safe, without risks to health, and adequate as regards facilities and arrangements for their welfare at work.

3. Except in such cases as may be prescribed, it shall be the duty of every employer to prepare and as often as may be appropriate revise a written statement of his general policy with respect to the health and safety at work of his employees and the organisation and arrangements for the time being in force for carrying out that policy, and to bring the statement and any revision of it to the notice of all of his employees.
4. Regulations made by the Secretary of State may provide for the appointment in prescribed cases by recognised trade unions (within the meaning of the regulations) of safety representatives from among the employees, and those representatives shall represent the employees in consultations with the employers under subsection (6) below and shall have such other functions as may be prescribed.
5. (Repealed.)
6. It shall be the duty of every employer to consult any such representatives with a view to the making and maintenance of arrangements which will enable him and his employees to cooperate effectively in promoting and developing measures to ensure the health and safety at work of the employees, and in checking the effectiveness of such measures.
7. In such cases as may be prescribed it shall be the duty of every employer, if requested to do so by the safety representatives mentioned in subsections (4) and (5) above, to establish, in accordance with regulations made by the Secretary of State, a safety committee having the function of keeping under review the measures taken to ensure the health and safety at work of his employees and such other functions as may be prescribed.

Statute 12.2

Section 7 of the Health and Safety at Work Act 1974: Duty of Employee

(a) to take reasonable care for the health and safety of himself and of others who may be affected by his acts or omissions at work.

(b) as regards any duty or requirement imposed on his employer or other person by or under any of the relevant statutory provisions to cooperate with him in so far as is necessary to enable that duty or requirement to be performed or complied with.

The duties set by the Health and Safety at Work Act 1974 are enforced through the criminal courts.

Abolition of crown immunity

Health authorities used to enjoy protection from the enforcement provisions of much legislation on the grounds that, as Crown bodies, they were immune from prosecution. However, this immunity was removed by the National Health Service (Amendment) Act 1986 sections 1 and 2 in respect of the food legislation and Health and Safety at Work Act 1974. Some immunities were, however, retained under Schedule 8 of the Act, including Employer's Liability (Compulsory Insurance) Act 1969 (see page 313). Basildon and Thurrock University Hospital Trust was found guilty of health and safety offences after a patient died when his head became trapped in the bars of his bed.[2]

Powers of the health and safety inspector and Care Quality Commission

Health and safety inspectors employed by the Health and Safety Executive have extensive powers to ensure that health and safety duties are implemented. These powers are set out in section 20 of HASWA. The inspector is able to issue improvement or prohibition notices that order the recipient to make equipment or premises safe or to cease a particular activity until the danger is removed. He also has the power to prosecute the authority in the magistrates' or Crown Court for a breach of the duties or regulations or failure to comply with the notice. In October 2007 in a prosecution brought by the Health and Safety Executive, a headmaster was fined £12,500 with legal costs of £7500 following the death of a 3-year-old pupil who fell down unguarded steps. It was held there was inadequate supervision for the children at playtime.[3] However, his appeal to the Court of Appeal succeeded and his conviction was quashed.[4] The Court of Appeal held that the risk which the prosecution had to prove was a real risk as opposed to a fanciful or hypothetical risk. The fact that risk was a part of everyday life went to the issue of whether the injured person was exposed to that risk by the conduct of the operation in question. The evidence suggested that there was no real risk of the kind statutorily contemplated. Unless it could be said that the child was exposed to a real risk by the conduct of the school, no question as to the reasonably practicable measures taken to meet risk arose. In another case,[5] a headmistress and four school staff were suspended after a boy died following an asthma attack in school (see chapter 22).

The Care Quality Commission has the authority to cancel the registration, issue a warning notice or prosecute a care provider under the Health and Social Care Act 2008, sections 29, 30 and 33, where the care provider fails to meet the requirements of the Health and Social Care Act (regulated Activities) Regulations 2014.

This includes meeting the requirements of regulation 15 that:

1. All premises and equipment used by the service provider must be—

    (a) clean,

    (b) secure,

    (c) suitable for the purpose for which they are being used,

    (d) properly used,

    (e) properly maintained, and

    (f) appropriately located for the purpose for which they are being used.

2. The registered person must, in relation to such premises and equipment, maintain standards of hygiene appropriate for the purposes for which they are being used.

The House of Lords has held that in criminal prosecutions against an employer following an accident at work, it was sufficient for the prosecution to prove merely a risk of injury arising from a state of affairs at work, without identifying and proving specific breaches of duty by the employer. Once that was done, a *prima facie* case of breach was established. The onus then passed to the employer to make good the defence of reasonable practicability.[6]

Could an individual nurse be prosecuted?

Yes, under the Health and Safety at Work Act 1974 Section 7 (see Statute Box 12.2), which places a duty on all employees in respect of health and safety. First, a nurse who, for example, failed to follow the correct practice in disposing of pressurised cans as a result of which an incinerator blew up, injuring a porter, could be prosecuted for breach of her duty under section 7 of the Act. Second, the nurse as manager will have responsibilities in advising on and implementing the NHS trust's duties under the Act and if they neglect these they could also be prosecuted personally. In Practical Dilemma 12.1 the ward sister and others responsible for failing to undertake a risk assessment and basic precautions could be prosecuted under Section 7 of the 1974 Act and the employer could be prosecuted for breach of its duties under Section 2 of the 1974 Act (see Statute Box 12.1).

Practical dilemma 12.1 Ward boiler

A ward kitchen has a water heater that is not fixed according to the regulations. The boiler is moved to a more convenient location. A lead from the boiler runs to a point a few feet away. A cleaner trips over the lead, the boiler falls on them and they are severely scalded. The Health and Safety Inspectorate investigates and considers prosecuting the ward sister and others responsible.

It is also a criminal offence for any person to interfere with health and safety measures (see Statute Box 12.4).

General health and safety duty of employer to non-employees

Under section 3 of the 1974 Act, the employer has a general duty of care to persons not in his employment. The employer has a duty to conduct his undertaking in such a way as to ensure, so far as is reasonably practicable, that persons not in his employment who may be affected thereby are not exposed to risks to their health and safety. This duty would therefore cover patients, visitors and the general public. The Court of Appeal refused to allow an appeal against conviction of offences under sections 3(1) and 33(1)(a) of HASWA when a boy of 7 went with his father and younger brother to an indoor pool operated by the defendants. There was a notice saying that children under 8 should be accompanied by an adult. The boy could not swim and was not wearing armbands. He went to part of the pool near the deep end and was seen under water and rescued by a member of the public. He survived but sustained severe brain damage. The pool owner argued that the accident had resulted from inadequate supervision by the boy's father: it was not the conduct of his undertaking which had exposed the boy to risk. However, the Court of Appeal held that the absence of parental supervision did not exonerate the defendant from responsibility. Absolute safety could not be guaranteed but what was required of the defendant was that the running of the swimming pool should be carried out in a way that ensured the safety, as far as was reasonably practicable, of all those who used it.[7] The implications of this case for paediatric wards and areas where children come with parents are obvious.

Statute 12.3
Section 20 of the Health and Safety at Work Act 1974

An inspector may, for the purpose of carrying into effect any of the relevant statutory provisions within the field of responsibility of the enforcing authority which appointed him, exercise the powers set out in subsection (2) below.

(i) The powers of an inspector referred to in the preceding subsection are the following, namely:

 (a) at any reasonable time (or, in a situation which in his opinion is or may be dangerous, at any time) to enter any premises which he has reason to believe it is necessary for him to enter for the purpose mentioned in subsection (1) above;

 (b) to take with him a constable if he has reasonable cause to apprehend any serious obstruction in the execution of his duty;

 (c) without prejudice to the preceding paragraph, on entering any premises by virtue of paragraph (a) above to take with him:

(i) any other person duly authorised by his (the inspector's) enforcing authority; and
(ii) any equipment or materials required for any purpose for which the power of entry is being exercised;

 (d) to make such examination and investigation as may in any circumstances be necessary for the purpose mentioned in subsection (1) above;

 (e) as regards any premises which he has power to enter to direct that those premises or any part of them, or anything therein, shall be left undisturbed (whether generally or in particular respects) for so long as is reasonably necessary for the purpose of any examination or investigation under paragraph (d) above;

 (f) to take such measurements and photographs and make such recordings as he considers necessary for the purpose of any examination or investigation under paragraph (d) above;

 (g) to take samples of any articles or substances found in any premises which he has power to enter, and of the atmosphere in or in the vicinity of any such premises;

 (h) in the case of any article or substance found in any premises which he has power to enter, being an article or substance which appears to him to have caused or to be likely to cause danger to health or safety, to cause it to be dismantled or subjected to any process or test (but not so as to damage or destroy it unless this is in the circumstances necessary for the purpose mentioned in subsection (1) above);

 (i) in the case of any such article or substance as is mentioned in the preceding paragraph, to take possession of it and detain it for so long as is necessary for all or any of the following purposes, namely:

(i) to examine it and do to it anything which he has power to do under that paragraph;
(ii) to ensure that it is not tampered with before his examination of it is completed;
(iii) to ensure that it is available for use as evidence in any proceedings for an offence under any of the relevant statutory provisions or any proceedings relating to a notice under section 21 or 22;

(j) if he is conducting an examination or investigation under (d) to require any person . . . to answer any questions as the inspector thinks fit and to sign a declaration of the truth of his answers . . .

(k) to require production of, inspect and take copies of any entry in any books or documents . . .

(l) to require any person to afford himself such facilities and assistance within that person's control or responsibilities as are necessary for him to exercise his powers;

(m) any other power which is necessary for the purpose of exercising any of the above powers.

Statute 12.4

Section 8 of the Health and Safety at Work Act 1974

No person shall intentionally or recklessly interfere with or misuse anything provided in the interest of health, safety or welfare in pursuance of any relevant statutory provisions.

The Court of Appeal has held[8] that, provided the employer has taken all reasonable care in laying down safe systems of work and ensuring that the employees had the necessary skill and instruction and were subject to proper supervision, with safe premises, plant and equipment, the employer was not guilty of an offence under section 3 of the 1974 Act if the employee were negligent and caused harm to others.

Safety Representatives and Safety Committees Regulations 1977 (SRSC)

These regulations brought into force the requirement in HASWA 1974 that employers should permit the safety representative appointed by the recognised trade union to inspect the workplace, get information held by the employer relating to health, safety or welfare and have paid time off for training and carrying out their functions. Each employer is required to set up a Health and Safety Committee to consider matters relating to health and safety. The Health and Safety Executive (HSE)[9] has published guidance for the Trade Union Congress known as the 'Brown Book' for training purposes.

Health and Safety (Consultation with Employees) Regulations 1996

These apply to those workplaces that are not covered by SRSC and require employers to consult with workers or their representatives on all matters relating to employees' health and safety. Guidance from the HSE is available on its worker involvement website.

Health and safety at work regulations

Regulations came into force on 1 January 1993 as a result of European Directives. These are shown in Box 12.1.

Box 12.1 — **Health and safety regulations that came into force on 1 January 1993**

1. Management of Health and Safety at Work Regulations 1992 (updated 1999)
2. Provision and Use of Work Equipment Regulations 1992 (updated 1998)
3. Manual Handling Operations Regulations 1992 (as amended 2002)
4. Workplace (Health, Safety and Welfare Regulations) 1992 (updated 1999)
5. Personal Protective Equipment at Work Regulations 1992 (updated 1999)
6. Health and Safety (Display Screen Equipment) Regulations 1992 (updated 1999)

The regulations shown in Box 12.1 are enforceable against all employers and employees (whether NHS or not). Many of these have now been updated and reissued. Codes of practice have been issued by the Health and Safety Commission. Failure to comply with the code is not in itself an offence, but can be used in evidence in criminal proceedings.

(For protection of the employee against dismissal in health and safety cases, see chapter 10.)

The Environmental Protection Act 1990 creates duties in relation to waste management.[10] Failure to comply with the waste management regulations could lead to prosecution, sanctions from the Care Quality Commission and professional conduct proceedings by the NMC.

Management of Health and Safety at Work Regulations 1999

These regulations require each employer to undertake a suitable and sufficient assessment of the risks to the health and safety of his employees. A code of practice has been approved in conjunction with these regulations.[11] This code does not have legal force, but has special legal status.

If an employer is prosecuted for a breach of health or safety law and it is proved that they did not follow the relevant provisions of the code, they will need to show that they have complied with the law in some other way or a court will find them at fault.

The guidance

The guidance emphasises that risk assessment must be a systematic general examination of work activity with a recording of significant findings rather than a *de facto* activity.

The definition of risk includes both the likelihood that harm will occur and its severity. The aim of risk assessment is to guide the judgement of the employer or self-employed person, as to the measures they ought to take to fulfil their statutory obligations laid down under the Health and Safety at Work Act 1974 and its regulations.

Suitable and sufficient is defined in the guidance as:

- able to identify the significant risks arising from or in connection with work
- able to identify appropriate sources of information and examples of good practice
- appropriate to the nature of the work and should identify the period of time for which it is likely to remain valid.

Recording

The 'record should represent an effective statement of hazards and risks which then leads management to take the relevant actions to protect health and safety'. It should be in writing, unless in computerised form, and easily retrievable. It should include:

1. a record of the preventive and protective measures in place to control risks;
2. further action required to reduce risk sufficiently; and
3. proof that a suitable and sufficient assessment has been made.

Principles that apply in risk assessment

The following principles apply in risk assessment:

1. If possible avoid the risk altogether.
2. Evaluate risks that cannot be avoided by carrying out a risk assessment.
3. Combat risks at source rather than by palliative measures.
4. Adapt work to the requirements of the individual.
5. Take advantage of technological and technical progress.
6. Implement risk prevention measures to form part of a coherent policy and approach. This will progressively reduce those risks that cannot be prevented or avoided altogether and will take account of the way work is organised, the working conditions, the environment and any relevant social factors.
7. Give priority to those measures that protect the whole workplace and all those who work there, and so give the greatest benefit.
8. Ensure that workers, whether employees or self-employed, need to understand what they must do.
9. The existence of a positive health and safety culture should exist within an organisation. This means that avoidance, prevention and reduction of risk at work must be accepted as part of the organisation's approach and attitude to all its activities. It should be recognised at all levels of the organisation, from junior to senior management.

The Court of Appeal[12] held that the duty of the employer to provide a suitable and sufficient risk assessment under Regulation 3 of the Management of Health and Safety at Work Regulations 1999[13] and training for its employees under Regulation 9 of the Provisions and Use of Work Equipment Regulations 1998[14] imposed a higher standard than the common law duty which incorporated reasonable foreseeability. The claimant worked for London Underground first as a guard and then as a driver and developed tenosynovitis in her shoulder owing to the strain from the prolonged use of the traction brake controller, known as the dead man's handle. The employer had a duty to provide adequate training, which included a duty to investigate the risks inherent in its operations, taking professional advice where necessary. The right approach to deciding whether the training was adequate for health and safety purposes was to examine whether the risk assessment was suitable and sufficient.

In a case on the Provisions and Use of Work Equipment Regulations 1998 Regulation 4 and 5, the court had to decide if the council was responsible for a ramp.

> **Case 12.1** **Smith (Jean) v Northamptonshire County Council [2008]**
>
> # Unsafe ramp[15]
>
> The Court of Appeal held that an employer was not liable for a slip on another's ramp. Mrs Smith was employed by the council as carer/driver and collected a client in a wheelchair from her home. When pushing the chair down the ramp, which had been installed by the NHS, she stepped on the edge and it gave way.
>
> The trial judge had held that Regulation 5 imposed **strict liability** on the council for maintaining the ramp as work equipment for use at work and found in favour of Mrs Smith. The Court of Appeal, however, allowed the Council's appeal and held that strict liability should only be imposed by clear language. For someone to have an obligation to maintain something it would normally have to be within his power to do so without obtaining someone else's consent. Strict liability should not flow out of a position in which there was no right and no responsibility to do that thing or insist on doing that thing for which strict liability was being imposed.
>
> The claimant appealed to the House of Lords but lost her appeal.[16] The House of Lords, in a majority judgment, held that the test to be applied was whether the work equipment was incorporated into and adopted as part of the employer's undertaking. It could not be said that the ramp was either incorporated into or adopted as part of the council's undertaking or under their control. They did not provide it or own it or possess it. They did not have any responsibility or indeed any right without more to repair it.

The House of Lords[17] held that a door-closing device could be work equipment for the purposes of Regulation 2 of the Provision and Use of Work Equipment Regulations,[18] so that a mechanic who was injured while repairing such a device could bring proceedings against his employer.

The Court of Appeal has held that earlier good industrial practice is no defence and whether a workplace was in fact made and kept safe was to be judged objectively without reference to what might earlier have been thought to be good practice.[19] The claimants held that they had suffered hearing loss in a knitwear factory.

The Workplace (Health, Safety and Welfare) Regulations (SI 1992 No. 3004) were breached by an employer when an accident occurred when a school caretaker pushing a trolley hit a protruding paving slab. The council was held liable in damages since it was in breach of the regulations. The council could not plead as a defence that it was a freak accident.[20]

Risk management and the nurse

For the most part, the nurse would share common health and safety hazards with other hospital, community or social services employees and thus models of risk assessment and management that applied to other health professionals would also apply to nursing. Thus hazards relating to the safety of equipment, cross-infection risks, safe working practices or to violence at work would all apply to nurses who should be involved in the system of the assessment of risk.

Each nurse should therefore be able to carry out a risk assessment of health and safety hazards in relation to colleagues, clients, carers and the general public.

Reporting of Injuries, Diseases and Dangerous Occurrences Regulations 1995 (RIDDOR), updated in 2012 and replaced in 2013

The regulations govern the reporting of injuries, diseases and dangerous occurrences. The 1985 regulations were replaced by new regulations that came into force on 1 April 1996.[21] There is now one set of regulations in place of the four sets under the 1985 regulations. The list of reportable diseases has been updated, as has the list of dangerous occurrences. It is legally possible for reports to be made by telephone to the Incident Contact Centre.[22] The 2013 regulations list specific injuries to workers which must be reported, replacing the major injury list of the 1995 regulations.[23]

Schedule 1 to the 2013 regulations lists the reporting and recording procedures, Schedule 2 lists the dangerous occurrences that are reportable, Schedule 3 sets out the diseases reportable offshore.

Regulation 12 of RIDDOR 2013 lays down the requirements in relation to record keeping of reportable events or diseases. These records must be kept for at least three years from the date on which they were made. The records must contain the details set out in Schedule 1 (see Box 12.2).

Box 12.2 **Contents of records kept under RIDDOR schedule 1 part 2**

1. Date and time of the accident or dangerous occurrence
2. Where accident suffered by a person at work: full name, occupation and nature of injury
3. Where accident suffered by a person not at work: full name of person, status, nature of injury, unless these are not known and it is not reasonably practicable to ascertain them
4. Place where the accident or dangerous occurrence happened
5. Brief description of the circumstances in which the accident or dangerous occurrence happened
6. Date on which the accident or dangerous occurrence was first notified or reported to the relevant enforcement authority
7. Method by which the accident or dangerous occurrence was first notified or reported

---

Schedule 1 part 2 also sets out the records required in the event of a reportable disease.

A record must be kept of any accident causing an injury which results in the worker being away from work or incapacitated for more than three days, but the incident does not have to be reported unless the incapacitation period exceeds seven days.[24] Further guidance on RIDDOR 2013 is available on the HSE website.

NHS Improvement (formerly the National Patient Safety Agency (NPSA))

The National Patient Safety Agency (NPSA) was established in 2001 following a report, *An Organisation with a Memory*,[25, 26] written by an expert group chaired by Professor Liam Donaldson, Chief Medical Officer, which had recommended setting up a national reporting system. The Expert Committee was established in February 1999 with the brief to 'examine the extent to which the National Health Service and its constituent organisations have the capability to learn from untoward incidents and service failures so that similar occurrences are avoided in the future. To draw conclusions and make recommendations.' The aim of the NHS mandatory reporting system was to log all failures, mistakes, errors and near misses in healthcare and to be in place before 2001. Since May 2006 all reporting organisations have been able to access their incident data and compare their profile with similar NHS organisations.

An alert issued by NPSA in March 2007 was concerned with safe practice with epidural injections and infusions.[27] The remit of the NPSA was extended in 2005 to include safety aspects of hospital design, cleanliness and food. It was also given the task of ensuring research was carried out safely through its responsibility for the National Research Ethics Service (NRES) (formerly the Central Office for Research Ethics Committees (COREC)). It is now part of NHS Improvement, which is tasked with learning from patient safety incidents.[28]

The NPSA was also responsible for the National Clinical Assessment Service (NCAS)[29] which is concerned with the performance of individual doctors and dentists and took over from NICE (see chapter 5) responsibility for the three confidential enquiries: into maternal death and child health; patient outcome and death; and suicide and homicide by persons with mental illness. NCAS is now part of NHS Resolution.[30]

Openness and Candour in the NHS

The government accepted a recommendation from the Francis Report for a duty of candour to encourage openness and transparency in health services, including nursing services, in an attempt to prevent a repeat of the deliberate concealment of poor care and negligence found in the Mid Staffordshire Hospital scandal (Department of Health 2014).

The Francis Report (2013) defines candour as the volunteering of relevant information to persons who have been harmed by the provision of services, whether or not the information has been requested and whether or not a complaint has been made. The duty places a legal obligation on nurses to report poor practice where patients have been harmed.

There are two forms of the duty that apply to nurses: an organisational duty that is imposed on the employing trust and a professional duty imposed on registered nurses.

Statutory organisational duty of candour

The organisational duty of candour is imposed on nurses working in England under the provisions of the Health and Social Care Act 2008 and the Health and Social Care Act 2008 (Regulated Activities) Regulations 2014. It applies to all health service bodies regulated by the Care Quality Commission (CQC), the statutory regulator for health services in England. Nursing services have been subject to these regulations since 1 April 2015.

The 2014 regulations introduce revised fundamental standards for health bodies registered with the CQC and include a duty of candour. The Health and Social Care Act 2008 (Regulated Activities) Regulations 2014, regulation 20 requires nursing services to act in an open and transparent way with patients in relation to their care and treatment. It imposes a general duty to be candid with patients whether or not there has been a complaint and seeks to encourage an open, honest culture.

In practice, the organisational duty of candour requires a nursing service to tell the patient or their representative about a notifiable patient safety incident as soon as is reasonably practicable after the incident.

Notifiable patient safety incident

A notifiable safety incident is defined as one where a patient suffered or could suffer unintended harm resulting in:

- death,
- severe harm,
- moderate harm, or
- prolonged psychological harm (experienced continuously for 28 days or more).

The definition of these terms is derived from the National Patient Safety Agency's *Seven steps to patient safety* (2004). This defines harm as:

- injury,
- suffering,
- disability, or
- death.

To meet the threshold for disclosure under the duty of candour the harm must be moderate or severe as set out in Box 12.3.[31]

Box 12.3 **National patient safety agency terms and definitions**

No harm

Impact prevented – Any patient safety incident that had the potential to cause harm but was prevented, resulting in no harm.

Impact not prevented – Any patient safety incident that ran to completion but no harm occurred to people receiving care.

Low Harm: Any patient safety incident that required extra observation or minor treatment and caused minimal harm, to one or more persons receiving care.

Moderate Harm: Any patient safety incident that resulted in a moderate increase in treatment and which caused significant but not permanent harm, to one or more persons receiving care.

Severe Harm: Any patient safety incident that appears to have resulted in permanent harm to one or more persons receiving care.

Death: Any patient safety incident that directly resulted in the catastrophic death of one or more persons receiving care.

Duty to give an explanation and apology

Once a notifiable patient safety incident has arisen with a patient the nursing service must give that patient a full explanation of what is currently known and details of any further inquiry to be carried out. The patient must also receive an apology. Both the explanation and apology must be made in person. The duty to explain and apologise includes a requirement to support the patient during this process. This might include the provision of an interpreter to ensure the patient understands the explanation and is able to ask questions of the nurse. It also includes the need to give emotional support to the patient.

Once the patient has received an explanation and apology the nursing service is required to provide the patient with a written note of the discussion and must ensure that a written notice of the incident and copies of correspondence are kept for later inspection by the CQC.

Statutory duties in wales, northern ireland and scotland

There is currently no equivalent statutory organisational duty of candour with the legal force of the one imposed in England in place in the other devolved health services but there are general duties for those services to be open and raise concerns.

In Wales a statutory duty of candour has been introduced by Part 3 of the Health and Social Care (Quality and Engagement) (Wales) Act 2020. Section 3 of the 2020 Act provides that:

- The duty of candour comes into effect in relation to an NHS body if it appears to the body that two conditions are met.
- The first condition is that a person to whom health care is being or has been provided by the body has suffered an adverse outcome.
- The second condition is that the provision of the health care was or may have been a factor in the service user suffering that outcome.
- An adverse outcome is described as a user experiences, or could experience, any unexpected or unintended harm that is more than minimal.

The Scottish organisational duty of candour is established by the Health (Tobacco, Nicotine etc. and Care) (Scotland) Act 2016 and the Duty of Candour Procedure (Scotland) Regulations 2018.

In Northern Ireland, a consultation on a statutory duty of candour was completed in 2021 but legislation to introduce the duty has yet to be passed by the Northern Ireland Assembly.

Professional duty of candour

In its response to the Francis Report (2013) the government made clear that a statutory organisational duty of candour alone was not enough to promote openness and honesty in the National Health Service. In the government's view it was critical to ensure that registered health professionals also had an individual duty of candour imposed on them.

Imposing a professional duty of candour on all registered health professionals, and this includes nurses, ensures a consistent approach to candour and the reporting of errors. A professional duty also ensures that those who seek to obstruct others in raising concerns will be in breach of their professional code and guilty of professional misconduct.

The Professional Standards Authority (PSA) oversees the regulation of health and social care professionals by regulating the professional regulators including the Nursing and Midwifery Council. The PSA were charged by the government to ensure clear and consistent guidance and standards for the duty of candour by the professional regulators.

The regulators of health and social care professionals have issued a joint statement on the professional duty of candour that establishes a common professional duty on registered health professionals even though it may be expressed in different ways in their statutory codes. The statutory regulators must promote the professional duty of candour expressed in the joint statement and hold registered professionals accountable against it.

The jointly agreed professional duty of candour requires that:

> Every healthcare professional must be open and honest with patients when something goes wrong with their treatment or care which causes, or has the potential to cause, harm or distress.
>
> *(General Chiropractic Council, et al. 2014)*

Nurse's professional duty of candour

The Nursing and Midwifery Council have implemented this joint statement on the requirements of a professional duty of candour as standard 14 of their Code. The standard requires that nurses must:

> Be open and candid with all service users about all aspects of care and treatment, including when any mistakes or harm have taken place.

To achieve this, a nurse must:

- act immediately to put right the situation if someone has suffered actual harm for any reason or an incident has happened which had the potential for harm
- explain fully and promptly what has happened, including the likely effects, and apologise to the person affected and, where appropriate, their advocate, family or carers, and
- document all these events formally and take further action (escalate) if appropriate so they can be dealt with quickly.

Guidance on the duty of candour

The Nursing and Midwifery Council and the General Medical Council (2015) have issued joint guidance on the implementation of their professional duty of candour. The guidance makes clear that:

- Openness and honesty begins before care and treatment and patients must be fully informed about their care and this includes the risks as well as the benefits of the options available.
- The professional duty of candour is not intended for circumstances where a patient's condition gets worse due to the natural progression of their illness. It applies when something goes wrong with a patient's care, and they suffer harm or distress as a result.
- When a nurse realises that something has gone wrong, and after doing what they can to put matters right, the nurse or someone from the healthcare team must speak to the patient. The most appropriate team member will usually be the lead or accountable clinician.
- Nurses must speak to the patient as soon as possible after they realise something has gone wrong with their care. There is no need to wait until the outcome of an investigation to speak to the patient, but the nurse should be clear about what has and has not yet been established.
- Nurses should apologise to the patient, who will expect to be told three things as part of that apology: what happened, what can be done to deal with any harm caused and what will be done to prevent someone else being harmed.
- Nurses must embrace a learning culture by reporting errors so that lessons can be learnt quickly and patients can be protected from harm in the future.

Protection of Employees who Report Health and Safety Hazards

Additional protection for staff who report health and safety hazards has been given by the Trade Union Reform and Employment Rights Act 1993 against dismissal in health and safety cases and was consolidated in the Employment Rights Act 1996 (see chapter 10). The Public Interest Disclosure Act 1998 was intended to strengthen protection given to employees who report health and safety hazards. (This is considered in chapter 4 under whistleblowing.)

Occupiers' Liability Acts 1957 and 1984

General principles

If a nurse is injured as a result of the state of the premises, she may be able to bring an action against the occupier who has a duty under the Occupiers' Liability Act 1957 to ensure that the premises are safe. The statutory duty is set out below. The occupier's duty to trespassers comes under the Occupiers' Liability Act 1984, which is considered below.

Statute 12.5
Sections 2(1) and (2) of the Occupiers' Liability Act 1957

Section 2(1) An occupier of premises owes the same duty, the 'common duty of care', to all his visitors, except in so far as he is free to and does extend, restrict, modify or exclude his duty to any visitor or visitors by agreement or otherwise. Section 2(2) The common duty of care is a duty to take such care as in all the circumstances of the case is reasonable to see that the visitor will be reasonably safe in using the premises for the purposes for which he is invited or permitted by the occupier to be there.

The duty under the Occupiers' Liability Act is owed to the visitor. This term 'visitor' includes the person who has express permission to be on the premises as well as the person who has implied permission to be there. Thus in the hospital context, the term 'visitors' will include employees, patients, friends and relatives visiting patients, contractors and suppliers and others who have a genuine interest in being there. If any of these persons were to be injured, for example, when plaster fell off the wall, they could claim compensation from the occupier.

Who is the occupier?

The occupier is the person who has control over the premises. This will usually be the owner of the premises, but not necessarily. There could be several occupiers, each having control over the premises and responsibilities for the safety of the building. For example, contractors might be working on hospital premises and both the NHS trust and the contractor could be regarded as occupiers for the purpose of the Act. A private house visited by a community nurse may be owner-occupied, in which case that person will be the occupier for the purposes of the Act. Alternatively, it could be under a tenancy agreement, in which case the landlord and the tenant will have different duties under this agreement regarding the upkeep and maintenance of the premises and could therefore be regarded as occupiers under the statutory provisions. Which occupier is liable for harm to a visitor will therefore depend on the cause of the injury.

Case 12.2 *Slade* v *Battersea HMC* [1955]

Slippery floor[32]

A visitor slipped on polish that had been put on the floor but not wiped off, which left the floor excessively slippery.

The visitor succeeded in obtaining compensation for the harm. The occupier had failed to take reasonable care for the safety of the visitor. (This was a case decided before the 1957 Act, but the result would be the same after 1957.) In a more recent case,[33] a woman sustained personal injuries when, late at night, she fell down a flight of stairs leading to a public lavatory for which the local authority (LA) was responsible. The premises were locked and the stairway was unlit. She admitted that she had drunk a relatively small amount of alcohol. She sued the LA on the grounds that they were occupiers of the premises and owed a duty of care to her. She lost the case on the grounds that she had voluntarily accepted the risk of injury by using the stairs in the darkness (*volenti non fit injuria*) and without taking proper care for her own safety. Further, the evidence from the A&E department showed that she had consumed a greater amount of alcohol than she had admitted in evidence. Even if the court were wrong on the voluntary assumption of risk, she would be contributorily negligent to a high degree.

Statute 12.6
Section 2(4)(a) of the Occupiers' Liability Act 1957

Section 2(4)(a) In determining whether the occupier of premises has discharged the common duty of care to a visitor, regard is to be had to all these circumstances, so that (for example): where damage is caused to a visitor by a danger of which he had been warned by the occupier, the warning is not to be treated without more as absolving the occupier from liability, unless in all the circumstances it was enough to enable the visitor to be reasonably safe.

What is the effect of a warning notice?

Section 2(4)(a) of the Occupiers' Liability Act 1957 is set out in Statute Box 12.6. The warning is not conclusive: if compliance with it is sufficient to prevent any harm to the visitor, then it will be effective as a defence in an action under the 1957 Act.

Practical Dilemma 12.2   Warning

An NHS trust is undertaking major renovation work to a corridor and puts up a warning notice saying 'Danger'. As a nurse walks along, she is struck by a piece of plaster falling from the ceiling.

If there were other precautions that the NHS trust could reasonably have taken, e.g. a safety net cordoning off the work area, then the NHS trust would probably be seen to have been in breach of its duty of care to the visitor subject to the possibility of contributory negligence by her. If, contrariwise, the notice said, 'Corridor closed – diversion' and indicated a different route that was practicable, then the occupier would have satisfied the duty under the Act. If, of course, the nurse ignored the notice, continued along the dangerous corridor and was injured, then it is probable that there would be no breach of duty by the NHS trust, since the notice was in all the circumstances enough to enable the nurse to be reasonably safe.

Independent contractors

Where independent contractors are brought on to site, the usual occupier or owner of the premises will not normally be liable for their safety (see Statute Box 12.7).

Privatisation of cleaning and catering services

What is the effect of the privatisation of services on the occupier's liability? Privatisation may lead to some complications, since where services are contracted out, there is likely to be dual occupation of premises, i.e. by the NHS trust and by the private company. Thus in the case of a contract for cleaning services, if an injury is caused to a visitor by the conditions of the premises, e.g. an uneven surface or falling plaster and the NHS trust has retained responsibility for such conditions, then the NHS trust would be responsible for the visitor's injuries. If, by way of contrast, the injuries were caused by the carelessness of any of the contractor's employees, then the contractor would be responsible for compensating the person injured as a result of the negligence under the principles of vicarious liability previously discussed in chapter 4. If, therefore, the employee of the cleaning firm has left the floor in a dangerous state and there are no warning notices and a nurse is injured as a consequence, she would sue the cleaning company because its employee had been negligent in the course of employment and had caused her foreseeable harm.

Statute 12.7
Section 2(4)(b) of the Occupiers' Liability Act 1957

Section 2(4)(b) When damage is caused to a visitor due to the faulty execution of any work of construction, maintenance or repair by an independent contractor employed by the occupier, the occupier is not to be treated without more as answerable for the danger, if in all the circumstances he had acted reasonably in entrusting the work to an independent contractor and had taken such steps (if any) as he reasonably ought in order to satisfy himself that the contractor was competent and that the work had been properly done.

Liability for children under the Occupiers' Liability Act 1957

It is expressly provided that all the circumstances must be taken into account in deciding whether the occupier is in breach of his duty of care under the Act (see Statute Box 12.8). The occupier can expect a lower standard of care from children and therefore additional precautions have to be taken where the presence of children can be foreseen.

Statute 12.8
Section 2(3) of the Occupiers' Liability Act 1957

Section 2(3) The circumstances relevant for the present purpose include the degree of care, and of want of care, which would ordinarily be looked for in such a visitor, so that (for example) in proper cases: an occupier must be prepared for children to be less careful than adults.

Case 12.3 *Jolley v Sutton LBC* [2000]

Playing about on a boat[34]

Sutton Borough Council were the owners and occupiers of the common parts of a block of council flats. A boat with trailer was brought on to the land and abandoned on a grass area where children played. The boat became derelict and rotten. The council put a notice on the boat that said: 'Do not touch this vehicle unless you are the owner.' Some boys planned to repair it in the hope that they could take it to Cornwall. They swivelled it round and lifted the bows on to the trailer so as to be able to get under the boat to repair the hull. They jacked the bows of the boat up. The boat fell on to the claimant, a boy of 14, as he lay underneath it attempting to repair and paint it. He sustained serious spinal injuries and became paraplegic.

The High Court judge awarded the claimant £633,770, taking into account contributory negligence of 25 per cent for the injuries he sustained. However, the Court of Appeal found in favour of the defendant since, although it was reasonably foreseeable that injuries could have occurred from playing on the boat, the injuries sustained were not reasonably foreseeable and therefore the defendants were not liable for them. The Council had not disputed that it was negligent, but argued that it was not liable because the accident was of a different kind from anything that it could have reasonably foreseen. The claimant appealed to the House of Lords, which upheld the appeal. The House of Lords held that ingenuity of children in finding unexpected ways of doing mischief to themselves and others should not be underestimated. Reasonable foreseeability was not a fixed point on the scale of probability. The Council was liable under the Occupiers' Liability Act 1957 and under section 2(3) had to take into account the fact that children would be less careful than adults. The Council had admitted that it should have removed the boat and the risk that it should have taken into account was that children would meddle with the boat and injuries would thereby occur. Clearly, following this judgment, liability depends on how the risk is framed.

Trespassers and Occupiers' Liability Act 1984

The Occupiers' Liability Act 1957 does not cover any duty towards trespassers. The courts recognised a limited duty of the occupier towards trespassers, particularly children, but subsequently statutory provision was made in the Occupiers' Liability Act 1984. Whether or not a duty is owed by the occupier to trespassers, in relation to risks on the premises, depends on the following factors (s. 1(3)):

- if the occupier is aware of the danger or has reasonable grounds to believe that it exists;
- if the occupier knows or has reasonable grounds to believe that the other is in the vicinity of the danger concerned or that he may come into the vicinity of the danger (in either case, whether the other has lawful authority for being in that vicinity or not); and
- the risk is one against which, in all the circumstances of the case, he may reasonably be expected to offer the other some protection.

In applying these factors to decide if a duty is owed to a trespasser, it would be rare for a duty to be owed to an adult. There is, however, more likely to be a duty owed to a child trespasser. For example, on hospital premises, if a child is expressly told that he may not go through a particular door or into another section of the hospital and he disobeys those instructions, then he becomes a trespasser for the purposes of the Occupiers' Liability Acts. It is likely that a duty would then arise under the 1984 Act.

Nature of the duty owed to trespassers

Once it is held that a duty of care is owed to a trespasser, section 1(4) of the 1984 Act defines the duty as shown in Statute Box 12.9.

Statute 12.9

Duty of Care to a Trespasser Under Section 1(4) 1984 Act

'The duty is to take such care as is reasonable in all the circumstances of the case to see that he does not suffer injury on the premises by reason of the danger concerned.'

The duty can be discharged by giving warnings, but in the case of children, these may have limited effect and depend on the age of the child.

The occupier has the right to request a person to leave the premises and if that person fails to leave he or she then becomes a trespasser and the occupier can use reasonable force in removing the trespasser. This rule does not apply to a motor vehicle.[35]

The nurse and premises in the community

Where a nurse is visiting private homes, the occupier may be the owner of the house who is also in occupation or the occupier may be a tenant. If the nurse is injured on the premises, it will depend on how the injury occurred as to who would be liable: thus, if she is injured as the result of a frayed rug, the person in occupation, whether tenant or owner, would be liable; if she were injured as a result of a structural defect, then the owner or landlord would be liable depending on the nature of the tenancy agreement.

The occupier has the right to ask any visitor to leave the premises. Should the visitor fail to leave, then she becomes a trespasser and the occupier can use reasonable force to evict the trespasser. If, therefore, the nurse should be asked by a client or carer to leave, she should go. Should she be concerned for the well-being of the client, she should ensure that social services are notified so that appropriate action can be taken under the Care Act 2014 or the Mental Health Act 1983. Where there is a clash between carer and client and the former asks her to leave and the latter for her to stay, the nurse has to decide on the basis of the specific circumstances: the rights of the client to occupation as compared with those of the carer and the specific needs of the client. Where she considers it prudent to leave the premises, she must discuss with her manager how best the client's needs can be met.

Consumer Protection Act 1987

Product liability

The Consumer Protection Act 1987 enables a claim to be brought where harm has occurred as a result of a defect in a product. It is a form of strict liability in that negligence by the defendant does not have to be proved. The Consumer Protection Act 1987 (Part 1), which came into force on 1 March 1988, gives a right of compensation against the producers and suppliers of products if a defect in the product has caused personal injury, death, loss or damage to property, without the requirement of showing that the defendant was at fault. This was introduced into this country following a European Directive dated 25 July 1985 (No. 85/3741/EEC). The Act applies to the Crown. The NHS trust itself could be a defendant in a product liability action since it is a producer of many products; it could also be liable as a supplier.

A product is defined as meaning any goods or electricity and includes a product that is comprised in another product, whether by virtue of being a component part or raw material or otherwise.

Defect

The definition of defect is shown in Statute Box 12.10. The defendant can rely on the fact that the state of scientific knowledge at the time was such that the defect could not have been discovered (i.e. 'the state of the art' defence or that the state of scientific and technical knowledge at the time the goods were supplied was not such that the producer of products of that kind might be expected to have discovered the defect).

Statute 12.10

Sections 3 and 4 of the Consumer Protection Act 1987

3 (1) Subject to the following provisions of this section, there is a defect in a product for the purposes of this part if the safety of the product is not such as persons generally are entitled to expect; and for those purposes 'safety', in

relation to a product, shall include safety with respect to products comprised in that product and safety in the context of risks of damage to property, as well as in the context of risks of death or personal injury.

(1) In determining for the purposes of subsection (1) above what persons generally are entitled to expect in relation to a product all the circumstances shall be taken into account, including:

(2) In determining for the purposes of subsection (1) above what persons generally are entitled to expect in relation to a product all the circumstances shall be taken into account, including:

   (a) the manner in which, and purposes for which, the product has been marketed, its get-up, the use of any mark in relation to the product and any instructions for, or warnings with respect to, doing or refraining from doing anything with or in relation to the product;

   (b) what might reasonably be expected to be done with or in relation to the product; and

   (c) the time when the product was supplied by its producer to another; and nothing in this section shall require a defect to be inferred from the fact alone that the safety of a product which is supplied after that time is greater than the safety of the product in question.

4 (1) In any civil proceedings by virtue of this part against any person ('the person proceeded against') in respect of a defect in a product it shall be a defence for him to show:

   (a) that the defect is attributable to compliance with any requirement imposed by or under any enactment or with any Community obligation; or

   (b) that the person proceeded against did not at any time supply the product to another; or

   (c) that the following conditions are satisfied, that is to say:
      (i) that the only supply of the product to another by the person proceeded against was otherwise than in the course of a business of that person's; and
      (ii) that Section 2(2) above does not apply to that person or applies to him by virtue only of things done otherwise than with a view to profit; or

   (d) that the defect did not exist in the product at the relevant time; or

   (e) that the state of scientific and technical knowledge at the relevant time was not such that a producer of products of the same description as the product in question might be expected to have discovered the defect if it had existed in his products while they were under his control; or

   (f) that the defect
      (i) constituted a defect in a product ('the subsequent product') in which the product in question has been comprised; and
      (ii) was wholly attributable to the design of the subsequent product or to compliance by the producer of the product in question with instructions given by the producer of the subsequent product.

How does product liability affect the nurse?

Practical Dilemma 12.3 — Needle injury

A nurse is giving an injection to a patient when the needle snaps and she is injured.

Under the Consumer Protection Act 1987, the nurse would need to discover from the supplier of the needle in the NHS trust (probably the *central sterile services department* (CSSD)) the producer of that particular needle. The supplier has a duty under section 2(3) to inform her of the name of the producer who will then be strictly liable to the nurse for causing her harm. If the CSSD is unable to provide her with that information, the CSSD could itself be liable to her. The nurse herself would have to show that there was a defect in the needle, i.e. that the safety was not such as persons generally are entitled to expect. This is defined in section 3(2) as including the manner in which and purpose for which the product has been marketed, the instructions and warnings accompanying it and what might reasonably be expected to be done with or in relation to it at the time it was supplied. In addition, the nurse has a remedy under the Employer's Liability (Defective Equipment) Act 1969. The nurse should also ensure that an adverse notice about the needles is made to the Medicines and Healthcare Products Regulatory Agency. An EU Directive[36] led to the introduction of regulations relating to sharp instruments in healthcare which came into force on 11 May 2013.[37] These require healthcare employers and contractors to follow rules relating to the use and disposal of medical sharps including the duty to ensure that the use of medical sharps at work is avoided so far as is reasonably practicable. The regulations also cover information and training, arrangements in the event of an injury and notification of injuries.

In a Scottish case a driver was awarded £3500 following a needle stick injury sustained during waste collection. The employers were found to be in breach of the Personal Protective Equipment at Work Regulations 1992.[38]

Timing

There is a 10-year time limit from the date of the supply of the product. The individual plaintiff must bring the action within three years of suffering the harm or having knowledge of the relevant circumstances. The Supreme Court refused to allow the substitution of the parent company more than 10 years after the product was circulated in a case where it was argued that a defect in the vaccine had caused brain damage.[39]

Naming the producer

What if the NHS trust department that supplied the goods cannot name the producer? The person who suffered the harm must ask the supplier to identify the producer or importer of the product in the EU and must make that request within a reasonable period after the damage has occurred and at a time when it is not reasonably practicable for the person making the request to identify those persons. If the health department supplying the goods fails to comply within a reasonable period after receiving the request, then the claimant is entitled to recover damages from the supplying department. All departments in an NHS trust that supply products to persons who suffer damage from them could thus become liable: the supplies department, pharmacy, cleaning, catering, CSSD, office equipment, works and buildings.

The implications of this are that department records must be sufficiently comprehensive and clear to provide the appropriate information to the person injured by the defect, in order that the claim can be made against the actual producer of the product rather than the supplier.

The nurse as supplier

Could the nurse ever be a supplier? In the course of their duty, a nurse certainly supplies many products to patients, other staff, visitors and contractors: drugs, food/drink, equipment, syringes, etc. Could they be a supplier for the purposes of this Act?

Practical Dilemma 12.4 — Supplying defective products

The nurse gives a patient a high-protein food to take home with him, which is defective, e.g. it has glass in it, and the patient is injured.

In most similar circumstances, it will be clear to the person suffering harm who the producers or trademark user are and it will therefore be reasonably practicable for the person suffering harm to identify the potential defendant. In other cases, the nurse will have obtained the goods from another department in the hospital, which would become the supplier for the purposes of the Act.

Product Liability (Consumer Protection Act 1987) and the Employer's Liability (Defective Equipment) Act 1969

The right of the employee to claim from the employer under the 1969 Act is unaffected by the provisions of the 1987 Act. Clearly, any person who has been injured by a defective product can use whichever remedy is likely to be most successful and in fact can bring an action using several different causes of action. The relationship between these two Acts is as follows:

1. The injured employee can obtain compensation from the employer under the 1969 Act only if there has been negligence by a third party.
2. The injured employee can obtain compensation from the employer as supplier only if he has not identified the producer under the 1987 Act.
3. The 1987 Act covers all persons suffering damage, i.e. patients, employees, visitors, etc. The 1969 Act relates only to employees.
4. The 1987 Act covers damages in the form of personal injury, death, loss or damage to property; the 1969 Act covers only loss of life, impairment of a person's physical or mental condition and any disease, not loss or damage to property.
5. Fault need not be established under the 1987 Act – only a defect in the product. However, the defence of what is known at the time is available.

Defences

Certain defences are available under section 4, which are shown in Statute Box 12.10.

What damage must the claimant establish?

Compensation is payable for death, personal injury or any loss of or damage to any property (including land) (s. 5(1)). The loss or damage shall be regarded as having occurred at the earliest time at which a person with an interest in the property had knowledge of the material facts about the loss or damage (s. 5(5)). Knowledge is further defined in section 5(6) and (7).

There have been few examples of actions being brought under the Consumer Protection Act 1987 in healthcare cases and only a handful of cases brought under it have been reported. One reported in March 1993[40] led to Simon Garratt being awarded £1400 against the manufacturers of a pair of surgical scissors that broke during an operation on his knee, with the blade being left embedded. A second operation was required to remove it. Had he relied on the law of negligence to obtain compensation, he would have had to show that the manufacturers were in breach of the duty of care that they owed to him. Under the Consumer Protection Act 1987, he had to show the harm, the defect and the fact that it was produced by the defendant.

In a case in 2001,[41] it was held that a claim brought under the Consumer Protection Act 1987 in respect of the infection by patients with hepatitis C contracted from blood and blood products used in blood transfusions could succeed. This decision may well lead to greater use of the Consumer Protection Act 1987 if personal injuries are caused, since negligence does not have to be established under the Act, only that there was a defect in the product that has caused the harm.

The General Product Safety Regulations 1994 require producers and distributors to take steps to ensure that the products they supply are safe, that they provide consumers with relevant information and warnings, and that they keep themselves informed about risks. The Consumer Protection (Distance Selling) Regulations 2000 provide protection for the consumer where contracts are made on the internet, through digital TV, by mail order, by phone or fax.

Medicines and Healthcare Products Regulatory Agency (MHRA)

The MHRA was established in April 2003 as an executive agency of the Department of Health and took over the functions formerly carried out by the Medical Devices Agency (MDA) and the Medicines Control Agency. It can be accessed via its website.[42] This section looks at its role in medical devices. (Consideration of its role in medicines can be seen in chapter 27.)

Medical devices

The MDA (now superseded by the MHRA) was established to promote the safe and effective use of devices. In particular its role was to ensure that whenever a medical device is used, it is:

1. suitable for its intended purpose;
2. properly understood by the professional user; and
3. maintained in a safe and reliable condition.

What is a medical device? Annex B to Safety Notice 9801 gives examples of medical devices.[43] It covers the following.

1. Equipment used in the diagnosis or treatment of disease, and the monitoring of patients, e.g. syringes and needles, dressings, catheters, beds, mattresses and covers, physiotherapy equipment.
2. Equipment used in life support, e.g. ventilators, defibrillators.
3. *In vitro* diagnostic medical devices and their accessories, e.g. blood gas analysers. (Regulations came into force in 2000 on *in vitro* diagnostic devices.)
4. Equipment used in the care of disabled people, e.g. orthotic and prosthetic appliances, wheelchairs and special support seating, patient hoists, walking aids, pressure care prevention equipment.

5. Aids to daily living, e.g. commodes, hearing aids, urine drainage systems, domiciliary oxygen therapy systems, incontinence pads, prescribable footwear.
6. Equipment used by ambulance services (but not the vehicles themselves), e.g. stretchers and trolleys, resuscitators.
7. Other examples of medical devices, including: condoms, contact lenses and care products, intrauterine devices.

Regulations[44] require that from 14 June 1998 medical devices placed on the market (made available for use or distribution even if no charge is made) must conform to 'the essential requirements', including safety required by law and bear a CE marking as a sign of that conformity. Although most of the obligations contained in the Regulations fall on manufacturers, purchasers who are positioned further down the supply chain may also be liable – for example, for supplying equipment which does not bear a CE marking or which carries a marking liable to mislead people.[45]

The CE marking is the requirement of the EC Directive on medical devices.[46] The manufacturer that can demonstrate conformity with the regulations is entitled to apply the CE marking to a medical device.

The essential requirements include the general principle that:

> A device must not harm patients or users, and any risks must be outweighed by benefits. Design and construction must be inherently safe, and if there are residual risks, users must be informed about them. Devices must perform as claimed, and not fail due to the stresses of normal use. Transport and storage must not have adverse effects. Essential requirements also include prerequisites in relation to the design and construction, infection and microbial contamination, mechanical construction, measuring devices, exposure to radiation, built-in computer systems, electrical and electronic design, mechanical design, devices which deliver fluids to a patient, function of controls and indicators.

The Medical Devices Directives of the EU were consolidated in regulations in 2002[47] and amended in 2007.[48] Part II of the 2002 regulations sets out the requirements for general medical devices; Part III covers active implantable medical devices and Part IV covers *in vitro* diagnostic medical devices. The regulations were amended in 2003 to cover the reclassification of breast implants,[49] in 2007 to cover the reclassification of total hip, knee and shoulder joints[50] in 2008[51] and in 2012.[52] The regulations are available on the UK legislation website.[53]

Exceptions to the regulations include:

1. Devices made especially for the individual patient ('custom made'). (Guidance note No. 9 of the MHRA covers this.)
2. Devices made by the organisation ('legal entity') using them. (Bulletin 18 of the MHRA gives guidance on such items.)

Non-CE-marked medical devices undergoing clinical investigation are now covered by the 2002 regulations and require approval from the MHRA and guidance is provided on its website.

Following Brexit, the UK government intended to replace the CE mark and certification with a UK equivalent. However, in 2023 the UK Parliament passed regulation extending the validity of the CE mark in the UK until a revised regulatory framework can be introduced. This is unlikely to be until at least Medical devices – extended acceptance of CE marked medical devices on the Great Britain market – GOV.UK (www.gov.uk) 2025.

The MHRA (formerly the MDA) has powers under the Consumer Protection Act 1987 to issue warnings or remove devices from the market.

Devices are divided into three classes according to possible hazards, Class 2 being further subdivided. Thus Class 1 has a low risk, e.g. a bandage; Class 2a has a medium risk, e.g. simple breast pump; Class 2b has a medium risk, e.g. ventilator; Class 3 has a high risk, e.g. intra-aortic balloon.

Any warning about equipment issued by the MHRA should be acted on immediately. Notices from the Agency are sent to regional general managers, chief executives of health authorities and NHS trusts, directors of social services, managers of independent healthcare units and rehabilitation service managers. Failure to ensure that these notices are obtained and acted on could be used as evidence of failure to provide a reasonable standard of care. Guidance on the management of medical devices for use by hospitals and community-based organisations (including social services) was issued in 2006.[54] The topics covered include: monitoring/audit; reporting adverse incidents; acquiring the most appropriate device; acceptance procedures for newly delivered devices; maintenance and repair; training; adequacy of manufacturer instructions, disposal and legal liability. In February 2004 the MHRA issued a warning about equipment misuse. Doctors and nurses had carried out procedures with improvised equipment which had resulted in cases where two infants had died after a wooden tongue depressor was used as a splint, and led to an infection. In another case the wrong kind of cot sides were fitted to a bed, leading to the death of an elderly patient from asphyxiation.[55]

Adverse incident reporting procedures

The Device Bulletin issued in 2006 covers adverse incident reporting procedures. Minor faults or discrepancies should also be reported to the MHRA. The website home page of the MHRA gives advice on reporting methods which can be online, or by email, post, fax or telephone.[56]

In 2014 the MHRA and NHS England worked together to simplify adverse incident reporting. Further information on the patient safety alert on improving medical device incident reporting and learning can be found on the website.[57] The initiative also covers alerts about medication errors (see chapter 27).

Liaison officer

The MHRA recommends that each healthcare organisation should appoint a medical devices management group which should include the MHRA medical device liaison officer to ensure that adverse incident reporting and MHRA information and advice are implemented. Specialist subgroups may be needed to make recommendations to this group. The liaison officer should have the necessary authority to:

1. ensure that procedures are in place for the reporting of adverse incidents involving medical devices to the MHRA;
2. act as the point of receipt for MHRA publications;
3. ensure dissemination within their own organisation of MHRA publications; and
4. act as the contact point between the MHRA and their organisation.

Single-use items

Where a supplier has labelled its product 'single use', then the official advice is that it should not be reprocessed and reused unless the reprocessor is able to ensure the integrity and safety in use of each reprocessed item and there is clear evidence of the effectiveness of the reprocessing operation.[58]

A pushchair company, Maclaren, paid compensation to more than 40 British children who suffered injuries in their buggies, with payments of between £10,000 and £25,000 depending on the severity of the injury. Maclaren stated that the agreement to pay out compensation was not an admission of liability but that it took children's safety very seriously.[59]

Revised EU regulations for medical devices were issued in 2017 but have a three-year transition period and do not come fully into force until 2020.[60]

Control of Substances Hazardous to Health 2002

The Control of Substances Hazardous to Health (COSHH) Regulations 1988 came into effect in 1989 and were replaced by amended regulations in 1996. New regulations came into force in November 2002,[61] replacing the 1999 regulations in order to comply with the EC Chemical Agents Directive, which set more detailed rules of compliance. The HSE has set up a COSHH website to provide guidance for employers[62] and has provided a brief guide to the regulations.[63] This guide sets out the eight stages of a COSHH assessment, which are shown in Box 12.4.

The regulations aim to control activities where exposure to substances could lead to disease or ill health, i.e. substances that are toxic, harmful, corrosive or irritant; the regulations also cover those that have delayed effects or are hazardous in conjunction with other substances. The employer must assess the risks and take appropriate action, e.g. providing protective clothing, information and training of staff. All health workers have responsibilities under the regulations relating to the Control of Substances Hazardous to Health. The nurse who uses different substances in her work should be specifically alert to the need to ensure that the regulations are implemented. New maximum exposure limits have been introduced. Further details of the regulations and guidance can be obtained from the Health and Safety Executive or from the COSHH website.

There must be clarity over who has the responsibility of carrying out the assessment. The guidance emphasises the importance of involving all employees in the assessment.

All potentially hazardous substances must be identified: these will include domestic materials such as bleach, toilet cleaner, window cleaner and polishes; office materials such as correction fluids as well as the medicinal products in the treatment room and materials and substances used in nursing.

Box 12.4 Stages in COSHH assessment

1. Work out what hazardous substances are used in your workplace and find out the risks from using these substances to people's health.
2. Decide what precautions are needed before starting work with hazardous substances.
3. Prevent people being exposed to hazardous substances, but where this is not reasonably practicable, control the exposure.
4. Make sure control measures are used and maintained properly and that safety procedures are followed.
5. If required, monitor exposure of employees to hazardous substances.
6. Carry out health surveillance where your assessment has shown that this is necessary or where COSHH makes specific requirements.
7. If required, prepare plans and procedures to deal with accidents, incidents and emergencies.
8. Make sure employees are properly informed, trained and supervised.

An assessment has to be made as to whether each substance could be inhaled, swallowed, absorbed or introduced through the skin or injected into the body (such as by needle).

The effects of each route of entry or contact and the potential harm must then be identified.

There must then be an identification of the persons who could be exposed and how.

Once this assessment is complete, decisions must be made on the necessary measures to be taken to comply with the regulations and who should undertake the different tasks. In certain cases, health surveillance is required if there is a reasonable likelihood that the disease or ill effect associated with exposure will occur in the workplace concerned. Nurses should be particularly vigilant about any substances used in their activities, including cleaning fluids, and ensure that a risk assessment is undertaken and its results implemented.

Managers should ensure that the employees are given information, instruction and training.

Records should show the results of the assessment, what action has been taken and by whom, and regular monitoring and review of the situation.

Corporate manslaughter and corporate homicide

As a consequence of the Corporate Manslaughter and Corporate Homicide Act 2007 it is possible for an organisation to which the Act applies to be prosecuted in the case of a death under both Health and Safety legislation and the 2007 Act. The jury can be instructed to find the accused organisation guilty of both offences. An organisation can be found guilty of an offence under the 2007 Act only if the way in which its activities are managed or organised by its senior management is a substantial element in the breach of duty of care owed by the organisation. Senior management means the persons who play significant roles in (i) the making of decisions about how the whole or a substantial part of its activities are to be managed or organised, or (ii) the actual managing or organising of the whole or a substantial part of those activities.

Common law duties: employer's duty

Direct Duty of Care for Safety of the Employee

Duty of the employer as an implied term of the contract of employment

As was seen in chapter 10, some of the terms in the contract of employment are implied by the law. These include the obligation of the employer to safeguard the health and safety of the employee by employing competent staff, setting up a safe system of work and maintaining safe premises, equipment and plant. The employee must obey the reasonable instructions of the employer and take reasonable care in carrying out the work. Thus the employee may have a claim for breach of contract by the employer if she has been injured as a result of failures on the employer's part in not providing the appropriate training or equipment. The employer's duty at common law is set out in Box 12.5.

Box 12.5 Employer's direct duty of care

At common law, the employer has an implied term in the contract of employment to look after the safety of the employee:

1. to ensure the premises, plant and equipment are safe
2. to provide competent staff
3. to establish a safe system of work

The employer's duty at common law to take reasonable care to safeguard the employees against the reasonably foreseeable possibility of harm arising from work-related disorders is paralleled by the duties laid down in the Health and Safety at Work Act 1974 and under the regulations relating to Manual Handling, the Management of Health and Safety at Work, Display Screen Equipment and the other regulations discussed above. Where several employers are involved in causing harm to an employee the House of Lords ruled, in a case where employees alleged that asbestos had caused mesothelioma, that liability was several only, i.e. each defendant employer was only responsible for its own contribution to the claimant's injuries.[64] This led to the Compensation Act 2006 which states that liability in such circumstances is joint and several and the Act has retrospective effect.

Effect of Failures by the Employer

Failure by the employer to take reasonable care of the health, safety or welfare of the employee could result in the following actions by the employee:

1. Action for breach of contract of employment;
2. Action for negligence, where the employee has suffered harm; or
3. Application in the employment tribunal for constructive dismissal, if it can be shown that the employer is in fundamental breach of the contract of employment.

It was reported in July 2014 that a care assistant had been murdered by a patient at Wotton Lawn Hospital in Gloucester, an acute mental health unit. An inquiry into the role of the employing trust in the death of the care assistant by the Health and Safety Executive found no breaches of health and safety law. There was no evidence to link the trust's management systems to the death and no further action was taken.[65]

Examples of cases brought in relation to the employer's duty of care at common law are given in Cases 12.5 and 12.6, relating to stress and manual handling, respectively.

There is an overlap between the direct duty of care of the employer for the safety of the employee and the duty of the employer as occupier under the Occupiers' Liability Act 1957. Thus in a case where a nurse is injured as a result of defects in the NHS trust's premises, she may have a cause of action under the Occupiers' Liability Act and also because of breach of the employer's common law duty to care for the employee.

Statute 12.11
Employer's Liability (Compulsory Insurance) Act 1969

Every employer carrying on any business in Great Britain shall insure against liability for bodily injury or disease sustained by his employees and arising out of and in the course of their employment.

'Business' includes a trade or profession and includes any activity carried out by a body of persons, whether corporate or unincorporate. There is a penalty for failure to insure.

Insurance by the Employer

The Employer's Liability (Compulsory Insurance) Act 1969 obliges all non-Crown employers to be covered by an approved policy of insurance against liability for bodily injury or disease sustained by an employee and arising out of and in the course of employment. By section 60 of the NHS and Community Care Act 1990, health authorities ceased to enjoy Crown immunity. However, Schedule 8 of the Act preserves immunity from this Act for health authorities and NHS trusts. The employers of a nurse working in the private sector or a practice nurse working for general practitioners are, however, bound by the Act.

Defective Equipment

If an employee has been injured as the result of defective equipment, an additional remedy may be available under the Employer's Liability (Defective Equipment) Act 1969. This is set out in Statute Box 12.12. The Act is binding on the Crown and enables the employee to obtain compensation from the employer if the injury has been caused by defective equipment supplied by the employer where a third party is to blame. Instead of the employee having the cost and hassle of obtaining compensation from the third party, that burden falls on the employer, from whom the employee can obtain direct compensation. Now that civil liability for breach of the health and safety regulations has been abolished (see s. 69 Enterprise and Regulatory Reform Act 2013), the Employer's Liability (Defective Equipment) Act is likely to become more significant for the injured employee who has been injured by defective equipment.

Statute 12.12
Employer's Liability (Defective Equipment) Act 1969

Factors which must be present

1. Personal injury by employee in the course of employment
2. As a consequence of a defect in equipment
3. Equipment provided by his employer for purposes of his business
4. Defect attributable wholly or partly to the fault of a third party (whether identified or not)

Action

1. Recover compensation from employer
2. Contributory negligence by employee may be raised as a defence (either full or partial)
3. Employer can recover contribution from third party (in contract or negligence)

Applies to the Crown.

Practical Dilemma 12.5   Faulty bed

A nurse is injured when a recently supplied bed, which she is raising by the foot pedal, breaks and falls on to her leg. It is discovered that there was a defect in the bed mounting that should have been spotted by the manufacturers before it left the factory.

The nurse could claim compensation from the NHS trust under the provisions of the Employer's Liability (Defective Equipment) Act 1969. The costs, problems and time associated with suing the manufacturers would then fall on the shoulders of the NHS trust. She also has an additional remedy under the Consumer Protection Act 1987.

Remedies available to an injured employee

The laws relating to health and safety are significant to nursing practice. The nurse themself may suffer from injuries at work and also has a significant responsibility to protect the health and safety of others, including colleagues, patients and visitors. Back injuries are seen almost as an occupational hazard for nurses and midwives; publicity has recently been given to the number of staff who are injured by violence at work, including work in the community; the hazards that a nurse faces in administering carcinogenic substances such as cytotoxic drugs are only now being appreciated and precautions (such as protective clothing and masks) are being laid down. The nurse has always faced the problem of contamination from infectious diseases, and the particular problems relating to HIV and infectious diseases and the role of the Health Protection Agency are considered in chapter 25. In this section, the remedies available to the nurse for injuries at work will be considered. The remedies can be seen in Figure 12.1. The nurse may be able to sue several different defendants.

Injuries Caused by Another Employee

Where a nurse has been injured as a result of the negligence of another employee, they can either sue the employee for compensation or they could bring an action against the NHS trust under the principles of vicarious liability.

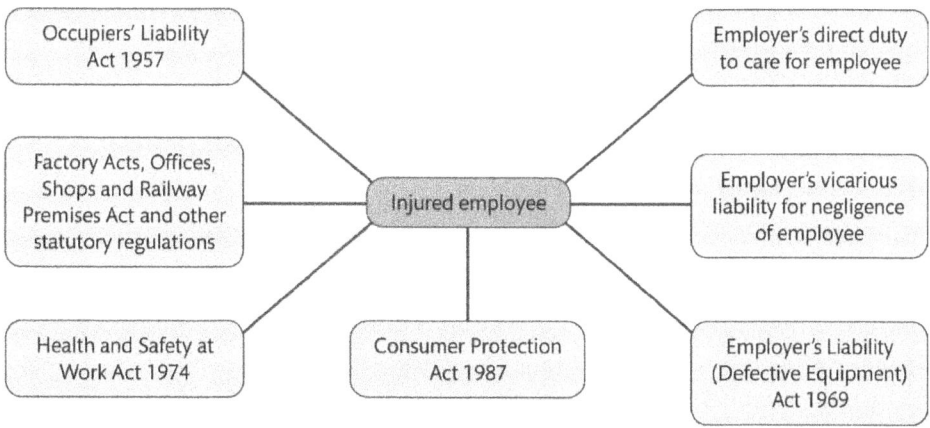

Figure 12.1   Remedies available to an injured employee

Practical Dilemma 12.6 — Wheelchair chaos

Two nurses, Mary and Jean, are working together in a ward for elderly mentally infirm patients. They are moving a patient from a chair into a wheelchair. As they do so, the wheelchair moves and Mary, in her endeavour to save the patient, takes the full weight and falls to the floor. She suffers a severe injury to her back and shoulder. An investigation reveals that Jean was responsible for ensuring that the wheelchair brake was safely on and her carelessness was responsible for Mary's injuries.

Mary can take one of the following paths:

1. She could sue Jean personally, since Jean is probably in breach of the duty of care she owes to Mary to ensure that reasonable steps are taken to prevent foreseeable harm to Mary. However, such an action is likely to be pointless unless Jean is insured for such liability or has sufficient funds to pay compensation to Mary.
2. She could sue the NHS trust for its vicarious liability for harm caused by the negligence of an employee. Jean is an employee, has been negligent and is acting in the course of employment. Mary would still have to establish that Jean was personally negligent, but this action has the advantage over suing Jean personally since the NHS trust should have the funds to pay compensation.
3. In addition, Mary could sue the NHS trust for breach of its duty of care to look after her safety as an employee. In this action, Mary would have to establish that the NHS trust itself was at fault, e.g. if it had failed to provide Jean with adequate training in carrying out such a manoeuvre.

In all three actions it will, of course, be a defence, complete or partial, that Mary was herself contributorily negligent (see chapter 6).

Liability of the Employer for Work Outside the Premises

In the following case, a health authority was held liable for failing to give adequate instruction to a young resident support worker.

Case 12.4 — *Fraser* v *Winchester HA* [1999]

Employer's liability for failing to give adequate instructions[66]

A resident support worker at a home for mentally and physically disabled residents was sent on a week's camping holiday with a patient without supervision or assistance. She had no training or instruction in the use of camping equipment. She suffered burns to her face and hands when, needing to cook an evening meal for the patient, she changed a cylinder on a gas cooker at the entrance to the tent and near to a lit candle. There was an explosion and the tent caught fire. The Court of Appeal agreed with the High Court finding that she should have been given instruction and better equipment, but held her one-third to blame because she realised the risk in what she did.

Special areas

Violence

Violence in the NHS against health service employees not just from strangers in the streets, but also from carers and clients, is an increasing phenomenon. Figures produced by the Department of Health in 2003[67] show that there was an estimated 116,000 violent incidents in the NHS (excluding general medical services), with 16 incidents per 1000 ambulance staff per month. The terms of service of general practitioners were changed to enable them to arrange for the removal from their list of any patient who threatened them with violence. Several assaults on staff have led to criminal prosecutions and inquiries. For example, in 1983,[68] a voluntary patient at a mental hospital was charged with assault occasioning actual bodily harm to an occupational therapist employed at the hospital. An occupational therapist was killed by a mentally ill patient in the Edith Morgan Unit at Torbay and an inquiry was set up.[69] A healthcare assistant was attacked in the grounds of a Bristol hospital,[70] in spite of the fact that there were security guards and improved lighting and closed circuit television as a result of a review four and a half years before. A young mental health worker, Ashleigh Ewing, was stabbed to death by a patient who had been discharged from psychiatric hospital. The patient was found guilty of manslaughter on the ground of diminished responsibility and ordered to be detained indefinitely in a secure unit. An Inquiry was set up by the North East Strategic Health Authority.[71] The charity Mental Health Matters was fined £30,000 for failing to protect Ashleigh Ewing, the support worker who had visited the patient unaccompanied. Of all hospital staff working for NHS trusts, midwives experience more harassment than any other professional group, including doctors, nurses and healthcare assistants.[72]

The Court of Appeal held in 2006 that the NHS trust had failed in its duty of care to six nursing staff who were assaulted by a patient in Rampton Hospital. The hospital had failed to carry out a risk assessment in accordance with the recommendations of the Tilt Report into Security in High Security Hospitals and as a consequence the staff were injured.[73]

Zero tolerance

In October 2000, the Department of Health announced new guidelines to tackle violence against NHS staff who are most at risk.[74] The guidelines cover risk assessment, crime prevention, protection of NHS staff in the community, techniques for dealing with abusive and potentially violent situations, training, reporting of incidents, the criminal justice system and support for victims.

The HSE has declared a zero tolerance policy on violence and assaults on staff in the NHS and set up a website[75] to provide information and advice. Guidance has been issued for managers in reducing violence to NHS staff. The RCN and NHS Executive have also published guidance on reducing the risks from violence and aggression in the community.[76] The Crime and Disorder Act 1998 established local crime and disorder reduction partnerships (CDRPs), led jointly by police and local authorities. They have a statutory responsibility to develop and implement a strategy to tackle crime and disorder in their area in consultation with health, education and the voluntary and private sectors. The 1998 Act was amended by the Police Reform Act 2002 to extend responsibility for implementing the strategy to the fire and police authorities and included PCTs in the partnerships. In spite of the efforts, the National Audit Office[77] reported in March 2003 that reports of violence against NHS staff had risen by 13 per cent over two years, with many incidents not being reported. The Secretary of State for Health therefore announced[78] the establishment of a new legal protection unit within the Department of Health to support private legal action against the attackers.

The NHS Security Management Service was established in April 2003 to take responsibility for all security management issues in the NHS, including violence to staff. It published a strategy placing violence against staff as a top priority and established mandatory reporting of incidents of violence. It is now incorporated into the NHS Counter Fraud and Security Management Service Division of the NHS Business Services Authority and has developed a programme of work from the Zero Tolerance Campaign.[79] In Wales the Welsh Assembly government has launched the All Wales NHS Violence and Aggression Training Passport and Information Scheme, and in Scotland the Scottish Executive is coordinating a Zero Tolerance Campaign. In September 2007 funding of £97 million was announced for further protection of NHS staff from violence: £29 million of this sum was to be used for safety alarms for lone workers and the remainder for training, additional local security management specialists, more prosecutions and a centralised reporting system to the NHS Security Management Service.[80] The Security Incident Reporting System allows NHS health bodies to report security incidents to NHS Protect. Its remit is to identify and tackle crime across the health service. The collected data assists NHS organisations to work to prevent further occurrences.[81] NHS Protect also hosts a safe and secure health facilities website to provide an information service on security.[82] Reference can also be made to a practical guide on dealing with violence in the NHS, by Paul Linsley.[83]

Remedies following violence

If a nurse has suffered harm as a consequence of violence, the remedies shown in Box 12.6 are available to her.

Box 12.6   Remedies following violence

1. Sue the aggressor personally for trespass to the person. (There is little point if they have no assets or income to pay the damages awarded.)
2. Sue the employer if she can establish that there has been a breach of the employer's duty of care to her.
3. Obtain compensation from the criminal courts following a successful prosecution of the assailant.
4. Claim compensation from the Criminal Injuries Compensation Authority.
5. The nurse could receive, if eligible, statutory sick pay, Whitley Council sickness pay and DSS benefits.

Practical Dilemma 12.7   Injuries in the A&E department

A patient with lacerations to the face and severe bruising is brought into the department by two friends. All three have been drinking heavily. Two nurses take the injured man into the treatment room and ask the others to stay in the waiting room or leave the hospital. They insist on following the patient and in the ensuing fracas a nurse is injured.

Suing the patient

Could the nurse sue the patient if she has been injured by an assault? Yes, the nurse would have a right of action against anyone who assaults her, but there are difficulties where the defendant is mentally disordered. The magistrates' courts have thrown out such cases as being inappropriate. If the defendant is prosecuted, then the magistrate or judge can make an order for compensation to be paid by the defendant to the injured person. If the nurse decides to bring civil proceedings for trespass to the person, the defendant may not have the resources to pay any compensation awarded by the civil courts. Alternatively (and probably preferably), the nurse could seek compensation from the Criminal Injuries Compensation Authority.

Suing the NHS trust or employer

The employer's duty extends to protecting the employee against reasonably foreseeable attacks from violent patients or even from violent visitors and trespassers. If the employer has failed in this duty, then the injured employee could sue the employer.

Practical Dilemma 12.8 — Mixed ward

A mental health nurse is on an acute mixed ward. Complaints have been made that, although this is a mixed ward, there are insufficient numbers of male nurses and thus the female nurses are often dealing with male patients on their own. A known aggressive male patient, without any warning or provocation, suddenly produces a razor and cuts a nurse badly on the face.

To obtain compensation from the NHS trust, the nurse must establish that another employee has been negligent in the course of employment and therefore the NHS trust is vicariously liable or that the NHS trust was itself directly at fault. To establish this, she would need to show that inadequate precautions were taken for her safety; that the risk of harm was reasonably foreseeable; that there were reasonable precautions that the authority could have taken and failed to take, e.g. male staffing, training in the handling of violent patients, special facilities for dealing with known aggressive patients, a special wing, an alarm system, a safe system for control of dangerous items. The injured nurse would also have to show a causal connection between the injuries she suffered and these failures on the authority's part, i.e. if she would still have been injured even had these precautions been taken, then the NHS trust would not be liable. In its defence, the NHS trust would have to establish either that such reasonable precautions had been provided — a dispute on the facts — or that even if such precautions had been taken, the injury would still have occurred. In addition, it might be able to show that the nurse failed to take reasonable care of her own safety, i.e. she was contributorily negligent. Some employers have argued that being injured by aggressive mentally ill patients is an occupational hazard for the nurse working with the mentally ill or handicapped and that there is a voluntary assumption of the risk of injury by the staff concerned (see chapter 6). However, it is not thought that this would provide a successful defence for an employer who was clearly at fault in respect of reasonable precautions in protecting the nurse from harm.

Criminal prosecution

Any aggression should be reported to the police and the Crown Prosecution Service will decide whether a public prosecution should commence. If the defendant is convicted, the magistrates or judge could make an order that criminal compensation is paid to the victim. There is evidence that public prosecutions for assault on NHS staff are increasing. In its response to the Healthcare Commission's NHS staff survey on violence and abuse against NHS staff by patients and relatives, the NHS Security Management Service stated that there had been a 1600 per cent increase in the number of prosecutions brought against those who assaulted NHS staff. If the assault has been notified to the police, the victim would be able to obtain compensation from the Criminal Injuries Compensation Authority, which is considered in chapter 2.

Self-defence

Can the nurse defend herself if attacked by a patient, visitor, trespasser or employee? Every citizen has the right of self-defence. In the above example, therefore, the nurse could use reasonable means to defend herself against an aggressor. What is meant by reasonable?

Practical Dilemma 12.9 Reasonable means

A nurse is faced by a patient who is approaching her with a knife. He is 6 feet tall, a stockily built man of 35 years. There are no other staff or competent patients in the room and there is no call system available. As he comes forward, she picks up a chair and hits him over the head with it. He is severely concussed and requires stitches. Could she successfully defend an action for assault brought by the patient? Has she acted reasonably in defending herself?

Reasonableness means, first, that the force used should be no more than is necessary to accomplish the object for which it is allowed (so retaliation, revenge and punishment are not permitted) and, second, the reaction must be in proportion to the harm that is threatened. Thus, all the circumstances must be taken into account: the contrast between the strength, size and expertise of the assailant and the defendant, and the type of harm with which the person is being threatened. Obviously, the greater the severity of the threatened danger, the more reasonable it is to take tougher measures. In assessing the reasonableness of the defence, account is taken of the fact that the defendant may have only a brief period to make up his mind what to do. Turning back to Practical Dilemma 12.9, if the nurse in question is tiny with no training in self-defence, the odds do seem to be stacked against her and may justify her use of the chair. All the circumstances must be taken into account, including the possibility of her retreating from the assault. Should the nurse be prosecuted and a trial take place in the Crown Court, it is for the jury to decide if the measures used in self-defence were reasonable in all the circumstances. The issue of violence and the community health worker is discussed in chapter 22.

Risk assessment

Monitoring of potentially violent situations is essential and the nurse should play her full part to bring any concerns to the attention of the management and ensure that action is taken. The employer has a duty to take reasonable care of the nurse in relation to reasonably foreseeable violence. A risk assessment could include the following questions.

1. *Is it possible to remove the risk altogether?* If the answer to this is 'yes' but, for example, only by stopping all home visits by nurses, this would not be reasonably practicable.
2. *What preventive action or protective measures can be taken?* The answer to this might include the provision of two-way radios, personal alarms or, in very dangerous areas or on visits to

clients who present a threat, nurses going in pairs or accompanied by another person. In the institutional setting, protective measures may include more staffing, higher levels of supervision of difficult-to-manage patients and special security measures.

3. *Has the nature of the risk changed?* (e.g. is the district more violent than it was formerly assessed to be? Has the nature and condition of patients in a hospital ward deteriorated?) Assess the extent of the success of the measures taken to prevent harm to nurses. Are any further measures necessary?

This type of analysis will not only relate to the nurses, but also to a wider assessment of all health professionals into which the nurse could have an input.

Practical Dilemma 12.10   Fear of violence

A nurse visited a patient in his home following a stroke. She felt threatened by his attitude, but found difficulty in defining exactly the reason for her fears. Should she record her concerns?

This is a situation with which many nurses could identify. There is almost an intuitive feeling of fear. However, the nurse would have a duty to ensure that her colleagues were warned of potential dangers and she might therefore record in her notes that it might be advisable for a second person to accompany the nurse for the next house call. The duty of confidentiality owed to the patient (see chapter 8) would be subject to an exception in the public interest where a nurse needed to warn colleagues about a fear of violence from a particular patient. Reference should be made to the guidance prepared by the Health and Safety Commission.[84] This gives practical advice for reducing the risk of violence in a variety of settings and emphasises the importance of commitment from the highest levels of management.

Domestic violence

It may sometimes come to the attention of nurses and particularly midwives that patients are possibly being subjected to violence at home. Clearly, if this involves a child, it is essential to ensure that child protection procedures are initiated and these are considered in chapter 13. Where it is an adult who is the victim, the tendency in the past has been to respect the confidentiality of the victim and leave it to that person to report it to the police. However, attitudes are changing and domestic violence is no longer seen as a private matter between individuals but a criminal act where society has responsibilities.[85] In June 2003 the Home Office issued a consultation paper[86] on ways to prevent and follow up domestic violence. The paper looked at three elements: prevention, protection and justice and support for victims. The Domestic Violence, Crime and Victims Act 2004 followed and was aimed at facilitating prosecutions and convictions. It made breach of a non-molestation order a criminal offence, created a new offence of causing or allowing the death of a child or vulnerable adult (extended in 2012 to causing or allowing serious physical harm (equivalent to grievous bodily harm) to a child or vulnerable adult).[87] The 2004 Act also defined a common assault as an arrestable offence for the purposes of the Police and Criminal Evidence Act 1984, thereby increasing the powers of the police and citizens in relation to such an offence. Provisions under Part 3 of the Act relating to victims required a Victim's Code of Practice to be issued by the Secretary of State to cover the services to be provided to a victim of criminal conduct. Failure to comply with the Code, although not an offence in itself, could be used in evidence in civil and criminal proceedings.[88] A revised code of practice for victims of violence came into operation on 10 December 2013.[89] It can be accessed online.[90]

In January 2011 the European Commission on Domestic Violence funded a two-year project called the Iceberg Project, which together with other projects known as Daphne, sought to contribute to the protection of children, young people and women from all forms of violence. The role of Coventry University in this project and its literature review is described by Susan Lees and colleagues.[91]

The Domestic Violence Disclosure Scheme is to be implemented following regional trials. Dubbed Clare's law (after Clare Wood was murdered by her boyfriend) her father campaigned for women to be able to ask the police if a man has a history of abuse. The scheme gives a 'Right to ask' to the family and a 'Right to know' to the police to give information. Critics of the scheme suggest that the money would be better spent on improving the basic police response to victims of domestic violence.[92]

A report by the HM Inspectorate of Constabulary commissioned by the Home Secretary stated that thousands of people are at risk of harm or even murder because of widespread police failure in England and Wales to tackle domestic abuse. Only 8 out of 43 forces were responding well to domestic abuse. The Home Secretary responded by saying that she expected the forces to implement the recommendations and she was establishing a new national oversight group which she would chair.[93]

(See chapter 18 for a discussion on elder abuse.)

Stress

Concern with stress at work is now recognised as part of the employer's duty in taking reasonable care of the health and safety of the employee. One of the first cases to recognise stress as a ground for compensation is shown in Case 12.5.

Case 12.5 *Walker v Northumberland County Council* [1994]

Stress at work[94]

A social worker obtained compensation when his employer failed to provide the necessary support in a stressful work situation when he returned to work following an earlier absence due to stress. The employer was not liable for the initial absence, but that put the employer on notice that the employee was vulnerable and its failure to provide the assistance he needed was a breach of its duty to provide reasonable care for his health and safety as required to do under the contract of employment.

In order to establish grounds for compensation for stress induced by work, an employee would have to show:

1. that he or she was under an unacceptable level of stress at work;
2. that the employer was aware of this situation;
3. that there was reasonable action that the employer could have taken to relieve this pressure;

4. that the employer failed to take that action; and
5. that as a result the employee has suffered a serious mental condition.

The Court of Appeal has clarified the law relating to compensation for stress at work in four appeals which were heard together.[95] In each one the employer appealed against a finding of liability for an employee's psychiatric illness caused by stress at work. Two of the claimants were teachers in public sector comprehensive schools, the third an administrative assistant at a local authority training centre and the fourth a raw material operative in a factory.

In determining whether the employer was liable or not, the Court of Appeal held that the ordinary principles of employer's liability applied to an allegation of psychiatric illness caused by stress at work. The threshold question was whether the particular kind of harm – an injury to health (as distinct to occupational health) that was attributable to stress at work (as distinct from other factors) – to the employee was reasonably foreseeable. Foreseeability depended on what the employer knew or ought reasonably to have known about the individual employee. Because of the nature of mental disorder, it was harder to foresee than physical injury, but might be easier to foresee in a known individual than in the population at large. An employer was usually entitled to assume that the employee could withstand the normal pressures of his job unless he knew of some particular problem or vulnerability. The test was the same whatever the employment: there were no occupations that should be regarded as intrinsically dangerous to mental health.

The relevant factors identified by the Court of Appeal in determining the reasonable foreseeability of stress were:

- nature and extent of the work done by the employee; and
- signs from the employee of impending harm to his health.

The employer was entitled to take at face value what he was told by an employee; he did not have to make searching enquiries of the employee or seek to make further enquiries of the employee's medical advisers. If there were indications of impending harm to health arising from stress at work and these indications were plain enough for any reasonable employer to realise that he should do something about it, the duty of the employer to take steps would be triggered. The employer could only be in breach of duty if he failed to take the steps which were reasonable in the circumstances, bearing in mind the magnitude of the risk of harm occurring, the gravity of the harm which might occur, the costs and practicability of preventing it and the justifications for running the risk.

The factors to be taken into account in determining what was reasonable action by the employer included:

- the size and scope of the employer's operation, its resources, and the demands it faced;
- the interests of other employees; and
- the need to treat other employees fairly (for example, in any redistribution of duties).

An employer could be reasonably expected to take steps which were likely to do some good, and the court was likely to need expert evidence on that. An employer who offered a confidential advice service, with referral to appropriate counselling or treatment services, was unlikely to be found in breach of duty. If the only reasonable and effective step would have been to dismiss or demote the employee, the employer would not be in breach of duty in allowing a willing employee to continue in the job. In all cases, therefore, it was necessary to identify the steps that the employer both could and should have taken before finding him in breach of his duty of care. The claimant had to show that the breach of duty had caused or materially contributed to the harm suffered. It was not enough to show that the occupational stress had caused the harm. Where the harm suffered had more than one cause, the employer should only pay for that proportion of the harm suffered that was attributable to his wrongdoing, unless the harm was truly indivisible. It was for the defendant to raise the question of apportionment. The assessment of damages would take account of any pre-existing disorder or vulnerability and of the chance that the claimant would have succumbed to a stress-related disorder in any event.

On the actual facts of the appeals before it, the Court of Appeal allowed the appeals by the employers in three cases and dismissed the appeal in the case of *Jones* v *Sandwell Metropolitan Borough Council*.

Subsequently, the House of Lords (in a majority decision) allowed an appeal from one of the employees,[96] holding on the facts of the case that the school's senior management team should have taken the initiative in making sympathetic enquiries about Mr Barber, head of the maths department, when he returned to work in June 1996 and in making some reduction in his workload to ease his return. In addition, his condition should have been monitored and, had it not improved, some more drastic action would have had to be taken.

In a subsequent case it was held that the mere fact that the employers had provided counselling services did not relieve them of the duty to take reasonable care of an employee who was being subjected to considerable stress because of overwork and a lack of clear management controls. The Court of Appeal dismissed the employer's appeal against the finding of a breach of the duty of care and the award of £134,000.[97]

A university head of department, who claimed that he was subject to deliberate harassment by the university and that his psychiatric illness was stress-induced, failed in his claim because the judge held that the evidence did not support the contention that he was the victim of organised and deliberate harassment and that the risk of injury was not foreseeable until May 1997, when his symptoms became evident and the university had not failed to take reasonable steps to address the situation. He lost his appeal to the Court of Appeal.[98]

A Court of Appeal decision[99] dismissed an employer's appeal against a finding that it had breached its duty of care to the employee. The Court of Appeal held that the judge had been right to find that the Post Office owed a duty of care to Young, given its knowledge that Young's psychiatric problems were work-related. The Post Office's failure to fully implement the agreed measures for Young's return to work were sufficiently serious to amount to a breach of that duty. Young was known to the Post Office to be both vulnerable, which meant that extra care should have been taken of him, and conscientious, which meant that he was likely to try to carry out his work without complaint. No finding of contributory negligence was therefore appropriate.

Nicola Adedeji, a mother of two, who miscarried while under stress after her employer refused her flexitime working, won her case against the City of London Corporation, owner of the Barbican Centre. Her compensation, which has not been reported, is likely to have exceeded £100,000 for sex discrimination and unfair dismissal.[100]

The Health and Safety Inspectorate issued its first enforcement notice for failure to protect staff from stress in August 2003 against the West Dorset Hospitals NHS Trust.[101] Failure to observe the enforcement notice would lead to prosecution. The trust was given six months to assess stress levels among its 1100 staff and introduce a new programme.

Stress reduction is one of eight key targets set by the HSE, which has set up a stress website[102] covering the reasons why stress must be tackled, management standards and good practice. It has also provided a guide on improving efficiency which shows how tackling stress at work can improve an organisation's efficiency and gives examples in case studies, many from the NHS where stress levels have been reduced. Guidance is also provided on managing stress by the RCN for employees[103] and employers[104] and for its shop stewards.[105] The latter guidance takes RCN representatives through the HSE's management standards and the process of conducting a stress risk assessment and details how RCN safety representatives can get involved in each stage of the risk assessment process. It includes a number of case studies highlighting how representatives have implemented the HSE standards in their own workplaces. It also provides guidance for assisting staff who have returned to work after stress-related absence.

NICE published guidelines on workplace well-being in 2009.[106] The guidelines were endorsed by MIND, encouraging employers to follow the guidelines and reduce workplace stress. The guidance of NICE aimed to help reduce the estimated 13.7 million working days lost each year due to work-related mental health conditions, including stress, depression and anxiety which were currently estimated to cost UK employers around £28.3 billion per year at current pay levels.

Manual Handling

Where a nurse has injured their back at work, they may have a claim against their employer for breach of the duty of care owed to them at common law or failure to implement the Manual Handling Regulations. In addition, the employer may be vicariously liable for harm caused by another employee. Alternatively, if their back has been injured as a result of a defect in a product (e.g. a hoist or bed), they may be able to bring a case against the supplier under the Consumer Protection Act 1987. This section will first consider the regulations relating to manual handling, the decided cases and then consider specific situations that cause concern to the nurse.

Case 12.6 *Boag v Hounslow [1994]*

Back injury[107]

On 24 July 1994 a nurse was awarded £205,000 for a back injury. The circumstances were that in November 1988, she and a colleague were trying to lift an elderly woman from a commode to a chair, when the patient's legs gave way. Owing to the lack of space, Mrs Boag was forced to twist her back to place the woman in the chair. The health authority, which admitted liability, agreed the out-of-court settlement shortly before the case was due to be heard. She was forced to give up her job and is regularly confined to bed. She attended a pain relief clinic and will probably never work again. Her husband had to take time off work to help with the two children.

Manual Handling Regulations

Regulations were introduced in 1992 as a result of an EC Directive and were amended in 2002.[108] The RCN and the National Back Pain Association, in their 'Guide to the Handling of Patients',[109] point out that there are discrepancies between the EC Framework Directive[110] and the UK regulations and that the former imposes a higher duty on employers closer to that of 'practicality' rather than 'reasonable practicability'. The regulations were amended in 2002 to add another paragraph on determining the appropriate steps to reduce the risk of injury.[111] The risk assessment must take into account that a worker may be at risk if he or she: is physically unsuited to carry out the task; is wearing unsuitable clothing, footwear or other personal effects; or does not have adequate or appropriate knowledge or training. Guidance on manual handling is given by the HSE.[112] The guidelines are not themselves the law and the booklet advises that the guidelines set out in Appendix 1 'should not be regarded as precise recommendations. They should be applied with caution. Where doubt remains a more detailed assessment should be made.' A short guide is provided by the HSE which can be downloaded from its website.[113]

The HSE has developed a manual handling assessment chart tool which can be downloaded from its website.[114] The HSE has also published case studies on how simple action can be taken to prevent back injuries. For example, the provision of bed rails enabled the best use of a patient's arm strength when being washed in bed.[115] It has also published in 2012 a brief guide for smaller organisations on manual handling at work. The RCN has also published guidance on manual handling in a variety of settings.[116]

Summary of manual handling regulations

The duty placed on the employer under the regulations can be summed up as follows.

1. If reasonably practicable, avoid the hazardous manual handling.
2. Make a suitable and sufficient assessment of any hazardous manual handling that cannot be reasonably avoided.
3. Reduce the risk of injury from this handling so far as is reasonably practicable.
4. Give general indications of risk and precise information on the weight of each load and the heaviest side of any load, where the centre of gravity is not positioned centrally.
5. Review the assessment if there are any changes in the circumstances.

It is in the interests of all nurses to ensure that the employer is reminded when a review becomes necessary under the above provisions.

The duty that is owed by the employer is owed not only to employees, but also to temporary staff such as agency or bank staff who are called in to assist. All such employees are entitled to be included in the risk assessment process, since, as has been seen, the assessment must take into account the individual characteristics of each employee. Nurses who are unusually small in height or not so strong as the average might require special provisions in relation to manual handling.

Provision and Use of Work Equipment Regulations 1998 (PUWER)

PUWER (as amended by 2002 regulations) replaces the earlier Provision and Use of Work Equipment Regulations 1992 and applies to all equipment, including lifting equipment, used at work. There is a new requirement to inspect work equipment where significant risk could result from incorrect installation or relocation, deterioration or as a result of exceptional circumstances and to record the results of those inspections (Reg. 6). PUWER places requirements on duty holders to provide suitable work equipment for the task (Reg. 4), information and instructions (Reg. 8), and training to people who use it (Reg. 9). It also requires measures to be taken concerning dangerous parts of machinery (Reg. 11), controls and control systems (Regs 14–18), stability (Reg. 20) and mobility (Regs 25–9). The House of Lords held that there had been a breach of Regs 4(1) and 20 of the 1998 PUWER Regulations when a ladder to a bunk in a production platform was not fixed and had not been replaced properly so that a worker fell when descending from the top bunk. The incident was a foreseeable situation.[117]

Lifting Operations and Lifting Equipment Regulations 1998 (LOLER)

These regulations came into force on 5 December 1998 and apply in all premises and work situations subject to the Health and Safety at Work Act 1974 and build on the requirements of the Provision and Use of Work Equipment Regulations 1998.

In its guidance on the application of the LOLER regulations, the Health and Safety Commission note that (paragraph 47):

> As hoists are used to lift patients, e.g. from beds and baths, in hospitals and residential homes, are provided for use at work and are lifting equipment to which LOLER applies, the duty holder, e.g. the NHS trust running the hospital or the owner of the residential home, must satisfy their duties under LOLER.

Enforcement of regulations on manual handling

What action can be taken if the employer ignores these regulations? The regulations are part of the health and safety provisions that form part of the criminal law. Infringement of the regulations can lead to prosecution by the Health and Safety Inspectorate. The Inspectorate has the power to issue enforcement or prohibition notices against any corporate body or individual.

Court decisions on manual handling

Carrying a microwave The Court of Appeal found in favour of an employee who had injured his back while carrying a microwave weighing between 15 and 20 kg.[118] The Court of Appeal found that:

- the employers had failed to assess the specific risk in relation to the particular task to be performed by the employee and was therefore in breach of the Manual Handling Regulations (Reg. 4(1)(b)(ii));
- the employers had failed to take appropriate steps to reduce the risk by failing to give the training recognised as being necessary to increase awareness of the risk and reduce instinctive responses;
- it was reasonably foreseeable that an employee would twist while supporting a lead; and
- failure to provide the appropriate training was therefore, on the balance of probabilities, a cause of the accident.

Carrying by ambulance crew The microwave case contrasts with another decision of the Court of Appeal in another manual handling case[119] where the Court held that the employers were not in breach of the directive or regulations on manual handling. King, an ambulance technician, suffered serious injuries carrying an elderly patient down the stairway of his home. He and his colleague had taken the patient down the stairway, which was narrow and steep, in a carry chair. He had been injured when forced for a brief moment to bear the full weight of the chair. The judge found in favour of the ambulance technician, holding that the employers were in breach of EC Directive 90/269 (Article 3(2)) and the Manual Handling Regulations and that the employers had acted negligently by discouraging employees in circumstances such as those in this particular case from calling the fire service to take patients from their homes.

Sussex Ambulance NHS Trust appealed against the finding. The Court of Appeal held that the NHS trust was not liable either under the Directive or under the Manual Handling Regulations. There was nothing to suggest that calling the fire service would have been appropriate in the case. The evidence showed that such an option was rarely used because it had to be carefully planned, took a long time and caused distress to the patient. There might be cases where calling the fire service would be appropriate, but that would depend on the seriousness of the problem, the urgency of the case and the actual or likely response of the patient or his/her carers and the fire service. King had failed to show that, given that possibility, more emphasis in training would have avoided his injuries. The ambulance service owed the same duty of care to its employees as did any other employer. However, the question of what was reasonable for it to do might have to be judged in the light of its duties to the public and the resources available to it when performing those duties. While the risks to King had not been negligible, the task that he had been carrying out was of considerable social utility.

Furthermore, Sussex Ambulance NHS Trust had limited resources so far as equipment was concerned. There was no evidence of any steps that the trust could have taken to prevent the risk and the only suggestion made was that it should have called on a third party to perform the task for it. Since calling the fire service was not appropriate or reasonably practicable for the purpose of the directive and the regulations, the Sussex Ambulance NHS Trust had not shown a lack of reasonable care. Accordingly, it had not acted negligently.

Newham General Hospital In contrast to the ambulance case, a nurse aged 36 years was awarded £420,000 in damages by the High Court for a crippling back injury caused by her lifting a patient at Newham General Hospital, East London.[120]

East Sussex case and human rights and manual handling In February 2003 the High Court gave judgment on a case, where the claimants raised the issue of their human rights not to be hoisted.[121] A and B were sisters born in 1976 and 1980 who suffered from profound physical and learning disabilities. They lived in the family home which had been specially adapted and equipped for them and were looked after on a full-time basis by their mother X and their stepfather Y. A dispute arose between the claimants and East Sussex County Council (ESCC), which provided community care services, over the extent to which moving and lifting should be done manually. ESCC's policy on manual handling did not permit care staff to lift A or B manually. The claimants, supported by the Disability Rights Commission, argued that ESCC's manual handling policies, as applied to A and B, were unlawful and unjustifiable, on the basis that they improperly failed to take into account the needs of the disabled people involved. Its policy was subsequently amended to make it clear that ESCC did not operate a blanket no lifting policy. The claimants argued that the application of the policy to the specific circumstances of A and B's care and the draft protocols prepared by the independent handling adviser were unlawful.

The judge considered the effect of sections 2 and 3 of the Health and Safety at Work Act 1974, the Manual Handling Operations Regulations 1992 and the Management of Health and Safety at Work Regulations 1999; decided cases on manual handling and the implications of the European Convention on Human Rights and the Charter of Fundamental Rights of the European Union. He emphasised that one must guard against jumping too readily to the conclusion that manual handling is necessarily more dignified than the use of equipment. Hoisting is not inherently undignified, let alone inherently inhuman or degrading. He identified the principles that applied and stated that, ultimately, the employer must balance the impact of the assessment on both carer and the disabled person.

This balancing exercise is to be resolved in the context of Article 8 by enquiring of each claimant whether the interference with his right to be respected is such as to be 'necessary in a democratic society'. Once the balance has been struck, if it comes down in favour of manual handling, then the employer must make the appropriate assessment and take all appropriate steps to minimise the risks that exist. The assessment must be properly documented and lead to clear protocols which cover all situations, including foreseeable emergencies and, in the case of patients such as A and B, events such as episodes of spasm and distress that might arise. The judge accepted that protocols developed by the employer cannot be too prescriptive. He emphasised that it was for ESCC to formulate its manual handling policy and to make the appropriate assessment in relation to A and B. Neither of those is a matter for the court. The making and drafting of the kind of assessments called for in a case such as this is outside the competence and expertise of the court. What the court can and should do is to assist ESCC by identifying the relevant legal principles.

The outcome of the case was that ESCC was required to complete with the assistance of the independent manual handling adviser the appropriate assessments and protocols. If these were not acceptable to the claimants, they could challenge them by way of judicial review.

Wolstenholme case In a case in Milton Keynes where Lorraine Wolstenholme, a disabled woman of 50, had slept in a wheelchair for 17 months after nurses stopped lifting her in case they were injured, a High Court judge ordered that arrangements for moving her had to be made by a specific date (19 December 2003).[122]

What remedies exist for compensation?

Section 47 of the Health and Safety at Work Act 1974 prevents breach of a duty under sections 2–8 of the Act being used as the basis for a claim in the civil courts. Breach of the regulations can no longer be the basis of a civil claim for compensation, as a consequence of section 69 of the Enterprise and Regulatory Reform Act 2013 unless the Regulations provide to the contrary. Regulations provide an exception for new or expectant mothers in respect of their rights under the Pregnant Workers Directive.[123] A nurse who suffered harm as a result of the failure of the employer to take reasonable steps to safeguard her health and safety could sue in the civil courts on the basis of the employer's duty at common law i.e. negligence by the employer would have to be shown, which is likely to be more difficult to prove than a breach of the regulations. The statutory duty to ensure the Act is implemented is paralleled by a duty at common law placed on the employer to take reasonable steps to ensure the employee's health and safety. Contracts of employment should state clearly the duty on the employer to take reasonable care of the employee's safety and also the employee's duty to cooperate with the employer in carrying out health and safety duties under the Act and at common law. It is, of course, in the long-term interest of the employer to prevent back injuries, thereby avoiding payment of substantial compensation to his injured employees and also reducing the incidence of sickness and absenteeism.

Training in risk management and manual handling

This is essential to ensure that staff have the understanding to carry out the assessments and to advise on lifting and the appropriate equipment. Regular monitoring should take place to ensure that the training is effective and the policies for review are in place. There is also a duty on the employer to ensure that staff who are not expected to be regularly involved in manual handling are aware of the risks of so doing. This was the decision in the case of *Colclough* v *Staffordshire County Council*,[124] where a social worker obtained compensation following a back injury caused by moving a client to safety. The council was liable because it failed to provide any training on risk awareness of the dangers of that situation. The implication of this decision is that even staff who are not expected to be involved in manual handling as part of their work, must be trained in risk awareness to protect them, should they ever be in the situation where they could be endangered through manual handling.

Lifting and instructing others

Nurses may be asked to instruct others such as carers, clients or other health or social service employees in the carrying out of the regulations on manual handling. Before they instruct others, they should be sure that they receive the necessary additional training to undertake the task of instruction, since failure to instruct competently could in itself give rise to an action in negligence, should harm occur as a result of negligent instructions.

Failures to instruct by agencies

Sometimes nurses become aware that agency staff have not been instructed in manual handling techniques. It would be reasonable practice in this situation for the nurses to ensure that senior management or the agency were informed so that steps could be taken to provide formal training for agency staff.

Therapeutic handling

It is sometimes argued that therapeutic lifting, e.g. in orthopaedic wards, to facilitate early mobilisation does not come under the manual handling regulations. There are, however, no grounds for this assertion. The definition of manual handling is:

> [A]ny transporting or supporting of a load (including the lifting, putting down, pushing, pulling, carrying or moving thereof) by hand or by bodily force.

This would, therefore, include therapeutic situations.

No lifting policy and therapeutic handling

The first requirement of any manual handling policy is to avoid any manual handling that could reasonably practically be avoided. Clearly, if this were to be implemented in the therapeutic regime, patients would never get mobilised following strokes and orthopaedic and other trauma. The nurse should ensure that a risk assessment is carried out that takes into account both the needs of the patient to become mobile and also dangers that staff face in promoting this mobilisation.

Lifting extremely heavy persons

This is of considerable concern to nurses. The National Institute for Health and Clinical Excellence defined morbid obesity as having a body mass index of more than 40 kg/m^2 or between 35 and 40 kg/m^2 with comorbidities.[125] An article on support for bariatric employees includes the case study of a nurse who weighed 27 stone but was assessed as medically fit for practice by the occupational health consultant.[126] The legal issues arising are considerable. Staff cannot cease to provide services for such persons, but the consequences in terms of costs and effort in minimising the risk of harm are considerable.

Sexual and Other Harassment and Bullying

It is essential that nurses are sensitive to the dangers of sexual harassment and make every effort to avoid potentially difficult situations. On the one hand, they must be aware of the sex discrimination laws (see chapter 10) and must ensure that they do not discriminate either directly or indirectly. On the other hand, they must ensure that they are chaperoned in any situation that could lead to accusations of harassment by the nurse or where the nurse themselves is at risk.

Protection from harassment act 1997

The Protection from Harassment Act 1997 can also provide some protection in the workplace, if an individual considers that they are subject to unreasonable unwanted attention.

The Act creates:

1. *a criminal offence of harassment* (section 1), which is defined as a person pursuing a course of conduct that amounts to harassment of another and that he knows or ought to know what amounts to harassment of the other (the reasonable person test is applied);
2. *a civil wrong*, whereby a person who fears an actual or future breach of section 1, may claim compensation including damages for anxiety and financial loss;
3. the right to claim an injunction to restrain the defendant from pursuing any conduct that amounts to harassment;
4. the right to apply for a warrant for the arrest of the defendant, if the injunction has not been obeyed;
5. *an offence of putting people in fear of violence*, where a person causes by his conduct another person to fear on at least two occasions that violence will be used against them;
6. *restraining orders* can be made by the court for the purpose of protecting the victim of the offence or any other person from further conduct amounting to harassment or to fear of violence.

Certain defences are permitted in the Act, including that an individual is preventing or detecting crime. Judy Veakins won her appeal after the County Court had dismissed her claim against her employers for damages for harassment under the Protection from Harassment Act 1997. She claimed that she was harassed at work by her supervisor for whose acts the company was vicariously liable. The company did not dispute vicarious liability if harassment was established. The Court of Appeal held that there was no reason why the Protection from Harassment Act could not be used for workplace harassment but the usual remedy for high-handed or discriminatory misconduct by or on behalf of an employer would be more fitting in the employment tribunal.[127] In another case the House of Lords held that the Act was not restricted to protection against stalking but had a wider application[128] and an employer could be vicariously liable for harassment caused by an employee. Those suffering from harassment as a result of discrimination may also have a cause of action under the Equality Act 2010 (see chapter 10).

Bullying at work

Research into bullying in an NHS community trust found that, of the 70 per cent of staff who responded to a questionnaire on bullying, 38 per cent reported being bullied in the previous year and 42 per cent reported witnessing the bullying of others. It was concluded that bullying was a serious problem.[129] There was a suggestion at the public inquiry into the deaths at Staffordshire Hospital, that bullying was a significant issue.

In a case in 1998, £100,000 was accepted in an out-of-court settlement by a teacher who alleged that he had been bullied by the head teacher and other staff, when he was teaching in a school in Pembrokeshire.[130] Dyfed County Council denied negligence. He suffered a minor breakdown in October 1996 and was returned to the same school, although he had asked for a transfer. He claimed that he was isolated, ignored and subjected to a series of practical jokes. He then suffered a second nervous breakdown. It was claimed that a support plan worked out for him by the council was not properly implemented. Another teacher was awarded £86,000 after being bullied, harassed and being subjected to unacceptable professional conduct.[131] The Barber decision (see page 322) was followed in a case where a police officer sued the Chief Constable for his vicarious liability for the actions of policemen who bullied and victimised the claimant. Since it was foreseeable that he could suffer psychological injury from their actions, he was awarded £18,000 general damages for the physical and mental injury he suffered.[132] Failure by an employer to take adequate steps to control bullying by a group of women of another female employee which led to a foreseeable risk of psychiatric injury led to a finding that he was vicariously liable for his employees' actions under the Protection from Harassment Act 1997 and also at common law. The employee was awarded £60,000 plus past and future loss and expenses.[133] A former police officer succeeded in a claim for personal injuries caused by the bullying by officers employed by the Chief Constable who was held vicariously liable. The injuries were foreseeable as a consequence of the treatment he received.[134]

The lessons for managers from these cases are obvious. Advice is given by Claire Walker on how to deal with bullying[135] and Jacqueline Grove gives some practical advice on how to recognise the signs of stress from bullying and provides a survival guide.[136] In August 2000 a teacher was paid £15,000 compensation for unfair dismissal after an education authority had ignored medical reports that the teacher was being bullied into a breakdown, and then dismissed him while on long-term sick leave. The teacher stated that he planned to seek civil compensation for personal injuries.[137] An RCN guide on harassment and bullying at work[138] emphasises that nurses should not tolerate harassment, but challenge it by reporting it and keeping records. A review on the literature on bullying at work from the Health and Safety Laboratory is available from the HSE website.[139] The aim of the project is to enable the HSE to develop guidance for organisations on primary interventions in relation to bullying. The Chartered Management Institute published a report on bullying at work in 2008[140] which showed that 70 per cent of those managers polled by the CMI had witnessed bullying in the past three years and 42 per cent had been bullied themselves. Root causes appeared to be lack of management skills, personality clashes and authoritarian management styles. ACAS has published leaflets on bullying for use by: (1) managers and employers; (2) employees; and (3) building a culture of respect.[141]

Repetitive Strain Injury (RSI)

This condition is also known as occupational overuse syndrome (OOS). Nurses should be aware, both for themselves and their patients, of the legal implications of RSI.

Even though, in an early case, a judge was quoted out of context as declaring that RSI has no place in medical books,[142] RSI has been recognised for the purpose of compensation in health and safety cases. A House of Lords' decision, however, may make it more difficult to obtain compensation for RSI.

On 25 June 1998 the House of Lords[143] rejected claims that a secretary, who was sacked after she developed a form of RSI, should be able to sue her employers. It overruled the Court of Appeal decision that Ann Pickford should be allowed to make a claim against Imperial Chemical Industries. The Court of Appeal had found that ICI was negligent in failing to warn her of the need to take breaks during her work using a word processor and gave her the right to take her case back to the High Court for an assessment of damages, which she estimated at £175,000. In a majority judgment (4 to 1), the House of Lords decided that ICI did not need to warn her about the dangers of RSI because typing took up only a maximum 75 per cent of her workload. To impose a warning that might cause more harm than good would be undesirable, since it might be counterproductive. The House of Lords questioned whether she had proved that the pain was organic in origin. She had been sacked in 1990 after taking long periods off work because of pain in both hands. She claimed that the injury had been caused by the very large amount of typing at speed for long periods without breaks or rest periods. The House of Lords said that it could reasonably have been expected that a person of her intelligence and experience would take rest pauses without being told.

It also held that RSI as a medical term was unhelpful. It covered so many conditions that it was of no diagnostic value as a disease. PDA4 (Prescribed Disease A4) had, however, a recognised place in the Department of Health and Social Security's list for the purposes of industrial injury, meaning a cramp of the hand or forearm due to repetitive movements such as those used in any occupation involving prolonged periods of handwriting or typing. The House of Lords held that the Court of Appeal should not have overruled the findings of the High Court judge, since he had ample evidence before him to justify his decision that in the plaintiff's case the giving of warnings was unnecessary, even though typists in another department had been given warnings. The Health and Safety Executive published guidance on RSI in March 2009, on upper limb disorders and on musculoskeletal low back pain in October 2010 which are available on its website.[144]

Smoking

The dangers of smoking both to the smoker and to those passive smokers in the vicinity have led to an increase in the number of workplaces and public areas where smoking is prohibited.

From July 2007 smoking has been banned in public places, which include hospitals.

In April 2002, NICE published guidance on the effectiveness of aids to smoking cessation.

Recently the sale of e-cigarettes has escalated, with controversy as to whether they should be banned on the grounds that in a non-smoking area it is difficult to distinguish an e-cigarette from a conventional cigarette. Those promoting e-cigarettes stress that they are far less dangerous to health.

Anti-smoking legislation

The Tobacco Advertising and Promotion Act 2002, banning press and billboard advertising of tobacco products in the UK, came into force on 14 February 2003 and provisions prohibiting sponsorship of sporting and other events by tobacco companies were being brought into force between July 2003 and July 2005. On 30 September 2003 new, more forceful, warnings in black and white have been compulsory on cigarette packets covering at least 30 per cent of the front of the packet and at least 40 per cent of the back. The warnings also include the NHS Helpline number (0800 169 0169).[145] Evidence that a ban on smoking in public places can improve health is seen from evidence of its effects in the US town of Helena.[146] Smoking in public places was banned for six months and researchers showed that, in comparison with earlier figures, the ban led to a 60 per cent reduction in heart attacks. The ban was lifted after a legal challenge. From July 2007 smoking in public places throughout the United Kingdom has been illegal. A consultation was launched in February 2007 to obtain views on raising the minimum legal age to purchase tobacco, and this was increased to 18 years in October 2007. The Chief Medical Officer has produced a series of video podcasts on smoking during pregnancy – these are available on the Department of Health website.[147] The EU on 30 November 2009 called on member states to adopt anti-smoking laws in public places, work places and public transport within three years. Patients at Rampton secure hospital failed in their argument that to ban smoking in a secure hospital was contrary to their human rights. The High Court held on 20 May 2008 that the ban on smoking was justified on health and safety grounds. The Court of Appeal in a majority judgment dismissed their appeal. The patients argued that the policy of prohibiting smoking in the premises of an NHS trust was a violation of their human rights as set out under Articles 8 and 14. The Court of Appeal held that although Rampton was the claimants' home, it was not a private home but a public institution operated as a hospital under section 4 of the 2006 Health Act which required all premises used by the public to be smoke-free by 1 July 2007.[148] Article 8 did not protect the right to smoke at Rampton. The dissenting judge Lord Keene held that the concept of personal autonomy which the Strasbourg court had adopted in *Pretty* v *United Kingdom*[149] was wide enough to incorporate a right to choose to smoke.

In contrast, in Scotland Charles McCann, a detained patient, won his case that a ban on smoking was contrary to his human rights. He was not, however, awarded the £3000 compensation he sought since it was held that he had saved more than £8000 in not being allowed to smoke.[150]

In September 2013 it was reported that the government was contemplating banning smoking in prisons.[151] The implementation of a phased smoking ban in prisons was fully implanted when the ban was extended to high security prisons in August 2017. The ban has since been blamed for the increase in violence in prisons in 2018.[152]

Healthcare Sharps Injuries

The Health and Safety Executive (HSE), the organisation that polices health and safety laws in the United Kingdom, undertook an inspection initiative aimed at gauging compliance with regulations seeking to prevent injuries from healthcare sharps in the NHS. Inspections were conducted in 40 NHS organisations across England, Scotland and Wales.[153]

Sharps or needlestick incidents are one of the most common causes of injury to staff, including nurses, in healthcare and they carry a serious risk of harm through the transmission of blood-borne infection.[154] Sharps incidents are the second most common cause of injury to NHS staff, marginally behind manual handling injuries.[155]

Sharps injuries occur when a sharp instrument such as a needle, scalpel or stitch cutter, penetrates the skin. If the sharp instrument is contaminated by blood, then transmission of infection is possible. The injuries can cause anxiety and distress to those affected and can, in the most serious cases, result in infection with blood-borne pathogens such as HIV or hepatitis B or C. It is known that at least four UK health workers have died as a result of occupationally acquired HIV and there have been a further 17 cases of health staff being infected with hepatitis C as a result of a sharps injury.[156]

Health and safety law

The Health and Safety Executive (HSE), have long been aware of the risk to health service staff from sharps incidents. They have taken action against employing NHS organisations for breaching health and safety laws following healthcare sharps injuries. In *R v Worcestershire Acute Hospitals NHS Trust* [2010] (Unreported, October 8) an NHS Trust pleaded guilty and was fined £12,500 with £9,000 costs when a trainee phlebotomist, taking blood from an infected patient, unmonitored, caught her wrist on the needle. An investigation by the HSE found the employee was not made aware of the patient's infection status and there were failures relating to risk assessments to blood-borne viruses, training and review of safe working practices.

General duties on the NHS to ensure the health and safety of staff are set out in the Health and Safety at Work etc. Act 1974 and its regulations including the:

- Safety Representatives and Safety Committees Regulations 1977[157] requiring that employers consult with safety representatives on matters affecting the health and safety of employees. This includes inspection of sharps injury reports and of work areas to ensure safe practice in the prevention of sharps injuries.
- Health and Safety (First Aid) Regulations 1981[158] requiring employers to provide adequate and appropriate equipment, facilities and staff to ensure employees receive immediate attention should a sharps injury occur at work.
- The Personal Protective Equipment at Work Regulations 1992[159] requiring employers to assess, select, provide and maintain personal protective equipment including the provision of suitable gloves, aprons and other equipment to minimise the risk of exposure to blood-borne infection.

- Reporting of Injuries, Diseases and Dangerous Occurrences Regulations 1995[160] requiring employers to report to the HSE occupationally acquired diseases, injuries and dangerous occurrences including known exposure to blood-borne infection following a sharps injury.
- Provision and Use of Work Equipment Regulations 1998[161] requiring employers to select and provide suitable work equipment and provide information and instruction on safe use including sharps bins, needles, scalpels and other sharps.
- Management of Health and Safety at Work Regulations 1999[162] placing a duty on employers to carry out risk assessments of all significant hazards in the workplace and provide employees with information on the risks to their health and safety and what preventative and protective measures are in place. This includes assessing the risk of sharps injuries and providing training to staff on minimising that risk.
- Control of Substances Hazardous to Health Regulations 2002[163] placing a duty on employers to identify any exposure to substances hazardous to health, assess the risk of exposure and put in place measures to control the exposure. That duty includes assessment of the risk of blood-borne infection from sharps injuries and controlling exposure through safety engineered devices, personal protective equipment and safe work systems that includes information and training for staff at risk of exposure. In *Skinner* v *Scottish Ambulance Service and others* [2004][164] Scottish appeal court judges ruled that cost grounds alone could not be used by employers as a lawful reason for not buying safer sharps devices.

Specific healthcare sharps regulations

Despite the wide range of general duties illustrated above, the number of sharps injuries in healthcare throughout the European Union continued to rise. In the United Kingdom alone there was a near 50 percent increase in the number of reported sharps injuries leading to an agreement on measures to prevent sharps injuries throughout the European Union.[165]

In the United Kingdom these measures were introduced into law by the Health and Safety (Sharp Instruments in Healthcare) Regulations 2013.[166]

Application of the regulations to nurses

The 2013 regulations apply to organisations whose primary activity is to manage and provide healthcare and including situations where employees provide care for people in their own homes. The regulations do apply to nursing services, and managers must ensure that risk assessments and arrangements to comply with the regulations take account of the circumstances that nurses work in, including arrangements for lone workers.

Duties under the 2013 regulations

The safe management of healthcare sharps is underpinned by existing health and safety legislation that emphasises the need to assess the risks, provide appropriate information and training, and consult with employees.

Health and Safety (Sharp Instruments in Healthcare) Regulations 2013 set out specific requirements that must be taken by healthcare employers and their contractors. The key change in approach in the regulations is on the prevention of unnecessary exposure to sharp instruments.

Prevention of exposure to sharps

The HSE recognises that nurses will continue to use instruments such as needles, scalpels and stitch cutters as they are essential tools in practice. However, the regulations require nurse managers and employers to ensure that sharp instruments are only used where they are absolutely necessary. Managers must audit the use of sharps and identify situations where their use can be excluded. The HSE cites an example of needles being used to collect urine samples from catheter bags when this is not necessary.[167] Nurse managers must also introduce needle-free equipment where it is available and reasonably practicable to do so (Health and Safety (Sharp Instruments in Healthcare) Regulations 2013, reg. 5).

Use of safer sharps

Where nurse managers do not consider it reasonably practicable to avoid the use of sharp instruments in a procedure then the 2013 regulation requires the use of safer sharps that incorporate protection mechanisms where it is reasonably practicable to do so. This might include the use of syringes and needles that have a shield that covers the needle after use.

Procedures for the safe use and disposal of sharps

Where such safer sharps are not available then safe procedures for working with and disposing of the sharp instrument must be in place. For nurses this will include a requirement for nurse managers to ensure safe procedures for the use and disposal of sharps provided by patients such as insulin syringes and needles that are kept in the patient's home.

Preventing the recapping of needles

Nurse managers must ensure that their staff do not recap needles and sharps unless a risk assessment demonstrates that it is required to prevent a risk. Where this is the case then devices such as needle blocks must be provided to control the risk of injury.

Sharps disposal containers

Clearly marked and secure containers must be provided and must now be placed close to where sharps are used together with instructions for nurses on how to safely dispose of the sharp. Nurse managers will now have to ensure the provision of suitable containers for use in a patient's home. A risk assessment will have to demonstrate that the type of sharp, portable sharp container and information for staff is appropriate for the environment the nurse is working in.

Information and training

The Health and Safety (Sharp Instruments in Healthcare) Regulations 2013, regulation 6(2)(3), place a duty on employers and their managers to work with safety representatives to develop information to be given to staff about the risks from sharps. The regulations require that such information covers:

- the risks from injuries involving medical sharps;
- relevant legal duties on employers and workers;
- good practice in preventing injury;
- the benefits and drawbacks of vaccination; and
- the support available to an injured person from their employer.

As well as the provision of information, nurse managers will have a duty to ensure that staff are given training on how to work safely with the sharps used by them in practice. The Health and Safety (Sharp Instruments in Healthcare) Regulations 2013, regulation 6(4), require that this training covers:

- the correct use of safer sharps;
- safe use and disposal of sharps used in practice;
- what to do in the event of a sharps injury; and
- arrangements for health surveillance and other procedures.

Duty to report sharps injury

Under the 2013 regulations, nurses have a duty to notify their employer of a sharps incident at work. Nurse managers must ensure that there are arrangements in place for the timely report of such injuries including arrangements for out of hours reporting. Managers must then record the incident and investigate the circumstances and causes of the incident. The investigation must be proportionate to the seriousness of the injury. A clean needle injury will not require as rigorous an investigation as an incident where there is exposure to blood-borne infection.

Where an injury is reported that has or might have exposed the nurse to blood-borne infection then immediate medical advice and post-exposure treatment and counselling must be available to that member of staff.

Duty to review procedures

The Health and Safety (Sharp Instruments in Healthcare) Regulations 2013, regulation 7(2), require employing organisations to review their procedures for the control of sharp risks by:

- evaluating the degree of compliance with the procedures;
- identifying areas where procedures are absent or inadequate;
- consulting with staff and their representatives; and
- evaluating sharps injury and incident data.

Findings of the inspection initiative

The main focus of the HSE inspection initiative[168] was to gather evidence to assess compliance with the Health and Safety (Sharp Instruments in Healthcare) Regulations 2013. Of the 40 organisations inspected some 34 were in breach of the 2013 regulations. These breaches were mainly in relation to the requirement for the safe use and disposal of sharps under regulation 5, information and training under regulation 6 and arrangements in the event of an injury under regulation 7 of the Health and Safety (Sharp Instruments in Healthcare) Regulations 2013.

Breaches in relation to the use and disposal of medical sharps included:

- a general failure to use safer sharps where reasonably practicable, or inconsistent use of safer sharps across the organisation. Initial reviews of sharps were often undertaken but this was not followed through over time or across the organisation, or employees were not represented on the steering group.
- some cases where inspectors found no sharps prevention strategy in place or organisations had failed to provide needles with safety mechanisms that were readily available such as hollow-bore hypodermic needles. There was still widespread use of non-safe devices including scalpels, winged IV cannula and other sharps.

- evidence of non-safe and safe sharps being stored together, leading to confusion for staff who were unsure which item to use.
- the need for better communication with procurement to ensure that only safer sharps were purchased and available, where reasonably practicable.
- a number of instances where the sharps bins were at low level and within reach of children; the temporary closures not being used; and sharps bins not located at point of use.
- used needles were left on a trolley or tray rather than being disposed of in a sharps bin.

Conclusions

A risk management strategy is at the heart of any policy relating to health and safety, not just for employees, but also for the clients and general public. Regular monitoring of the implementation of a risk management policy should ensure that harm is avoided and that a quality service is maintained for the public. This should be accompanied by clear, comprehensive documentation. The Health and Safety Executive has continued to implement its strategy for workplace health and safety in Great Britain to 2010 and beyond. However, there is still much room for improvement within the NHS. It is clear that there is no room for complacency and there is a strong imperative for the NHS to improve the health and safety of the working environment as well as the health, safety and welfare of the workforce. The effect of Lord Young's recommendations on the NHS and the 'compensation culture' and the implications of the Francis Inquiry on the culture of the NHS in relation to safety remain to be seen. Also unknown are the implications of the change in law so that breach of the Health and Safety regulations ceases to be the basis for a civil action for compensation. (Infection control is considered in chapter 25.)

Reflection questions

1. The Health and Safety at Work Act 1974 is enforced through the criminal courts. The employer's duty to care for the safety of his employees exists at common law. What is meant by these two statements and what is the difference in the enforcement provisions of each?
2. Who is the occupier of premises owned by the NHS trust and used by general practitioners?
3. All the circumstances must be taken into account in deciding whether the occupier is in breach of his common duty of care. What does this mean? Explain the statement in relation to an accident caused to an infant patient who slipped on a pool of water on the floor in the ward.
4. A nurse is injured while lifting a patient because the nurse assisting her suddenly let go and the injured nurse was left supporting the whole weight. What remedies, if any, does the injured nurse have and how could she claim compensation?
5. If a nurse is injured as the result of defective equipment, in what ways could she obtain compensation and what action should be taken?
6. What records should be kept in relation to any health and safety incident or in connection with claims under Part 1 of the Consumer Protection Act 1987?

Further exercises

Ask to see (if you have not already received one) a copy of your NHS trust's or employer's health and safety policy. How is this policy reflected in your working conditions?

References

[1] www.dailymail.co.uk/health/article-2110208/NHS-staff-cash-accidents-work--4k-slipping-potato.html
[2] News item, *The Times*, 27 February 2010
[3] Russell Jenkins, Head fined over fall that led to boy's death, *The Times*, 29 September 2007
[4] *R v Porter,* The Times Law Report, 9 July 2008; [2009] EWCA Crim 1271
[5] Joanna Sugden, Headmistress and four school staff are suspended over boy's asthma death, *The Times*, 25 March 2010
[6] *R v Chargot and others*, The Times Law Report, 16 December 2008
[7] *R v Upper Bay Ltd*, The Times Law Report, 28 April 2010
[8] *R v Nelson Group Services (Maintenance) Ltd*, The Times Law Report, 17 September 1998 CA
[9] www.hse.gov.uk
[10] Richard Griffith, Management of clinical waste, *British Journal of Midwifery*, 22(2):145–6, February 2014
[11] Health and Safety Commission, Management of Health and Safety at Work, Approved Code of Practice and Guidance, HMSO, London, 2000
[12] *Allison* v *London Underground Ltd*, The Times Law Report, 29 February 2008
[13] Management of Health and Safety at Work Regulations 1999 SI 1999/3242
[14] Provisions and Use of Work Equipment Regulations 1998 SI 1998/2306
[15] *Smith (Jean)* v *Northamptonshire County Council*, The Times Law Report, 24 March 2008
[16] *Smith (Jean)* v *Northamptonshire County Council*, The Times Law Report, 21 May 2009
[17] *Spencer-Franks* v *Kellog Brown and Root Ltd and Another*, The Times Law Report, 3 July 2008 HL
[18] Provision and Use of Work Equipment Regulations 1998 SI 1998/2306
[19] *Baker and others* v *Quantum Clothing and others*, The Times Law Report, 18 June 2009 CA
[20] *Craner* v *Dorset County Council*, The Times Law Report, 27 February 2009
[21] Health and Safety Executive, *A Guide to the Reporting of Injuries, Diseases and Dangerous Occurrences Regulations 1995*, HSE Books, 1999
[22] 0845 300 99 23. The HSE information line is 0845 345 0055
[23] RIDDOR Regulations 2013 SI 2013/1471
[24] Reporting of Injuries, Diseases and Dangerous Occurrences (Amendment) Regulations 2012 SI 2012/199
[25] Department of Health, An Organisation with a Memory: report of an expert group chaired by Professor Liam Donaldson, Chief Medical Officer, Department of Health
[26] Copies are available from The Stationery Office, PO Box 29, Norwich NR3 1GN or from the Department of Health website at www.gov.uk
[27] National Patient Safety Agency, Patient Safety Alert No. 21: Safer Practice with Epidural Injections and Infusions, NPSA, March 2007

28 https://improvement.nhs.uk/resources/learning-from-patient-safety-incidents
29 www.ncas.nhs.uk
30 https://resolution.nhs.uk/annual-report-and-accounts-201617
31 National Patient Safety Agency (2004) *Seven steps to patient safety*. London: NPSA
32 *Slade* v *Battersea HMC* [1955] 1 WLR 207
33 *Dobell* v *Thanet* DC, 22 March 1999, Current Law, August 2000, No. 527
34 *Jolley* v *Sutton London Borough Council*, The Times Law Report, 24 May 2000; [2000] 3 All ER 409
35 *R* v *Burns*, The Times Law Report, 10 June 2010
36 2010/32/EU implementing the framework agreement on prevention from sharp injuries in the hospital and healthcare sector
37 The Health and Safety (Sharp Instruments in Healthcare) Regulations 2013 SI 2013/645
38 *McPake* v *SRCL* Ltd [2013] CSOH 157
39 *O'Byrne* v *Aventis Pasteur MSD Ltd*, The Times Law Report, 27 May 2010 Supreme Court
40 B. Dimond, Protecting the consumer, *Nursing Standard*, 7(243):18–19, March 1993
41 *A and Others* v *National Blood Authority and Another (sub nom Re Hepatitis C Litigation)*, The Times Law Report, 4 April 2001; [2001] 3 All ER 289
42 www.mhra.gov.uk/
43 MDA SN 9801, Reporting Adverse Incidents Relating to Medical Devices, January 1998
44 SI 1994/3017, Medical Devices Regulations 1994 came into force 1 January 1995, mandatory from 14 June 1998. Directive 93/42/EEC
45 Medical Devices Agency Bulletin, Medical Device and Equipment Management for Hospital and Community-based Organisations, MDA DB 9801, January 1998
46 Directive 93/42/EEC 1993 concerning medical devices
47 The Medical Devices Regulations 2002 SI 2002/618
48 The Medical Devices Regulations 2007 SI 2007/400
49 SI 2003/1697
50 SI 2007/400
51 SI 2008/2936
52 SI 2012/1426
53 www.legislation.org.uk
54 Device Bulletin DB 2006(05) Managing Medical Devices, MHRA
55 www.mhra.gov.uk/; *Nursing and Midwifery Council News*, 5 February 2004
56 MHRA Device Bulletin DB 2007(01), Reporting Adverse Incidents and Disseminating Medical Device Alerts, available from www.mhra.gov.uk
57 www.england.nhs.uk/2014/03/20/med-devices
58 MDA, The Reuse of Medical Devices Supplied for Single-Use Only, MDA, London, 1995
59 Valerie Elliott, Pushchair company pays out for children's injuries, *The Times*, 7 May 2010
60 Regulation (EU) 2017/745 Of The European Parliament And Of The Council of 5 April 2017 on medical devices, amending Directive 2001/83/EC, Regulation (EC) No 178/2002 and Regulation (EC) No 1223/2009 and repealing Council Directives 90/385/EEC and 93/42/EEC; https://eur-lex.europa.eu/legal-content/EN/TXT/HTML/?uri=CELEX:32017R0745&from=EN
61 Control of Substances Hazardous to Health (COSHH) Regulations 2002, SI 2002/2677
62 www.coshh-essentials.org.uk
63 HSE, COSHH: A brief guide to the Regulations, INDG136, revised April 2005
64 *Barker* v *Corus* (UK) Plc [2006] UKHL 20; [2006] 3 ALL ER 785

65 www.shponline.co.uk/no-breaches-found-hse-hospital-stabbing
66 *Fraser* v *Winchester Health Authority*, The Times Law Report, 12 July 1999 CA
67 Department of Health, Survey of Violence, Accidents and Harassment in the NHS, 15 September 2003
68 *R* v *Lincolnshire (Kesteven) Justices, ex parte Connor* [1983] 1 All ER 901 QBD
69 L. Blom-Cooper, H. Hally and E. Murphy, *The Falling Shadow – One Patient's Mental Healthcare 1978–1993*, Duckworth, London, 1995 (report of an inquiry into the death of an occupational therapist at Edith Morgan Unit, Torbay, 1995)
70 Chris Mahoney, Scene of HCA attack was secure, *Nursing Times*, 96(6):5, 10 February 2000
71 Andrew Norfolk, Freed patient stabbed health worker to death on home visit, *The Times*, 23 October 2007
72 Nursing and Midwifery Council News, 9 January 2004
73 *Bucks* and *others* v *Nottinghamshire NHS Trust* [2006] EWCA Civ 1576
74 Department of Health, Guidance on Tackling Violence, October 2000; NHS Response Line 0541 555455
75 www.hse.gov.uk
76 Royal College of Nursing and NHS Executive, Safer Working in the Community, Order No. 000920, RCN and NHS Executive, September 1998
77 National Audit Office, A Safer Place to Work: protecting NHS hospital and ambulance staff from violence and aggression, NAO, 2003; www.nao.gov.uk/publications/nao_reports/02–3/0203527es.pdf
78 Sam Lister, Ministers to fund action on abusive patients, *The Times*, 15 April 2003
79 www.cfsms.nhs.uk/. Free phone line 0800 028 40 60
80 Department of Health press release, 25 September 2007
81 www.nhsbsa.nhs.uk
82 www.sshf.nhs.uk
83 P. Linsley, *Violence and Aggression in the Workplace: a practical guide for all healthcare staff*, Radcliffe Publishing, Oxford, 2006
84 Health and Safety Commission, *Violence and Aggression to Staff in Health Services*, HSE Books, 1997
85 B. Dimond, Domestic violence and the midwife: can you report it?, *British Journal of Midwifery*, 11(8):557–61, August 2003
86 Home Office, Safety and Justice: the government's proposals on domestic violence, Home Office, June 2003; webarchive.nationalarchives.gov.uk
87 The Domestic Violence, Crime and Victims (Amendment) Act 2012 section 5
88 Dimond, Protecting victims of domestic violence, *British Journal of Midwifery*, 13(2):105, February 2005
89 B. Domestic Violence, Crime and Victims Act 2004 (Victims' Code of Practice) Order 2013 SI 2013/2907
90 www.gov.uk/government/publications/the-code-of-practice-for-victims-of-crime
91 S. Lees and D. Phimister *et al.*, Domestic violence: the base of the iceberg, *British Journal of Midwifery*, 21(7):493–8, July 2013
92 Danielle Sheridan, Pride and sadness of father who fought for 'Clare's Law', *The Times*, 26 November 2013
93 Dominic Casciani, Police fail abuse victims says HMIC report, *The Guardian*, 27 March 2014
94 *Walker* v *Northumberland County Council*, The Times Law Report, 24 November 1994 QBD
95 *Hatton* v *Sutherland; Barber* v *Somerset County Council; Jones* v *Sandwell Metropolitan Borough Council; Baker* v *Baker Refractories Ltd*, The Times Law Report, 12 February 2002, [2002] EWCA 76, [2002] 2 All ER 1

[96] *Barber* v *Somerset County Council*, The Times Law Report, 5 April 2004 HL
[97] *Daw* v *Intel Corp (UK) Ltd* [2007] EWCA Civ 70; [2007] 2 All ER 126, (2007) 104(8) LSG 36
[98] *Foumeny* v *University of Leeds* [2003] EWCA Civ 557; [2003] ELR 443
[99] *Young* v *Post Office* [2002] EWCA Civ 661; (2002) IRLR 660
[100] Steve Bird, Work-stress mother who miscarried wins her case against Barbican bosses, *The Times*, 22 December 2007
[101] Simon de Bruxelles, Oliver Wright and Helen Rumbelow, Bosses will be fined for workers' stress, *The Times*, 5 August 2003
[102] www.hse.gov.uk/stress
[103] Royal College of Nursing, Managing your Stress, Order No. 001481, RCN, March 2001
[104] Royal College of Nursing, Working Well – a call to employers, Order No. 001595, RCN, March 2002
[105] Royal College of Nursing, Work-related Stress. A good practice guide for RCN representatives, Order No. 003531, RCN, 2009
[106] National Institute for Health and Clinical Excellence, Promoting Mental Wellbeing Through Product and Healthy Working Conditions: guidance for employers, NICE, 2009
[107] *Boag* v *Hounslow and Spelthorne Health Authority*, The Times Law Report, 25 July 1994
[108] Health and Safety (Miscellaneous Amendments) Regulations, 2002 SI 2002/2174
[109] Royal College of Nursing and the National Back Pain Association, Guide to the Handling of Patients, NBPA with the RCN, 4th edition, 1997
[110] EC Directive 90/269/EEC on the minimum health and safety requirements for the manual handling of loads (fourth individual directive within the meaning of Article 16(1) of Directive 89/391/EEC)
[111] Health and Safety (Miscellaneous Amendments) Regulations 2002, SI 2002/2174, paragraph 4
[112] Health and Safety Executive, Manual Handling Operations Regulations 1992 (as amended), Guidance on Regulations, L23 (third edition), HSE, 2004
[113] HSE, Getting to Grips with Manual Handling: a short guide, INDC143, revised June 2006
[114] www.hse.gov.uk/msd/mac
[115] HSE, Handling Home Care: achieving safe, efficient and practical outcomes for care workers and clients, HSG225, HSE Books (no date)
[116] RCN, Code of Practice for Patient Handling, Order No. 804, reprinted October 2007; RCN, Safer Staff, Better Care: RCN manual handling training guidance and competencies, Order No. 001975, February 2003; RCN, Introducing a Safer Patient Handling Policy, Order No. 000603, revised March 1999; RCN, Changing Practice, Improving Health – an integrated back injury prevention programme for nursing and care homes, Order No. 001255, August 2001
[117] *Robb* v *Salamis (M&I) Ltd* [2006] EWHL 56; [2007] 2 All ER 97
[118] *O'Neil* v *DSG Retail Ltd*, The Times Law Report, 9 September 2002; [2002] EWCA 1139; [2003] ICR 222
[119] *King* v *Sussex Ambulance NHS Trust* [2002] EWCA 953; [2002] ICR 1413
[120] News item, £420,000 award, *The Times*, 17 October 2002
[121] *R (on the application of A and B, X and Y)* v *East Sussex County Council (The Disability Rights Commission: an interested party)* Case No. CO/4843/2001, 10 February 2003
[122] News item, *The Times*, 19 November 2003
[123] The Health and Safety at Work Act 1974 (Civil Liability) (Exceptions) Regulations 2013 SI 2013/1667

[124] *Colclough* v *Staffordshire County Council*, 30 June 1994, Current Law, 208, October 1994
[125] National Institute for Health and Clinical Excellence (2002), Guidance on surgery for morbid obesity
[126] Jane Charlton and Julian M Pearce (2007) Supporting bariatric employees, *The Column*, 19(1):12–16
[127] *Veakins* v *Kier Islington Ltd*, The Times Law Report, 13 January 2010
[128] *Majrowski* v *Guy's and St Thomas's NHS Trust* [2006] UKHL 34; [2007] 1AC 224; [2005] ICR 977
[129] Lyn Quine, Workplace bullying in NHS community trust: staff questionnaire survey, *British Medical Journal*, 318(25):228–32, January 1999
[130] Victoria Fletcher, Teacher 'bullied by staff' wins £100,000, *The Times*, 17 July 1998
[131] Tony Hatpin, Teacher bullied by head awarded £86,000, *The Times*, 18 November 2003
[132] *Clark* v *Chief Constable of Essex* [2006] EWHC 2290; (2006) 103(38) LSG 32
[133] *Green* v *DB Group Services (UK) Ltd* [2006] EWHC 1898; [2006] IRLR 754
[134] *Clark* v *Chief Constable of Essex* [2006] EWHC 2290
[135] Claire Walker, Bullied to death, *Nursing Times*, 96(18):26–8, 4 May 2000
[136] Jacqueline Grove, Survival and resistance, *Nursing Times*, 96(18):26–8, 4 May 2000
[137] Paul Wilkinson, Teacher wins payout over school clash, *The Times*, 9 August 2000
[138] RCN, Bullying and Harassment at Work: a good practice guide for RCN negotiators and healthcare managers, Order No. 000926, reprinted October 2002; RCN, Dealing with Bullying and Harassment – guide for RCN members, Order No. 001301, January 2001; RCN, Dealing with Bullying and Harassment – guide for nursing students, Order No. 001497, August 2002
[139] Johanna Beswick *et al.*, Bullying at Work: a review of the literature, WPS/06/04, Health and Safety Laboratory, 2006
[140] Chartered Management Institute (2008) Bullying at Work: the experience of managers, CMI
[141] www.acas.org.uk
[142] *Mughal* v *Reuters Ltd* [1993] IRLR 571
[143] *Pickford* v *Imperial Chemical Industries Plc*, The Times Law Report, 30 June 1998 HL
[144] www.hse.gov.uk
[145] Department of Health press release 2003/0362, 30 September 2003
[146] News item, Smoking ban 'boosts health', *The Times*, 2 April 2003
[147] Chief Medical Officer, Smoking During Pregnancy, DH, June 2007
[148] *R (E)* v *Nottinghamshire Healthcare NHS trust* and *R (N)* v *Secretary of State for Health*, The Times Law Report, 10 August 2009
[149] *Pretty* v *United Kingdom* [2002] ECHR 427
[150] Dave Finlay, Patient wins fight against smoking ban at Carstairs, *Herald Scotland*, 28 August 2013
[151] Richard Ford, Smoking to be banned in prisons, *The Times*, 20 September 2013
[152] http://theconversation.com/smoking-bans-are-sparking-a-rise-in-violence-and-disorder-in-uk-prisons-83990
[153] Health and Safety Executive (2016) *Prevention and management of sharps injuries: Inspection of NHS Organisations*, retrieved from www.hse.gov.uk/healthservices/needlesticks/prevention-management-sharps-injuries.pdf
[154] NHS European Office (2013) *Briefing: Protecting healthcare workers from sharps injuries*, retrieved from www.nhsemployers.org/SiteCollectionDocuments/pdf
[155] National Audit Office (2003) *A safer place to work, Improving the management of health and safety risk to staff in NHS Trusts. Report compiled by the comptroller and auditor general HC-623*, retrieved from www.nao.org.uk/wp-content/uploads/2003/04/0203623.pdf

[156] NHS European Office (2013) *Briefing: Protecting healthcare workers from sharps injuries*, retrieved from nhsemployers.org/SiteCollectionDocuments/Protecting_healthcare_workers_from_sharps_injuries_KL_20130507.pdf
[157] Safety Representatives and Safety Committees Regulations 1977 (SI 1977/500)
[158] Health and Safety (First Aid) Regulations 1981 (SI 1981/917)
[159] Personal Protective Equipment at Work Regulations 1992 (1992/2966)
[160] Reporting of Injuries, Diseases and Dangerous Occurrences Regulations 1995 (1995/3163)
[161] Provision and Use of Work Equipment Regulations 1998 (1998/2306)
[162] Management of Health and Safety at Work Regulations 1999 (SI 1999/3242)
[163] Control of Substances Hazardous to Health Regulations 2002 (SI 2002/2677)
[164] *Skinner* v *Scottish Ambulance Service and others* [2004] Scot (D) 17/7 (Court of Session)
[165] Council Directive 2010/32/EU of 10 May 2010 implementing the Framework Agreement on prevention from sharp injuries in the hospital and healthcare sector concluded by HOSPEEM and EPSU [2010]
[166] Health and Safety (Sharp Instruments in Healthcare) Regulations 2013 (SI 2013/645)
[167] Health and Safety Executive (2013) *HSE Health Service Information sheet 7 Health and Safety (Sharp Instruments in Healthcare) Regulations 2013, Guidance for employers and employees*, retrieved from www.hse.gov.uk/pubns/hsis7.pdf
[168] Health and Safety Executive (2016) *Prevention and management of sharps injuries: Inspection of NHS Organisations*, retrieved from www.hse.gov.uk/healthservices/needlesticks/prevention-management-sharps-injuries.pdf

Part II
Specialist Areas

Chapter 13
Children and Young Persons

This chapter discusses

- Consent to treatment
- Safeguarding children
- Parental care and the nurse
- Disciplining a child
- Education of children in hospital
- Adolescents
- Deprivation of liberty of children and young persons
- Court proceedings and the child or young person

Introduction

In addition to the basic principles of law discussed in the first part of this book, those who nurse children and young persons must also be aware of several special legal provisions that apply to those under 18 years. (In some hospitals, children over 16 years are cared for in adult wards, in others there are special adolescent units.) The Human Rights Act 1998 gives rights to the child (see the website of this book), as does the United Nations Convention on the Rights of the Child (1989).[1] While the UN Convention is not directly enforceable in the UK (unlike the European Convention on Human Rights), the extent to which the UK complies with the Convention is monitored on a biannual basis. The Children Act 1989 has provided a framework for the provision of services for children in need and sets out the basic principles to be followed in determining the welfare of the child. There have been significant developments in the protection of children following the inquiries into the deaths of Victoria Climbié (which led to the Children Act 2004) and of Baby P (the Laming recommendations followed). The Department of Health has provided guidance on the welfare of children and young people in hospital[2] and the Audit Commission investigated the care of children in hospitals in 1993.[3] The RCN has published the results of a study into children's nursing and acute healthcare service provision that found a high level of non-adherence to national recommendations.[4] It followed this with a report in July 2001[5] and also guidance for nurses of children on a philosophy of care[6] and a position statement on children and young people.[7] Subsequently it published a toolkit for practice nurses in caring for children[8] and guidance on clinical practice and competencies across a range of conditions.

In 2014 the RCN published updated guidance on child abuse.[9] The British Medical Association has provided guidance on consent and the child.[10] The Royal College of Paediatrics and Child Health (RCPCH) has published guidance on many aspects of child protection, including *Child Protection Companion: Guidance for Clinicians on how to recognise and manage child abuse and neglect* (2006); *Safeguarding Children and Young people: roles and competencies for health care staff* (2006), an Intercollegiate document outlining the competencies required for healthcare staff to safeguard children and young people; *Child Protection Confidentiality: responsibilities of doctors in child protection cases with regard to confidentiality* (February 2004); an updated version of its *Fabricated and Induced Illness by Carers* (2009); *Involving Children and Young People in Health Services* (2011) and guidelines and standards for clinical practice on a range of topics. All these publications are available from the RCPCH website.[11]

In September 2013 the President of the Royal College of Paediatrics and Child Health stated that children in Britain were more likely to die from diseases or infections such as asthma, pneumonia and meningitis than elsewhere in Western Europe and 2000 children die needlessly every year due to poor NHS care.[12] A letter was sent by the RCPCH and the chief executive of Public Health England to every Council in the country urging local authorities to take action to tackle the unacceptable variation in the quality of care for children and young people and reduce health inequalities.

Consent to treatment

At age 18 and over, adults, if mentally competent, are able to make all decisions in relation to their medical care. They can also consent to being participants in research programmes and this applies whether the research is seen as being in their therapeutic interests or not. Prior to 18 years, several different provisions apply.

The 16- and 17-Year-Old

Treatment

Under section 8 of the Family Law Reform Act 1969, the child of 16 or 17 can give a valid consent to treatment. The provisions of this section are set out in Statute Box 13.1 below. These two subsections cover most eventualities as far as consent to treatment is concerned for the 16- and 17-year-old. Treatment is defined widely and would cover all nursing care. There is a presumption that, like the adult, the young person of 16 or 17 is capable of giving consent. This presumption is now contained in the Mental Capacity Act 2005 (which applies to those over 16 years) section 1(2), which states that a person must be assumed to have capacity unless it is established that he lacks capacity. Under section 2(4) of the MCA any question whether a person lacks capacity within the meaning of this Act must be decided on the balance of probabilities.

The approach to consent to treatment for a minor refined by Sir James Munby in *An NHS Trust* v *X* [2021][13] as was summarised in this way:

(1) Until the child reaches the age of 16 the relevant inquiry is as to whether the child is Gillick competent.

(2) Once the child reaches the age of 16:
   (i) the issue of Gillick competence falls away, and
   (ii) the child is assumed to have legal capacity (the right in law) to consent to treatment in accordance with section 8 of the Family Law Reform Act 1969, unless
   (iii) the child is shown to lack mental capacity as defined in section 2(1) of the Mental Capacity Act 2005.

In *Bell & Anor* v *The Tavistock And Portman NHS Foundation Trust* [2020][14] the High Court held that:

In respect of a young person aged 16 or over, the legal position is that there is a presumption of capacity arising from section 8 of the Family Law Reform Act 1969. As is explained in re W (A Minor) (Medical Treatment: Courts Jurisdiction) [1993], that does not mean that a court cannot protect the child under its inherent jurisdiction if it considers the treatment not to be in the child's best interests.

Consent to research

It should be noted that the Family Law Reform Act does not cover consent to take part in research unless it can genuinely be considered to be part of the treatment. Thus a 16-year-old suffering from a disorder where there is no clearly proven successful method of treatment might well asked to consent to a new, untried form of treatment as part of a research project. If the presumption that the individual has the mental capacity to give consent stands and it is clearly in the patient's therapeutic interests and if there are no undue risks, then such a proposal would be covered by the words of the section. If, however, there was at hand a proven successful method of treatment, but the child was approached to see if he would agree to take part in a research programme where there were considerable risks that may or may not be of benefit to him, it is likely

---

Statute 13.1
Sections 8(1) and (2) of the Family Law Reform Act 1969

Section 8(1) The consent of a minor who has attained the age of 16 years to any surgical, medical, or dental treatment, which in the absence of consent would constitute a trespass to his person will be as effective as it would be if he were of full age; and where a minor has by virtue of this section given an effective consent to any treatment, it shall not be necessary to obtain any consent for it from his parent or guardian.

Treatment is defined very widely (Section 8(2)). In this section, 'surgical, medical, or dental treatment' includes any procedure undertaken for the purposes of diagnosis and this section applies to any procedure (including in particular the administration of an anaesthetic) which is ancillary to any treatment as it applies to that treatment.

that such a treatment would not be covered by the Family Reform Act (though it may be covered by the Mental Capacity Act 2005 and its provisions relating to research and mental incapacity (see chapter 17)). Similarly, where a child or a young person of 16 or 17 is asked to participate in research which is of no benefit to him, consent cannot be given under the provisions of the Family Law Reform Act 1969, but could be given under the Mental Capacity Act 2005, if the young person lacked the requisite mental capacity and was over 16 years. In February 2014 NICE stated that children should be taking part in clinical trials since it is an important factor that has contributed to improved survival rates of childhood cancers. NICE published new guidance on 27 February 2014 (see chapter 27).

Refusal to have treatment

Case 13.1   Re W

Anorexia nervosa and the 16-year-old[15]

A 16-year-old girl under local authority care suffered from anorexia nervosa. She refused to move to a specialist hospital. The Court of Appeal held that the Family Law Reform Act 1969 section 8 did not prevent consent being given by parents or the court. While she had a right to give consent under the Act, she could not refuse treatment that was necessary to save her life.

In a 2014 case Mr Justice Hayden made a 16-year-old girl a **ward of court** and temporarily ordered that she should have no contact with her mother. The girl 'A' weighed 5½ stones and had been in hospital for a year, vomiting up to 30 times a day. Her mother objected to plans to tube feed her. The judge was told that her condition was critical and her body had started shutting down. The judge authorised reasonable force and sedation to be used in inserting the tube in her nostril. The mother, however, felt that the doctors must have missed some other reason for her condition.[16]

In another case[17] (*An NHS Foundation Trust* v *P*) the hospital was granted a declaration of lawfulness to enable it to treat a 17-year-old against her wishes following an overdose of paracetamol even though a psychiatrist declared her mentally competent to give consent to treatment. Her parents gave consent to treatment but she refused. The court found that the girl had capacity to make decisions as to medical treatment but that in balancing the competing factors there could be no hesitation in concluding that the balance fell firmly in favour of overriding her wishes. Her Article 8 rights had to be taken into account but here they were outweighed by her rights under Article 2. The court was under a positive duty to protect a person whose life was at risk.

Emergencies

The Act does not prevent any emergency action being taken to save the life of a child who is unconscious or unable to give consent. Thus a 16-year-old who is wheeled into the A&E department in an unconscious state can be given emergency treatment in the same way that a patient of any age would be treated. The professional providing this emergency treatment would be protected against any allegation of trespass to the person by the defence that he or she was acting in an emergency in the person's best interests under the Mental Capacity Act 2005. For a younger person the health professional could rely on the Children Act 1989 Section 3(5).

Parallel consent

Section 8 of the Family Law Reform Act can also be interpreted as giving power to parents to give a valid consent on behalf of their child of 16 or 17. This is because a third subsection of this section states:

> **Section 8(3): Nothing in this section shall be construed as making ineffective any consent which would have been effective if the section had not been enacted.**

One interpretation of this is that the fact that the child of 16 or 17 can now give a valid consent to treatment does not mean that consent by the parents on behalf of the child ceases to be effective. Prior to the 1969 Act, a parent could give a valid consent on behalf of his child up to adulthood and this right is not affected by the Act. Thus there exists a parallel right to consent: both the parents and the child of 16 or 17 could give consent. This is unlikely to cause difficulties except in those rare occasions where there is a dispute between the child and the parent. Whose views does the doctor or nurse take?

Practical dilemma 13.1   Clash between parent and child

A girl of 17 who had recently become a Jehovah's Witness was involved in a car crash. She was just conscious as she was wheeled into the A&E department and made it clear that she did not wish to be given a blood transfusion. Her parents were notified of the crash and told of her statement. However, not sharing her religious views, they said they would give their consent if blood was necessary to save her life. The consultant wishes to know the legal situation.

The fact that section 8(3) preserves the right of the parent to give consent means that, legally, the doctor could rely on that consent as a defence against any action for trespass to the person subsequently brought by the girl. Prior to section 8 of the Family Law Reform Act being passed, parents had the right to give consent and this right continues. However, to go against the wishes of the young girl is a serious situation and ideally the dispute should be brought to court. What if the doctor took notice of the girl's refusal, did not give blood and as a consequence the girl died? Could the parents then sue the doctor for negligence? The answer is that such a case would probably be unsuccessful, but much would depend on the circumstances – for example, the mental competence of the daughter in refusing blood; whether she understood the full implications; her general and specific capacity to give a valid consent.

Where there is a clash, the doctor has the choice of following the wishes of the child or the parents: if the position were reversed and the parents were Jehovah's Witnesses and the daughter consented to having blood, there would be no difficulties; he could rely on her consent under section 8(1) and if the girl were unconscious he could act in an emergency to save her life, whatever the views of the parents. However, where it is the child of 16 or 17 who is withholding consent and the parents wish to give it, many would argue that it is the doctor's duty to save life and he should rely on the parents' consent under section 8(3). The point was considered by the courts in *Re W*[18] where the court overruled the child's refusal (see Case 13.1). Were such a dispute to arise and where time permits, the best procedure to follow would be a reference to the court under the Children Act 1989. If time did not permit a court application, the ruling in the case of *An NHS Foundation Trust* v *P* discussed above[19] could be followed and her Article 2 right to life be seen to take precedence over her Article 8 rights.

A significant amendment to the law on the detention of young persons of 16 and 17 in psychiatric hospitals by the Mental Health Act 2007 (section 43 amending section 131 of the 1983 Act) meant that from October 2008 parents are no longer able to give consent to the admission of young persons of 16 and 17 who refuse to or are incapable of giving consent to admission. The Mental Capacity Act 2005 which came into force between April and October 2007 covers those over 16 years who lack the mental capacity to make decisions because of an impairment or a disturbance in the functioning of the mind or brain. It requires those who make decisions on behalf of those who lack mental capacity to act in the best interests of that person. Young persons of 16 or 17 who have the requisite mental capacity would not come within the provisions of the Act and disputes over their care would be heard by the Family Court. The Court of Protection can make orders and directions in relation to those who lack mental capacity in relation to both property and financial matters as well as personal welfare. Where a person under 16 years is unlikely to have the requisite mental capacity after 16 years, then an order can be made in respect of such a person. For example, if a boy of 14 received compensation following a road accident which caused serious brain damage, the Court of Protection could give directions for the use of that compensation. There are provisions in the Mental Capacity Act 2005 to facilitate the transfer of cases between the Family Division of the High Court and the Court of Protection to ensure that cases are heard in the most appropriate forum.

Children Under 16 Years

The Children Act 1989 requires the court to have regard to 'the ascertainable wishes and feelings of the child concerned considered in the light of their age and understanding' (section 1(3)(a)) in deciding whether to make specific orders under the Act. Certain sections require, if the child has sufficient understanding, the child's consent to be given, before the child can be asked to submit to a medical or physical examination.

Case 13.2   *Re E*

Refusal of blood by 15-year-old[20]

A youth aged 15 years 9 months was suffering from leukaemia and required a blood transfusion as part of his treatment. Both he and his parents were devout Jehovah's Witnesses and refused to give consent. The health authority applied for him to be made a ward of court and for a declaration that the treatment could proceed. The judge held that the youth was intelligent enough to take decisions about his own well-being, but that he did not have a full understanding of what the blood transfusions would involve. The welfare of the child was the first and paramount consideration. Although the court should be very slow to interfere in a decision the child had taken, the welfare of the child led to only one conclusion: that the hospital should be at liberty to treat him with blood transfusions. The judge therefore gave leave to the hospital authority to give treatment, including blood transfusion, and the consent of the patient and his parents was dispensed with.

In a case similar to *Re E*, a girl of 15 years suffered from thalassaemia and had been kept alive by monthly blood transfusions and injections. She and her mother began to attend meetings of Jehovah's Witnesses and subsequently refused to accept blood transfusions. The judge decided that the treatment could be authorised on the grounds that it was in her best interests and the court had the power to overrule a competent child's refusal of treatment. He did, however, find that the girl was not Gillick-competent because she lacked emotional maturity.[21] The High Court applied the Gillick principle to a case where parents were not informed that an abortion was to be carried out on a competent girl under 16 years[22] (see chapter 14). The European Court of Human Rights has stated that taking blood samples and intimate photographs of a girl of nine without her parents' consent was a breach of Article 8.[23]

The principle that the courts must act in the best interests of the child can be seen in those cases where parents disagreed over whether their children should receive the MMR vaccination which are considered in chapter 25.

A trust applied for a declaration that a general anaesthetic could be used to insert a gastrojejunal tube and investigate why the stomach was not functioning normally. The child was seven years old with cerebral palsy and related medical and developmental complications. The parents agreed to the procedures but did not wish J the paediatric surgeon to operate. The Family Court granted the application and refused to dictate to the hospital who should carry out the procedures.[24]

Non-parents

The Children Act 1989 section 3(5) provides that a person who (a) does not have parental responsibility for a particular child, but (b) has care of the child, may (subject to the provision of this Act) do what is reasonable in all the circumstances of the case for the purpose of safeguarding or promoting the child's welfare. It is suggested that this would include giving consent to necessary emergency treatment in the absence of the parents. In addition, professional staff would have a duty of care to take action to save life in such circumstances.

Case 13.3 *Re R (A minor: wardship: consent to medical treatment)* [1991] 4 All ER 177 CA

Compulsory treatment for mental disorder

The court gave permission for psychiatric medication to be given to a girl aged 15 against her will. Her mental health had deteriorated and she was placed in an adolescent psychiatric unit. Her condition fluctuated between periods of lucidity. The Court of Appeal held that she was not mentally competent owing to the fluctuating nature of her mental illness.

Kennedy and Grubb[25] have suggested in discussing the reasoning of the Court of Appeal that: 'It is more respectful of patients' autonomy to interpret incompetence so as to include the manic depressive and the anorexic (where appropriate) rather than regard them as apparently competent and then do wholesale violence to the law's commitment to the rights of decision-making of the competent.'

Children's rights: can children give consent themselves?

If the child is mature and capable of understanding the situation and it is not possible to contact the parents, the child can give a valid consent and this principle is emphasised in the Children Act 1989. This issue was considered in the Gillick case on the narrow issue of advice and treatment for family planning. However, the principles established by the House of Lords cover a much wider area.

| Case 13.4 | *Gillick* v *West Norfolk and Wisbech AHA and the DHSS* [1985] |

The Gillick case[26]

Mrs Gillick questioned the lawfulness of a DHSS circular, HN(80)46, which was a revised version of part of a comprehensive *Memorandum of Guidance* on family planning services issued to health authorities in May 1974 under cover of circular HSC(IS)32. The circular stated that in certain circumstances a doctor could lawfully prescribe contraception for a girl under 16 without the consent of the parents. Mrs Gillick wrote to the acting administrator formally forbidding any medical staff employed by the Norfolk AHA to give 'any contraceptive or abortion advice or treatment whatever to my . . . daughters whilst they are under 16 years without my consent'. The administrator replied that the treatment prescribed by a doctor is a matter for the doctor's clinical judgement, taking into account all the factors of the case. Mrs Gillick, who had five daughters, then brought an action against the AHA and the DHSS seeking a declaration that the notice gave advice that was unlawful and wrong and that did or might adversely affect the welfare of her children, her right as a parent and her ability properly to discharge her duties as a parent. She sought a declaration that no doctor or other professional person employed by the health authority might give any contraceptive or abortion advice or treatment to any of her children below the age of 16 without her prior knowledge and consent.

She failed before the High Court judge, succeeded in her appeal before the Court of Appeal, and the DHSS and health authority then appealed to the judicial committee of the House of Lords, then the United Kingdom's highest Court (now replaced by the Supreme Court). The Lords decided by a majority of three to two against Mrs Gillick. The majority held that in exceptional circumstances a doctor could provide contraceptive advice and treatment to a girl under 16 without the parents' consent. The circular was therefore upheld.

Lord Fraser stated the exceptional circumstances, which are set out in Box 13.1. Many questions still remain uncertain. Can it be assumed that a mature child under 16 can give a valid consent to any form of treatment and research? What efforts must be made to obtain the parents' consent? For what can a child give consent: a few stitches; an anaesthetic; an abortion? Clearly the competence of the child must match the nature of the decision to be made: a young child may be able to agree to having stitches in his leg, but not to brain surgery. It is an overwhelming requirement that decisions must be made in the best interests of the child. The paramount consideration is the welfare of the child.

> **Box 13.1 Exceptional circumstances set out in the Gillick case**
>
> 1. The girl would, although under 16, understand the doctor's advice
> 2. He could not persuade her to inform her parents or allow him to inform the parents that she was seeking contraceptive advice
> 3. She was very likely to have sexual intercourse with or without contraceptive treatment
> 4. Unless she received contraceptive advice or treatment her physical or mental health or both were likely to suffer
> 5. Her best interests required him to give her contraceptive advice, treatment or both without parental consent

What is the position where the child is a mother? If she has the mental competence, does she have the legal capability of giving consent for her child to be treated or is it necessary to obtain the consent of her own parents, i.e. the baby's grandparents? As an example, many health visitors treating the child of an underage mother protect themselves by obtaining both the consent of the underage mother and also of a grandparent. From the cautious words of the majority judges sitting on the Gillick case in the House of Lords, it would appear that, provided the underage mother had the requisite mental competence to consent to treatment on the child's behalf, this would be a valid consent.

Another interpretation of section 8(3) of the Family Law Reform Act 1969 is that statutory powers given to a child of 16 or 17 to give a valid consent do not remove the ability of the mature child below 16 years to give a legally valid consent to treatment.

Where a child is refusing life-saving treatment, the test of Gillick competence will not be the only factor in determining the case, as Case 13.5 shows. In this case, the ruling in *Re W* was followed.

Case 13.5 *Re L*

Refusal by 14-year-old Jehovah's Witness[27]

A 14-year-old girl had sustained extensive and severe burns. Her life was considered to be at risk unless she underwent surgical treatment, which involved the possibility of a blood transfusion, although, as a practising Jehovah's Witness, she felt unable to consent to this. Her clearly expressed refusal was consistent with two earlier advance directive/release forms that she had completed, the last being only two months before her injuries. The hospital applied for leave to administer blood and blood products in the course of essential treatment without her consent.

The court granted the application on the grounds that:

1. She could not be said to be Gillick-competent. (Information had been withheld from her about the horrible death brought on by the onset and spread of gangrene, if blood were not transfused; and she had led a sheltered life, very much under the influence of the family.)
2. Even had she been found to be Gillick-competent, the extreme gravity of the case would, nevertheless, be sufficient basis for the order to be made.

A young person under 16 years could in theory rely on Article 3 of the European Convention on Human Rights (see the website of this book) or on Article 9 and his or her freedom to practise a specific religion to justify his or her refusal of life-saving treatment in conjunction with Article 14 and the right not to be discriminated against in the recognition of the Convention rights. However, the younger the age, the less likely the courts would be to find in favour of the youngster.

Clash between parents and child under 16

A case is considered in chapter 15 (Case 15.1) where a 15-year-old child's refusal to have a transplant was overruled by the court[28] together with cases where the wishes of the child were respected.

Overruling the parent

While parents have the power in law to give consent to the treatment of the child, this is not an absolute power. If their consent or their refusal to give consent is considered to be against the best interests of the child, then the court can intervene.

Case 13.6 In re D [1976]

Sterilisation of a mentally handicapped girl[29]

A girl of 11 years of age suffered from Sotos syndrome, the symptoms of which included accelerated growth during infancy, epilepsy, general clumsiness, an unusual facial appearance and behaviour problems, including emotional instability, certain aggressive tendencies and some impairment of mental function. The mother, taking the advice of the consultant paediatrician that her daughter would remain substantially handicapped and that she would always be unable to care for herself or look after any children, discussed with the obstetrician the possibility of her daughter being sterilised. An operation was arranged. However, before it was performed, the educational psychologist applied for the girl to be made a ward of court. Mrs Justice Heilbron, who heard the case, was not convinced that the operation was in the best interests of the girl and so ordered that the operation should not proceed.

It can be seen from this case how fortuitous it was that the case ever came before the courts. Had it not been for the strongly held views of the educational psychologist, the operation could well have gone ahead. This should not be so in the future. In a House of Lords' case,[30] where the judges agreed to a sterilisation proceeding on 'Jeanette', they made it clear that, in future, every such case of a sterilisation on a mentally handicapped child should receive the approval of the court before it proceeded. In that case, they did not make the distinction between therapeutic and non-therapeutic sterilisation, which Mrs Justice Heilbron had made *in re D*. In theory, every case of sterilisation on a child should come before the courts, even though the operation is performed because of the presence of a malignancy. This is further discussed in chapter 14.

The important point for children's nurses is that if they feel that a particular procedure or treatment agreed between the parents and the medical staff is not in the best interests of the child, then the nurse should raise it with her senior management who could, if necessary, arrange for the matter to be brought before the courts.

In a dispute between a family and the doctors, violence erupted on the wards as the family fought to prevent morphine, which would depress the respiratory functions, being administered to their child.

Case 13.7 *R v Portsmouth Hospitals NHS Trust ex p Glass* [1999]

Dispute over treatment[31]

A boy of 13 was severely disabled with only a limited lifespan. The mother wished him to receive whatever medical treatment was necessary to prolong his life. Following an incident in which the hospital gave the child morphine against the mother's wishes, family members resuscitated the child and prevented him from dying. There was a complete breakdown of trust between the family and the hospital. The mother sought a declaration as to the course doctors in the hospital should take if the boy were admitted for emergency treatment and disagreements arose as to the treatment to be given to or withheld from the child. The judge refused the mother's application for judicial review and she appealed to the Court of Appeal.

The Court of Appeal held that it would be inappropriate to grant a declaration in anticipation and indicate to doctors at a hospital what treatment they should or should not give in circumstances that had not yet arisen. The best course was for the parents of a child and the medical staff to agree on the approach to be taken for the treatment of that child, but if that were not possible and a grave conflict arose, then the actual circumstances must be brought before the court so that the court could resolve what was in the best interests of the child in the light of the facts existing at that time. The principles recognised by the Court of Appeal were as follows:

1. Sanctity of life;
2. Non-interference by the courts in areas of clinical judgement in the treatment of patients where that could be avoided;
3. Refusal of the courts to dictate appropriate treatment to a medical practitioner, subject to the court's power to take decisions in the child's best interests;
4. Treatment without consent, save in an emergency, was a trespass to the person; and
5. The court would interfere to protect the interests of a minor or a person under a disability.

The Court of Appeal dismissed the appeal.

Ms Glass subsequently appealed to the European Court of Human Rights, which held that the failure of the NHS trust to seek a declaration from the court before administering diamorphine to her son without her consent and in writing him up for do not resuscitate (DNR) instructions without her knowledge was a breach of her Article 8 rights.[32]

Members of the family were prosecuted for their violence in the hospital.

DNA and parental consent

Concerns have been expressed by the Human Genetics Commission about parents giving consent to their children's DNA being tested on the grounds that this could infringe their rights to take health decisions for themselves when they are adults. Such tests should be confined to cases where there is an immediate and compelling medical reason[33] (see chapter 21).

Transplants and the interests of the child

Practical dilemma 13.2 — Sisterly transplants

Mary, aged seven years, had an incurable blood disease and was found to be compatible only with her younger sister Janet, who was four years old. The parents therefore agreed that Janet would provide a bone marrow transplant for Mary. Staff Nurse Bryant was concerned by the legalities of the proposed transplant.

The parents have the right to consent to any treatment that is in the interests of the child (subject to any statutory limitations). However, in this case, there is a clash between the interests of Mary and the interests of Janet. Any operation, no matter how small, involves some risk to the patient and Janet would be put at risk for the benefit of Mary. In the case of a bone marrow transplant, it could be argued that the risk is so small and the psychological benefit for Janet when she becomes older so immense that it would be inhuman not to allow Janet to be a donor. If she were asked, she would probably agree herself, although her capacity to understand would be very limited. The situation would come under the legislation relating to transplants from live donors and the provisions of the Human Tissue Act 2004 (see chapter 15). The situation that would arise if Janet were mentally incapacitated and in an institution is discussed in chapter 16.

A further extreme example of using one child for the benefit of another arose in October 2000 when it was reported from the USA that parents had had a baby selected by *in vitro* fertilisation (IVF) who would provide compatible bone marrow for treating their daughter who suffered from a serious blood disorder.[34] The Human Fertilisation and Embryology Authority has stated that IVF is available for parents who wish to ensure that the selected embryo will be a match for an existing child. This situation is now covered by the Human Fertilisation and Embryology Act 2008 and is considered in chapter 21.

In 1993 the court held that a blood transfusion should be given to a premature baby girl who suffered from respiratory distress syndrome and whose parents were Jehovah's Witnesses. The order authorising medical treatment was to be made under the court's inherent jurisdiction rather than pursuant to the Children Act 1989.[35]

In 2000 the future of conjoined twin girls came before the Court of Appeal.[36] The Court of Appeal decided that the operation could proceed.

Withholding of consent by parents

Where the parents refuse to give consent to treatment, which the doctors determine is in the best interests of the child, then there is a well-tried procedure for taking the appropriate action. No child should die because the parents have unreasonably refused their consent to a necessary treatment. In March 2014 a judge gave permission for a baby boy to have blood transfusions during an operation despite his parents' objections. The parents were Jehovah's Witnesses and the judge was told that the baby had no long-term prospect of survival without cardiac surgery. The parents had agreed to the surgery but not to a blood transfusion.[37]

Practical dilemma 13.3 — Blood transfusion

Eric, aged three years, is admitted with an operable tumour. The neurologist reassures the parents and says that Eric can be saved. The parents say that on religious grounds they could not agree to Eric's having a blood transfusion. Mr Sharpe, the neurosurgeon, replies that he would not be prepared to carry out such an operation with such a restriction, as it is highly likely that blood would be required in the operating theatre. The parents therefore refuse their consent to the operation. Since the tumour is operable, the neurosurgeon cannot let the child die, so he has two options. He can either proceed and justify his action on the basis that he is acting in the best interests of the child in an emergency; or he can arrange for an application to be made to the court for Eric to be made a ward of court, and for the operation to be ordered to proceed.

In the case of an emergency, when there is insufficient time to obtain a declaration from the court, essential action must be taken to save the life of the child, if that is clinically in the best interests of the child.

Case 13.8 — *In re B (A Minor)* [1981]

Down's syndrome[38]

A child who was born suffering from Down's syndrome and an intestinal blockage required an operation to relieve the obstruction if she were to live for more than a few days. If the operation were performed, the child might die within a few months, but it was probable that her life expectancy would be 20–30 years. Her parents, having decided that it would be kinder to allow her to die rather than live as a physically and mentally handicapped person, refused consent to the operation. The local authority made the child a ward of court and, when a surgeon decided that the wishes of the parents should be respected, they sought an order authorising the operation to be performed by other named surgeons. The judge in the High Court decided that the wishes of the parents should be respected and refused to make the order. The local authority took the case to the Court of Appeal, which said that the operation should proceed.

The court decided that the question before it was whether it was in the best interests of the child that she should have the operation and not whether the parents' wishes should be respected. Since the effect of the operation might be that the child would have the normal lifespan of a person with Down's syndrome, and since it had not been demonstrated that the life of such a person was of such a nature that the child should be condemned to die, the court would make an order that the operation be performed.

One significant case in which the courts did not follow the medical views was where parents refused to permit a liver transplant to take place on their toddler. The Court of Appeal held that in the very specific circumstances of the case (the parents lived abroad and as health professionals they believed the transplant not to be in the best interests of the child) the transplant would not be ordered against their wishes.[39] (See chapter 15 for further discussion on transplants and consent.)

The court will review any decision where parents are withholding consent or giving consent and decide whether the treatment should be given in the light of the best interests of the child. It is open to any interested party to ask the court to determine this question when he or she is concerned at what is proposed or not proposed.

Parents have a legal duty to care for their children. Where they fail to obtain medical treatment, they could be guilty of a criminal offence. A father was convicted of manslaughter and imprisoned and the mother given a suspended sentence for failing to give their diabetic daughter insulin.[40] The couple refused to allow their diabetic daughter to receive modern medicine because of their religious beliefs. In September 2002 a couple were jailed for starving their tortured 2-year-old daughter to death.[41] In March 2014 parents pleaded guilty to manslaughter after their 5-month-old baby died of rickets caused by severe vitamin D deficiency. They had failed to seek proper medical care because of their religious beliefs despite the advice of their relatives.[42] The father was jailed for 3 years and the mother for 2 years 3 months. A serious case review by Bexley Safeguarding Children's Board found that it was a preventable death and a number of opportunities to protect the baby were missed. The GP should have been aware of the importance of breastfeeding mothers to take vitamin D supplements and this would have been even more relevant in this case. The health visitor's visit was considered extraordinarily optimistic and the parents were seen to be very cooperative.

The Board also found a lack of any agency checks, which if undertaken would likely have provided a more complete picture of the risks.[43]

Letting die

The Down's syndrome case (Case 13.8) above raises the issue of whether it is permissible in law to allow a severely handicapped child to die or even assist them to die. In what circumstances does the doctor cease to have a duty to keep the child alive? Certainly, as the case of *In re B* shows, the views of the parents are not the deciding factor. The point was raised in the case of Dr Arthur, who was prosecuted for murder (later changed to attempted murder), since he prescribed, with the consent of the parents, the substance DF118 for a Down's syndrome baby who also suffered from severe abdominal abnormalities. A jury acquitted him.[44]

The law does not recognise any form of euthanasia, but in practice it is left to the discretion of the medical staff to determine the extent of heroic medicine that is justified for severely handicapped babies. This discretion is reviewable in the courts. It is not an easy situation for medical staff and the Royal College of Paediatrics and Child Health has published guidelines to assist practitioners,[45] as has the British Medical Association.[46] This issue is discussed further in the section on special care baby units and in chapter 28 in relation to adults.

In a Northern Ireland case (*A Health and Social Care Trust* v *M and others*[47]) the court ruled that a five-month-old baby with catastrophic and irreversible brain damage could be removed from a ventilator and made the subject of palliative care only. The father had obtained expert evidence which suggested that neuro-stimulation would assist the boy and the Trust's application for the ventilation to be withdrawn should be refused or adjourned for at least two weeks. Such evidence was contradicted by the other experts.

It can be seen from these cases that any decision to withdraw or withhold life sustaining treatment from critically sick children must be made in the child's best interests (*Camden LBC* v *R (A Minor) (Blood Transfusion)* [1993][48]).

The test for best interests with critically ill children is firmly based in common law and has been developed by the courts as cases have been brought for judgment over the last 30 years. Over that time the courts have had the opportunity to consider each aspect of the care of critically ill children and the test for best interests has become ever more sophisticated and extends beyond a mere balancing of the risks and benefits of continued treatment.

In the early cases we have seen that the notion of a best interest adopted by the courts was limited to the likely life expectancy of the child if life sustaining treatment were to be given (see *Re B (A Minor) (Wardship: Medical Treatment)* [1981][49] above).

Some ten years later the court refined the determination of a best interest to include the pain and suffering the child would have to endure. In *J (A Minor) (Child in Care: Medical Treatment)* [1993][50] a profoundly brain damaged child with a very short life expectancy was not thought to be benefitting from treatment and both the parents and medical team sought an order allowing them to curtail treatment. The court held that denial of treatment to prolong life could only be sanctioned when in the best interests of the child. The test that applied was based on an assessment of the quality of life of the child and their future pain and suffering in relation to the lifesaving treatment.

No absolutist test

In *J (A Minor) (Child in Care: Medical Treatment)* [1993] it was argued that in the case of critically ill children an absolutist test should be applied. That is, doctors and nurses should have a duty to continue life sustaining treatment right up to the death of the child. The court, however, found that even where the patient was a critically ill child it was never the case that doctors and nurses had to continue giving treatment even where it was clearly futile. What the court called the absolutist test would never apply.

A decision of the Court of Appeal in *Re T (A Minor) (Wardship: Medical Treatment)* [1997][51] saw much broader, welfare, family and other non-medical factors adopted as part of the determination of a critically ill child's best interests. T was born with a lifethreatening liver defect requiring a liver transplant if the child was to live. His mother refused consent as she considered it was in the child's best interests not to suffer stressful and painful invasive surgery. The judge at first instance considered medical evidence that the chances of success were good and held that the mother's refusal to accept the unanimous advice of the doctors was not the conduct of a reasonable parent.

The Court of Appeal held that the judge had erred in his approach to best interests as he had not weighed in the balance reasons against the treatment which might be held by a reasonable parent on much broader welfare and family grounds than a clinical assessment of the likely success of the treatment.

In *A NHS Trust* v *MB and Mr & Mrs B* [2006] similar grounds were used to justify the continuation of treatment in the case of a terminally ill child who was unable to breathe unaided since birth and required positive pressure ventilation. The NHS trust argued that his quality of life was so low and the burdens of living so great that it was in his best interests to withdraw all forms of ventilation. His parents however, argued that a tracheostomy should be performed to enable long term ventilation.

In common with all cases concerning children the court held that the child's welfare was their paramount consideration (Children Act 1989 s.1). The court considered the quality and value to the child of his relationship with his family and found it was not in his best interests to discontinue ventilation with the inevitable result that he would die. He had age-appropriate cognition, a relationship of value with his family, and other pleasures from sight, touch and sound. Those benefits were precious and real and the routine discomfort, distress and pain did not outweigh those benefits.

However, the court also held that to undergo procedures that went beyond ventilation such as cardio-pulmonary resuscitation, administration of intravenous antibiotics and blood sampling should not be provided unless the medical team thought it clinically appropriate.

A decision on a critically sick child's best interests must be determined on wider grounds than benefits and risks of continued treatment. To make this determination it is necessary to discuss the child's best interests with the parents.

Referring the matter to court

Where parents strongly oppose the giving or withholding of treatment then, unless the situation is urgent, the matter will need to be referred to the court for a decision. Failing to seek the courts approval in these circumstances would be a breach of the child's right to respect for a private and family life under article 8 of the European Convention on Human Rights.

In *Glass* v *United Kingdom* [2004][52] a severely physically and mentally disabled baby, argued that his right to physical integrity under the European Convention on Human Rights 1950 Art. 8 had been breached when on his readmission with respiratory failure, the hospital insisted that he was dying and that diamorphine should be given to relieve his distress. His mother disagreed and objected to the proposed treatment in the belief that it would harm his chances of recovery. Despite her objection diamorphine was administered but his condition improved and he returned home.

The European Court of Human Rights found that treatment contrary to his mother's wishes breached the baby's right to physical integrity under Article 8 as the hospital had failed to seek the High Court's approval for the proposed treatment.

Permissive declarations

When the court's approval for a plan of care is sought the method used to authorise treatment is by way of a declaration where the court declares that the proposed treatment is lawful. A declaration is binding on the parties before the court and doctors and nurses are bound by their terms.

The courts are aware that a declaration may restrict a health professional's ability to exercise their clinical judgement. To avoid such a situation the court resorts to the use of a permissive declarations (*A NHS Trust* v *MB and Mr & Mrs B* [2006])[53]. In a permissive declaration the court authorises the withholding of treatment at the discretion of the care team. In *Re Wyatt (A Child) (Medical Treatment: Continuation of Order)* [2005][54] the intervention of the court was sought in respect of the medical treatment of a critically ill child who had also developed an intermittent rasping cough and a viral infection. The only intervention would be intubation and ventilation but the doctors argued that it would not be in her best interests as essentially it would be futile. The parents were of the view that if she were ventilated she would recover.

The court made it clear that in the best interests of the child the care team should be able to refrain from having to intervene by way of intubation and ventilation. The authority was granted by way of a permissive not mandatory declaration so that at the moment the decision arose the care team could exercise their clinical judgment, in the child's best interests, as to whether to withhold the treatment or not.

Safeguarding children

The children's nurse needs to be aware of the possibility that injuries or illness in a child may have been caused by another person. This applies not just to bruising or lacerations, but also to undernourishment and other ailments, including psychological damage. The possibility of sexual abuse must also be borne in mind if the relevant symptoms are present. The parents have a legal duty to provide care for their dependent children under section 1(1) of the Children and Young Persons Act 1933.

The nurse is confronted by the following problems. What action should she take if she suspects a child of being the object of abuse of any kind? What are the potential consequences for her if she is mistaken? What powers does she have to prevent a parent removing a child from the ward when the child has been placed under an emergency section of the Children Act? What would her position be in relation to a court hearing? Does she have to make a statement to the police?

Practical dilemma 13.4   Child abuse?

Jane, a girl of six months, was admitted to the children's ward with a suspected chest infection. She was immediately placed on antibiotics and sputum samples taken. While the nurse was changing her, she noticed some bruising to the upper legs and a possible burn mark on her back. The nurse pointed these marks out to the junior doctor, who suggested that the registrar should be called in, as it was possible that these marks were the result of abuse.

A procedure for dealing with suspected child abuse should be available on every ward. If child abuse is suspected, the nurse should be particularly vigilant in not leaving the child unattended with the parents. In addition, it is quite likely that she could be called on to give evidence to the court as to the nature of the relationship and interaction between the parents and the child in hospital and also as to the physical and mental state of the child on admission. It is essential, therefore, that their record keeping should be detailed and clear to enable them to answer questions at some later time. Where cot death is feared, a new procedure was introduced in January 2004 following the acquittal of several mothers who were imprisoned for killing their babies. The consent of the Director of Public Prosecutions must be obtained where the prosecution of parents is contemplated in respect of the death of a young child, in order that the possibility of cot death can be ruled out. The acquittals resulted from the discrediting of evidence of Munchausen syndrome by proxy relied on by the expert witness Professor Sir Roy Meadows, a paediatrician.

Statute 13.2
Children Act 1989: protection of children

A Part IV	Care and supervision order, Sections 31–42
B Part V	Protection of children, Sections 43–52
C Part XII	Miscellaneous and general, Section 100 Restriction of wardship; jurisdiction of High Court still exists in emergency situations
Section 43	Child assessment order
Section 44	Orders for emergency protection of children
Section 45	Duration of emergency protection orders
Section 46	Removal and accommodation of children by police in cases of emergency
Section 47	Local authority's duty to investigate
Section 48	Powers to assist in discovery of children who may be in need of emergency protection
Section 49	Abduction of children in care
Section 50	Recovery of abducted children
Section 51	Refuges for children at risk
Section 52	Risk and regulation relating to emergency protection order

---

The social services department of the local authority can apply for a child assessment order or an order for the emergency protection of the child under Part V of the Children Act 1989 to care for the child initially, pending the outcome of the full proceedings for the care of the child.

The orders that can be made in respect of a child suspected of being abused are contained in the Children Act 1989, set out in Statute Box 13.2. Failure by a local authority to take reasonable precautions to prevent abuse can lead to payment of compensation. In September 2007 Hackney agreed, in an out-of-court settlement, to pay £100,000 to a woman of 39 years and her two younger siblings, because it failed to remove them as children from their abusive home.[55] Jake Pierce won £25,000 compensation because of failures by social services. A social services department had returned him to the care of his parents without making a proper assessment and the court held that this fell short of the standard of practice to be expected of a reasonably competent local authority and it was therefore negligent. Pierce had been subjected to almost daily beatings by his parents and was kept in squalid conditions.[56] The House of Lords considered the nature of the duty of care owed by a local authority to children under the Children (Leaving Care) Act 2000 in a case where it held the duty of care owed by the local authority's children's services unit to look after a homeless child could not be fulfilled by referring the child to the homeless persons unit.[57]

The Court of Appeal held in July 2013 that for the purposes of section 23C(4) of the Children Act 1989 as amended by the Children (Leaving Care) Act 2000 a child who had been in care up to the age of 18 was entitled to have his educational expenses met by the local authority and these included university tuition fees.[58]

Further provisions relating to the transition for children to adult care and support are made in the sections 58–66 of the Care Act 2014 and shown in Statute Box 13.3.

Statute 13.3
Sections 58–66 Care Act 2014

58 Assessment of a child's needs for care and support
59 Child's needs assessment: requirements etc.
60 Assessment of a child's carer's needs for support
61 Child's carer's assessment: requirements etc.
62 Power to meet child's carer's needs for support
63 Assessment of a young carer's needs for support
64 Young carer's assessment: requirements etc.
65 Assessments under sections 58 to 64: further provision
66 Continuity of services under other legislation

Working Together to Safeguard Children

This is a guide to inter-agency working to safeguard and promote the welfare of children. Strengthened guidance was published in 2018[59] to reflect changes to the law introduced by the Children and Social Work Act 2017. This amends the Children Act 2004 and replaces local child safeguarding boards with safeguarding partners for local authority areas in England.

The three safeguarding partners, police, health and councils, are required to make joint safeguarding decisions to meet the needs of local children and families. Senior police, council and health leaders will jointly be responsible for setting out local plans to keep children safe and will be accountable for how well agencies work together to protect children from abuse and neglect. The new *Working Together to Safeguard Children* guidance is aimed at all professionals who come into contact with children and families and includes guidance on current threats to child protection, such as sexual and criminal exploitation, gangs and radicalisation.

Key changes to guidance and law include:

- equal duties placed on the police, clinical commissioning groups (CCGs) and local authorities to work together on safeguarding decisions and to promote children's welfare;
- greater accountability on senior leaders for each agency: the council Chief Executive, the accounting officer of a CCG and the Chief Officer of Police;
- strengthening expectations on schools and other educational settings that they must cooperate with the multi-agency safeguarding arrangements;
- extending safeguarding responsibilities to sports clubs and religious organisations in recognition of their important role in working with and protecting children and young people;

- new duties on CCGs and councils to carry out reviews of child deaths, instead of children's services, in line with evidence that only a small number of these incidents relate to safeguarding concerns; and
- better reviews of complex or nationally-important cases, and improving identification of the lessons learnt from these, led by the new Child Safeguarding Practice Review Panel chaired by Edward Timpson that replace Serious Case Reviews.

Duties in the Children Act 1989 that require inter-agency cooperation include:

> **Section 27 enables a local authority to request help from: any local authority; any local education authority; any local housing authority; any health authority and any person authorised by the Secretary of State or, in Wales, the National Assembly. The request must be responded to.**
>
> **Under Section 47, a duty is placed on such organisations or persons to help a local authority with its enquiries in cases where there is reasonable cause to suspect that a child is suffering or is likely to suffer significant harm.**

Where a child had been assaulted by one or other of two people, the court was not required to identify which one was the perpetrator.[60]

Following the inquiry conducted by Lord Laming into the death of Victoria Climbié[61] the Department of Health published a detailed response, 'Keeping Children Safe',[62] and this was followed by a single source document for safeguarding children.[63] This document aimed to provide a single set of advice for all those involved in the care of children, which replaced local guidance. It was followed by a Green Paper, 'Every Child Matters',[64] published in September 2003. The Green Paper focused on four main areas:

1. supporting parents and carers;
2. early intervention and effective protection;
3. accountability and integration – locally, regionally and nationally; and
4. workforce reform.

Five outcomes were considered as key to well-being in childhood and later life: being healthy, staying safe, enjoying and achieving, making a positive contribution and achieving economic well-being.

A Children's Commissioner (one was already appointed in Wales) has been established as an independent champion for children. (The functions set out in section 2 of the Children Act 2004 are replaced by section 107 of the Children and Families Act 2014.) In addition, legislation to create a Director of Children's Services accountable for local authority education and children's social services was proposed. A Minister for Children, Young People and Families has been created in the Department for Education. The Children Act 2004 provides the legal underpinning for 'Every Child Matters' and its provisions are shown in Box 13.2. Significant features include the new Local Safeguarding Children Boards, and the duty on local authorities to appoint a Director of Children's Services and a lead member for children's services. Regulations for the Local Safeguarding Children Boards were issued in 2006[65] and amended in 2010.[66]

The Children and Families Act 2014 makes provision on the adoption and contact (Part 1); family justice (Part 2); those with special educational needs (Part 3 – supplemented by regulations[67]); childcare (Part 4); welfare of children (Part 5); the Children's Commissioner (Part 6); statutory rights to leave and pay; time of work, antenatal care and flexible working (Parts 7–9) (See chapter 10) and General Provisions (10).

Concerns were expressed by Ofsted in 2014 that another Climbié abuse case could be forthcoming because of the large unknown private fostering arrangements which are not reported to local authorities (LA) as required by law.[68]

Box 13.2 Provisions of the Children Act 2004

Part 1 Children's Commissioner

Part 2 Children's services in England

    Cooperation to improve well-being

    Arrangements to safeguard and promote welfare

    Information databases

    Local Safeguarding Children Boards: establishment, functions, procedure and funding

    Children and young people's plans

    Director of children's services

    Lead member for children's services

    Inspections of children's services

Part 3 Children's services in Wales

Following the Lord Laming inquiry into the death of Victoria Climbié, the Joint Chief Inspectors have reported on safeguarding arrangements for children and young people in England. The Healthcare Commission contributed to the third Joint Chief Inspectors' Report on Safeguarding Children, published in October 2008. The Children's Inspectorate is now the Office for Standards in Education and Social Care and it reviews the work of Local Safeguarding Children Boards. Section 11 of the Children Act 2004 places a statutory duty on key people and bodies to make arrangements to safeguard and promote the welfare of children. The Department for Children, Schools and Families (DCSF) issued statutory guidance on the duty in 2005 and a revised version was published in April 2007. Part 1 of the guidance sets out the arrangements that are likely to be common to all or most of the agencies concerned. Part 2 deals with implementation in each particular agency to which the Section 11 duty applies. The DCSF stated that:

These arrangements require all agencies to have:

- **senior management commitment to the importance of safeguarding and promoting children's welfare;**
- **a clear statement of the agency's responsibilities towards children, available for all staff;**
- **a clear line of accountability within the organisation for work on safeguarding and promoting the welfare of children;**

- service development that takes account of the need to safeguard and promote welfare, and is informed, where appropriate, by the views of children and families;
- training on safeguarding and promoting the welfare of children for all staff working with, or in contact with, children and families;
- safe recruitment procedures in place;
- effective inter-agency working to safeguard and promote the welfare of children; and
- effective information sharing.

In 2010 the DCSF was replaced by the Department of Education (DE).

The RCN has published guidance on child protection and the nurse[69] and emphasises the need of each trust to have a designated or named nurse for child protection, have child protection procedures in place and have a defined policy on raising concerns about colleagues. A self-assessment tool for child protection arrangements for clinicians was updated and relaunched by the Healthcare Commission in 2004 and is available from the CQC website. Guidance was provided in 2007 for practitioners and managers to help them identify and deal with abuse which may be linked to a belief in spirit possession. The guidance followed the research report on child abuse linked with accusations of possessions and witchcraft published in June 2006.[70]

The case of Baby P

Baby P died in Haringey as a result of appalling abuse, despite being seen on over 60 occasions by health professionals, social services staff, police and others. He was known to be at risk. The Director of Children's Services was dismissed. (She eventually was awarded £679,452 by the Court of Appeal for unfair and unlawful dismissal, the Department of Education being required to contribute to that sum because the then Secretary of Education had issued unlawful directions to Haringey about her future.)

The GP who saw Baby P eight days before his death was found guilty by the GMC of a serious breach of a professional duty for not acting upon the visible signs of child abuse. Lord Laming was invited to report on the failings which had led to Baby P's death. Lord Laming's report,[71] published on 12 March 2009, put forward 52 recommendations for improving child protection services, some of which are shown in Figure 13.1. A consultant paediatrician, Dr Kim Holt, who raised concerns about the clinic that sent Baby P home to die, sued the NHS for compensation after complaining that she was forced out of her job and suffered a nervous breakdown.[72] She has subsequently received an apology from Great Ormond Street hospital and in 2014 was appointed as a professional adviser to the CQC.

Figure 13.1 Recommendations from Lord Laming's report in March 2009

- National agency to oversee reform implementation. Cabinet minister responsible for success
- Social work students must get child protection training and work experience before starting their job
- Increased quality of degrees; introduction of a children's social worker postgraduate qualification
- Court fees for applying to take children into care should be scrapped if they affect decisions
- Ofsted inspectors examining children's social services to have child protection experience
- A national strategy to address recruitment problems
- Guidelines on caseloads
- Directors with no child protection experience should appoint an experienced social work manager to support them

Lord Laming found that many authorities had failed to adopt the reforms recommended in the Victoria Climbié Inquiry in 2000. In February 2009 it was reported that two-thirds of hospitals fail to conduct routine checks on injured children suspected of being at risk, despite warnings after the death of Baby P.[73] There have been many official reports into the circumstances surrounding the death of Baby P. Two have been carried out by Haringey Council itself; the Audit Commission on children's services reported on 4 March 2009 and the Laming Report on Baby P was published on 12 March 2009. The Healthcare Commission's investigation of the NHS care surrounding Baby P was published by the CQC in May 2009.[74] This report found systematic errors in how the NHS trusts dealt with the case of Baby P and made recommendations to the trusts involved. These included:

- The NHS trusts should ensure that their staff are clear about child protection procedures and have received safeguarding training to an appropriate level.
- A sufficient number of appropriately qualified paediatric staff should be available when required, in line with established guidelines.
- The adequacy of consultant cover should be reviewed at one hospital.
- All four NHS trusts need to establish clear communication and working arrangements with relevant social services departments and, in particular, ensure that there is no delay in establishing contact between agencies once a safeguarding referral has been made to social services.
- The trusts must ensure that appropriate arrangements are in place to enable:
  - safeguarding supervision;
  - staff to attend multi-agency child protection case conferences;
  - appropriate training to be undertaken;
  - signing off the trusts' own declarations against core standards, assuring themselves that they can do so and do so adequately.

The Baby P case shows that coordination between the various services involved meant that no one took control and that there were serious failures by doctors and health visitors to detect evidence of non-accidental injuries. There were also poor links between health and social services. As a consequence of government action, £60 million was made available to bring about changes in child protection. These changes included all children's services directors being sent for compulsory training in the realities of frontline social work under plans to drive up standards in child protection that were announced on 13 March 2009.[75]

The government's initial response to Laming was published in 2009 and a year later, in March 2010, it published a progress report.[76] It looked at National Leadership in the form of a Cabinet forum on which four key Secretaries of State sat; the appointment of a Chief Adviser on the Safety of Children; the establishment of a National Safeguarding Delivery Unit (NSDU); the setting up of safeguarding national indicators and targets and revisions to *Working Together to Safeguard Children*. It also reviewed the system for regulation and inspection and the role of the CQC (see chapter 5). It considered the revised guidance for Area Child Protection Officers on investigating child abuse and safeguarding children and the comprehensive toolkit for forces to incorporate into practice. A table sets out a comparison of Laming's recommendations in 2009, the Government's response in May 2009 and the progress in March 2010. An annex provides a template for serious case review executive summaries. *Working Together to Safeguard Children* was updated in the light of the recommendations.

Criticism of the care system was made by the cross-party Children, Schools and Families Select Committee on 20 April 2009. The Committee called for a new national framework of fees and allowances for foster parents, who look after about two-thirds of the 60,000 children in the care system, in order to attract and retain better families. Other criticisms related to the fact that many children left care at 16 years, encouraged by local authorities on financial grounds, yet this was the time when they could go off the rails, and of the lack of training of staff in care homes. Care should become a positive experience for the child. The House of Commons Education Committee held in March 2014 that children in residential care should not be placed more than 20 miles from their own homes.

A review of the culture and barriers within the care of children was chaired by Sir Ian Kennedy who reported in September 2010[77] and made significant recommendations on how the services should be radically revised. One of its conclusions was that GPs and nurses should receive extra training in the care of children as a matter of urgency because young people's welfare is such a priority for the NHS. The RCPCH welcomed the report and said that the challenge was how the Kennedy Report would fit in with the other changes proposed by the government that affect children.[78]

Many of the findings in Kennedy's report were incorporated into the Department of Health's plans for the health of children and young people.[79] This emphasises the importance of ensuring that decisions are made with the family; that information is available on an age-specific basis; services should be child-centred; and respecting the wishes of the Gillick-competent child.

In November 2010 the cross-party Public Accounts Committee found that following the Baby P case the children's family court service was unable to cope with the surge of children being taken into care and did not have a contingency plan to deal with the influx of cases.[80]

In April 2010 it was reported that following an Audit Commission finding that children's services in Doncaster Council were not fit for their purpose, the government was prepared to use statutory powers to appoint commissioners and take over the running of the Council.[81] The Audit Commission had sent inspectors into the borough after two brothers of 10 and 11 in the care of social services were sentenced for an attack on children aged 9 and 11.

Any nurse must also be alert to the possibility of a colleague causing harm to a patient. This is considered in the section on whistleblowing in chapter 4. The RCPCH published guidance in 2009 on fabricated or induced illness by carers which is available on its website. Other issues that arise in relation to non-accidental injury include disclosure of confidential information (this is covered in chapter 8) and giving evidence before the court (covered in chapter 9).

The case of Daniel Pelka

A serious case review was set up following the death of Daniel Pelka, aged four, who had been starved and battered to death by his mother and stepfather, both of whom were convicted of his murder and given life sentences. The report was published on 17 September 2013 and found that numerous opportunities were missed by social workers, the police, teachers and doctors all of whom had contact with Daniel and his family. No single agency or individual was blamed for the death. The report called for improvements in the identification and reporting of domestic abuse and better reporting by schools of injuries to children. There was no record of any conversation held with Daniel about his home life, his experiences, his wishes and his feelings. The report is available on the Coventry website.[82] It emphasised the importance of integrating the lessons which had been learnt into safeguarding practice. *The Times* in its leader[83] stated that if one adult had taken responsibility then he might be still alive and suggested that a named social worker should be assigned to every at-risk child in the country and be responsible for his or her welfare.

A report by the Coventry Safeguarding Children Board found that health professionals had delayed passing on information and that there were unacceptable delays in circulating the minutes of a strategy meeting that looked at a broken arm suffered by Daniel in 2011.[84] On 21 March 2014 an Ofsted Report found that children's services at Coventry City Council remained inadequate: their leadership, management and governance were condemned and Ofsted questioned the effectiveness of the local children safeguarding board.[85]

Section 1 of the Children and Young Persons Act 1933 has been amended to widen the offence of failing to care for a child under sixteen. A person over sixteen also now commits the offence of neglect if they are intoxicated through drink or drugs and suffocate a child under three as a result of sharing a bed with them. The amendment was introduced by the Serious Crime Act 2015, section 66.

Child sex abuse: mandatory reporting

Following the scandals of mass sex abuse and grooming of girls in Rotherham and Rochdale the Home Affairs Select Committee published a damning report on 10 June 2013 recommending changes to the law and suggesting that the government should examine creating a mandatory duty for every professional to report suspicions of child sex abuse.[86] The government responded in September 2013[87] to each of the recommendations. It was not, however, considering any plans to introduce mandatory reporting of child abuse and neglect, given the robust reporting procedures already in place under *Working Together to Safeguard Children*. It stated that there is sufficient legislation and statutory guidance to tell professionals what should happen if they are concerned about a child. However, on 9 July 2014 the Prime Minister announced that a statutory duty to report suspected child abuse cases was under consideration.

Mandatory reporting of child abuse has been supported by the Children's Commissioner Maggie Atkinson and by Sir Keir Starmer, the former Director of Public Prosecutions. A private GP who had failed to report sex abuse claims about two children, aged four and six, and who said that he did not wish to read about procedures for safeguarding children was struck off by the GMC.[88]

A report published by Kids Company and the Centre for Social Justice think-tank called for a royal commission on child protection. It feared that budget cuts have left children subject to 'unscrupulous and illegal practices' by local authorities who order social workers to downgrade the dangers children are facing so that they can be given cheaper forms of help or none at all.[89] Kids Company have launched an Independent Children's Task Force chaired by Sir Keir Starmer (see above) to redesign children's social care and mental health services.

Liability of Local Authorities for Abuse of Children

Recent cases have held the local authority (LA) liable in respect of failures to take action to prevent abuse and in making negligent adoption and fostering arrangements. In 2001 the ECHR overruled the House of Lords' decision that the LA was not liable in negligence or for breach of statutory duty to children who had been abused by their parents.[90] The ECHR held that the local authority had a duty of care to the children, whose Article 3, 6 and 13 rights had been breached.[91] Two people who had been abused as children by their stepfather succeeded in their claim that the LA had failed to provide an appropriate means of obtaining a determination of their allegations. These allegations were that the LA had failed to protect them from serious ill treatment[92] and therefore were in breach of Article 13. (Article 13 requires there to be an effective remedy before a national authority for any breach of human rights notwithstanding that the violation has been committed by persons acting in an official capacity.) (Article 13 is not included in Schedule 1 of the Human Rights Act 1998 (see the website of this book).) On the facts, there was no breach of Article 3. In contrast, in another case the ECHR held that where the LA failed to protect children from sexual abuse by the stepfather, the LA was in violation of Article 3 and Article 13 and was held liable to pay damages.[93] In another case against a local authority, this time by a couple who adopted a violent child, the couple won their case that they should have been notified by the LA of the boy's serious and emotional behavioural difficulties.[94] The court held that the LA could be held vicariously liable for negligence by its employees in failing to fulfil their duty of care owed to those who might foreseeably be injured if the duty was carelessly exercised. Research conducted by the Fostering Network suggested that over half of foster parents had been given inadequate information about the children in their care which had put themselves and their own children at risk.[95]

Errors in identifying child abuse and human rights

There have been misdiagnoses of child abuse. For example, in one case,[96] following a case conference, a baby was taken into care on the basis of medical evidence that suggested that a spiral fracture of her femur was evidence of non-accidental injury. Subsequently, it was discovered that the baby suffered from brittle bone disease and the child was returned to the parents nine months after the hospital admission. The parents sued and action was also brought in the name of the child arguing a case of negligence, and breach of Article 8 of the European Convention on Human Rights. The claims failed on the grounds that the child had suffered no injury for which the law recognised a remedy; a duty of care was not owed by the defendants to the parents (the doctor owed a duty of care to the child and his obligations within the multidisciplinary process militated against the doctor owing any additional duty to the parents in relation to the diagnosis which commenced such a process) and to hold the doctor liable to the parents would cut across the statutory scheme set up for the protection of the child. The Human Rights Act came into force on 2 October 2000, was not retrospective and the cause of action arose in September 1998 and June 1999. In one case[97] in East Berkshire, a mother was suspected of Munchausen syndrome by proxy when her son suffered from allergic reactions following birth and he was placed on the 'at risk' register. However, it was subsequently discovered that he did have allergy problems. The mother claimed compensation on the grounds that the original diagnosis was made negligently. The House of Lords held that it would not be fair, just or reasonable to impose a duty of care on a doctor in respect of a negligent clinical diagnosis where there was a concurrent and potentially conflicting duty of care towards a child patient. No duty of care was owed to the parents. However, in 2010 the ECHR held that a duty of care was owed to parents and there were breaches of the European Convention on Human Rights.[98] The parents who had failed in their applications before the House of Lords[99] succeeded in their claim for compensation.

In the case of *MAK and RK v the UK* the ECHR held that the taking of blood samples and intimate photographs of a girl aged nine without her parents' consent violated Article 8 of the European Convention on Human Rights, which guaranteed the right to respect for private and family life (see the website of this book). There was also a violation of Article 13 because of the absence of an effective remedy. The ECHR ordered the UK to pay MAK (the mother) €2,000 and RK €4,500 and €15,000 jointly for their costs. The circumstances of the case were that bruising was noticed on the girl's skin and the paediatrician suspected abuse by the father. The paediatrician delayed in referring the girl to a dermatologist who diagnosed a rare skin disease.[100]

Surrey County Council social workers who enlisted the help of the police in removing a child of one from her parents were criticised by Mrs Judge Theis who held that the claims against the parents were not borne out by the evidence and social workers had misunderstood many issues. The girl had been born with heart problems and required surgery at 10 days old. She was in hospital for 11 months and the parents were taught how to care for her and coped for months with round the clock care regime, with professional support until concerns were raised about their care of the girl.[101]

In another case, Mrs Justice Pauffley said that she was profoundly alarmed at the discovery that family courts were effectively in cahoots with social services through clandestine arrangements which undermined the independence of the justice system. Courts were routinely removing children from their mothers into care without adequate investigation.[102]

The Court of Appeal in a decision involving two cases deplored failures, particularly by public bodies such as a local authority, to comply with court orders.[103] In the cases parents had appealed or opposed adoption orders and the local authorities had failed to comply with the orders.

In another case the ECHR held that failure by the LA to conduct a risk assessment, resulting in a child being placed with foster parents, was a breach of the Article 8 rights of the parent (AD) and the child (OD).[104] The paediatricians had noticed several fractures to the child's ribs and concluded that they were sustained non-accidentally, dismissing the possibility that the child might have brittle bone disease. Subsequently, the child was found to have brittle bone disease and normal handling could have caused the fractures. The Court of Appeal held that the LA did not owe a duty of care and there was no evidence that the child had suffered any actionable damage.[105] The ECHR found that there was both a breach of Article 8 rights and also Article 13 since the mother had no effective remedy for her complaints contrary to Article 13.

As a result of these cases it is now clear that the LA does have a duty of care to potential foster parents to ensure a risk assessment is carried out and to parents accused of child abuse to ensure that other causes of a child's injuries are examined prior to a child being taken into care.

Protection of Children Act 1999

This Act requires organisations to refer persons considered unsuitable to work with children to the Department of Health for inclusion on their list (see chapter 10).

Parental care and the nurse

Practical dilemma 13.5   Mum knows best

The children's ward at Roger Park Hospital introduced a scheme for mothers and other relatives to undertake some of the tasks in caring for the children. Originally, the scheme covered only the day-to-day routine care of dressing, feeding, bathing and amusing the child. Subsequently, however, it was extended to nursing and extended-role tasks, including the care of nasal-gastric feeding and intravenous medication. The reason for this extension was that several of the mothers of long-term chronically ill children undertook all these tasks in the community. The nurse or doctor had the task of ensuring that the mother had the appropriate training and the necessary equipment.

Mrs Tait agreed to give her four-year-old child, Robin, who had a chronic lung condition, the appropriate drugs intravenously every six hours. She had undertaken several such treatments on her own before and was familiar with the routine and procedure. On the ward, she was given the keys to help herself to the necessary drugs. This was contrary to the accepted practice but was permitted because it was felt that she could be trusted. She gave Robin the 8.00 a.m. treatment without problems. She had to leave the hospital in the afternoon but told another parent that she would be back for the afternoon treatment. Unfortunately, she did not return until 3.30 p.m. because of an unexpected traffic holdup. Robin was with some other children watching *Teletubbies*. Mrs Tait immediately went to the staff nurse to get the keys to draw up the drugs for the next treatment. She took the boxes from the cupboard and started to make up the syringes. She then took Robin into the single room to give him his treatment. As she was giving the medication, Robin became very ill and she called for help. It was then discovered that the afternoon dose had already been given to Robin and although this had been written up into his notes, the nurse who did so was at tea when Mrs Tait returned and she herself did not check Robin's notes as it was never her practice to do so. Robin suffered severe renal failure as a result of an overdose of an antibiotic. Is the accident entirely the mother's fault or does the nurse carry some responsibility?

What is the situation where responsibilities like this are divided between several people? In legal terms, it is probably true to say that the care of the child in hospital is primarily the responsibility of the nurse under the clinical supervision of the medical staff. In a sense, the nurse is delegating to the mother those duties that she is capable of performing and probably performs on her own at home. The nurse should only delegate those tasks that she feels the mother is competent to perform and, in addition, she should ensure that the mother (or, of course, any other relative, friend or volunteer) has the correct amount of training and supervision to undertake the task safely. The nurse would be responsible in negligence if she delegated an unsuitable task to the mother or failed to provide her with the appropriate instructions or gave her inadequate supervision. If, however, the nurse has satisfied all those requirements and something still goes wrong because the mother makes a mistake, then it would be the mother's responsibility for any harm caused to the child as a result of the mistake.

In the above situation, there is clearly a failure in communication between nurse and mother. It would have been preferable to set up a procedure whereby the mother was told to look at the drug chart, to fill it in when she gave the drugs to the child and also to check that the drugs had not already been given. She should also be supervised in her administration of the drugs. It is questionable whether the mother should have been allowed direct access to the medicines. Clearly, the nurse would be at fault in failing to set up this procedure and the supervision, and the mother would bear some responsibility for failing to check that they had been given, although in mitigation it could be said that the person responsible for the ward at the time she returned should have known the child had already had his medication and informed the mother accordingly. The problems relating to supervision and instructing others are dealt with more fully in chapter 23. The RCN has provided guidance on administering intravenous therapy to children in the community.[106] The Department of Health has published an NHS childcare strategy to provide affordable and accessible quality childcare and is attracting more staff to work in the NHS. Further information is available from the DH website.

Disciplining a child

Practical dilemma 13.6   The nurse *in loco parentis*

Adam was a bright seven-year-old who appeared totally undaunted by his stay in hospital for a hernia operation. Unfortunately, his mother could spend very little time with him as she had two younger children and her husband was overseas. Once Adam had recovered from the immediate effects of his operation, he was uncontrollable. He wandered around the wards into the single-bed wards, ignoring all the nurses' instructions and delighting in disobeying them. In one of the single rooms, a child was being barrier nursed with suspected meningitis. Staff Nurse James saw Adam about to enter this room and in her anxiety and her impatience with him, she hit him hard on the leg. Adam screamed and other nurses came running. Staff Nurse James was disciplined by the senior nurse and Adam's mother said that she was going to make a formal complaint against the nurse and the hospital. Staff Nurse James argued that in the circumstances there was little else she could have done to prevent Adam entering that room and, in any case, she had the powers of a parent to discipline a child who needed to be controlled.

The ECHR has ruled that severe corporal punishment to discipline children was a breach of Article 3 of the European Convention on Human Rights.[107] In the case, a stepfather had beaten a nine-year-old boy on several occasions with a garden cane. The stepfather had been prosecuted for assault occasioning actual bodily harm, but had been acquitted by the jury who accepted his defence that the caning had been necessary and reasonable to discipline the boy. The ECHR held that ill treatment must attain a minimum level of severity if it is to fall within the scope of Article 3. It depended on all the circumstances of the case, such as the nature and context of the treatment, its duration, its physical and mental effects and, in some instances, the sex, age and state of health of the victim. In finding that there had been a breach of Article 3, it awarded the boy £10,000 against the UK government and costs. The UK government acknowledged that the UK law failed to provide adequate protection to children and should be amended. Subsequently, guidance was issued by the government on the use of corporal punishment against children. Guidance for good practice in restraining, holding still and containing children has been issued by the RCN.[108] The Joint Committee of House of Lords and House of Commons,[109] in monitoring the UK compliance with the UN Charter on the Rights of the Child, considered that the retention in UK use of the defence of 'reasonable chastisement' is incompatible with the provisions of Article 19 of the Convention. Subsequently, the Children Act 2004 was enacted and section 58 is shown in Statute Box 13.4.

> ## Statute 13.4
> ### Section 58 Children Act 2004
>
> 1. In relation to any offence specified in subsection (2) below, battery of a child cannot be justified on the ground that it constituted reasonable punishment.
> 2. The offences referred to in subsection (1) are:
>   (a) An offence under Section 18 or 20 of the Offences against the Person Act 1861 (wounding and causing grievous bodily harm)
>   (b) An offence under Section 47 of that Act (assault occasioning actual bodily harm)
>   (c) An offence under Section 1 of the Children and Young Persons Act 1933 (cruelty to persons under 16).
> 3. Battery of a child causing actual bodily harm to a child cannot be justified in any civil proceedings on the ground that it constituted reasonable punishment.
> 4. For the purposes of subsection (3) 'actual bodily harm' has the same meaning as it has for the purposes of Section 47 of the Offences against the Person Act 1861.
> 5. In Section 1 of the Children and Young Persons Act 1933, omit subsection (7) (Section 1(7) made any parent or person having lawful control or charge of a child to administer punishment an exception to the offence of assaulting or wilfully ill-treating a child).

The effect of this section is that a parent who causes harm to his or her child and is prosecuted under the Offences Against the Person Act 1861 sections 18, 20 or 47 or under the Children and Young Persons Act 1933 section 1 cannot use a defence that the battery constituted reasonable punishment. The same applies in civil proceedings where actual bodily harm is caused.

In 2007 the Children's Commissioner for England called for a complete ban on smacking children[110] as a consultation on the effect of the change in the law was initiated. As a result of the review the Children's Minister ruled out a total ban on smacking children on 26 October 2007.[111] In March 2010 Sir Roger Singleton, Chief Adviser on the Safety of Children, published an independent report on 'Physical punishment: improving consistency and protection', which made three recommendations:

1. The current ban on physical punishment in schools and other children's settings should be extended to include any form of advice, guidance, teaching, training, instruction, worship, treatment or therapy and to any form of care or supervision which is carried out other than by a parent or member of the child's own family or household;
2. The government should continue to promote positive parenting strategies and effective behaviour management techniques directed towards eliminating the use of smacking. Parents who disapprove of smacking should make this clear to others who care for their children; and
3. The development of appropriate safeguarding policies in informal education and learning organisations should continue to be promoted. Legal changes which flow from adoption of these recommendations will need to be communicated effectively.

The government of the time accepted these recommendations.

It therefore follows that corporal punishment should not be used when acting in the place of the parents. In the above example, Staff Nurse James has acted unlawfully and other methods of control would have been preferable. There were other ways of stopping Adam entering the room other than hitting him and, in the circumstances, it seems more likely that she lost her temper and was unreasonable.

A respect for the rights of the child and good nursing practice would advocate no use of physical force against a patient. A nurse faces both criminal and civil proceedings against her personally if she uses corporal punishment on a patient. She would, however, be entitled to use reasonable force to protect herself or other people by restraining the child if she or others were threatened with violence. The implications of this for staffing levels are clear and the degree of unruliness in children and the extent of parental help could affect the level of staffing required. Guidance on the use of restraint and therapeutic holding in the care of children and young people is provided by the RCN.[112] Training for staff in coping with unruly children is essential.

In Wales the Children (Abolition of Defence of Reasonable Punishment) (Wales) Act 2020 makes any form of physical punishment, including smacking, unlawful. Similarly, in Scotland the Children (Equal Protection from Assault) (Scotland) Act 2019 makes it unlawful to physically punish a child in Scotland.

Adolescents

Some hospitals have set up adolescent units for those between 13 and 16/17 years so that special provisions can be made for those in this group. Difficult problems can arise, as Practical Dilemma 13.7 illustrates.

Practical dilemma 13.7 — Refusal to obey the rules

David, aged 15, suffered from cystic fibrosis and required regular IV antibiotic treatment. Roger Park Hospital had set up a specialist unit for youngsters suffering from cystic fibrosis, and rules had been laid down about the conduct of the patients. David frequently took his own discharge from hospital, returning with alcohol, and staff also feared that he was taking soft drugs. They tried to reason with him but he was not cooperative. His parents said that he should be made to comply with the hospital regime. What is the law?

In Practical Dilemma 13.7, the managers of the unit are entitled to lay down the terms on which patients and visitors may enter. If David is Gillick-competent, then he could agree an understanding with the unit that he will be admitted for treatment only on the basis of accepting the rules that have been laid down. If he refuses to agree to those conditions, including the prohibition on alcohol, then he could be told that he cannot be treated in the unit. In law his parents could give consent to his having treatment, but it is difficult for staff to maintain IV treatment if the young person is objecting to having it. In the long term, it may be possible for the CF patients and other patients with chronic conditions to agree on the 'house rules' and how they are to be implemented and thus bring peer pressure to bear on David. It is essential that the unit manager makes clear that the rules, especially relating to alcohol and illegal drugs, are enforced and those who do not accept the conditions cannot be cared for there. Where the adolescent is over 16 years and lacks capacity to give consent to a specific decision, the Mental Capacity Act 2005 would now apply. Action can be taken in the best interests of the young person. If there is a dispute about the lack of capacity or what would constitute 'best interests' for a particular patient, an application could be made to the Court of Protection. (See chapter 7 for further consideration of the Mental Capacity Act 2005.) The RCN has published several papers providing guidance for members on caring for adolescents. They include 'Adolescent Transition Care. Guidance for nursing staff',[113] which aims to secure a seamless transition for those with chronic diseases from children's to adult services. The RCN has also published 'Adolescence: boundaries and connections', which is an RCN guide for working with young people.[114] This guide resulted from an RCN survey which highlighted the need for person-centred, adolescent care. It includes practical tips that nurses can use in their daily work and addresses issues such as adolescent development, confidentiality, consent and local resources. It also includes comments from young people themselves. The RCN Adolescent Forum has developed information to offer guidance to nurses involved in caring for the needs of young people covering consent to treatment, primary care and nurse training.[115]

Deprivation of liberty of children and young persons

Concern that children and young persons could be deprived of their liberty in hospitals and other care setting were confirmed by the United Kingdom Supreme Court in *Cheshire West and Chester Council* v *P* [2014].[116] In this case the Supreme Court held that a 17-year-old, who was an inpatient in an NHS unit for adolescents with learning disabilities and challenging behaviour, was confined to the unit and so deprived of her liberty. Since the Supreme Court ruling in *Cheshire West* the courts have been asked to consider the cases of other minors in care settings to determine whether they too were deprived of their liberty.[117]

It is essential that nurses working with children and young people inform their practice by reference to these cases and seek authorisation where a minor is being deprived of their liberty.

Minors

The United Nations Convention on the Rights of the Child (1989)[118] defines a child as 'every human being below the age of 18 years . . . unless national laws recognise the age of majority earlier'. In the United Kingdom, by convention, the courts refer to all persons under 18 as minors with those under 16 referred to as children and 16- and 17-year-olds as young persons. No minor is a wholly autonomous being and a person, usually a parent, with parental responsibility can make decisions in relation to the minor until they reach majority at 18 (Children Act 1989, section 2).

Deprivation of Liberty

The European Convention on Human Rights[119] guarantees a limited right to liberty under article 5. A person cannot be deprived of their liberty unless it is in accordance with the situations set out in the article and is authorised by law.

Determining whether the restrictions imposed on a minor amount to a deprivation of liberty is an essential requirement for nurses working with children and young persons. The European Court of Human Rights (ECtHR) in *Storck v Germany ECHR 406* (2005)[120] held that three elements had to be satisfied for a minor to be deprived of their liberty:

- An objective element;
- A subjective element; and
- Imputability to the state.

Objective deprivation of liberty

In *Storck* the ECtHR held that the question of whether a minor was objectively deprived of their liberty depended on whether the minor was confined in a particular place for more than a negligible length of time. In *Cheshire West and Chester Council v P* [2014] the UK Supreme Court held that an objective deprivation of liberty depended on the specific situation of the minor but the acid test for determining whether that situation satisfied the *Storck* objective component was whether the minor was under the continuous supervision and control of those caring for them and was not free to leave the place where they were accommodated.

Two elements arise from the acid test:

- Continuous supervision and control – where the minor is subject to an enduring period of observation and is continuously required to follow instruction, seek permission or have another undertake a task on their behalf; and
- Not being free to leave – where the minor cannot pack their bags and move to alternative accommodation without permission.

Restriction and deprivation of liberty

The Courts accept that it is not uncommon for restrictions to be placed on a minor, particularly a younger child to ensure their safety and to discipline the child. These restrictions do not amount to a deprivation of liberty. There is a clear distinction between an objective deprivation of liberty, and a mere restriction on liberty of movement (*Re K (A Child) (Secure Accommodation Order: Right to Liberty)* [2001]).[121]

In *Re A-F (Children) (Care Orders: Restrictions on Liberty)* [2018][122] a deprivation of liberty does not arise because a parent or other person *in loco parentis*:

- makes it a rule that a child of tender years is not to leave the house unless accompanied by some suitable person; or
- an exasperated parent has sent a naughty child to his room and told him to stay there for two hours; or
- a rebellious teenager has been grounded or subjected to a parentally enforced curfew, even where this is enforced by locking a door.

Age can also be a determinative component of the *Storck* objective element of a deprivation of liberty. In *Cheshire West and Chester Council v P* [2014] the Supreme Court held that the situation of a young child does not involve a confinement even where the acid test appears to be met. Lord Kerr in Cheshire West suggested that a three-year-old child must be restrained for his or her own safety if walking near a busy road, or playing near a bonfire. Such restraint would be unlawful if exercised over an adult but would be lawful, and required of any nearby adult, if exercised over the child.

For there to be a restriction that amounts to confinement meeting the *Storck* objective element there needs to be an interruption or curtailment of the freedom of action normally ascribed to a child of that age and understanding.

In *Re B* [2017][123] an eleven-year-old boy with autistic spectrum disorder accommodated in a residential unit and assessment centre where he was:

- subject to supervision from a distance (he was not followed but staff were always aware where he was and what he was doing);
- not left alone with the other child in the placement;
- always accompanied when out in the community;
- subject, from time to time, to the removal and/or limitation of access to a computer and Xbox; and
- subject to numerous specialist methods used by staff to deal with his behaviour, including physical restraint.

The Court held that while some of the restrictions would be in place for any child of B's age there were significant restrictions that did amount to an objective deprivation of liberty including:

- effectively being under 24-hour watch, i.e. he was never left unsupervised with the other young person in the placement;
- having restricted and supervised contact with his parents and siblings; and
- being physically restrained on a significant number of occasions due to his physically challenging behaviour, which included assaults on staff and a need for an increased staff presence.

The subjective element

The second element of a *Storck* determination of a deprivation of liberty requires that the person has not subjectively agreed to the restrictions they are under. In *Nielsen* v *Denmark (33488/96) (2000)*[124] the ECtHR held that a parent could consent to restrictions that amounted to an objective deprivation of liberty on behalf of a minor if it was a reasonable exercise of their parental responsibility. A parent could therefore consent on behalf of a child to restrictions that would otherwise be an objective deprivation of liberty.

For those aged 16 or 17 the UK Supreme Court held in *Re D (a child)* [2019][125] that it would not be a reasonable exercise of parental responsibility to consent to arrangements that amounted to a deprivation of liberty of a minor who was 16 or 17. The young persons were entitled to the protection of the ECHR and any deprivation of liberty would need to be authorised by the court of protection.

In many cases involving restrictions and restraint of a minor under 16 in hospital, a deprivation of liberty would not arise if the nurse obtained the consent of a person with parental responsibility. That requirement does, however, highlight limits to the use of consent.

A foster carer does not generally have parental responsibility that would enable the carer to provide a valid consent for the purpose of the *Storck* subjective element. Similarly, where a child is subject to a care order (interim or final) then neither the local authority nor the parents can exercise parental responsibility in such a way as to provide a valid consent that meets the *Storck* subjective element.

Imputability to the state

The reason why a local authority or the parents of a child cannot consent to what would otherwise be a deprivation of liberty where there is a care order is the involvement of the state in the exercise of parental responsibility over the minor.

In *AB (A Child) (Deprivation of Liberty: Consent)* [2015][126] the Court found that while it might be appropriate for a parent to consent to restrictions on a minor that amount to a deprivation of liberty, where the minor was subject to a care order such consent would be outside the zone of parental responsibility. The state could not consent to a deprivation of liberty and so the local authority would be unable to consent to the restrictions even where the court had granted parental responsibility as part of the care order. As all three elements of *Storck* are met, there will be a deprivation of liberty that will need to be authorised to be lawful.

The National Deprivation of Liberty Court

In response to the increasing numbers of applications to the family division of the High Court requesting authorisation of a child under 16's deprivation of liberty, the president created a specialist National Deprivation of Liberty Court that launched in 2022.

The number of applications requesting the High Court exercise its inherent jurisdiction to authorise a child's deprivation of liberty rose from 108 case in 2017 to 579 cases in 2021 (Roe 2021)[127].

The aim of the National Deprivation of liberty Court is to develop expertise in cases where children with complex needs and those at risk of significant harm are subject to restrictions that amount to a deprivation of liberty. This Court does not hear cases relating to adults or minors under 16 who lack mental capacity.

Authorising the deprivation of liberty of a child

Local authorities would generally deprive a child of their liberty through the use of secure accommodation orders obtained from a court under section 25 of the Children Act 1989 or section 119 of the Social Services and Wellbeing (Wales) Act 2014. The Children (Secure Accommodation) Regulations 1991[128] and the The Children Secure Accommodation (Wales) Regulations 2015[129] extend the use of secure accommodation to hospitals.

Local authorities can only make use of secure accommodation in suitably registered children's homes. Hospitals and other health service premises can make use of the power without having to pre designated the accommodation as secure but can only use it for 72 hours in any 28 day period before requiring authorisation from a court (*Re B (A Minor) (Treatment and Secure Accommodation)* [1997])[130].

The inherent jurisdiction of the High Court

The limited availability of registered secure accommodation and the complex needs of the children requiring restrictions to protect them from significant harms means that secure accommodation orders are not suitable or not available in many cases.

Where a child with complex mental or physical health needs is deprived of their liberty in accommodation that is not secure accommodation then a judge of the family division of the High Court can authorise the deprivation of liberty by exercising their inherent jurisdiction (*Re D* [2017][131]). The Court can exercise its inherent jurisdiction where it has reasonable cause to believe that the child would otherwise suffer significant harm (Children Act 1989, section 100(4)).

In *Re X* [2016][132] the Court held that a judge exercising the inherent jurisdiction of the court, with respect to minors, has the power to direct that the minor shall be placed and remain in a specified institution such as a hospital or residential unit. The courts powers extend to authorising the minor's deprivation of liberty and the use of reasonable force to ensure the minor remains there.

In *Re X* [2016] a 10-year-old boy with autism spectrum disorder and a learning disability put himself in dangerous situations that required him to have constant supervision and periods of physical restraint in the specialist unit where he was accommodated. The Court accepted that the restrictions were necessary to promote his welfare and protect him from harm and did amount to a deprivation of liberty. The court also accepted that it would not be appropriate to move the minor to a unit that provided secure accommodation and his needs were being fully met in the specialist unit. The Court authorised the deprivation of liberty by exercising the inherent jurisdiction.

The national deprivation of liberty court now hears such cases to ensure consistency and to develop the expertise of judges. Since its introduction it has hear some 854 children have been subject to an application for a deprivation of liberty authorisation.

In its analysis of the cases the **Nuffield Family Justice Observatory (2023)**[133] the applications are made because of an immediate and severe risk to the child compounded by a lack of suitable accommodation registered to care for children with complex needs in secure accommodation. This requires the national deprivation of liberty court to authorise deprivations of liberty in unregistered placements such as hospitals and residential homes in fifty percent of cases.

Typical of the complex cases heard by the national deprivation of liberty court is *Re J (Deprivation of Liberty: Hospital)* [2022][134] where The court considered whether to authorise the continued deprivation of liberty of a 13-year-old girl at a hospital pending her transfer to a bespoke placement.

The girl was subject to an interim care order. Lack of provision for children with complex needs, resulted in her being accommodated in a hospital for three months. She had no mental or physical health requirement for inpatient treatment and the hospital environment was not suitable for her needs. Her mother was unwilling and unable to accommodate her, a foster placement was not viable, secure accommodation was not suitable and a children's home would not accept her due to her behaviour. The local authority had identified a rented property at which care could be provided and would allow her to continue school. The girl was subject to continual confinement, she did not and could not consent to them and the restrictions were imputable to the state.

The Court held that a local authority could place a child in a hospital. However, the court had to be satisfied that it was necessary, proportionate and in the child's best interests for authorisation to be given. There was no alternative place for her and the restrictions amounting to the deprivation of her liberty had been needed to keep her safe whilst living at the hospital.

A hospital was not a suitable place for a 13-year-old girl who had no need for treatment. However, due to the national lack of resources to accommodate and care for children with complex needs, that appeared to be the only place where she could live until the local authority was able to arrange and have ready the proposed bespoke placement. Remaining at the hospital during the transition to the new placement would afford her some stability at least.

Conclusions

It is clear from the cases of Baby P and Daniel Pelka that the reforms to child protection following the Children Act 2004 have not been effective in preventing deaths of children, even when these cases were well known to health and social care professionals. Figures released to the *Sunday Times* under the Freedom of Information Act in 2013 suggested that up to 110 deaths had occurred from neglect or abuse at home in the six years following the Baby P case.[135] The Alexis Jay Independent Inquiry into the child sexual exploitation in Rotherham between 1997 and 2013 raises major concerns about child protection safeguards and the accountability of senior officers in the local authority and police. The Labour government prior to the coalition government had published a 10-year Children's Plan which included a comprehensive review of Child and Adolescent Mental Health Services, the primary school curriculum, speech and language therapy and special educational needs, the development of Master's level qualifications for all new teachers, a national plan to tackle child obesity, a review of poor housing and a Youth Crime Action Plan.[136] The coalition government published its vision for child services[137] and it remains to be seen the extent to which this can be implemented at a time of considerable cuts in public expenditure. There will continue to be considerable pressure on nurses working with babies, children and adolescents in this high-profile, challenging area of nursing. The Children, Schools and Families Act 2010 Part 2 gives the media enhanced access to family proceedings which are thus likely to receive more publicity. The Children and Families Act 2014 (Part 2) makes significant changes to improve the operation of the family justice system. In private family law, couples are required to attend a family mediation, information and assessment meeting before being able to apply for certain orders, both separated parents should be involved in the children's lives if that is safe and consistent with the welfare of the child. A child arrangements order replaces residence and contact orders. In public law a maximum 26-week time limit is set for completing care and supervision proceedings, with the possibility of an extension of up to eight weeks at a time if necessary to resolve proceedings justly. The Court of Appeal has held that there was no longer a supposed 'rule' that where two parents had parental responsibility for a child, neither could unilaterally change the child's habitual residence. What was required was a factual inquiry tailored to the circumstances of an individual case.[138]

Reflection questions

1. What is the difference between a child of 15 and one of 16 years as far as consent to treatment is concerned? What is the effect of the Family Law Reform Act 1969 Section 8?

2. Consider the extent to which your department allows parents to take part in the care of children in hospital. What additional responsibilities does this place on the nurse?

Further exercises

1. Examine the UN Charter on the Rights of the Child. What impact does this have on the care of the child in hospital?
2. Obtain a copy of your NHS trust's procedure on the care of suspected non-accidental injury cases and familiarise yourself with it.
3. If you were faced with a very disobedient child, how would you control them?
4. Access the procedures for child protection prepared by your organisation and familiarise yourself with their implications for your work.

References

1. P.R. Ghandhi, *Blackstone's International Human Rights Documents*, 3rd edn, Oxford University Press, Oxford, 2003
2. Department of Health, Welfare of Children and Young People in Hospital, HMSO, London, 1991
3. Audit Commission, Children First: a study of hospital services, HMSO, London, 1993
4. Royal College of Nursing, Children's Services: acute health care provision, Order No. 001055, RCN, June 1999
5. Royal College of Nursing, Children's Services: acute health care provision, Order No. 001156, RCN, July 2001
6. Royal College of Nursing, Children and Young People's Nursing: a philosophy of care guidance for nursing staff, Order No. 002012, RCN, April 2003
7. Royal College of Nursing, Preparing Nurses to Care for Children and Young People, Order No. 001997, RCN, April 2003; Royal College of Nursing, Signpost Guide for Nurses Working with Young People, Order No. 002021, RCN, April 2003
8. Royal College of Nursing, Getting it Right for Children and Young People. A self-assessment toolkit for practice nurses, 002 77725, RCN, April 2006
9. Royal College of Nursing, Safeguarding Children and Young People – every nurse's responsibility, order No. 004542 RCN, 2014
10. British Medical Association, Consent, Rights and Choices in the Healthcare for Children and Young People, BMA, 2001
11. www.rcpch.ac.uk
12. Sarah-Kate Templeton, Poor NHS care 'kills 2,000 children', *Sunday Times*, 29 September 2013
13. *An NHS Trust v X* [2021] EWHC 65 (Fam)
14. *Bell & Anor v The Tavistock And Portman NHS Foundation Trust* [2020] EWHC 3274 (Admin)
15. *In re W (A Minor: medical treatment)* [1992] 4 All ER 627
16. *An NHS Foundation Trust v A, M, P, and A Local Authority* [2014] EWHC 920
17. *An NHS Foundation Trust v P* [2014] EWHC 1650 (Fam)
18. *In re W (A Minor: medical treatment)* [1992] 4 All ER 627
19. *An NHS Foundation Trust v P* [2014] EWHC 1650 (Fam)
20. *Re E (A Minor: wardship: medical treatment)* [1993] 1 FLR 386 FD
21. *Re S (A minor: consent to medical treatment)* [1994] 2 FLR 1065
22. *R (On the application of Axon) v Secretary of State* [2006] EWHC 37 Admin
23. *MAK and RK v UK* [2010] 363 ECHR
24. *TM (Medical Treatment) Re* [2013] EWHC 4103 Fam

[25] Ian Kennedy and Andrew Grubb, *Medical Law*, Butterworths, London, 2000
[26] *Gillick v West Norfolk and Wisbech AHA and the DHSS* [1985] 3 All ER 402 Refusal of blood by 15-year-old[*
[27] *Re L (Medical treatment: Gillick competency)* [1999] 1 Med L Review 58; [1998] 2 FLR 810
[28] *Re M (Medical treatment: consent)* [1999] 2 FLR 1097
[29] *In re D (A Minor: wardship, sterilisation)* [1976] 1 All ER 327
[30] *In re B (A Minor: wardship, sterilisation)* [1987] 2 All ER 206
[31] *R v Portsmouth Hospitals NHS Trust ex p Glass* [1999] 2 FLR 905; [1999] Lloyd's Law Rep Med, 367
[32] *Glass v United Kingdom*, The Times Law Report, 11 March 2004, ECHR
[33] Mark Henderson, DNA tests may threaten your child's rights, *The Times*, 4 August 2010
[34] Damian Whitworth, Joy of the family in front line of science, *The Times*, 5 October 2000
[35] *In re O (A Minor: medical treatment)* [1993] 4 Med LR 272
[36] *In re A (Minors: conjoined twins: medical treatment)*, The Times Law Report, 10 October 2000
[37] News item, *The Times*, 4 March 2014
[38] *In re B (A Minor)* [1981] 1 WLR 1421
[39] *Re C (A Minor) (medical treatment – refusal of parental consent)* [1997] 8 Med LR 166 CA also known as *Re T* [1997] 1 All ER 906
[40] News item, *The Times*, 29 October 1993
[41] Michael Horsnell, Couple jailed for starving tortured daughter to death, *The Times*, 21 September 2002
[42] Leila Haddou, Parents jailed for manslaughter of baby who had rickets, *Guardian*, 28 February 2014
[43] https://media.inzu.net/2acc977c715cd84d14a75f01032546ad/mysite/downloads/105_FinalOverviewReportBABYF.pdf
[44] *R v Arthur* (1981) 12 BMLR 1
[45] Royal College of Paediatrics and Child Health, Withholding or Withdrawing Life Saving Treatment in Children: a framework for practice, RCPCH, September 1997 (reissued in 2004)
[46] British Medical Association, Withholding and Withdrawing Life-prolonging Medical Treatment, 2nd edn, BMA, 2000
[47] *Health and Social Care Trust v M and others* [2014] NIFam 3
[48] *Camden LBC v R (A Minor) (Blood Transfusion)* [1993] 2 FLR 757
[49] *Re B (A Minor) (Wardship: Medical Treatment)* [1981] 1 WLR 1421
[50] *J (A Minor) (Child in Care: Medical Treatment)* [1993] Fam 15
[51] *Re T (A Minor) (Wardship: Medical Treatment)* [1997] 1 WLR 242 (CA)
[52] *Glass v United Kingdom* [2004] 1 FLR 1019
[53] *A NHS Trust v MB and Mr & Mrs B* [2006] EWHC 507
[54] *Re Wyatt (A Child) (Medical Treatment: Continuation of Order)* [2005] EWCA Civ 1181
[55] Clare Dyer, £100,000 for abused siblings council failed to take into care, *Guardian*, 17 September 2007
[56] *Pierce v Doncaster Metropolitan Borough Council*, The Times Law Report, 27 December 2007
[57] *R (G) v Southwark London Borough Council*, The Times Law Report, 4 June 2009
[58] *R (Kebede and Another) v Newcastle City Council*, The Times Law Report, 28 October 2013

[59] https://assets.publishing.service.gov.uk/government/uploads/system/uploads/attachment_data/file/729914/Working_Together_to_Safeguard_Children-2018.pdf
[60] *In re D (Children) (Care proceedings: Preliminary hearing)*, The Times Law Report, 25 August 2009
[61] www.victoria-climbie-inquiry.org.uk
[62] Department of Health, Keeping Children Safe, Stationery Office, London, 2003
[63] Department of Health, What To Do if You're Worried a Child is Being Abused, DH, 2003; webarchive.nationalarchives.gov.uk
[64] Department of Health, Every Child Matters, Green Paper, September 2003
[65] Local Safeguarding Children Boards Regulations 2006 SI 2006/90
[66] Local Safeguarding Children Boards Regulations 2010 SI 2010/622
[67] The Special Educational Needs and Disability Regulations 2014 SI 2014/1530
[68] Ruth Gledhill, Private fostering may cause 'a new Climbié', *The Times*, 25 January 2014
[69] Royal College of Nursing, Child Protection: every nurse's responsibility, Order No. 002045, RCN, June 2003; available on www.rcn.org.uk
[70] Both reports are available from the website www.everychildmatters.co.uk
[71] Lord Laming, The Protection of Children in England. A Progress Report, London, Stationery Office, 2009
[72] David Rose, Doctor who raised alarm at Baby P clinic sues Great Ormond St to get her job back, *The Times*, 20 September 2010
[73] David Rose, Hospitals fail to check children at risk, despite Baby P, *The Times*, 19 February 2009
[74] Care Quality Commission (2009) Review of the involvement and action taken by health bodies in relation to the case of Baby P, CQC, London
[75] Rosemary Bennett, Child services chiefs to be retrained in family risks, *The Times*, 12 March 2009
[76] HM Government, The Government's Response to Lord Laming; One Year On, March 2010, Stationery Office
[77] Ian Kennedy, Getting it Right for Children and Young People: overcoming cultural barriers in the NHS so as to meet their needs, DH, 2010
[78] David Rose, Doctors need more childcare training says Baby P review, *The Times*, 17 September 2010
[79] Department of Health, Achieving Equity and Excellence for Children, DH, 2010
[80] Rosemary Bennett, Children's court service 'could not cope with Baby P aftermath', *The Times*, 11 November 2010
[81] Andrew Norfolk, A rotten borough: Government set to take over Doncaster's broken council, *The Times*, 20 April 2010
[82] www.coventrylscb.org.uk
[83] Editorial, Missing Persons, *The Times*, 17 September 2013
[84] Ruth Gledhill, Delays left Daniel, 4, to be beaten to death by parents, *The Times*, 6 February 2014
[85] Ruth Gledhill, Coventry child services 'still inadequate', *The Times*, 22 March 2014
[86] House of Commons Home Affairs Committee, Child sexual exploitation and the response to localised grooming, Second report of session 2013–14 HC 68-1
[87] Home Department, Child sexual exploitation and the response to localised grooming, Government Response Cm 8705, September 2013
[88] Dominic Kennedy, 'Arrogant' doctor is struck off for not reporting sex claims, *The Times*, 21 January 2014
[89] Rosemary Bennett, Budget cuts leave children open to abuse and neglect, *The Times*, 24 June 2014

90. *X and others* v *Bedfordshire CC* [1995] 3 All ER 353
91. *Z and others* v *United Kingdom* [2001] ECHR 333 (Application no 29392/95)
92. *DP and JC* v *United Kingdom* (Application No. 38719/97), The Times Law Report, 23 October 2002 ECHR; [2003] IFLR 50
93. *E and Others* v *United Kingdom* (Application No. 33218/96), The Times Law Report, 4 December 2002 ECHR
94. *A and Another* v *Essex County* Council, The Times Law Report, 24 January 2003
95. Rosemary Bennett, Foster parents not told if they are caring for abusive children, *The Times*, 15 September 2009
96. *RK and MK* v *Oldham NHS Trust*, Lloyd's Rep Med 1 [2003] 1
97. *JD* v *East Berkshire Community NHS Trust, North Staffordshire Hospital NHS Trust and Others*, Lloyd's Rep Med 1 [2003] 9; [2005] UKHL 23; [2005] 2 All ER 443
98. *MAK and RK* v *United Kingdom*, Application Nos 45901/05 and 40146/06, The Times Law Report, 19 April 2010 ECHR; [2010] ECHR 363
99. *D* v *East Berkshire Community Health NHS Trust*; *MAK* v *Dewsbury Healthcare NHS Trust*; *RK* v *Oldham NHS Trust* [2005] 2 AC 373
100. *MAK and RK* v *UK*, The Times Law Report, 19 April 2010 ECHR; [2010] ECHR 363
101. News item, *The Times*, 8 August 2013
102. Frances Gibb, Family court judges are in cahoots with social workers, *The Times*, 19 February 2014
103. *In re W (A child) (Adoption: leave to oppose making of adoption order)* and *In re H (A child) (Adoption: leave to oppose making of adoption order)*, The Times Law Report, 13 January 2014
104. *AD and OD* v *United Kingdom*, The Times Law Report, 2 April 2010 [2010] ECHR 340
105. *D* v *Bury MBC*, The Times Law Report, 24 January 2006 [2006] 1 WLR 917
106. Royal College of Nursing, Administering Intravenous Therapy to Children in the Community Setting – guidance for nursing staff, Order No. 001244, RCN, October 2001
107. *A* v *The United Kingdom* (100/1997/884/1096) judgment on 23 September 1998; (1999) 27 EHRR 611
108. Royal College of Nursing, Restraining, Holding Still and Containing Children, Order No. 000999, RCN, March 1999
109. Joint Committee on Human Rights, The UN Convention on the Rights of the Child, HL Paper 117 (incorporating HL Paper 98.i and ii of 2003), HC 81 (incorporating HC 1103-I of 2001–02 and 81-I of 2002–03), Stationery Office, London, 2003
110. Francis Elliott, Parents face total smacking ban as rules are reviewed, *The Times*, 16 June 2007
111. News item, Total smacking ban is ruled out, *The Times*, 26 October 2007
112. Royal College of Nursing, Restrictive physical intervention and therapeutic holding for children and young people, Order No. 003753, RCN, London, April 2010
113. Royal College of Nursing, Adolescent Transition Care. Guidance for nursing staff, 002 313, RCN, London, July 2004 updated in 2013
114. Royal College of Nursing, Adolescence: boundaries and connections. An RCN guide for working with young people, 003256 RCN, London, August 2008
115. Royal College of Nursing, Caring for Young People: guidance for nursing staff, 001824 RCN, 2013
116. *Cheshire West and Chester Council* v *P* [2014] UKSC 19
117. *R. (on the application of Ferreira)* v *HM Senior Coroner for Inner South London* [2017] EWCA Civ 31

[118] United Nations (1989) *Convention on the Rights of the Child adopted under General Assembly resolution 44/25*

[119] Council of Europe (1950) *European Convention on Fundamental Human Rights and Freedoms Rome: Council of Europe*

[120] *Storck v Germany* 61603/00 [2005] ECHR 406

[121] *Re K (A Child) (Secure Accommodation Order: Right to Liberty)* [2001] Fam 377

[122] *Re A-F (Children) (Care Orders: Restrictions on Liberty)* [2018] EWHC 138 (fam)

[123] *Re B* [2017] EWFC B93

[124] *Nielsen v Denmark* (33488/96) (2000) ECHR 81

[125] *Re D (a child)* [2019] UKSC 42

[126] Roe A. (2021) What do we know about children and young people deprived of their liberty in England and Wales? An evidence review available on the Nuffield Family Justice Observatory Website at https://www.nuffieldfjo.org.uk/resource/children-and-young-people-deprived-of-their-liberty-england-and-wales

[127] Children (Secure Accommodation) Regulations 1991 ((1991/1505))

[128] The Children Secure Accommodation (Wales) Regulations 2015 (W. 298)

[129] *Re B (A Minor) (Treatment and Secure Accommodation)* [1997] 1 FLR 767

[130] *Re D* [2017] EWCA Civ 1695

[131] *Re X* [2016] EWFC B31

[132] Nuffield Family Justice Observatory (2023) National deprivation of liberty court: Latest data trends – February 2023 available on the Nuffied Family Justice Observatory Website at https://www.nuffieldfjo.org.uk/resource/national-deprivation-of-liberty-court-latest-data-trends-february-2023

[133] *Re J (Deprivation of Liberty: Hospital)* [2022] EWFC 121

[134] *AB (A Child) (Deprivation of Liberty: Consent)* [2015] EWHC Fam 3125

[135] George Arbuthnott, And still they die: up to 110 since Baby P, *Sunday Times*, 27 October 2013

[136] The Children's Plan, Building Brighter Futures, Department for Children, Schools and Families, December 2007, www.dfes.gov.uk/publications/childrensplan/downloads/The_Childrens_Plan.pdf (last accessed 25 January 2008)

[137] Department of Health, Achieving Equity and Excellence for Children, DH, 2010

[138] *In re H (Children)(Custody Rights: Jurisdiction)*, The Times Law Report, 8 August 2014

Chapter 14

The Nurse and Gynaecology

This chapter discusses

- Abortion
- Sterilisation
- Female circumcision

Introduction

This chapter considers the areas of particular concern to the nurse who specialises in gynaecology. For convenience, the chapter also includes the law relating to vasectomies within the topic of sterilisation. For issues relating to fertilisation and IVF, see chapter 21. Reference should also be made to chapter 13 for the law relating to consent by the young person to abortion, sterilisation and family planning and to chapter 16 on the law relating to those with learning disabilities.

Abortion

General Principles

Although the unborn child is not a legal personality and cannot sue or be sued until it is born, its existence is protected in law by the Offences Against the Persons Act 1861, section 58 of which makes it an offence to administer drugs or use instruments to procure a miscarriage, and section 59 which prohibits other activities to procure a miscarriage. In addition, under the Infant Life Preservation Act 1929, it is an offence to destroy the life of a child capable of being born alive. The Infant Life Preservation Act 1929 provides that any person who, with intent to destroy the life of a child capable of being born alive, by any wilful act, causes a child to die before it has an existence independent of its mother, shall be guilty of felony, to whit, of child destruction. Twenty-eight weeks' gestation was *prima facie* evidence that the child was capable of being born alive. However, these acts are subject to the Abortion Act 1967 as amended by the

Human Fertilisation and Embryology Act 1990. An abortion that satisfies the legal requirements laid down in this Act is not an offence. Under section 5(1) of the Abortion Act, no offence under the Infant Life Preservation Act 1929 takes place if the abortion is carried out by a registered medical practitioner who terminates a pregnancy in accordance with the provisions of the Act. If these legal requirements are not satisfied, then abortion is an offence that carries a maximum sentence of life imprisonment. The provisions of the Act as amended are set out in Statute Box 14.1.

Statute 14.1

Provisions of the Abortion Act 1967 Sections 1(1) and 5(2) (As Amended by the Human Fertilisation and Embryology Act 1990)

1(1) [A] person shall not be guilty of an offence under the law relating to abortion when a pregnancy is terminated by a registered medical practitioner if two registered medical practitioners are of the opinion, formed in good faith:

(a) that the pregnancy has not exceeded its 24th week and that the continuance of the pregnancy would involve risk, greater than if the pregnancy were terminated, of injury to the physical or mental health of the pregnant woman or any existing children of her family; or

(b) that the termination is necessary to prevent grave permanent injury to the physical or mental health of the pregnant woman; or

(c) that the continuance of the pregnancy would involve risk to the life of the pregnant woman, greater than if the pregnancy were terminated; or

(d) that there is a substantial risk that if the child were born it would suffer from such physical or mental abnormalities as to be seriously handicapped.

5(2) . . . in the case of a woman carrying more than one foetus, anything done with intent to (a) procure her miscarriage of any foetus is authorised by that section if—

(a) the ground for termination of the pregnancy specified in subsection (1)(d) of that section (*see above*) applies in relation to any foetus and the thing is done for the purpose of procuring the miscarriage of that foetus, or

(b) any of the other grounds for termination of the pregnancy specified in that section applies.

Account may be taken of the pregnant woman's actual or reasonably foreseeable environment in deciding whether there is a risk of injury to health under paragraph (a) (s. 1(2)). In December 2003[1] a curate was given approval to have a judicial review of a case where a woman had a late abortion because her fetus had a cleft palate. The curate, who herself had had three operations to correct a congenital jaw defect, argued that a cleft palate did not come within the provisions of section 1(1)(d) of the Abortion Act. Subsequently, the police carried out an investigation and in March 2005 the Crown Prosecution Service stated that they had decided not to prosecute because they were satisfied that the doctors involved had acted in good faith.

The abortion must be carried out in an NHS hospital or a place specifically approved by the Secretary of State or Minister of Health for the purposes of the Act. Emergency provisions are set out in Statute Box 14.2.

New abortion guidance and procedures were published in May 2014 by the Department of Health. It emphasises the following points:

- abortion on the grounds of gender alone is not lawful;
- the expectation that two doctors when certifying that an abortion meets the criteria set out in the Act, must consider the individual circumstances of the woman and be prepared to justify their decision;
- it is good practice for at least one of the doctors to have seen the pregnant woman before reaching a decision about the termination;
- pre-signing of statutory abortion certificates prior to consideration of a woman's circumstances is not compliant with the Act; and
- doctors have a legal duty to report all abortions to the Chief Medical Officer.

Statute 14.2
Emergency Provisions

The provisions set out in Statute Box 14.1, including the requirement to have two registered medical practitioners, do not apply in an emergency when a registered medical practitioner is of the opinion, formed in good faith, that the termination is immediately necessary to save the life or to prevent grave permanent injury to the physical or mental health of the pregnant woman.

Conscientious objection to participation in an abortion

The Abortion Act is one of the few examples where a professional can lawfully refuse to take part in an activity on the grounds of a conscientious objection. Thus section 4 states that:

> [N]o person shall be under any duty, whether by contract or by any statutory or other legal requirement, to participate in any treatment authorised by this Act to which he has a conscientious objection: Provided that in any legal proceedings the burden of proof of conscientious objection shall rest on the person claiming to rely on it.

This right is, however, subject to section 4(2):

> Nothing in subsection (1) of this section shall affect any duty to participate in treatment which is necessary to save the life or to prevent grave permanent injury to the physical or mental health of a pregnant woman.

The extent of the protection from being involved in an abortion was considered by the courts in Case 14.1.

Case 14.1 — R v Salford Health Authority ex parte Janaway [1988]

The letter[2]

Mrs Janaway, a medical secretary, refused to type a letter referring a patient from a general practitioner to a consultant with a view to a possible termination of pregnancy. She was a Roman Catholic who believed strongly that abortion was morally wrong. The genuineness of her belief was never in dispute. She was asked to type the letter and refused on the basis that she was protected by section 4 of the Abortion Act. She was dismissed by the health authority and subsequently applied for judicial review of the health authority's decision. This was refused and she therefore appealed.

The Court of Appeal held that she was not entitled to claim the protection of section 4 of the Act. It could not be said that by typing the letter she was participating in any treatment authorised by the Act, neither could typing such a letter be regarded as a criminal offence prior to the Abortion Act so that it could be regarded as now being protected by the provisions of the Act. The House of Lords dismissed Mrs Janaway's appeal.

Case 14.2 — Doogan and Anor Re Judicial Review [2012] (Glasgow case)

Midwife managers and termination of pregnancy

Two midwives in Glasgow launched an appeal against a court decision that they had to supervise abortions regardless of their conscientious objection. The judge in the Scottish Court of Session[3] told the midwives Mary Doogan and Connie Wood, both labour ward sisters, that the conscience clause in the Abortion Act would exempt them from hands-on involvement in abortions but as senior midwives they had to accept management instructions to oversee abortions performed by other midwives on the labour ward. Their costs were being underwritten by the Society for the Protection of Unborn Children[4]. They won their appeal.

However, the Supreme Court held that the conscientious objection clause only applied to actual hands-on looking after and treatment, but the midwives could take their case to the employment tribunal to determine their claim to exercise their religious beliefs without discrimination (*Doogan and Another* v *Greater Glasgow and Clyde Health Board* [2014] UKSC 68).[5]

Nurses' participation in prostaglandin abortions

Case 14.3	*RCN* v *The Department of Health and Social Security* [1981]

Prostaglandin drip[6]

The Royal College of Nursing brought a case on behalf of its members against the DHSS because members had complained that they were often left on wards to supervise (sometimes for several days) a patient who was having a prostaglandin-induced abortion. The doctor would set up the drip and then the nurse would undertake the care of the patient. The RCN queried the legality of this in the light of the wording of the Act that the pregnancy should be terminated by a registered medical practitioner. The RCN questioned, in particular, advice given in a DHSS letter and circular relating to the procedures that might be performed by an appropriately skilled nurse or midwife.

In Case 14.3, the House of Lords decided on a majority of three to two that the DHSS advice did not involve the performance of unlawful acts by members of the RCN. Lord Diplock's views are set out in Box 14.1.

Box 14.1	Lord Diplock's view in the case of *RCN* v *DHSS* [1981] 1 All ER 545

In the context of the Act what was required was that a registered medical practitioner – a doctor – should accept responsibility for all stages of the treatment for the termination of the pregnancy. The particular method to be used should be decided by the doctor in charge of that treatment; he should carry out any physical acts, forming part of the treatment, that in accordance with accepted medical practice were done only by qualified medical practitioners, and should give specific instructions as to the carrying out of such parts of the treatment as in accordance with accepted medical practice were carried out by nurses or other hospital staff without medical qualifications. To each of them the doctor or his substitute should be available to be consulted or called in for assistance from beginning to end of the treatment. In other words, the doctor need not do everything with his own hands; the subsection's requirements were satisfied when the treatment was one prescribed by a registered medical practitioner carried out in accordance with his directions and of which he remained in charge throughout.

This decision has considerable significance for the scope of professional practice. It could be argued that even where a statute expressly places responsibilities on a registered medical practitioner, the law is still followed when that activity is delegated to another healthcare professional acting under the aegis of the registered medical practitioner. This is the view taken by those who argue that the legislation allows nurses to perform surgical abortions.[7] The possibility of extending the nurse's role in abortions is considered below under future reforms to the abortion law. The scope of professional practice is considered in chapter 23.

When is an abortion illegal?

The simple answer is: under any circumstances other than those permitted under the 1967 Act as amended by the 1990 Act. It is specifically provided that no offence is committed under the Infant Life Preservation Act 1929 if the provisions of the 1967 Act are followed (section 5 as amended by the 1990 Act). The amendments to the 1967 Abortion Act limit termination to 24 weeks or less, but only for section 1(1)(a). Subsections (b), (c) and (d) give no time limit (see Statute Box 14.1). It was reported in May 2007[8] that a woman who had a backstreet abortion when she was 7½ months' pregnant was convicted on a charge of child destruction under the Infant Life Preservation Act 1929 as re-enacted in the Crimes Act 1958. A body was never found.

A man was jailed for two years after secretly giving his pregnant partner miscarriage-inducing drugs. He pleaded guilty to administering poison or other noxious things to procure a miscarriage under section 58 of the Offences Against the Person Act 1861.[9]

The Abortion Act does not permit abortion on grounds of the sex of the foetus, yet statistics seemed to show that there was an imbalance in the expected sex ratio of female to male foetuses compared with the actual ratio was particularly notable for mothers born in Pakistan, Bangladesh and Afghanistan.[10] In the light of these findings Sarah Wollaston, a GP and MP for Totnes, has suggested that the decision to tell parents the sex of their baby at 12 weeks or 20-week scans should be reviewed.

Being born alive

Practical dilemma 14.1   Birth or abortion?

Jodie Spencer was 15 and her pregnancy was discovered only at a late stage. From the information provided by her and from his own medical examination, the doctor judged her to be about 22 weeks pregnant. He agreed that a termination should proceed and he arranged for her to see a second doctor, who agreed with him. Jodie was immediately admitted for a termination. However, because of unforeseeable delays on the ward, this was not commenced for another week. When the foetus was expelled it appeared to cry out and the nurse felt that it was breathing. She did not know what to do. The doctor told her to put the remains in the bucket for incineration. She was reluctant to do this, however, since she felt it to be a child capable of surviving. Where does the law stand?

If it is clear that there is a live birth, then all reasonable steps should be taken to preserve its life, otherwise there could be a prosecution for murder or manslaughter. A prosecution was brought against Dr Hamilton when an abortion produced a live foetus.[11] However, the case did not proceed beyond the committal proceedings. In the above situation, Practical Dilemma 14.1, if it is apparent that the aborted foetus is breathing and viable, then he or she should be transferred to a special care baby unit. Failure to do so could be grounds for a charge of attempted murder. In addition, of course, even if the child were to die shortly afterwards, it would still have to be registered as a live birth.

Rights of the foetus

Whether or not the foetus had a right to life under Article 2 of the European Convention on Human Rights was considered in a French case heard before the European Court of Human Rights.[12] A doctor thought a woman (who was pregnant) was attending clinic for the removal of a contraceptive coil, and ruptured the amniotic sac, as a result of which the pregnancy had to be terminated. The claimant alleged that the failure of France to have a criminal remedy for killing a foetus was a breach of the foetus's Article 2 rights. The ECHR held that the foetus was not a person and therefore not directly protected by Article 2, but it was left open as to whether the foetus could claim a version of right to life under the Article and the EU countries could decide the question themselves. Three Irish women alleged that the laws against termination of pregnancy breached their rights by putting their health at risk in forcing them to go abroad for terminations. The ECHR held that the three women's complaints concerning the abortion laws in Ireland under Articles 8, 13 and 14 were admissible. In the case of C (who had become pregnant while suffering from a rare form of cancer and feared for her own life and that of the child if she continued with the pregnancy and was therefore compelled to go abroad for a termination), it held that there had been a violation of Article 8.[13] In another Irish case an Indian dentist died when she was refused an abortion as she miscarried. At the inquest the jury held that she died as a result of medical misadventure. The coroner recommended that Ireland's Medical Council should say exactly when a doctor can intervene to save the life of a pregnant woman.[14] In 2018 The Republic of Ireland held a referendum on changing the constitution to begin the path of legalising abortion in line with most European countries, including England and Wales. Northern Ireland did not permit abortions unless under exceptional circumstances, where the woman's life is at risk, or there is a permanent or serious risk to her physical and/or mental health. In June 2018, the Supreme Court of the United Kingdom held that the law of Northern Ireland was incompatible with Article 8 of the European Convention on Human Rights. However, the claimant did not have legal standing to bring the case and therefore the court only provided a non-binding opinion that an incompatibility existed. However, this case plus campaigns to change the law led to Northern Ireland changing the law on abortions via the Northern Ireland (Executive Formation etc) Act 2019 and the Abortion (Northern Ireland Regulations, 2020, 2021 and 2022.[15] Abortions can be provided for any reason up to 12 weeks gestation. After 12 weeks the reasons for abortion are the same as for the rest of the UK, and are available up to 23 weeks and 6 days of pregnancy.

In English law, the foetus is not a person in the eyes of the law and is not simply part of the mother[16] and cannot be made a ward of court.[17]

Negligence in failing to detect abnormality

In a case in 1991,[18] the plaintiff had an ultrasound scan when she was about 26 weeks pregnant. The radiographer queried a possible abnormality of the spine, but the consultant decided that there was no firm evidence of abnormality justifying further action. The baby was born and found to be suffering from spina bifida. The mother claimed that the defendants were negligent in not ascertaining the possibility of abnormality and thus enabling her to have an abortion. Her claim failed since (under the Abortion Act 1967, i.e. prior to the 1990 amendments) it would have been illegal to have carried out an abortion at that stage, since the baby would have been capable of being born alive within the meaning of the 1929 Act.

If similar facts were to occur now, compensation would be payable if the mother were able to establish negligence, since there is no longer any time limit for securing a termination if there is a substantial risk that if the child were born it would suffer from such physical or mental abnormalities as to be seriously handicapped.

Challenge by the putative father

Case 14.4 *C v S* [1987]

Father's intervention[19]

An Oxford student whose girlfriend became pregnant sought to stop the abortion on the grounds that the foetus, of between 18 and 24 weeks, was viable and that the abortion would thus be an offence under the Infant Life Preservation Act 1929. In this case, the pregnant woman was given medication to terminate the pregnancy shortly after the time that conception must have occurred. It was assumed that the medication had been effective. She subsequently took anti-depressant drugs and underwent two chest X-rays, one of which was taken without any shielding to protect a foetus. Any of these treatments could have harmed the foetus. When she discovered that she was still pregnant, she obtained the two necessary signatures for abortion. The father brought the court action.

The Court of Appeal decided that the foetus was not capable of being born alive and therefore the termination of the pregnancy would not constitute an offence under the 1929 Act. The medical evidence showed that the cardiac muscle would be contracting and that there would be signs of primitive movement. It was said that these were real discernible signs of life. But the foetus would never be capable of breathing, either naturally or with the aid of a ventilator. Since the amendment to the Abortion Act 1967, the viability of the foetus is no longer in issue. In a Scottish case in 1997,[20] a father was refused an injunction to restrain his wife from having an abortion.

Husband's attempt to stop an abortion

Case 14.5 *Paton v Trustees of British Pregnancy Advisory Service* [1978]

Husband's rights

In Case 14.4, the putative father was not married to the mother, but it might be asked whether, if he were married, it would give him any rights to prevent the abortion going ahead. This point came before the courts when Mr Paton asked the court to prevent his wife going ahead with a termination. Two doctors had signed that the termination should proceed. Mr Paton claimed that, as the father of the child, he had a right to apply to the court for the termination to be stopped.[21]

The court, however, disagreed. It held that, provided the requirements of the Act were met, then the husband did not have any right in law to prevent the abortion proceeding. He had no *locus standi* before the court. Mr Paton took his case to the European Commission on Human Rights,[22] arguing that the life of the foetus is protected under Article 2 of the European Convention on Human Rights (right to life) and also the father's rights were protected under Article 8 (the right of respect for family life). He failed in both his arguments.

Right to an abortion

An abortion refused

Practical dilemma 14.2 — An enforced child

After having two children, Joanne Edwards considered her family to be complete. They moved to a larger house with a huge mortgage and Joanne took a part-time job to help pay for the additional loan and the extras: meals out and holidays. She was horrified when she discovered that she might be pregnant. Joanne became severely depressed and visited her GP. He was very reassuring, stating that she could have an abortion and within a few days she was referred to a consultant obstetrician. He listened to her case and then informed her that he did not consider that she satisfied the requirements of the Abortion Act and that he would therefore be unable to write a medical recommendation. Joanne's depression became worse and she was unable to work. Eventually, her husband suggested that she should seek another opinion. She was reluctant to do so, not believing that it would be of any value. Eventually, however, under pressure from her husband she paid privately to see another specialist, who informed her that in his opinion she did meet the Act's requirements. However, since she was now 23 weeks pregnant, he would be unwilling to propose an abortion since the pregnancy was too far advanced for an abortion to be performed safely and at this late stage he believed that it could constitute an offence under the Act. Joanne eventually had the child, but is seeking compensation against the first specialist. Is she likely to succeed?

Joanne does not have an absolute right to an abortion. To obtain compensation, she would have to prove that, in making his assessment of her present or foreseeable physical or mental health, the specialist was negligent in failing to take into account factors that approved medical practice would have expected him to have taken into account, and that his assessment had been made negligently. She may get some support from her GP but, of course, it was open to him to refer her to another doctor at an earlier stage. Indeed, the GP's failure to refer her to a second consultant might in itself give rise to a claim of negligence against the GP. However, if the first consultant's report had been adamant that there was no greater risk in proceeding with the pregnancy, then the GP could argue that there was no negligence on his part in accepting that view as the likely prevailing one and therefore a further referral was not justified.

Women may be dependent on the personal views of the doctors when they seek a termination of pregnancy. However, to establish negligence by a GP, there must be clear evidence that the GP failed to follow a reasonable standard of care in advising about arrangements for termination. In one case,[23] a woman visited her GP to seek a termination of pregnancy. She did not know that the GP was opposed to abortion on ethical and religious grounds. The woman alleged that the GP, by stating that it was too late and that it would not be recommended, effectively prevented her from having an abortion and was therefore in breach of the duty of care owed to her. The GP referred her to an abortion counsellor, who told her of a private clinic at which an abortion could be obtained. She continued with the pregnancy and following an antepartum haemorrhage gave birth to a brain-damaged child. Her claim against the GP was dismissed on the grounds that in the light of the contemporaneous records and what she and her boyfriend had said in other contexts, the evidence showed that she had changed her mind and gone on to arrange antenatal care.

A woman who changed her mind about having an abortion was paid £27,500 in an out-of-court settlement by an NHS trust which ignored her attempts to withdraw her consent.[24]

There is concern that the availability of abortions varies according to where you live and therefore women who would satisfy the legal requirements of the Abortion Act 1967 may not receive a termination. A survey conducted by the Abortion Law Reform Association[25] in December 1999 showed that obtaining an abortion on the NHS depended on criteria such as whether you have had one before, your age, finances and whether you have been using contraception. The Royal College of Obstetricians and Gynaecologists[26] has recommended a maximum waiting time of 21 days from first doctor consultation to the surgical procedure and that 14 days should be the aim. This is clearly an area where NICE could make recommendations for uniformity of NHS provision across the country. (See chapter 5 on the work of NICE.) The House of Commons Scientific and Technology Committee recommended in October 2007 that the inequality across the country should be eradicated.

The RCN has provided guidance on abortion care for nurses, midwives and public health nurses.[27] The guidance aims to provide clear and accurate information for nurses; to improve knowledge about abortion and abortion care; to empower nurses to develop their roles in abortion care; and to protect the public by identifying relevant legislation and standards of care. The guidance was also updated in 2024 to reference people who are pregnant but do not identify as a woman.

In 2022 the total number of abortions for women resident in England and Wales was 251,377 which was the highest rise since the Abortion Act 1967 was implemented, representing a 17 per cent increase from 2021. The rate for women between 25 and 29 was 21.8 per 1000. The NHS funded 98 per cent of the abortions, of which over half took place in the independent sector under NHS contract. Ninety per cent of abortions were carried out at under 13 weeks gestation, 80 per cent were under 10 weeks. Medical abortions accounted for 65 per cent of the total: In 2022, 4,729 abortions were carried out under Ground E (risk that the child would be born with a disability).[28] Figures produced in May 2014 showed that more over-35s than teenagers need unwanted pregnancy help. Marie Stopes International reported in April 2014 that one in four women who has an abortion goes on to have another. It urged greater investment in sex and relationship education in schools and more investment in contraceptive training for health professionals. NICE has recommended that women should get the morning-after pill in advance and issued contraceptive guidance for young people under 25 in 2014 (see chapter 13).

A study carried out by the Universities of Southampton and Kent found that half of those women who had an abortion after 12 weeks did not know that they were pregnant for at least two months and a further quarter only discovered their pregnancies at three months or later; two in five said that their periods had continued.[29]

Independent sector organisations that wish to provide abortion services must obtain registration from the Care Quality Commission and comply with the national minimum standards and regulations for independent healthcare and the procedures for the approval of independent sector places for the termination of pregnancy. In 2005 the Chief Medical Officer investigated a complaint that the British Pregnancy Advisory Service (BPAS) broke the law relating to late abortions by advising a Spanish clinic. His report[30] concluded that BPAS had not broken the law, but the investigation raised a number of issues around access to abortions, training of staff and information for women. Recommendations for primary care trusts (now clinical commissioning groups) are contained in a letter he wrote to PCTs and Strategic Health Authorities.[31] Considerable controversy arose when Channel 4 announced that it was running advertisements for Marie Stopes International, a charity that carries out about 65,000 abortions a year.[32] In December 2009, three women living in Ireland challenged the strict laws against abortion in Ireland before the European Court of Human Rights. They claimed that the laws violated their human rights.

Other related offences

The Offences Against the Person Act 1861 section 58 makes it an offence to administer drugs or use instruments to procure an abortion. When a woman is charged, it must be shown that she is pregnant. This is not necessary when another person is charged with an offence. Section 59 of the 1861 Act makes it an offence to supply or procure any poison or any instrument or any other thing knowing that it is to be used with intent to cause a miscarriage whether or not the woman is with child. The Court of Appeal held in 2010 that where a husband duped his wife into going to have an abortion, he was not guilty of an offence under section 59 of the Offences against the Person Act 1861.[33] The facts were that Ahmed's wife, who was three months pregnant, only spoke Urdu and was told by her husband that she was attending the clinic to have a minor operation to remove blisters from her ovaries, which were endangering her baby. The medical staff, who had been told by the husband that it was his wife's wish to have an abortion, were concerned that she was having a termination at a late stage and arranged for an interpreter before carrying out the termination. Only then did the wife realise that an abortion had been arranged. The Court of Appeal held the *actus reus* (see chapter 2) of section 59 had not been met (i.e. supplying or procuring of an instrument) and he could not be guilty of an offence under that Act, nor was there any other offence known to law with which he could have been properly convicted.

If the requirements of the Abortion Act are complied with, the provisions of the 1861 Act would not apply. Section 60 of the 1861 Act makes it an offence to conceal the birth of a child. Mr Reginald Dixon[34] was prosecuted under section 58 of the Offences Against the Person Act 1861 when he continued carrying out a hysterectomy after discovering during the operation that the patient was pregnant. The patient subsequently said that had she known she would have wanted to keep the baby. He defended the charge on the grounds that he had acted in good faith to preserve the woman from grave permanent injury to her mental health within section 1(1)(b) of the Act. He was acquitted by the jury.

Dr Bourne, a gynaecologist, was prosecuted under section 58 of the 1861 Act after he had terminated the pregnancy of a 14-year-old girl who had been raped. He was found not guilty on the ground that his action was taken to preserve the life of the mother.[35] This situation is now covered by the emergency provisions of the Abortion Act 1967 (as amended).

The courts have considered whether the post-coital contraception pill came under the abortion laws. In *R v Dhingra*,[36] charges against a doctor under section 18 of the Offences Against the Person Act 1861 for inserting an intrauterine device (IUD) were dismissed on the grounds that preventing implantation could not be interpreted as a miscarriage, and in *R (Smeaton) v Secretary of State for Health*[37] the claim by the Society for the Protection of Unborn Children that the sale of the morning-after pill without prescription was an offence under the 1861 Act was rejected.

Termination of one of multiple pregnancy

The Human Fertilisation and Embryology Act 1990 section 37 added a further amendment to the Abortion Act 1967 to cover the situation where one or more foetus(es) in a multiple pregnancy is terminated. The termination may be justified either to protect the health or life of the mother or where there is a substantial risk that if the child were born it would suffer from such physical or mental abnormalities as to be seriously handicapped (i.e. s. 1(1)(d)). (See statute Box 14.1.)

Confidentiality and illegal abortions

Practical dilemma 14.3 — To tell or keep quiet

Pam Reynolds is admitted in an emergency to the A&E department with severe bleeding. She is transferred to the gynaecology ward where it is clear to nursing and medical staff that she had probably tried to obtain an illegal abortion, although Pam herself is silent as to what happened. It is the third time this month that there has been such an admission and the gynaecologist suspects that one person may be responsible. Does he or the nursing staff have any duty in law to inform the police?

The simple answer is that there is no statute that places a duty on anyone to report a crime of causing a miscarriage or an offence under the Infant Life Preservation Act. If, of course, the police had heard of the illegal abortion and had begun to investigate, then they would be able to subpoena witnesses or obtain information for their enquiries under the procedures laid down under the Police and Criminal Evidence Act 1984. What about notifying them before they are aware of the possible crime? Some would argue that the doctor has a public duty to inform the police in such circumstances; that it is in the public interest for him to disclose the information, but until the law is changed, this is not obligatory by law, but a nurse may have a professional duty to act in the public interest under NMC guidance. (For those offences that must be reported to the police, see chapter 8.)

Notification

The Abortion Regulations 1968, as amended by subsequent regulations, place a duty on the practitioner to notify the Chief Medical Officer (CMO) on the appropriate forms, but restricts disclosure to anyone other than:

- an authorised officer of the DH;
- the Registrar General;
- the Director of Public Prosecutions;
- the police;
- for the purposes of criminal proceedings;

- bona fide scientific research;
- to any practitioner with the consent of the woman; and
- at the request of the president of the General Medical Council for the purpose of investigating whether there has been serious professional misconduct.

Regulation 3[38] requires a certificate of opinion to be given in writing by the registered medical practitioners. Regulations which came into force in 2002[39] amend the notification provisions, enabling it to take place by electronic means and enabling a person authorised by the CMO who is engaged in setting up, maintaining and supporting the computer system to be notified of the abortion. A new Schedule sets out the information to be supplied. Amendments to the Regulations in 2008[40] take account of the appointment of an independent Statistics Board and notification to the National Statistician.

Consent by a pregnant person under 16 years

If a girl of 14 seeks an abortion, do her parents have to consent on her behalf? The answer depends on the competence of the girl and what is in her best interests. Assuming that the girl is not in the care of the local authority and is seeking an abortion, then provided that she has the capacity to make the decision, she could give a valid consent under the Gillick principles discussed in chapter 13 on children's nursing. In the Axon case the High Court upheld the right of a young person under 16 to keep information relating to a prospective abortion from the knowledge of the parents.[41] The High Court upheld the guidance given by Lord Fraser in the House of Lords in the Gillick case and maintained that it did not breach Article 8 of the ECHR (see chapter 13). What, however, if the girl's own parents wanted her to have the child and promised that they would care for it; could they refuse to allow the termination to proceed?

Case 14.6   *In re P (A Minor)* [1981]

Whose choice?[42]

The mother was 15. She already had a son of twelve months and had been in care since she was 13 following a conviction for theft. She lived in a mother and child unit with schooling facilities and was then twelve weeks pregnant. Her own parents objected to the abortion (as they had done during the first pregnancy). Her father offered to take care of his grandson and leave the daughter with the new baby. As a Seventh Day Adventist, he opposed the termination of life on religious grounds. He also thought that the girl would live to regret the decision she had taken. He was convinced that she was still a child and that she should not be allowed to take a decision that she could subsequently regret.

The child was placed under the wardship jurisdiction of the court and Mrs Justice Butler-Sloss ordered that the termination of the pregnancy should proceed. The judge was clearly influenced by the wishes of the girl, who had set her mind on the termination and had not, in fact, contemplated that it might not proceed. She discussed the matter with the girl and formed the opinion that she was of a strong personality and mature views. The judge also held that, on the facts, the risks to the health of the mother and the interests of the existing child satisfied the requirements of the 1967 Act. The grandparents' objections were thus overruled and they were accorded no rights in the matter. In this case, of course, the child was already in the care of the local authority. Where this is not so, it may be the practice for the parents of the pregnant girl to sign the consent form for a termination. Probably, too, if there is a clash between the rights of the mother and the grandparents, the latter may put pressure on the girl to agree to an abortion since she may well be dependent on their help in bringing up the child. Should a health professional become aware of such a conflict between an under-aged child and her parents, she could take action to ensure that the matter was determined by the court under the Children Act 1989.

Abortion and those lacking mental capacity

Under 18 years old

The parents have the right to make decisions on behalf of the minor provided that they are acting in the best interests of the child. The welfare of the child is the paramount consideration. The principles discussed in relation to the sterilisation of the minor by the House of Lords in *In re B* would thus apply. It is considered necessary to obtain the approval of the court. Where a young person is over 16 years and lacks the mental capacity to make his or her own decisions, this situation would now come under the Mental Capacity Act 2005.

Adult person lacking mental capacity

Case 14.7 *T v T* [1988]

The mother with learning disabilities[43]

The defendant was a woman aged 19 who was epileptic with severe learning disabilities. She was totally dependent on others and was cared for by her mother. She became pregnant and termination of pregnancy was recommended by the medical advisers on the grounds that there would be complications associated with that condition and that she would be incapable of providing and caring for a child. The doctors also recommended that she should be protected from any further pregnancies by being sterilised. The doctors were, however, unwilling to carry out the abortion or sterilisation operation without authorisation. The mother thus applied to the court for a declaration that the procedures could be carried out lawfully.

The court held that the situation was not covered by the Mental Health Act 1983 consent to treatment provisions (see chapter 19), neither did a guardian under the Act have the power to give consent. The court was prepared to grant the declaration requested and declared the proposed treatment lawful and therefore a defence to any action for trespass to the person. The doctors would be carrying out the treatment in the interests of the patient as part of their duty of care to the patient. The court also held that it no longer had a power to act as *parens patriae* (a kind of wardship jurisdiction) and the court could therefore not give consent itself. (It held that this power had been repealed in 1959 and should be reinstated. A subsequent case,[44] however, has held that the courts did have the power to make decisions on the day-to-day care of mentally incapacitated adults. This case is considered in chapter 16.) The circumstances set out in Case 14.7 would now be covered by the Mental Capacity Act 2005.

Mental Capacity Act 2005

The Mental Capacity Act 2005 which came into force in October 2007 provides that where a person over 16 years lacks the capacity required to make a specific decision, then action must be taken in her best interests according to the statutory provisions. The Court of Protection has jurisdiction over matters of personal welfare as well as property and finance. Were the situation in Case 14.7 to occur now, once it had been established that the pregnant woman lacked mental capacity, or where her capacity was disputed, an application would be made to the Court of Protection for a declaration as to what was in her best interests. If her mental capacity were in dispute, then the Court of Protection could determine whether she was able to make her own decisions. (The Act is discussed in chapter 7.)

In the case of *Re P*[45] the solicitor who was one of P's deputies queried whether P had capacity in relation to whether to continue with her pregnancy or have an abortion. Hedley J held that she manifestly lacked litigation capacity but did have capacity in relation to continuing the pregnancy. Generally courts and health officials should not try to decide whether P would be able to bring up a child but should instead concentrate on whether the pregnancy itself is in her best interests (the reasoning being that once the child is born, if the mother does not have the ability to care for a child, society had perfectly adequate processes to deal with that). The judge also stated that the purpose of the mental capacity legislation is not to dress an incapacitated person in cotton wool but to allow them to make the same mistakes that all other human beings are able to make and not infrequently do.

In another case[46] the judge held that a woman compulsorily detained under the Mental Health Act had the capacity to decide to have a termination. 'It would be a total affront to the autonomy of this patient to conclude that she lacks capacity to the level required to make this decision.'

Future reforms to the abortion law

There are pressures at present to revise the abortion laws: there are those who maintain that the 24-week time limit should be reduced and claim that their case is supported by fetal scans; there are those who wish to facilitate earlier abortions and give more responsibility to nurses. The British Pregnancy and Advisory Service recommended in 2006 that there should be legal reforms to allow nurses to prescribe the abortion pill to women within the first nine weeks as a responsible back-up to contraception.[47] The BMA at its meeting in June 2007 was not prepared to support nurses and midwives being allowed to conduct early abortions but it did vote that only one doctor's signature should be required in the first nine weeks. In October 2007 the Science and Technology Committee of the House of Commons published a comprehensive report on the scientific developments relating to the Abortion Act 1967.[48] Among its recommendations it held that:

- there was no evidence on the basis of fetal viability rates below 24 weeks which would justify the reduction of the abortion limit below 24 weeks;
- it considered that there were grounds for the enhancement of the nurse's role in relation to terminations, particularly in relation to signing the HAS 1 form and carrying out early surgical abortions;
- consideration could be given to amending the Act to enable the second stage of early medical abortion to be self-administered in a woman's home;

- NICE should be responsible for clinical guidelines on abortion provision, including health risks associated with abortion; and
- the government should consider ways of ensuring that all those who offer pregnancy counselling services make the guidelines available or indicate clearly in their advertising that they do not support referral for abortion.

In 2024 the RCN updated its guidance on the nurse and termination of pregnancy and sets out the role of the nurse and the legal limitations.[49]

Sterilisation

Sterilisation of a minor with learning disabilities

Case 14.8 *In re B (A Minor: Wardship Sterilisation)* [1987]

Sterilisation[50]

Jeanette was 17 years old, but was described as having a mental age of five or six. Her mother and the local authority, which held a care order on her, advised by the social worker, the gynaecologist and a paediatrician, considered it vital that she should not become pregnant. She had been found in a compromising situation in her residential home. She could not be relied on to take or accept oral contraceptives. Jeanette was likely to move to an adult training centre at the age of 19 and it would not be possible to provide her with the degree of supervision she had at present.

The House of Lords decided that the paramount consideration was the interests of the girl and, taking account of all the medical evidence, decided that it was in her interests to be sterilised. They made no distinction between non-therapeutic and therapeutic care of the child and recommended that in future all such cases should come before the courts. The Mental Capacity Act 2005 applies to those over 16 years and from 1 October 2007 consideration of whether a sterilisation was in the interest of a girl of 17 years would come before the Court of Protection. Cases concerning children under 16 years would be heard under the Children Act 1989 by the Family Division of the High Court. However, the Mental Capacity Act 2005 facilitates transfers to and from the Court of Protection and High Court.

Sterilisation of an adult with learning disabilities

The House of Lords in the Jeanette case discussed above declared their decision before Jeanette reached 18, so they did not consider the law in relationship to the adult mentally handicapped person. This was considered in the case of *T v T* (Case 14.7), but that decision was taken in the High Court. The view of the House of Lords on this situation was given in the case of *In re F v West Berkshire Health Authority*.

In this case, the court had to decide whether the sterilisation of a mentally handicapped woman, F, aged 35, would be unlawful because of her lack of capacity to give her consent to the operation. Mr Justice Scott Baker in the Family Division granted a declaration that it was in the best interests of F to have the operation. He stated that there was a problem when, because of a mental condition, a patient was unable to give any meaningful consent to treatment for a physical condition. If he did nothing, a doctor could be said to be negligent; if he operated, he, *prima facie*, committed the tort of battery. The law's answer to this was that a professional was not liable if he acted in good faith and in the best interests of the patients. The Court of Appeal upheld this decision. The House of Lords confirmed the power at common law for a doctor to act in the best interests of the patient incapable of giving consent. The court also had an inherent jurisdiction to make declarations on the lawfulness of such treatment. Court involvement in cases of sterilisation was highly desirable as a matter of good practice.[51] A practice note was issued providing guidance on the procedure that should be followed for making medical and welfare decisions on behalf of adults lacking capacity.[52] The Mental Capacity Act 2005 would now apply and such issues would be heard before the Court of Protection.

There can be disputes over what the best interests of a patient are and in a more recent case the Court of Appeal held that it was in the interests of a woman of 29 with severe learning disabilities to be fitted with an IUD rather than undergo a subtotal hysterectomy. The judge had failed to give proper weight to the unanimous medical evidence that supported the less invasive coil treatment.[53] In a case involving male sterilisation, the Court of Appeal held that it was not in the best interests of a man with learning disabilities to have a vasectomy, which his mother wanted to take place.[54] The Court of Appeal held that the best interests of the patient encompassed medical, emotional and all other welfare issues. In relation to sterilisation, the best interests of a man were not the equivalent of the best interests of a woman because of the obvious biological differences. This contrasts with the case of DE where the Court of Protection agreed that a vasectomy could be carried out on a 36-year-old with learning disabilities[55] (see chapter 16).

The situation in Case 14.8 would now be covered by the Mental Capacity Act 2005. Where serious decisions have to be made on behalf of a person lacking the requisite mental capacity, an application would have to be made to the new Court of Protection to determine the best interests of that person. The Mental Capacity Act requires decisions to be made in the best interests of an adult who lacks the requisite mental capacity.

Unsuccessful sterilisations

Case 14.9 Emeh v Kensington and Chelsea and Westminster Health Authority [1985]

Unwanted pregnancy[56]

Mrs Emeh, a mother of three children, underwent an operation for sterilisation in May 1976. In January 1977 she discovered that she was 20 weeks pregnant. She refused to have an abortion. She then gave birth to a child with congenital abnormalities who required constant medical and parental supervision. She claimed damages for the unwanted pregnancy and the birth and upkeep of the child. The trial judge held that the operation had been performed negligently and she could therefore recover damages for the time before she discovered the pregnancy, but since she refused to have an abortion, she was not entitled to the costs thereafter apart from the cost of undergoing the second sterilisation operation. Mrs Emeh appealed to the Court of Appeal and won.

The Court of Appeal held that since the avoidance of a further pregnancy was the object of the sterilisation operation, it was unreasonable after the period of pregnancy that had elapsed to expect the claimant to undergo an abortion. Her failure to do so was not unreasonable. She was therefore entitled to recover damages for her financial loss caused by the negligent performance of the sterilisation operation. She was awarded £7000 for loss of future earnings, £3000 for pain and suffering up to the trial and £10,000 for future loss of amenity and pain and suffering that will occur during the life of the child.

This decision is to be welcomed since it reverses an earlier decision.[57] The mother's refusal to have an abortion was not an unreasonable one and it could not be used as a reason to limit the damages payable. It has recently been confirmed in a decision of the House of Lords (see the McFarlane[58] case, Case 14.10) that arranging an adoption or abortion was not a requirement of the parents following the diagnosis of an unwanted child: 'There was no legal or moral duty to arrange an abortion or an adoption of an unplanned child.'

In another case,[59] a woman was sterilised when she was four weeks pregnant, a fact unknown to herself and the surgeon. The health authority accepted liability and damages of £96,631 were awarded, which included the future cost of caring for and educating the child. A pregnancy test should have been carried out before the operation for sterilisation was performed. Subsequently, the issue as to whether there should be compensation for bearing a healthy (but unplanned child) has come before the House of Lords.

Unplanned pregnancies

Unplanned healthy baby

The House of Lords has stated that compensation is not payable for the costs in bringing up a healthy child. In *McFarlane and Another* v *Tayside Health Board*[60], the House of Lords laid down the principles that should apply to any assessment.

Case 14.10 *McFarlane and Another* v *Tayside Health Board* [1999]

Unplanned pregnancy – compensation for healthy baby[61]

Mr and Mrs McFarlane had four children and Mr M agreed to have a vasectomy. Six months after the operation, he was advised that the sperm counts were negative and he could dispense with contraceptive precautions. Mrs M subsequently became pregnant and gave birth to a healthy daughter. They brought proceedings for damages for the cost of rearing the child and the pain and suffering by Mrs M in carrying and giving birth to her. Her claim was dismissed initially on the ground that such damages were irrecoverable in principle. The appeal succeeded and it was held that the couple should be given the opportunity to prove their loss and damage. The health board appealed to the House of Lords.

The House of Lords held that where medical negligence resulted in an unwanted pregnancy, and the birth of a healthy child, the parents were not entitled to recover damages for the costs of rearing that child, but the mother was entitled to recover damages for the pain and distress suffered during the pregnancy and in giving birth and for the financial loss associated with the pregnancy. Damages for the cost of bringing up a healthy baby were irrecoverable since it was not fair, just or reasonable to impose liability for such economic losses on a doctor or his employer. Lord Steyn held that it was morally unacceptable to allow such a claim having regard to the principle of distributive justice, which focused on the just distribution of burdens and losses among members of a society.

Unplanned baby with disabilities

In the McFarlane case, the House of Lords were considering the birth of an unplanned healthy baby. However, different considerations would arise if the unplanned baby were to be disabled. In the case of *Nunnerley and Another* v *Warrington Health Authority and Another*[62] (held before the decision of the McFarlane case was known), the mother was given negligent advice that led to the unwanted birth of a disabled child. The High Court judge held that the claim for damages should not be limited to the costs of the care which they themselves had a legal duty to provide, but damages were payable for the cost of care beyond 18 years. The judge held that the normal principle of compensation should apply, i.e. the claimants were entitled to be put in the position that they would have been in but for the wrong done to them and they were therefore entitled to compensation beyond the child's eighteenth birthday.

In another case,[63] M gave birth to a baby with Down's syndrome. The doctor had failed to inform her of the results of a routine scan that indicated that she was likely to give birth to a child suffering from Down's syndrome. M said that had she been informed of the results of the scan, then she would have chosen a termination. Liability was admitted and she was awarded £118,746. The High Court judge held that the ruling in *McFarlane* v *Tayside Health Authority* was confined to the birth of a healthy baby. This principle was followed in *Hardman* v *Amin*[64] where a doctor misdiagnosed rubella as tonsillitis in a pregnant woman, who therefore did not have a termination. The doctor subsequently admitted negligence. The mother successfully claimed the costs of the upbringing of a severely disabled baby.

In *Gaynor and Vincent* v *Warrington HA and Liverpool HA*,[65] where damages were sought for the birth of an unplanned child, who was disabled, the Court of Appeal held that it would be contrary to the general rules of the law of negligence and damages to enforce a cut-off when a child reached the age of 18 years. There was a considerable body of family law that indicated that the liability of the defendants towards a disabled child and the parents who cared for that child should continue beyond the age of 18. In another case a sterilisation operation was carried out when the claimant was pregnant and the defendant was deemed negligent in not carrying out a pregnancy test and advising about a termination. The baby suffered from disabilities following the mother's exposure to bacteria during childbirth. The defendant was held to be responsible for the foreseeable and disastrous consequences of performing her services negligently and therefore liable for the costs of bringing up a disabled child.[66] In the case of *Parkinson* v *St James and Seacroft University Hospital NHS Trust*,[67] the Court of Appeal held that the extra expenses associated with bringing up a child with a significant disability could be claimed.

Unplanned baby to a mother with disabilities

Case 14.11 — Rees v Darlington Memorial Hospital NHS Trust [2003]

Unplanned pregnancy – compensation for healthy baby to a blind mother[68]

Mrs Rees suffered a severe and progressive visual disability such that she felt unable to discharge the ordinary duties of a mother. She therefore wished to be sterilised and made her wishes known to a consultant employed by the defendants. The operation was performed negligently. She bore a healthy and normal child and sought damages for his upbringing. The Court of Appeal (in a majority decision) held that she was entitled to the additional costs attributable to her disability. The defendant appealed to the House of Lords.

The House of Lords allowed the appeal, and, following the unanimous decision in *McFarlane* v *Tayside Health Board*[69] held that a disabled mother who gave birth to a normal, healthy child after a failed sterilisation operation could not recover by way of damages the extra costs of rearing him which were referable to her disability. However, she was a victim of a legal wrong which it was appropriate to recognise by the award of a conventional sum. This was put at £15,000 to be added to the award for pregnancy and birth.

Failure to warn of risks of pregnancy

There have been cases where no negligence in the performance of the operation has been proved, but compensation has been claimed on the grounds that the patient was not warned that there was a possibility of the operation being reversed and the patient becoming fertile or pregnant. This occurred in the following case.

Case 14.12 — Gold v Haringey HA [1987]

No warning[70]

Mrs Gold, who had two children, decided when she became pregnant again that she would not have any more children. She was referred to the consultant obstetrician who suggested sterilisation, but did not discuss the possibility of the husband having a vasectomy which had a slightly lower failure rate, neither did he discuss the risk of failure with her. The sterilisation operation was performed the day after the birth of the child, but was not a success and Mrs Gold gave birth to a fourth child. She sued the health authority for negligence because she had not been warned of the risk of failure and the statement that the operation was irreversible was a negligent misrepresentation.

Initially Mrs Gold was awarded £19,000 damages on the grounds that, although the operation had not been negligently performed, the defendants had been negligent in failing to warn her of the possibility of failure of the operation. The defendants appealed and the Court of Appeal allowed the appeal for the following reasons.

1. The standard of care required of the medical practitioner was the same as that required of members of the profession, i.e. the ordinary skilled member of that profession who exercised and professed that special skill (see chapter 3 for further details on this standard). Where medical advice had been given, the standard of care required did not depend on the context in which it was given, but on whether there was a substantial body of doctors who would have given the same advice. Since, in 1979, a substantial body of responsible doctors would not have warned her of the risk of failure of the sterilisation operation, the health authority was not liable in negligence.

2. The statement that the operation was irreversible could not reasonably be constructed as a representation that the operation was bound to achieve its objectives. Mrs Gold therefore lost the case.

The Court of Appeal made it clear that it did not accept any distinction between advice given for a therapeutic procedure and that for a non-therapeutic procedure. The same standard should be applied to both, i.e. the Bolam Test.

Private healthcare

What if the case concerns an operation carried out in the private sector? Do any different principles apply? The significant difference between NHS care and private care is that there is a contract between patient and hospital in the provision of private care and failure to perform a satisfactory operation could lead to claims for breach of contract as well as a claim for negligence. In the case of *Thake v Maurice*, the High Court awarded compensation for failure to warn the husband and the wife about the risks of the sterilisation failing. The Court of Appeal[71] decided that the standard of care required in the law of negligence would be the same as the standard to be given under a private contract for healthcare:

> **The reasonable man would have expected the defendant to exercise all the special care and skill of a surgeon in that specialty; he would not in my view have expected the defendant to give a guarantee of 100 per cent success. (Neill LJ)**

Similar arguments could not be used in an NHS context since there is no contractual relationship between an NHS patient and the health authority or doctor. The possibility of action arising from failed sterilisations has led to much more meticulous wording of the agreement and warnings in relation to the possibilities of failure.

Where a child is born as a result of a failed sterilisation the legal situation is as follows:

(a) The costs of bringing up a healthy child are not payable (*McFarlane v Tayside Health Board*);

(b) Any extra costs directly due to the child being significantly disabled are payable (*Parkinson v St James and Seacroft University Hospital NHS Trust*);

(c) The mother can claim damages for the pain and suffering of the pregnancy and childbirth and financial loss (*McFarlane* v *Tayside Health Board*); and

(d) A disabled mother is entitled to a set award of £15,000 in recognition of the harm that she has suffered (*Rees* v *Darlington*).

(The sterilisation of a child under 16 is considered in chapter 13, which also considers the law relating to contraceptive advice for the under-16-year-old.)

Rights of the spouse

There is no legal requirement that if a person wishes to be sterilised the agreement of his or her spouse or partner must be obtained. Clearly, however, joint discussion with the couple of the implications is desirable.

Practical dilemma 14.4   The husband says 'no'

Audrey Rich was expecting her seventh child. Her eldest child was 10 years old and they lived with the husband in a four-bedroomed council house. She felt she could not cope with any further pregnancies and sought advice as to the possibility of being sterilised after the birth of the seventh. An appointment was arranged with the obstetrician for Audrey and Steve, but Steve refused to attend, claiming that he would never give his consent to Audrey's being sterilised. Audrey went on her own to see the obstetrician, who told her that he could not carry out the operation without her husband's consent.

There is no duty in law to obtain the consent of the spouse before sterilising the partner. In the past, there was a legal duty when the husband had a right of consortium and could sue any person who caused him to lose this right. However, this right to sue for loss of consortium was repealed by the Administration of Justice Act 1982 section 2(a). The woman has never enjoyed such a right; the House of Lords refused to extend it to women in 1952.[72] There may be considerable advantages in obtaining a signature to say that the spouse knows of the intended operation, since if this is obtained the doctor is less likely to be summoned as a witness in divorce proceedings where one spouse is alleging that the operation was performed without his/her knowledge. However, a form signifying knowledge of the operation is very different from a form of consent.

In the situation outlined above, Audrey could obtain a solicitor's letter confirming the law, but this, of course, does not place any duty on the doctor to perform the operation. She could request referral to a doctor who would perform the operation or even apply to the health authority for assistance. Ultimately, she could seek a judicial review from the court of the refusal to perform the operation and obtain a declaration that such an operation could proceed without the husband's consent.

Female circumcision

Under the Prohibition of Female Circumcision Act 1985 female circumcision was a criminal offence. There was, however, evidence that some girls from ethnic minorities were being taken overseas to be circumcised. This led to the 1985 Act being replaced by the Female Genital Mutilation Act 2003 (FMG), which strengthens the law against female genital mutilation (FGM). Under Section 1(1) of this Act it is a criminal offence for any person to:

> [E]xcise, infibulate or otherwise mutilate the whole or any part of a girl's labia majora or labia minora or clitoris.

The word 'girl' includes woman. Section 1(1) is subject to section 1(2), which states no offence is committed by an approved person who performs:

(a) a surgical operation on a girl which is necessary for her physical or mental health; or

(b) a surgical operation on a girl who is in any stage of labour, or has just given birth, for purposes connected with the labour or birth by an approved person.

An approved person is defined as:

(a) in relation to an operation falling within subsection 1(2)(a), a registered medical practitioner;

(b) in relation to an operation falling within subsection 1(2)(b), a registered medical; practitioner, a registered midwife, or a person undergoing a course of training with a view to becoming such a practitioner or midwife.

There is also no offence if a person performs a surgical operation falling within section 1(2)(a) or (b) outside the UK and exercises functions corresponding to those of an approved person.

Section 1(5) states that for the purpose of determining whether an operation is necessary for the mental health of a girl, it is immaterial whether she or any other person believes that the operation is required as a matter of custom or ritual.

Section 2 makes it an offence for a person to aid, abet, counsel or procure a girl to excise, infibulate or otherwise mutilate the whole or any part of her own labia majora, labia minora or clitoris.

Under section 3, it an offence to aid, abet, counsel or procure a person who is not a UK national or permanent UK resident to do a relevant act of female genital mutilation outside the UK. An act is a relevant act of female genital mutilation if it is done in relation to a UK resident and it would constitute an offence under section 1. Exceptions in relation to surgical operation and childbirth by approved persons apply. The Act also extends the offences to any act done outside the UK by a UK national or permanent resident.

Ann Clwyd, the Labour MP who introduced the legislation leading to the 2003 Act, complained at the lack of prosecutions under the legislation. A report suggested that African village elders were being flown into the UK to circumcise young girls.[73] The Metropolitan police offered £20,000 to anyone giving information which leads to successful prosecution for female genital mutilation.[74] The House of Lords overruled a Court of Appeal decision that held that a 19-year-old from Sierra Leone was not protected by the asylum laws since she did not belong to a particular social group fearing prosecution. The House of Lords held that the fear of genital mutilation if she were to return enabled her to stay in Britain.[75] Baroness Hale stated that female genital mutilation is in breach of international human rights law and standards. A campaign for a worldwide ban on female genital mutilation was launched at the United Nations in September 2010.[76]

The lack of prosecutions has led to widespread efforts to eradicate FGM.

In 2013 the International Development Select Committee of the House of Commons recommended better enforcement of the 2003 Act in the UK to provide greater protection for girls.[77] The government responded in September 2013 but disagreed with the Select Committee's recommendation on an up-to-date binding document requiring all service providers to play their part. The government considered that the existing cooperation between departments and the integrated approach to tackling FGM was successful. A helpline was set up by the NSPCC to assist those fearing genital mutilation on 24 June 2013.[78] A coalition of medical royal colleges and civil society groups published a report in 2013 stating that about 66,000 women in Britain have undergone FGM yet there has never been a prosecution. As many as 23,000 girls were currently at risk, mainly from African communities. The report urged that there should be a national campaign similar to the ones on HIV and domestic violence to highlight the problem.[79] Between October and December 2017 there were 65 female genital mutilation protection orders applied for to the family court, and of these 59 were made. Any person who suspects a child/woman is at risk can apply for an order, which includes the nurse. If someone breaches the order, he or she can be prosecuted under the Female Genital Mutilation Act 2003.[80]

In 2014 it was stated that government discussions were taking place with teaching unions to require teachers to report suspicions of FGM being planned. International Development Minister Lynne Featherstone, while spearheading the campaign to reduce FGM, was shocked that 8 in 10 teachers had received no child protection training in FGM.[81] In July 2013 it was announced that eight police files on alleged female genital mutilation had been passed to the Crown Prosecution Service with a view to bringing the first prosecutions in the UK.[82] One of the cases ended up in court, that of Dhanuson Dharmasena who was accused of illegally stitching up a mother after she had given birth, therefore re-doing the FGM she had received as a 6-year old in Somalia. However, he was acquitted of all the charges, as there were systematic hospital failings in not noticing the previous FGM, and it was accepted that Dr Dharmasena had in fact saved the life of the patient. In October 2023, the Crown Prosecution Service secured the conviction of a woman who was assisting in FGM. This was the first successful conviction of FGM in the UK.[83]

In January 2014 a conference was held to launch a report[84] which confronted the lack of prosecutions for FGM in comparison with France where over 100 prosecutions have been brought. The report's author pressed for mandatory reporting by health professionals, teachers and others to report suspected cases to the authorities immediately. The former Director of Public Prosecutions Sir Keir Starmer agreed, saying that the authorities had been too passive over a crime that annually put at risk an estimated 65,000 girls under the age of 13. See also the work of the campaigning GP Dr Phoebe Abe.[85] In March 2014, in a submission to the Home Affairs Select Committee, the Ministry of Justice suggested that a new civil court order could be created to be used by a young girl who fears being subjected to FGM. Breach of the order would lead to the violator being brought to court and jailed for 2 years for contempt of court. These recommendations were accepted, and these orders came into effect in July 2015, inserting a new section 5A into the Female Genital Mutilation Act 2003.

Well-known figures such as the Duchess of Cornwall and Baroness Ruth Rendell have supported the campaign to eradicate FGM, while charities such as FORWARD, Daughters of Eve and the NSPCC are all giving publicity to the campaign against FGM. In 2014 the then Mayor of London Boris Johnson urged hospitals to share details of victims of FGM with the police and social services, and on 17 March 2014 he recommended that the law should be changed to make it obligatory for health professionals to report FMG. In February 2014 the Secretary of State for Education met with campaigners to discuss ways of combating FGM through the schools and agreed to warn all head teachers about the risk of pupils being subjected to FGM.[86] Again, these recommendations have been accepted by Parliament and it is now mandatory for health and social care professionals and teachers to report suspected FGM cases. This mandatory reporting forms part of section 5B of the Female Genital Mutilation Act 2003. Failure to report concerns can lead to the practitioner being referred to their professional regulator, thus in the case of nurses the NMC. Healthcare assistants and teaching assistants, or those in an unregulated role currently have no duty to report concerns, although they may through their employment contracts be obligated to report suspected cases. It was reported on 20 March 2014 that nearly 4000 women had been treated in London hospitals since 2009 for complications following FGM.

The police are working with the UK Border Agency to stop parents suspected of taking their daughters overseas for FGM and there are proposals that overseas aid should not be given to countries which allow the practice of FGM.

In May 2014 the Medical Practitioners Tribunal Service, which is part of the GMC found a doctor guilty of offering to assist in arranging FGM following a *Sunday Times* undercover operation.[87]

Conclusions

Decisions relating to abortion and sterilisations for adults who lack the mental capacity to make their own decisions now go to the Court of Protection and the decisions are made in accordance with the Mental Capacity Act 2005. This Act creates a framework for the law relating to sterilisation or abortion and other decisions on behalf of those adults who lack the requisite mental capacity. The debate on changing the law on abortion is ongoing, with those in favour seeking to remove the rule that two doctors are required to authorise the abortion and suggesting that a nurse should be able to prescribe an abortion pill and carry out early surgery for termination, and those against arguing that the 24-week time limit should be reduced to 21 weeks (Nadine Dorries presented a Bill to Parliament calling for the limit to be reduced to 21 weeks in November 2006). However, the discussions on abortion in Parliament during the debates on the Human Fertilisation and Embryology Bill did not lead to any changes to the 24-week time limit. There is also controversy as to whether termination on grounds of the gender of the child, irrespective of any sex-linked genetic condition should be made illegal.[88] Because of the controversial nature of the subject, pressure for legislative change is likely to continue.

Reflection questions

1. What is the legal situation if an aborted fetus is found to be breathing?
2. What do you consider should be the registered nurse's role in the termination of pregnancy?
3. What information do you consider should be given to a patient before his or her consent is given to an operation for sterilisation? What are the legal requirements? (See also chapters 7 and 16).

Further exercises

1. Obtain a set of the documentation that has to be completed when an abortion is performed and examine the legal requirements as shown in these forms.
2. What forms are completed in your hospital when an operation for sterilisation is performed? Can you see any significant differences in the form completed by the patient and the form (if any) completed by the spouse?
3. What is your duty as a registered nurse if you suspect a girl/woman has undergone or is at risk of female genital mutilation?

References

[1] *Jepson* v *Chief Constable of West Mercia* [2003] EWHC 3318
[2] *R* v *Salford Health Authority ex parte Janaway*, The Times Law Report, 2 December 1988; [1988] 3 All ER 1079
[3] *Doogan and Anor Re Judicial Review* [2012] ScotCS CSOH 32
[4] www.spuc.org.uk
[5] *Doogan and Anor* v *NHS Greater Glasgow and Clyde Health Board* [2013] ScotCS CSIH 36; [2014] UKSC 68
[6] *Royal College of Nursing* v *The Department of Health and Social Security* [1981] 1 All ER 545
[7] Nigel Hawkes, Law allows unsupervised nurses to carry out abortions, says surgeons, *The Times*, 27 March 2007
[8] Nick Britten, Jury convicts mother who destroyed foetus, *Daily Telegraph*, 27 May 2007
[9] Simon de Bruxelles, Boyfriend gave his partner drugs to make her miscarry, *The Times*, 31October 2013
[10] Hannah Devlin, Illegal abortions 'explain boy-girl ratio imbalance', *The Times*, 16 January 2014
[11] *R* v *Hamilton*, The Times Law Report, 16 September 1983
[12] *Vo* v *France* [2004] 2 FCR 577 (ECHR)
[13] *A B and C* v *Ireland* [2010] ECHR 2032
[14] Rosemary Bennett, Jury backs coroner's call for change to Ireland's confused abortion rules, *The Times*, 20 April 2013
[15] NIDirect (2024) Abortion Services, https://www.nidirect.gov.uk/articles/abortion-services
[16] *Attorney-General's Reference* (No. 3 of 1994) [1998] AC 245
[17] *In re F (in utero)* [1988] 2 All ER 193
[18] *Rance and Another* v *Mid Downs Health Authority and Another* [1991] 1 All ER 801
[19] *C* v *S* [1987] 1 All ER 1230
[20] *Kelly* v *Kelly* [1997] SLT 896
[21] *Paton* v *Trustees of British Pregnancy Advisory Service* [1978] 2 All ER 987
[22] *Paton* v *UK* (1980) 3 EHRR 408
[23] *Barr* v *Matthews* (2000) 52 BMLR 217
[24] Clare Dyer, Cash settlement for woman who changed her mind on abortion, *Guardian*, 30 July 2007
[25] Kathryn Godfrey, Abortion by postcode, *Nursing Times*, 95(48):30–1, December 1999

26 Royal College of Obstetricians and Gynaecologists, Report on Abortions, RCOG, 2000
27 Royal College of Nursing, Termination of Pregnancy and Abortion care. RCN clinical guidance., 011 285, RCN, 2024
28 Department of Health, Abortion Statistics England and Wales 2017, DH, June 2018
29 Rosemary Bennett, Half of late abortions are for women who didn't notice they were pregnant, The Times, 19 April 2007
30 Department of Health, An Investigation into the British Pregnancy Advisory Service Response to Requests for Late Abortion, DH, September 2005
31 Chief Medical Officer Letter, 21 September 2005, Gateway Reference 5463, DH
32 Rosemary Bennett, Fury as TV advert for abortion advice gets go ahead, *The Times*, 20 May 2010
33 *R v Ahmed*, The Times Law Report, 6 September 2010
34 *R v Dixon* (Reginald) (1995) unreported
35 *R v Bourne* [1939] 1KB 687
36 *R v Dhingra* (1991) unreported
37 *R (Smeaton) v Secretary of State for Health* [2002] EWHC 610, [2002] 2 FCR 193
38 Abortion Regulations 1991, SI 1999/490
39 Abortion (Amendment) (England) Regulations 2002, SI 2002/887
40 Abortion (Amendment) Regulations 2008, SI 2008/735
41 *R (On the application of Axon) v Secretary of State* [2006] EWHC 37 Admin
42 *In re P (A Minor)* [1981] 80 LGR 301
43 *T v T* [1988] 1 All ER 613
44 *In re F (Adult: Court's Jurisdiction)*, The Times Law Report, 25 July 2000
45 *Re P (Abortion)* [2013] EWHC 50; [2013] MHLO (mental health law online) 1 (COP)
46 *Re SB (A patient, capacity to consent to termination)* [2013] EWHC 1417
47 Lewis Smith, Abortion should be made easier for women says charity, *The Times*, 28 November 2006
48 Science and Technology Committee, Scientific developments relating to the Abortion Act 1967, 12th Report Session 2006–7, HC 1045–1, October 2007
49 Royal College of Nursing, Termination of pregnancy: an RCN nursing framework, 2013
50 *In re B (A Minor: Wardship Sterilisation)* [1987] 2 All ER 206
51 *In re F v West Berkshire Health Authority* [1989] 2 All ER 545
52 Practice Note [2001] 2 FCR 569, Adult lacking capacity; enquiries@offsol.gsi.gov.uk
53 *Re S (Sterilisation: patient's best interests)* [2000] 2 FLR 389
54 *Re A (Male sterilisation)* [2000] 1 FLR 549
55 *An NHS Trust v DE* [2013] EWHC 2562 (Fam)
56 *Emeh v Kensington and Chelsea and Westminster Health Authority* [1985] 2 WLR 233
57 *Udale v Bloomsbury AHA* [1983] 2 All ER 522
58 *McFarlane and Another v Tayside Health Board* [1999] 4 All ER 961 HL
59 *Allen v Bloomsbury Health Authority and Another* [1993] 1 All ER 651
60 *McFarlane and Another v Tayside Health Board* [1999] 4 All ER 961 HL; [2000] 2 AC 59
61 Ibid.
62 *Nunnerley and Another v Warrington Health Authority and Another, The Times Law Report*, 26 November 1999; [2000] PIQR 069
63 *Rand v East Dorset HA* [2000] Lloyd's Rep Med 181
64 *Hardman v Amin* [2000] Lloyd's Rep Med 498
65 *Gaynor and Vincent v Warrington HA and Liverpool HA* [2003] 7 Lloyd's Rep Med 365 CA
66 *Groom v Selby* [2001] EWCA Civ 1522; [2002] PIQR P201 CA

[67] *Parkinson* v *St James and Seacroft University Hospital NHS Trust* [2001] EWCA Civ 530
[68] *Rees* v *Darlington Memorial Hospital NHS Trust, The Times Law Report*, 21 October 2003 *HL*; [2003] UKHL 52; [2002] 2 All ER 177 CA
[69] *McFarlane* v *Tayside Health Board* [1999] 4 All ER 961 HL; [2000] 2 AC 59
[70] *Gold* v *Haringey HA* [1987] 2 All ER 888
[71] *Thake* v *Maurice* [1986] QB 644; [1984] 2 All ER 513
[72] *Best* v *Samuel Fox and Co.* [1952] 2 All ER 394
[73] Nicola Woolcock, Parents fly in African village elders to circumcise their young daughters, *The Times*, 23 October 2006
[74] Helen Pidd, Met's unique £20,000 reward to stop mutilation of women, 11 July 2007
[75] *Secretary of State for the Home Department (Respondent)* v *Fornah (FC) (Appellant)* [2006] UKHL 46
[76] www.banfgm.org
[77] International Development Select Committee of the House of Commons 2013, Violence against women and girls 2013-4, Second session 2013-4 HC 107
[78] 0800 028 3550
[79] Chris Smyth, Health workers asked to look out for tortured girls, *The Times*, 4 November 2013
[80] Ministry of Justice, Family Court Statistics Quarterly, England and Wales, Annual 2017 including October to December 2017, 29 March 2018, MoJ
[81] Marie Woolf, Teachers monitor girls for mutilation, Sunday Times, 12 January 2014
[82] James Gillespie and Hannah Summers, First female mutilation cases weighed up, *Sunday Times*, 7 July 2013
[83] Sandra Laville 'Doctor found not guilty of FGM on patient at London hospital' *The Guardian*, 4 February 2015
[84] Julie Bindel, An unpunished crime: the lack of prosecutions for female genital mutilation in the UK, New Culture Forum, 2014, www.newcultureforum.org.uk/home/pdf/fgm_report.pdf
[85] Lucy Bannerman, 'I was so shocked. This has to stop', *The Times*, 25 January 2014
[86] Lucy Bannerman, Gove urges schools to fight female mutilation, *The Times*, 26 February 2014
[87] News item, *The Times*, 28 May 2014
[88] Lucy Bannerman, 'Sex selection is a myth', insists campaigner who defends right to abort a female foetus, *The Times*, 21 September 2013

Chapter 15
Acute Care

This chapter discusses

- Civil liability procedures and practices in theatre
- The theatre nurse and the scope of professional practice
- Accidents in the theatre
- Consent in the theatre
- Recovery room nursing
- Transfusions and blood contamination
- Organ transplantation
- Intensive care units: resource pressures
- Review of critical care services

Introduction

This chapter looks at the acute care and the hi-tech end of nursing, where developments in equipment and technology constantly challenge the registered nurse to keep up to date in maintaining her professional competence. This is also an area where demarcations between different registered health professionals change as the workplace demands. New statutes on transplant law and human tissue and mental capacity change the legal framework within which the nurse functions. Like the ward nurse, the theatre nurse is constantly concerned with the possibility of litigation and also with the problems of her role in relation to the surgeons, the operating department assistants and the anaesthetists. These areas and the others to be covered in this chapter are set out above. Reference should also be made to chapter 23 on the scope of professional practice and chapter 28 on the law relating to death and inquests and the need to report to the coroner if a patient dies on the operating table or shortly afterwards.

Civil liability procedures and practices in theatre

Professional liability

Practical dilemma 15.1 — Lost swab

Staff Nurse French was the scrub nurse for a hernia operation performed by a registrar. They were running late and still had two patients left on the morning list. The afternoon list was due to start in 10 minutes. Just before the registrar sutured the patient's wound, he asked for a swab count. Staff Nurse French checked the 34 used swabs, which had been hung on the rack, and six unused swabs and two unopened packs with the operating department practitioner. She confirmed that those were the only ones in use and the patient was sewn up. A few days later, just before the patient would normally have been discharged, he reported violent pains and became seriously ill. It was decided to X-ray the patient prior to returning him to theatre. The X-ray showed up a swab. The relatives of the patient were told what had happened and they made it clear that they would seek compensation. An internal investigation was commenced to see if the cause of this error could be found. The conclusions were that there was an extra swab in one of the packs and this had not been spotted when the staff nurse opened and counted them. A dispute then ensued between the registrar and the staff nurse over liability for the incident. The staff nurse claimed that, as she had checked the swabs in front of the registrar, he should accept responsibility for it; the registrar stated that, as the staff nurse had clearly counted wrongly, it was entirely her responsibility and, in addition, the unscrubbed runner nurse had made a second check.

In a dispute like this, the patient would be able to argue that this is a case of *res ipsa loquitur* and the burden should pass to the NHS trust to show that they were not negligent. (This is discussed in chapter 6.) The case of *Wilsher* v *Essex Area Health Authority*[1] laid down the principle that the courts do not accept any concept of team liability (see chapter 4 Case 4.3). The NHS trust itself could be directly liable and, in addition, each individual professional could be liable for what they personally did or failed to do and would be judged according to the standards expected of them, but the employer would accept vicarious liability.

The actual proportion of responsibility in a case like the above would obviously depend on the actual facts of what went wrong. When the swabs were unpacked, were they properly checked to ensure that none were stuck together? What was the accepted approved practice that the doctor and the nurse should have followed? Were there any justifiable reasons why this need not have been followed? In addition, there might be some liability on the part of the manufacturer as well., Health bodies accept responsibility for the negligence of doctors and dentists while acting in the course of employment. This also applies to NHS trusts. It is, therefore, less important how liability between nurse and doctor is shared, since the compensation will be paid to the patient by the employer, because of its vicarious liability for the negligence of its employees. It is important, however, to allocate responsibilities through procedures and policies to ensure that similar harm does not occur again. It is essential that procedures are in place to prevent such incidents arising.

There have been some very rare cases where, although the scrub nurse points out that a swab is unaccounted for, the surgeon still proceeds with stitching up the patient. This may be justifiable in particular cases if the patient's condition is deteriorating and there is a greater risk in keeping him under the anaesthetic than in taking the risk of the swab still being inside him. It would be very different if the surgeon were simply ignoring the nurse's count without any justification. The proportion of liability between nurse and surgeon thus depends entirely on the individual facts of the case.

Policies and practices

Practical Dilemma 15.1 illustrates the importance of having clear policies and codes of practice as to the responsibility of each person in theatre, so that there is no overlap. In a situation where the patient is unable to correct any wrong assumptions, it is essential that these codes cover every possible danger. The responsibility for the identification of the patient, the nature of the operation to be performed, including the identification of the part of the body or limb to be operated on, must all be clearly allocated so that there can be no errors. Many of these procedures may be repeats of checks already made at ward level, but they cannot be omitted on that account in theatre. If any such cases came to court, the judge would expect evidence on what the procedure should have been and what in fact took place.

There are many implications for theatre nurses: they should clearly be familiar with the procedures and implement them, resisting any unjustifiable shortcuts whatever the pressure. In addition, their records should be detailed and meaningful so that if there is a query about the care in the theatre, then they are able to refer to a comprehensive account of what took place. Booklets produced by organisations such as the Medical Defence Union and the Medical Protection Society and professional associations, such as the Royal College of Nursing,[2] the British Association of Critical Care Nurses[3] and the Association for Perioperative Practice[4] (formerly the National Association of Theatre Nurses), cover procedures for admission, labelling and ward procedure, lost swabs and instruments and other causes of potential hazards (see Figure 15.1). 'A Step Guide to Improving Operating Theatre Performance',[5] prepared by the NHS Modernisation Agency, was sent to all NHS trusts in 2006 to reduce cancelled operations and to optimise theatre use. It drew on best practice across the country.

In 2003 the National Institute for Health and Care Excellence (NICE) published interventional procedures guidance covering eight clinical areas to protect patients and to support health professionals when performing innovative surgical procedures. For four of the procedures, NICE advised that the data appear adequate to support their use; in the other four, there was uncertainty and in such cases NICE advised that patients are kept fully informed and that clinicians monitor and audit the results of the procedures they undertake carefully. Guidelines issued by NICE in respect of specific surgical procedures are available from its website[6] (see chapter 5).

In 2000 the wrong kidney was removed from a patient in Prince Philip Hospital, Llanelli. In the subsequent report of the inquiry by the Commission for Health Improvement[7] into that incident, it was found that there were serious faults in the marking of X-rays and significant recommendations were made. A trial of the two surgeons involved began at Cardiff Crown Court, but the prosecution failed to establish that the removal of the wrong kidney caused the death of the patient and the jury was ordered by the judge to acquit the defendants. Subsequently, professional conduct proceedings were held by the General Medical Council.

Potential hazards in operating theatres

- Allergies not marked on notes
- Units of blood not checked
- Nerves over bony surfaces damaged
- Eyes exposed to harm
- Sharp and powered tools used dangerously
- Faulty gauges on pneumatic cuffs, faulty monitors
- Tourniquets left on too long and skin necrosis beneath tourniquet cuffs
- Spirit solutions used with cautery
- Hot instruments and hot water in tubing
- Water mattresses overheating
- Diathermy burns
- Uninsulated electrodes
- Misplaced footswitch
- Faulty alarms and faulty equipment

Figure 15.1 Potential hazards in the operating theatre

The Action Against Medical Accidents[8] reported that since 2004 there had been 283 claims against NHS trusts after surgical instruments or other foreign bodies had been left inside patients following surgery. Four million pounds was paid in compensation for such incidents.[9] The National Patient Safety Agency issued a patient safety alert on correct site surgery with recommended action to be taken by the NHS in March 2005[10] and a fact sheet on patient safety in anaesthetics and theatres is available on its website. In June 2012 the functions of the NPSA were transferred to NHS England.

In May 2013 a Freedom of Information request by *The Times* revealed that over 750 patients over the past four years had suffered from serious mistakes in surgery in England. These included 322 of foreign objects left inside patients, 214 cases of surgery on the wrong side of the body, 73 cases of tubes being inserted in the lungs instead of the stomach or veins and 58 cases of wrong implants or prostheses being fitted. These cases are known as 'never events' and according to Mike Durkin, Director of Patient Safety for NHS England 'even one is too many in any week, in any day in any hospital'.[11] The Department of Health produces an annual list of 'never events', i.e. incidents which are considered unacceptable and eminently preventable. Data covering never events from 1 February to 31 March 2018 revealed some 76 never events including 30 wrong site surgeries and 16 retained foreign objects post procedure, 5 misplaced naso- or orogastric tubes and 5 wrong implant procedures.[12]

A surgeon, Dr Siddiqui, was struck off after the GMC found that he had failed to address concerns over the past four years. He had made a series of errors leaving patients worse off: seven patients suffered care below the standard expected and six cases were seriously below the expected standard.[13]

Two surgeons at Imperial College and the Royal Brompton Hospital are under investigation by the GMC over alleged poor care of a patient with a rare life-threatening condition.[14]

Further information and guidance on anaesthetic, theatre and recovery room procedures can be obtained from the British Anaesthetic and Recover Nurses Association (BARNA)[15] and from the Association for Perioperative Practice.[16]

The theatre nurse and the scope of professional practice

There is little uniformity in the tasks that nurses are expected to perform in theatre. The duties of a scrub nurse can depend on the personal preferences of an individual surgeon, the employment of operating department practitioners (ODPs) and on whether the hospital is a teaching hospital. Anaesthetic nurses may also have a variety of duties: for example, in some theatres they may be expected to draw up the drugs in syringes for the anaesthetist to check; in others, the anaesthetist might do this themselves. The nurse's role will also depend on the existence of and the duties performed by the ODP. Some of the tasks they perform will be regarded as expanded-role duties in which they might have been trained on a post-registration training course. In its report *Anaesthesia under Examination*,[17] the Audit Commission made significant recommendations on anaesthetic and pain management services, and suggested that there was considerable scope for the role expansion of many of the different professional groups who work in theatres. The report illustrates how problems can arise when interdisciplinary team working breaks down. It puts forward practical suggestions on how trusts can improve anaesthetic and pain relief services. ODPs are now a registered profession under the aegis of the Health and Care Professions Council. The scope of professional practice of the theatre nurse should take into account the role of the ODP (see chapter 23). In 2014 the HCPC published new standards of proficiency for ODPs.[18] The NPSA has published a safety leaflet on teamwork, including teamwork in surgery, which is available on its website.[19] While expanded roles are of increasing significance it is essential that basic skills are not neglected. In 2013 the National Confidential Enquiry into Patient Outcome and Death found that one in five patients had a problem caused by an IV drip being administered wrongly and many have died. As a consequence of this finding NICE produced draft clinical guidelines on intravenous fluid therapy in hospitals.[20] In July 2013 following the death of a patient during an operation in the cardiac department at Croydon University Hospital an argument broke out between the consultant and the hospital management: the former alleging that no one had told the doctors performing surgery that a specialist nurse had been suspended and was not available; the NHS trust saying it did not accept claims of bad management.[21]

Accidents in the theatre

An incident book should be kept to record accidents and other mishaps in theatre and the recovery room, and accidents and other untoward incidents should be reported to the chief executive or their assigned officer. There may be opposition from some medical staff over the necessity to record untoward incidents, but the nurse has a duty to ensure that records are maintained on incidents that cause harm: diathermy burns, an unintentional cut and the more serious incidents such as operating on the wrong side of the patient or even on the wrong patient. A policy of disclosure to the patient should be encouraged. However, it is not for the nurse to notify the patient; this is the consultant's or manager's duty. The National Patient Safety Agency (NPSA), now NHS Improvement, set up a national reporting system of adverse healthcare incidents so that lessons could be learnt and accidents prevented. An association has been established for assistants in surgical practice (National Association of Assistants in Surgical Practice), which has set up a website to support members.[22] It also runs workshops and conferences to provide professional development to assistants in surgical practice, including non-medically qualified practitioners. Its code of practice and clinical milestones for the surgical care practitioner can be seen on its website. See also the website for the Association of Perioperative Practitioners for guidance on standards.[23] Examples of negligence in surgery include a surgeon who lied to a patient, telling her that he had removed a brain tumour and then lied frequently to cover it up.[24] Another surgeon, Ian Paterson, performed four unnecessary breast operations on a woman and an inquiry found that he had performed more than a thousand inappropriate or unnecessary surgeries on women over a 17-year period. The slowness of the managers to take action against him was criticised in a review led by Sir Ian Kennedy which reported in December 2013.[25]

A surgeon who engraved a patient's liver with his initials was suspended by the University Hospitals Birmingham NHS Foundation Trust.[26] The patient has subsequently asked for the surgeon to be reinstated.[27] The surgeon was found guilty of assault in January 2018 and fined £10,000 and ordered to do 120 hours of unpaid work.[28]

In June 2008 a new safety checklist for surgical teams was launched by the World Health Organization (WHO). Several studies had shown that in industrial countries major complications occur in 3–16 per cent of inpatient surgical procedures, and permanent disability or death rates are about 0.4–0.8 per cent, according to the WHO. The checklist, which is being backed by NHS Improvement, was drawn up using evidence from eight pilot sites, including one based at St Mary's Hospital in London. Use of the checklist in pilot sites has increased the rate of adherence to receive proven standards of surgical care from 36 to 68 per cent and in some hospitals to almost 100 per cent. Further information and the checklist are available on the WHO website.[29] A paper published in the *New England Journal of Medicine* showed that use of the WHO checklist reduced the rate of deaths and surgical complications by more than one-third across all eight pilot hospitals. The rate of major inpatient complications dropped from 11 per cent to 7 per cent, and the inpatient death rate following major operations fell from 1.5 per cent to 0.8 per cent.[30]

In May 2013 a report from Imperial College London showed that patients who have operations on a Friday are almost 50 per cent more likely to die than those who have operations on a Monday.[31] The authors suggested that the root cause was that over the weekend when patients were recuperating senior doctors were often unavailable, nursing staff were fewer and testing services reduced. *The Sunday Times* initiated a campaign in 2013 to ensure that hospitals were properly staffed 24 hours a day, seven days a week.

As part of the initiative to improve NHS standards the NHS England Medical Director Sir Bruce Keogh recommended that all consultants should devise ways of publicly measuring their performance. The press has tended to focus on death rates, but these are not necessarily an effective measure since low numbers of operations means that chance factors overwhelm the influence of surgeon performance on the number of deaths.[32] He set up a Forum in February 2013 to look at 'NHS Services, Seven Days a Week'. The findings were published in December 2013 which showed that the increased risk of mortality at the weekend could be as high as 11 per cent on a Saturday and 16 per cent on a Sunday. He set out 10 new clinical standards describing the standard of urgent and emergency care all patients should expect seven days a week, each supported by clinical evidence and developed in partnership with the Academy of Medical Royal Colleges. He recommended that they should be adopted by the end of the 2016/17 financial year. The NHS Improving Quality (NHSIQ) report *NHS Services Open Seven Days a Week: Every Day Counts*, the forum summary report and the Board paper are accessible on the website of NHS England.[33]

The Director of Patient Experience at NHS England, has recommended that doctors should take more responsibility for hospital food and drink, since hospital meals are absolutely crucial to patient care.[34]

Consent in the theatre

Some particular problems arise in relation to consent in the theatre. One is the failure of ward staff to ensure that the appropriate forms have been filled in before the patient is sent to theatre. Consider Practical Dilemma 15.2.

Practical dilemma 15.2 — Validity of consent

Paula Green was admitted to hospital for a biopsy of the breast. It was intended that, should there be any malignancy, a mastectomy would be carried out immediately. Paula was given the pre-medication by the ward staff and brought to theatre. When the theatre sister was checking through the records, she noticed that there was no consent form. The anaesthetist, who had begun to prepare Paula for the operation, said that he had seen Paula on the ward the previous day and knew there was no doubt that she wanted this to be carried out and that she might still be able to put her signature to a form. The theatre sister was very concerned about this. The surgical registrar then apologised and said that he had spoken to Paula about the operation and that she knew the implications of it. However, when he had visited the ward, he had run out of consent forms. He had intended returning to the ward to get Paula's signature but had been distracted and had completely forgotten about it. He saw no reason not to proceed with the operation and argued that Paula would be far more upset if the operation did not proceed and she returned to the ward without it than for the operation to go ahead without her signature. What should the theatre sister do?

Consent after pre-medication

In chapter 7, it was pointed out that consent can be given in a variety of forms: in writing, by word of mouth, by implication. These are all equally valid in law. It could be argued, therefore, that the fact that Paula had given her consent to the registrar means that that can be relied on and therefore the operation can proceed. However, consent in writing is infinitely superior as a form of evidence. Imagine that Paula's operation proceeded. When the biopsy was analysed, a malignancy was discovered and the surgeon therefore proceeded with a mastectomy. On recovery, however, Paula denied that she had any idea that this was a likely possibility and had she known she would have preferred to have had radiotherapy. This possibility cannot be discounted and in such a situation it would be far better for Paula to return to the ward and, when the pre-medication has worn off, to agree in writing that the operation can proceed. One can imagine certain circumstances where there would be such considerable risks in postponing the operation that, on balance, the advantages to the patient are in favour of proceeding rather than returning the patient to the ward. In such cases, there could be an action for negligence if harm were caused by this delay. However, these would be unusual circumstances. In general, it would be wiser to ensure that the patient has signed a consent form and has had all the risks and implications explained to her. Sending the patient back to the ward, although undoubtedly leading to a furious complaint from a rightly indignant patient, has several long-term advantages: the ward staff will be less likely to give the patient a pre-medication before checking whether the consent forms have been signed and the doctors will know that they cannot get by with a casual approach to patients' rights.

A more difficult situation which occasionally occurs is where the patient themselves, after pre-medication and prior to the general anaesthetic, asks the surgeon if something else could be 'sorted out', e.g. an in-grown toe nail, a cyst, etc. What is the surgeon to do? It would seem churlish for them to say, 'No. I must have your consent in writing for that and since you have been pre-medicated you are incapable of giving a valid consent.' Contrariwise, if the surgeon agrees to proceed and undertakes the additional task and there are some unforeseen or unmentioned side effects, then litigation may result. Compensation was paid to a patient when she changed her mind about an abortion, but this was ignored and the termination was carried out[35] (see chapter 14).

Consent refused

Practical dilemma 15.3   What the eyes don't see . . .

An adult Jehovah's Witness patient makes it clear that he will agree to a particular operation only on the understanding that he will not be given blood (see chapter 7, Figure 7.1). The surgeon agrees to operate on that basis, but does intend that, if blood is needed, the patient will be given it anyway and will be none the wiser. The operation proceeds. The patient begins to haemorrhage and the surgeon instructs that blood should be given. Somehow the patient discovers what has happened and sues the NHS trust for trespass to the person.

In this case, it is clear that there has been a trespass to the person since the patient was given blood contrary to his express instructions and any deliberate intention to mislead the patient by the surgeon was a breach of professional conduct. The patient should, therefore, be entitled to substantial damages. Only if there were any doubt about the mental capacity of the patient and therefore the possibility that he was incapable of making a decision, could the judge consider that the actions were justified in the best interests of the patient under the Mental Capacity Act 2005. (See the case of *Re MB*, which is considered in chapter 7.) To avoid the possibility of court action, a surgeon could advise that they are not prepared to operate with restrictions on their discretion and if the patient refused to give an unrestricted consent, then they would not be operated on. (Note the case of *Malette* v *Shulman*, where blood was given to an unconscious card-carrying patient (see in chapter 7 Case 7.6).)

Other restrictions that the patient may also wish to impose on the surgeons are often refused; thus it should be made clear that the operation will not be performed by a particular surgeon or that there will be a specified anaesthetist or that any particular procedure will be followed. It is now recommended that the forms contained in the Department of Health's guidance on consent to examination and treatment[36] should be used prior to any operation. (These are discussed in chapter 7.)

Even though the patient has consented to a particular operation and is therefore prevented from bringing an action for trespass to the person, it might well be that if harm occurs, the patient will complain that they have not been informed of this possibility and side effects and that, had they known, they would not have gone ahead with it. This possibility is discussed in connection with the Montgomery case (see chapter 7).

One important point must be emphasised, however. The patient, in signing the consent form, is consenting to an action that without their consent would count as a trespass to their person. They are also consenting to undergo the risks of those unforeseen chances that, no matter how much care is taken, can still occur. They are not consenting to negligence or to the possibility that harm could occur to them because a nurse or doctor is careless or because the procedures are not followed correctly or inadequate precautions are taken to ensure that the patient will be safe.

Sometimes it might be pointed out to the patient that a particular operation is experimental and they might expressly agree to undergo the additional risk of this unknown procedure, but they still do not consent to the possibility of a failure to follow approved accepted practice.

Other difficulties in relation to consent to treatment are considered in the chapters relating to consent generally (chapter 7), children's nursing (chapter 13), gynaecology (abortion and sterilisations) (chapter 14), learning disabilities (chapter 16), the older person (chapter 18), psychiatric nursing (chapter 19) and A&E departments (chapter 20).

There have been successful claims by patients who have brought action on the grounds that, while under the anaesthetic, they were conscious of activities around them and suffered agonising pain, but were unable to move. Research published in 2007 suggested that about 1 in 14,000 patients who had a general anaesthetic experienced awareness if certain risk factors were present. If these risk factors were not present the rate reduced to 1 in 42,000 patients.[37] The Royal College of Anaesthetists has published risk information leaflets. Section 8 of these covers awareness during general anaesthesia. The fifth edition was published in 2014 and showed that 51 per cent of incidents led to distress and 41 per cent to long-term psychological harm. A woman received £30,000 in compensation from Coventry City Hospital when she woke up during abdominal surgery. The consultant anaesthetist later admitted that he had changed his usual procedure and stopped the anaesthetic too early.[38] Clearly, nurses should be vigilant for any sign that the patient is not properly anaesthetised.

Recovery room nursing

This is often under the control of the consultant anaesthetist. Recovery nurses will usually have post-registration training in recovery nursing. The training includes developing the skills, expertise and knowledge to detect possible adverse side effects resulting from the anaesthetic drugs. They must be trained to act speedily in an emergency, and staffing ratios assume even greater importance than in some other areas. It is essential that they are clear as to their competence in a wide area.

Another interesting facet of the law in this area is the fact that nurses may hear confidential information from the semi-conscious patient that would come under the principles discussed in chapter 8. Similarly, it is essential that nurses do not discuss the patient or any other patient in front of any of the semi-conscious patients in the recovery room since there are many accounts of patients who have overheard what staff have said and have been very upset by this. The nurse's duty of care obviously includes the duty of foreseeing what could harm a patient in this context and taking reasonable precautions to prevent that occurring.

Transfusions and blood contamination

In an attempt to reduce transfusion errors, the British Committee for Standards in Haematology, Blood Transfusion Task Force, RCN and the Royal College of Surgeons of England[39] produced the first clinical guidelines on blood transfusion. If hospitals implement them and provide the necessary resources and training, transfusion errors should be reduced. Guidance has also been provided by the NPSA.[40] An NHS Blood and Transplant (NHSBT) organisation was set up in 2005 as a special health authority. It combines the roles of the National Blood Authority and UK Transplant with a remit of increasing the quality, safety and supply of donated blood, organs and tissues and increasing the effectiveness of blood and transplant services. New regulations on blood safety require annual reports on serious adverse events and reactions to be made by blood establishments, hospital blood banks and facilities where blood transfusions take place.[41] Following the review of arm's-length bodies, the NHSBT remained an independent arm's-length body, but its Bio Products Laboratory was transferred into a Department of Health-owned limited company.[42] Further information on the NHSBT including its strategic plan for 2013–2018 can be found on its website.[43] The Serious Hazards of Transfusion Report for 2013 showed that errors were the largest cause of adverse transfusion incidents and urged a redesign of the transfusion process by mapping and audit, locally and nationally.

Criticisms were made of the waiting times and inefficiencies of the blood donor clinics with 1 in every 80 persons being sent away for non-medical reasons, an increase of 40 per cent compared with two years ago.[44] The criticism has led to the suggestion that the NHS Blood and Transfusion Service should become a charity.[45]

Compensation for being infected with contaminated blood

Before the disease of AIDS was recognised in this country as a possible killer, many haemophiliacs were given contaminated blood and have since become HIV positive. To succeed in an action for compensation in respect of the harm caused by being given contaminated blood, they would need to be able to show that those professionals providing the blood should have tested it for AIDS and were in breach of their duty of care in failing to do so and that this failure was contrary to the standard accepted practices of the time. It is unlikely that those who were originally infected could show this and therefore they have been dependent on government *ex gratia* payments and charity to assist them. The government paid compensation to them, but the agreement included a waiver to prevent them from taking action over other blood-borne viruses that they might contract in the future. This waiver was challenged by a haemophiliac who claimed that he was infected with hepatitis C virus from a blood transfusion. Any person receiving contaminated blood now, which has not been properly tested, would have a *prima facie* case of negligence and might also be able to obtain compensation under the Consumer Protection Act[46] (see chapter 12). In August 2003 the Secretary of State announced that £100 million was being made available to compensate people who had been infected with hepatitis C from contaminated blood products. The numbers include 2800 haemophiliacs who were infected through contaminated clotting agents they were given during the 1970s and 1980s. The details of the scheme were announced in January 2004:[47] from April 2004 patients who were alive on 29 August 2003 and who had been infected with hepatitis C after being given blood by the NHS before September 1999 were to receive an initial lump sum of £20,000. This included those who had contracted hepatitis C through someone infected with the disease. Those with more advanced stages of illness were to receive a further £45,000. However, the widows of haemophiliacs who had died from the disease were excluded from the compensation.

In 2018 the Infected Blood Inquiry began to examine why men, women and children in the UK were given infected blood or infected blood products; the impact on their families; how the authorities (including government) responded; the nature of any support provided following infection; questions of consent; and whether there was a cover-up.[48]

The inquiry's final report was published in May 2024 and NHS Blood and Transplant have set up an implementation group to develop an action plan to put into effect the recommendations of that report.[49]

Initial compensation for the victims of the infected blood scandal will receive an initial payment of some £100,000 while final compensation is calculated. This could be up to £2 million is some cases.[50]

Organ transplantation

Transplants from deceased persons

The Human Tissue Act 2004 covers the use of organs from living or dead donors.

Practical dilemma 15.4 A transplant opportunity?

A youth of 23 years is knocked down in a road traffic accident. He has no identification on him and appears to be unaccompanied. He is brought into hospital by the ambulance crew and is resuscitated. He is maintained on the ventilator, but the prognosis is poor. Transplant teams are anxious to remove his lungs, heart, kidneys and liver and an ophthalmologist would like to make use of his eyes. The police are asked to notify the relatives as soon as possible. They are advised by the surgeon that the organs should be removed within half an hour of death. The youth is kept on a positive pressure ventilator. Can his organs be used for transplant on diagnosis of death before the relatives are contacted? What difference would it make if he were found to be carrying a donor card?

The Human Tissue Act 2004 now applies to the situation in Practical Dilemma 15.4. The procedure relating to the diagnosis and certification of death (see chapter 28) must be followed. Death must be certified by registered medical practitioners who are not connected with the transplant team. Where the dying person has not indicated his wishes, then any person whom he has nominated to act on his behalf can give consent to the organ donation. The nomination can be oral or in writing, with stipulations about witnesses and only adults can be nominees. Where there has been no such nomination, then a person in a qualifying relationship such as a partner or other relative or friend can give consent. Section 27(4) of the Act sets out a hierarchy of persons who are defined as in a qualifying relationship, beginning with spouse or partner and ending with friend of long standing. If there is no donor card or if the dying person has not registered as an organ donor nor made a nomination, then the person in a qualifying relationship must be contacted. If, however, the dying person has been registered as an organ donor with the NHS organ donor register[51] or is carrying a donor card, then that would count as a valid consent for the removal of the organs.

Keeping the patient ventilated

Section 43 of the Human Tissue Act 2004 states that where part of a body (i.e. of a deceased person) lying in a hospital, nursing home or other institution is or may be suitable for use for transplantation, it shall be lawful for the person having the control and management of the institution:

(a) to take steps for the purpose of preserving the part for use for transplantation; and

(b) to retain the body for that purpose.

However, the authority given under this section only extends to the taking of the minimum steps necessary for the purpose mentioned in that provision, and to the use of the least invasive procedure. The authority can include that of the coroner.[52] Once it has been established that consent making removal of the part for transplantation lawful has not been, and will not be, given, then the authority under this section ceases to apply.

Transplants from living donors

Special provisions apply to a situation where a potential donor is alive, as Practical Dilemma 15.5 illustrates.

Practical dilemma 15.5   Live donation

A nurse cares for a renal patient aged 23. She has been on dialysis for a number of years, but has been advised that a kidney transplant is urgently required. Her mother has offered to be a donor and seeks the advice of the nurse over whether such an offer would be accepted.

Under section 33 of the Human Tissue Act 2004 it is a criminal offence to remove any transplantable material from the body of a living person intending that the material be used for the purpose of transplantation. However, in certain circumstances approval can be given by the Human Tissue Authority to the transplantation of organs (or part of organs), bone marrow and peripheral blood stem cells from living persons. Regulations drawn up under the Human Tissue Act specify the strict conditions which must be satisfied.[53] The prohibition on transplants from a live donor is lifted under Regulation 11 if specific conditions are satisfied. The conditions which must be satisfied include the following.

1. A registered medical practitioner who has clinical responsibility for the donor must have caused the matter to be referred to the Human Tissue Authority.
2. The Authority must be satisfied that no reward has been or is to be given and consent has been given for the removal of the transplantable material or it is otherwise lawful.

3. The Authority must take into account the report of the interviews with the donor (or person who gave consent) and the recipient when making its decision.
4. The authority must give notice of its decision to:
   (a) the donor (or any person acting on his behalf);
   (b) the recipient (or any person acting on his behalf); and
   (c) the registered medical practitioner who referred the matter to the Authority.
5. One or more qualified persons must have conducted separate interviews with each of the following:
   (a) the donor;
   (b) if different from the donor, the person giving consent; and
   (c) the recipient;
   and (unless the transplant is the result of a court order) reported to the Authority on the following matters:
   (a) any evidence of duress or coercion affecting the decision to give consent;
   (b) any evidence of an offer of a reward; and
   (c) any difficulties of communication with the person interviewed and an explanation of how those difficulties were overcome.
6. The following matters must be covered in the report of the interview with the donor and, where relevant, the other person giving consent:
   (a) the information given to the person interviewed as to the nature of the medical procedure for, and the risk involved in, the removal of the transplantable material;
   (b) the full name of the person who gave that information and his qualification to give it; and
   (c) the capacity of the person interviewed to understand:
      (i) the nature of the medical procedure and the risk involved, and
      (ii) that the consent may be withdrawn at any time before the removal of the transplantable material.
7. A person is qualified to conduct an interview if:
   (a) he appears to the Authority to be suitably qualified to conduct the interview;
   (b) he does not have any connection with any of the persons to be interviewed, or with a person who stands in a qualifying relationship to any of those persons, which the Authority considers to be of a kind that might raise doubts about his ability to act impartially; and
   (c) in the case of an interview with the donor or other person giving consent, he is not the person who gave the information to those people.

In Practical Dilemma 15.5 the mother of the renal patient should make known her intention to the doctor in charge of the patient, who can ensure that the appropriate referral is made to the Human Tissue Authority and the procedure would then be set in place. She may of course not prove to be a match. However, it is possible for her to take part in a paired or pooled donation. In October 2007 there was a report of a paired donation, i.e. twinned kidney transplant between couples, where a potential donor from couple A was matched with a recipient from couple B and the partner of the recipient was matched with the partner of the donor A. It is therefore possible for the mother to be matched with another recipient whose relative was a potential donor and match for her child. Regulation 13 requires that where the donor is a child, an adult who lacks the capacity to give consent or the case involves a paired donation, pooled donation or non-directed altruistic donation, then a panel of no fewer than three members of the Human Tissue Authority must make the decision on whether approval should be given. Procedures are in place for requiring the HTA to review its decision over a transplant (Regulations 13 and 14). Transitional provisions covered organ transplants between genetically related persons.[54]

It was reported in November 2013 that a hospital in Colombo, Sri Lanka was offering kidney transplants to UK patients despite the law banning the sale of human organs.[55]

Dispute over resources is holding back the possibility of hand transplants. Clinical commissioning groups are refusing to finance the operations, claiming that it is the responsibility of NHS England which pays for specialist care.[56]

Transplant and consent by the recipient provisions

Transplants and children

The principles of consent (considered in chapter 7) apply to the recipient of the transplant. If the person is mentally competent and over 18 years, then they can give consent or refuse. If the person is under 18 years, then the principles that are discussed in chapter 13 on children apply. In the following case, the mother consented to the child's transplant, but the child refused.

Case 15.1 *Re M (Medical Treatment: Consent)* [1999]

Child refusing a transplant[57]

A 15-year-old girl refused to consent to a transplant that was needed to save her life. She stated that she did not wish to have anyone else's heart and she did not wish to take medication for the rest of her life. The hospital, which had obtained her mother's consent to the transplant, sought leave from the court to carry out the transplant.

The court held that the hospital could give treatment according to the doctor's clinical judgement, including a heart transplant. The girl was an intelligent person whose wishes carried considerable weight, but she had been overwhelmed by her circumstances and the decision she was being asked to make. Her severe condition had developed only recently and she had had only a few days to consider her situation. While recognising the risk that for the rest of her life she would carry resentment about what had been done to her, the court weighed that risk against the certainty of death if the order were not made.

In contrast to Case 15.1 when Hannah Jones, who was terminally ill with leukaemia, refused a heart transplant on the grounds that she would prefer to die with dignity, her parents respected her wishes and, despite doctors reporting the case to the child protection officers, no application was made to court to enforce a transplant. After interviewing the child, the child protection officer accepted that her wishes should prevail.[58] It was subsequently reported that she had changed her mind and agreed to go on to the waiting list.[59] Similarly, Liam Gawthorpe who was born with a heart defect and pulmonary hypertension, refused a heart and lung transplant when he was 11 years old and again when he was 18 because he wanted to enjoy the time he had left. His parents accepted his wishes.[60]

Transplants from mentally incapacitated persons

Where a transplant from a mentally incompetent person is being considered and the person is unable to give consent, the sole question for the courts is what is in the interests of the donor. This situation arose in the American case of *Hart* v *Brown* where the donor and recipient were identical twin girls. The court approved the parental request to transfer a kidney from one to the other. One of the main justifications was that, medically, such a graft was more likely to be successful and another justification was that, if they refused to allow the donation, the donor might, in later life, feel guilty at not being allowed to be a donor.[61] In another American case (*Strunk* v *Strunk*),[62] a kidney transplant was authorised to proceed from an institutionalised adult with the mental capacity of a six-year-old to his brother who was terminally ill with kidney trouble. The court accepted the medical evidence that there was a strong emotional bond between the brothers and the mentally incompetent person would suffer a severe traumatic experience if the brother died.

In England, the courts have discussed whether a mentally and physically impaired younger sister could give bone marrow to her older sister who was suffering from a serious blood condition.[63] The court held that it was in the younger sister's best interest for her to give bone marrow to her older sister and the risks to her were minimal. The important issue was that it is the interests of the donor that have to be considered, not the interests of the recipient. It can be a criminal offence for parents to fail to take appropriate action for the care of their children.

The situation of transplants from a person lacking the requisite mental capacity is now covered by the Human Tissue Act 2004 and the Regulations made under that Act.[64] The transplant could only take place if it were clearly in the best interests of the proposed donor and if it were approved by a panel of at least three members of the Human Tissue Authority.

Liability arising from transplants

Practical dilemma 15.6 | **Diseased organs**

A patient received a kidney transplant and was subsequently told that it was HIV-infected. It was discovered that this was unknown to the doctors and family of the deceased patient. Does the patient who received the kidney have any rights of action?

In the above situation, there is a duty of care, according to the reasonable professional standard for the transplant team, to ensure that the kidney is reasonably safe for transplant. In determining whether this duty of care had been fulfilled, note would be taken of the timescale within which any tests would have to take place. The possibility of the patient being able to sue under the Consumer Protection Act 1987 depends on whether the organ could be defined as 'goods' under that Act and whether the transaction could be seen as in the course of business. Since the Human Organ Transplant Act 1989 (now consolidated in the Human Tissue Act 2004) prohibits commercial dealings, it could be argued that organ transplantation is not in the course of business. However, the activities of hospitals and health organisations would be defined as in 'the course of business'. National heart and lung transplant standards have been published by the National Specialist Commissioning Advisory Group[65] in 2006 to ensure that patients receive services that match the evidence on best care available. These standards replace those issued in September 2002. A businessman claimed £14 million compensation from an NHS trust when an operation for him to donate a kidney to his father went wrong, causing catastrophic damage to his remaining kidney. The NHS trust accepted liability, but disputed the damages claimed which the victim said were loss of earnings because he was unable to set up a pharmaceutical market research company.[66] He was awarded £6.7 million in damages.

Other concerns which are considered in chapter 28 include the decision not to resuscitate a patient and consent for the use of organs and tissues and in what circumstances machines can be switched off.

The EU Organ Donation Directive has been written into UK law through the Quality and Safety of Organs intended for Transplantation Regulations 2012[67] which were amended in 2014.[68] Each transplant unit and the NHSBT are required to have a licence to perform any of the activities regulated under the 2012 regulations which cover procurement activities and transplantation activities. For further details see the Organ Donation and Transplantation website.[69] Under the regulations it is a statutory duty to report a serious adverse event and adverse reaction (SAEAR) to the NHSBT. Further information can be found on the organ donation website.[70]

Encouraging donors

The government launched *Saving Lives, Valuing Donors* in July 2003 which was a 10-year framework to encourage people to donate organs and tissues. The progress was reviewed in 2004.[71] This was followed by many initiatives governmental as well as personal to increase the number of organs available for donation, including the appointment of a task force by the Department of Health to investigate improvements to the transplant services reported in January 2008.[72] It made recommendations on increasing the number of transplant coordinators, strengthening the network of retrieval teams, identifying potential donors sooner and mandatory training of critical care staff. The taskforce rejected the option of presumed consent for organ donation. The Nuffield Council on Bioethics published a consultation paper in April 2010 which explored ways of encouraging organ and tissue donation. Other suggestions came from research at the John Radcliffe Hospital in Oxford which suggested that requests for donations were more likely to be successful when the request was separated from the announcement of death and when a transplant coordinator accompanied the doctor.

The Welsh Government took the decision in 2010 to introduce 'presumed consent' to organ donation[73] and in 2013 Wales became the first country in the UK to introduce a system of presumed consent for organ donation.[74] The Act imposes upon Ministers in Wales the duty to promote transplantation, and it provides that in the absence of express provision in relation to consent, consent will be deemed to have been given in most cases. Deemed consent does not apply to those under 18 years, those who have lived in Wales for less than one year, and people who lacked capacity to understand that consent could be deemed in the absence of express consent. Doctors will therefore have the right to remove people's organs when they die unless they have registered an objection. Its introduction will be studied carefully in the rest of the UK to analyse its effect on the numbers of organs available for transplant and upon public opinion.

Waiting lists for kidney donors may be reduced as a result of recent research which suggests that kidneys from dead donors may be viable.[75] Provided that kidneys can be transplanted within

12 hours from non-heart-beating donors, they are as safe and as effective as those from someone whose heart is still beating but is brain-dead.

In 2013 a Facebook campaign led to a 21-fold rise in those signing up as organ donors.[76] Since its launch in May 2013 almost 1 million more people have joined the donor register. Facebook users are encouraged to describe themselves as organ donors. A suggestion that people should be able to jump the queue for a transplant if they are on the organ donor register to boost donation rates among ethnic minorities was made by Dr Sharif, a kidney consultant at Queen Elizabeth Hospital Birmingham.[77]

Retention of organs

Considerable public concern was raised when it was learnt that human organs from children who had died had been retained at Bristol Royal Infirmary. New guidance was considered necessary when, during the inquiry into allegations of professional misconduct in carrying out paediatric heart surgery, it was learnt that more than 11,000 children who had died in the past 40 years had had their organs used for research in British hospitals without the explicit consent of their parents.

At the same time, concerns were raised about the retention of human brains and spinal cords at the Walton Centre, Liverpool, and of children's organs at Alder Hey Hospital. The Report of the Royal Liverpool's Children's Inquiry (chaired by Michael Redfern QC)[78] on the retention of organs and body parts was published on 30 January 2001. Its publication coincided with three other publications:

1. *A report of a census of organs and tissues retained by pathology services in England carried out by the Chief Medical Officer*[79]
2. *The removal, retention and use of human organs and tissue from post-mortem examination: advice from the Chief Medical Officer*[80]
3. *Consent to organ and tissue retention at post-mortem examination and disposal of human materials.*[81]

The inquiry found that thousands of children's body parts had been collected at the hospital, some going back to before 1973. Most, however, were retained after 1988 when Professor Richard Van Velzen was appointed to the Department of Pathology and there was a huge increase in the number of organs removed and retained.

In response to the Redfern Report, the Secretary of State set up a Retained Organs Commission under the chairmanship of Professor Margaret Brazier. It was a special health authority which had the responsibility of overseeing the return of tissues and organs from collections around the country, ensuring that collections were accurately catalogued, providing information on collections throughout the country, ensuring that suitable counselling was available, acting as an advocate for parents if problems arose, advising on good practice in this area and handling enquiries from families and the public. On completion of its work it ceased to exist in March 2004.

Legal action by parents who had suffered as a result of the removal and retention of organs from their dead children in a group litigation action was initiated and the court agreed that the legal costs would be capped at £506,500.[82] On 26 March 2004 the High Court ruled, in respect of three test cases, that where hospitals had illegally removed the organs in post-mortem examinations without the parents' consent, parents could claim damages if they had suffered psychological injury.[83] Damages of £2750 were awarded in one of the test cases; the other two lost.

As a consequence of these developments the Human Tissue Act 2004 was passed which made it an explicit requirement that the informed consent of the parents or relatives must be obtained for the post mortem to be carried out (unless required by a coroner) and for the removal and retention of organs or tissues and the introduction of criminal offences for failure to obey the laws. These are discussed below.

'Human Bodies, Human Choices'

A consultation paper, 'Human Bodies, Human Choices', was published in July 2002,[84] which invited feedback on the principles to apply to the removal, retention and storage and use of organs. It was followed by proposals for new legislation on human organs and tissue, which were published in September 2003.[85]

Human Tissue Act 2004

The Human Tissue Act 2004 gave legal effect to the recommendations of the consultation paper and to the European Tissue Directive,[86] which was implemented in 2007.[87] The Act regulates the removal, storage and use of human organs and other tissues for specified purposes, specifies the appropriate consent for children and adults; creates a criminal offence in relation to the removal without appropriate consent; establishes a Human Tissue Authority and a licensing regime, arranges for the publication of codes of practice and sets up inspectorates for anatomy and pathology and of organ and tissue for human use. In addition, it makes provision for the use of DNA and creates an offence relating to non-consensual analysis of DNA, with specified exceptions. The government did not support any legal change to allow a person's organs to be donated automatically on their death unless they or their family had specifically asked otherwise, i.e. presumed consent for organ donation was not included in the Act. However, the Chief Medical Officer of the DH called in July 2007 for the introduction of an 'opt-out' system and a review was carried out. Further information is available from the website[88] of the Human Tissue Authority on which the codes of practice can be found.

In May 2007 a man became the first person to be convicted under the Human Tissue Act for trying to sell his kidney online for £24,000 in order to pay for his gambling debts.[89]

Intensive care units: resource pressures

There is national concern over the pressure placed on intensive care beds, often highlighted during flu epidemics. Thus in the winter of 2003/04 a warning was given by the Intensive Care Society in its report *Critical Insight* that critical care units across the country would face an inevitable bed shortage as the flu season began.[90]

An Audit Commission report[91] on intensive care units pointed out: 'It does not make sense to respond to pressures created in cheaper areas of the hospital by increasing the number of the most expensive beds.' The report found that critical care beds were not always used appropriately and 'critical care units can become the backstop of a poorly performing hospital'. It gave as an example of inappropriate use the fact that almost one-third of hospitals place extra strain on critical care beds, and bear unnecessary extra costs, by nursing patients with epidurals for pain relief after major surgery within critical care units. The Audit Commission report found that there were great variations in the resources deployed: 'Some units employ twice as many nurses as others have in order to have, for example, five direct care "bedside" nurses on duty at any time . . . Yet the cost of neither nurses nor doctors is related to mortality differences between units.' It suggests that there should be national research to record more scientifically the benefits offered by one-to-one nursing. The Intensive Care Foundation was founded in 2003 by the Intensive Care Society to facilitate and support the highest quality collaborative care research in the UK. Further information on its activities and also of the role of the Intensive Care Society can be found on the latter's website.[92]

Practical dilemma 15.7 Inadequate staffing

During a flu epidemic, there was considerable pressure on ITU beds and operations were being postponed because of the inability to offer patients follow-up in ITU. During this crisis, an extra bed was used in ITU, although the staffing numbers were not increased. Sarah Roberts was attempting to look after her own patient as well as cover for another patient, when the nurse was on break. Unfortunately, she administered the wrong dose of a drug and the patient died.

Sarah could face criminal proceedings for acting with a lack of professional care. If it can be shown that she is guilty of such gross professional recklessness and negligence that it amounts to a criminal offence, she could be found guilty of the manslaughter of the patient. Account would be taken of the pressure she had been placed under and the extent to which she had fulfilled her professional duty to the NMC under its Code by drawing the crisis situation to the notice of senior management and taking other appropriate action. (The legal issues relating to resources are considered in chapter 4.)

Review of critical care services

Following the Audit Report, an expert group was set up to review critical care services. Its report,[93] *Comprehensive Critical Care*, was published in 2000 along with a review of adult critical care nursing.[94] The Comprehensive Critical Care Report recommended a modernisation programme to develop consistent and comprehensive critical care services. Four levels of care were identified:

Level 0 normal acute ward care;

Level 1 acute ward care, with additional advice and support from critical care team;

Level 2 more detailed observation or interventions, e.g. patients with a single failing organ system; and

Level 3 advanced respiratory support alone or basic respiratory support together with support of at least two organ systems.

The report highlighted the need for action in four areas:

1. a hospital-wide approach to critical care;
2. a networked service;

3. workforce development; and

4. better information with all critical care services, collecting reliable management information and participating in outcome-focused clinical audit.

In 2013 NHS England published detailed plans to meet increases in demand for critical care service. It aimed to coordinate a strategic response to increasing demand and capacity pressures in critical care during winter months. It is available on its website.[95]

Other major concerns of relevance to the intensive care nurse include definition of the scope of her professional practice. The DH launched a document called the *Recruitment and Retention of Staff in Critical Care* on 4 June 2004. This is considered in chapter 23 and the same basic principles that are discussed there apply to the intensive care nurse. Other aspects relating to death are considered in chapter 28. A telephone survey was conducted by the RCN[96] that provided an analysis of the role of the nurse in intensive care and illustrated considerable differences in the functioning of nurses in ICUs and considerable flexibility of roles between doctors and nurses. These findings were confirmed by the report of the Audit Commission, which is considered above. In 2003 RCN published guidance on nurse staffing in critical care which includes consideration of the measuring of patient dependency, the role of critical care nurses, supervisory shift leaders, flexible working and other significant issues.[97] It has also published information on staffing levels for children's services, including paediatric intensive care[98] and in 2007 provided guidance on safe nurse staffing levels in critical care.[99]

In 2008 the DH (in conjunction with representatives from the British Association of Critical Care Nurses, the Intensive Care Society, the Intercollegiate Board for Training in Intensive Care Medicine and the Royal College of Nursing Critical Care Forum) published guidance on the role of an advanced critical care practitioner. It covers: how the role should function within the critical care team; the benefits of introducing the role in clinical practice; and a national framework of education and competence for the role within recognised standards of practice. It also published a National Education and Competence Framework for assistant critical care practitioners. Both documents are available on the DH website. Several universities offer a Masters Course in Advanced Critical Care Practice. Information on the national association of critical care practitioners is available on the website for the Faculty of Intensive Care Medicine.[100]

Conclusions

It is inevitable that standards in acute care will be one of the main areas of litigation. In addition, the work within operating theatres and the efficiency of surgical wards are central to any major success in the reduction of waiting lists and the decrease of litigation. Standards across all health service areas are subject to inspection by the Care Quality Commission (CQC) and all staff must be aware of recommendations from the National Institute for Health and Care Excellence. Significant changes have resulted from developments in the scope of professional practice of the nurse and from the recognition of the operating practitioner as a health professional registered under the Health Professions Council. The Human Tissue Act 2004 has made significant changes to the laws relating to many of the issues covered in this chapter. The shortage of organs for transplant continues to be of major concern and the effect of the law in Wales which presume consent to donation will be closely watched. The proposal that the HTA should be amalgamated with the Human Fertilisation and Embryology Authority (HFEA) into the Regulatory Authority for Tissue and Embryos (RATE) was dropped by the Government following criticism by the Joint Parliamentary Scrutiny Committee reviewing the Human Fertilisation and Embryology (Draft) Bill (see chapter 21). However, the review of arm's-length bodies has recommended that eventually both the HFEA and the HTA should be reorganised, with their functions being transferred to the CQC or the Health and Social Care Information Centre.[101] For the present they remain as separate organisations.[102]

Reflection questions

1. How do the provisions of the Health and Safety at Work Act (see chapter 12) affect the theatre manager?
2. Procedures do not provide the solution to every eventuality. In what circumstances do you consider a nurse would be justified in deviating from a specified procedure (see chapter 3)?
3. How do the basic principles of consent to treatment affect the work of the surgical ward and theatre nurse (see chapter 7)?
4. What are the main provisions of the Human Tissue Act on the law on consent to donate organs? What are the advantages and disadvantages of introducing an opt-out system?
5. Examine the role of the consultant nurse in ITU. What safeguards should exist to protect the patient?

Further exercises

1. Look back over the records that you have made on a patient who was in hospital several weeks before. If you were now to be challenged on any aspect of your care in that case, how useful and comprehensive would your notes be? Are there any obvious gaps on which you should have kept a record and are there any faults in the record keeping? (Refer to chapter 9.)
2. How do the principles relating to the scope of professional practice affect the nurse working in the areas considered in this chapter (see chapter 23)?
3. Obtain a copy of the incident book that is kept in the theatre in which you work and consider how some of these incidents could have been avoided.
4. Over a period of 2 weeks, list the legal problems that you have encountered in your work in an intensive care unit or transplant unit and refresh your memory of the basic principles of accountability.
5. Relatives often have very fixed views on the outcome they wish for the seriously ill patient. Prepare a short paper outlining the basic principles of consent that apply in order to clarify the situation for relatives. Refer to the Mental Capacity Act 2005 (see chapters 7 and 28).

References

1. *Wilsher* v *Essex Area Health Authority* [1986] 3 All ER 801 CA
2. www.rcn.org.uk
3. www.baccn.org.uk
4. www.afpp.org.uk
5. Department of Health, A Step Guide to Improving Operating Theatre Performance, 2002, case studies published in 2005
6. www.nice.org.uk
7. Commission for Health Improvement, Report on Prince Philip Hospital Llanelli, 15 November 2000
8. www.avma.org.uk
9. News item, Surgical instruments left inside patients, *The Operating Theatre Journal*, 201, June/July 2007, www.orme.org.uk
10. National Patient Safety Agency, Patient safety alert No. 06, March 2005
11. Martin Barrow, Hundreds of patients suffer after serious mistakes during surgery, *The Times*, 10 May 2013
12. https://improvement.nhs.uk/documents/2613/Never_Events_1_February_to_31_March_2018_.pdf
13. News item, *The Times*, 22 February 2014
14. Jack Grimson, *The Sunday Times*, 2 February 2014
15. www.barna.co.uk
16. www.afpp.org.uk
17. Audit Commission, Anaesthesia under Examination: the efficiency and effectiveness of anaesthesia and pain relief services in England and Wales, Audit Commission, 17 December 1997
18. www.hcpc-uk.org/aboutregistration/standards/standardsofproficiency
19. National Patient Safety Agency, Patient Safety Division Teamwork for Safety: why we need it, and how we do it (no date)
20. NICE, 21 May 2013
21. News item, Absent nurse death, *The Times*, 6 July 2013
22. www.naasp.org.uk
23. www.afpp.org.uk
24. Lindsay McIntosh, Surgeon 'lied to patient that he had removed her brain tumour', *The Times*, 8 August 2013
25. Solihull Hospital, Kennedy Breastcare Review on www.heartofengland.nhs.uk
26. Dominic Kennedy, Trust suspends top surgeon who 'engraved liver', *The Times*, 26 December 2013
27. News item, *The Times*, 17 February 2014
28. https://theguardian.com/uk-news/2018/jan/12/surgeon-burned-initials-livers-two-patients-fined-simon-bramhall-assault-transplant
29. www.who.int
30. Haynes, A. B. *et al.*, A Surgical Safety Checklist to Reduce Morbidity and Mortality in a Global Population, *New England Journal of Medicine*, 360:491–9, January 2009
31. Chris Smyth, Fatal Friday: how risk of dying after operation soars towards the end of the week, *The Times*, 29 May 2013
32. Chris Smyth, Death-rate tables 'are not the best way to identify bad surgeons', *The Times*, 5 July 2013
33. www.england.nhs.uk
34. Chris Smyth, Doctors 'must put meals at heart of hospital care plans', *The Times*, 25 November 2013

[35] Clare Dyer, Cash settlement for woman who changed her mind on abortion, *The Guardian*, 30 July 2007
[36] Department of Health, Good Practice in Consent Implementation Guide, DH, 2001, 2nd edn, 2009
[37] Pollard *et al.*, Intra-operative awareness – a review of 3 years' data, *Anesthiology*, 106:269–74, 2007
[38] Buss, C., I felt surgeon cut into my stomach, *Leicester Mercury*, 22 January 2013
[39] British Committee for Standards in Haematology, Blood Transfusion Task Force, RCN and the Royal College of Surgeons of England, The administration of blood and blood components and the management of transfused patients, *Transfusion Medicine*, 9(3):227–38, 1999
[40] National Patient Safety Agency, Right Patient, Right Blood – new advice for safer blood transfusions, November 2006
[41] Blood Safety and Quality Regulation, SI 2005/50 (amended SI 2006/2013 and SI 2007/604)
[42] Department of Health, Liberating the NHS: Report of the arm's-length bodies, London, Crown, 2010
[43] www.nhsbt.nhs.uk
[44] Chris Smyth, Blood donors turned away by clinics' incompetence, *The Times*, 14 January 2014
[45] Mike Hudson, Giving Blood, Letter to the Editor, *The Times*, 15 January 2014
[46] *A and Others* v *National Blood Authority and Another (sub nom Re Hepatitis C Litigation)*, The Times Law Report, 4 April 2001; [2001] 3 All ER 289
[47] Department of Health press release 2004/0025, Details of Hepatitis C ex gratia payment scheme announced
[48] www.infectedbloodinquiry.org.uk
[49] Infected Blood Inquiry (2024) Reports available at https://www.infectedblood inquiry.org.uk
[50] UK Government (2024) Infected blood compensation scheme available at Infected Blood Compensation Scheme Summary - GOV.UK (www.gov.uk)
[51] www.uktransplant.org.uk/ukt
[52] Coroners and Justice Act 2009, Schedule 21 paragraph 50 adding subsection 5A to section 43 of the Human Tissue Act 2004
[53] Human Tissue Act 2004 (Persons who Lack Capacity to Consent and Transplants) Regulations 2006, SI 2006/1659
[54] Human Tissue Act 2004 (Commencement No. 5 and Transitional Provisions) (Amendment) Order 2006/2169
[55] Robin Pagnamenta and John Simpson, Cash for kidneys offer lures Britons, *The Times*, 12 November 2013
[56] News Item, Cash row is blocking hand transplants, says surgeon, *The Times*, 28 December 2013
[57] *Re M (Medical Treatment: consent)* [1999] 2 FLR 1097
[58] Simon de Bruxelles, Girl wins fight to turn down transplant, *The Times*, 11 November 2008
[59] Simon de Bruxelles, Change of heart by girl, 14, who fought for the right to die, *The Times*, 21
[60] News Item, Battling teenager refuses transplant, *The Times*, 27 August 2013
[61] *Hart* v *Brown* 289 A 2d 386 Conn 1972
[62] *Strunk* v *Strunk* 445 SW 2d 145 (Ky App) 1969
[63] *Y (Adult Patient: transplant: bone marrow) Re* (1996) BMLR 111; (1996) 4 Med LR 204
[64] Human Tissue Act 2004 (Persons who Lack Capacity to Consent and Transplants) Regulations 2006, SI 2006/1659

65 Available on the DH website at www.gov.uk
66 News item, Man sues NHS for £14m after botched surgery, *The Times*, 3 November 2010
67 Quality and Safety of Organs intended for Transplantation Regulations 2012 SI 2012/1501
68 Quality and Safety of Organs intended for Transplantation Regulations 2014 SI 2014/1459
69 www.odt.nhs.uk
70 www.organdonation.nhs.uk
71 Department of Health, Saving Lives, Valuing Donors: A transplant framework for England – one year on, DH, 2004
72 Department of Health, Organs for transplants: A report from the Organ Donation Taskforce, Stationery Office, 2008
73 News item, Consent presumed, *The Times*, 14 July 2010
74 Human Transplant (Wales) Act 2013
75 David Rose, Wait for transplants may be cut as study finds kidneys from dead donors are viable, *The Times*, 19 August 2010
76 Whipple Tom, Facebook pokes its users into signing up as organ donors, *The Times*, 18 June 2013
77 Smyth Chris, Transplant 'for donors first', *The Times*, 21 August 2013
78 Department of Health, The Royal Liverpool's Children's Inquiry Report, DH, 30 January 2001
79 Chief Medical Officer, A Report of a Census of Organs and Tissues Retained by Pathology Services in England, DH, January 2001
80 Department of Health, The Removal, Retention and Use of Human Organs and Tissue from Post-Mortem Examination: advice from the Chief Medical Officer, DH, January 2001
81 Department of Health, Consent to Organ and Tissue Retention at Post-Mortem Examination and Disposal of Human Materials, DH, January 2001
82 *AB and Others* v *Leeds Teaching Hospitals NHS Trust and in the Matter of the Nationwide Organ Group Litigation* [2003] Lloyd's Rep Med 7 355
83 *AB and Others* v *Leeds Teaching Hospitals NHS Trust and Another*, The Times Law Report, 12 April 2004
84 Department of Health and Welsh Assembly, Human Bodies, Human Choices: a consultation report, July 2002
85 Department of Health and Welsh Assembly, Proposals for New Legislation on Human Organs and Tissue, September 2003
86 Tissue Directive 2004/23/EC
87 Human Tissue (Quality and Safety for Human Application) Regulations, SI 2007/1523
88 www.hta.gov.uk
89 Stephanie Condron, Gambler tried to sell his kidney online, *Daily Telegraph*, 11 May 2007
90 Oliver Wright and Christian Barby, Critical care beds shortage 'certain' when flu strikes, *The Times*, 26 November 2003
91 Audit Commission, Critical to Success: the place of efficient and effective critical care services within the acute hospital, Audit Commission, 1999
92 www.ics.ac.uk
93 Department of Health, Comprehensive Critical Care Report of an Expert Group, DH, 2000
94 Department of Health, The Review of Adult Critical Care Nursing Report to the Chief Nursing Officer, DH, 2000
95 www.england.nhs.uk/commissioning/ccs

[96] Royal College of Nursing, The Nature of Nursing Work in Intensive Care, Order No. 000728, RCN, May 1997
[97] 002172, RCN, September 2003
[98] 001976, RCN, February 2003
[99] 001976, RCN, October 2007
[100] www.ficm.ac.uk
[101] Department of Health, Liberating the NHS: Report of the arm's-length bodies, London, Crown, 2010
[102] www.gov.uk/government/publications/arms-length-bodies/our-arms-lengths-bodies

Chapter 16

Learning Disabilities and Safeguarding People

This chapter discusses

- Acting in the best interests of a mentally incapacitated adult
- Deprivation of Liberty Safeguards (DoLS) (Bournewood)
- Carers
- Court of Protection and Code of Practice
- White Paper *Valuing People*
- Safeguarding vulnerable adults
- Sexual relations and related issues
- Property
- Direct payments
- Registration and inspections

Introduction

While some persons with learning disabilities may also suffer from a mental disorder (just as they might have physical disabilities and illnesses and come under the chapters on gynaecology (chapter 14) or acute care (chapter 15)), the definition of mental disorder in the Mental Health Act 1983 (as amended by the 2007 Act) excludes learning disabilities on its own. Only if the learning disability is associated with abnormally aggressive or seriously irresponsible conduct on the person's part will it come within the statutory definition of mental disorder and could lead to detention under the Mental Health legislation. Mental disorder is considered in chapter 19. NICE has published various guidelines (many of which have been updated in 2017 and 2018) for looking after people with learning disabilities.[1] Those with learning disabilities have exactly the same rights as others. If they are assessed as having the requisite mental capacity to make a specific decision, then they have the right of autonomy or self-determination. Where a person with learning disabilities also has a mental illness, then he or she may come within the provisions of the Mental Health Act 1983. Where a person with learning disabilities lacks the requisite mental capacity to make a specific decision, then he or she would come under the provisions of the Mental Capacity Act 2005. People with learning disabilities can also rely upon the rights set out in the European Convention on Human Rights (see the website of this book). The Equality Act 2010 is discussed in chapter 10 and recognises many of the rights set out in the United Nations Convention on the rights of persons with disabilities (signed in 2006) which is available on the internet.[2] The topics discussed in this chapter are shown above.

Acting in the best interests of a mentally incapacitated adult

Case 16.1 *In re F (Adult: Court's Jurisdiction)* [2000]

Care of incapable adults at risk of harm[3]

T, an 18-year-old girl with an intellectual age of five to eight, lacked the capacity to make decisions about her future. The local authority sought to invoke the inherent jurisdiction of the court under the doctrine of necessity to obtain directions as to where T should live and to supervise her contact with her natural family, principally her mother. The mother challenged the power of the court to make such a ruling, on the grounds that its former parens patriae jurisdiction had lapsed in 1959. The Court of Appeal held that in the present conflict, where serious questions hung over the future care of T if returned to her mother, there was no practicable alternative to intervention by the court.

In Case 16.1 it was held that it was essential that T's best interests should be considered by the High Court and there was no impediment to the judge hearing the substantive issues involved in the case. Lord Justice Sedley specifically stated that this conclusion did not conflict with the European Convention for the Protection of Human Rights and Fundamental Freedoms[4] (see the website of this book). The House of Lords in the *Re F* (1989)[5] case recognised the powers that existed at common law which enabled professionals and carers to make decisions on behalf of those lacking the mental capacity to make decisions in their best interests. In a third case,[6] a young man (S), born in 1984 with velo-cardio-facial syndrome with severe global developmental delay and bilateral renal dysplasia, was assessed as having a cognitive functioning age of about five to six. His dialysis catheter became infected and there was concern over what treatment would be in his best interests. The then President of the Family Division, Dame Elizabeth Butler-Sloss, held that:

- The fundamental principle of the sanctity of life was of particular relevance in this case where the existing and proposed treatment options were crucial to sustain S's life.
- As S lacked capacity to make decisions about his medical treatment and there was disagreement between S's family and the treating clinicians, it was the duty of the court to decide, in

an exercise addressing medical, emotional and all other welfare issues, what was in his best interests.

- Just because a person could not understand treatment it was wrong to say that he could not have it: it was crucial that S, who suffered from serious mental in addition to physical problems, should not be given less satisfactory treatment than a person who had full capacity to understand the risk, pain and discomfort inseparable from major surgery.

- It was in S's best interests that he should continue to receive dialysis as long as some form of that treatment was working and providing him with a reasonable quality of life; when haemodialysis was no longer effective, he should move to peritoneal dialysis; dialysis via an arteriovenous fistula should not be ruled out but should be considered in consultation with learning disability experts once S had settled into the adult renal unit and an adult way of life; a kidney transplant should not now be carried out as it was not clear that he would enjoy a longer lifespan with a transplant; but if, in future, medical reasons were in favour of a transplant, it should not be rejected on the grounds of S's inability to understand the purpose and consequences of the operation or concerns about his management.

These three cases preceded the implementation of the Mental Capacity Act 2005 which replaced the common law by statutory provisions for decision making on behalf of those mentally incapacitated adults who were unable to make their own decisions.

Mental Capacity Act 2005

This Act, which came fully into force in October 2007, provides a statutory definition of mental incapacity and sets out the steps to be taken in determining the best interests of a person who lacks the requisite mental capacity (see chapter 7). It requires, in the absence of informal carers or others who can be consulted about a person's best interests, an independent mental capacity advocate (IMCA) to be appointed where decisions relating to serious medical treatment, accommodation or protection measures are being considered. (In the latter case, an IMCA can be appointed even if there are informal carers.) In 2014 the Court of Protection ruled that a woman suffering from autistic spectrum disorder and borderline learning difficulties lacked the capacity to make her own decisions and that physically invasive medical procedures, i.e. a Caesarean, were in her best interests. She had already had five children who were in care and her third child who was born secretly at home was believed to have been fed on packet soup for his first week and was in a dehydrated and malnourished state when taken into care.[7]

In determining the capacity of a person with learning disabilities it must be emphasised that the capacity to consent must be related to the actual decision being made, that acquiescence does not necessarily mean consent and that if capacity is considered to be lacking then the decision must be made in the best interests of the person.

Restraint

Under the Mental Capacity Act 2005 restraint can only be used where a person reasonably believes that it is necessary to do so in order to prevent harm to the person who lacks the requisite mental capacity and where the act of restraint is a proportionate response to (a) the likelihood of P's suffering harm, and (b) the seriousness of that harm. As a consequence of amendments to the Mental Capacity Act 2005 introduced by the Mental Health Act 2007, safeguards have been introduced where a person lacking the requisite mental capacity is deprived of his or her liberty. These were introduced as a result of the decision of the European Court of Human Rights in the

Bournewood case (see page 424). (See also the discussion on restraint in chapter 18 in relation to the elderly and in chapter 19 in relation to the mentally disordered.)

In a case (*LA* v *A*, page 477 ref 81) concerning a married couple, both with learning disabilities, who were opposed to contraception, the local authority sought a declaration that Mrs A lacked capacity to decide whether to use contraception and that it would be in her interests to be required to receive it. The judge ruled that she lacked the capacity to make a decision about contraception, that her refusal was not the product of her own free mind and that she lacked the ability to use or weigh the information given to her. He refused, however, to make a declaration that it was in her best interests for contraception to be given by force, and quoted from Lady Hale in the case of *R* v *Broadmoor Special Hospital Authority*[8] where she had stated that where an incapacitated person was actively opposed to a course of action, 'the benefits which it holds for him will have to be carefully weighed against the disadvantage of going against his wishes, especially if force is required to do this'.

Case 16.2 — **ZH (A Protected Party) v Commissioner of Police of the Metropolis, Liberty and Another Intervening [2013]**

Restraint of an autistic boy was inhuman[9]

The Court of Appeal held that physical restraint of a vulnerable teenage boy who was autistic, epileptic and lacked understanding of what was happening to him, carried out by police officers with handcuffs and leg restraints, and his detention in a cage in a police van, were capable of constituting inhuman or degrading treatment contrary to Article 3 and a deprivation of liberty in breach of Article 5 of the European Convention on Human Rights. The boy had been taken by carers to the local swimming baths. He became fixated by the water and did not move. The manager called the police. The boy was still standing beside the pool, but jumped in fully clothed when the police arrived. He was removed from the water by lifeguards and the police took him into custody as described above. The restraint and detention lasted about 45 minutes.

The Bournewood Case

The House of Lords in the Bournewood[10] case considered the question of whether a mentally incapacitated person, incapable of giving consent to admission, could be held at common law in a psychiatric hospital and not placed under the Mental Health Act 1983 (see Case 16.3). It decided that section 131 of the Mental Health Act 1983 did not require a mentally disordered person to have the capacity to consent to admission as an informal patient. However, the application against this decision to the ECHR succeeded and the UK government was required to introduce changes. The result was that the Mental Capacity Act 2005 was amended to make provision for the deprivation of liberty of such persons (which are known as the Deprivation of Liberty Safeguards (DoLS) under schedule A1 of the Mental Capacity Act 2005).

> ### Case 16.3   *L v United Kingdom* [2004] (The Bournewood Case)
>
> **Lack of capacity to consent to admission[11]**
>
> L, an adult with learning disabilities, was informally admitted to a mental health unit. He was not detained under the Mental Health Act 1983. His carers asked for his discharge, but his psychiatrist considered that it was not in his best interests to be discharged and that he should remain in hospital. The carers challenged the legality of this decision. They lost in the High Court, but the Court of Appeal held that section 131 of the Mental Health Act required a person to have the mental capacity to agree to admission; a person lacking the requisite capacity should be examined for compulsory admission under the Act. The House of Lords upheld the appeal of the NHS trust, holding that an adult lacking mental capacity could be cared for and detained in a psychiatric hospital, using common law powers. Subsequently, an application was made to the ECHR, which held that there was a breach of his Article 5 right to liberty.

As a consequence of the Bournewood case, changes to the law were necessary to ensure compliance with the Human Rights Act 1998 (see chapter 1). Article 5 of the European Convention on Human Rights, which is set out in Schedule 1 in the Human Rights Act 1998, states:

> **Everyone has the right to liberty and security of person. No one shall be deprived of his liberty save in the following cases and in accordance with a procedure prescribed by law.**

Included in the 'following cases' under (e) are 'persons of unsound mind'. However, the fact that mentally incapacitated adults could under the House of Lords' Bournewood ruling be detained without being placed under the Mental Health Act 1983 was not a procedure prescribed by law. The Bournewood amendments to the Mental Capacity Act 2005 were therefore necessary to provide protection for such persons when a restriction of liberty was required in their best interests.

Deprivation of Liberty Safeguards (DoLS) (Bournewood)

The Mental Health Act 2007 amended the Mental Capacity Act 2005 to introduce the safeguards necessary to justify loss of liberty of residents in hospitals and care homes. These are known as the Deprivation of Liberty Safeguards (DoLS). The DoLS regulations came into force on 3 November 2008[12] together with the regulations relating to the appointment of the relevant person's representative.[13] The DoLS are set out in the new Schedule A1 to the Mental Capacity Act as introduced by the Mental Health Act 2007 and can be found in a briefing paper available from the Department of Health.[14] Please note that the Department of Health is now referred to as the Department of Health and Social Care (2018), and this department is responsible for England only. If you are resident in any of the other UK nations you will need to access the equivalent departments for those respective legislatures.

The following situations should be kept distinct:

(a) Where a patient requires treatment for mental disorder, and is objecting to that treatment, an application should be made under the Mental Health Act 1983 as amended by the 2007 Act.

(b) Where a patient is suffering from mental disorder and requires restriction of his or her liberty for which detention under the Mental Health Act is inappropriate, because they are compliant with their treatment, then the DoLS apply.

(c) Where a person lacks the mental capacity to make his or her own decisions, the Mental Capacity Act applies and limited restraint may be used (see chapter 18).

Who is Covered by the Deprivation of Liberty Safeguards?

- Those over 18 years;
- Those who suffer from a disorder or disability of mind (as defined in the Mental Health Act 1983) (see chapter 19);
- Those who lack the capacity to give consent to the arrangements made for their care; and
- Those for whom such care (in circumstances that amount to a deprivation of liberty within the meaning of Article 5 of the European Convention on Human Rights) is considered after an independent assessment to be a necessary and proportionate response in their best interests to protect them from harm.

The DoLS Code of Practice published by the Ministry of Justice[15] sets out the following circumstances where the use of the Deprivation of Liberty Safeguards may be indicated:

- Where restraint is used to admit a person or to prevent their leaving;
- Where movement is controlled for a significant period;
- Where a request for discharge by relatives is refused;
- Where an individual is prevented from having social contact because of restrictions placed on access by others; and
- Where continuous supervision and control has led to a loss of autonomy by an individual.[16]

What Procedures are Required?

1 Application for authorisation

The care home or hospital, i.e. the managing authority, must identify a client/patient as lacking capacity and who risks being deprived of his or her liberty. It must apply to the supervisory body, i.e. the local authority in which the client/patient was ordinarily resident, for the authorisation of deprivation of liberty.

2 Assessments required

1. Age assessment – client/patient must be over 18 years.
2. Mental health assessment – client/patient must be suffering a mental disorder.
3. Mental capacity assessment – client/patient must lack the capacity to decide whether to be admitted to or remain in the hospital or care home.
4. Eligibility assessment – the client/patient must:
    (a) Not be detained under the Mental Health Act;
    (b) Not be subject to a conflicting requirement under the Mental Health Act;
    (c) Not be subject to powers of recall under the Mental Health Act;
    (d) Not be subject to a treatment order in hospital to which the client/patient objects.
5. Best interests assessment – the authorisation would be in the client/patient's best interests and is a proportionate response to the likelihood of suffering harm and the seriousness of that harm.
6. There is no conflict between the authorisation sought and a valid decision by a donee of a lasting power of attorney or a deputy, nor with a valid and applicable advance decision made by the client/patient.

3 Appointment of representative for the client/patient

If the best interests assessor concludes that the client/patient has the capacity to appoint his or her own representative, then they can do this. Otherwise the best interests assessor can appoint a representative. If the assessor notifies the supervisory body that a representative has not been appointed, then it can appoint a representative who can be paid to act as the client's/patient's representative.

4 Authorisation granted

If all the assessments are satisfactory then authorisation by the supervisory body can be granted for the deprivation of the client's/patient's liberty for up to twelve months. An urgent authorisation can be issued for a maximum of seven days by the managing authority while it awaits a decision on a standard authorisation by the supervisory body.

5 Review and monitoring

The supervisory body should keep under review the client's/patient's deprivation of liberty and the whole process of the assessments and authorisation will be monitored to ensure that all the required procedures were followed.

The DoLS were first considered by the court in the case of *GJ* v *the Foundation Trust*.[17] In this case the court had to consider whether GJ was 'ineligible to be deprived of liberty by the MCA'. The judge considered the historical background to DoLS and the relationship between the Mental Health Act and the Mental Capacity Act and DoLS. He concluded that in the case before him the deprivation of liberty of GJ, who suffered from mental disorder and also diabetes, was justified under DoLS. He considered that if the nature of the treatment for which deprivation of liberty was required was essentially for physical health problems then it would not be appropriate for the patient to be detained under the Mental Health Act (which can only authorise treatment for mental disorder).

In May 2014 the Court of Appeal held that a man who lacked mental capacity as a result of serious brain injury which led to his leading a chaotic life as an alcoholic could be detained in his best interests in a care home for the purpose of receiving care and treatment.[18] His appeal against the decision not to terminate the standard authorisation to deprive him of his liberty was turned down. See also the case where a judge upheld a woman's application to return home and overruled the DoLS authorisation (see chapter 28).[19]

The case of G v E & Ors[20] (see Case 16.7, page 500) under the Court of Protection is an example of the complexity which can arise in such situations. In this case the local authority was held to be at fault in moving a person to different accommodation without carrying out a DoLS assessment. Ben Troke and Neil Ward explore the complexities and as yet unanswered questions relating to DoLS.[21] Further information on DoLS can be found on the Alzheimer's Society's website[22] which provides a PDF fact sheet.

The CQC undertakes an annual report on Deprivation of Liberty Safeguards which can be accessed on its website.[23] The conclusions in its report for 2011/12 were that there was still confusion around the precise definition and thresholds for deprivation (as opposed to restriction) of liberty. Recent court decisions have ruled that there is no universal definition. Decisions can only be made on individual circumstances. The relationship between care, appropriate restrictions of liberty, the Deprivation of Liberty Safeguards and the wider Mental Capacity Act has become complex and potentially confusing. It recommended that health and social care providers operating the DoLS system should give the highest priority to improve understanding and practice of the MCA.

Fundamental flaws in the protection provided by the Mental Capacity Act and DoLS were found by the House of Lords in its report published in March 2014[24] on the post-legislative scrutiny of the Mental Capacity Act 2005.

See also the case of An NHS Trust v Dr A [2013][25] on DoLs and deprivation of liberty in a hunger strike which is considered in chapter 7. In March 2014 the Supreme Court ruled on the test of mental capacity for the purpose of bringing an action and ruled that a settlement agreed without a litigation friend being appointed was invalid[26] (see chapter 7).

Case 16.4

P (by his Litigation Friend the Official Solicitor) v Cheshire West and Cheshire Council and Anor [2014][27]

Two sisters with learning disabilities and a man with cerebral palsy brought an action stating that the Deprivation of Liberty Safeguards had not been applied to them. The Court of Appeal ruled that they were not deprived of their liberty, because their freedom was inherently restricted because of their disabilities and their lives in their homes were not significantly different from their previous circumstances. The Supreme Court held that vulnerable people with dementia and other disabilities have the same human right to physical liberty as the rest of the human race as guaranteed by Article 5 of the European Convention on Human Rights. It considered how a deprivation of liberty should be defined, seeing the acid test as being whether a person is under the complete supervision and control of those caring for her and is not free to leave the place where she lives. The following are not relevant: the person's compliance or lack of objection, the relative normality of the placement, and the reason or purpose behind a particular placement. There should be no confusion between the question of the quality of the arrangements which have been made and the question of whether these arrangements constitute a deprivation of liberty. Lady Hale stated that a gilded cage is still a cage and suggested that there must be a regular review to ensure that the restrictions on their liberty are justified. The Supreme Court also heard the case of *P and Q* v *Surrey County Council (subnom Re MIG and MEG)* and in a majority verdict held that there was a deprivation of liberty. P and Q were sisters with substantial learning disabilities and lacked the capacity to make decisions about their care and where they lived. They were moved from the family home in 2007, P to to a family home with a devoted foster mother and Q to a specialist residential home. The Court of Appeal had held that neither was deprived of her liberty.[28]

Following the UK Supreme Court decision in *Cheshire West* (Case 16.4), the Department of Health and Social care issued a note on the implications of both the Cheshire and Surrey County Council judgments for those responsible for the assessment and authorisation of deprivation of liberty, the care of individuals and those responsible for policies and procedures.[29]

The note recommended that the revised test for determining a deprivation of liberty be applied (i.e. the person is under continuous supervision and control and is not free to leave, and the person lacks capacity to consent to these arrangements). It stated that deprivation of liberty can still occur in domestic settings. Suggested action included relevant staff familiarising themselves with the provisions of the Mental Capacity Act 2005, particularly the five principles and specifically the least restrictive principle (see chapter 7); being alert to any restrictions and restraint; reviewing existing care and treatment plans; exploring alternative ways of providing care and treatment to identify less restrictive means; and ensuring that, if unavoidable, any deprivation of liberty is authorised. Local Authorities are advised to review their allocation of resources to ensure they meet their legal obligations in the light of the Supreme Court judgment. As a consequence of this decision the Vice-President of the Court of Protection estimated that many thousands more cases will come to the Court of Protection to have their detention authorised.[30]

In its state of care report for 2022/23 the CQC reported that the number of applications to deprive a person of their liberty under the safeguards rose to over 300,000 in England.[31]

The Steven Neary case (see case 16.5) illustrates the difficulties of local authorities in using DoL safeguards.[32]

See also the case of *MH* v *United Kingdom*[33] where the European Court of Human Rights suggested that DoLS may not be a sufficient defence against an alleged breach of Article 5(4) if the person lacks capacity and is not represented. (See chapter 19 for a consideration of the case.)

Case 16.5 *London Borough of Hillingon* v *Neary* [2011]

Steven Neary, who suffered from autism and severe learning disabilities was taken into respite at the request of his father for a few days in December 2009. He remained there until December 2010 against both his and his father's wishes. The father and son contended that the LA's actions were unlawful. The LA claimed that initially the father had consented to the stay and thereafter Steven was kept in the home lawfully as a result of using Deprivation of Liberty Safeguards. Mr Justice Jackson held that the DoLS authorisations relied upon flawed assessments. The LA had failed to accept the principle that all other things being equal Steven should have been cared for by his family, they had failed to appoint an independent mental capacity advocate speedily and had delayed in referring the matter to the Court of Protection. The LA therefore had breached Steven's rights under Articles 8, Article 5(1) and 5(4). The judge held that 'there is an obligation on the State to ensure that a person deprived of liberty is not only entitled but enabled to have the lawfulness of his detention reviewed speedily by a court'.

In 2012 a local authority sought a declaration relating to restrictions which had been put in place on the liberty of G, a 57-year-old man who resided in a private care home. He suffered from a number of mental disorders, including childhood autism, dissocial personality disorder and paedophilia and lacked the capacity to make decisions concerning his care needs. Restrictions included strip searching, and monitoring of correspondence and telephone conversations. The Court of Protection granted the declaration and stated that the restrictions were sufficiently detailed in the scope of their safeguards and complied with Article 8.[34]

Carers

The implementation of the Mental Capacity Act 2005 has major implications for carers of those with learning disabilities. Their role in the decision-making process where a person lacks the mental capacity to make a specific decision has been clarified. Information which they can give about the mentally incapacitated person's past wishes and feelings, views, beliefs and any other relevant information must be passed to the decision maker to determine the best interests of the mentally incapacitated person. While the Act does not stipulate that informal (i.e. unpaid) carers are required to follow the guidance in the Code of Practice, it suggests they would find the advice of considerable help.[35] The Care Act 2014 recognises the right of the carer to be assessed and supported (see chapter 22).

Independent Mental Capacity Advocates (IMCA)

Where a relative or friend is not available to be consulted in the process of determining the best interests of a person lacking the requisite mental capacity, the Mental Capacity Act 2005 requires the appointment of an IMCA in specified circumstances. These include where serious medical treatment is being considered and where accommodation is being arranged by the NHS or social services. Under the regulations[36] drawn up under the Mental Capacity Act 2005 an IMCA should be appointed in an adult protection case even though relatives or informal carers are available. Further information on the IMCA can be found in the author's work.[37]

Refusal to Grant Accommodation

The rights of relatives to refuse to take back a client who has been in respite care also need to be considered. In the case of an adult person suffering from mental impairment, if the relatives refuse to take the person back home this is their right and they cannot be compelled to look after him or her. Health and social services professionals would have to look for other accommodation for the client.

Protection of the Autonomy of the Client

Conversely it may happen that an extremely diligent parent/carer is unwilling to allow a son or daughter with learning disabilities to leave home and enter sheltered accommodation. In one case a mother had been placed under an **injunction** not to visit her son who had been moved to alternative accommodation. The Court of Appeal ruled that the injunction should be lifted as it was not appropriate to threaten her with imprisonment, but the case illustrates the difficulties of 'letting go'.

Case 16.6   Local Authority X v MM [2007][38]

The local authority (LA) brought the case seeking orders that M lacked capacity to conduct litigation, make decisions as to where she should reside, determine with whom she should have contact, manage her own affairs or enter into marriage. It also wanted a declaration that it was in M's best interests to reside in supported accommodation and to have limited contact with K, her partner. M was a vulnerable adult who suffered paranoid schizophrenia and learning disabilities. She had been with K for 15 years. The LA received information that K was intending to move M from her supported accommodation and disengage from psychiatric services. They therefore applied for an interim injunction to prevent M being moved from her supported accommodation or to have unsupervised contact with K.

The capacity to consent to sexual intercourse has been considered by the Supreme Court in *A Local authority and JB* [2021][39] see case 16.7.

Case 16.7   A local authority v JB [2021] UKSC 52

A 38 year old man with an autistic spectrum disorder and impaired cognition appealed against a decision that he lacked capacity to engage in sexual relations.

The UK Supreme Court held that when formulating the matter to be decided under section 2(1) of the Mental Capacity Act 2005 it was appropriate to consider whether the person could engage in sexual relations rather than merely consent to sexual relations as it concerned initiating the sexual activity rather than consenting to relations proposed by another person.

This important ruling has modified the information a person must understand, retain use and weigh to have capacity to engage in sexual relations. This includes:

- The nature and character of the sexual act including its mechanics
- That the other person must be able to consent and does consent to the sexual activity

- That they can say yes or no to sexual relations and can decide whether or not to engage
- That a foreseeable consequence of intercourse between a man and a woman of child bearing age is that the woman may become pregnant
- That sexual activity carries risks to health particularly sexually transmitted infections and the risk can be reduced by wearing a condom

Court of Protection and Code of Practice

The Court of Protection was established as a superior court of record by the Mental Capacity Act.[40] It has the power to make decisions about both personal welfare and property and affairs for a person who lacks the requisite mental capacity and can make declarations about advance decisions (see chapter 28). It also has ultimate control over those appointed under a lasting power of attorney (see chapter 18). Court-appointed deputies replaced the previous system of receiverships and have extended powers to include welfare and healthcare matters as well as financial and property affairs. There is now a single integrated framework for making personal welfare decisions, healthcare decisions and financial decisions on behalf of those lacking the requisite mental capacity, as recommended by the Law Commission in 1995.[41] The Court can make both one-off orders and also appoint a deputy with continuing powers. Under section 15 of the Mental Capacity Act it can make declarations on:

(a) Whether a person has or lacks capacity to make a decision specified in the declaration.
(b) Whether a person has or lacks capacity to make decisions on such matters as are described in the declaration.
(c) The lawfulness or otherwise of any act (which includes an omission and course of conduct) done, or yet to be done, in relation to that person.

Examples of (c) might include deciding whether the withholding or withdrawing of medical treatment is in the best interests of P.

In 2014 the Court of Protection exercised its supervisory powers when it heard an application by a local authority for breach of an order made by the court. The partner (Lindsey M who had a drink problem) of a mentally incapacitated man PW broke an order that she should not have contact or seek to go into the property of PW. The judge deferred sentence to give Lindsey M a chance to show that she could comply with the order.[42]

Significant changes in the way the Court of Protection works followed the increase in workload arising from the decision of the Supreme Court in the Cheshire west case (see Case 16.4). A clearer regional structure rather than ad hoc regional sittings together with greater openness in its hearings have been implemented. Even before the Cheshire west decision, its workload had increased by 30 per cent in the preceding four years. In the figures for 2023 the number of applications to the Court under the Mental Capacity Act 2005 had increased by a quarter compared to 2022 with the Court making some 58,530 orders during that year.[43] Guidance on the publication of judgments was issued in 2014.[44]

A Code of Practice providing guidance on the Mental Capacity Act 2005 was prepared by the Department of Constitutional Affairs (now the Ministry of Justice) and is available online.[45] A supplementary code was published to provide guidance on the Deprivation of Liberty Safeguards.[46]

Case 16.8   G v E & Ors [2010]

Decision making by the Court of Protection[47]

E (aged 19) suffered from a rare and very complex genetic condition known as tuberous sclerosis and as a result had a severe learning disability. An application was brought by E's sister, G. The respondents to the application were E himself by his litigation friend, the Official Solicitor; the local authority in whose area E resides; and F, a woman with whom E resided for over 10 years, initially as a foster carer under section 20 of the Children Act 1989 and subsequently under an adult placement until he was removed by the local authority in April 2009. G asked for the following issues to be determined:

(i) whether E has capacity to make decisions;

(ii) whether it is in his best interests to return to live with F or whether he should be cared for in a residential care home and, if so, which care home;

(iii) what contact provision should be made for G and/or F if E does not return home;

(iv) whether the local authority has unlawfully detained E in breach of Article 5 of the European Convention for the Protection of Human Rights and Fundamental Freedoms and/or the Deprivation of Liberty Safeguards under the Mental Capacity Act 2005 and/or Article 6 of the convention;

(v) whether the local authority has interfered with E's right to a home and/or to family life under Article 8 of the convention;

(vi) whether E should receive damages from the local authority and the amount of such damages for breach of Articles 5, 6 and/or 8;

(vii) whether the local authority should bear the costs of this claim.

In an interim hearing in March 2010 the judge had to determine the following issues:

1. whether E is currently deprived of his liberty; and
2. what is in E's best interest with regard to residence and contact pending the final hearing, listed for July 2010.

He held that E lacked the mental capacity to make his own decisions; that the local authority had unlawfully deprived E of his liberty and infringed his Article 5 rights by placing him in accommodation without seeking authorisation under the Deprivation of Liberty Safeguards or seeking an order of the Court of Protection. It was also in breach of his Article 8 rights by removing him from the protection of F's care without proper authorisation. E was to stay in his present accommodation until the full hearing in July 2010. An appeal against the Court of Protection ruling failed.[48]

Appointment of Deputy

The Court of Protection can make a single order or appoint a deputy in relation to a matter within its jurisdiction, which includes personal welfare as well as finance and property. Section 16 makes provisions for the Court of Protection to make decisions and for the appointment of deputies. The deputy must act on behalf of the patient in accordance with the principles set out in the

Mental Capacity Act 2005, in the best interests of the patient (see chapter 7) and within the powers granted him or her by the Court of Protection. The deputies can be given powers (with specified limitations) over matters of personal welfare which extend in particular to:

- deciding where P is to live (where a deputy makes a decision on this, it is subject to the restrictions on deputies);
- deciding what contact, if any, P is to have with any specified persons (the deputy has no power to make an order prohibiting a named person from having contact with P); and
- giving or refusing consent to the carrying out or continuation of a treatment by a person providing healthcare for P.

A deputy cannot give a direction that a person responsible for P's healthcare allows a different person to take over that responsibility: only the Court of Protection has that power. Where the deputy is given powers over a person's property and affairs, they could include the following:

- the control and management of P's property;
- the sale, exchange, charging gift or other disposition of P's property;
- the acquisition of property in P's name or on P's behalf;
- the carrying on, on P's behalf, of any profession, trade or business;
- the taking of a decision which will have the effect of dissolving a partnership of which P is a member;
- the carrying out of any contract entered into by P;
- the discharge of P's debts and of any of P's obligations, whether legally enforceable or not;
- the settlement of any of P's property, whether for P's benefit or for the benefit of others;
- the execution for P of a will (unless P is under 18 years old) (subject to restriction on deputies);
- the exercise of any power (including a power to consent) vested in P whether beneficially or as trustee or otherwise; and
- the conduct of legal proceedings in P's name or on P's behalf.

The Code of Practice identifies the following list as duties to be followed by the court-appointed deputy.[49] It notes that when agreeing to act as deputy whether in relation to welfare or financial affairs, the deputy is taking on a role which carries powers that s/he must use carefully and responsibly. The standard of conduct expected of deputies involves compliance with the following duties as an agent and with the statutory requirements:

- To comply with the principles of the Act
- To act in the best interests of the client
- To follow the Code of Practice
- To act within the scope of their authority given by the Court of Protection
- To act with due care and skill (duty of care)
- Not to take advantage of their situation (fiduciary duty)
- To indemnify the person against liability to third parties caused by the deputy's negligence
- Not to delegate duties unless authorised to do so
- To act in good faith

- To respect the person's confidentiality
- To comply with the directions of the Court of Protection.

To be appointed as a deputy an individual must be 18 years or over. An individual of at least 18 years or a trust corporation can be appointed as a deputy in respect of powers relating to property and affairs. The deputy must give consent to the appointment. The holder of a specified office or position may be appointed as deputy. Two or more deputies could be appointed to act jointly or jointly and severally. (Jointly means that they act together in making decisions and exercising the powers; severally means that they act as individuals separately.)

The deputy is entitled to be reimbursed out of P's property for his reasonable expenses in discharging his functions. In addition, if the court so directs when appointing the deputy, the deputy can receive remuneration out of P's property for discharging his functions. The court can give the deputy powers to take possession or control of all or any specified part of P's property and to exercise all or any specified powers in respect of it, including such powers of investment as the court decides.

The Office of Public Guardian acts as supervisor of the deputy and any complaints about the conduct of a deputy can be made to that Office. Further information on the role of the deputy, the Office of Public Guardian and the Court of Protection can be obtained from the Ministry of Justice website.[50] See also Bridgit Dimond's work.[51]

White Paper Valuing People

The White Paper *Valuing People – a New Strategy for Learning Disability for the 21st Century*[52] (which held that long-term hospitals were not an appropriate home environment for people with learning disabilities) recognised four key principles as lying at the heart of the government's proposals: rights, independence, choice and inclusion. The White Paper was described by the government as taking a lifelong approach, beginning with an integrated approach to services for disabled children and their families, and then providing new opportunities for a full and purposeful adult life. The proposals were intended to result in improvements in education, social services, health, employment, housing and support for people with learning disabilities and their families and carers. The White Paper estimated that there were about 210,000 people with severe learning disabilities and about 1.2 million with a mild or moderate disability. It set out the following proposals:

- New national objectives for services for those with learning disabilities
- A new Learning Disability Development fund
- A new central implementation support fund
- Disabled children and their families to be an integral part of the Quality Protects Programme, the Special Educational Needs Programme of Action and the Connexions Service
- Development of advocacy services to assist them in having as much choice and control over their lives as possible
- Supporting carers by implementing the Carers and Disabled Children Act 2000 and by funding the development of a national learning disability information centre and helpline in partnership with Mencap

- Improving health of those with learning disabilities by providing the same rights of access to mainstream health services as the rest of the population by appointing health facilitators, ensuring registration with a GP and a health action plan for each client
- Giving greater choice over where they live with more appropriate accommodation
- More local day services to assist them in leading a full and purposeful life
- New targets for increasing numbers of people with learning disabilities in work
- Raising of standards and quality of services provided for those with learning disabilities, including training and qualifications for care staff through a learning disability awards framework
- Effective partnership working through Learning Disability Partnership Boards.

To implement these changes, a Learning Disability Task Force was set up to advise the government, supported by an Implementation Support Team to promote change at regional and local level. In December 2007 the Department of Health published a consultation document 'Valuing People Now',[53] which set out the next steps on the Valuing People policy and its delivery. It saw the main priorities for 2008–2011 to be personalisation; what people do during the day; better health; access to housing and making sure that change happened. The wider agenda would include an emphasis on advocacy and human rights; partnership with families; ensuring all those with learning disabilities were included; working with the criminal justice system and the department of transport and local groups to ensure those with learning disabilities can become full members of their local communities; providing the same opportunities as others in the transition from childhood to adulthood and supporting those who work with those with learning disabilities. The consultation ended in March 2008 and a summary of the responses was published by the government in 2009.[54] One of the conclusions was that:

> There were consistent worries about whether Valuing People Now will make a real difference to people's lives, particularly in terms of funding and legislative 'teeth'. Many respondents felt that Valuing People Now was strong on vision but short on the detailed implementation plans to make the vision a reality, particularly compared to the 'view from the ground' that many respondents were experiencing.

A report published in 2008 gave stark evidence of the discrimination suffered by those with learning disabilities in accessing healthcare[55] and showed the extent of the challenge in ensuring equality of healthcare provision for those with learning disabilities. In 2016 guidance entitled *Connect for Change* was issued by the Royal College of Nursing, which continued to criticise the number of learning disability clients still under hospital-based care rather than being cared for in a community setting.[56] The situation in Practical Dilemma 16.1 is probably not unusual.

Practical dilemma 16.1   Not worth bothering about

Stan had fallen from a first-floor window in his community home and was taken to A&E by his carer. He had very limited speech and was unable to explain where he hurt and screamed when the doctor tried to examine him. The doctor suggested that the carer should take him home and give him paracetamol and a hot drink and return to the A&E department if it looked as though he had a fracture or any other serious problems. What action should the carer take?

Clearly the carer should try to ensure that Stan receives the reasonable standard of care which any person is entitled to in the A&E department and if the approved practice would have been to take X-rays and even admit overnight, then Stan is entitled to that standard. His difficulties in speaking should not be used by clinicians as a reason to provide a lower standard of care. The carer should try and make it clear to the doctor that Stan should be treated as an ordinary patient and that his learning disabilities should not be used as an excuse to refuse him a reasonable standard of care.

Other examples can be given where, because of a failure to X-ray, fractures are not diagnosed, or there is a failure to offer screening (e.g. cervical, breast, etc.) facilities which would be available to those with mental capacity. In a case reported to the author by an occupational therapist, the suggestion was made that a client with learning disabilities, who was non-verbal and autistic and whose fingers in her hand had curled tightly into her palm, getting tighter over recent years, should have her tendons cut. Her fingernails were growing into her palm, causing a lot of pain, and she was referred to a plastic surgeon who suggested that the tendons in her fingers should be cut. The usual practice would have been for the hand gradually to be opened up using a splint. The occupational therapist protested, pointing out that she still used her hands, and made good use of her thumb and little finger to manipulate objects.[57] In such conflicts where a health professional is aware that a patient/client with learning disabilities is not receiving an acceptable standard of care, an application can be made to the Court of Protection which has the power to appoint a deputy.

Distressing accounts abound on the ill-treatment of those with learning disabilities. The Health Service Ombudsman reported on a case where the hospital missed every opportunity to save the life of a woman with learning disabilities. She had been admitted to Basildon Hospital in Essex in 2009 with suspected pneumonia but had to wait five days to see a respiratory consultant. Staff failed to administer antibiotics immediately and did not consider moving her to a high dependency unit. Her parents who had complained to the Ombudsman felt that she had been denied adequate care because of her learning disabilities.[58]

The mother of an autistic boy placed a bug in his toy to catch foul-mouth carers. He came home from a respite stay spouting four-letter words. She handed the recordings to police and officials at Rhondda Cynon Taf council and four members of staff at Nantgwyn care home in Aberdare, South Wales were given formal warnings.[59]

Confidential Inquiry into Premature Deaths of People with a Learning Disability

It is a sad reflection on the impact of the White Paper and subsequent documents that the Confidential Inquiry (commissioned by the Department of Health in 2010) reported in 2013 that one third of the deaths investigated could have been prevented if good quality healthcare had been provided. The Mencap website provides a summary of the report.[60] In a formal response to the report the Department of Health admitted unacceptable inequalities and said that it would look at making a series of improvements around coordination, record keeping and best practice.

Mencap stated that it was hugely disappointed that key recommendations in the report were ignored.[61] A spokesman stated that over 1200 children and adults with learning disabilities continue to die unnecessarily in England every year because of discrimination in the NHS.

Crossing Service Provision Boundaries

Individuals do not of course fit into neat categories and all health professionals must be aware of the dangers of failing to treat the whole person and ignoring problems which do not fit into a specific form of service provision. These individuals are often vulnerable but can be excluded from support mechanisms owing to having the 'wrong' diagnosis to access services. For example, teenagers who have a dual diagnosis of learning disability and mental disorder may not come within any particular service. The Child and Adolescent Mental Health Service may not see a child with an IQ of 60 or less; the paediatric services may not work with major mental health issues. Any registered nurse who is involved in the care of a child or a person with learning disabilities would have a legal responsibility to ensure that all the appropriate services from other agencies and departments were involved and may herself become the coordinator of care for a particular client. The law requires that a reasonable standard of care is provided for the client, irrespective of the different service providers he or she may come under. Failures to cooperate across service boundaries were evident in the Baby P case discussed in chapter 13.

The Joint Committee on Human Rights published its report *A Life like Any Other? Human Rights of Adults with Learning Disabilities* on 6 March 2008.[62] The Joint Committee put forward 81 conclusions and recommendations for the government and other organisations on ensuring that the human rights of those adults with learning disabilities were respected. The government responded to the report in May 2008,[63] outlining the action it intended taking in relation to each recommendation, including the review of the *Valuing People* plan and the importance of the role of the Equality and Human Rights Commission in safeguarding the human rights of those with learning disabilities. Both the Joint Committee's Report and the Government Response can be accessed on the parliamentary website.[64] See also the DH publication on a review of human rights and equality of opportunity in mental health and learning disabilities.[65] In October 2010 the High Court held that there was no statutory obligation on a local authority to maintain a statement of special educational needs or to fund a young person to continue in secondary education beyond the age of 19 years to complete his A levels. Section 2(5) of the Education Act 1996 could not be interpreted to impose a duty on behalf of a young person over 19.[66]

Safeguarding vulnerable adults

A new Safeguarding Vulnerable Adults Policy and a protocol for joint working between the Office of the Public Guardian (OPG) and local authorities was launched in December 2008.[67] This policy provides a framework for delivering the OPG's role in safeguarding vulnerable adults, as the Mental Capacity Act 2005 introduced a statutory duty for the Public Guardian to supervise, investigate concerns and regulate court-appointed deputies. The policy is supported by the OPG's *Safeguarding Vulnerable Adults: Procedures and Guidance* document. The protocol for joint working outlines the respective roles that the OPG, the Court of Protection and local authorities play in adult protection, ensuring that areas of overlap can be harmonised. The agencies work together to help prevent and respond to abuse, by sharing information and following principles laid down in the guidelines. To view the policy, protocol and guidelines, see the OPG website.[68] The Safeguarding Vulnerable Groups Act 2006 and the Disclosure and Barring Service is considered in chapter 10 and other safeguarding provisions in chapter 18.

Sexual relations and related issues

Implicit in the concept of normalisation is the view that those suffering from learning disabilities should be able to participate in sexual activity according to their mental understanding. See the case of *A Local Authority* v *JB* [2021] discussed above in relation to the mental capacity to consent to having sexual relations.

Protection by the Criminal Code

The law protects those who do not have the capacity to give consent to sexual intercourse. It was an offence for a man to have unlawful sexual intercourse with a woman who had a learning disability under the Sexual Offences Act 1956 section 7 and 8. This has now been repealed and replaced by the criminal offences under the Sexual Offences Act 2003. It was a defence if a man is able to prove that he did not know and had no reason to suspect that the woman had a learning disability. In the case of *R* v *Hudson*,[69] the Court of Criminal Appeal allowed the appeal of the defendant against conviction on the grounds that a subjective test should have been applied to determine whether he had reason to suspect this.

The Sexual Offences Act 2003 repealed the provisions of section 128 of the Mental Health Act 1959 which made it an offence for a man on the staff of or employed by a hospital or mental nursing home to have extramarital sexual intercourse with a woman who is receiving treatment for mental disorder in that hospital or home either as an outpatient or an inpatient.

Under the Sexual Offences Act 2003 the following offences are created in relation to carers:

Section 38 care worker: sexual activity with a person with mental disorder;

Section 39 care worker: causing or inciting sexual activity;

Section 40 care worker: sexual activity in the presence of a person with mental disorder; and

Section 41 care worker: causing a person with a mental disorder to watch a sexual act.

Section 42 includes in the definition of care worker a person who has functions in a home in the course of employment which have brought him or are likely to bring him into regular face-to-face contact with the person with mental disorder. The definition also covers the situation where the patient is receiving NHS independent hospital or clinic services and the person has functions to perform in the course of employment. Those who regularly have face-to-face contact with clients as a result of providing care, assistance or services to them in connection with their mental disorder, whether or not in the course of employment, also come within the definition.

Where a person with learning disabilities is suspected of a crime it is important that the Code of Practice C (revised 2023) under the Police and Criminal Evidence Act (see chapter 2)

is followed and that before a person with learning disabilities is interviewed by the police he/she is represented by an appropriate adult (i.e. a relative, guardian or other person responsible for their care or custody; someone experienced in dealing with mentally disordered or mentally vulnerable people who is not a police officer or employed by the police, or failing these, some other responsible adult aged over 18 who is not a police officer or employed by the police).

The Mental Capacity Act (s. 44(2)) creates an offence to ill-treat or wilfully neglect a person who lacks capacity (see chapter 18). If a health care professional ill-treats or wilfully neglects a person with a learning disability they will be committing an offence under section 20 of the Criminal Justice and Courts Act 2015.

Reform of the Mental Capacity Act: Liberty Protection Safeguards

The Mental Capacity (Amendment) Act 2019 is seeking to introduce a simpler process to the current system with respect to Deprivation of Liberty Safeguards (DoLS). The proposed reforms to DoLS include:

- More involvement with the families, and swifter access to assessments;
- The process to be less onerous upon carers, people, families and the local authorities;
- Allowing the NHS rather than local authorities to make decisions regarding their patients, allowing for greater efficiency and accountability; and
- Remove repeat assessments and authorisations when someone moves between a care home, hospital and ambulance as part of their treatment.

The aim of the 2019 Act is to make the authorisation of a deprivation of liberty less bureaucratic and complex. It is anticipated that DoLS will be abolished and Liberty Protection Safeguards introduced in their place but the government has delayed its implementation several times.

Sterilisation

As a result of the case of *Re D* in 1976[70] (where a mother sought a declaration that her daughter, a sufferer of Sotos syndrome, could be sterilised), it became a requirement that those seeking a non-therapeutic sterilisation (i.e. one which was not required for the physical health of the patient) should first obtain a declaration of the court. In the *Re D* case the judge refused to permit the sterilisation of a girl of 11 years since it was not established that the child would not have the ability to make a decision for herself at a later date. On the other hand, in Jeanette's case[71] the House of Lords gave its approval to the sterilisation of a girl of 17 years who suffered from learning disabilities and her parents consented to the sterilisation. In the case of *Re F*[72], the House of Lords declared that it would be lawful to sterilise a woman who lacked the capacity to consent if it were in her best interests and the doctors acted in accordance with their professional practice standard.

The situation is now covered by either the Children Act 1989 or the Mental Capacity Act 2005. Where the person is under 16 years an application for sterilisation would be made to the Family Division of the High Court. Where the person is over 18 years an application could be made to the Court of Protection. A young person of 16 or 17 could be referred to either court as appropriate. If there is a request from a relative that the person be sterilised then the professional should raise this issue with the multi-disciplinary team and ensure that, if necessary, an application is made to the appropriate court. The decision to sterilise a child is one of the most significant which can be taken and it is essential that any health professional who is involved in the court proceedings and the evidence which is required should follow the principles considered in chapter 13 in relation to children. In relation to adults, the Code of Practice on the Mental Capacity Act (issued by the Department of Constitutional Affairs and now available from the website of the DCA's successor, the Ministry of Justice[73]) notes in paragraph 8.22:

> **that cases involving non-therapeutic sterilisation will require a careful assessment of whether such sterilisation would be in the best interests of the person who lacks capacity and such cases should continue to be referred to the court.**

A local authority sought a declaration from the Court of Protection regarding the best interests of K who was 21 years with Down's syndrome and an associated mild/moderate learning disability. Her parents wished her to be sterilised. A best interests meeting between the parents, LA and staff from the NHS trust decided that a non-therapeutic sterilisation was not in her best interests. The parents indicated that they were taking K abroad. The LA brought proceedings seeking a declaration in relation to contraception and sterilisation and an injunction not to remove K from the jurisdiction. The LA and Official Solicitor commissioned a report from a gynaecology expert who stated that sterilisation was not in K's best interests and was not the least restrictive option. The Court of Protection laid down the principles and procedure which should apply when non-therapeutic sterilisation was being considered. Such a decision was so serious that the Court of Protection should make it. In the actual case the CoP stated that any issue of non-therapeutic sterilisation should be brought back before the court so that those who were responsible for K's care were clear about the requirements going forward.[74]

In the case of *Re A* a mother applied for a declaration that a vasectomy was in the best interests of A, her son (who had Down's syndrome and was borderline between significant and severe impairment of intelligence), in the absence of his consent. After balancing the burdens and benefits of the proposed vasectomy to A, the Court of Appeal held that the vasectomy would not be in A's best interests.[75] In August 2010 Justice Bodey of the Court of Protection[76] refused to grant an order forcing a woman with a low IQ to have compulsory contraception. He stated that such a plan had shades of social engineering. The facts were that a married woman of 29 years who had an IQ of 53 had two children who had been put up for adoption. The council applied for the order because her violent and bullying husband wished her to have more children and they considered that such an order would be in her best interests.[77]

In August 2013 the Court of Protection heard an application for a vasectomy to be permitted on DE. The NHS trust with the support of the parents, GP and local authority applied to the court to allow a vasectomy on DE a 36-year-old with learning disabilities who already had a son born in 2010.[78] The court heard that DE did not want to become a father again and another child could cause him psychological harm. Experts stated that DE had the capacity to consent to sexual relationships but not to making decisions about contraception. Mrs Justice Eleanor King in a reserved decision ruled that a vasectomy could take place since it was in his best interests not to have another child. Mencap welcomed the decision but stated this decision should not be seen as a green light for other applications for sterilisation in respect of people with a learning disability.[79]

Abortion

A person with learning disabilities who has the capacity to give a valid consent could sign the form for an abortion to be carried out provided that the requirements of the Abortion Act 1967 (as amended by the Human Fertilisation and Embryology Act 1990) are met. Where the adult with learning disabilities lacks capacity, then the Mental Capacity Act 2005 would apply. The Code of Practice (paragraphs 6.18–6.19) points out that some treatment decisions are so serious that they must be made by the Court of Protection and it includes within this category termination of pregnancy in certain circumstances. The court has also given guidance on when certain termination of pregnancy cases should be brought before the court.[80]

Property

The legal issues relating to property are considered in chapter 24. Those with learning disabilities are vulnerable to exploitation and the duty of care owed to them would include the duty to take care of their property. Any moneys belonging to the client and handled by staff must be strictly accounted for and records kept. Facilities should be provided for cash or other valuables to be safely stored, and care should also be taken to prevent one client misappropriating property belonging to another. The Court of Protection has a remit to make decisions on behalf of mentally incapacitated adults in respect of personal welfare and property and financial decisions. A deputy could be appointed to make decisions in relation to any property or financial interests of an adult lacking mental capacity. The jurisdiction of the Court of Protection is normally restricted to those over 16 years but where it is anticipated that the lack of the requisite mental capacity could continue beyond 16 years then it can hear cases involving persons who are younger than 16 years. For example, if a child was severely injured in a road accident which led to serious brain damage and received a payment for several million pounds as a consequence, the Court of Protection could hear an application relating to his case since the disability would persist beyond 16 years. A man with learning disabilities sought judicial review of the cutting of services by his council and its failure to fulfil its public service duties under section 149 of the Equality Act 2010. The Court of Appeal agreed that he had made out both grounds of appeal, but that since the council's budget had now expired it would not grant him any relief since that would effectively require the council to rewrite a now expired budget from an earlier year which would be detrimental to good administration.[81] (See chapter 24 for discussion of maladministration of the property of residents in homes run by Mencap.)

Direct payments

Direct payment for personal care was introduced in 1997. On 1 April 1997 the Community Care (Direct Payments) Act came into force which enabled social services departments to make payments in cash instead of kind to certain groups in receipt of community care. This enables a person to purchase their own care. However, the local authority originally retained its discretion and could not be compelled to offer cash rather than services. The level of payment must be sufficient to enable the recipient to buy the services that the payments are intended to cover. New regulations came into force in 2003[82] under which there is now a duty to make direct payments to an eligible individual who appears to be capable of managing a direct payment by himself or with such assistance as may be available to him. (Persons listed in regulation 2 were ineligible but these regulations were replaced in 2009,[83] which reduced the categories of exclusion. Schedule 2 to the 2009 regulations excludes those under drug or alcoholic treatment or rehabilitation regimes imposed under criminal justice legislation.) If a person meets the criteria for direct payments and has had a community care assessment then the services needed are identified and he or she then has the choice of using the local social services or using the money provided to buy services from an alternative provider. In the DH circular 'Transforming Social Care' in January 2008,[84] it was estimated that only 54,000 out of a potential million recipients were receiving direct payments. The circular aimed at increasing the numbers of persons receiving direct payments or individual budgets.

An analysis of the purchase of assistive devices by older people who had fallen and called 999 ambulance showed that 54 per cent had purchased their own devices such as walking frames and bath boards, spending on average £700 each. The authors concluded that as social services' direct payments allow people to manage their own care packages, more people will be buying direct and may be looking for advice.[85]

Changes were introduced by sections 31–33 of the Care Act 2014 (England only) which are shown in Statute Box 16.1.

Statute 16.1
Care Act 2014 Sections 31–33

1. This section applies where—
   (a) a personal budget for an adult specifies an amount which the local authority must pay towards the cost of meeting the needs to which the personal budget relates, and
   (b) the adult requests the local authority to meet some or all of those needs by making payments to the adult or a person nominated by the adult.
2. If conditions 1 to 4 are met, the local authority must, subject to regulations under section 33, make the payments to which the request relates to the adult or nominated person.
3. A payment under this section is referred to in this Part as a 'direct payment'.
4. Condition 1 is that—
   (a) the adult has capacity to make the request, and
   (b) where there is a nominated person, that person agrees to receive the payments.
5. Condition 2 is that—
   (a) the local authority is not prohibited by regulations under section 33 from meeting the adult's needs by making direct payments to the adult or nominated person, and
   (b) if regulations under that section give the local authority discretion to decide not to meet the adult's needs by making direct payments to the adult or nominated person, it does not exercise that discretion.

6. Condition 3 is that the local authority is satisfied that the adult or nominated person is capable of managing direct payments—
   (a) by himself or herself, or
   (b) with whatever help the authority thinks the adult or nominated person will be able to access.
7. Condition 4 is that the local authority is satisfied that making direct payments to the adult or nominated person is an appropriate way to meet the needs in question.

32 Adults without capacity to request direct payments

1. This section applies where—
   (a) a personal budget for an adult specifies an amount which the local authority must pay towards the cost of meeting the needs to which the personal budget relates, and
   (b) the adult lacks capacity to request the local authority to meet any of those needs by making payments to the adult, but
   (c) an authorised person requests the local authority to meet some or all of those needs by making payments to the authorised person.
2. If conditions 1 to 5 are met, the local authority must, subject to regulations under section 33, make the payments to which the request relates to the authorised person.
3. A payment under this section is referred to in this Part as a 'direct payment'.
4. A person is authorised for the purposes of this section if—
   (a) the person is authorised under the Mental Capacity Act 2005 to make decisions about the adult's needs for care and support,
   (b) where the person is not authorised as mentioned in paragraph (a), a person who is so authorised agrees with the local authority that the person is a suitable person to whom to make direct payments, or
   (c) where the person is not authorised as mentioned in paragraph (a) and there is no person who is so authorised, the local authority considers that the person is a suitable person to whom to make direct payments.
5. Condition 1 is that, where the authorised person is not authorised as mentioned in subsection (4)(a) but there is at least one person who is so authorised, a person who is so authorised supports the authorised person's request.
6. Condition 2 is that—
   (a) the local authority is not prohibited by regulations under section 33 from meeting the adult's needs by making direct payments to the authorised person, and
   (b) if regulations under that section give the local authority discretion to decide not to meet the adult's needs by making direct payments to the authorised person, it does not exercise that discretion.

▶

7. Condition 3 is that the local authority is satisfied that the authorised person will act in the adult's best interests in arranging for the provision of the care and support for which the direct payments under this section would be used.
8. Condition 4 is that the local authority is satisfied that the authorised person is capable of managing direct payments—
   (a) by himself or herself, or
   (b) with whatever help the authority thinks the authorised person will be able to access.
9. Condition 5 is that the local authority is satisfied that making direct payments to the authorised person is an appropriate way to meet the needs in question.

33 Direct payments: further provision

1. Regulations must make further provision about direct payments.
2. The regulations may, in particular, specify—
   (a) cases or circumstances in which a local authority must not, or cases or circumstances in which it has the discretion to decide not to, meet needs by making direct payments;
   (b) conditions which a local authority may or must attach to the making of direct payments;
   (c) matters to which a local authority may or must have regard when making a decision of a specified type in relation to direct payments;
   (d) steps which a local authority may or must take before, or after, making a decision of a specified type in relation to direct payments;
   (e) cases or circumstances in which an adult who lacks capacity to request the making of direct payments must or may nonetheless be regarded for the purposes of this Part or the regulations as having capacity to do so;
   (f) cases or circumstances in which an adult who no longer lacks capacity to make such a request must or may nonetheless be regarded for any of those purposes as lacking capacity to do so;
   (g) cases or circumstances in which a local authority making direct payments must review the making of those payments.
3. A direct payment is made on condition that it be used only to pay for arrangements under which the needs specified under section 25(2)(a) in the care and support plan or (as the case may be) the support plan are met.
4. In a case where one or more of conditions 1 to 4 in section 31 is no longer met or one or more of conditions 1 to 5 in section 32 is no longer met, the local authority must terminate the making of direct payments.
5. In a case where a condition specified under subsection (2)(b) or the condition mentioned in subsection (3) is breached, the local authority—
   (a) may terminate the making of direct payments, and
   (b) may require repayment of the whole or part of a direct payment (with section 69 accordingly applying to sums which the local authority requires to be repaid).

Direct Payments: Health Care

Under section 11 of the Health Act 2009, direct payment for healthcare was introduced into the NHS (ss. 12A–12D of the National Health Service Act 2006).

Regulations for the NHS Direct Payments came into force in June 2010[86] relating to the setting up of pilot schemes for providing direct payments in accordance with a care plan, for their monitoring and review and for the repayment of the payments in specified circumstances. In 2013 the pilot schemes were ended and the direct payments for healthcare extended across England.[87] Amendments were subsequently made to enable an individual living in the same household, a family member or a friend to be paid to provide care using part of a patient's direct payment in exceptional circumstances and which were omitted in error.[88]

Complaints about non-NHS providers of direct payment services for healthcare have been added to the jurisdiction of the Health Service Commissioner.[89]

Between 2009 and 2013 personal health budgets were piloted in over 60 sites across England. The government published a response[90] to the consultation on direct payments for healthcare in 2013. It concluded that with a phased implementation process, personal health budgets and direct payments for healthcare will pave the way to a more person-centred future for the NHS.

This led to new regulations in 2013[91] while regulations relating to the pilot schemes were repealed.[92] These specify the persons to whom or in respect of whom the direct payments can be made, those excluded (these include those subject to drug or alcohol rehabilitation requirements, or subject to youth rehabilitation orders), the nomination of a person to receive the payment on the patient's behalf (reg. 6), the requirements in relation to a care plan and care coordinator (reg. 8) and the provision of information, advice and support in connection with the making of the direct payment. The conditions which must be complied with are set out in regulation 10 and regulation 14 covers the monitoring and review of direct payments. Regulations 15–17 cover the repayment, recovery and stopping of direct payments. A person lacking the requisite mental capacity may under regulation 5 be the recipient of a direct payment if that person has a representative who consents to the making of a direct payment order and the health body making the grant must have regard to whether it is appropriate for a person with that person's condition, and the impact of that condition on the person's life and whether a direct payment represents value for money. The representative must agree to act on the patient's behalf, act in the best interests of the patient, be responsible contractually for the payment, use the direct payment in accordance with the care plan and comply with relevant provisions of the regulations.

Amendments were made to the 2013 regulations requiring a health body to reconsider a decision not to make a direct payment and to give reasons for the decision. The amending regulations also reinstate provisions in earlier regulations but omitted in error for an individual living in the same household, a family member or a friend to be paid to provide care using part of a patient's direct payment in very limited circumstances.[93]

In the case of *Morgan* v *Phillips*,[94] the defendant in a road traffic accident argued unsuccessfully that the amount of direct payments should be taken into account in calculating the compensation for future care costs.

Registration and inspections

Community homes for those with learning disabilities come under the aegis of the Care Quality Commission (see chapter 5) which replaced the Healthcare Commission, the Mental Health Act Commission and the Commission for Social Care Inspection in April 2009. A scandal was reported in Cornwall where significant failings were found at Buddock Hospital (a unit for 14 patients with severe disabilities). The Healthcare Commission carried out a national audit of learning disability services and then consulted on a three-year plan.[95] The three-year plan envisaged:

- Audit of all inpatient care being provided for learning disability service users across the NHS and independent sector, including commissioning arrangements;
- Investigation into long-stay hospitals to ensure that they are providing a safe and acceptable service;
- Review of the care of people with learning disabilities who are placed outside their local area away from family and friends;
- Increase the accessibility of the Commission's services so that people with a learning disability can better raise complaints and concerns about their care; and
- Establish champions at the regional offices of the Healthcare Commission responsible for monitoring services for people with a disability.

Full reports by the CQC on its inspections of individual care homes for those with learning disabilities can be found on its website.[96] It uses the following criteria in its inspections: treating people with respect and involving them in their care; providing care, treatment and support that meets people's needs; caring for safety and protecting them from harm; staffing and management. The Winterbourne View Hospital Report is considered in chapter 5.

In December 2006, as a result of the Equality Act 2006, public bodies were placed under a new disability equality duty to ensure that their organisations had a policy to identify and eradicate discrimination against disabled people. Public authorities are required to carry out six duties:

- To promote equality of opportunity between disabled and other persons
- To eliminate discrimination that is unlawful under the Disability Discrimination Act 1995
- To eliminate harassment related to their disabilities
- To promote positive attitudes
- To encourage participation in public life and
- To take account of their disabilities, even where that involves them more favourably than other persons.

It remains to be seen how effective this duty is in relation to those with learning disabilities. (The legislation is now re-enacted in the Equality Act 2010 (see chapter 10).)

Conclusions

The Mental Capacity Act 2005 and the Deprivation of Liberty Safeguards have provided a significant framework in the protection of those with learning disabilities. It is clear from the reports of the Care Quality Commission that much still should be done to ensure reasonable standards of care and the protection of their rights and this is now being reflected by the introduction of a Mental Capacity Bill currently progressing through parliament. NHS England issued guidance in 2012 on learning disabilities for clinical commissioning groups to assist them in commissioning high quality, cost-effective general and specialist health services for those with learning disabilities.[97] It is available on the Improving Health and Lives website (a website belonging to Public

Health England specifically for the care of learning disabilities).[98] A report published in 2010[99] showed that less than 50 per cent of calls to the police following anti-social behaviour against the disabled, especially those with learning disabilities, received a response. (Such behaviour led to the suicide of a mother, Fiona Pilkington, who killed her disabled daughter in 2007.) There are clearly still major challenges ahead for nurses working within this specialist field.

Reflection questions

1. A girl with learning disabilities aged 19 years has been admitted for an abortion and you hear that she is to be sterilised. You feel that the decision has been rushed and should be delayed. What action could be taken? How would your answer differ if she were 15 years old? (See also chapter 14.)

2. A young man with severe learning disabilities has been admitted for an appendectomy. You are aware that there is a dispute between his elderly parents and the social workers over his long-term accommodation, since the social workers wish him to be placed in a community home for those with learning disabilities. What is the law which applies to the situation and what role could you have in the discharge planning and a decision being made?

3. Decisions on behalf of those adults lacking the requisite mental capacity to make their own decisions must be made in their best interests. What is meant by this? Draw up a table showing the stages to be followed in the decision-making process (see chapter 7).

Further exercises

1. What are the implications of the Mental Capacity Act 2005 for the making of decisions on behalf of those who have severe learning disabilities? (See also chapter 7).
2. As a community nurse who has specialised in the care of those with learning disabilities you are concerned that one client is given very little freedom and is often placed in a restraining chair which he cannot get out of. You consider that the community home is acting illegally. What action would you take and what is the law which applies to the situation?
3. Reflect upon any client/patient with severe learning disabilities whom you have cared for and consider the legal issues which arose in their care.

References

[1] www.nice.org.uk/guidance/population-groups/people-with-learning-disabilities#panel-pathways
[2] www.un.org
[3] *In re F (Adult: court's jurisdiction)*, The Times Law Report, 25 July 2000; [2000] 2 FLR 512

[4] European Convention for the Protection of Human Rights and Fundamental Freedoms 1953, Cmd 8969
[5] *F v West Berkshire Health Authority* [1989] 2 All ER 545
[6] *A Hospital NHS Trust v S, DG (S's father) and SG (S's mother)* [2003] Lloyd's Rep Med 3 137
[7] *The Mental Health Trust and Anor v DD and Anor* [2014] EWCOP 11
[8] *R v Broadmoor Special Hospital Authority* [2002] 1 WLR 419
[9] *ZH (A protected party) v Commissioner of Police of the Metropolis, Liberty and another intervening* [2013] EWCA 69 Court of Appeal, The Times Law Report, 12 April 2013
[10] *R v Bournewood Community and Mental Health NHS Trust ex p L* [1998] 3 All ER 289; [1999] AC 458
[11] *L v United Kingdom* (Application No. 45508/99) [2004] ECHR 720, The Times Law Report, 19 October 2004
[12] The Mental Capacity (Deprivation of Liberty: Standard Authorisations, Assessments and Ordinary Residence) Regulations 2008, SI 2008/1858
[13] The Mental Capacity (Deprivation of Liberty: Appointment of the Relevant Person's Representative) Regulations 2008, SI 2008/1315
[14] Department of Health Briefing Sheet, Bournewood, November 2006, Gateway Reference 6794
[15] Ministry of Justice, Mental Capacity Act 2005, Deprivation of Liberty Safeguards: Code of Practice 2008
[16] Ministry of Justice and Department of Health (2008) Impact assessment of the Mental Capacity Act 2005 – deprivation of liberty safeguards to accompany the code of practice and regulations, Ministry of Justice, London
[17] *GJ v The Foundation Trust* [2009] EWHC 2972 (Fam)
[18] *RB (by his litigation friend, the Official Solicitor) v Brighton and Hove City Council*, The Times Law Report, 12 June 2014
[19] *Re M (Best interests: Deprivation of Liberty)* [2013] EWCOP 3456
[20] *G v E & Ors* [2010] EWHC 621 (Fam)
[21] Ben Troke and Neil Ward, Are we just playing with DoLS? *British Journal of Healthcare Management*, 16(11):536–40, 2010
[22] www.alzheimers.org.uk
[23] www.cqc.org.uk
[24] House of Lords Select Committee, Mental Capacity Act 2005: post legislative scrutiny, HL Paper 139 March 2014
[25] *NHS Trust v Dr A* [2013] EWHC 2442 CoP
[26] *Dunhill v Burgin* [2014] UKSC 18, The Times Law Report, 28 March 2014
[27] *P (by his litigation friend, the Official Solicitor) v Cheshire West and Cheshire Council and Anor* [2014] UKSC 19
[28] *P and Q v Surrey County Council* [2011] EWCA Civ 190
[29] Department of Health, Deprivation of Liberty Safeguards, 28 March 2014
[30] Frances Gibb, The sun should shine in on such heart-wrenching cases, *The Times*, 10 July 2014
[31] Care Quality Commission (2023) Deprivation of liberty safeguards available on the CQC Website at https://www.cqc.org.uk/publications/major-report/state-care/2022-2023/dols
[32] *London Borough of Hillingdon v Neary and another* [2011] EWCOP 1377
[33] *MH v United Kingdom* [2013] ECHR 1008
[34] *J Council v GU* [2012] EWHC 3531 CoP
[35] Code of Practice, Mental Capacity Act 2005, Department of Constitutional Affairs, February 2007, available on the website of the Ministry of Justice at www.gov.uk

[36] The Mental Capacity Act 2005 (Independent Mental Capacity Advocates)(Expansion of Role) Regulations 2006, SI 2006/2883
[37] B. Dimond, *Legal Aspects of Mental Capacity*, Blackwell Publishing, Oxford, 2007
[38] *Local Authority X* v *MM* [2007] EWHC 2003 Fam
[39] *A local authority* v *JB* [2021] UKSC 52
[40] Sections 45–56 Mental Capacity Act 2005
[41] Law Commission Report No. 231, Mental Incapacity, Stationery Office, London, 1995
[42] *W (Court of Protection order)* [2014] EWCOP B8
[43] Ministry of Justice (2023) Family Courts statistics to December 2023 available on the MoJ Website at https://www.gov.uk/government/statistics/family-court-statistics-quarterly-october-to-december-2023/family-court-statistics-quarterly-october-to-december-2023#mental-capacity-act---court-of-protection
[44] Practice Guidance (CP: Transparency in the Court of Protection: Publication of judgments) [2014] 1 WLR 235
[45] Ministry of Justice www.gov.uk
[46] Ministry of Justice, Mental Capacity Act 2005, Deprivation of Liberty Safeguards: Code of Practice 2008
[47] *G* v *E & Ors* [2010] EWHC 621 (Fam)
[48] *G* v *E* [2010] EWCA 822 Civ
[49] Code of Practice, Mental Capacity Act 2005, Department of Constitutional Affairs, February 2007, Paragraph 8.56
[50] Ministry of Justice www.gov.uk
[51] B. Dimond, *Legal Aspects of Mental Capacity*, Blackwell Publishing, Oxford, 2007
[52] Department of Health, White Paper, Valuing People: a new strategy for learning disability for the 21st century, Cm 5086, March 2001, Stationery Office
[53] Department of Health, White Paper, Valuing People Now – from progress to transformation – a consultation on the next three years of learning disability policy, DH, London
[54] HM Government, Summary of Responses to the Consultation on Valuing People Now: from progress to transformation, 2009
[55] Jonathan Michael, Healthcare For All: report of the independent inquiry into access to healthcare for people with learning disabilities, 2008, www.iahpld.org.uk/health-care.final
[56] Royal College of Nursing, Connect for Change: An update on learning disability services in England, February 2016, RCN, London
[57] B.C. Dimond, *The Legal Aspects of Occupational Therapy*, 3rd edn, Wiley Blackwell, Oxford, 2010
[58] News item, Disability woman who died after 'appalling' care, *The Times*, 21 May 2013
[59] News item, Mother bugs son's toy to catch foul-mouthed carers, *The Times*, 4 July 2013
[60] www.mencap.org.uk
[61] Chris Smyth, Anger over 'lack of leadership' on death toll of patients with learning disabilities, *The Times*, 13 July 2013
[62] Joint Committee on Human Rights, A Life Like Any Other? Human Rights of Adults with Learning Disabilities, Seventh Report of session 2007–8 HL Paper 40-1/HC73-1; www.publications.parliament.uk
[63] Government Response to the Joint Committee on Human Rights, A Life Like Any Other? Human Rights of Adults with Learning Disabilities, Cm 7378, Stationery Office
[64] www.publications.parliament.uk
[65] Department of Health, Human rights and equality of opportunity, Bamford Review of Mental Health and Learning Disabilities, DH, London, 2006
[66] *R (B)* v *Islington London Borough Council*, The Times Law Report, 6 October 2010

67. Department of Health and Welsh Assembly Government, Mental Capacity Act Update Edition 20, February 2009
68. www.gov.uk/government/organisations/office-of-public-guardian
69. *R v Hudson* [1965] 1 All ER 721
70. *Re D (A Minor) (Wardship: Sterilisation)* [1976] 1 All ER 327
71. *Re B (A Minor) (Wardship: Sterilisation)* [1987] 2 WLR 1213
72. *F v West Berkshire Health Authority and another* [1989] 2 All ER 545; also reported as *Re F*
73. Ministry of Justice www.gov.uk
74. *A Local Authority v K* [2013] EWHC 242
75. *Re A (Medical Treatment: male sterilisation)* (1999) 53 BMLR 66
76. *A Local Authority v A & Anor* [2010] EWHC 1549 (Fam)
77. David Sanderson, Judge vetoes forced contraception, *The Times*, 20 August 2010
78. *A NHS Trust v DE* [2013] EWHC 2562 (Fam)
79. David Brown, Judge orders sterilisation for man with learning disabilities, *The Times*, 17 August 2013
80. *D v An NHS Trust (Medical Treatment: Consent: Termination)* [2004] 1 FLR 1110
81. *Regina (Hunt) v North Somerset Council*, CA, The Times Law Report, 20 November 2013
82. The Community Care, Services to Carers and Children's Services (Direct Payments) (England) Regulations 2003 SI 2003/762
83. The Community Care, Services for Carers and Children's Services (Direct Payments) (England) Regulations 2009, SI 2009/1887 amended by The Community Care, Services for Carers and Children's Services (Direct Payments) (England) Regulations 2013 SI 2013/2270
84. Department of Health, Transforming Social Care, January 2008
85. P.A. Logan, A. Murphy, A.E.R. Drummond, S. Bailey *et al.*, An investigation of the number and cost of assistive devices used by older people who had fallen and called a 999 ambulance, *British Journal of Occupational Therapy*, 70(11):475–8, 2007
86. National Health Service (Direct Payments) Regulations 2010 SI 2010/1000
87. National Health Service (Direct Payments) Regulations 2013 SI 2013/1617
88. National Health Service (Direct Payments) (Amendment) Regulations 2013 SI 2013/2354
89. Section 12 Health Act 2009
90. Department of Health, Consultation on Direct Payments for Healthcare: Government Response, DH, 2013
91. The National Health Service (Direct Payments) Regulations 2013 SI 2013/1617
92. The National Health Service (Direct Payments) Regulations 2013 SI 2013/1563
93. The National Health Service (Direct Payments) Regulations 2013 SI 2013/2354
94. *Morgan v Phillips* [2006] All ER (D) 189 March
95. Healthcare Commission, Three-year plan for adults with learning disabilities, Stationery Office, 2005
96. www.cqc.org.uk
97. NHS England, Improving the Health and Wellbeing of People with Learning Disabilities: an Evidence-based Guide for clinical commissioning groups, October 2012
98. www.improvinghealthandlives.org.uk
99. HM Inspectorate, Constabulary Review of Antisocial Behaviour, HMIC, 2010

Chapter 17
Nurse Educator and Researcher

This chapter discusses

- NMC and standards in education
- Record keeping by teachers
- Liability for instructing others
- Hearing about unsound practices
- Employment law
- Legal aspects of research
- Health Research Authority (HRA)
- Confidentiality
- Consent
- Health Education England

Introduction

Law is relevant to the role of the nurse educator in several respects. Lecturers have been involved in litigation in respect of what they have taught, how it was taught and when. NHS employees and nurse lecturers should be familiar with the differences and implications. The legal issues arising from research are also relevant to the lecturer. They need also to be concerned with all the general aspects of the law covered in the first part of this book – not only in relation to their own position, but also because they might have to teach some of it!

NMC and standards in education

Guidance on the standards for the preparation of teachers of nursing, midwifery and health visiting was provided by the UKCC[1] and developed by the NMC[2] with revised arrangements for the introduction of standards for practice teachers. The Higher Education Academy developed a national professional standards framework for teaching and supporting learning in higher education in 2006 which complemented the NMC standard to support learning and assessment in practice which applied from 2007. The HE Academy was asked to accredit the NMC standard so that NMC teachers could be recognised by the HE Academy. From 2006 all teachers new to teaching in HE must have a teaching qualification.[3] Pre-registration and post-registration standards set by the NMC and the NMC quality assurance arrangements for education are considered in chapter 11.

Good character and good health

To obtain registered status, students must not only pass the academic and practical requirements of the course, but they also need a declaration by the head of the college (or department) of nursing that there is no reason why the student is not eligible to be placed on the NMC Register. This places a clear duty on the lecturers to ensure that any information that indicates that the person would be unsuitable should be brought to the attention of the head of the college or department of nursing. This requirement is particularly important in the light of the recommendations of the Clothier Inquiry into Beverly Allitt. The report[4] recommended that those with a history of personality disorder should not be taken into nursing (see chapter 5). The NMC conducted a consultation on how registrants should certify their character and health for the purposes of re-registration, and published guidance on good health and good character in 2006 as an Appendix to Annexe 2 of circular NMC 06/16. This was revised in 2008 and updated in 2015.[5] The guidance sets out the law, defines what is meant by good character and good health, and presents several scenarios to illustrate the decisions which have to be made. It states that:

> **Good character is important and is central to the Code 2015 (updated in 2018) in that nurses and midwives must be honest and trustworthy. Good character is based on an individual's conduct, behaviour and attitude. It also takes account of any convictions, cautions and pending charges that are likely to be incompatible with professional registration. A person's character must be sufficiently good for them to be capable of safe and effective practice without supervision.**

> **Good health is necessary to undertake practice as a nurse or midwife. Good health means that a person must be capable of safe and effective practice without supervision. It does not mean the absence of any disability or health condition. Many disabled people and those with health conditions are able to practise with or without adjustments to support their practice.**

The Guidance also considers what is meant by reasonable adjustments to enable a person to practise safely without supervision.

Research published in February 2014 showed that patients have a significantly better chance of surviving on wards where more nurses have degrees.[6] Anne Marie Rafferty, Professor of Nursing Policy at King's College London and the lead British author on the study published in the

Lancet, said that the findings were a vindication of NHS England's decision in September 2013 to require all nurses to have a bachelor's degree.

Record keeping by teachers

Practical dilemma 17.1 — Instruction in lifting – the evidence

Beryl Sharp, a nurse tutor, received a request from her hospital claims manager to provide her with the information she had given to a staff nurse on a lifting course. It appeared that this staff nurse had sustained a serious back injury at work and was suing the NHS trust for a breach in its direct liability to take care of her safety. The claim was likely to amount to a considerable sum, since the prognosis was poor and she was unlikely to be able to return to work in the foreseeable future. The NHS trust was defending the claim on the grounds that the ward was adequately staffed and that the staff nurse had been given instruction in lifting. It now required evidence of that fact from Beryl. Fortunately, Beryl was a hoarder – a fact frequently greeted with derision by her colleagues. She never threw anything out and was able to go through her records and find the series of seminars that had been organised on lifting. She had both the dates and the names of participants, including the names of those who had failed to attend. She had not given the seminar herself: a physiotherapist had done the teaching. Beryl had simply organised it as part of her work as an organiser for continuing education. She checked her records and could find no record that the particular staff nurse had attended. In fact, she was able to see that she was included in the list of those who were supposed to attend, but was not present at a seminar and that 'sick' had been written against her name. There was no evidence that she had been invited to attend a subsequent seminar, although another three were held in the following months.

One can imagine that this information would disappoint the hospital claims manager in providing information to defend the staff nurse's claim. However, it is not completely fatal to any defence of the claim, since it might well be that the staff nurse had received appropriate training in lifting during her pre-registration nurse training. In addition, there may be some element of contributory negligence in that the staff nurse herself failed to ensure that she was included on another seminar once she had returned from sick leave.

Such a request gives rise to many further questions for the nurse lecturer. How long must records be kept? What sort of detail is necessary? It will be recalled from the section in chapter 6 dealing with the time limits for bringing a court action that in a case of negligence the action must be brought within three years of the negligent incident (unless the victim is under 18 years old, under a disability or, in cases where she was not aware of the fact of the negligence or the existence of harm, within three years of such information becoming available). A period of retention of seven years is therefore likely to cover most eventualities apart from these exceptions. In addition, it could be argued that in those areas where regular retraining and revision study days are necessary, if several years have elapsed since the opportunity to go on to a course, then the

NHS Trust or Health Board is at fault in not providing a revision course. The information that should be retained is set out in Box 17.1.

> **Box 17.1** **Information that should be kept by the nurse tutor**
>
> Names of those who should have attended the sessions
> Names of those who did attend
> Times and dates of the sessions
> Content of the sessions and who did the teaching
> Grades of achievement where there was any assessment

Records are, of course, kept of the content, standard and timetable of pre-registration students, and it is not difficult to extend this to the post-pre-registration courses.

Liability for instructing others

In chapter 3, there is an explanation of the duty of care owed by those who are instructing others so that if harm were to occur as a result of negligent instructions, the tutor can be sued by the person who has suffered the harm. This applies not just to the classroom situation, but also to all those situations where advice is given in circumstances where the person receiving it can be expected to act on it. If the advice has been given negligently, then an action in negligence for breach of a duty of care may follow.

Practical dilemma 17.2 — Negligent instructions

Beryl Sharp acted as the course tutor on some of the post-basic courses. She ran one course, that of training nurses in the adding of drugs to IVs, and failed to mention that, according to the local guidelines, the first dose of the drug to be added to the IV should always be given by a doctor. One of the staff nurses who had been at that session and had been deemed competent to give IV drugs returned to the ward and was instructed that a patient who was already on an intravenous drip had been written up for an IV drug. At the appropriate time, the staff nurse prepared the drug, checked it with another nurse, and added it to the drip according to the instructions she had been taught on the course. The patient reacted violently against the drug and a doctor was summoned urgently. An inquiry was then held to find out why the first dose of this drug had been administered by a nurse and not by a doctor. It was the local policy for the doctor to administer the first dose of a drug intravenously. It then emerged that Beryl Sharp had failed to point out this requirement in her teaching on the course.

In this situation, the victim is a patient. In other cases, the victim could be the person who received the negligent information or advice. Where a patient is the victim, the claim is relatively simple: they would show that they had suffered harm as a result of a negligent act of an employee acting in the course of employment and therefore that the employer is vicariously liable for the harm. Alternatively, the individual employee could be sued as personally liable for the harm. In such a case, the employee may bring her own action against the tutor who was negligent in the instructions that she gave. In this type of action, the following facts would have to be shown:

1. A duty of care was owed by the instructor to the student and to a third party injured by the student.
2. There was a breach of this duty since the instructions were given negligently.
3. As a reasonably foreseeable consequence of this breach, the person has suffered harm (this might be personal injury, but it could also include financial loss or loss or damage to property).

It is essential that the person harmed can show that this harm was caused by the negligence of the tutor. If it were unreasonable for the person to rely on the instruction by the tutor, then compensation would not be payable on the basis of the tutor's negligence. The defendant might be able to show that there was no negligence since the latest NICE guidelines on intravenous fluid therapy[7] do not require the first dose to be given by a registered medical practitioner.

Hearing about unsound practices

If a lecturer in the college of nursing discovers from their learners about staff who are guilty of unacceptable practices or ill treatment of patients, what action should the nurse lecturer take? Should they investigate the allegation and, if challenged, say why? Should they keep their source secret? Should they report their suspicions to nurse management? Obviously, there can be no single answer since much depends on the circumstances. If, for example, the learner has witnessed ill treatment of a patient by a member of staff on a ward, then the learner should be encouraged to write a statement setting out exactly what they have seen and the nurse lecturer should ensure that appropriate action is taken by nurse management, at the same time protecting the learner from any victimisation. (Refer to whistleblowing and the Public Interest Disclosure Act 1998 considered in chapter 4.) If the nurse witnesses a procedure being carried out on the wards that is not in line with present-day safe practices, the nurse lecturer could arrange appropriate revision courses with in-service training officer colleagues.

Conflicts could also arise where the college has been teaching students the basic principles of patients' rights, e.g. consent to treatment, and as a result the student encounters difficulties with some medical staff. There could be criticism of the lecturers and of the college for its teachings. Such a situation indicates the importance of very close contact between the college and the NHS trust. The college of nursing should not, however, be seen as a policing machine for the hospital. By the same token, it has an essential part to play in maintaining the highest standards of nursing care in cooperation with the managers. Close integration of nurse clinical teaching and practice is essential.

Calls for a duty of candour arising from the Francis Report, and subsequent actions taken, are discussed in chapter 12.

Employment law

Students

Learners were once both employees and students. Following the introduction of Project 2000, learners are students, usually attached to a college of education. The college negotiates an agreement with accredited hospitals for the clinical placements (now known as practice learning opportunities). In theory, students are supernumerary to the workforce, but inevitably, especially in the last years of training, the hospitals and community services may exploit their services. There is no right in the learning contract for the student to insist on employment once they are qualified. There may, however, be a contractual relationship between the institution and the student: the institution agrees to prepare the student for a particular qualification and the student agrees to arrange payment and follow the requirements of the course. Andrew Croskery, a student who obtained a 2:2 degree in electrical engineering, sued the University of Belfast because he felt that had he had the appropriate supervision he would have obtained a 2:1 degree. His application for judicial review was heard on 25 September 2010 but failed on the grounds that the case should remain exclusively within the jurisdiction of the University's own appeal body.[8]

Dismissal on grounds of absenteeism or course failure

Since the student is not an employee, if they should be dismissed during the course on the grounds of absenteeism or failing course assessments or examinations, then the student's remedy is an appeal through the appeal mechanisms of the university. These should have clear guidelines on the rules that operate in these circumstances and these procedures should be carefully followed. There is a contractual relationship between the student and the university that is enforceable in law.

Practice learning opportunities

There is normally a memorandum of agreement between colleges providing clinical training and the hospitals and community trusts providing practice learning opportunities. This agreement should cover the issue of liability for the actions of the students if they cause harm to others through negligence. Since the students are not employees of the unit providing practice learning opportunities, the units can argue that they are not vicariously liable for the actions of students. In addition, the agreement should cover liability for harm to the student. Prior agreement between the university and the organisation providing the practice learning opportunities can resolve such issues and also cover the topic of supervision of the student and clinical instruction. The NMC has published a fact sheet on practice placement opportunities across borders within the UK.[9]

Contractual rights of lecturers

Lecturers, tutors and clinical instructors are, of course, under a contract of employment whether their employer is a university/higher education institution or an NHS organisation, and they are obliged to observe the express and implied terms of the contract of employment (see chapter 10). In addition, they are entitled to expect that their employer will recognise its contractual obligations under the contract of employment. A memorandum of understanding for joint staff of universities and NHS organisations was agreed in March 2007 and can be downloaded.[10] It was prepared in response to the VAT tribunal ruling in April 2005 in a case involving the University of Glasgow and HM Revenue and Customs. The memorandum sets out the NHS and university understanding of the role of joint staff, clarifies selected duties and responsibilities of their employers, documents established practice in respect of these staff and confirms that such arrangements are outside the scope of VAT.

Legal aspects of research

Research-based practice is an essential requirement of professional care. An analysis of the role and importance of research in midwifery practice is equally applicable to all areas of nursing.[11] The National Institute for Health and Care Excellence (see chapter 5) seeks to identify and publish recommended clinically effective practice that has a strong research basis. The Department of Health initiated in 2006 a programme for research in the NHS called Best Research for Best Health.[12] The five-year strategy and its implementation plans, prepared by the National Institute of Health Research[13] (NIHR), can be downloaded from its website. The NIHR has established a School for Social Care Research. The NIHR was established in 2006 and funded through the Department of Health to improve the health and wealth of the nation through research. It has four main strands:

- NIHR Faculty: supporting individuals carrying out and participating in research;
- NIHR Research: commissioning and funding research;
- NIHR Infrastructure: providing facilities for a thriving research environment; and
- NIHR Systems: creating unified, streamlined and simple systems for managing research and its outputs.

In 2010 the White Paper *Equity and Excellence: Liberating the NHS* was published as a vision for the NHS. It emphasised the core role of research in the NHS; the role of the NHS Commissioning Board (NHS England) in promoting research; the importance of clinical research and the NIHR; and the success of NIHR clinical research networks.

In January 2011 the Academy of Medical Sciences made recommendations in relation to medical research regulation[14] suggesting the establishment of a new arm's-length body (now the Health Research Authority); facilitating NHS trusts' timely approval of research studies; improving the UK environment for clinical trials; providing access to patient data that protects individuals' interests; and embedding a culture that values research within the NHS. A Research Support Service was launched by the NIHR in May 2011.

Standard 6 of the NMC Code[15] requires that nurses:

Always practise in line with the best available evidence

To achieve this, [nurses] must:

- make sure that any information or advice given is evidence-based, including information relating to using any healthcare products or services, and
- maintain the knowledge and skills you need for safe and effective practice.

The nurse is increasingly likely to be involved in research, either conducting it themselves or being involved in the care of patients who are the subjects of a research project. Often a research project is an integral part of a management course or post-registration qualification and they will be expected to prepare a dissertation or project that shows some original material and analysis. In addition, there may well be researchers coming into their department or ward: they should in either case be aware of the many legal issues that arise. Some of the basic problems relate to consent by the patient, confidentiality and disclosure of the findings, safety of the researcher and liability for any volunteer in a drugs research programme. The conduct of research and the rights of the research subject are set out in the Declaration of Helsinki, which was reproduced as an appendix in the Department of Health's guidance for local research ethics committees, originally issued in 1991.[16] New guidance on research ethics committees was issued in July 2001[17] and updated in 2005.[18] Since 2011 they have come under the remit of the NHS Health Research Authority. A European Directive[19] on clinical trials has been incorporated into legislation[20] and is summarised in Box 17.2. The directive became law domestically via The Medicines for Human Use (Clinical Trials) Regulations 2004.

Box 17.2 EC Directive 2001/20/EC

On the implementation of good clinical practice in the conduct of clinical trials on medicinal products for human use

Article 1 Aim of the Directive:

- To establish specific provisions regarding the conduct of clinical trials, including multi-centre trials on human subjects involving medicinal product as defined by Article 1 of Directive 65/66/EEC
- Good clinical practice to be identified and complied with
- To adopt and if necessary revise principles of good clinical practice and detailed guidance to be published by the Commission
- All clinical trials to be designed, conducted and reported in accordance with the principles of good clinical practice

Article 2 Definitions

Article 3 Protection of clinical trial subjects

Article 4 Clinical trials on minors

Article 5 Clinical trials on incapacitated adults not able to give informed legal consent

Article 6 Ethics Committee

Article 7 Single opinion

Article 8 Detailed guidance to be published by Commission

Article 9 Commencement of a clinical trial

Article 10 Conduct of a clinical trial

Article 11 Exchange of information

Article 12 Suspension of the trial or infringements

Article 13 Manufacture and import of investigational medicinal products

Article 14 Labelling

Article 15 Verification of compliance of investigational medicinal products with good clinical and manufacturing practice

Article 16 Notification of adverse events

Article 17 Notification of serious adverse reactions

Article 18 Guidance concerning reports

Article 19 General provisions

Article 20 Adaptation to scientific and technical progress

Article 21 Committee procedure

Article 22 Application

Article 23 Entry into force 4 April 2001

Whilst the above was incorporated into The Medicines for Human Use (Clinical Trials) Regulations 2004, after Brexit minor changes have been made to the 2004 regulations via The Medicines for Human Use (Clinical Trials) (Amendment) (EU Exit) Regulations 2019.

In addition, a researcher would be required to observe the rights set out in the European Convention on Human Rights, which, since 2 October 2000, are actionable in this country (see chapter 1). Where the nurse becomes aware that the rights of the patient are not being protected by the researchers, he or she would have a professional duty to raise this with senior management and, if no action were taken, to make use of the whistleblowing provisions of the Public Interest Disclosure Act 1998 (see chapter 4). Reference can be made to the author's chapter exploring the legal implications of research.[21]

Control of a research programme

Practical dilemma 17.3   Gagged

Ann Jones, a ward sister, was on a management course that required her to complete a dissertation. She chose as her subject the consequences of the privatisation of cleaning services and studied one hospital where the services were contracted out to a private firm and another hospital where direct labour ancillary staff were used. Her conclusions were that privatisation led to a lower standard of cleaning, a less hygienic environment for patients, and nursing staff undertaking more cleaning work because the private firm sent cleaners to the wards for only a short proportion of the day. Just before she was due to submit the dissertation for her diploma, her nursing director heard of it and asked to see it. She has now been told that her findings are politically unacceptable, that she cannot present it to the college and that she must commence a totally different topic of research.

This situation gives rise to many legal issues. In this situation, the researcher is also an employee. She therefore has responsibilities to her employer. Even if she were an independent researcher funded from outside the institution that is the subject of the research, she might well have had to agree to a clause that the research findings have to have the prior approval of the institution before the research results can be published. As an employee, she would be expected to obey the reasonable orders of the employer. Is it reasonable in these circumstances for the researcher to be silenced? The answer would depend on more detailed facts: for example, was it only because the results were unwelcome that they are being suppressed? Was the basis of her data collection and statistical analysis sound? If there is no criticism to be made of her method and findings other than that they are embarrassing, it could be argued that the same principles apply here as apply in the situation discussed in chapter 7 relating to reporting on negligence by a colleague or some other form of unacceptable practice. Where management itself fails to take action, i.e. when all the internal procedures for improving the situation have been used to no avail, then it would not be considered unreasonable to take the matter to a higher authority, initially within the organisation and, if necessary, ultimately outside, but this obviously depends on the findings and the reasons for prohibiting publication.

The Public Interest Disclosure Act 1998 can be used to ensure that any person properly reporting health and safety concerns or criminal matters is protected from victimisation (see chapter 4). In November 2003 a university criminologist, who was conducting research into assisted suicides by people with AIDS, was awarded £62,000 by a committee of academic enquiry into the actions of Exeter University because Exeter University withdrew a written promise to give him legal backing should a court order him to disclose the names of those to whom he had spoken.[22] He had been forced to abandon his research, because he promised those involved in helping him that he would protect their identities. Simon Singh was sued for libel by the British Chiropractic Association for writing about 'bogus treatments' and found liable by the High Court.[23] However, he succeeded in his appeal but had to meet his own costs of £200,000. There were calls for libel laws to have no place in genuine scientific research. Subsequently the Defamation Act has provided a public interest defence to such cases.

Research Ethics Committees (RECs)

The researcher must ensure that she receives the proper approval before beginning any research. In some cases, this might mean obtaining the approval of a local ethics committee. Where this authority is received, it would be more difficult to prohibit publication of the results purely on the grounds of embarrassment at the findings.

Research involving patients or patient information may not be started until ethical approval has been obtained. It is the personal responsibility of the person named as principal investigator to apply for approval by the REC and this person retains responsibility for the scientific and ethical conduct of the research.

In 2011 (updated 2012) the UK Health Departments published the policy document 'Governance Arrangements' for research ethics committees which set out what is expected from research ethics committees that review research proposals relating to areas of the UK Health Departments' responsibility. The policy applies to all four parts of the UK and covers the principles, requirements and standards for research ethics committees, including their remit, composition, functions, management and accountability. This was replaced in

2020 with the Governance Arrangements for Research Ethics Committees (2020) (updated in 2021).

The Care Act 2014 section 112(2) defines a research ethics committee as

a group of persons which assesses the ethics of research involving individuals; and the ways in which health or social care research might involve individuals include, for example

(a) by obtaining information from them;

(b) by obtaining bodily tissue or fluid from them;

(c) by using information, tissue or fluid obtained from them on a previous occasion; and

(d) by requiring them to undergo a test or other process (including xenotransplantation).

The Health Research Authority is required to publish a document, called 'the REC policy document', which specifies the requirements which it expects research ethics committees it recognises or establishes to comply with, and to monitor their compliance with those requirements.

United Kingdom Ethics Committee Authority (UKECA)

In May 2004, the UK Ethics Committee Authority (UKECA), composed of UK health ministers, was created as the body responsible for establishing, recognising and monitoring RECs to review clinical trials of medicines under the EC Directive. Information on the work of UKECA can be found on the Health Research Authority website.[24] A Central Office for Research Ethics Committees (COREC – now National Research Ethics Service (NRES)) was set up to work on behalf of the Department of Health, to coordinate the development of the RECs, manage multi-centre research ethics committees (MRECs) and provide advice on policy, operational matters and training. COREC acted for UKECA in providing advice/assistance to these committees. An ad hoc advisory group was set up to review the operation of NHS RECs and reported in June 2005.[25] COREC was placed under the National Patient Safety Agency in 2005 and relaunched as the National Research Ethics Service (NRES) in March 2007. The NRES had a dual mission: to protect the rights, safety, dignity and well-being of research participants; and to facilitate and promote ethical research that is of potential benefit to participants, science and society. The National has since been removed from the name and it is now called RES.

Health Research Authority (HRA)

The review of arm's-length bodies proposed that the future of the NRES should be considered as part of the wider Academy of Medical Science's review of research regulation with a view to moving this function from the NPSA into a single research regulatory body.[26]

Subsequently in 2011 the NHS Health Research Authority was established as a Special Health Authority to protect and promote the interests of patients and the public in health research and to streamline the regulation of research. The National Research Ethics Service (NRES) was a core function and directorate within the Health Research Authority.

The Care Act 2014 (ss. 109–116 and Schedule 7) established HRA as a body corporate, non-departmental public body, with responsibility for the UK-wide Research Governance Framework. It is responsible for Research Ethics Committees, the Gene Therapy Advisory

Committees and the Confidentiality Advisory Group which advises on section 251 of the NHS Act 2006. The RECs are managed through the NRES. (Further information on the HRA can be found on its website.[27])

The main functions of the HRA (under s. 110) are:

(a) functions relating to the coordination and standardisation of practice relating to the regulation of health and social care research (see section 111);

(b) functions relating to research ethics committees (see sections 112 to 115);

(c) functions as a member of the United Kingdom Ethics Committee Authority (see section 116 and the Medicines for Human Use (Clinical Trials) Regulations 2004 (S.I. 2004/1031)); and

(d) functions relating to approvals for processing confidential information relating to patients (see section 117 and the Health Service (Control of Patient Information) Regulations 2002 (S.I. 2002/1438)).

Its main objectives in exercising its functions are:

(a) to protect participants and potential participants in health or social care research and the general public by encouraging research that is safe and ethical; and

(b) to promote the interests of those participants and potential participants and the general public by facilitating the conduct of research that is safe and ethical (including by promoting transparency in research).

It is required to publish guidance on good practice in the management and conduct of health and social care research. Under section 112 it must ensure that research ethics committees it recognises or establishes provide an efficient and effective means of assessing the ethics of health and social care research.

Confidentiality

Where use is made of personal information, access to it and disclosure of it in such a form that the individuals can be identified is subject to the provisions of the General Data Protection Regulation (GDPR) (see chapter 8). This means that if the data are not exempt from any of the provisions of the GDPR and if they are to be used in addition for research, then they must also be registered for research use. Even where the data are not automated, they would still come under the provisions of the GDPR, which applies to both computerised and manually held data. This means that they may be disclosed only in those exceptional circumstances outlined in chapter 8.

Difficulties can arise for the researcher where information is obtained that has nothing to do with the research, i.e. it is simply doing the research that has given the opportunity to gain this information. The General Medical Council states that information can be given by practitioners about their patients for the purpose of research, but the patient's consent should be sought or the information provided in an anonymous form.[28] The Patient Information Advisory Group (PIAG) was set up under section 61 of the Health and Social Care Act 2001 to consider proposals for the use of patient-identifiable information. The PIAG was replaced by the National Information and Governance Board for Health and Social Care (NIGB),[29] which was established under section 157 of the Health and Social Care Act 2008. NIGB was subsequently replaced by HRA. Further information can be obtained from the HRA website.[30]

Practical dilemma 17.4 Silence or disclosure?

Sandra James, a staff nurse, was conducting a research project into the care of a post-operative surgical patient. She was interested in the rate of infection, length of stay, convalescent care and the nature of community care. Her research therefore required visits to the patients' homes. One of her patients, Glenda Mitchell, had been operated on for gallstones. She was in hospital for seven days and was then discharged to her home. Her cohabitee had taken a few days off work to care for their three-year-old daughter. While Sandra was visiting the home, she was surprised to see that the child was very frightened of her and was withdrawn and hostile. Sandra tried to talk to her and touch her and noticed severe bruising and pinch marks on the child's legs.

In a suspected case of non-accidental injury, there is a clear justification for disclosing confidential information in the interests of the child. In a case like this, Sandra might try to persuade the mother to explain the child's bruising and, if this were unsatisfactory, she should ensure that appropriate action is taken to protect the child, e.g. arranging for the health visitor to visit, initiating the non-accidental injury (NAI) procedure or even bringing in the NSPCC.

Whatever action she takes along these lines would be protected from any litigation for breach of confidentiality on the grounds that the public interest justified it. In one case,[31] the House of Lords stated that the NSPCC was entitled to maintain the secrecy of the names of its informants, even if they had been malicious. This decision is based on public policy because it is essential that people are prepared to report potential incidents of child abuse. If, however, the facts of this situation are changed slightly and instead of a potential NAI case a potential crime against property is suspected, e.g. stolen goods are seen in the house, many professionals would feel that their professional duty of confidentiality must be maintained.

Consent

Unfortunately, not all research subjects are notified that they are to be included in a research project and their consent is not always obtained to the participation. Even in randomised controlled trials of drugs, patients should be informed that they have the right to refuse to take part. If the treatment is therapeutic rather than pure research, then in exceptional circumstances it could be argued that the doctor's right of therapeutic privilege (discussed by the House of Lords in the Montgomery[32] case (see chapter 7)) applied and there are special circumstances to justify not informing the patient of that fact. The right of therapeutic privilege could be relied on only in exceptional circumstances and the presumption is that the patient's consent should be obtained.

The basic legal principles are as follows: consent to participate in research should be given freely by an adult, mentally competent person and should be preceded by sufficient relevant information about serious harmful side effects as approved practice would require the professional to give the patient. Where research is contemplated on minors, it should proceed only if it is in the subject's interests and the benefits substantially outweigh any potential harm and the research is approved by the REC. The question as to whether parents have the right to consent to non-therapeutic research on their children is discussed in chapter 13. The RCN has provided guidance on obtaining consent for research[33] and also on research ethics.[34] The Duff Report (which followed the tragedy at Northwick Park where six volunteers developed multiple organ failure while trying out a new drug) recommended that participants in clinical drug trials should be given information on how adverse events should be reported.[35]

Concern has been raised about a controversial research project where paramedics give heart attack victims either placebo injections or adrenaline to test the effectiveness of adrenaline. The trial will not allow for consent to be obtained through the usual means. The study is being led by the University of Warwick. Ethical approval has been given by the Oxford research ethics committee.[36] There are concerns that adrenaline could be doing more harm than good and needed to be tested.

Consent and the mentally incapacitated adult

In a case in 2003 Judge Butler-Sloss gave approval to treatment being carried out on two teenagers suffering from variant Creutzfeldt-Jakob disease even though the treatment had not yet been tested on humans. Their parents gave consent.[37] This situation involving research on those lacking the requisite mental capacity to give consent is now covered by the Mental Capacity Act 2005 (apart from clinical trials). The Act enables research to be carried out, but only if stringent conditions are met. These are set out in sections 30–34 of the Act and shown in Box 17.3.

Box 17.3 Conditions for research on those lacking mental capacity set by the Mental Capacity Act

- The research is connected with an impairing condition affecting P (the person lacking mental capacity) or its treatment
- An impairing condition is defined in section 31(3) as a condition which is (or may be) attributable to, or which causes or contributes to, the impairment of, or disturbance in the functioning of, the mind or brain
- There must be reasonable grounds for believing that the research would not be as effective if carried out only on, or only in relation to, persons who have the capacity to consent to taking part in the project
- 5a The research must have the potential to benefit P without imposing on P a burden that is disproportionate to the potential benefit to P or
- 5b be intended to provide knowledge of the causes or treatment of, or of the care of persons affected by, the same or a similar condition
- If 5(b) applies and not 5(a), there must be reasonable grounds for believing:
   (a) that the risk to P from taking part in the project is likely to be negligible, and
   (b) that anything done to, or in relation to, P will not:
      (i) interfere with P's freedom of action or privacy in a significant way, or
      (ii) be unduly invasive or restrictive
- There must be reasonable arrangements in place for ensuring that the requirements of consulting carers and additional safeguards are met.

Regulations[38] cover the situation where an adult who had given consent to participation in research lost the requisite mental capacity during the research project. The Department for Constitutional Affairs (now absorbed in the Ministry of Justice) has provided a Code of Practice on the implementation of the Mental Capacity Act 2005,[39] which is available on the Ministry of Justice website.[40] The provisions of the Mental Capacity Act 2005 do not apply to research which comes under the Clinical Trial Regulations.

Consent to research and statutory provisions

The Department of Health has prepared guidance on consent by a legal representative on behalf of a person not able to consent under the Medicines for Human Use (Clinical Trials) Regulations 2003. Where there are any risks to the adult, an application to court would probably have to be made. Where there are no risks, the local research ethics committee (LREC) should be made aware of the lack of mental capacity of the research subjects. Failure to obtain consent to research or to give the necessary information could render the researcher liable to action. The Human Fertilisation and Embryology Act 1990 (as amended by the Human Fertilisation and Embryology Act 2008) prevents research taking place on an embryo after the first 14 days from fertilisation. Section 3 of the amended 1990 Act places prohibitions on the use of human embryos and section 4 prohibits activities in connection with genetic material not of human origin and stipulates activities which a research licence cannot authorise (see chapter 21).

The law on the removal, storage and use of organs and tissue was changed by the Human Tissue Act 2004 as the result of the scandal at Bristol Royal Infirmary when, during an inquiry into allegations of professional misconduct in carrying out paediatric heart surgery, it was learnt that more than 11,000 children who had died in the past 40 years had had their organs used for research in British hospitals without the explicit consent of their parents. (The law relating to the removal, retention and storage of organs and tissue is discussed in chapter 15.)

In 2013 the National Institute for Health Research launched the campaign 'It's OK to ask' to encourage patients who are undergoing treatment for a medical condition to ask their doctor about clinical research and whether taking part in a study might be right for them. The campaign asks patients to give feedback to the NIHR via its Facebook page or by telephone.

Liability for volunteers in research

Practical dilemma 17.5   Guinea-pig

Benjamin Robinson was a medical student who was very short of money because he sent part of his grant home to his family each week. He heard of a research project being undertaken in the pharmaceutical department and offered his services. Because he was anxious to be accepted, he failed to tell the medical officer in charge of the research that he had suffered from glandular fever as a child. He subsequently took drugs to test out the toxicity of a drug for migraine. A few weeks later, he had a heart attack and died. Is there any liability for his death by the NHS trust and/or the research team?

At present there is no law that the volunteer should automatically obtain compensation for harm that occurs as a result of the research participation. The Pearson Report of 1978[41] recommended that volunteers in medical research should be compensated on a no-fault basis, but this has not been implemented through legislation. At present, the Association of the British Pharmaceutical Industry (ABPI) has prepared guidelines for the provision of compensation to victims of research and supports through a written agreement with each research subject that any subjects who have been harmed as a result of participation in a drugs trial will be compensated on a strict liability basis without proof of negligence. This is a voluntary agreement, but would normally be a part of the protocol of the research project approved by the LREC. Apart from this scheme, as the law stands at present, the volunteer who is harmed as a result of participation in a research project can obtain compensation only on the basis of negligence, i.e. he must establish that a duty of care was owed to him, this has been broken, and as a reasonably foreseeable result of this breach the subject has suffered some harm.

Applying these principles here, it is hoped that the pharmaceutical company undertaking the research would compensate Benjamin's family on a **strict liability** basis. If the pharmaceutical company failed to pay up, then the family would have to show that in one way or another the researchers were negligent; for example, the researchers failed to give Benjamin a proper medical examination or the design of the research was faulty and reasonably foreseeably dangerous to the volunteers. There is little evidence of that here and, in addition, Benjamin, by concealing his previous illness, would have been contributorily negligent and therefore considered to a certain extent to be responsible for what happened.

It is possible that if it can be established that Benjamin was harmed as the result of a defect in a product, then the Consumer Protection Act 1987 applies and Benjamin's family can obtain compensation under these provisions against the producer or supplier. This is considered in greater length in chapter 12. Much of the debate on liability would hinge on whether at the time of production the producer should have realised that there was a defect in the product.

Another possible defence against such a claim is the possibility of alleging that Benjamin, by volunteering willingly, assumed the risks of such an event occurring. This is known as the defence of *volenti non fit injuria* and is explained in more detail in chapter 6. In order to rely on this as a defence, it would have to be shown not only that Benjamin knew of the risks, but also that he consented willingly to run them and agreed to waive all claim for compensation as a result.

Fraud in research

There is a danger that the pressure to undertake research and provide significant results could lead to fraudulent research practices. For example, it was discovered that a cancer specialist had fabricated the results of his research into the efficacy of a chemotherapy drug.[42] Failure by a practitioner registered with the NMC to follow sound and honest research principles could be seen as evidence of unfitness to practise and lead to their being struck off the Register.

Health and safety of the researcher

Exactly the same principles of health and safety apply to the researcher as apply to other employees, i.e. the employer owes a duty of care at common law to ensure that they are provided with a safe environment, a safe system of work and competent staff. Where the researchers are not employees, the occupier of the premises on which they are working would still be expected to uphold the duty of care for their safety under the Occupiers' Liability Act 1957. It could be, however, that as specialists they would be expected to be aware of those risks that arise from their particular tasks and the NHS trust would not be liable for harm resulting from that. The provisions of the Health and Safety at Work Act 1974 would also apply (see chapter 12).

Research publication and libel

A decision by the Court of Appeal and new legislation in the Defamation Act 2013 in relation to the publication of research should remove from researchers the fear of a libel action over their findings. Dr Simon Singh, a science writer, successfully defended an action for libel brought against him by the British Chiropractic Association (BCA). The BCA had won in the High Court, the judge holding that Singh's comments about chiropractic were factual assertions rather than expressions of opinion, which meant that he could not use the defence of fair comment. The Court of Appeal overruled the High Court, holding that his criticism of the BCA's medical claims was honest opinion and he was entitled to the defence of fair comment. The Court of Appeal held that 'scientific controversies must be settled by the methods of science rather than by the methods of litigation'.[43] (See also chapter 29.) However, threats of defamation action against Dr Dalia Nield, who has cast doubts on the efficacy of a breast-enhancing cream, suggested that the Court of Appeal has not resolved the issue.[44] Amendments to the Defamation Act which would introduce a stronger public interest defence and thus protect discussions about science, evidence and healthcare from defamation actions were included by Parliament in the Defamation Act 2013.

Health Education England

A special health authority known as Health Education England (HEE) was established in 2012. HEE describes itself as responsible for the education, training and personal development of every member of the healthcare workforce in England. It was abolished by the Care Act 2014 and replaced by a non-departmental corporate body of the same name with functions and constitution set out in sections 96 to 102 and Schedule 5 of the Care Act 2014. Further information on its role can be found on its website.[45] It was based on proposals outlined in *Liberating the NHS*[46] and most of its provisions extend to England and Wales. HEE has the responsibility for carrying out the Secretary of State's functions in relation to the planning and delivery of education and training. It is required under section 98 to exercise its functions with a view to ensuring that a sufficient number of persons with the skills and training to work as healthcare workers for the purposes of the health service is available to do so throughout England. It is also required (s. 99) to exercise its functions with a view to securing continuous improvement:

(a) in the quality of education and training provided for healthcare workers, and

(b) in the quality of health services.

It must also promote:

(a) research into matters relating to such of the activities listed in section 63(2) of the Health Services and Public Health Act 1968 (social care services, primary care services and other health services) as are relevant to HEE's functions, and

(b) the use in those activities of evidence obtained from the research.

It must also exercise its functions with a view to securing that education and training for healthcare workers is provided in a way which promotes the NHS Constitution.

The Secretary of State must publish before the start of each financial year a document which specifies the objectives and priorities that the Secretary of State has set for HEE for that year in relation to the education and training to be provided for healthcare workers. The Secretary of State must also publish at intervals of not more than three years a document (called the 'Education Outcomes Framework') which specifies the outcomes that the Secretary of State has set for HEE to achieve having regard to those objectives and priorities. In its turn HEE must publish a document which specifies the objectives and priorities that it has set, for the period specified in the document, for the planning and delivery of education and training to healthcare workers, and specifies the outcomes that HEE expects to achieve in that respect during that period having regard to those objectives and priorities and provides guidance for Local Education Training Boards. Section 101 sets out the matters to which HEE must have regard in performing its functions. These matters include:

(a) the likely future demand for health services and for persons with the skills and training to work as healthcare workers for the purposes of the health service,

(b) the sustainability of the supply of persons with the skills and training to work as such,

(c) the priorities that providers of health services have for the education and training of persons wishing to work as such,

(d) the mandate (see chapter 5) published under section 13A of the National Health Service Act 2006,

(e) the objectives of the Secretary of State in exercising public health functions (as defined by section 1H of that Act),

(f) the priorities that the National Health Service Commissioning Board has for the provision of health services,

(g) documents published by the Secretary of State under section 100(1), (2) or (3),

(h) the desirability of promoting the integration of health provision with health-related provision and care and support provision,

(i) the desirability of enabling healthcare workers to switch between different posts relating to health provision, health-related provision or care and support provision, and

(j) such other matters as regulations may specify.

HEE is required to make arrangements to obtain advice from those who have an interest in the provision of education and training for healthcare workers and must receive representations from health service providers, users, carers, healthcare workers, regulatory bodies and those providing education and training.

Local Education and Training Boards (LETBs)

Under section 103–7 and Schedule 6 of the Care Act 2014 the HEE must appoint committees for areas in England, each of which is to be called a Local Education and Training Board. The main function of an LETB is to exercise on HEE's behalf its functions to plan and deliver education for healthcare workers and ensure sufficient skilled healthcare workers in the health service in its area. It is required to publish an education and training plan and arrange for the commissioning of the necessary provision which will be funded by HEE. Further information on the role of LETBs and the location of each can be found on the NHS Employers' website.[47] The Secretary of State may specify a tariff setting approved prices in respect of education and training.

Conclusions

The content of nurse education and training and how it should be taught have come sharply into focus following criticisms of nursing care in the inquiry into Stafford Hospital (see chapter 5). A suggestion by the government that prospective nurses should be compelled to spend up to a year with hands-on care to avoid a repeat of the Stafford Hospital scandal was greeted by the Royal College of Nursing as a waste of public money, unworkable and having no benefit to patients[48] and was not supported by the well-known NHS commentator Professor Alan Glasper.[49] Subsequently, a survey carried out by the National Nursing Research Unit at King's College London found that almost 90 per cent of nurses found that they were too busy to carry out basic simple tasks such as comforting distressed patients, preventing bed sores and giving the right drugs. Minimum staffing levels were called for.[50] In his first week in office, the new Chief Inspector of Hospitals, Professor Sir Mike Richards, stated that nursing numbers needed to rise if quality of service was to be maintained. He said that the ability of nurses to provide compassionate care has been undermined through being overworked on understaffed wards.[51] In May 2014 NICE issued guidance on nurse staffing, but stopped short of giving recommended staffing levels. Statutory safe staffing levels have been introduced in Scotland and Wales.[52]

The controversy as to how to bring back compassion into nursing has many implications for those working in nurse education. They need to take part in the debate as to whether the abandoned role of state enrolled nurse should be reintroduced, what should be the content of nurse education and what should be the balance between teaching in the classroom and practical work on the wards. In addition nurse tutors should be at the forefront of research into staffing levels and measuring patient dependency. It is too early at this stage to gauge the value and implications of the HEE and the LETBs. The dispute over restrictions on using patient information and research projects is considered in chapter 8.

Reflection questions

1. How could a nurse lecturer defend themselves if a nurse who is accused of causing harm to the patient blamed the teaching that they had received in the nurse training college?
2. What records do you currently keep on your teaching programmes? Review the period for which you keep them and their content in the light of this chapter.
3. What records do you keep in respect of external lecturers who are invited to teach in your department? How would you defend a case where an employee was suing for back injury and the manual handling training was carried out in your department?
4. In what ways does cooperation exist between the nurse training school and the wards and departments to ensure that the nurses' training meets the standards of approved accepted practice?
5. Researchers state that they are carrying out research on those who are unable to give consent. What protection does the Mental Capacity Act 2005 apply to such participants?

Further exercise

1. Prepare a procedure for initiating a research proposal, for obtaining the necessary approvals, for envisaging any possible difficulties in carrying it out and for publishing the results.

References

[1] UKCC, Standards for the Preparation of Teachers of Nursing, Midwifery and Health Visiting, UKCC, March 2000
[2] Nursing and Midwifery Council, Revised arrangements for the introduction of standards for practice teachers, Circular 08/2007
[3] Nursing and Midwifery Council, Higher Education Academy Membership A–Z, advice sheet, NMC, March 2006
[4] Clothier Report, The Allitt Inquiry: an independent inquiry relating to deaths and injuries on the children's ward at Grantham and Kesteven General Hospital during the period February to April 1991, HMSO, London, 1994
[5] Nursing and Midwifery Council, Good Health and Good Character: guidance for educational institutions, NMC, 2015; https://nmc.org.uk/globalassets/sitedocuments/registration/character-and-health-decision-making-guidance.pdf
[6] Oliver Moody, Graduate nurses increase patients' survival chances, *The Times*, 26 February 2014
[7] NICE, Intravenous fluid therapy: Quality standard consultation, May 2013
[8] *Croskery* v *Belfast University* NINHC/QB/2010/129; www.idras.ac.uk
[9] Nursing and Midwifery Council, Guidance for arranging practice placement experience for students from other UK countries, QA Fact sheet P/2004, April 2010, NMC
[10] Department of Health, Gateway Clearance Reference 7984, March 2007; www.bma.org.uk
[11] Lois Rowland and Charlotte Jones, Research midwives; importance and practicalities, *British Journal of Midwives*, 21(1):60–64, January 2013
[12] Department of Health, Best Research for Best Health, DH, 2006
[13] www.nihr.ac.uk
[14] www.nihr.ac.uk
[15] Nursing and Midwifery Council (2015) The Code: Professional standards of practice and behaviour for nurses and midwives, NMC, London
[16] Department of Health, Guidance for Local Research Ethics Committees, DH, 1991 (HSG(91)5)
[17] www.hra.nhs.uk
[18] Department of Health, Research Governance Framework for Health and Social Care, 2nd edn, 2005
[19] EC Directive 2001/20/EC
[20] Medicines for Human Use (Clinical Trials), SI 2004/1031 (Amended SI 2006/1928 and SI 2006/2984)
[21] B. Dimond, Legal issues, chapter 9 in Louise de Raeve (ed.) *Nursing Research: An Ethical and Legal Appraisal*, London and Philadelphia, Baillière Tindall, 1996
[22] Simon de Bruxelles, Academic awarded £62,000 for broken promise, *The Times*, 21 November 2003
[23] *British Chiropractic Association* v *Simon Singh* [2009] EWHC 1101
[24] www.hra.nhs.uk

25. Department of Health, Report of the Ad Hoc Advisory Group on the Operation of NHS Research Ethics Committees, June 2005
26. Department of Health, Liberating the NHS: Report of the arm's-length bodies, London, Crown, 2010
27. www.hra.nhs.uk
28. General Medical Council, Confidentiality, GMC, London, 1995
29. www.hra.nhs.uk
30. Ibid.
31. *In re D* v *NSPCC* [1977] 1 All ER 589
32. *Montgomery* v *Lanarkshire Health Board* [2015] UKSC 11
33. Royal College of Nursing, Informed consent in health and social care research, 002267, 2nd edition, RCN, 2011
34. Royal College of Nursing, Research Ethics: RCN guidance for nurses, 003138, RCN, 2011
35. Duff Report, Expert Group on Phase 1 Clinical Trial, December 2006, Stationery Office
36. Alice Hutton, Paramedics to give heart attack victims placebo injections, *The Times*, 13 August 2014
37. *Simms* v *Simms* [2003] 1 All ER 669
38. The Mental Capacity Act 2005 (Loss of Capacity during Research Project) (England) Regulations 2007, SI 2007/679
39. Code of Practice, Mental Capacity Act 2005, Department of Constitutional Affairs, February 2007
40. Ministry of Justice; www.gov.uk
41. Pearson Report, Royal Commission on Civil Liberty and Compensation for Personal Injury, Cmnd 7054, HMSO, London, 1978
42. Lois Rogers, Cancer 'cure' doctor admits bogus research, *The Sunday Times*, 13 February 2000
43. *British Chiropractic Association* v *Singh CA*, The Times Law Report, 23 April 2010
44. News item, Doctor faces libel action, *The Times*, 11 November 2010
45. www.hee.nhs.uk
46. Department of Health, Liberating the NHS: Developing the healthcare workforce from design to delivery, 2012
47. www.nhsemployers.org
48. Martin Barrow, Nurses dismiss 'stupid' plan to make them go back to basics, *The Times*, 22 April 2013
49. Alan Glasper, A year as a healthcare assistant a prerequisite?, *British Journal of Nursing*, 22(9):536–7, 2013
50. Chris Smyth, Nurses are 'too busy to provide basic care', *The Times*, 30 July 2013
51. Tom Whipple, Overworked nurses 'too busy to care', *The Times*, 20 July 2013
52. Health and Care (Staffing) (Scotland) Bill 2018 and Nurse Staffing Levels (Wales) Act 2016

Chapter 18

Legal Aspects of the Care of Older People

This chapter discusses

- Rights to care
- National Service Framework for Older People
- Intermediate care
- Consent to treatment
- Force, restraint and assault
- Medication and the confused older patient
- Dementia
- Standard of care
- Risk management
- Abuse of older people
- Mental Capacity Act 2005 and decision making for the mentally incapacitated adult

Introduction

It is a truism that every elderly person is different. The fact that a person is over 60 or 70 or 80 or 90 says absolutely nothing else about them. Standards of health, loneliness, housing, finance, mobility and capability are as varied as with any other age group. All that can be said of them as a group is that it is more likely than not that they will be faced with some problems – social, economic, health or others – and that these are more likely to be multiple problems, interrelated, with one triggering off another. For example, it might be that an older person living on their own has limited mobility and therefore finds it difficult to get to the shops. They thus do not feed themselves properly, and come under the hospital's care as a result of lack of proper nourishment. Figures produced by NHS Digital show that the average age of patients has been increasing steadily for many years, and patients over the age of 45 increased by nearly 44 per cent (from

6.9 million to 9.9 million) between 2005/06 and 2015/16. Provision against discrimination on grounds of age is now included in the Equality Act 2010. The government has provided guidance on banning age discrimination in services.[1] (Age discrimination laws relating to employment are discussed in chapter 10.) In addition, older people can claim discrimination in respect of their human rights as set out in the European Convention on Human Rights as a result of Article 14 (see chapter 1). All that has been said of the general principles of negligence and vicarious liability applies equally to the nurse who cares for older people. Discrimination issues may also arise in the care of older people from black and minority ethnic communities or from ageism, and these must also be addressed.[2] The Equality Act 2010 has recognised the right not to suffer combined discrimination. Section 14 protects against combined discrimination where (1) a person (A) discriminates against another (B) if, because of a combination of two relevant protected characteristics, A treats B less favourably than A treats or would treat a person who does not share either of those characteristics. Discrimination on grounds of age could thus be linked with discrimination on grounds of: disability; gender reassignment; race; religion or belief; sex; or sexual orientation.

In February 2007 Age Concern noted that ageism is the most common form of discrimination in the UK. Its survey revealed that more than three times more people have been the victims of ageism than any other form of discrimination.[3] Older people are the highest users of acute services in the NHS.[4] There are particular difficulties that the nurse who cares for older people is more likely to encounter than other nurses and these are considered in this chapter. In 2008 the RCN published a resource pack for students learning to work with older people[5] and a mentorship A5 card designed to explain the positive benefits of mentorship for those caring for older people to raise standards of care.[6]

There are, in addition, problems relating to the property and possessions of older people and these are dealt with in chapter 24. In chapter 28, there is a discussion on the law relating to the making of wills and other aspects of dealing with death. Those nurses who care for older people in the community should refer to chapter 22 for coverage of that topic. Those caring for older people who have mental incapacity should refer to chapter 19. Advance decisions are considered in chapter 28.

Rights to care

There are no laws that set a cut-off point at which interventions for older people are not justified. On the contrary, the human rights legislation and the Equality Act 2010 would prohibit discrimination on the grounds of age. In the past, for example, there have been occasions where ambulances have been told to take patients over 65 to an elderly care/general medical ward rather than to a coronary care unit; where a non-resuscitation policy has been based on the age of the patient rather than their physical condition and prognosis; where they have been refused surgical treatment because of their age. Age UK reports that such discrimination is still occurring.[7] Research published in December 2013 suggested that there was a culture of ageism in the NHS since the elderly were being denied hip and knee replacements as the NHS attempted to save £20 billion.[8] A BBC article on its website found that age discrimination might be preventing older people over 65 from having access to much needed surgery,[9] indeed older lung cancer patients are six times less likely to be offered potentially life-saving surgery than younger people.[10] In January 2013 Macmillan Cancer Support reported that doctors were discriminating against older patients in cancer care and in a survey of 101 oncologists 81 per cent would offer chemotherapy for a high risk breast cancer patient of 68, but only 47 per cent would do so for an identical patient of 73.[11]

Such discrimination has no legal basis. There are in law no age limits for accessing treatment. The only criteria are the prognosis of the patient and the extent to which further investment in their health is justified in terms of the benefit that it would bring to that individual. The Equality Act 2010 recognises age as one of eight characteristics to be protected against discrimination (see chapter 10). A tool has been designed to identify whether or not age discrimination is occurring in hospital, primary care and social care.[12] Discrimination of the grounds of age would be a breach of Article 14 of the European Convention on Human Rights (see the website of this book) when linked with violation of another Article. However, in one case the High Court held that it was not a breach of Article 8(1) of the European Convention on Human Rights, or, if it was, it was justified under Article 8(2), when a local authority closed a day centre, because it was working well below full capacity and the cost savings would release resources for domiciliary care. The local authority had not acted irrationally.[13]

A plea to retain a specialism of old age psychiatric services was made by a group of distinguished health professionals to the editor of *The Times*[14] who argued that a misunderstanding of the age discrimination laws will lead to a much worse service for elderly people.

National Service Framework for Older People

The Social Services Inspectorate report on improving older people's services[15] in 2001 showed that local authorities were expanding their services to promote independence through prevention and rehabilitation. This was in accordance with the philosophy of the National Service Framework (NSF) for Older People[16] published by the Department of Health in 2001, which was a 10-year plan for improving health and care services for older people in England. Guidance was issued in March 2001.[17]

The NSF for Older People was:

A strategy to ensure fair, high quality, integrated health and social care services for older people. It is a 10-year programme of action linking services to support independence and promote good health, specialised services for key conditions, and culture change so that all older people and their carers are always treated with respect, dignity and fairness.

The eight standards cover the following areas:

Standard 1	Rooting out age discrimination
Standard 2	Person-centred care
Standard 3	Intermediate care
Standard 4	General hospital care
Standard 5	Stroke
Standard 6	Falls
Standard 7	Mental health in older people
Standard 8	Promotion of health and active life in older age.

Each standard set out its aim, defined the standard and identified its rationale and the key interventions. In addition, a timetable of milestones was set by which specific targets must be achieved.

A booklet on medicines and older people was also published to ensure that older people gained maximum benefit from medication and did not suffer unnecessarily from illness caused by excessive, inappropriate or inadequate consumption of medicines. The NSF also identified how the standards were to be implemented at local level and the national support that would underpin the standards. The National Institute for Health and Care Excellence (NICE) had an important role to play in ensuring that the standards were based on clinically effective research-based practice.

In March 2014 the Chief Executive of NICE Sir Andrew Dillon stated that 'age would inevitably be a factor (in assessing new drugs) as the young have more years left to contribute. Elderly people would not be denied new drugs because NICE plans would raise the number of treatments approved.'[18] The NSF for Older People was underpinned by a programme of research commissioned by the Policy Research Programme and Service and Delivery Organisation Programme.[19] The Care Quality Commission (replacing the Healthcare Commission (i.e. CHAI) and the Commission for Social Care Inspection (CSCI)) ensured through inspections that the standards were implemented across health and social services. In addition, progress overall was initially overseen by the NHS Modernisation Board and the Older People's Taskforce. A progress report on the NSF was issued by the National Director for Older People's Health in November 2004, entitled *Better Health in Old Age*.[20] In 2007 the Department of Health and the National Director for Older People issued a review outlining the next steps in implementing the NSF.[21] It looked at three themes: dignity in care, joined-up care and healthy ageing, and considered 10 programmes for progress with a review of the available resources. In 2008 the Department of Health published an overview report on research to support the NSF for Older People.[22] It identified the demographic significance of older people and considered the progress in implementing some of the initiatives (for example, it concluded that reimbursing hospitals for delayed discharges was no longer a necessary policy in England) and set out new areas for research. The National Director for Older People also published in 2007 guidance on a change of direction in the provision of services for older people by bringing the services closer to their homes.[23] Additional guidance was issued on specific standards.

The priorities for the second phase of the 10-year programme for the NSF for Older People were set out by the Department of Health in April 2006 and can be downloaded from the DH website.[24] In October 2010 it was announced that paramedics were in a pilot trial to give drugs to stroke victims before they reach hospital to reduce high blood pressure and reduce the damage from the stroke.[25]

The National Service Framework for Older People (NSFOP) has been discontinued. It was replaced in 2013 with the formation of NHS England. However, the NSFOP played a crucial role in setting quality standards for health and social care services for older people, emphasising respect, prevention, specialist care, and promoting healthy lifestyles.

Updates on health-related studies and research for older people can be found on the NHS website.[26]

In Wales there is a Strategy for Older People, published in 2013 by the Welsh Government which is closely aligned to the Social Services and Well-being (Wales) Act 2014 that examines elderly person's well-being in the context of the social, financial and environmental aspects of their lives. In 2016/17 the Scottish Government provided funding of over £535,000 to older people's organisations to assist in tackling barriers to independent living, and significant resources are being provided to address loneliness and social isolation. In Wales, Scotland and Northern

Ireland there is an Older People's Commissioner to champion the rights of older people, especially at government level. To date (2018), no such role exists in England.

The National Service Framework (NSF) for Long-term Conditions 2005

In 2005 the DH published a strategy setting five key outcomes for people with long-term conditions.[27] It pointed out that one in three of the population suffers from a long-term condition and the number of people with a long-term condition was expected to rise by 23 per cent over the next 25 years. A revised edition of the compendium on long-term conditions first issued in 2004 was published in 2008.[28]

The NSF for long-term conditions sets out 11 quality requirements in health and social care services:

1. A person-centred service;
2. Early recognition followed by prompt diagnosis and treatment;
3. Emergency and acute management;
4. Early and specialist rehabilitation;
5. Community rehabilitation and support;
6. Vocational rehabilitation;
7. Providing equipment and accommodation;
8. Providing personal care and support;
9. Palliative care;
10. Support for family and carers; and
11. Care during admission to hospital.

Other initiatives to improve the services for older people include the Dignity in Care campaign, launched in November 2006, which aimed to ensure that older people are treated with dignity when using health and social care services. It wished to create a zero tolerance of lack of dignity in the care of older people in any care setting. In 2007 the Healthcare Commission carried out a review of acute services to ensure that older people are treated with dignity and respect.

The National Service Framework for Long Term Conditions (NSF) has also been discontinued by NHS England and its Long Term conditions strategy.[29]

Intermediate care

Intermediate care has been described[30] as a core element of the government's programme for improving services for older people. In conjunction with improvements to community equipment services, home care support and related services, it should enable increased numbers of older people to maintain independent lives at home.

To come within the definition of intermediate care, services must meet *all* of the following criteria:

- they are targeted at people who would otherwise face unnecessarily prolonged hospital stays or inappropriate admission to acute inpatient care, long-term residential care or continuing NHS inpatient care;

- they are provided on the basis of a comprehensive assessment, resulting in a structured individual care plan that involves active therapy, treatment or opportunity for recovery;
- they have a planned outcome of maximising independence and typically enabling patients/users to resume living at home;
- they are time-limited, normally no longer than 6 weeks and frequently as little as 1–2 weeks or less; and
- they involve cross-professional working, with a single assessment framework, single professional records and shared protocols.

Various models are used, including rapid response, hospital at home, residential rehabilitation, supported discharge and day rehabilitation, discharge to assess and reablement.. The 2001 guidance suggested that intermediate care should last no longer than six weeks with discretion in individual cases. The 2009 guidance recognised the short-term nature of intermediate care but recommended the need for flexibility and avoiding unrealistic expectations. Sanctions against local authorities that fail to provide discharge arrangements for an older person in hospital, thereby blocking a bed, are provided under the Community Discharge (Delayed Discharges) Act 2003, which is discussed in chapter 22. A fact sheet (Number 76) published by Age Concern in May 2018 gives the current situation on intermediate care and reablement.[31] See also the Hospital 2 Home resource pack which is considered in chapter 22.

Consent to treatment

Practical dilemma 18.1 An operation at 90?

Gwen Ash was admitted to hospital suffering from severe abdominal/chest pain. Gwen was intermittently competent. There were days when she recognised Amy, her daughter, and others where she did not, but instead abused Amy when she came to visit her. The physician diagnosed a hiatus hernia. There was considerable debate over the best method of treatment. Initially, a strict diet and medication were proposed, but there were signs that this was not working when Gwen started bleeding internally. The physician asked Amy to come in and see him to talk about Gwen's future care. He said that possibly the only long-term course of treatment was an operation. However, at Gwen's age there were considerable risks in undertaking this. Although she was in a reasonably good state of health, she might not withstand the operation. Amy was in a dilemma, not knowing whether to sign the form of consent on Gwen's behalf. She attempted to explain the position to Gwen. Gwen grasped the fact that she would have to have an operation. She made it clear to Amy that she had had a good life and did not want to be cut open now. Amy also spoke to the ward sister who explained that Gwen was in very good health and would probably survive the operation, but, of course, one could not be 100 per cent sure. What should Amy do?

In Practical Dilemma 18.1, if Gwen is assessed as lacking the requisite mental capacity to make a decision about the operation, the Mental Capacity Act 2005 would apply. Does Gwen lack mental capacity?

It could well be that in her more lucid moments she is capable of understanding what is happening to her and of giving a valid consent or refusal. At other times, she may well be far removed from reality. If the doctor obtains her signature on a form consenting to the operation in one of these rational spells, can he rely on it when she becomes mentally confused? The answer is probably yes. Section 2(2) of the Mental Capacity Act 2005 states that 'It does not matter whether the impairment or disturbance is permanent or temporary'. Provided that Gwen has the mental capacity at the time she gives consent to the operation, that would be a valid consent. It is essential, however, that only a reasonable time elapses between the signing of the form and the operation being carried out and the operation must clearly be in the interests of the patient. What is reasonable? Certainly not as long as a year, but possibly up to three months. It depends on the operation to be performed and whether the circumstances remain exactly as they were when the patient signed the form.

If Gwen is incapable of making a decision when the operation is required, then under the Mental Capacity Act 2005 (in the absence of an advance decision in which Gwen when mentally capable had set out her wishes as to what should happen in this situation (see chapter 28)), action must be taken in her best interests. The steps set out in the Mental Capacity Act 2005 in determining the best interests of Gwen must be followed (see chapter 7). If the operation for a hiatus hernia is seen as serious medical treatment then there must be consultation with carers over what Gwen would have wished, and what her feelings, views, values and beliefs would have been in order to determine her best interests. In the absence of such persons to consult it would be necessary to appoint an independent mental capacity advocate. (This appointment is not necessary here because her daughter Amy can be consulted.) Advance decisions or living wills are considered in chapter 28.

Case 18.1 London Borough of Redbridge v G [2014]

In February 2014 the local authority (LA) applied to the court for a declaration that G an elderly lady lacked the requisite mental capacity to make her own decisions and were concerned at the influence of C, a live-in carer, and F, another carer over her. Russell J made a declaration of incapacity in relation to the relevant decisions and that proceedings in relation to her welfare and in particular her residence with C should continue in the Court of Protection.[32] Subsequently her carers C and F were involved in public protests outside Ilford town hall to protest about the involvement of the LA in G's care. There was a dispute as to whether G herself wished to be in contact with the press. Cobb J ordered an assessment to be made about G's mental capacity to communicate directly with the press and for the interim determined that it was probably not in G's best interests to be in communication with the press. He also made an interim order that C and F should facilitate visits by the LA social workers.[33] Sir James Mumby in the Court of Protection held that G's Article 8 rights not to be involved with the press took precedence over Article 10 rights of the press. He refused the application of Associated Newspapers Ltd to be joined as a party to the case.[34]

In a case decided in July 2014 Mr Justice Cobb of the Court of Protection decided that it was in the best interests of a patient with dementia to continue to stay in a care facility despite the recommendation of the social worker that she would be happier at home. The judge held that the patient (who was German and had moved to the UK after the Second World War) was physically well cared for, and had a social life readily at hand.[35]

Force, restraint and assault

Caring for confused older patients raises concerns about what action can be taken in fulfilment of the duty of care, when treatment is being refused contrary to the best interests of the patient or when they are at risk of harm and need to be restrained. Useful guidance is provided by the RCN on restraint and rights, risks and responsibilities.[36] Anyone using restraint of any sort must ensure that their actions are compatible with Article 3 of the Human Rights Convention, which is discussed in chapter 1 and can be found on the website of this book. Advice is also given by the Department of Health entitled *Positive and Proactive Care: reducing the need for restrictive interventions*, which provides guidance for when or when not to use restraint. Where an adult lacks the mental capacity to make their own decisions a limited form of restraint can be used under the Mental Capacity Act (MCA) 2005. Under Section 5 of the MCA restraint cannot be used unless two conditions are satisfied. These are:

- that the decision maker must reasonably believe that it is necessary to do the act in order to prevent harm to the client/patient, and
- that the action is a proportionate response.

Proportionate means that the act of restraint is proportionate to both the likelihood of harm to the client/patient and the seriousness of the harm.

The use of restraint is defined as including both the decision maker using or threatening to use force to secure the doing of an act which the client/patient resists and also restricting the mentally incapacitated person's liberty of movement, whether or not he or she resists.

Examples of justified restraint might include pulling a person back from crossing in front of a car or moving a person away from an open window. The Mental Capacity Act was amended to enable a person's liberty to be restricted in circumstances where the use of mental health legislation was not justified or possible. These amendments, known as the Deprivation of Liberty Safeguards (DoLS) were made to fill what was known as the Bournewood gap and they are considered in chapter 16. The Supreme Court has ruled that the severely disabled are entitled to the same protection from the DoLS as are applicable to others.[37] The case is considered in chapter 16 (see Case 16.4) and is likely to lead to many more applications to the Court of Protection.

Examples of Bad Practice

The Parliamentary Joint Committee on Human Rights in August 2007[38] found that more than a fifth of care homes have been found to be failing basic standards of care for privacy and dignity. Its recommendations are considered in chapter 22.

Four care workers were found guilty of ill-treatment or neglect of elderly residents at a nursing home and three were imprisoned the other given a community order.[39]

In 2013 there were 109,000 referrals to social services last year of suspected elder abuse a rise of 2000 on 2012. A quarter of cases involved a spouse, partner or family member and the abuse ranged from neglect to physical violence.[40] The charity Action on Elder Abuse is concerned at the government's slowness in acknowledging the problem.

A report by the Good Care Guide stated that staff at a care home tied an elderly lady to a chair to stop her wandering.[41] It found that more than a quarter of families had claimed that relatives had suffered poor treatment in care homes or by carers in their own home.

Restless Patients

Practical dilemma 18.2 — The wanderer

One further difficulty that the staff had with Gwen (described in Practical Dilemma 18.1) was that she could never stay in one place. She always liked to be on the move. Her restlessness took her all around the hospital where she was well known and those with time on their hands would eventually bring her back to the ward. Unfortunately, building work started on site and the contractors were asked to take special care in crossing hospital roads. The director of nursing instructed Gwen's ward manager to keep her on the ward because of the danger. The ward manager could not be sure that someone was always available to keep an eye on Gwen and, rather than lock the ward door and imprison all the patients, she decided to use a restrainer on Gwen so that every time Gwen tried to get out of her chair a belt, which was fastened around Gwen and to the chair, rang a bell and prevented Gwen from leaving the chair. Amy visited Gwen and was distressed to see this form of restraint; Gwen herself protested about it. What is the legal position?

To restrict a person's movement without lawful authority so that they have no way of escape is a form of false imprisonment. This effectively is what Gwen is – imprisoned. Limited restraint could be used under the Mental Capacity Act, as described above. However, any form of restraint which could be seen as a breach of Article 5 and a person's right to liberty and security of person must comply with either the Mental Health Act 1983 (as amended) or the Deprivation of Liberty Safeguards enacted by amendments to the Mental Capacity Act 2005 and introduced to fill the Bournewood gap.

The form of restraint used by the ward manager would appear to be neither temporary nor reasonable. What alternatives are available to the ward staff, given that they have a duty to care for Gwen and to prevent her exposure to danger? Adequate staffing to keep an eye on each person is obviously one possibility, but given present-day economic constraints and nurse staffing levels it may not be a realistic option. Another possibility is the use of more volunteers to supervise certain patients. One suggestion is to change the locks so that it takes some ingenuity to open the door without the help of the ward staff, although this is not a happy compromise, and may still be viewed as a deprivation of liberty in that the staff may need to assist, and therefore remain effectively in control of the locks. In this case, a Deprivation of Liberty Safeguard assessment is still required. Electronic tagging devices can also be used, so that if a patient wearing such a device goes through an exit, then a bell warns the staff, but again an assessment is required. Even if there are no contractors onsite, there may be other dangers such as a main road nearby, a stream in the grounds, etc. If unreasonable methods of restraint are used, for example locking someone in their room, this could be a violation of the patient's human rights as set out in Article 3, 'No one shall be subjected to torture or to inhuman or degrading treatment or punishment', or under Article 5.

Where staff consider that some form of restraint is necessary to control very aggressive older patients, they should obtain advice on the application of the Mental Capacity Act 2005 and the Deprivation of Liberty Safeguards. (See chapters 7 and 16 or the Mental Health Act 1983, chapter 19.) The Alzheimer's Society suggest that electronic tagging should be offered to dementia sufferers to allow their relatives to locate them quickly should they wander off. The Society advised that, where possible, permission should be sought from the sufferer, perhaps in advance, before he or she has reached the later stages of dementia.[42]

Control at Night

At night, bed rails are often used to prevent patients climbing or falling out of bed. In one sense, where the older person is clearly struggling against them, these represent a form of restraint. By the same token, they may in some circumstances be justified and indeed necessary where the patient is very confused and restless. Failure to use them might lead to action against the authority for failing in its duty of care for the patient. However, the potential danger of the patient trying to climb over the cot sides and causing himself harm must always be borne in mind. A risk assessment has to be carried out on whether the use of cot sides in each individual situation is justified and safe. Records should be kept of this risk assessment. Information is available from the Medicines and Healthcare Products Regulatory Agency (MHRA) (see chapter 12) on the use of bed safety rails.[43] Its Device Bulletin in 2006,[44] updated in December 2013 provides guidance on the use of bed rails which are not supplied by the bed manufacturer, the need for a full risk assessment on the suitability of using a bed rail and general guidance on their use.

A man died when his head became trapped in bed rails when in hospital. The NHS Trust was fined £533,334 after admitting to failing to provide safe care to the man.

Daily Care

Practical dilemma 18.3   Chiropody case

One form of treatment that Gwen could not tolerate was having her toenails cut. She was abusive to the podiatrist, who found it very difficult to keep her nails in reasonable order. The podiatrist asked the ward manager if she would hold Gwen down while she attempted to cut her nails. The ward manager was not happy with this suggestion and felt that they should first seek medical guidance as it might be preferable to cut the nails when Gwen was mildly sedated. What is the legal position?

Chapter 7 discusses consent to treatment where it is stated that touching another person without their consent or some other lawful authority is a trespass to their person. Does the fact that Gwen needs to have her toenails cut constitute lawful authority? The answer to this is, in general, no. However, the fact that Gwen lacks the capacity to give a valid consent may well justify the professionals taking some action to care for her. As has been seen earlier, professionals are justified in acting in the best interests of a patient incapable of making his or her own decisions under the Mental Capacity Act 2005. This is quite clear if the patient is unconscious. In considering podiatry, we are not talking of something that is, at least initially (although it may well be ultimately), a life-saving procedure. In addition, there are numerous nursing tasks and social tasks such as bathing, hair washing and brushing to which patients like Gwen may well object. In theory, of course, to brush Gwen's hair without her consent is a trespass to her person. There may be occasions when Gwen can be persuaded to have it done and will not struggle against it. However, inevitably, there may come a time when Gwen needs to have something done despite her protests. In such cases restraint may be used, providing the conditions set out in the Mental Capacity Act as described above are satisfied. If the level of restraint required is such that it could infringe her rights under Article 5 of the European Convention on Human Rights, then it may be necessary to consider using the Deprivation of Liberty Safeguards resulting from the Bournewood case.

Medication and the confused older patient

The above principles apply equally to the administration of medication. The majority of patients in general and mental health hospitals and care settings are on some form of medication, but only a few of them are under a section (about 5–10 per cent of psychiatric patients). There are many occasions when, through a variety of reasons ranging from justifiable ones to pure cussedness or confusion, they reject the tablets, injections or liquid. What does the nurse do? Obviously, where the patient is capable of making that decision, their refusal should be respected. But this is rarely the case. Often the patient is in Gwen's situation: intermittently or permanently confused. The provisions of the Mental Capacity Act which enable action to be taken in the best interests of the person lacking the capacity to make decisions can be applied (see chapter 7).

In 2007 the NMC published[45] standards for medicines management which included the administration of medicines by covert means. This is discussed in chapter 27 on medicines.

Practical dilemma 18.4   Resistance in the elderly

On one occasion Gwen made it clear that she would not have her medication, which was prescribed as a sedative and for her heart condition. As an informal patient, could she be forced to take the medication since it was for her benefit and she lacked the mental capacity to make a reasoned judgement over whether she should be taking it?

It is necessary in a situation such as Practical Dilemma 18.4 for a clear assessment to be made of Gwen and whether she lacks mental capacity to make a decision about her medication and whether or not she is suffering from mental disorder. If Gwen is assessed as lacking the mental capacity to decide whether she should take medication, then she would come under the provisions of the Mental Capacity Act 2005 and action must be taken in her best interests. The provisions of the Act are set out in chapter 7 and also considered in chapter 16. If she is assessed as suffering from mental disorder then consideration should be given as to whether she should be detained under the Mental Health Act 1983 (as amended) and given compulsory treatment under Part 4 of the Act (see chapter 19). The answer to the question in Practical Dilemma 18.4 is that as an informal patient lacking the requisite mental capacity to determine whether or not to take medication, she could be compelled to take medication if it was considered to be in her best interests.

Medication may sometimes be used as a form of restraint. There are considerable dangers in so doing and the practice may be declared illegal under Article 3 of the Human Rights Convention (see chapter 1 and the website of this book) on the grounds that it is degrading or inhuman treatment. A line has to be drawn between medication that is in the best interests of a mentally incompetent patient (and could therefore be given under the Mental Capacity Act) and medication that is for other purposes. The latter would be unlawful. In January 2004 a House of Commons Health Committee Investigation into elder abuse reported that more than half of the care homes for older people were failing to administer old people's medication properly. Only 45 per cent of homes met minimum standards. The situation found by the Joint Committee in August 2007 on elder abuse in care homes suggested that standards had not improved. A review carried out for the Department of Health in November 2009[46] found that over 144,000 patients suffering from dementia were being given anti-psychotic drugs unnecessarily. The Care Services Minister undertook to appoint a national clinical director for dementia to conduct an audit of GPs' and hospital doctors' prescribing of anti-psychotic drugs. The review considered that their use could be reduced by two-thirds.

An expert report from the Royal College of Physicians on the feeding of patients at the end of life concluded that care homes were insisting on feeding residents with feeding tubes because there are not enough staff to provide conventional feeding.[47]

Dementia

The National Audit Office reported in 2007 that too little is being done to deal with the growing problem of dementia care. Its report stated that Britain was slow to diagnose cases and lagged behind other European countries in providing care. According to the Alzheimer's Society, there are around 850,000 people living with dementia in the UK, and it is estimated that by 2025, this figure will rise to around 1 million (2017 figures).[48]

In July 2014 the number of people known to have dementia rose by almost two-thirds in seven years following a big push to tell sufferers that they have the disease.[49] A survey in 2009 by the Alzheimer's Society found that dementia patients over 65 years were kept in hospital too long and received disgraceful care that worsened their condition.[50] Many patients were malnourished, dehydrated or unable to return home.

In January 2008 the Public Accounts Committee of the House of Commons published a report on improving services and support for people with dementia.[51] The report came to the following conclusions:

1. Dementia affects over 560,000 people in England, costs about £14 billion a year but has not been an NHS priority.
2. Unlike cancer and coronary heart disease, there is no single individual with responsibility or accountability for improving dementia services. The DH should appoint a Senior Responsible Officer.
3. Between a half and two-thirds of people with dementia never receive a formal diagnosis. Diagnosis should always be made, regardless as to whether interventions are available, and could be assisted if GP practices had greater support from mental health services, if the Royal College of General Practitioners developed a dementia care pathway, and by the Institute of Innovation and Improvement promulgating good diagnostic practice.
4. There is a poor awareness among the public and some professionals of dementia and what can be done to help people with the disease. DH should commission a dementia awareness campaign.
5. People with dementia require support from multiple health and social care providers but this is often difficult to manage. On diagnosis, people with dementia and their carers should

be given a single health or social care professional contact point (e.g. a social worker or community psychiatric nurse) to improve the coordination of care.

6. Carers save the taxpayer £5 billion a year, yet between a half and two-thirds of all carers do not receive the carer's assessment to which they are entitled. The DH should emphasise to local health organisations and their social care partners that they need to develop an action plan which gives priority to assessing and meeting the needs of carers and develop a commissioning toolkit to demonstrate the cost benefits of the different options for providing support, including respite and domiciliary care.

7. Sixty-two per cent of care home residents are currently estimated to have dementia but less than 28 per cent of care home places are registered to provide specialist dementia care. CSCI (now the Care Quality Commission) should assess staff qualifications and training as part of its review of the quality of care for people with dementia, and local mental health teams should use the finding when allocating resources to community psychiatric teams.

8. Hospital Care for people with dementia is often not well managed, increasing the risk of longer stays, admission to a care home and deterioration in the patient's health. Hospitals should routinely undertake a mental health assessment. Care records should be shown to paramedics, so that an informed decision on admission to hospital or to care home can be made.

Following the Public Accounts Committee report the DH promised that a National Dementia Strategy would be developed. As part of an awareness campaign on dementia, the Alzheimer's Society published in 2008 a booklet 'Worried about your Memory' to assist in the identification of Alzheimer's which is available from its website.[52]

The Department of Health published its dementia strategy in February 2009.[53] The key objectives are shown in Figure 18.1. Experts say that dementia will affect at least 1.4 million people and cost the economy £30 billion a year within a generation. The implementation plan published by the DH at the same time as the strategy recognised that all areas would not be able to implement the strategy within five years. Therefore seven key priority outcomes were identified that were likely to need focused attention for early delivery:

- Early intervention and diagnosis for all;
- Improved community personal support services;
- Implementing the New Deal for Carers;
- Improved quality of care for people with dementia in general hospitals;
- Living well with dementia in care homes;
- An informed and effective workforce for people with dementia; and
- A Joint Commissioning strategy for dementia.

Dementia care was allocated £150 million for the first two years of the five-year strategy. The Alzheimer's Society welcomed the initiative but was surprised that research was not a fundamental component of the strategy and was disappointed that the review of anti-psychotic drugs had been delayed.

A report published on 17 March 2009 by a firm of health and social care analysts, Laing and Buisson, which surveyed 6000 care homes, found that training was 'fragmented and ad-hoc' with a third of homes failing to provide staff with specialist instruction. The need for the implementation of the national strategy was obvious.

- **Objective 1: Improving public and professional awareness and understanding of dementia.** Public and professional awareness and understanding of dementia to be improved and the stigma associated with it addressed. This should inform individuals of the benefits of timely diagnosis and care, promote the prevention of dementia, and reduce social exclusion and discrimination. It should encourage behaviour change in terms of appropriate help-seeking and help provision.
- **Objective 2: Good-quality early diagnosis and intervention for all.** All people with dementia to have access to a pathway of care that delivers: a rapid and competent specialist assessment; an accurate diagnosis, sensitively communicated to the person with dementia and their carers; and treatment, care and support provided as needed following diagnosis. The system needs to have the capacity to see all new cases of dementia in the area.
- **Objective 3: Good-quality information for those with diagnosed dementia and their carers.** Providing people with dementia and their carers with good-quality information on the illness and on the services available, both at diagnosis and throughout the course of their care.
- **Objective 4: Enabling easy access to care, support and advice following diagnosis.** A dementia adviser to facilitate easy access to appropriate care, support and advice for those diagnosed with dementia and their carers.
- **Objective 5: Development of structured peer support and learning networks.** The establishment and maintenance of such networks will provide direct local peer support for people with dementia and their carers. It will also enable people with dementia and their carers to take an active role in the development and prioritisation of local services.
- **Objective 6: Improved community personal support services.** Provision of an appropriate range of services to support people with dementia living at home and their carers. Access to flexible and reliable services, ranging from early intervention to specialist home care services, which are responsive to the personal needs and preferences of each individual and take account of their broader family circumstances. Accessible to people living alone or with carers, and people who pay for their care privately, through personal budgets or through local authority-arranged services.
- **Objective 7: Implementing the Carers' Strategy.** Family carers are the most important resource available for people with dementia. Active work is needed to ensure that the provisions of the Carers' Strategy are available for carers of people with dementia. Carers have a right to an assessment of their needs and can be supported through an agreed plan to support the important role they play in the care of the person with dementia. This will include good-quality, personalised breaks. Action should also be taken to strengthen support for children who are in caring roles, ensuring that their particular needs as children are protected.
- **Objective 8: Improved quality of care for people with dementia in general hospitals.** Identifying leadership for dementia in general hospitals, defining the care pathway for dementia there and the commissioning of specialist liaison older people's mental health teams to work in general hospitals.
- **Objective 9: Improved intermediate care for people with dementia.** Intermediate care which is accessible to people with dementia and which meets their needs.
- **Objective 10: Considering the potential for housing support, housing-related services and telecare to support people with dementia and their carers.** The needs of people with dementia and their carers should be included in the development of housing options, assistive technology and telecare. As evidence emerges, commissioners should consider the provision of options to prolong independent living and delay reliance on more intensive services.
- **Objective 11: Living well with dementia in care homes.** Improved quality of care for people with dementia in care homes by the development of explicit leadership for dementia within care homes, defining the care pathway there, the commissioning of specialist in-reach services from community mental health teams, and through inspection regimes.
- **Objective 12: Improved end of life care for people with dementia.** People with dementia and their carers to be involved in planning end of life care which recognises the principles outlined in the Department of Health End of Life Care Strategy. Local work on the End of Life Care Strategy to consider dementia.
- **Objective 13: An informed and effective workforce for people with dementia.** Health and social care staff involved in the care of people who may have dementia to have the necessary skills to provide the best quality of care in the roles and settings where they work. To be achieved by effective basic training and continuous professional and vocational development in dementia.

Figure 18.1
Objectives of the National Dementia Strategy from the DH, February 2009

- **Objective 14: A joint commissioning strategy for dementia.** Local commissioning and planning mechanisms to be established to determine the services needed for people with dementia and their carers, and how best to meet these needs. These commissioning plans should be informed by the World Class Commissioning guidance for dementia developed to support this Strategy and set out in Annex 1.
- **Objective 15: Improved assessment and regulation of health and care services and of how systems are working for people with dementia and their carers.** Inspection regimes for care homes and other services that better assure the quality of dementia care provided.
- **Objective 16: A clear picture of research evidence and needs.** Evidence to be available on the existing research base on dementia in the UK and gaps that need to be filled.
- **Objective 17: Effective national and regional support for implementation of the Strategy.** Appropriate national and regional support to be available to advise and assist local implementation of the Strategy. Good-quality information to be available on the development of dementia services, including information from evaluations and demonstrator sites.

In 2013 the DH launched 'Making a Difference in Dementia: Nursing Vision and Strategy' using the 6 Cs of care, compassion, competence, communication, courage and commitment to emphasise the strategic role of the nurse.[54] Subsequently, a G8 Conference held in London agreed that dementia should be curable by 2025. New treatments were to be fast tracked for approval as part of an international action plan. A global dementia envoy was to be appointed to keep the condition high on the political agenda and to ensure international research efforts are properly coordinated.[55] UK spending on dementia research is to be doubled over the next decade (to reach £130 million by 2025). The CQC has initiated a programme of inspections of hospitals and care homes to check how people with dementia are treated.[56] Following a survey the Alzheimer's Society reported that one in three dementia sufferers leaves home only once a week and one in ten only leave home once a month. It urged the need to change attitudes and build awareness in the community.[57] A report from the Rush University Medical Centre in Chicago suggested that Alzheimer's is responsible for almost as many deaths as heart disease or cancer, but is unreported on death certificates which list the immediate cause of death such as pneumonia rather than the underlying cause.[58]

A report in October 2013 by the Leonard Cheshire Disability Charity stated that many elderly people were being forced to choose between going thirsty and going to the lavatory because more home care visits last for only 15 minutes. The charity has started a campaign to end the scandal of the 15-minute care visit.[59] In April 2014 the director of social care at the CQC stated that care visits to dementia patients that lasted 15 minutes or less were 'ineffective, inappropriate and unsafe'. A new inspection regime was being introduced which would penalise care companies who supplied this type of visit to patients with dementia.[60]

A report in 2014 by Baroness Kingsmill criticised the fact that the 1.8 million care workers for the elderly were underqualified, undertrained and paid below the minimum wage which led to the frail and elderly not receiving the help they required.[61] (See chapter 23 and healthcare support workers.)

The National Dementia Strategy was to be replaced by a new 10 year plan from the Department of Health and Social care in 2022 with the aim of reducing preventable dementia and to ensure timely diagnosis of dementia. Sadly, the plan has yet to be published despite the DHSC predicting that some 1.6 million people will be living with dementia by 2040.

Dementia and other Legal Issues

A person suffering from dementia may involve a nurse in many other legal areas; for convenience a guide to the relevant chapters is given below.

- The Mental Capacity Act – see chapters 7 and 16;
- The Mental Health Acts 1983 and 2007, compulsory admission, guardianship, powers of the nearest relative, supervised community treatment order and Section 117 – see chapter 19;
- Deprivation of Liberty Safeguards – see chapter 16;
- Safeguarding adults issues – see below and also chapter 10;
- Financial management and the Court of Protection – see chapters 16 and 24;
- Powers of deputy and the Office of Public Guardian – see chapters 16 and 24;
- Lasting powers of attorney – see below in this chapter and chapter 24;
- Advance decisions/Living wills – see chapter 28.

Standard of care

Practical dilemma 18.5 An unknown break

Fred, a patient, aged 75, recovering from an orthopaedic operation, was occasionally restless in the night. On one such occasion, he fell out of bed. The nurse in charge rushed to his aid and with the help of the other night nurses, she put him back in bed. Fred appeared none the worse, was happy to have a cup of tea and then he settled down. The next morning, the nurse in charge was about to mention to the day shift that Fred had had a disturbed night, but did not give them the details as they were distracted by a patient with a query. A few days later, Fred was seen to be avoiding putting any weight on his left leg. He was examined, sent for X-ray and a fracture diagnosed. His son asked how this had happened. However, no one could recall any incident in the day and the night staff had not entered the earlier incident in the records or reported an accident. An investigation was then initiated.

Even if the nurse in charge considered on reasonable grounds that there was no need to call the doctor out in the night, her failure to ensure that the incident was reported to the doctor on the following morning and her failure to arrange for a doctor to examine Fred was clearly not in accordance with approved practice. In addition, she failed to give to the day staff a full account of the night's events so that they were unable to ensure that the appropriate action was taken. The nurse in charge compounded these omissions by failing to fill in an accident report. Unless there are any other mitigating factors in an incident like this, Fred would undoubtedly have a possible claim for compensation against the negligent nurse and therefore against the NHS trust for its vicarious liability for their employee. Compensation is unlikely to amount to very much, since it would cover only the additional days of pain and suffering because the fracture had not been diagnosed earlier (unless, of course, the nurses were negligent in failing to put cot sides up and prevent the original fall). However, if it is discovered that those few days' delay have had considerable effects on the long-term prospects for Fred's recovery, then, clearly, compensation would be greater. The nurse in charge would obviously face disciplinary proceedings and also fitness to practise investigations. In its annual report for 2002/03, the NMC highlighted the fact that many cases heard by its Professional Conduct Committee related to poor practice in the care of older people and vulnerable patients. This category made up almost 30 per cent of complaints during 2002/03. Two of the four cases it describes in detail in its report are concerned with practitioners' failure to deal appropriately with older patients who had falls. A survey by Age UK (a merger of Age Concern and Help the Aged) found that almost one in three nurses would not trust the NHS to care for a malnourished elderly relative. It found that elderly people were not helped with feeding, with unopened food trays being removed without any questions.[62] Age UK's evidence is supported by figures provided by the National Confidential Enquiry into Patient Outcome and Death published in November 2010, which showed that only a third of elderly patients received good hospital care and, for one-fifth, surgery was so delayed that it impaired recovery. In June 2013 NICE published clinical guidance on preventing falls in older people.[63] In May 2014 the chair of NICE, David Haslam, criticised the care of thousands of elderly patients who were dumped onto an unthinking conveyor belt of NHS care and made to endure operations and medications they do not need. He said that NICE was attempting to reverse the behaviour.

In November 2013 it was reported that nurses had forgotten a patient aged 84 over a weekend.[64] The case was revealed by the Patients Association which stated that the NHS was struggling to provide basic care and was in desperate need of reform. It appeared that the patient had been admitted with a suspected fractured hip and had suffered a stroke, had been prescribed 17 different drugs, but was left to lie in urine and had not been offered food or water for a day. She died a few days later following discharge.

In another tragic death, managers refused to allow paramedics to enter the room of a stroke victim in a care home because it breached company policy.[65] A telephone operator refused to let the paramedics have the code to a wall-mounted safe containing the master key because it was not confirmed that it was a paramedic calling.

Pressure Ulcers

It is accepted that the breakdown of tissue is not confined to older patients, but since they may be more vulnerable to pressure ulcers, this subject is discussed in this chapter. Many years ago the possibility of suffering from pressure ulcers was believed to be an inevitable result of long-term immobilisation. Now, however, pressure ulcers are seen as evidence of negligence by those providing the care and inevitably are therefore likely to result in litigation. Public Health England states on its website that the cost of treating a pressure ulcer is between £1214 and £14,108. Pressure ulcers in older patients are often associated with a fivefold increase in mortality. In-hospital mortality in this age group is 25–33 per cent.[66] In recent years awards have been made of £32,000[67] and £14,000[68] and where death results from the inadequate care that leads to pressure ulcers, manslaughter charges could be brought.[69] Disciplinary proceedings by the employer and fitness to practise proceedings could also be brought against those who have failed to act according to appropriate standards. NICE has prepared guidelines on pressure ulcer risk management and prevention[70] that will be updated as the research basis for best practice improves. Eventually NICE guidance is likely to be incorporated into the Bolam Test of reasonable professional practice. In July 2010 the National Patient Safety Agency (NPSA) (now incorporated within NHS England) announced that it was adopting a zero tolerance approach in relation to pressure ulcers and it provided guidance on prevention.[71] Pressure ulcers were one of the 10 key areas of clinical activity chosen by NPSA for 2010. There may be disputes over which hospital, care home or other establishment is responsible for the breakdown of tissue, and documentation of the examination of a patient on admission (or discharge) and of the risk assessment and management undertaken would be essential to establish which institution and staff were liable for the patient's condition. Prevention and management of pressure ulcers is one of the fundamental areas of patient care for which the Department of Health has identified essence of care benchmarks, first published in 2001 and revised in 2010[72] (see chapter 3). In Wales the essence of care benchmarks are referred to as the fundamentals of care, and include pressure ulcers as one of those fundamentals of care.

Winter Crises

An agreement was made between the government and the Red Cross, the RVS and Age UK to provide over 5000 trained volunteers to ease the elderly winter crisis in 2013. Volunteers were to act as part of triage schemes to try to reroute people away from A&E and to provide support possibly reducing admissions.[73] However, Jeremy Hunt said subsequently that it was up to individual hospitals to approach the charities and most of the fund to help hospitals prepare for the winter had been allocated and the £38 million was rejected.[74] NHS England urged neighbours, forming an army of good Samaritans, to help the elderly during the winter. Charities criticised the plan as being ludicrous and an ill-thought-through idea.

An Audit of Intermediate Care found that almost no more of the services were being offered in 2013 than the previous year. Yet the pressure to fill existing intermediate care capacity with people leaving hospital appears to have worsened with 70 per cent of (intermediate care) beds now occupied by people coming off the wards.[75]

Continuing Care of Older People

In December 1997, the UKCC published a policy paper on the continuing care of older people.[76] Among its recommendations were: that the UKCC should recognise that the central features of the nursing role in continuing care are holistic assessment, health promotion and the ability to work in multi-professional partnership with clients, their carers and other agencies; that specialist practitioners, in particular community nurses and health visitors, be actively involved in all continuing care settings; and community nurses and health visitors have a key role in the assessment of older people for continuing care services and in ongoing assessment and review following placement. The NMC in its professional conduct annual report for 2002/03 placed emphasis on the practitioners' duty of care to older patients and clients. The NMC published guidance for the care of older people. Lack of services following the discharge of older people was highlighted by the Royal Voluntary Service which reported that one in 10 elderly people discharged from hospital arrives home to an empty house with no help.[77] Fifteen per cent of over-75s are readmitted within 28 days of discharge. A report from Age Concern in 2014 found that the number of people receiving council care had dropped considerably with only 896,000 receiving help with washing, dressing and eating despite an increase in the numbers of over-65s by 1 million. The amount spent on social care for older people had dropped by £1.2bn (15.4 per cent) since 2010.[78]

The Equality and Human Rights Commission (EHRC) reported in October 2013 that elderly people are being put at risk of neglect and abuse by overstretched home care workers who are paid less than the minimum wage.[79]

In 2011 the EHRC published a report[80] on an inquiry into older people and human rights in home care[81] which recommended that it should:

(a) address gaps in the legal and regulatory framework (e.g. definition of public function under s. 73 Care Act 2014 extends the protection of the human rights convention and the Care Act 2014 places duties on local authorities to promote individual well-being);
(b) address lack of awareness among local authorities about what human rights obligations mean in practice;
(c) address the lack of awareness about human rights and care entitlements among older people and their families;
(d) ensure that there are better arrangements in place to detect threats to human rights in home care; and
(e) address the status of home care workers.

Many of these recommendations have been implemented in the Care Act 2014 which is considered in chapter 22.

Registered homes

The Royal Commission[82] recommended that a National Care Commission should be set up to monitor trends, including demography and spending, to ensure transparency and accountability in the system, to represent the interests of consumers and set national benchmarks, now and in the future. The Care Standards Act 2000 set out a new framework for regulation of the independent healthcare sector and most social care. A National Care Standards Commission was established. This was subsequently abolished and its health registration and inspection functions transferred to CHAI (i.e. the Healthcare Commission) and its social services registration and inspection functions transferred to the Commission for Social Care Inspection. From 1 April 2009 the Care Quality Commission is one regulatory authority, with enhanced powers, combining the Healthcare Commission, the Mental Health Act Commission and the Commission for Social Care Inspection (see chapters 5 and 22). The CQC standards for quality and reports of its inspections of individual homes can be found on its website.[83] From 2013 it has tightened up its inspections and appointed professionally qualified inspectors with expertise in specific areas.

Risk management

It is recognised that if vulnerable clients are to lead lives with a reasonable quality then certain risks must be faced. Thus it would be less risky keeping clients in an institution rather than taking them out for walks or other activities. The report[84] on the responses to the government's Green Paper on 'Independence, Well-being and Choice'[85] points out that 'Care cannot and should not strive to be 100 per cent risk free'. It recognised that there is a balance to be struck between enabling people to have control over their lives and ensuring that they are free from harm, exploitation and mistreatment. The Green Paper sought to encourage a more open debate about risk management. The feedback showed that there was support for the development of a risk management framework to include guidance and training to provide staff with the support they needed to operate in a new culture which favoured greater exposure to risk. The White Paper *Our Health, Our Care, Our Say*, published in 2006,[86] emphasised choice and control as critical components of the future strategy for health and social care. It gave a commitment to developing a national approach to risk management. Subsequently the Department of Health issued a guide to independence, choice and risk.[87] The guide can be downloaded from the National Archives website.[88] The guide provided a risk management framework for use by everyone involved in supporting adults using social care within any setting, including NHS staff working in multidisciplinary or joint teams. It states that:

> The governing principle is that people have the right to live their lives to the full as long as that doesn't stop others from doing the same. By taking account of the benefits in terms of independence, well-being and choice, it should be possible for a person to have a support plan which enables them to manage risks and to live their lives in ways which best suit them.

The DH also developed a supported decision tool template which was designed to guide and record the discussion when a person's choices involve an element of risk. This can be adapted to fit into local formats or used as a stand-alone tool.

Abuse of older people

In 2007 the National Centre for Social Research and King's College London reported on a two-year study which showed that almost 350,000 pensioners were abused or neglected in their own homes by carers (family members were responsible for 51 per cent). Campaigners called for new laws to give social workers the same rights of entry as they have where child abuse is suspected.[89]

The Health and Social Care Information Centre published figures on cases of abuse against the elderly in October 2013 which suggested a 28 per cent rise in alerts to local authorities to the year ending March 2013 from the year before. Campaigners are seeking a tightening of the law to ensure that elder abuse is taken as seriously as child abuse and prosecutions are made earlier.[90] Sections 42–47 of the Care Act 2014 places a duty on local authorities to safeguard adults at risk of abuse or neglect. The Disclosure and Barring Service (which replaced the Criminal Bureau and Independent Safeguarding Authority) processes checks on people seeking employment with children or vulnerable adults (see chapter 10).

In 2013 the Department of Health published an updated policy statement on safeguarding adults who are vulnerable to abuse and neglect. It is available on the government website.[91] It sets out the following principles of safeguarding adults:

- empowerment
- prevention
- proportionality
- protection
- partnership, and
- accountability,

and shows how these should be implemented by the various organisations involved in the care of the vulnerable and has a useful bibliography of related guidance.

The Care Act 2014 (England only) sections 42–45 and Schedule 2 made further provision in relation to Safeguarding Adult Boards and is shown in Statute Box 18.1.

Statute 18.1
Care Act 2014 Sections 42–5
Safeguarding adults at risk

Section 42

(1) This section applies where a local authority has reasonable cause to suspect that an adult in its area (whether or not ordinarily resident there)—
   (a) has needs for care and support (whether or not the authority is meeting any of those needs),
   (b) is experiencing, or is at risk of, abuse or neglect, and
   (c) as a result of those needs is unable to protect himself or herself against the abuse or neglect or the risk of it.

(2) The local authority must make (or cause to be made) whatever enquiries it thinks necessary to enable it to decide whether any action should be taken in the adult's case (whether under this Part or otherwise) and, if so, what and by whom.

(3) 'Abuse' includes financial abuse; and for that purpose 'financial abuse' includes—
  (a) having money or other property stolen,
  (b) being defrauded,
  (c) being put under pressure in relation to money or other property, and
  (d) having money or other property misused.

Section 43

Each local authority must establish a Safeguarding Adults Board (an 'SAB') for its area with the objective of helping and protecting adults in its area in cases of need. The way in which an SAB must seek to achieve its objective is by coordinating and ensuring the effectiveness of what each of its members does. An SAB may do anything which appears to it to be necessary or desirable for the purpose of achieving its objective.

Section 44

(1) An SAB must arrange for there to be a review of a case involving an adult in its area with needs for care and support (whether or not the local authority has been meeting any of those needs) if—
  (a) there is reasonable cause for concern about how the SAB, members of it or other persons with relevant functions worked together to safeguard the adult, and
  (b) condition 1 or 2 is met.

(2) Condition 1 is met if—
  (a) the adult has died, and
  (b) the SAB knows or suspects that the death resulted from abuse or neglect (whether or not it knew about or suspected the abuse or neglect before the adult died).

(3) Condition 2 is met if—
  (a) the adult is still alive, and
  (b) the SAB knows or suspects that the adult has experienced serious abuse or neglect.

(4) An SAB may arrange for there to be a review of any other case involving an adult in its area with needs for care and support (whether or not the local authority has been meeting any of those needs).

(5) Each member of the SAB must cooperate in and contribute to the carrying out of a review under this section with a view to—
  (a) identifying the lessons to be learnt from the adult's case, and
  (b) applying those lessons to future cases.

Section 45 sets out the right of the SAB to obtain information from persons providing specified conditions are met.

Code of Practice

Each local authority should have in place a code of practice to protect older people from abuse. An agreed procedure should be followed where there are concerns that an older person may be subject to abuse. Community nurses should obtain a copy of their local code of practice if they have reason to fear that one of their patients is subject to abuse, whether physical, sexual, emotional or financial. Box 18.1 sets out the steps that a community nurse should follow. Age UK has been running a campaign to prevent elder abuse and further details and leaflets can be obtained from its website.[92] A confidential helpline has been set up by Action on Elder Abuse[93] which also provides guidelines for health and social workers in detecting and preventing elder abuse, available on its website.[94]

Box 18.1 **Guidelines for action in abuse of older people**

1. Find out if the local authority has a procedure for the protection of vulnerable adults where abuse is suspected. If so, follow this procedure. Ensure you document your concerns and action.
2. In the absence of a procedure, seek the advice and guidance of senior management. Information can also be obtained from the Action on Elder Abuse helpline.
3. Keep clear records of the facts on which your suspicions are based.
4. Check if the circumstances set out in section 135(1) of the Mental Health Act 1983 (see chapter 19) appear to be present.
5. Report your concerns to the appropriate social worker, suggesting, if appropriate, a community care assessment under section 47 of the NHS and Community Care Act 1990.
6. Ensure that the patient's general practitioner is also notified of your concerns.

Legal Protection

The Domestic Violence Crime and Victims Act (DVCV Act) 2004 requires persons living in a household where there is a child or vulnerable adult to take reasonable steps to prevent the unlawful death of that person. Reasonable steps suggested by Counsel and Care[95] would include:

- reporting suspicions of abuse to the police;
- contacting local social services;
- making sure that any injuries are treated promptly;
- explaining concerns to the GP; and
- contacting an organisation such as Action on Elder Abuse.

The DVCV Act defines a vulnerable person as:

> **any person aged 16 or over whose ability to protect himself from violence, abuse or neglect is significantly impaired through physical or mental disability or illness, through old age or otherwise.**

In addition, under the Mental Capacity Act 2005 it is a criminal offence under section 44(2) to ill-treat or wilfully neglect a person who lacks capacity. The Act applies to a person (D) who has the care of a person (P) who lacks, or whom D reasonably believes to lack, capacity; to the donee of a lasting power of attorney, or an enduring power of attorney created by P; or to a deputy appointed by the court for P. In one of the first prosecutions under section 44(2), the owner and the manager of a Southampton care home were sentenced: the former to a 30-week jail sentence suspended for 18 months and a fine of £27,000, costs of £25,000 and 200 hours' community service; and the latter to 200 hours' of community service. Nine residents of the 34-bedded care home were found in urine-soaked beds, malnourished, dehydrated and some with bed sores.[96] Four care staff from Hillcroft Nursing Home in Lancashire were charged and convicted under the MCA for ill-treatment or neglect of a person who lacks capacity under the Mental Capacity Act in November 2013.[97] The judge stated that lack of proper management allowed a culture to develop where (abusive) conduct was allowed to carry on. A registered nurse failed in her appeal against her conviction for wilfully neglecting a person who lacked capacity under section 44 of the Mental Capacity Act 2005. She had failed to apply cardiac pulmonary resuscitation to a patient and by the time the ambulance arrived, he had died. The Court of Appeal held that the judge had been right to direct the jury that the offence of wilful neglect could be made out even if failure to act was the result of panic. Neglect was wilful if a nurse or medical practitioner knew that it was necessary to administer a piece of treatment but deliberately decided not to do so because she could not face it.[98] In contrast, in another case under section 44(2) the Court of Appeal ruled that the appeal of a registered nurse (N) against her conviction should succeed. She cared for a former resident in a care home run by her who now lived in a property owned by N. The Court of Appeal held that the judge had misdirected the jury over the issue of autonomy and the nature of wilful neglect. The Court of Appeal stated that section 44 did not create an absolute offence. Therefore, actions or omissions, or a combination of both, which reflected or were believed to reflect the protected autonomy or the individual needing care did not constitute wilful neglect.[99]

Details of the Safeguarding Vulnerable Groups Act 2006 and subsequent developments can be found in chapter 10.

Long-term funding of care for older people together with the Dilnot Report is considered in chapter 22. Direct payments for health and social care are considered in chapter 16.

Mental Capacity Act 2005 and decision making for the mentally incapacitated adult

The Mental Capacity Act 2005 provides a statutory definition for mental incapacity and those acting on behalf of those lacking the requisite mental capacity must act in those persons' best interests. The Act also makes provision for advance decisions (see chapter 28). The Act also provides for a lasting power of attorney to be granted to a donee, which can include the power to make decisions on treatment and care, once the donor loses the requisite mental capacity. The Court of Protection has been established which has a wider jurisdiction and can make decisions on personal welfare and appoint deputies to make decisions. (See chapters 16 and 24 and the Court of Protection and property.) In Scotland, the Adults with Incapacity (Scotland) Act 2000 covers the situation of decision making on behalf of incapacitated adults.

Lasting Powers of Attorney

A lasting power of attorney (LPA) is a statutory form of power of attorney recognised in section 9 of the Mental Capacity Act. By means of this power of attorney the donor (P) confers on the donee (or donees) or the attorney(s) authority to make decisions about all or any of the following:

(a) P's personal welfare or specified matters concerning P's person welfare, and
(b) P's property and affairs or specified matters concerning P's property and affairs, and this includes authority to make such decisions in circumstances where P no longer has capacity.

Different forms are available for the two kinds of LPA, i.e. a property and affairs LPA and a personal welfare LPA.

The 'donor' is the person granting the power (known in the legislation as 'P'); and the 'donee' or the 'attorney' is the person who is given the power. The 'instrument' is the document granting the power and the conditions on which it is given.

The power to make care and welfare decisions only comes into force when the donor no longer has the mental capacity to make his or her own decisions. This contrasts with the donation of powers in relation to finance and property, where the actual delegation can take place when the donor still has the requisite mental capacity.

To create a valid LPA, the conditions laid down in section 10 must be complied with. These are as follows:

- It must be registered in accordance with the provisions of Schedule 1;
- It must be registered at the time when P executes the instrument;
- P has reached 18; and
- P has capacity to execute it.

Since October 2007, enduring powers of attorney cannot be created. Those which exist, however, can continue to be valid (they cannot cover matters of personal welfare) but it is possible for the donor, if he or she has the requisite mental capacity, to replace the enduring power of attorney with a lasting power of attorney. Further information and the requisite forms can be obtained from the Office of Public Guardian.[100] The Court has held that while an attorney appointed under a lasting power of attorney can appoint a replacement, a replacement attorney cannot appoint a replacement.[101] A lasting power of attorney was revoked by the Court of Protection. It had been granted by an elderly lady (H), who resided in a care home, to her daughter. The Office of Public Guardian raised concerns about the failure to pay care home fees: the fact that the daughter was giving her very little pocket money; a credit card and overdraft had been applied for in H's name; and unaccounted transfers and frequent cash withdrawals had been made from H's accounts. H lacked the capacity to revoke the LPA and it was appropriate for the Court to revoke it on her behalf and appoint a deputy. Her Article 8 rights were not infringed since the revocation and appointment of a deputy was a proportionate response for the protection of her rights.[102]

Conclusions

There have been a plethora of statements of policy and guidelines and initiatives on the care of the older person. They include 'A Vision for Social Care' in November 2010 published by the government; Partnerships for Older People were funded by the Department of Health to improve services for older people. Between 2006 and 2009, 29 pilot schemes were set up and an evaluation of their effectiveness, published in October 2009. Yet there are major issues which still need resolving in the care of older people. The first is the demographic time bomb with the numbers of those over 60 increasing in comparison with those of working age and the consequent problems of meeting the costs of their care. The Coalition government set up a Commission to explore all the previous White Papers and make recommendations on the future funding. Secondly, it is still abundantly clear that the elderly suffer abuse and low standards of care. In September 2007 the Healthcare Commission called upon NHS hospitals to step up efforts to provide dignity in care to older people[103] and *Equality in Later Life* was published in 2009. However, there still appears to be a gulf between the exhortations of public bodies and the reality of the standards provided. Every registered health professional has a professional duty to ensure that there is greater respect for the dignity and privacy of the older person. The Mental Capacity Act 2005, including the Deprivation of Liberty Safeguards and the European Convention of Human Rights, have provided the framework for the protection of the rights of those incapable of making their own decisions and protecting themselves, but much still needs to be done to ensure that the law is enforced. The contribution of the elderly to the costs of their care and their entitlement to continuing health care are considered in chapter 22.

Reflection questions

1. A crucial factor in the care of older people is the extent to which the patient is mentally capable and able to make decisions. Look at the Mental Capacity Act 2005 and determine how the definition of incapacity can be applied to your patients (see also chapter 7).
2. What particular precautions should you take when caring for older patients who are distressed and presenting with challenging behaviour?

Further exercises

1. To what extent do you consider the nurse should be the advocate for the patient and to what extent do you think that this role can be left to relatives?
2. Obtain a copy of your NHS trust/health board's summary of accidents to patients and analyse those relating to older patients. To what extent do you consider some of these accidents could have been prevented if different procedures had been adopted by the carers or by the NHS trust/health board itself?

References

1. www.gov.uk
2. Royal College of Nursing, The Nursing Care of Older Patients from Black and Minority Ethnic Communities, Order No. 000860, RCN, April 1998
3. www.ageuk.org.uk
4. Healthcare Commission, Review of dignity in care, 2007
5. Royal College of Nursing, An Ageing Population: education and practice preparation for nursing students learning to work with older people. A resource pack for nursing students 003222, RCN, March 2008
6. Royal College of Nursing, An Ageing Population: Mentorship, an A5 card for nursing students 003230, RCN, March 2008
7. Ageisim and Age Equality 2013, www.ageuk.org.uk
8. Tom Knowles, NHS 'rations' ops for aged in bid to cut £20 billion, *The Times*, 7 December 2013
9. Nick Triggle, NHS surgery 'age discrimination', *BBC News*, 3 July 2014
10. News item, *The Times*, 9 June 2014
11. Chris Smyth, Doctors are blamed for elderly cancer care, *The Times*, 24 January 2014
12. Department of Health, NSF for Older People: Age Discrimination Benchmarking, 2003
13. *R (On the application of Bishop) v Bromley LBC* [2006] EWHC 2148; (2006) 9 CCL Rep 635
14. Dr James Warner et al., Letter to Editor, *The Times*, 24 January 2014
15. Department of Health Social Services Inspectorate, Improving Older People's Services, DH, 2001
16. Department of Health, National Service Framework for Older People, DH, 2001
17. Department of Health, Intermediate Care, HSC 2001/01; LAC(2001)12
18. Chris Smyth, Lives of young 'more valuable to society', *The Times*, 27 March 2014
19. Department of Health; www.gov.uk
20. Professor Ian Philip, National Director for Older People's Health, Better Health in Old Age, DH, November 2004
21. Department of Health, A New Ambition for Old Age, DH, 2007
22. Department of Health, Health and Care Services for Older People: overview report on research to support the National Service Framework for Older People, DH, 2008
23. Department of Health, A Recipe for Care – not a single ingredient, DH, 2007
24. Department of Health, A New Ambition for Old Age: next steps in implementing the National Service Framework for Older People, DH, 2006
25. Sam Lister, Stroke victims to be treated with drugs by paramedics, *The Times*, 29 October 2010
26. www.nhs.uk
27. Department of Health www.gov.uk
28. Department of Health, Raising the Profile of Long Term Conditions Care: a compendium of information, DH, 2008
29. NHS England (2023) Long Term Conditions available on the NHS England Website at https://www.england.nhs.uk/ourwork/clinical-policy/ltc/
30. Department of Health, Intermediate Care, HSC 2001/01; LAC(2001)1, updated 2009
31. www.ageuk.org.uk
32. *London Borough of Redbridge v G and others* [2014] EWHC 485
33. *London Borough of Redbridge v G and others* [2014] EWCOP 959
34. *London Borough of Redbridge v G and others* [2014] EWCOP 1361

35 *UF v X County Council and others (No. 2)* [2014] EWCOP 18
36 Royal College of Nursing, Let's talk about restraint: rights, risk and responsibility, Order No. 003208, RCN, April 2008
37 *P (by his litigation friend the Official Solicitor)* v *Cheshire West and Cheshire Council and Anor* [2014] UKSC 19
38 House of Lords and House of Commons Joint Committee on Human Rights of Older People in Healthcare, 18th Session, 2006–7, HL 156-1/HC 378-1, August 2007
39 Tom Knowles, Carers jailed for abusing the elderly, *The Times*, 11 January 2014
40 Rosemary Bennett, Give police power to stop family abuse of elderly, *The Times*, 6 March 2014
41 Rosemary Bennett, Carers tied grandmother to a chair, *The Times*, 16 January 2014
42 Rosemary Bennett, Electronic tags to track dementia patients, *The Times*, 27 December 2007
43 Are You Sleeping Safely? An event to help you use bed safety rails wisely, www.mhra.gov.uk
44 Medicines and Healthcare Products Regulatory Agency, Safe Use of Bed Rails, DB 2006(06), 2006
45 NMC, Standards for medicines management, NMC, 2007
46 Sube Banerjee, Report on the prescribing of anti-psychotic drugs to people with dementia, November 2009, DH
47 Sam Lister, Care home patients given feeding tubes 'to save on staffing', The Times, 6 January 2010
48 www.alzheimers.org.uk
49 Chris Smyth, Dementia diagnoses soar by 60%, *The Times*, 31 July 2014
50 News item, *The Times*, 17 November 2009
51 House of Commons Committee of Public Accounts, Improving Services and Support for People with Dementia Sixth Report of Session 2007–8 HC 228, Stationery Office, 2008
52 www.alzheimers.org.uk
53 Department of Health, Living Well with Dementia: A National Dementia Strategy, DH, February 2009
54 Department of Health, Making a Difference in Dementia: Nursing Vision and Strategy, DH, 2013
55 Chris Smyth, G8 leaders promise to end tragedy of dementia, *The Times*, 12 December 2013
56 Chris Smyth, Cameron to double case for dementia, *The Times*, 11 December 2013
57 Chris Smyth, Help free Alzheimer's 'prisoners' says charity, *The Times*, 3 September 2013
58 Hannah Devlin, Alzheimer's kills just as many as cancer but figures go unrecorded, *The Times*, 6 March 2014
59 www.leonardcheshire.org
60 Rosemary Bennett, Watchdog attacks rushed care visits, *The Times*, 28 April 2014
61 Baroness Kingsmill, Taking Care: an independent report into working conditions in the Care Sector, 2014; www.yourbritain.org.uk
62 Age Concern, Still hungry to be heard, Age Concern, 2010
63 NICE Falls (CG161) 2013
64 Tom Knowles, Nurses 'forgot' patient, 84, over weekend, *The Times*, 28 November 2013
65 Tom Knowles, Stroke victim died after home barred paramedics, *The Times*, 19 November 2013
66 Public Health England, Guidance: Pressure ulcers: applying all our health, 2015; www.gov.uk

67 *Castle* v *Kings Healthcare NHS Trust (2000) AVMA Medical Legal Journal*, 6(6):251–2
68 *P* v *Hillingdon Hospital NHS Trust (2000) AVMA Medical Legal Journal*, 6(6):253
69 www.nmc.org.uk
70 National Institute for Health and Clinical Excellence, NICE Guideline on Pressure Ulcers (CG179), NICE, April 2014
71 www.npsa.nhs.uk
72 Department of Health, Essence of Care, Stationery Office, 2010
73 Jill Sherman, NHS volunteers offer to ease elderly winter crisis, *The Times*, 14 November 2013
74 Jill Sherman, Charities attack NHS plea to visit elderly, *The Times*, 28 November 2013
75 Chris Smyth, Tide of elderly patients add to strain, *The Times*, 13 November 2013
76 Abigail Masterson, UKCC Policy Paper No. 1: the continuing care of older people, UKCC, December 1997
77 Rosemary Bennett, After hospital the old suffer again, *The Times*, 5 December 2013
78 www.ageuk.org.uk; 6 March 2014
79 Rosemary Bennett, Overstretched care workers 'put elderly in danger', *The Times*, 8 October 2013
80 EHRC, Close to Home: An Inquiry into older people and human rights in home care 2011; www.equalityhumanrights.com
81 www.equalityhumanrights.com
82 Royal Commission, With Respect to Old Age, Stationery Office, London, March 1999
83 www.cqc.org.uk
84 Department of Health, Responses to the Consultation on Adult Social Care in England: analysis of feedback from the Green Paper Independence, Well-being and Choice, DH, 2005
85 Department of Health, Green Paper, Independence, Well-being and Choice, DH, 2005
86 Department of Health, Our Health, Our Care, Our Say: a new direction for community services, DH, 2006
87 Department of Health, Independence, Choice and Risk: a guide to best practice in supported decision making, DH, 2007
88 www.nationalarchives.gov.uk
89 National Centre for Social Research and King's College London, The UK Study of Abuse and Neglect, June 2007
90 Rosemary Bennett, Disturbing rise in cases of abuse against the elderly, *The Times*, 5 October 2013
91 www.gov.uk
92 www.helptheaged.org.uk
93 Action on Elder Abuse Helpline, Freephone 0808 808 8141
94 www.elderabuse.org.uk
95 www.counselandcare.org.uk
96 Rosemary Bennett, Women convicted of wilful neglect at filthy care home for the elderly, *The Times*, 7 August 2010
97 BBC News, Lancashire, 10 January 2014
98 *R* v *Patel (Parulben)* [2013] EWCA Crim 959
99 *R* v *Nursing (Ligaya)* [2012] EWCA Crim 2521
100 Ministry of Justice www.gov.uk
101 *Public Guardian* v *Boff* [2013] WTLR 1349
102 *Harcourt Re sub nom Public Guardian* v *A* [2012] WTLR 1779
103 Healthcare Commission, Caring for Dignity: a national report on dignity in care for older people while in hospital, 27 September 2007

Chapter 19

Nursing People with Mental Health Problems or Learning Disability

This chapter discusses

- Informal patients
- Patients detained under mental health legislation
- Holding power of the nurse
- Compulsory detention of an informal inpatient
- Compulsory admission
- Definition and role of nearest relative
- Role of the approved mental health professional
- Informing the patient and relatives
- Consent to treatment provisions
- Community provisions

Introduction

This chapter cannot cover all the law relevant to the nursing of those with mental health problems or a learning disability.[1] The intention is to deal with some of the more common dilemmas faced by these nurses through the case study approach and to include in the diagrams a summary of some of the main points of the Mental Health Act 1983 (as amended by the Mental Health Act 2007). This Act is the main legislation covering the detention of the mentally disordered and for the most part replaces the Act of 1959, which, by the end of the 1970s, was seen as failing to protect the rights of the mentally disordered. The chapter also considers the amendments introduced by the Mental Health Act 2007. Chapter 16 considers the amendments to the Mental Capacity Act 2005 (known as the Deprivation of Liberty Safeguards (DoLS)) which were introduced as a result of the Bournewood case where the European Court of Human Rights criticised the reliance on common law for restricting the liberty of those unable to give a valid consent (the Bournewood gap). Reference should be made to the Code of Practice of the Department of Health on the Mental Health Act.[2] The NMC has republished guidelines for mental health and learning disabilities nursing[3] and also guidance for the nursing, midwifery and health visiting contribution to the continuing care of people with mental health problems.[4] The legislation must be read in conjunction with the Articles of the European Convention on Human Rights (see chapter 1 and the website of this book). For example, in 2003 the House of Lords ruled that conditional discharge under section 73 of the Mental Health Act 1983 was not incompatible with the European Convention on Human Rights.[5] In 2002 the High Court held that a same-sex couple should be recognised as having the same rights as heterosexual cohabitees and therefore after six months' cohabitation the partner would be treated as the nearest relative.[6] Article 2 and the right to life came under scrutiny in relation to the duties of NHS trusts when the daughter of a detained patient who had committed suicide on a railway line claimed that the trust was in breach of Article 2. The case was heard on the preliminary issue as to the proper test to be used to establish a breach of Article 2. The court held that the correct test was one of gross negligence of the kind sufficient to sustain a charge of manslaughter. Using this test the daughter had no reasonable chance of succeeding in her claim and the trust's application for summary judgment striking out the claim succeeded.[7] (See, however, Case 19.1.) In 2013 the European Court of Human Rights held that the extradition of a prisoner suffering from paranoid schizophrenia to the USA where he might be held at the Administrative Maximum Facility in Colorado would be inhuman or degrading treatment because the detention conditions would be likely to exacerbate his condition and his extradition would therefore be a violation of Article 3.[8] In 2013 the Supreme Court held that the Secretary of State had acted unlawfully when he declined to exercise his statutory discretion to refer the case of a detained patient to a mental health review tribunal for review in circumstances where the patient had a right to make an application for herself.[9]

Informal patients

Britain has the highest number of people claiming employment benefits for mental health conditions in the developed world as mental illness costs the UK economy £70 billion each year.[10]

The vast majority (well over 90 per cent) of patients who are cared for in psychiatric hospitals are not detained. They have either given consent to admission or, if they lack the mental capacity to consent to admission, they are treated under the provisions of the Mental Capacity Act 2005 (which replaces the common law powers recognised by the House of Lords in the *Re F* case[11]) (see chapter 7). Some patients may be deprived of liberty and come within the Deprivation of Liberty Safeguards which are discussed in chapter 16. (See also chapter 18 and restraint and the elderly.) The implementation of the Mental Capacity Act 2005 in 2007 saw the common law power to act in the best interests of a mentally incapacitated adult replaced by the statutory provisions (see chapters 16 and 7).

Nature of the duty of care owed to the informal patient

Case 19.1 Duty owed to the informal patient[12]

Melanie Rabone, aged 24, had a history of depression and had attempted suicide several times. She agreed to be admitted to hospital voluntarily and two days later her father expressed grave concern about her condition and told staff that she should not be discharged. Despite this information a consultant psychiatrist agreed to give her home leave for two days at her request and she hanged herself the next day. The High Court held that the NHS had no duty under the Human Rights Act to protect Melanie because she was not a detained patient. The remedy for clinical negligence was an action for negligence and the claimants had already settled a negligence action.[13] The Court of Appeal upheld this decision. However, the Supreme Court held unanimously that she was entitled to the same duty of care as a patient detained under the Mental Health Act. The Trust should have taken reasonable steps to protect her even though she was a voluntary patient.

A coroner condemned an NHS mental health team who had refused to admit a girl to the Antelope House mental health unit in Southampton on the grounds that she was an attention seeker. Three hours later she committed suicide.[14]

The National Confidential Inquiry into Suicide and Homicide by People with Mental Illness 2017[15] shows that the number of suicides by mentally ill people has fallen but more could be done by NHS trusts in the implementation of improved risk assessments and monitoring.

Patients detained under mental health legislation

Only about 5–10 per cent of psychiatric patients are at any one time detained under the mental health legislation. However, the numbers are increasing: the CQC reported in 2018 that mental health detentions were at a record high.[16] Detentions were up 40 per cent in 10 years. The next section gives an account of the main statutory provisions of the Mental Health Act 1983 (as amended by the Mental Health Act 2007) that apply to the detention and treatment of such patients. The Court of Appeal has ruled that there is no statutory or public policy reason for an absolute bar on the provision of facilities recommended by or consistent with the recommendations of the responsible clinician, which might be available at a price, within or without the NHS system. A detained patient was entitled to pay for his care and treatment.[17]

Fundamental principles

The Mental Health Act 2007 amends the Mental Health Act 1983 to require the Secretary of State to include in the Code of Practice (prepared under section 118 of the 1983 Act) a statement of principles. Each of the following matters must be addressed in this statement:

(a) respect for patients' past and present wishes and feelings,

(b) respect for diversity generally including, in particular, diversity of religion, culture and sexual orientation (within the meaning of section 35 of the Equality Act 2006, as amended by the Equality Act 2010),

(c) minimising restrictions on liberty,
(d) involvement of patients in planning, developing and delivering care and treatment appropriate to them,
(e) avoidance of unlawful discrimination,
(f) effectiveness of treatment,
(g) views of carers and other interested parties,
(h) patient well-being and safety, and
(i) public safety.

The Secretary of State shall also have regard to the desirability of ensuring the efficient use of resources and the equitable distribution of services.

Definition of mental disorder

No person may be compulsorily detained under the Mental Health Act 1983 unless they are suffering from a mental disorder as defined in the Act. The definition as revised by the 2007 Act is:

any disorder or disability of the mind.

(The previous classifications of mental illness, mental impairment and psychopathic disorder are no longer used in the statutory definition.)

Learning disability (which is defined as 'a state of arrested or incomplete development of the mind which includes significant impairment of intelligence and social functioning') is not considered to be mental disorder, other than for detentions for assessment, unless the disability is associated with abnormally aggressive or seriously irresponsible conduct on the person's part (see chapter 16).

Dependence on alcohol or drugs is not considered to be a disorder or disability of the mind for the purposes of the definition of mental disorder.

Holding power of the nurse

Practical dilemma 19.1 — To stop or let go

Bill Smith, an informal patient in a psychiatric hospital, admitted three weeks before, wakes up at 3.00 a.m. and starts abusing nursing auxiliary Mavis Jones who is on her own, Staff Nurse Rachel Robinson having just gone for her break. Bill starts throwing furniture around and is threatening to leave the ward. Mavis contacts the night operator and asks for immediate help. What is her legal position in relation to Bill? Rachel Robinson returns with a charge nurse. They telephone for the responsible clinician and are informed that he will not be able to arrive until 9.30 a.m. What are their legal powers?

Statute Box 19.1 sets out the main points of the holding power of the nurse laid down by section 5(4) of the Act. As a nursing auxiliary, Mavis is not a prescribed nurse for the purposes of using the holding power under the Mental Health Act. The only nurses designated as prescribed nurses under the Act are those who have been trained in mental illness or learning disabilities. She does, however, have the health carer's duty to act in an emergency to save life. She also has the powers of the citizen to effect an arrest on the limited occasions set out in the Police and Criminal Evidence Act. If she feared for the life of Bill were he to be allowed to leave hospital immediately or for the life of anyone else, she could legally prevent his leaving the ward in an emergency. Rachel Robinson would be regarded as a prescribed nurse if she were registered as a nurse with an entry in the Register indicating that the nurse's field of practice is either mental health nursing, or learning disabilities nursing.[18] She can exercise the holding power set out under section 5(4) of the Mental Health Act 1983 if the conditions set out in Statute Box 19.1 are present. If all these requirements are present, then Rachel has the power to detain Bill for up to six hours. As soon as the appropriate medical practitioner arrives, however, the holding power will cease.

Statute 19.1
Section 5(4) of the Mental Health Act 1983

1. The patient is receiving treatment for mental disorder.
2. The patient is an inpatient.
3. It appears to the prescribed nurse that the patient is suffering from mental disorder to such a degree that it is necessary for his health or safety or for the protection of others for him to be immediately restrained from leaving the hospital.
4. It is not practicable to secure the immediate attendance of a practitioner who could exercise the powers under section 5(2).

Rachel must fill in the appropriate forms and ensure that these are taken to the managers of the hospital immediately. Procedures vary: in some hospitals, it is the practice for the hospital manager to be on call for such purposes; in others, this duty is delegated to the nurse manager on duty at night and weekends. If the doctor arrives and decides that Bill should be detained under section 5(2), then whatever part of the holding power has elapsed before his arrival will become part of the 72 hours' detention.

From the situation described here, it is apparent that the appropriate doctor will not be able to arrive within the six hours. In this case, it is essential for the doctor to exercise his powers of nomination under section 5(3) so that another medical practitioner (or approved clinician) can act as nominee and see Bill at the earliest possibility. (The 2007 Act amendments introduced the 'approved clinician' who can be a health professional, other than a doctor, who has had the appropriate training.)

This situation gives rise to other questions. Must Rachel remain with Bill personally even though she is due off duty at 7.30 a.m.? There is no requirement in the Act that Rachel should stay. The fact that Bill is under a holding power should, of course, be made clear to the senior nurse on the shift that takes over from Rachel. In particular, she should be informed of the time of commencement of the holding power and, if a doctor or the approved clinician, fails to arrive, the time when the holding power is due to end.

What powers does Rachel have in relation to Bill? Could Bill, for example, forcibly be given some medication for which he has been written up? The Act gives Rachel the power to restrain Bill from leaving hospital. She does not have power under the Mental Health Act to compel Bill to have treatment. **Informal** patients or those who have been placed under short-term detention orders covered by sections 5(2), 5(4) and section 4 are specifically excluded from the compulsory treatment provisions of Part 4 of the Act.

What if Bill runs off during the period of the holding power – can he be brought back? Section 18(5), by implication, allows Bill to be brought back as long as the time limit for the holding power has not elapsed. Section 18(1) (as amended by the 2007 Act) enables a patient who is absent without leave to be taken into custody and returned to the hospital by any **approved mental health professional**, by any officer on the staff of the hospital, by any constable or by any person authorised in writing by the managers of the hospital.

Could the holding power be used if Bill were an inpatient in a general hospital? From the requirements listed above, it is clear that Bill must be receiving treatment for mental disorder. It is, of course, possible for Bill to be admitted for surgery while still under treatment for a mental disorder and in this case the holding power could be exercised, but only if the nurse had the appropriate registration.

Compulsory detention of an informal inpatient

What would happen in a general hospital if a patient became severely mentally disordered? Temporary emergency measures could be taken to save life: either the life of the patient or of others. In addition, it is possible for any registered medical practitioner or approved clinician in charge of the patient to exercise the powers under section 5(2).

This section applies to an inpatient in a hospital. There is no requirement that he should be having treatment for mental disorder. The registered medical practitioner or approved clinician in charge of the patient's treatment must consider that an application ought to be made under the Act for the admission of the patient to hospital. He then furnishes the managers with a report to that effect and the patient may then be detained in the hospital for a period of 72 hours from the time the report is furnished.

In such circumstances on a general ward, it would also be possible to make use of the powers under section 4. In this case, it would be necessary for the nearest relative or an approved mental health professional to make the appropriate application for admission.

Compulsory admission

Table 19.1 sets out the section numbers and requirements for each section that enable compulsory admission to take place and the length of detention. The requirements in relation to the two medical recommendations are set out in Box 19.1.

In the case of *MH* v *United Kingdom*[19] a severely disabled adult with Down's syndrome was removed under section 135 and detained for assessment under section 2 which she did not challenge within 14 days. Her mother as nearest relative applied to discharge her but it was barred, and when she objected to a proposed guardianship order proceedings were commenced to displace her as nearest relative. As a consequence MH was detained for six months rather than the maximum 28 days. MH argued that Article 5(4) was violated since the right to challenge her

Table 19.1 Compulsory admission provisions

Section	Duration (up to)	Applicant	Medical requirements	Other requirements
4 Emergency admission for assessment	72 hours	Approved mental health professional or nearest relative	1 recommendation only stating that patient is suffering from mental disorder and stating the provisions of Section 2 exist (see below)	Applicant must have personally seen patient within 24 hours before the application. Admission must be of urgent necessity
2 Admission for assessment	28 days	Approved mental health professional or nearest relative	2 medical recommendations: (a) patient is suffering from mental disorder of a nature or degree which warrants detention in hospital for assessment and; (b) he/she ought to be so detained in the interests of his/her own health or safety or with a view to the protection of others	Applicant must personally have seen patient within the period of 14 days ending with the date of the application
3 Admission for treatment	6 months, renewable for a further 6 months, then for a period of 1 year	Approved mental health professional or nearest relative	2 medical recommendations: (a) patient is suffering from mental disorder of a nature or degree which makes it appropriate for him/her to receive medical treatment in hospital and (b) repealed by 2007 Act (c) it is necessary for the health or safety of the patient or for the protection of others that he/she should receive such treatment and it cannot be provided unless he/she is detained under this section and (d) appropriate medical treatment is available	As above under section 2. Approved mental health professional must consult with nearest relative before making an application unless this would not be reasonably practicable or would involve unreasonable delay. The application cannot be made if the nearest relative objects

(continued)

Section	Duration (up to)	Applicant	Medical requirements	Other requirements
37 Hospital order without restrictions	6 months, renewable for a further 6 months, then for a period of 1 year	Order can be made by Crown Court in case of person convicted of an offence punishable by imprisonment or by magistrates: (a) if convicted of offence punishable on summary conviction with imprisonment or (b) if person is suffering from mental disorder and magistrates are satisfied that he committed the crime	2 doctors required to give oral or written evidence that: (a) offender is suffering from mental disorder of a nature or degree which makes it appropriate for him/her to be detained for medical treatment and appropriate medical treatment is available for him (b) repealed by 2007 Act (c) the court is of the opinion, having regard to all the circumstances, that the most suitable method of disposing of the case is by means of a hospital order	
41 Restriction order (imposed in conjunction with hospital order section 37)	For a specified period	Crown Court that has made a hospital order can impose a restriction order. Magistrates' court cannot make a restriction order but can send offender over 14 to Crown Court for a restriction order to be made	As for section 37; at least 1 of the 2 doctors must give evidence orally before the court	

detention was ineffective if she lacked the ability to instruct solicitors. The House of Lords[20] had held that Article 5(4) did not require every case to be considered by a court and the scheme was capable of being operated compatibly. The automatic extension of time as a result of the displacement proceedings suggested that the Secretary of State should make a tribunal reference as soon as possible. The European Court of Human Rights held that MH's Article 5(4) rights were violated in relation to the initial 28 days of detention but not thereafter.

The nearest relative's claim that the exclusion of the relative's right to apply to a tribunal (s. 66) following the extension of a patient's detention under section 29(4) was a violation of her human rights was rejected.[21]

The Court of Appeal held that making a restriction order was the responsibility of the judge, irrespective of the views of the medical practitioners.[22]

Box 19.1 Requirements for the two medical recommendations of section 12 (as amended by 2007 Act)

1. Practitioners must have personally examined the patient either together or separately, but where they have examined the patient separately not more than 5 days must have elapsed between the days on which the separate examinations took place.

2. One of the medical recommendations must be from a practitioner approved by the Secretary of State for such purposes as having special experience in the diagnosis or treatment of mental disorder and unless that practitioner has previous acquaintance with the patient, the other practitioner should have, if practicable.

2A. A registered medical practitioner who is an approved clinician shall be treated as also approved for the purposes of this section under subsection (2) above as having special experience as mentioned there.

3. No medical recommendation shall be given for the purposes of an application mentioned in subsection (1) above if the circumstances are such that there would be a potential conflict of interest for the purposes of regulations under section 12A below.

5. After that section insert—

12A Conflicts of interest

1. The appropriate national authority may make regulations as to the circumstances in which there would be a potential conflict of interest such that—

    (a) an approved mental health professional shall not make an application mentioned in section 11(1) above;

    (b) a registered medical practitioner shall not give a recommendation for the purposes of an application mentioned in section 12(1) above.

> 2. Regulations under subsection (1) above may make—
>   (a) provision for the prohibitions in paragraphs (a) and (b) of that subsection to be subject to specified exceptions;
>   (b) different provision for different cases; and
>   (c) transitional, consequential, incidental or supplemental provision.
> 3. In subsection (1) above, 'the appropriate national authority' means—
>   (a) in relation to applications in which admission is sought to a hospital in England or to guardianship applications in respect of which the area of the relevant local social services authority is in England, the Secretary of State;
>   (b) in relation to applications in which admission is sought to a hospital in Wales or to guardianship applications in respect of which the area of the relevant local social services authority is in Wales, the Welsh Ministers.
> 4. References in this section to the relevant local social services authority, in relation to a guardianship application, are references to the local social services authority named in the application as guardian or (as the case may be) the local social services authority for the area in which the person so named resides.
>
> These provisions also apply to the two medical recommendations for guardianship.

The Mental Health (Approved Functions) Act 2012 gave retrospective validation to the power to approve practitioners or clinicians under the Mental Health Act 1983 and ensure the lawfulness of any detention or other action which was taken on the basis that a valid power to approve existed. This was required because four strategic health authorities had unlawfully delegated the exercise of their approval powers to NHS trusts.

Definition and role of nearest relative

The nearest relative has an important role to play and has to be given specific information; this task often falls on the nurse. The definition of nearest relative and the hierarchy is given in Statute Box 19.2, which also sets out the powers of the nearest relative.

Statute 19.2
Section 26(i) of the Mental Health Act 1983

Definition and powers of the nearest relative

Definition: the highest in the following hierarchy:

- relative who ordinarily resides with or cares for the patient
- husband or wife or civil partner
- son or daughter

> father or mother
> brother or sister
> grandparent
> grandchild
> uncle or aunt
> nephew or niece.
>
> Preference is given in relatives of the same description to the whole blood relation over the half-blood relation and the elder or eldest regardless of sex.
>
> Husband and wife include a person who is living with the patient as the patient's husband or wife and has been so living for not less than 6 months. A person other than a relative with whom the patient ordinarily resides for a period of not less than 5 years shall be treated as if he were a relative.
>
> Power of nearest relative:
>
> 1. To apply for the admission of the patient for assessment, for assessment in an emergency, for treatment and for guardianship.
> 2. To be informed about the approved mental health professional's application to admit patient for assessment.
> 3. To be consulted about the approved mental health professional's proposed application for treatment and to object to it.
> 4. To be given information about the details of the patient's detention, consent to treatment, rights to apply for discharge, etc. (but subject to the patient's right to object to this information being given).
> 5. To discharge the patient after giving 72 hours' notice in writing to the managers.
> 6. To apply to a mental health review tribunal under sections 16, 25 and 29.

Role of the approved mental health professional

Table 19.2 sets out the main tasks of the **approved mental health professional** (AMHP) (which replaces the **approved social worker** as a result of the amendments in the Mental Health Act 2007). Only mental health professionals who have completed the appropriate training (and are not registered medical practitioners) can be recognised as approved for the purposes of the Act. While the Act allows the nearest relative to be an applicant for compulsory admission under sections 2, 3, 4 and 7, in practice the applicant will usually be the approved mental health professional and this is the preferred procedure. The Court of Appeal held that the scope of the legal duty of the AMHP should be considered at a full hearing in allowing the appeal of a patient against the refusal of his application for leave to bring proceedings (under s. 139(2)) against local authorities for the failures of two AMHPs to discharge their duties under the Act. The patient argued that the AMHPs, among other failures, should have assessed the suitability of the unit to which the patient was to be transferred.[23]

Table 19.2 Role of the approved mental health professional

Duty	Details
Duties of the approved mental health professional	
Section 11(3) Inform nearest relative of admission of patient and of nearest relative's right to discharge	1. In admission for assessment (sections 2 and 4) 2. Before or within a reasonable time after an application for admission for assessment is made 3. Such steps as are practicable to inform the person appearing to be the nearest relative
Section 11(4) Consult nearest relative on admission for treatment or guardianship and discontinue application if nearest relative notifies objection	1. Consultation with person appearing to be the nearest relative of the patient 2. Unless it appears that in the circumstances such consultation is not reasonably practicable or would involve unreasonable delay
Section 13(1) To apply for admission or guardianship order if satisfied application ought to be made and is of the opinion that it is necessary or proper for application to be made by him	1. In respect of patient within the area of local social services authority by whom he is appointed 2. Must have regard to wishes expressed by relatives of patient or any other relevant circumstances that are necessary or proper for application to be made by him
Section 13(2) To interview patient in suitable manner and satisfy himself that detention in a hospital is in all the circumstances of the case the most appropriate way of providing the care and medical treatment of which the patient stands in need	1. Before making application for admission to hospital
Section 13(4) To take patient's case into consideration with a view to making an application for admission. If he decides not to make an application he will inform the nearest relative in writing of his reasons	1. If nearest relative so requires local social services authority of area in which patient resides, authority must direct approved mental health professional as soon as practicable
Section 14 To provide report on social circumstances	1. Where patient admitted to hospital an application by nearest relative other than section 4 2. Managers must as soon as practicable give notice of that fact to local social services authority for area in which patient resided immediately before his admission
Section 117 Duty of district health authority and of local social services authority to provide or arrange for the provision of aftercare services	1. Applies to patients detained under section 3 or admitted under hospital order (section 37) or transferred under transfer direction (sections 47 or 48) who cease to be detained and leave hospital 2. Authorities must cooperate with relevant voluntary agencies 3. Aftercare services to be provided until such time as the authorities are satisfied that the person concerned is no longer in need of such services

Informing the patient and relatives

Informing the patient

The task of explaining the patient's legal rights to them once a detention order has been imposed often falls on the nurse.

Statute 19.3
Section 132 of the Mental Health Act 1983

Informing the patient

The managers of the hospital in which a patient is detained under the Act must:

1. Take such steps as are practicable to ensure the patient understands:
   - under which provisions of the Act he is for the time being detained and the effect of that provision
   - what rights of applying to a mental health review tribunal are available to him in respect of his detention under that provision, and
   - the effect of certain provisions of the Mental Health Act including the consent to treatment provisions, the role of the Care Quality Commission (formerly the Mental Health Act Commission) and other provisions relating to the protection of the patient.

2. The steps to inform the patient must be taken as soon as practicable after the commencement of the patient's detention under the provision in question.

3. The requisite information must be given to the patient in writing and also by word of mouth.

Practical dilemma 19.2 — Information

Edna Johns, an informal patient in a psychiatric hospital, became very disturbed and aggressive in the early hours of the morning, threatening to kill herself and wishing to leave hospital. Staff Nurse Thomas, a registered mental nurse (RMN), on learning that the responsible medical officer would take at least 30 minutes to arrive on the ward, decided to exercise the holding power under section 5(4). When the appropriate doctor arrived, he decided to detain Edna under section 5(2). Within the next 48 hours, the approved mental health professional applied for admission under section 3 on the recommendation of Edna's doctor and a second recommendation. What duties exist in relation to informing Edna?

The duties set out under section 132 are illustrated in Statute Box 19.3. Forms are available covering the information to be given under each section. Often the nursing staff have the task of giving out the forms and telling the patient about the provisions. It is vital that it is recorded that the patient has been informed since it is a statutory duty and there should be evidence that the statutory duty has been carried out.

In Edna's case, she will have been placed under three separate sections in less than 72 hours. She must be given the relevant information each time the section is imposed and will be given a different form each time. Section 132 requires the information to be given as soon as practicable after the commencement of the section. 'Practicable' must take into account the patient's physical and mental ability to take in what is said. To stand over a screaming or even unconscious patient reading them their rights would not seem to be a proper fulfilment of the statutory duty.

Informing the relatives

Where the patient is too disturbed to take in the information, the statutory duty to inform the nearest relative assumes even greater importance. Section 132(4) requires the managers to furnish the person appearing to them to be the patient's nearest relative with a copy of any information given to the patient, in writing, under the duty outlined above. The steps for this must be taken when the information is given to the patient or within a reasonable time thereafter. The patient has the right of veto and can request that this information is not given. Reasonable time here would seem to imply that it is not necessary to phone Edna's relative in the middle of the night to inform them of the exercise of the holding power, but this should be done as soon as possible the next day.

Consent to treatment provisions

Treatment is defined in section 145 of the Mental Health Act 1983 (as amended by the 2007 Act) as including 'nursing, psychological intervention, and specialist mental health habilitation, rehabilitation and care'. Any reference in the Act to medical treatment for mental disorder refers to medical treatment with the purpose of alleviating, or preventing a worsening of, the disorder or one or more of its symptoms or manifestations. In the case of *MD* v *Nottinghamshire Healthcare NHS Trust* it was held that the treatment did not have to lower the risk of the patient being less dangerous to come within the statutory definition[24] and that appropriate treatment was available at Rampton hospital.

Statute Box 19.4 and Box 19.2 set out the main provisions.

Long-term detained patients

Under the provision of Part 4 of the Mental Health Act 1983, those patients who are detained under long-term detention provisions (e.g. sections 2, 3, 37 and 41) can in certain circumstances be given compulsory treatment. For these patients, the Act covers all possible treatments for mental disorder, both in emergency and non-emergency situations. The provisions are set out in the Statute Box 19.4 below.

Statute 19.4
Sections 57, 58 and 63 of the Mental Health Act 1983

1. Treatments involving brain surgery or hormonal implants can only be given with the patient's consent, which must be certified and only after independent certification of the consent and of the fact that the treatment should proceed (section 57).

2. Treatments involving electroconvulsive therapy or medication where 3 months or more have elapsed since medication was first given during that period of detention can only be given either (a) with the consent of the patient and it is certified by the patient's own approved clinician in charge of the treatment or another registered medical practitioner appointed specifically for that purpose that he is capable of understanding its nature, purpose and likely effects, or (b) the registered medical practitioner appointed (not being the responsible clinician or the approved clinician in charge of the treatment in question) has certified in writing that the patient is not capable of understanding the nature, purpose and likely effects of that treatment or has not consented to it, but that . . . the treatment should be given (section 58) (as amended by the 2007 Act, see Box 19.3).

3. All other treatments: these can be given without the consent of the patient provided they are for mental disorder and are given by or under the direction of the approved clinician in charge of the treatment (section 63).

Box 19.2 Consent to treatment: urgent treatments

These can be given according to the degree of urgency and whether they are irreversible or hazardous.

Any treatment	which is immediately necessary	to save the patient's life
Treatment which is not irreversible	if it is immediately necessary	to prevent serious deterioration
Treatment which is not irreversible or hazardous	if it is immediately necessary	to alleviate serious suffering
Treatment which is not irreversible or hazardous	if it is immediately necessary and represents the minimum interference necessary	to prevent the patient from behaving violently or being a danger to himself or others

Irreversible is defined as 'if it has unfavourable irreversible physical or psychological consequences' and hazardous is defined as 'if it entails significant physical hazard'.

A new section 62A has been added to the Mental Health Act 1983 to enable treatment to be given to those community patients who have been recalled. The patient is to be treated as if he had remained liable to be detained since the making of the community order.

Electroconvulsive therapy (ECT) and other specified treatments

Amendments were made to section 58 of the Mental Health Act 1983 by section 27 of the Mental Health Act 2007 to cover electroconvulsive therapy (ECT) and other treatments specified in regulations. A person shall not be given such treatments unless he or she falls within certain specified conditions. These conditions include those listed in Box 19.3.

Box 19.3 Section 58A

Specified conditions for treatments

1. The patient is at least 18, has consented to the treatment and his capacity to consent has been certified by the approved clinician in charge of it or by the appointed registered medical practitioner
2. The patient is under 18, has consented to the treatment and an appointed registered medical practitioner (not being the approved clinician in charge of the treatment) has certified in writing the patient's capacity to consent and that it is appropriate for the treatment to be given, or
3. An appointed registered medical practitioner (not being the responsible clinician or approved clinician in charge of the treatment) has certified in writing:
   (a) that the patient is not capable of understanding the nature, purpose and likely effects of the treatment; but
   (b) that it is appropriate for the treatment to be given and
   (c) that giving him the treatment would not conflict with:
      (i) an advance decision which the registered medical practitioner concerned is satisfied is valid and applicable, or
      (ii) a decision made by a donee or deputy or by the Court of Protection.

Before a certificate is given in circumstance 3, the appointed registered medical practitioner must consult two persons who have been professionally concerned with the patient's medical treatment; one must be a nurse and the other neither a nurse nor a registered medical practitioner. In addition, neither shall be the responsible clinician or the approved clinician in charge of the treatment in question.

Role of the nurse

What is the role of the nurse in consent to treatment provisions? Under the provisions of sections 57 and 58, the independent registered medical practitioner, in determining whether the treatment should proceed, must consult with a nurse and another professional who have been professionally concerned with the patient's medical treatment. The independent doctor must record the fact that they have consulted these two persons. Interestingly, however, there is no requirement on the form that the doctor should actually record their opinions, so it could well happen that both the nurse and the other professional counselled against, say, ECT, but that the doctor still recommended ECT. A disagreement is unusual, but it is advisable for the nurse, whether there is agreement or not with their views, to ensure that the advice they gave is recorded clearly and comprehensively.

Challenges to compulsory treatment

A detained patient challenged the fact that she had been given treatment against her will, arguing that the judge should not have concluded that although there was a body of responsible medical opinion that the statutory test for medication had not been satisfied, it was in her best interests and necessary for the purposes of Article 3 that the proposed treatment should be administered. The Court of Appeal dismissed her appeal, holding that the standard of proof that medical necessity was shown is not the criminal standard, but it has to be convincingly shown, and whether the treatment satisfies the Bolam Test is a necessary but not a sufficient condition of treatment in a patient's best interests. Determining best interests may involve choosing the best option between what may be a number of options, all of which satisfy the Bolam Test. Even where there is a responsible body of opinion that the proposed treatment is not in the patient's best interests and is not medically necessary, it does not follow that it *cannot* be convincingly shown that the treatment proposed is in the best interests or medically necessary.[25]

Ian Brady, a former detained patient at Ashworth Hospital, wished to go on hunger strike and challenged the responsible medical practitioner's decision that he could be force-fed[26] on the grounds that it was contrary to his human rights. In the judicial review hearing the court held that his decision to go on hunger strike was a symptom of his personality disorder. He was therefore mentally incapacitated and his doctor had a duty to act in his best interests by feeding him. Unlike the Broadmoor patient C[27] (see chapter 7 Case 7.3), he was incapable of weighing up risks and benefits. In 2013 Brady was again in the news when he applied to a Mental Health Review Tribunal for transfer to prison (where he wished to commit suicide) and spoke personally at the hearing which was not held in private. The Tribunal refused the application, stating that he should remain at Ashworth Hospital since he suffered from a mental disorder which is of a nature and degree which makes it appropriate for him to continue to receive medical treatment. The publicity given to Brady was condemned by family and friends of his victims.[28]

The case of an Iranian doctor who went on hunger strike is considered in chapter 7.[29]

Seclusion

There is no provision in the Mental Health Act 1983 relating to seclusion. Placing a detained patient under seclusion was challenged by judicial review as being contrary to Article 3 of the European Convention on Human Rights, i.e. 'inhuman and degrading treatment or punishment'.[30] The High Court held that seclusion is capable of infringing a patient's rights under Article 3; it did not per se amount to a breach of those rights. Seclusion could also be negligent, **Wednesbury unreasonable** or a breach of Article 8 of the European Convention on Human Rights. Whether in fact seclusion amounts to inhuman or degrading treatment will depend on the circumstances of the particular case and will involve consideration of any intention to humiliate or debase the position of the alleged victim, the consequences of the treatment and the availability of resources. A power to seclude can be implied within the provisions of the Mental Health Act 1983 if there is a 'self-evident and pressing need' for that power. Seclusion did not amount to false imprisonment or a breach of Article 5 of the European Convention on Human Rights. Seclusion was not medical treatment for the purposes of the Act since it is not used to alleviate or prevent the deterioration of an illness or its symptoms or to enable treatment to be given, but its use is authorised to ensure that control is maintained over patients. The court held that there was no infringement of the patient's rights when he was secluded and the fact that there was a departure from the Code of Practice on the Mental Health Act did not affect the duration or conditions of the claimant's seclusion, which was not unlawful. In 2012 the European Court of Human Rights held that Ashworth's seclusion policy was foreseeable and in accordance with the law for the purposes of Article 8 of the ECHR, which gave a qualified right to respect for private and family life. Nor did it violate Article 5 and the right to liberty and security of person.[31]

Physical illness

These provisions on consent to treatment would thus appear to cover all eventualities concerning the long-term detained patient. However, there is a gap in relation to treatment for physical illness which in the case of a patient lacking mental capacity would be heard by the Court of Protection.

Practical dilemma 19.3   Appendicitis

Paul, a severely depressed patient, had been detained under section 3 for two months. One morning, he complained of severe stomach pains. He was sick, with a high temperature. Paul was taken to the 'sick' ward for the treatment of physical illnesses within the mental hospital and was diagnosed as suffering from appendicitis. It was recommended that an operation be performed immediately. When Paul heard this, he immediately said there was no way in which he would agree to the operation. What is the legal position?

If Part 4 of the Act is seen as applying only to the treatment of mental illness, then its provisions are irrelevant in these circumstances. Alternatively, it could be argued that if brain surgery can be undertaken under section 62 to save the life of a patient (and this may cover informal patients, since they are covered by the provisions of section 57), where the treatment is given for a mental disorder, then the words 'any treatment' in section 62 can cover not only treatment for mental disorder, but also treatment for physical disorders. If the purpose is to save life, then section 62(1)(a) covers the situation. This is a logical view, but it has not gained universal acceptance. The alternative is to say that the situation is not covered by Part 4 of the Act and therefore the provisions of the Mental Capacity Act 2005 would apply. These provisions enable treatment to be given without the patient's consent as part of the doctor's duty of care to the patient, but only if the patient lacks the requisite mental capacity to decide. In cases prior to the implementation of the MCA, *In re C* 1994[32] (see Case 7.3), a Broadmoor patient's refusal to have an amputation was upheld by the court. In the case of *B v Croydon Health Authority*, the Court of Appeal held that compulsory feeding by tube came under section 63.[33] There have also been several cases where a pregnant woman detained under the Mental Health Act 1983 has been compelled to undergo a Caesarean under section 63 of the Act.[34] This has been disputed by the Court of Appeal in *Re MB*.[35] It is clear that if a detained patient, suffering from mental disorder, has the mental capacity to understand the proposed treatment and the implications of his or her refusal, then the court would not order the treatment to proceed unless it could clearly be seen to be treatment for the mental disorder and therefore comes within section 63. This was the situation in the case of JB who suffered from schizophrenia, but was held to have the mental capacity to refuse a life-saving amputation of her leg[36] (see chapter 7). If, however, the patient lacks the mental capacity to refuse treatment in his or her best interests, treatment could lawfully be given under the Mental Capacity Act 2005. There are considerable advantages in securing a declaration of the Court of Protection that it is lawful to provide the treatment. In a case in 2010 a woman with longstanding schizophrenia was suffering from a prolapsed uterus. She refused treatment believing that there was a conspiracy on the part of medical personnel to subjugate and experiment upon her, if not kill her. The court was informed that if not treated, the condition could become life threatening. She required sedation, surgery and a period of recovery in hospital. The Judge Mrs Justice Macur accepted that it was in her best interests to be treated and for the court to sanction the deprivation of liberty.[37]

Section 63 came under consideration in the case of *Nottinghamshire Healthcare NHS Trust v RC*[38] where a patient who self-harmed was refusing a blood transfusion. He had made an advance decision refusing blood transfusions because of his religious beliefs. The doctor considered that the advance decision could be overridden because of section 63 but wished to secure the protection of a court declaration that her decision was lawful. The judge postponed a decision until the patient could be brought to court because of the importance of the issues including Article 2 (right to life), freedom of religion (Article 9) and respect for private life (Article 8). The full hearing decided that RW had capacity to refuse blood transfusions, the advance decision was valid and applicable, the self-harming was a symptom or manifestation of mental disorder, so a blood transfusion would be treatment under section 63. It would be an abuse of power to impose a blood transfusion given his current capacity and the advance decision.[39] In contrast, in a case in July 2014 the Court of Protection declared that a mentally ill woman, detained at a specialist hospital, who was not capable of making decisions about her treatment could have a hysterectomy in her best interests and necessary restraint could take place.[40]

Independent mental health advocates (IMHA)

The Mental Health Act 2007 amends the Mental Health Act 1983 to make provision for independent mental health advocates (IMHAs) to be available to help qualifying patients. Regulations[41] have been drawn up to specify the circumstances in which the IMHAs should be appointed and the conditions for their approval. New sections 130A, B, C and D are inserted into the 1983 Act to cover the details of these appointments, the qualifying patients and the information to be given to the IMHA. Guidance for commissioners of IMHAs was published in 2008.[42] This covers the framework for an IMHA service, the appointments of IMHAs and engagement with patients. Appendices include the regulations, relevant part of the Code of Practice and a model service specification. Supplementary guidance on access to patient records under section 130B of the Mental Health Act 1983 for IMHAs was published in April 2009.[43] This gives guidance to record holders and to IMHAs on when patient records can be withheld from IMHAs and the restrictions on IMHAs when disclosing information to the patient. For example, an IMHA must not pass on information which would not have been disclosed to the patient because of a risk of serious harm.

Short-term detained patients and informal patients

Short-term detained patients and informal patients are not covered by the Part 4 treatment provisions of the Mental Health Act. There is only one exception to this: informal patients are specifically covered by the provisions of section 57 relating to brain surgery and hormonal implants and by the relevant provisions of sections 59, 60 and 62. As far as section 57 is concerned, this means that brain surgery for mental disorder or hormonal implants cannot be given without the safeguards set out above. The short-term detained patient is not explicitly covered, but there would appear to be no reason why he should not receive the same protection.

As far as all other treatments are concerned, one has to look outside the Act for the law relating to consent to treatment and this is set out in chapter 7. Since only some 5–10 per cent of mentally ill and mentally handicapped patients are under the detention of the Mental Health Act 1983, the vast majority of patients are outside the basic provisions of the Act. Those who lack the requisite mental capacity to make specific decisions would come under the provisions of the Mental Capacity Act 2005 (see chapters 7 and 16).

Community provisions

The philosophy behind the Mental Health Act 1983 is that a patient should be compulsorily detained in hospital only if informal admission is not an option and if alternative services in the community cannot be provided. There were very few community provisions in the 1983 Act except for guardianship, section 17 (leave), and section 117 (aftercare). The Mental Health Act 2007 amended the Mental Health Act 1983 to make provision for a community treatment order which replaces aftercare under supervision (supervised discharge).

Guardianship

Practical dilemma 19.4   How much control?

Paul has been under a guardianship order for three months. He lives with his mother, the guardian, and attends a day centre three times each week. He sees the community psychiatric nurse (CPN) regularly, both at the centre and also at home, and is on substantial levels of medication. One day, he decides not to take the drugs. His mother pleads with him, but is unable to persuade him to take them. She informs the CPN who also attempts to persuade Paul, but is unsuccessful. His behaviour deteriorates and he becomes more aggressive. His mother asks if there is any way in which he could be compelled to take the drugs as she fears that he will ultimately have to be readmitted. Is there a way?

The answer is that the Mental Health Act 1983 excludes from the provisions relating to consent to treatment those patients on guardianship orders. There are three statutory powers in relation to guardianship and these are set out in section 7 (see Statute Box 19.5).

There are no means of enforcing the guardianship powers over the patient other than the right of returning the patient to the specified place if he absconds. The ultimate sanction is possibly the knowledge that if the patient does not cope in the community, then he is likely to be admitted to hospital. It is not, however, good professional practice to use this as a threat. Apart from gentle professional persuasion, there is no way to force a patient to take drugs. The Mental Health Act 2007 has introduced a community treatment order, and this is an option for patients who have been detained under section 3.

Statute 19.5
Statutory powers of the guardian under the Mental Health Act 1983 Section 7

1. The power to require the patient to reside at a place specified by the guardian.
2. The power to require the patient to attend at places and times specified for the purpose of medical treatment, occupation, education and training.
3. The power to require access to the patient to be given at any place where the patient is residing to any responsible clinician, approved mental health professional or any person specified.

Section 17 Leave

A detained patient can be given leave of absence by the responsible medical officer in charge of the patient. The leave does not have to be in writing, but good practice as recommended by the Code of Practice of the Department of Health[44] suggests that there should be a written record of the leave granted and the terms on which it is granted. Section 17 leave can be used as part of the care plan of the patient towards ultimate discharge from the section and from the hospital. Thus a patient on section 17 leave can be required to stay in residential accommodation. However, the patient cannot be charged for residential accommodation he is required to stay in as a condition of Section 17 (see Statute Box 19.6). Section 17 leave can be withdrawn at any time on the written instructions of the responsible clinician. Any nurse responsible for a patient would have to assess the patient prior to leave commencing, so that there were no grounds for preventing the leave taking place. The Mental Health Act 2007 supplements section 17 to provide for community treatment orders and inserts after section 17(2) the following (2A): 'But longer-term leave may not be granted to a patient unless the responsible clinician first considers whether the patient should be dealt with under section 17A instead.'

Section 117 Aftercare services

A statutory duty is placed on the health body and local authority (LA) in conjunction with the voluntary sector to provide or arrange for the provision of aftercare services for the patient. This duty continues until such time as the health body and LA consider that the patient is no longer in need of the services that they can provide. The duty cannot end if the patient is under a community treatment order (see Statute Box 19.6). The section applies to patients who have been detained under sections 3, 37, 47 and 48. However, the duty to provide a community care assessment under section 47 of the National Health Service and Community Care Act 1990 applies to these patients and also to patients detained under other sections of the Act (e.g. sections 2, 4, 5(2) and 5(4)) and to informal patients. The Care Act 2014 defines aftercare services as:

(a) meeting a need arising from or related to the person's mental disorder, and
(b) reducing the risk of a deterioration of the person's mental condition, and, accordingly, reducing the risk of the person requiring admission to a hospital again for treatment for mental disorder.

A new section 117A enables regulations to be made which require a LA to provide or arrange for the provision of accommodation which is the preference of the person with the person paying any extra cost which results. The LA can discharge its duty under this section by making direct payments.

The duties under section 117 cannot be forced on the patient, who may refuse to accept the treatment plan or services provided. This therefore led to concerns that patients were being released from psychiatric care without adequate supervision in the community. The case of Christopher Clunis, who killed Jonathan Zito, and the case of Ben Silcock, who was mauled in a lion's den, reinforced these fears. Some local authorities had been charging patients on a means-tested basis for residential accommodation provided under section 117. The Court of Appeal[45] made it clear that where accommodation is provided under section 117 for a patient, then a local authority may not provide it under section 21 or charge for it under section 22 of the National Assistance Act 1948. Where patients are required to live in residential accommodation under section 17, then they are entitled to this accommodation as an aftercare service under section 117 when discharged from detention under the Act and cannot therefore be charged for it. Section 117 does not cover patients detained under section 2, 4, 5(2) or who were informal.

Community Treatment order (CTO)

The provisions on aftercare under supervision, or supervised discharge introduced by the Mental Health (Patients in the Community) Act 1995 were replaced by the community treatment order introduced by section 32 of the Mental Health Act 2007 which added new sections 17A, 17B, 17C, 17D, 17E, 17F and 17G into the Mental Health Act 1983.

Statute 19.6

New Sections 17A, 17B, 17C, 17D, 17E, 17F and 17G of the Mental Health Act 1983

Under section 17A the responsible clinician may by order in writing discharge a detained patient from hospital subject to his being liable to recall in accordance with section 17E.

Under 17A(4) the responsible clinician may not make a community treatment order unless—

(a) in his opinion, the relevant criteria are met; and
(b) an approved mental health professional states in writing—
   (i) that he agrees with that opinion; and
   (ii) that it is appropriate to make the order.

(5) The relevant criteria are—
   (a) the patient is suffering from mental disorder of a nature or degree which makes it appropriate for him to receive medical treatment;
   (b) it is necessary for his health or safety or for the protection of other persons that he should receive such treatment;
   (c) subject to his being liable to be recalled as mentioned in paragraph (d) below, such treatment can be provided without his continuing to be detained in a hospital;
   (d) it is necessary that the responsible clinician should be able to exercise the power under section 17E(1) below to recall the patient to hospital; and
   (e) appropriate medical treatment is available for him.
(6) In determining whether the criterion in subsection (5)(d) above is met, the responsible clinician shall, in particular, consider, having regard to the patient's history of mental disorder and any other relevant factors, what risk there would be of a deterioration of the patient's condition if he were not detained in a hospital (as a result, for example, of his refusing or neglecting to receive the medical treatment he requires for his mental disorder).

17B Conditions for a community treatment order

(1) A community treatment order shall specify conditions to which the patient is to be subject while the order remains in force.
(2) But, subject to subsection (3) below, the order may specify conditions only if the responsible clinician, with the agreement of the approved mental health professional mentioned in section 17A(4)(b) above, thinks them necessary or appropriate for one or more of the following purposes—
   (a) ensuring that the patient receives medical treatment;
   (b) preventing risk of harm to the patient's health or safety;
   (c) protecting other persons.
(3) The order shall specify—
   (a) a condition that the patient make himself available for examination under Section 20A below; and
   (b) a condition that, if it is proposed to give a certificate under Part 4A of this Act that falls within section 64C(4) below in his case, he make himself available for examination so as to enable the certificate to be given.
(4) The responsible clinician may from time to time by order in writing vary the conditions specified in a community treatment order.
(5) He may also suspend any conditions specified in a community treatment order.
(6) If a community patient fails to comply with a condition specified in the community treatment order by virtue of subsection (2) above, that fact may be taken into account for the purposes of exercising the power of recall under section 17E(1) below.
(7) But nothing in this section restricts the exercise of that power to cases where there is such a failure.

17C Duration of community treatment order

A community treatment order shall remain in force until—

(a) the period mentioned in section 20A(1) below (as extended under any provision of this Act) expires, but this is subject to sections 21 and 22 below;

(b) the patient is discharged in pursuance of an order under section 23 below or a direction under section 72 below;

(c) the application for admission for treatment in respect of the patient otherwise ceases to have effect; or

(d) the order is revoked under section 17F below, whichever occurs first.

17D Effect of community treatment order

(1) The application for admission for treatment in respect of a patient shall not cease to have effect by virtue of his becoming a community patient.

(2) But while he remains a community patient—

   (a) the authority of the managers to detain him under section 6(2) above in pursuance of that application shall be suspended; and

   (b) reference (however expressed) in this or any other Act, or in any subordinate legislation (within the meaning of the Interpretation Act 1978), to patients liable to be detained, or detained, under this Act shall not include him.

(3) And section 20 below shall not apply to him while he remains a community patient.

(4) Accordingly, authority for his detention shall not expire during any period in which that authority is suspended by virtue of subsection (2)(a) above.

17E Power to recall to hospital

(1) The responsible clinician may recall a community patient to hospital if in his opinion—

   (a) the patient requires medical treatment in hospital for his mental disorder; and

   (b) there would be a risk of harm to the health or safety of the patient or to other persons if the patient were not recalled to hospital for that purpose.

(2) The responsible clinician may also recall a community patient to hospital if the patient fails to comply with a condition specified under section 17B(3) above.

(3) The hospital to which a patient is recalled need not be the responsible hospital.

(4) Nothing in this section prevents a patient from being recalled to a hospital even though he is already in the hospital at the time when the power of recall is exercised; references to recalling him shall be construed accordingly.

(5) The power of recall under subsections (1) and (2) above shall be exercisable by notice in writing to the patient.

(6) A notice under this section recalling a patient to hospital shall be sufficient authority for the managers of that hospital to detain the patient there in accordance with the provisions of this Act.

▶

17F Powers in respect of recalled patients

(1) This section applies to a community patient who is detained in a hospital by virtue of a notice recalling him there under section 17E above.

(2) The patient may be transferred to another hospital in such circumstances and subject to such conditions as may be prescribed in regulations made by the Secretary of State (if the hospital in which the patient is detained is in England) or the Welsh Ministers (if that hospital is in Wales).

(3) If he is so transferred to another hospital, he shall be treated for the purposes of this section (and section 17E above) as if the notice under that section were a notice recalling him to that other hospital and as if he had been detained there from the time when his detention in hospital by virtue of the notice first began.

(4) The responsible clinician may by order in writing revoke the community treatment order if—

  (a) in his opinion, the conditions mentioned in section 3(2) above are satisfied in respect of the patient; and

  (b) an approved mental health professional states in writing—

    (i) that he agrees with that opinion; and

    (ii) that it is appropriate to revoke the order.

(5) The responsible clinician may at any time release the patient under this section, but not after the community treatment order has been revoked.

(6) If the patient has not been released, nor the community treatment order revoked, by the end of the period of 72 hours, he shall then be released.

(7) But a patient who is released under this section remains subject to the community treatment order.

(8) In this section—

  (a) 'the period of 72 hours' means the period of 72 hours beginning with the time when the patient's detention in hospital by virtue of the notice under section 17E above begins; and

  (b) references to being released shall be construed as references to being released from that detention (and accordingly from being recalled to hospital).

17G sets out the effect of revoking a community treatment order

Statute 19.7

Sections 20A and 20B of the Mental Health Act

Section 20A Community treatment period

A community treatment order shall cease to be in force on expiry of the period of six months beginning with the day on which it was made and this period is referred to in this Act as 'the community treatment period'. The community treatment period may be

> extended for a period of six months and then on for further periods of up to one year at a time. Section 20A subsections 4–10 set out the conditions for renewal and the procedure to be followed.
>
> ### 20B Effect of expiry of community treatment order
>
> When the community treatment order expires, the community patient shall be deemed to be discharged absolutely from liability to recall under this Part of this Act, and the application for admission for treatment ceases to have effect.

An NHS foundation trust failed in its appeal against the decision of a tribunal to make a deferred discharge for a patient (who was diagnosed as suffering from paranoid schizophrenia) from a community treatment order. The tribunal found that she had been symptom free for three years. The Trust claimed that she had a history of improving, failing to take her medication and then deteriorating. The Upper Tribunal held that if the statutory conditions were not present, the patient had to be discharged from the CTO. 'She might be a classic revolving-door patient, but she was entitled to be free from control when the door was open outwards.'[46]

Treatment provisions for those on a community treatment order (CTO)

The Mental Health Act 2007 inserts into the Mental Health Act 1983 a new Part 4A which sets out the provisions for the treatment of community patients who are not recalled to hospital. Sections 64A–K set out the conditions on which treatment can be given in the community: 64D enables treatment to be given to an adult who lacks the requisite capacity, if specified conditions are met, but force may not be used; 64G enables emergency treatment to be given to patients lacking the capacity or competence to give consent and under this section force can be used, provided certain conditions are met and the treatment is to prevent harm to the patient and the force must be a proportionate response to the likelihood of the patient suffering harm and to the seriousness of that harm. Amendments were made to 64C and 64E under section 299 of Health and Social Care Act 2012 to vary the certificate requirement where the patient has capacity to consent to the treatment and has consented, with the effect that the approval of a Second Opinion Appointed Doctor (SOAD) will not generally be necessary if the patient is consenting to the treatment in question. If the patient withdraws his or her consent, then the appropriate certificate will be required. However, if the approved clinician in charge of the treatment considers that the discontinuance of the treatment, or of treatment under the plan, would cause serious suffering to the patient then the approved clinician can continue to give treatment. Electroconvulsive therapy may not be given without the consent of a patient, who has the requisite capacity, unless it is an emergency situation.

Failures in the community

The dangers of release from prison without an assessment of the prisoner's mental health were shown in the case of Phillip Simelane, a paranoid schizophrenic, who, following release from prison without supervision, killed Christina Edkins, a teenager on a bus. He admitted manslaughter on the grounds of diminished responsibility.[47] At present, the authorities have no power to place prisoners who had served less than 12 months under supervision. Legislation to change this is being introduced.

In another tragic case a woman was killed by her former partner who suffered from mental illness. Rachel Slack had driven Andrew Cairns to the police station where he was detained under the Mental Health Act. He was subsequently released by mental health workers who found no major mental illness. He killed himself after killing Rachel and her 23-month-old son. The inquest jury found that there were failures by the police to impress upon the mother the risk of serious injury or death.[48]

Section 135(1) Removal to place of safety

Statute Box 19.8 sets out the basic provisions of this power of the approved mental health professional. The section has been amended by the Policing and Crime Act 2017, Chapter 4, allowing a constable to hold a person at the premises where they are found – if they are a place of safety – instead of removing the person.

Statute 19.8
Mental Health Act 1983 Section 135(1) and (4)

(1) If it appears to a **Justice of the Peace**, on information on oath laid by an approved mental health professional, that there is a reasonable cause to suspect that a person believed to be suffering from mental disorder

   (a) has been, or is being, ill-treated, neglected or kept otherwise than under proper control, in any place within the jurisdiction of the justice; or

   (b) being unable to care for himself, is living alone in any such place

   the justice may issue a warrant authorising any constable to enter, if need be by force, any premises specified in the warrant in which that person is believed to be, and, if thought fit, to remove him to a place of safety with a view to the making of an application in respect of him under Part 2 of this Act, or of other arrangements for his treatment or care.

1(A) If the premises specified in the warrant are a place of safety, the constable executing the warrant may, instead of removing the person to another place of safety, keep the person at those premises for the purpose mentioned in subsection (1).

(4) In the execution of a warrant issued under section 135(1) a constable shall be accompanied by an approved mental health professional and by a registered medical practitioner (as amended by Police and Criminal Evidence Act 1984 Schedule 6 para 26 and the Mental Health Act 2007).

Amendments to section 135 by the 2007 Act (adding sections 135(3A) and (3B)) enable a patient to be transferred to one place of safety and from there to one or more other places of safety. The duration of detention at the place of safety cannot now exceed 24 hours under the provisions of the Mental Health Act 1983, section 135 (3ZA).

Section 136 Removal of mentally disordered persons without a warrant

Section 136 of the 1983 Act allowed a police officer to remove a person who appeared to be suffering from a mental disorder and in immediate need of care and control from a place to which the public have access, to a place of safety so they can be assessed for detention under Part 2 of the Act.

A place of safety for the purpose of sections 135 and 136 is defined by section 135(6) as:

- residential accommodation provided by a local social services authority under [Part 1 of the Care Act 2014 or Part 4 of the Social Services and Well-being (Wales) Act 2014],
- a hospital as defined by this Act,
- a police station,
- an independent hospital or care home for mentally disordered persons, or
- any other suitable place the occupier of which is willing temporarily to receive the patient.

There has been considerable concern over the use of section 136 since the documentation has been inadequate; the police have not always recorded the details as to when they have used this section; and when the patient has been brought to hospital, the details have not always been recorded by the hospital staff and managers. Many hospitals have now designed their own forms for this purpose that record the date and time the patient arrives and the number and name of the constable who brings the patient in. In April 2014 the Department of Health initiated a consultation on sections 135 and 136 to examine whether changes to primary legislation would improve outcomes for people experiencing a mental health crisis. Amendments to section 136 were introduced by the Policing and Crime Act 2017 (see below).

The police in England and Wales used the power 28,271 times in 2016, including 1124 instances where the patient was a child.[49] Police cells were used as the place of safety 2,100 times in 2016, including 43 occasions where the patient was a child. Criticism of the use of police cells as a place of safety, particularly for children; confusion over the definition of a place to which the public have access for the purpose of section 136; and delays in conducting mental health assessments, have resulted in significant amendments to both sections 135 and 136 of the Mental Health Act 1983 by the Policing and Crime Act 2017, Part 4, Chapter 4. The amendments, that came into force in December 2017, impact on the police's use of the sections, the selection of a place of safety and the timeliness of Mental Health Act assessments.

Amendments under the Policing and Crime Act 2017

One of the enduring criticisms and sources of challenge under section 136 is the requirement that a police officer can only use the power if the person in need of immediate care or control is in a place to which the public have access. Confusion over the meaning of that term has been the subject of several challenges in court.[50]

The amendment introduced by the Policing and Crime Act 2017, section 80 now allows a police officer to exercise the power in any place other than a dwelling or a non-communal yard, garden, garage or outhouse used in conjunction with that dwelling. The police officer is also entitled to enter a permitted place by force if necessary. This amendment gives greater flexibility to the police to act more quickly where the person is on private property, other than a private dwelling, such as a place of work, a roof or on railway property, where currently they require a warrant under section 135 before they enter.[51]

The Policing and Crime Act 2017, section 80 now gives police officers the option of keeping the person at the place of detention if it is a place of safety.

Before exercising the power under section 136, the police officer is required, if practicable, to consult with a:

- doctor,
- nurse,
- AMHP, or
- paramedic or occupational therapist (under the Mental Health Act 1983 (Places of Safety) Regulations 2017).

To be practical, mental health providers will have to ensure that the police have the contact details of the relevant practitioner to be consulted.

The Policing and Crime Act 2017, section 81 allows a private dwelling to be used as a place of safety where both the patient and the occupier of the property consent to its use.

Criticism of the use of police cells as a place of safety for children resulted in the new section 136A introduced into the Mental Health Act 1983 that forbids the use of police cells as a place of safety for anyone under 18 years. It also gives the Secretary of State the power to make regulations to limit the use of police cells as places of safety for adults detained under sections 135 and 136 of the Act. These requirements are set out under the Mental Health Act 1983 (Places of Safety) Regulations 2017.

Mental health providers will have to ensure that they have suitable, age-appropriate accommodation available as places of safety for those under 18 detained under sections 135 and 136 of the Mental Health Act 1983. A boy suffering a mental health crisis was forced to spend four hours overnight at a 24-hour McDonald's restaurant because there were no other places of safety available for the police to take him to.[52]

Duration of detention

The duration of detention for both section 135 and 136 have been reduced to 24 hours from the previous 72 hours. That initial detention period of 24 hours can be extended for a further 12 hours with the approval of the responsible doctor if the condition of the patient makes it necessary. Where the person is being held in a police station as a place of safety then any extension must also be approved by a senior police officer of the rank of superintendent or above (Policing and Crime Act 2017, section 82). The maximum period of 36 hours brings the police powers under the Mental Health Act 1983 into line with the length of detention that can be authorised by a senior police officer under the Police and Criminal Evidence Act 1984.

Mental health providers will have to ensure that AMHPs and suitably qualified doctors are available to undertake Mental Health Act assessments and make arrangements for the ongoing care and treatment of the patient within the new 24-hour limit. As the threshold for extending the duration of detention is based on the condition of the patient rather than the availability of staff and suitable hospital placement it is essential that there is a clear policy in place for the timely management of patients who require further care and treatment as required under the Mental Health Act 1983 codes of practice for England and Wales (Department of Health 2015; Welsh Government 2016).

Protective searches

The Policing and Crime Act 2017, section 83 clarifies the circumstances where a police officer may lawfully search a person subject to the police powers under sections 135 and 136 of the

Mental Health Act 1983. A police officer can search a person held under sections 135 and 136 if the officer has reasonable grounds for believing that the person has a dangerous item concealed on them that presents a danger to the person or others. The search is limited to that necessary to discover the item and is limited to a search of outer clothing and mouth.

Mental Health Units (Use of Force) Act 2018

Parliament passed the Mental Health Units (Use of Force) Act in November 2018 that requires:

- Mental health hospitals in England to actively take steps to reduce the use of force against patients, including by providing better training on managing difficult situations.
- Better data to be collected on the use of restraint and Police to wear body cameras when called to mental health settings, which can be used in evidence.

This Act, referred to as Seni's Law, was introduced following the death of Seni Lewis who died after being restrained on a mental health ward by 11 police officers. At the inquest into his death, the restraint used was deemed to be excessive, unreasonable and disproportionate.

Time limits for mental health review tribunals

Table 19.3 illustrates the time limits for applying to the tribunal, the powers of the tribunal, and the applicants. A major innovation of the 1983 Act was that the managers must automatically refer a patient to the tribunal if they have failed to apply themselves. There must be a tribunal hearing at least once every three years. Every child under 18 must be referred by the managers every year if he or she has not themselves applied.

Table 19.3 Applications to mental health review tribunals

Section	Patient	Nearest relative	Manager
2 or 4	Applications by patients within first 14 days of detention	No application by nearest relative	Application by manager under 2007 Act amendments
3	Application by patient within first 6 months of detention, once within second 6 months, then annually	Yes, within 28 days of being informed that responsible medical-officer has issued report barring discharge of patient When an order is made appointing a nearest relative under section 29 On reclassification of patient under section 16	Automatic referral if tribunal has not considered case within first 6 months of detention, thereafter if tribunal has not considered case within previous 3 years (1 year if patient is under 18)
37	Yes, once within second 6 months of detention, then annually	Yes, once within second 6 months of detention, then annually	Automatic if the case has not been considered by tribunal within previous 3 years (1 year if patient is under 18)
41	Yes, once within second 6 months of detention, then annually	No application by nearest relative	Automatic referral by Home Secretary if tribunal has not considered case within the preceding 3 years

Role of managers

The managers are given certain statutory duties under the Act (set out in Box 19.4). Of these, all can be delegated by the NHS trust board, except the duty to hear an application from a patient for discharge. In this case, the NHS trust is empowered to appoint a subcommittee for hearing such applications.

Box 19.4 **Role of managers**

1. To accept a patient and record admission (section 140).
2. To give information to detained patient (section 132) and community patient (section 132A).
3. To give information to nearest relative (section 132(4)) and inform him of discharge (section 133(1)) or of detention (section 25(2)).
4. To discharge patient (section 23(2)(b)). Powers may be exercised by any three or more members of the authority (section 23(4)).
5. To refer patient to mental health review tribunal (section 68 as amended by the Mental Health Act 2007).
6. To transfer patient (section 19(3), section 19(1a) reg. 7(2) and reg. 7(3)).
7. To give notice to local social services authority specifying hospitals in which arrangements are made for reception in case of special urgency of patients requiring treatment for mental disorder (section 140).

Definition of managers

NHS trust, PCT or NHS Foundation Trust or special health authority responsible for the administration of the hospital (section 145).
All powers can be delegated by manager to the officers except for (4) above: discharging the patient. Special provisions apply to NHS Foundations Trusts.

Care Quality Commission

Box 19.5 illustrates the powers of the Care Quality Commission in relation to mental health legislation. From April 2009 the Mental Health Act Commission (MHAC) was merged with the Healthcare Commission and the Commission for Social Care Inspection into the Care Quality Commission, a new regulatory body with enhanced powers (see chapter 5). The CQC Mental Health Act report for 2016/17[53] is available on its website.

Box 19.5 Powers of the Care Quality Commission in relation to mental health legislation

1. Duty to draft and monitor Code of Practice.
2. Prepare a biennial report to Parliament.
3. Review any decision at a special hospital to withhold a postal packet or its content.[54]
4. Carry out on behalf of the Secretary of State duties in relation to the review of the exercise of powers and discharge of duties under the Act, visiting and interviewing detained patients and hearing complaints from detained patients.
5. Exercise duties and appointment of second-opinion doctors in relation to Part 4, consent to treatment provisions.

Mentally ill patients and the European Convention on Human Rights

Several patients have won cases in Strasbourg for breach of their rights as set out in the European Convention on Human Rights, including the case of Bournewood (discussed in chapter 16). In one case,[55] the European Court of Human Rights held that the UK was in breach of Article 5 of the European Convention on Human Rights because for a considerable period of time the patient was not lawfully detained. Several mental health review tribunals had given the patient a deferred conditional discharge under section 73 of the Act, but discharge had been delayed because the local authority had been unable to find suitable supervised hostel accommodation. After 2 October 2000, those who allege that their human rights have been infringed have been able to bring action in the courts of the UK, instead of going to Strasbourg (see chapter 1 and the website of this book).

Conclusions

The changes effected by the Mental Capacity Act 2005 and the implementation of the amendments to the Mental Health Act 1983 by the Mental Health Act 2007 are now well established and the relatively new community treatment order is being increasingly used. The UK at the present time is facing changes in its incapacity and disability benefits all of which make the position of the mentally disordered more vulnerable. At the same time, plans to reduce the prison population by keeping drug addicts and the mentally ill out of jail will lead to more patients being treated for their psychiatric disorders and addiction in the community. The challenges facing health professionals and organisations concerned with their care are immense. Whilst reform of the Mental Health Act is overdue, the Mental Health Bill was shelved by the Government in 2023. It remains to be seen if this will be resurrected by the new Labour Government, elected in July 2024.

Reflection questions

1. Contrast the rights of the informal patient and compare these to the statutory rights of the patient detained under mental health legislation.
2. Analyse the provisions for giving compulsory treatment to those patients detained under the Act.

Further exercises

1. Study the restraint and seclusion policy in your hospital and consider the extent to which its implementation can remain within the law, in particular the Human Rights Act. (See the website of this book.)
2. Ask to see the latest report of the Care Quality Commission on your hospital.
3. In what ways would informal patients benefit from coming under the jurisdiction of the Care Quality Commission?
4. What is meant by Deprivation of Liberty Safeguards? Find out how they are applied in your hospital, residential home or private clinic. (See chapter 16.)

References

[1] See B. Dimond and F. Barker, *Mental Health Law for Nurses*, Blackwell Scientific Publications, Oxford, 1996
[2] Department of Health, Code of Practice on the Mental Health Act 1983, HMSO, 3rd edn, London, 1999
[3] Nursing and Midwifery Council, Guidelines for Mental Health and Learning Disabilities Nursing (originally published by UKCC), NMC, April 1998
[4] UKCC, The Nursing, Midwifery and Health Visiting Contribution to the Continuing Care of People with Mental Health Problems: a review and UKCC action plan, UKCC, 2000
[5] *R (H) v Secretary of State for the Home Department and Another* [2003] UKHL 59
[6] *R (on the application of SSG) v Liverpool County Council, the Secretary of State for Health and LS (interested party)* [2002] EWHC Admin 2803 (4000)
[7] *Savage v South Essex Partnership NHS Foundation Trust* [2006] EWHC 3562; The Times Law Report, 16 February 2007
[8] *Aswat v United Kingdom* (Application No. 17299/12) ECHR, The Times Law Report, 24 April 2013
[9] *R (Modaresi) v Secretary of State for Health and others*, The Times Law Report, 8 August 2013
[10] Kate Gibbons, Mental illness costs Britain £70bn a year, *The Times*, 11 February 2014
[11] *In re F v West Berkshire Health Authority* [1989] 2 All ER 545
[12] *Rabone and another v Pennine Care NHS Trust* [2012] UKSC 2

13 *Rabone and another* v *Pennine Care NHS Trust*, The Times Law Report, 14 October 2010
14 James Gillespie, Suicide girl branded a 'waste of space' by NHS, *Sunday Times*, 15 September 2013
15 University of Manchester, National Confidential Inquiry into Suicide and Homicide by People with Mental Illness, 2017
16 www.cqc.org.uk/sites/default/files/20180123_mhadetentions_report.pdf
17 *Coombs* v *Dorset NHS Primary Care Trust* [2013] EWCA Civ 471
18 The Mental Health (Nurses) (England) Order 2008, SI 2008/1207
19 *MH* v *United Kingdom* [2013] ECHR 1008
20 *MH* v *United Kingdom* [2006] AC 441
21 *MA* v *Secretary of State for Health* [2012] UKUT 474
22 *R* v *Parkins (John Robert)* [2012] EWCA Crim 856
23 *DD* v *Durham CC* [2013] EWCA Civ 96
24 *MD* v *Nottinghamshire Healthcare NHS Trust* [2010] UKUT 59
25 *R (on the application of N)* v *Doctor M and Others* [2003] Lloyd's Rep Med 2 81
26 *R* v *Collins ex p Brady* (2001) 58 BMLR 173; [2000] Lloyd's Rep Med 355
27 *Re C (Adult: refusal of medical treatment)* [1994] 1 All ER 819; (1993) 15 BMLR 77
28 Sean O'Neill and Russell Jenkins, Missing victim's family condemns court 'Brady Show', *The Times*, 29 June 2013
29 *An NHS Trust* v *Dr A* [2013] EWHC 2442 CoP
30 *S* v *Airedale National Health Service Trust* 1 [2003] Lloyd's Rep Med 21
31 *Manjaz* v *United Kingdom* (application No 2913/06) ECHR, The Times Law Report, 9 October 2012; [2012] ECHR 1704
32 *Re C (Adult: refusal of medical treatment)* [1994] 1 All ER 819; (1993) 15 BMLR 77
33 *B* v *Croydon Health Authority*, The Times Law Report, 1 December 1994
34 *Tameside and Glossop Acute Services Trust* v *CH* [1996] 1 FLR 762; *Norfolk and Norwich (NHS) Trust* v *W* [1996] 2 FLR 613
35 *Re MB (An Adult: medical treatment)* [1997] 2 FLR 426
36 *Heart of England NHS Foundation Trust* v *JB* [2014] EWHC 342
37 *An NHS Foundation Trust* v *D* [2010] EWHC 2535
38 *Nottinghamshire Healthcare NHS trust* v *RC* [2014] EWCOP 1136
39 *Nottinghamshire Healthcare NHS trust* v *RC* [2014] EWCOP 1317
40 News item, *The Times*, 23 July 2014
41 Mental Health Act 1983 (Independent Mental Health Advocates) (England) Regulations SI 2008/3166
42 National Institute for Mental Health in England, Independent Mental Health Advocacy: guidance for Commissioners, DH, 2008
43 Department of Health, Independent Mental Health Advocates: supplementary guidance on access to patient records under Section 130B of the Mental Health Act 1983, 2009
44 Department of Health, Code of Practice of the Mental Health Act 1983, Stationery Office, London, 1999
45 *R* v *Richmond LBC ex parte Watson and Other Appeals* [2001] 1 All ER 436
46 *CNWL NHS Foundation Trust* v *H-JH* [2012] UKUT 210
47 Danielle Sheridan, Fiona Hamilton and Richard Ford, Violent schizophrenic who stabbed girl to death was freed without supervision, *The Times*, 3 October 2013
48 Danielle Sheridan, Police failed to warn mother of murder risk from ex-partner, *The Times*, 23 October 2013
49 National Police Chiefs' Council (2016) National Police Chiefs' Council Lead for Mental Health Use of Section 136 of the Mental Health Act 1983 in 2015–16 (England and

50 Wales) available from NPCC at www.npcc.police.uk/documents/S136%20Data%202015%2016.pdf
50 *May* v *DPP* [2005] EWHC 1280; *Harriot* v *DPP* [2005] EWHC 965; *R* v *Roberts* [2003] EWCA Crim 2753
51 Explanatory notes to the Policing and Crime Act 2017 (2017) available from TSO at www.legislation.gov.uk/ukpga/2017/3/pdfs/ukpgaen_20170003_en.pdf
52 https://bbc.co.uk/news/uk-wales-politics-44398142
53 Care Quality Commission, Monitoring the Use of the Mental Health Act 2016/17, available at https://cqc.org.uk/sites/default/files/20180227_mhareport_web.pdf
54 Care Quality Commission (Additional Functions) Regulations 2009, SI 2009/410; SI 2011/1551 as amended by SI 2013/1413
55 *Stanley Johnson* v *The United Kingdom* [1997] series A 1991 VII 2391

Chapter 20

Accident and Emergency, Outpatients, Genito-Urinary Departments and Day Surgery

This chapter discusses

- Accident and emergency department
- Outpatients department
- Genito-urinary medicine
- Day surgery

Introduction

This chapter explores non-inpatient facilities which all raise similar legal issues in relation to dealing with workload pressures and confidentiality, and are increasingly becoming the focus of political attention. In particular, the spotlight has been cast over the future of A&E services (also referred to as unscheduled services), which have been at the centre of a number of proposals for reform.

Accident and emergency department

In recent years, the role of the nurse in the A&E department (sometimes referred to as the Emergency Department or ED) has undergone a fundamental change, not just as a result of the transfer of many activities formerly undertaken by medical staff to nurses, but as a result of the nurse taking on a wider sphere of responsibility and working within new parameters and developing a new specialty of A&E nursing. The role of the nurse practitioner includes the provision of immediate care to patients and the determination of priorities for care (triage). The legal implications of the expanded role of the nurse are considered in chapter 23.

Strategy for A&E units

In 2010 the National Audit Office published a highly critical report on deficiencies in the treatment of patients suffering major trauma.[1] It pointed out that hundreds of people who suffer serious injuries are dying because of poor care and that despite the many criticisms of trauma services since 1988 no improvements have taken place.

Major Trauma Networks were introduced in 2010 and this has led to an increase of 20 per cent in the survival rate for patients who have suffered multiple trauma in serious accidents, for example head injuries, stab wounds or major car accidents, but there has been criticism that rehabilitation services for civilians have lagged behind in comparison with the resources available for armed services personnel, such as the Help for Heroes Rehabilitation Complex at Headley Court.[2] There are at present 22 major trauma centres in England.

Proposals were put forward in November 2013 by the Medical Director of NHS England Sir Bruce Keogh to create two-tier A&E services. About 40–70 units would be designated as Major Emergency Centres, which would treat serious conditions such as heart attacks, major accidents and strokes. These recommendations were made in the light of the fact that 40 per cent of patients do not need A&E care, with 25 per cent visiting A&E because they could not get a GP appointment. These patients could be treated through contact with NHS 111 (replacing NHS Direct), or through contact with pharmacists. Blue light ambulances will ensure that the appropriate patients are transferred to the major emergency centres, bypassing local A&E centres.[3] In June 2014 the National Director for Acute Episodes of Care at NHS England, Professor Keith Willett, said that there was resistance to these centralisation changes and thousands of patients have died needlessly because of this damaging reluctance to accept changes in the NHS.[4]

Managing the workload

Many initiatives have been introduced to speed up the treatment of patients and avoid extensive waiting times.

In September 2007 NICE issued a clinical guideline on the triage, assessment, investigation and early management of head injury in infants, children and adults, which is available on its website.

The Department of Health published guidance in 2007 prepared by the Urgent Care Pathway Group on best practice for older people with complex needs. This identified best clinical practice in the three areas of falls, confusional states and hip fractures, and provided audit indicators for the ambulance service and for A&E.

The 'See and Treat' initiative from the Modernisation Agency's Emergency Services Collaborative aimed to assess and treat patients with minor complaints as soon as they arrive, rather than asking them to wait. The key principle was that the first clinician to see the patient is able to assess, treat and discharge them safely.[5]

The Department of Health set a target of four hours for waiting times for emergency care, but recognised that there were clinical exceptions to this.

The target setting was followed by a joint document prepared by the Royal Colleges of Surgeons and Physicians, the Faculty of Accident and Emergency Departments, the British Association for Emergency Medicine and the Department of Health's Clinical Director for Emergency Access on 'Reforming Emergency Care'.[6]

The coalition government announced in June 2010 that the target waiting time of four hours in A&E was to be abolished since it lacked clinical justification. Instead the focus was to be on outcomes and the clinical evidence to identify what directly contributes to delivering the best possible results for patients. However, in December 2013 the four-hour waiting time was still being used as a target and Dame Barbara Hakin, Chief Operating Officer of NHS England, expressed disappointment that in the biggest A&E units only 92.9 per cent were seen within four hours, below the 95 per cent target.[7]

A report published on 5 July 2010 by the Nuffield Trust stated that the NHS was being put under unsustainable pressure by the increase in the number of emergency admissions to hospital. Many patients admitted in an emergency stayed less than a day, suggesting that doctors were admitting people with low clinical need. The Director of the Nuffield Trust said that politicians needed the courage to close beds and increase the focus on primary care services.[8]

In October 2013 the College of Emergency Medicine published the paper *Stretched to the Limits* outlining the challenges faced by emergency consultants. Sixty-two per cent of those who responded stated that their current jobs were unsustainable.[9]

The lack of A&E doctors has led to A&E staff being lured with £40,000 bonuses.[10]

The CQC in its annual report published in November 2013 suggested that 1 in 10 people over 75 have been rushed to hospital needlessly in the past year. More than half a million people over 65 were admitted as an emergency for conditions that could have been treated at home. Avoidable admission rates were up by almost a third over the past five years.[11]

The Medical Director for NHS England warned in January 2014 that NHS funds given to LAs to help older people to stay healthy and therefore reduce the pressure on A&E departments were being diverted to fill potholes. In 2015 £2 billion was taken from the NHS budget to be used to help older people stay healthy.[12]

Criticisms have been made about the effect of competition in the NHS on the viability of A&E departments[13] and Professor Keith Willett, who is conducting a review of emergency services, says that the effect of the new NHS pricing policy has led to an adversarial relationship between hospitals. The NHS England review has resulted in plans led by the Urgent and Emergency Care Delivery Group to help hospitals and A&E departments keep waiting times in check.[14] Further information on the Delivery Group can be found on the NHS website.[15]

In May 2013 the CQC chair, David Prior, urged widespread closure of hospital beds and investment in community care. He stated that too many patients were arriving in hospital as emergencies, when they should have been dealt with by GPs, social care or other services. The leader in *The Times* on 22 May 2013 suggested that the absence of GP services out of hours means that huge pressure is being put on hospital A&E departments by patients who have no need to be there. Then subsequently a further *Times* leader on 25 July 2013 spoke of a looming crisis with the problems in A&E being a harbinger of a struggle to come for the NHS, in the light of a report by the Health Select Committee of the House of Commons that the government's plans to relieve pressure on A&E units in England were not good enough.[16] Only one in six of all hospitals had the recommended level of consultant cover and too many were unable to manage the use of beds and the discharging of patients, the committee reported. In September 2013 the chief executive of the NHS Confederation stated that 'The warning signs are clear; the time for stop-gap solutions has passed . . . As a society, we need to drastically change how we regard hospital-based A&Es.'[17] In June 2013 NHS England commissioned a review of unscheduled care to explore how best to deliver emergency health services in the future.[18] One initiative to ease pressure on A&E departments put forward by the Health

Secretary was that healthcare for elderly people should be centralised with the plan being made compulsory from 2014 with the aim of reducing the number of older people being admitted to hospital.[19]

Local initiatives

Since a considerable proportion of A&E patients are there as the result of alcohol abuse another option was to treat such patients outside the A&E unit. A letter to *The Times* from the Professor of Oral and Maxillofacial Surgery at Cardiff University[20] pointed to the experience in Cardiff where using information from A&E patients injured as a result of violence to target locations and times of violence has cut violence-related A&E attendances. This initiative was supported by the opening of a late-night alcohol treatment centre in a city-centre chapel where intoxicated people can be taken by friends, street pastors and ambulances and cared for by nurse practitioners in a place of safety until they have sobered up. This has reduced A&E attendances and waiting times significantly. In addition, the professor noted that the introduction of minimum alcohol prices also has the potential to reduce demands on A&E. The growing trend of underage drinking and their being sent to A&E departments was highlighted in an investigation by BBC Radio 5 Live. There were 293 admissions of under-11s, up a third on 2011 for alcohol-related problems in 2012. Twenty thousand children a year use NHS services to deal with substance addiction, of whom a third are there because of alcoholism.[21]

National Audit Office Report 2013

In October 2013 the National Audit Office published a report on emergency admissions to hospital.[22] This stated that many emergency admissions to hospital are avoidable and many patients stay in hospital longer than is necessary. The NAO recommended both short- and long-term strategies to address staffing shortages in A&E. The Department of Health and NHS England, the NAO said, should address barriers to seven-day working in hospitals, such as the consultants' contract, which gives consultants the right to refuse to work outside 7 a.m. to 7 p.m. Monday to Friday. They should also explore how key patient information can be shared between health organisations. The DH, NHS England and Monitor should consider how best to align incentives across the health system to reduce emergency admissions. NHS England should review the suitability of the measure for delayed discharge. The report can be accessed on the NAO website.[23]

The Public Accounts Committee reported in March 2014 that there was no clear plan in the NHS to end a chronic shortage of A&E doctors. Nearly one fifth of consultant posts in emergency departments were either vacant or filled by locums in 2012.[24] It made several recommendations including requiring the Department of Health and NHS England to create a strategy to deal with levels of performance; reforming the overall system for funding urgent and emergency care; and considering all available options to address immediate and longer-term shortage of A&E consultants. Figures from the College of Emergency Medicine suggested that 1 in 25 consultants left the NHS in 2013, three times as many as the year before. A spokesman for the DH said that many doctors returned to the NHS with experience which would benefit patients.[25] At the same time a poll by Healthwatch England showed that 1 in 5 people had attended an A&E for non-urgent care. Its chairwoman Anna Bradley suggested that people should not be blamed for going to the wrong place: 'Until the health and care sector offers a more consumer-friendly experience, things are unlikely to improve.'[26] These figures were supported by research at Imperial College London which found that more than 1 in 4 visits to the A&E happen because patients could not see a GP.[27]

NHS 111 Service

An investigation has claimed that local NHS 111 Services, which have replaced NHS Direct (see chapter 5), have inadequate numbers of qualified staff and have sent ambulances out for minor ailments such as hangovers, coughs, colds and cat scratches.[28] The Medical Director of NHS England Professor Sir Bruce Keogh suggested that patients should phone the NHS 111 phone line before they went to A&E. This may help divert many of them to out-of-hours services and relieve pressure on A&E departments.[29] Early teething problems beset the early stages of NHS 111 when NHS Direct pulled out of providing urgent care lines in 11 of the 46 areas.[30]

The nurse has a clear role in improving these services and it is essential that the training for expanding the scope of her professional practice should be in place. (The scope of professional practice of the nurse is considered in chapter 23.)

Emergency workers legislation

Emergency workers are often exposed to challenging situations, and will be assisting and treating patients and relatives who are often in an anxious state. Any hindrance in this duty can have dire consequences for the patient, thus the Emergency Workers (Obstruction) Act 2006 makes obstructing or hindering certain emergency workers (or those persons assisting emergency workers) from responding to emergency circumstances a criminal offence. The definition of emergency worker includes a person employed by (or by an organisation supplying services to) an NHS body in the provision of ambulance services or of a person providing services for the transport of organs, blood, equipment or personnel made at the request of an NHS body. The Home Office expanded upon categories of persons covered by the Act to include all fire and rescue services and those under contract as well as volunteers who provide an ambulance service on behalf of a Health Service.

The Assaults on Emergency Workers (Offences) Act 2018 created a specific offence of common assault or battery against a nurse who provides NHS care or other emergency workers who exercising the functions of such a worker (section 1(1)). Police and prosecutors now charge under the provisions of the 2018 Act where the complainant is a nurse.

Where common assault or battery is committed against a nurse or other emergency worker the maximum sentences are now double those imposed for common assault against a member of the public which under the provisions of the Criminal Justice Act 1988, section 39 stands at 6 months imprisonment. The Assaults on Emergency Workers (Offences) Act 2018, section 1(2) provides for a maximum sentence of 12 months imprisonment and/or an unlimited fine when the perpetrator is found guilty either in a magistrate's court or a crown court.

Acting in the exercise of functions as an emergency worker

For the aggravated version of common assault and battery against an emergency worker to be charged the victim has to have been acting or functioning as an emergency worker at the time of the offence. The Assaults on Emergency Workers (Offences) Act 2018 does not define acting in the exercise of functions as an emergency worker so it will be necessary for the police and prosecutors to identify and nurses to provide evidence of what they were doing at the time they were assaulted to demonstrate to the court that this element of the offence is satisfied.

Aggravating factor for more serious offences

As well as creating a discrete offence of assault and battery against an emergency worker the Assaults on Emergency Workers (Offences) Act 2018, section 2 also creates statutory aggravating factors for more serious offences committed against nurses and other emergency workers. Courts must consider the offending to be more serious when committed against a nurse and that it merits an increase in the sentence. The court must say in open court that committing the offence against a nurse or other emergency worker was an aggravating factor when sentencing the perpetrator (Crown Prosecution Service 2018).[31]

This statutory aggravating factor applies to:

- Threats to kill;
- Wounding with intent to cause grievous bodily harm;
- Malicious wounding;
- Administering poison etc.;
- Causing bodily injury by gunpowder etc.;
- Using explosive substances etc. with intent to cause grievous bodily harm;
- Assault occasioning actual bodily harm;
- Sexual assault;
- Manslaughter; and
- Kidnapping.

The courts also have the discretion to treat other offences against a nurse or other emergency worker as an aggravating factor even though the offence is not specifically mentioned in section 2 of the 2018 Act.

Assault on a nurse

A man who assaulted a nurse who was trying to provide to another patient pleaded guilty to three counts of common assault against an emergency worker under section 1 of the 2018 Act. The man had been drinking with a relative but was admitted to the emergency department after falling when drunk and sustaining a cut to the head. After examination and treatment, he was thought to be sleeping off his intoxication when he assaulted the nurse by grabbing her wrists and pushing her by the shoulders before punching and then kicking hospital security officers.

He was sentenced to a night time curfew from 7 p.m. to 7 a.m. for eight weeks, a 12-month community order and ordered to pay £150 compensation to each of his victims by magistrates (Hull University Teaching Hospitals 2019).[32]

Assaults continue to rise

Despite the creating of a specific criminal offence and statutory aggravating factors for more serious offences, initial figures show that the Assaults on Emergency Workers (Offences) Act 2018 has had little impact as a deterrent against assaults on emergency workers including nurses. Some 4000 assaults against emergency workers were reported in the six months following the introduction of the 2018 Act and tougher sentencing alone will not deter patients from assaulting nurses (Martin and Camber 2019).[33]

Further information is available on the government website.[34]

Pressure of work – legal issues

Practical dilemma 20.1 Priorities under pressure

The A&E department was unusually pressurised one weekend: staff shortages due to a flu epidemic and cutbacks because of an attempt to reduce overspending left only a skeleton staff. Unfortunately, there was a particularly horrific pile-up on the motorway in the fog. Twelve people were brought in with varying levels of seriousness. One of them, David Lewis, a boy of 10, appeared to be suffering mainly from shock and bruises. He complained of a sore wrist. His mother was advised to take him home and give him a few paracetamol, a hot drink and, after a good night's sleep, he would be fine. The next day, however, it was learned that he had died during the night after inhaling vomit.

There is every possibility in this case that the mother will make an official complaint and possibly take legal action. Normally, it is not a successful defence to an action for negligence that the staff were under pressure (see Case 4.10), if it can be established that they failed to follow the approved accepted practice in relation to the care of the patient. Dealing with children is particularly difficult, since they cannot always correctly identify the site of any pain and discomfort. The possibility of head injury does not appear to have been considered in this case and this would be subject to investigation. Was the mother told the correct way of caring for the boy? The legal position is as follows:

1. There is a duty to care for the boy.
2. It must be established by the parents that the staff failed to follow the accepted approved practice.
3. This failure reasonably foreseeably led to the death of the boy.

The workload in an A&E department is extremely erratic. One moment there can be few demands, the next there may be a major incident or a sudden influx of patients and the pressure is on. What is the standard of care in such circumstances? Even though the nurses and doctors are under extreme pressure, each patient is still entitled to expect the appropriate standard of care. Thus it would still be actionable if a fracture remained undiagnosed or if a head injury were to be missed. However, the courts would take into account the pressure on the staff if priorities had to be set over who should be treated first. It would be open to the court to examine the basis of these priorities. In chapter 4, the case of *Deacon* v *McVicar*[35] (Case 4.11) is considered. In this case, a patient alleged that she should have been seen earlier and the court was prepared to examine the records of other patients who were in the ward at the time to see if they were making demands on the staff at that time. These principles would apply to the policy of triage, i.e. the professional staff have to take all due care in treating the patients and, where priorities have to be decided on, this must be according to approved accepted practice. There is no doubt that, in general, pressure of work does not justify a lower standard of care for the patient. It may, in addition, lead to a successful action against the NHS trust itself if it can be established that the authority failed to provide adequate resources and training for the patients to be cared for safely. It may be necessary in emergencies for staff to undertake tasks that they are not properly trained to do. If so, it is a question of balancing one risk against another, i.e. the risk of not being treated at all against the risk of harm arising because the only available person to treat the patient has not had sufficient training. Inevitably, the only way of coping with wide variations in demand is either to bring in additional staff to meet peaks of demand or for patients with less severe conditions to wait until staff are available to assist. Even though waiting for a long time would probably not result in a successful legal action, the complaints procedure might be used for those who consider that they have waited an unacceptable length of time. To prevent such claims, clear standards of communication with patients must be drawn up and implemented to ensure that patients are fully apprised of the situation.

The parents of a nine-year-old girl alleged that Hull Royal Infirmary failed to diagnose a broken leg and sent her home after six hours with no X-rays and told her to keep trying to walk on it. Subsequently she was given an X-ray and a spiral fracture was diagnosed.[36]

Ambulance services

A CQC report[37] on ambulance services in London found that there were not enough qualified, skilled and experienced staff to meet people's needs, and action was needed on staffing and the safety, availability and suitability of equipment. A 21-year-old woman died after an ambulance crew (unqualified student paramedics) who were dispatched unsupervised by London Ambulance Service, failed to treat her or take her to hospital. The coroner found that there was a gross failure to provide basic medical attention and ruled that neglect contributed to the death of Sarah Mulenga.[38] Data from NHS England in December 2013 showed that ambulances were missing the 999 response target with variations across the country.[39] See the *Kent* v *Griffiths* case for an illustration of the liability of the ambulance service[40] (see chapter 3 Case 3.1).

Giving information to patients

Additional precautions must thus be taken to ensure that, where the patient is not detained overnight, they have sufficient information to recognise any signs and symptoms that suggest a return to the hospital or to the general practitioner for further consultation and examination. Most hospitals already have pre-printed leaflets covering warnings in relation to head injuries, care of plaster, the need for anti-tetanus and other potential dangers. There is a need to stress, by word of mouth also, the importance of a patient following these instructions. If a patient ignored the instructions, having had clear advice from the staff, there is unlikely to be any blame on the part of the staff and certainly there may be a large element of contributory negligence on the part of the patient. Where information is given by word of mouth to the patient, one frequent concern of the staff is, 'How can I prove what I said since it is only the patient's word against mine?' This is always a dilemma in negligence cases, since no matter how strong the defendant's case would appear to be on paper, it still has to be proved through witnesses to the satisfaction of the courts. It is here that good record keeping is extremely important. If the nurse notes that the patient was given the relevant information, this does not in itself prove that the relevant information was provided since the records do not necessarily reflect what actually took place, but it does indicate the existence of a system where the nurse is more likely than not to have given the requisite information. In addition, of course, any witness who can recall the events and substantiate what the nurse was saying will undoubtedly help the nurse in any hearing they may have to attend. An additional precaution where it is essential to emphasise the importance of following the correct advice is for the patient to be asked to sign that they have understood the importance of obeying the instructions and have received written instructions (see also chapter 4).

Relationship between the duty of care owed by the GP and by the A&E department

Another difficulty that arises in the A&E department is the extent to which the department is used, inappropriately as far as the operational policy of the A&E department is concerned, as a GP surgery or health centre. The replacement of GP out-of-hours services by deputising services has led to an increase in the use of A&E departments for minor illnesses and injuries and some departments are coping with this by setting up a primary care facility within the A&E department.

Practical dilemma 20.2 — Minor ailments

A patient came into the A&E department complaining of a pain in his ear. He was registered by the admission clerk and seen by a nurse, who then told him to wait to see the doctor. The doctor asked him how long he had had the pain and the man said that he had had it for about three days. He was asked if he had been to see his GP and he said that he was not sure who his GP was. The doctor suggested that he should go to see his GP and that he should not have come to the A&E department which was for emergency treatment of a serious kind. The man was very reluctant to go and very upset. It was subsequently learnt that he was admitted to the district general hospital with mastoid meningitis and an inquiry was established to find out why he had not been diagnosed in the A&E department.

The general principle would appear to be that once a patient comes through the doors, a duty of care is owed and the patient should not be sent away without an adequate examination. The words 'through the doors' are important, since a duty of care is not owed in a vacuum. It is perfectly possible for a hospital to say 'we do not accept A&E patients here' and refuse to treat a patient. However, once a hospital accepts a patient for attention, then a duty of care would arise to ensure that this patient receives the appropriate standard of care, even though it might mean arranging the transfer of the patient to another hospital or advising the patient to see his own GP. The Primary Care Foundation was commissioned by the Department of Health in May 2009 to carry out a study across England of the different models of primary care operating within or alongside emergency departments. It was asked to provide a viable estimate of the number of patients who attend emergency departments with conditions that could be dealt with elsewhere in primary care. It estimated that around half of the services across the country have some form of primary care service working with the emergency department. Its recommendations are particularly important for commissioners and providers of primary care and A&E services. It emphasised the importance of breaking down the barriers between primary care and emergency care clinicians and between the different organisations that employ the staff. Good joint working should be promoted.[41]

Extent of duty of care

> **Practical dilemma 20.3** **Referral for what?**
>
> A patient was referred to the A&E department by the GP for X-ray because she had fallen and sustained a severe injury and considerable bruising to her leg. The doctor arranged for her to be X-rayed and it was found to be negative. The patient mentioned to the doctor that she was very short of breath and thirsty. However, only her leg was examined. She subsequently discovered that she was suffering from diabetes and claimed that the doctor should have diagnosed this.

This is another situation that raises the extent of the duty of care owed by the hospital staff to the patient. If the GP refers a patient for a very specific purpose, which is carried out, can it then be said that the patient should have been given a full examination so that other significant defects could have been detected? The answer must obviously depend on the particular circumstances and what the reasonably accepted approved practice is.

The clinical nurse specialist in the A&E department

Increasingly, protocols are being developed for a nurse specialist to work within the A&E department, seeing patients who are not examined by a doctor, prescribing on a limited scale and performing an expanded range of activities. The legal issues arising from this scope of professional practice and the appointment of modern matrons in A&E departments are considered in chapter 23. A significant development in the A&E modernisation programme was the appointment of clinical nurse specialists (see chapter 23), now referred to in many places as an Advance Nurse Practitioner (ANP). Most Nurse Practitioners are able to prescribe from the full formulary, and diagnose and discharge patients.

Pressure to disclose confidential information

The basic principles relating to the disclosure of confidential information are discussed in chapter 8. In that chapter, two examples are given of requests for information in A&E departments. Staff are under particular pressure in this respect, since they are likely to be hounded by both the police and the press in order that sensitive and personal information can be disclosed. In very prescribed circumstances, the health professions owe a duty to act in the public interest, and this duty may take precedence over the duty of confidentiality owed to the patient (see chapter 8). Guidance is provided in the Code (NMC, 2015). The statutory powers of the police under the Police and Criminal Evidence Act enable, in cases of serious arrestable offences, a special procedure to be followed to compel the production of personal information and human tissue which would otherwise be protected from disclosure. Whatever the local policy on disclosure to the police, in the end it must be the individual professional's decision, since that individual may have to justify to the patient why confidentiality was not maintained.

Practical dilemma 20.4 — Road traffic accidents

The police are entitled to know the names and addresses of those who have been involved in a road traffic accident. This does not mean, however, that the media are also entitled to know these names or to know the condition of the patient. If the patient gives consent (and possibly the relatives, although this is more doubtful), then the information can be disclosed. If, however, this consent is refused, the hospital spokesperson must remain silent as far as the disclosure of any confidential information is concerned. Once again, practice varies and there is an absence of court cases to settle the issue. For example, some hospitals allow a condition report to be given to the press without obtaining the consent of the patient, e.g. 'Of the ten persons injured in the motorway pile-up on Tuesday, one has since died, three have been discharged, four are comfortable and two are on life support machines.' There are few who would see this as a breach of confidence. Anyone (and this includes medical staff) who is aware of information about people involved in a road accident where personal injuries occurred has a duty to ensure that the police are notified.[42]

Patients' records come under the provisions of the General Data Protection Regulation 2016 and are, of course, subject to close controls over disclosure (see chapter 8). NHS trusts and Health Boards should appoint a Data Protection Compliance Manager to oversee standards of confidentiality within the organisation. Any concerns could be raised with that person for further investigation and, if needed, appropriate action should be taken if confidentiality is breached without reasonable grounds.

Outpatients department

Excessive waiting

Practical dilemma 20.5 — Waiting

Bruce was self-employed and time was money. He had been suffering from a severe pain and his doctor had referred him to the consultant surgeon querying gallstones or cholecystitis. He was sent an appointment to see the surgeon at 9.30 a.m. in outpatients. Because he had an important meeting that afternoon, which could involve him in a lot of valuable work, he phoned the clerk, who assured him that the clinic ended at lunchtime. When he got to the clinic, he discovered that 30 people had been booked in for 9.30, most of whom had arrived before him. As he sat chatting, he discovered that others who had been booked in for 12.00 noon had come early, since they were seen in the order of arrival and not according to appointments. He settled down for a long wait and then was told at 1.00 p.m. that the surgeon had had to rush off to theatre to cover for a colleague who had been taken ill, but that if Bruce waited, the doctor would see him when the operation was over. Bruce said that he could not wait as he had a very important meeting. The clerk replied that if he went away he would be treated as a 'did not attend' and would have to take his place in the queue being seen in outpatients. He would not be able to give him an appointment for at least another three months. Bruce insisted on seeing the ward manager.

Oddly enough, there seems to be no legal grounds for bringing an action against an NHS trust for causing excessive waiting in outpatients or in A&E departments. The Department of Health had set down targets to reduce waiting in A&E departments, but these were enforced through the complaints system, rather than through legal action. In private practice there would be a contract between professional and client, and it could be more clearly argued that there was a breach of contract when a client was kept waiting an unreasonable length of time. However, in NHS care, there is no contract between the patient and the NHS trust or between the patient and the professional, and the patient who is aggrieved at having to wait an unreasonably long time would have to argue that there was a breach of the duty of care owed to the patient under the laws of negligence that has caused him some loss or harm – a loss or harm that is compensatable under the law. There have been actions when patients have waited excessively long periods of time for inpatient treatment. However, no action has been brought in relation to a long wait within the department itself. Such a complaint is more likely to be investigated by the hospital management and be reviewed by the Health Service Commissioner (i.e. Ombudsman) (see chapter 26). The Health Service Commissioner has investigated many complaints of unreasonable waiting times in A&E, outpatients and other departments. The procedure for handling complaints is considered in chapter 26. The NHS Constitution (see the website of this book) makes the following patient pledge:

> **The NHS also commits: to provide convenient, easy access to services within the waiting times set out in the Handbook to the NHS Constitution.**

The NHS Handbook to the Constitution sets 18 weeks from the date of referral to starting consultant-led treatment for non-urgent conditions and a maximum of 2 weeks from GP referral to be seen by a cancer specialist where cancer is suspected. Page 29 of the Handbook sets other waiting time targets. Both the NHS Constitution and the Handbook can be downloaded from the government website.[43] The main means of enforcing such a pledge would appear to be through the complaints mechanism.

In Practical Dilemma 20.5, when the ward manager is confronted by a very disgruntled patient he or she should ensure that the facts given by the clerk are accurate. It is unlikely, for example, that a patient who has been kept waiting in the way in which Bruce has should be treated as a 'did not attend'. If so, the system is manifestly unjust. The manager should be able, with cooperation from the doctor, to arrange for Bruce to be seen much earlier. In addition, he or she may be able to arrange a compromise by asking Bruce to attend the meeting and to return that same day. Certainly he or she should be able to take the heat out of the situation, explain the problems fully to Bruce, work out some acceptable solution and, of course, apologise to him for what has happened. This is not law, but it is good practice. However, there are many such occasions where the patient may or may not have a right of action in law where skilled counselling and cooperation with the patient prevents a situation developing into a court action or Health Service Ombudsman's inquiry. The RCN has provided a guide for competencies for advanced nurse practitioners.[44]

The Care Quality Commission published a briefing paper in 2010[45] on a survey of outpatients. In general there was an improvement in waiting times, cleanliness and the information given to patients. However, the results show that there is considerable room for improvement in the service provided. The survey carried out by the CQC in 2011 found that there was an improvement from the results of the 2009 survey.[46]

Mistaken identity

Practical dilemma 20.6 The wrong notes

Ward manager Bailey was short staffed in the outpatients department and the situation was made worse by a strike among the coordinators. However, the consultants were adamant that the clinics should continue. She called out for one patient, Handel Thomas, to come to the diabetic clinic. She checked that he was from The Marina, Fish Street, and he said he was. He was asked if he had brought any samples with him and he replied: 'No, no one told me to.' He was then taken in to see the consultant. He was given a very full investigation and was asked how often he injected his insulin. He was a little surprised at this and replied that he had never been told to use insulin.

After considerable confusion, during which time Handel was getting very disturbed, it emerged that there was another Handel Thomas in Fish Street. This Handel James Thomas lived at number 45 and was due to be seen in the eye clinic; the other Handel, Handel David Thomas from 2 Fish Street, should have been seen in the diabetic clinic.

In circumstances like this, there has been clear negligence by the manager in failing to check that she was taking the right patient to be seen and by the doctor who also did not check. However, apart from causing distress to the patient and a breach of confidentiality of information about the other patient, no harm has been caused to either, so it is not a case that is likely to end up in the courts. However, the potential implications of this type of mistake are terrifying and the tightest control must be kept over patient identification. Unfortunately, one cannot always rely on patients to point out the error since they can become institutionalised and frightened at the prospect of challenging the professionals, and stories abound as to what they are prepared to submit to by mistake. A news item in June 2014 reported that a pensioner died three hours after doctors operated on the wrong lung at the William Harvey Hospital in Kent.[47]

Genito-urinary medicine

Confidentiality

In a sexual health department (formerly known as the VD clinic, GUM Clinic or the 'special clinic'), strict confidentiality must be maintained. This section looks at some of the problems and pitfalls that can arise over confidentiality in this context and also at the statutory provisions.

Practical dilemma 20.7 A reasonable request

Mr Grey had just visited the sexual health clinic and samples had been taken. He was told that the results would be available by the Thursday of the following week. He was naturally anxious and, since he lived some 40 miles from the clinic, he phoned up late Thursday morning to find out the results. He gave his name and the nurse asked for his clinic number. She explained that it was on his card. He said that he had lost his card. She therefore told him that she would be unable to give him the result over the phone. He asked if that meant that the results were positive. She said not at all, but because of the principles of confidentiality, she could neither confirm that someone of that name had attended the clinic nor could she give any results over the phone without the clinic number. He became very angry, pointing out the inconvenience that he would suffer if he had to drive the 40 miles there and back, especially if the results were negative. She told him that she could not change the rules. He threatened to complain about her attitude and report her.

There is no doubt that the nurse is correct in not divulging information without being absolutely certain that she is talking to the patient. There are possible ways out of this dilemma. One would be for the nurse to phone a number that had already been given by the patient to the clinic for the notification of the results. The other would be to ensure that all patients are warned of the strict rules of confidentiality from the outset of their care so that they know the rules are firmly adhered to for their own protection, even in circumstances that cause them great inconvenience such as the one above.

A similar difficulty can be seen in Practical Dilemma 20.8.

Requests for information by a spouse

Practical dilemma 20.8 Spousely concern

A man phoned the sexual health clinic saying that he was the husband of Mrs Robinson, a patient who had an appointment at the clinic that afternoon. He said that she had lost her appointment card and forgotten the time and, since he was giving her a lift, could they let him know the time of the appointment?

This is the sort of request that few staff in a general outpatients department would hesitate to respond to helpfully. Yet, if confidentiality is to be preserved, it is essential that the person answering the phone does not admit to the fact (if this is indeed the case) that there is a patient of such a name attending the clinic.

Tracing

Obviously, it is essential that, as far as possible, any people who have been in contact with someone who is infected should be traced and advised to have tests. It is important that this be done without revealing the name of the contact. A form is completed to assist the clinic. If original contacts can be persuaded to advise their contacts to have a check, this is preferable to their receiving a call out of the blue.

Venereal disease regulations

These regulations (National Health Service (Venereal Diseases) Regulations 1974 Section 1 No. 29 (as amended by SI 1982 No. 288)) ensure that any information about any sexually transmitted disease is kept confidential.

In 2000, Directions[48] were issued for England only, which came into force on 1 April 2001 revoking earlier Directions of 1991. The 2000 Directions require:

> Every NHS trust and Primary Care Trust to take the necessary steps to secure that any information capable of identifying an individual obtained by any of their members or employees with respect to persons examined or treated for any sexually transmitted disease shall not be disclosed except—
>
> (a) for the purpose of communicating that information to a medical practitioner, or to a person employed under the direction of a medical practitioner in connection with the treatment of persons suffering from such disease or the prevention of the spread thereof, and
>
> (b) for the purpose of such treatment or prevention.

However, since the passing of the Health and Social Care Act 2012 these directions are largely redundant and only apply to remaining NHS Trusts. The Government is not renewing the directions, and confidentiality in relation to sexual health will follow generic confidentiality principles.

The National AIDS Trust (NAT) published in 2009 a booklet on confidentiality in healthcare for people living with HIV which is available on its website.[49]

It was suggested in the case of *X v Y and Another* (1988)[50] that AIDS came within the scope of the VD regulations. See chapter 25 for a consideration of the legal issues in AIDS and infectious diseases.

Day surgery

The NHS Plan saw an increase in day surgery as a means of helping the NHS achieve its targets of treating more patients faster and was therefore a key strand of NHS modernisation and predicted that 75 per cent of all elective operations would be carried out as day cases. In 2001 the Audit Commission considered that day surgery units were not being used to their maximum capacity.[51] An operational guide was published by the Department of Health[52] to improve efficiency in day surgery units with funds made available from the NHS Modernisation Programme. Some of the problems identified by the Audit Commission and the British Association of Day Surgery included:

- inappropriate and inefficient use of units (e.g. treating patients who could be cared for in a treatment room or outpatients);
- poor management and organisation, especially in relation to the flow of patients;
- clinicians' preference for inpatient surgery;
- mixing of inpatients and day cases on the same list, leading to cancellations due to theatre overruns; and
- failure to recognise day surgery as a priority.

All those areas of law that are the concern of inpatient care also apply to those working in day surgery. However, there are additional problems that can arise from the speed of turnover, the fact that patients are seen for a very short time and that significant decisions have to be made urgently. For example, crucial decisions have to be made about whether an operation is to proceed following the necessary tests; should the patient be admitted after surgery or could he/she be allowed to go home, and what information has to be given to the patient before the patient returns home. The pressure of work, the speed of patient throughput and the risk of harm arising means that clear protocols are necessary to ensure that patients receive a satisfactory standard of care and that they and their carers are given essential information pre- and post-surgery. Practical Dilemma 20.9 is only one of the situations where complaints and litigation can arise. Reference must be made to earlier chapters setting out basic principles of law. Benchmarking tools were introduced in 2004 by the Modernisation Agency in relation to day surgery so that trusts could assess their performance and learn of best practice across the country. Research at Salford University into the psychological impact of conscious day surgery found that more contact with nurses could help reduce patient anxiety. It suggested that if nurses met patients before the surgery and provided information about the operation and the anaesthesia this would help reduce anxiety in the majority of patients.[53] The Healthcare Commission reviewed services for day surgery in 2005 and concluded that there was scope to do much more day surgery within the capacity already available.[54] Figures published by the NHS Institute for Innovation and Improvement (now NHS Improvement) showed that only cataract care came anywhere near the potential national day case rate.[55] The use of Better Care, Better Value indicators reveal the potential to make significant cash or resource savings while improving quality by greater use of day surgery.[56] *Converting the Potential into Reality* (2009) sets out 10 steps a provider can take to realise the benefits of Better Care, Better Value indicators.

Practical dilemma 20.9　Day surgery

Barbara was called for day surgery to have an operation for carpal tunnel syndrome. The operation was to be performed under a local anaesthetic. She was told to arrive by 9.00 a.m. even though she would be the last on the list. She waited for two hours before she was seen by a nurse, who then booked her in and told her that she should not have had any breakfast. Barbara queried this, as a general anaesthetic was not planned. The nurse said it was a precaution in case the operation could not be performed under a local anaesthetic. At 2.30 p.m. she was taken down for surgery and told that she must stay in the ward until 6.00 p.m. She asked for and was given a cup of tea at 4.00 p.m. Apart from that, she had no food or drink. No instructions were given to her for postoperative care. She considers that she has been treated poorly. What rights does she have?

This situation is more likely to lead to a complaint than to litigation. There is the possibility of a claim under Article 3 of the Convention on Human Rights (see chapter 1 and the website of this book) in that she may have been given degrading or inhuman treatment. She is unlikely to benefit from civil litigation for compensation, unless there is long-term harm as a result of the failure to give her post-operative and post-discharge instructions. For example, if she should have been advised not to drive a car after the operation and, as a result of this omission, she was involved in an accident, then there would appear to be a breach of the duty of care owed to her. However, these deplorable circumstances might well be the subject of a complaint and of the argument that the pledges and rights recognised in the NHS Constitution were not respected.

Conclusions

The crises within A&E departments continue to place considerable pressure upon nursing staff. The importance of the nurse practitioner and clinical specialist role assumes greater significance as the shortage of A&E consultant specialists continues. At the same time patient expectations continue to rise. There are likely to be an increasing volume of complaints. There is evidence that the potential for day surgery instead of inpatient care has not yet been fully realised. Current plans put forward by the Chief Executive of NHS England for smaller hospitals to be retained are likely to lead to some imaginative use of Skype and the sharing of doctors and greater cooperation between health service providers.

Reflection questions

1. Does the nurse (or doctor) who works in the A&E department have a duty in law to assess the priority to be given to a patient and could he or she be held liable in the civil courts for failures in making that assessment?
2. Can a patient be lawfully refused treatment in an A&E department and be referred instead to their GP?
3. What remedy does a patient who has waited an excessive amount of time in the A&E department or the outpatients department have?
4. What precautions might be taken to preserve medical confidentiality in the A&E department in relation to:
   (a) the press
   (b) the police
   (c) other staff?

Further exercises

1. Do you consider that the spouse of a patient suffering from a sexually transmitted disease should have a right to be told of the spouse's medical condition? What is the law on this?
2. What remedies does a member of staff have who has been injured by a drunken patient in the A&E department? (See also chapter 12.)
3. In what way does the duty of staff in A&E departments differ from the duty of those on the wards in relation to the care of the patient's property? (Refer also to chapter 24.)

4. A patient is admitted into the A&E department with severe bleeding. His clothes have to be cut from him and because they are badly soiled they are sent for incineration. He subsequently complains that there was £300 in the pocket of his jacket. What is the liability of the hospital or of the A&E staff? (Refer to chapter 24.)
5. A clinical nurse specialist who works in day surgery is asked if she would like to apply for a nurse consultant post in this speciality. What differences would she anticipate in these two roles? (Refer also to chapter 23.)

References

[1] National Audit Office, Major Trauma Care in England, Report by the Comptroller and Auditor General HC 213 Session 2009–10, Stationery Office, London, 2010
[2] Kaya Burgess, We need trauma centres for civilians, say doctors, *The Times*, 3 February 2014
[3] Chris Smyth, A&E reform plan suggests two-tier care, *The Times*, 13 November 2013
[4] Chris Smyth, Resistance to change in NHS 'has cost thousands of lives', *The Times*, 1 July 2014
[5] Department of Health press release 2004/0058, Making See and Treat Work for Patients and Staff, 2004
[6] Royal College of Physicians, Reforming Emergency Care, May 2005
[7] Chris Smyth, Busy A&Es missing waiting target, *The Times*, 14 December 2013
[8] Sam Lister, Alarm at rise in emergency admissions, *The Times*, 5 July 2010
[9] www.collemergencymed.ac.uk
[10] Sarah-Kate Templeton and Kevin Dowling, Hospitals lure A&E staff with £40,000 bonus, *The Sunday Times*, 25 August 2013
[11] Chris Smyth, Rise in 'avoidable' A&E admissions for over 75s, *The Times*, 22 November 2013
[12] Chris Smyth, Councils 'will steal NHS cash for potholes', *The Times*, 22 January 2014
[13] Alison Pollock, Why A&E departments are fighting for their life, *The Guardian*, 14 January 2014
[14] www.england.nhs.uk
[15] www.nhs.uk
[16] House of Commons Select Committee, Urgent and Emergency Services 2nd Report 2013; www.publications.parliament.uk
[17] Chris Smyth, Hospitals face another 'war zone' winter as Hunt admits it will be tough on A&E, *The Times*, 11 September 2013
[18] NHS England, High quality care for all, now and for future generations: transforming urgent and emergency care services in England 2013; www.england.nhs.uk/wp-content/uploads/2013/06/urg-emerg-care-ev-bse.pdf
[19] NHS England, High quality care for all, now and for future generations: transforming urgent and emergency care services in England 2013; www.england.nhs.uk/wp-content/uploads/2013/06/urg-emerg-care-ev-bse.pdf
[20] Chris Smyth, Elderly to have one contact point on health to ease A&E pressures, The Times, 13 May 2013 Letter to the Editor, *The Times*, 10 June 2013
[21] Tom Whipple, Hundreds of drunk under-11s sent to A&E, *The Times*, 30 September 2013
[22] National Audit Office, Emergency admissions to hospital: managing the demand, HC 730, Stationery Office, 2013
[23] www.nao.org.uk

24. Public Accounts Committee 46th Report: Session 2013/4 Emergency Admissions to Hospitals March 2014; www.parliament.uk
25. Chris Smyth, A&E pressure drives consultants to quit Britain in record numbers, *The Times*, 9 June 2014
26. Chris Smyth, No plan to deal with lack of A&E doctors, *The Times*, 4 March 2014
27. Oliver Moody, Lack of GP appointments drives millions to A&E, *The Times*, 30 June 2014
28. Channel 4 *Dispatches*: NHS undercover broadcast, 29 July 2013
29. Chris Smyth, A&E 'phone before you go' plan, *The Times*, 18 June 2013
30. Chris Smyth, 111 Service future in doubt after NHS Direct pulls out, *The Times*, 30 Jul 2013
31. Crown Prosecution Service (2018) Assaults on Emergency Workers (Offences) Act 2018 available on the CPS Website at https://www.cps.gov.uk/legal-guidance/assaults-emergency-workers-offences-act-2018
32. Hull University Teaching Hospitals (2019) Warning after man is placed under curfew for assaulting nurse and security staff available on the Hull University Teaching Hospitals Website at https://www.hey.nhs.uk/news/2019/04/09/warning-after-man-is-placed-under-curfew-for-assaulting-nurse-and-security-staff/
33. Martin A. and Camber R. (2019) Revealed: More than 20 emergency workers are assaulted every day while on the line of duty in Wild West Britain available on the Mail online Website at https://www.dailymail.co.uk/news/article-7343089/More-20-emergency-workers-assaulted-day-line-duty.html
34. www.gov.uk
35. *Deacon* v *McVicar and Another*, 7 January, available on Lexis (1984) QBD
36. News item, A&E 'told girl with broken leg to go home and walk', *The Times*, 30 July 2013
37. Care Quality Commission, London Ambulance Service NHS Trust Inspection Report, 22 December 2012
38. Sarah-Kate Templeton, Patient died in care of unqualified paramedics, *The Sunday Times*, 12 May 2103
39. News item, Ambulances missing 999 response target, *The Times*, 7 December 2013
40. *Kent* v *Griffiths and Others*, The Times Law Report, 23 December 1998; The Times Law Report, 10 February 2000; [2000] 2 All ER 474
41. David Carson et al., *Primary Care and Emergency Departments*, Primary Care Foundation, March 2010
42. *Hunter* v *Mann* [1974] 1 QB 767
43. www.gov.uk
44. RCN Competences: Advanced Nurse Practitioners – an RCN guide, 003207, RCN 2012
45. Care Quality Commission, Supporting Briefing Note: issues highlighted by the 2009 survey of people attending NHS outpatient departments in England, CQC, 2010
46. www.cqc.org.uk
47. News item, 'Wrong lung' tragedy, *The Times*, 6 June 2014
48. NHS Trusts and PCTs (Sexually Transmitted Diseases), Directions 2000
49. www.nat.org.uk
50. *X* v *Y and another* [1988] 2 All ER 648
51. Audit Commission, Report on Day Surgery, AC, 2001
52. Department of Health, Day Surgery – operational guide, DH, 2002
53. News item, Salford research shows day surgery patients need more contact with nurses, *The Operating Theatre Journal*, 229, October/November 2009
54. Healthcare Commission, Acute hospital portfolio review: Day Surgery, 2005
55. www.institute.nhs.uk
56. www.institute.nhs.uk

Chapter 21

Human Fertility and Genetics

This chapter discusses

- Artificial insemination
- Human Fertilisation and Embryology Act 1990 as amended by 2008 Act
- *In vitro* fertilisation (IVF)
- Embryos
- Confidentiality
- Surrogacy
- Conscientious objection
- Genetics
- Gene therapy and genetic diagnosis
- Gender selection
- Genetic screening and testing
- Cloning

Introduction

Nurses are increasingly likely to be caring for patients in clinics and on the wards who are receiving treatment in connection with problems of fertility. Medical technology has made vast strides in this field and frequently outpaces the law. This chapter provides guidance on the current legislation relating to artificial insemination by donor, embryo implantation, surrogacy and genetic engineering. The legal problems that arise from sterilisation and family planning are considered in chapter 14 and those relating to organ and tissue removal, donation and storage in chapter 15. Genetic research using human tissue is considered in chapter 17. The Warnock Committee[1] considered the need for legislation across this field and its recommendations led to the Human Fertilisation and Embryology Act 1990 which introduced statutory controls in relation to reproductive medicine. Subsequent scientific developments after 1990 inevitably led to calls for new legislation. A White Paper[2] was published in December 2006 following extended consultation, and a draft Human Tissue and Embryos Bill was published in May 2007 and subjected to scrutiny by a committee of both Houses of Parliament. The government response to the Joint Committee's report was published in October 2007[3] and is shown in Box 21.1. Subsequently, the Human Fertilisation and Embryology Act 2008 was enacted and implemented.

> **Box 21.1** Government response to joint committee on the draft human tissue and embryos bill
>
> The government:
>
> - accepted the recommendation to retain the two separate authorities (Human Fertilisation and Embryology Authority and Human Tissue Authority), but would look at the scope for the two authorities to streamline legislation;
> - welcomed the recommendation that primary care trusts and Foundation trusts implement NICE guidance on minimum levels of IVF treatment, and accepted that although this is not a matter for legislation, the DH was funding a three-year programme of work (being carried out by Infertility Network UK) that aims to reduce inequalities in the provision of IVF;
> - agreed that the use of inter-species embryos for research could be put before Parliament, with the power given to the Regulator to permit or refuse licences in relation to all inter-species embryos;
> - agreed that a permitted embryo could only be implanted if it was from the genetic material of a woman and a man, and not from two women;
> - agreed that selecting for saviour siblings should not be limited to 'life-threatening' conditions, but only to 'serious' conditions;
> - sex selection should only be for medical reasons in accordance with current HFEA policy;
> - use of an embryo for research involving altering the genetic structure of the embryo could proceed within the 14-day period;
> - where embryos have been created using donor gametes, and a woman no longer wished to consent to the storage of the embryo, the clinic would not have to notify the donor;
> - whether it was in the best interests of a mentally incapacitated person to take gametes for storage should be left to the professional judgement of the clinicians;
> - the need for a father should be removed but the general duty to take account of the welfare of the child should be included in primary legislation;
> - there should be a time limit on the period of storage of gametes or embryos and this should be increased from 5 to 10 years but be subject to review;

- people intending to marry or cohabit or enter a civil partnership should be entitled to contact the HFEA to see whether they are related as a result of donor insemination, but the consent of both parties is required for this information to be provided;
- HFEA, which holds a register of all donor treatment since 1990, will be able to run the voluntary contact register which covered donor treatment preceding the 1990 Act;
- those of 16 years and over can obtain non-identifying information from HFEA, but the age limit of 18 years for those wishing to obtain identifying information is to be retained;
- putting the fact of donor conception on a birth certificate involves issues of privacy, human rights and data protection and will be kept under review;
- facilitating counselling for persons seeking donor information from the HFEA is important and will be included in discussions between the government and the HFEA on its annual business plan and priorities;
- the provision in the draft Bill for not allowing sex selection for non-medical purposes in sperm-sorting kits is to be removed since it relates to a potential development and it will be kept under review; and
- the possibility of bringing surrogacy within the remit of the HFEA would be considered.

Artificial insemination

Artificial insemination by husband (AIH)

If a married couple require help in conception such that the husband's semen is artificially transferred to the wife, the law would see the outcome of this as being identical with natural conception. As far as such aspects as inheritance, legal guardianship of the child, etc. are concerned, there is no difference between the artificially and the naturally conceived child. However, the involvement of a third person raises the possibility of other legal issues. For example, it is possible that if a pathology laboratory is involved, there could be a mix-up over the semen and the woman could be given semen from someone other than her husband. With genetic coding, it would now be possible to prove that the child is not the husband's, although, of course, it must be remembered that in order to succeed in a negligence action it must be established that there was a causal link between the negligent act and the harm caused (the woman could have had sex with a third person). Some have opposed AIH on moral grounds, since it is an unnatural form of conception, but the Warnock Committee[4] were of the view that it was an acceptable form of treatment except where a widow used semen that had been stored in a semen bank. They felt that insemination after the husband's death could lead to profound psychological problems for the child and the mother. The Warnock Committee considered that there was no need or even practical possibility of formal regulation of AIH, but recommended that it should be administered by or under the supervision of a medical practitioner.

No licence is required under the 1990 Act for artificial insemination by the husband. Neither is one required for AIP (artificial insemination of an unmarried woman with her partner's sperm). Neither AIH nor AIP requires the use of donated gametes. However, a licence would be required if the sperm is processed or stored. GIFT (gamete intrafallopian transfer) does not require a licence if the egg and sperm come from the woman and her partner/husband. Basic partner treatment services (i.e. treatment services that are provided for a woman and a man together without using (a) the gametes of any other person, or (b) embryos created outside the woman's body), are excluded from the licence and information provisions.

Following amendments made to the 1990 Act by the 2007 regulations,[5] a licence is required under the 1990 Act in respect of non-medical fertility services. Non-medical fertility services are any services that are provided, in the course of a business, for the purpose of assisting women to carry children, but which are not medical, surgical or obstetric services. This would cover internet-based businesses that arrange for donated sperm to be delivered to women at home for self-insemination.

The European Court of Human Rights held that the refusal of access to artificial insemination facilities to a life-term prisoner was a disproportionate action by the state and a breach of his Article 8 rights[6] (see chapter 1).

Artificial insemination by donor (AID)

Where the donor is not the husband, problems over legitimacy, rights to inheritance and the duties of the husband in relation to the child arise. A report from the Archbishop of Canterbury in 1948 recommended that AID should be made a criminal offence. The Feversham Report set up by the government in 1960 recommended that AID should be discouraged. The opposite has happened. In 1973 a panel under the chairmanship of Sir John Peel recommended the setting up of accreditation centres for AID, but this has not taken place. In an early case[7] (preceding the legislation of 1990), regarding the rights of the father, the father and mother had entered into an agreement that the girl would be artificially inseminated by him and then she would hand over the child on payment of £3000. She refused to hand the child over and the trial judge gave the father limited rights of access. The Court of Appeal, however, gave him no rights of access.

Artificial insemination by donor is not unlawful, but, in contrast to the child born from AIH, the child born as a result of AID is illegitimate and the husband of the mother has no parental rights and duties in relation to the child, unless he accepts the child as a child of the family. The donor could be held responsible for the maintenance of the child and could apply to the court for access or custody. A consultation paper was published by the government in 1986. Following this, a child who is born to a woman as the result of artificial insemination by someone other than her husband is treated as the child of the parties of that marriage. This is enacted by section 27 of the Family Reform Act 1987. The main condition is that the marriage must be in existence at the time. Proof to the satisfaction of the court that the other party to the marriage did not consent to the insemination will prevent this provision arising. This means that the burden is placed on the husband to show that the insemination was performed without his consent. This provision came into force in April 1988 and applies only to children born subsequently. Sections 33 to 38 of the 2008 Act cover the definition of mother and father in cases involving assisted reproduction.

In a significant decision, a gay man who had provided sperm for the artificial insemination of a woman on the basis that they would share in the child's upbringing (neither was in a gay relationship at the time) won his application to have joint parental rights over the child. The mother had denied him access to his son, two years old, at the time of the court hearing.[8] In another case where a child was conceived to a partner in a lesbian relationship by having sexual intercourse with a man, the man was given parental responsibility subject to a preamble and specified conditions by the Family Division of the High Court.[9] In a case in 2010 in the Court of Appeal a lesbian mother and the gay father disputed residency rights. (The father wished for shared residency, but the mother argued that the residency order should be made in favour of herself and her partner who had jointly been the children's (a boy of nine and girl of seven) primary carers since birth.) The CA held the father should have residency rights for 152 days of the year.[10] In a recent case the donor of sperm to a lesbian couple was not to be excluded from the life of his son and the woman failed in her attempt to prevent any contact between the father and son. The judge said that the father had rights of his own and that the baby would benefit from his input.[11] In a case in March 2014 the Court of Appeal overruled a family court decision that the genetic mother could not share residence of twin girls born from artificial insemination. The genetic mother had donated eggs to her lesbian lover but sole residence was awarded to the birth mother. The Court of Appeal upheld the challenge of the genetic mother and said that the case must be sent back to the county court.[12]

In another case in 2013 there was a dispute between the woman and the father of the child as to whether the child was born as a result of sperm donation according to him (Mr F) or sexual intercourse according to her.[13] If the child was the result of sexual intercourse F would be the legal parent of the child and had a duty to provide for the child financially. If F was a sperm donor then the question of parentage depended on the effect of section 35 of the Human Fertility and Embryology Act 2008. (Section 35: the husband of a woman who conceives following embryo or egg and sperm donation, where the sperm is not his, is deemed to be the father of the child unless he did not consent to the fertilisation.) M's husband was 30 years older than M. The judge concluded on the evidence (he found that both M and F had lied) that F was the biological and legal parent of the child. In the dispute over costs (M had paid £300,000) the judge held that the legal father should pay the husband's costs and the mother's costs with a reduction of 25 per cent to take account of her misconduct.

Anonymity of donors

There were two years of consultation on whether donors should be entitled to keep their anonymity or whether the offspring from donated gametes had a right to know the donors. A summary of the public consultation is available on the internet. In July 2003 the HFEA called for the removal of laws protecting the anonymity of all future sperm and egg donors, and acknowledged the fundamental right of donor offspring to have knowledge of their genetic origins. In a report in *The Times*,[14] Baroness Warnock admitted that she had been wrong to recommend that anonymity should be preserved. Two cases held that Britain was violating Article 8 of the European Convention on Human Rights by depriving children of the right to obtain knowledge of their personal identity. Legislation to give children of sperm, embryo and egg donors the right to find out about their parents was proposed by the government in January 2004[15] and led to new rules[16] to lift anonymity from future donors and allow donor-conceived children to access the identity of their donor when they reach 18 years coming into force on 1 April 2005. As a consequence, those who donated sperm, eggs or embryos after 1 April 2005 are, by law, identifiable. Any person born as a result of donation after this time is entitled to request and receive their donor's name and last known address, once they reach the age of 18. These rules do not have retrospective effect. Neither do they create financial or legal obligations on the donor for the child. From October 2023, the first cohort of DCI's (Donor Conceived Individuals) are able to apply for identifiable donor information. The HFEA issued guidance on the disclosure of information relating to gamete donation in 2004 following the new disclosure rules.[17] It lists the disclosures to donors which are permissible as long as the disclosure could not lead to the identification of a person whose identity should be protected. The information which could be disclosed includes telling a donor whether a live birth has resulted from the donation and, if so, the number of such births. Further information is available from the HFEA website. The lifting of anonymity has led to a shortage of donors and the HFEA has considered raising the payment to egg and sperm donors from £250 to £800, although as at 2024 this has not been the case.[18] Following a consultation paper, the Code of Practice section 13A was amended in April 2012 to cover the payment of donors. Centres may pay sperm donors a fixed sum of £35 per clinic visit (maximum of 10 visits, thus a maximum payment of £350, and egg donors can be compensated with a fixed sum of £750 per cycle of donation. For further details see the HFEA Code of Practice section 13A interpretation of mandatory requirements.

The laws relating to disclosure of genetic parentage are now contained in section 31ZA added to the 1990 Act by section 24 of the 2008 Act.

Safety of tissue and cells

Concern has been expressed by the HFEA over the purchase of sperm over the internet. It was announced in January 2004 that the first baby had been born to a lesbian couple following conception by sperm obtained via the internet. New rules came into force in July 2007[19] relating to standards on quality and safety for the donation, procurement, testing, processing, preservation, storage and distribution of tissues and cells which were set out in an EU Directive in 2004.[20] Internet sperm providers must therefore be licensed by the HFEA or have a third party agreement with a licensed centre to ensure standards of quality and safety of the sperm. The announcement that an IVF clinic was raffling a human egg to promote its new baby profiling service led to understandable concern[21] and a discussion on whether the law should permit a marketplace in human material.[22] In the UK donors can only receive reasonable expenses for their gifts and fixed sums as set out above.

Human Fertilisation and Embryology Act 1990 as amended by 2008 Act

The 1990 Act was passed to implement the recommendations of the Warnock Committee.[23] A summary of the provisions of the 1990 Act (as amended) is set out in Statute Box 21.1. It covered three main areas of activity:

1. licensed treatments, i.e. any fertility treatment that involves the use of donated eggs or sperm, or embryos created outside the body (i.e. IVF);
2. storage of eggs, sperm and embryos;
3. research on human embryos.

Statute 21.1

Provisions of the Human Fertilisation and Embryology Act 1990 as amended by the 2008 Act

1. Definition of terms 'embryo' and 'gamete' revised in 2008.
2. Specific activities prohibited: some completely; others without a licence (see Statute Box 21.2).
3. Human Fertilisation and Embryology Authority established with the function of:
   - reviewing information about embryos and advising Secretary of State
   - publicising services provided to public by HFEA or in pursuance of licences
   - providing advice and information
   - other functions specified in regulations
   - monitor committees to grant licences
   - giving directions
   - providing an annual report
   - maintaining a statement of general principles
   - promoting compliance with legal provisions and Code of Practice
   - carrying out its duties effectively, efficiently and economically.
4. Licences for treatment, storage, research and conditions of holding licence.
5. Code of practice to be issued by HFEA subject to Secretary of State's approval.
6. Definition of 'mother' and 'father'.
7. Register of information to be kept by HFEA with restriction on disclosure.
8. Amendments to Surrogacy Arrangements Act 1985 by providing that no surrogacy arrangement is enforceable by or against any of the persons making it.
9. Changes to Abortion Act 1967 (see chapter 14).
10. Protection of those with conscientious objection.
11. Powers of enforcement given to HFEA including power to enter premises.
12. Offences established.

Statute 21.2

Prohibited Activities

3 Prohibitions in connection with embryos

(1) No person shall bring about the creation of an embryo except in pursuance of a licence.

1(A) No person shall keep or use an embryo except—
  (a) in pursuance of a licence, or
  (b) in the case of –
    (i) the keeping, without storage, of an embryo intended for human application, or
    (ii) the processing, without storage, of such an embryo in pursuance of a third party agreement.
1(B) No person shall procure or distribute an embryo intended for human application except in pursuance of a licence or a third party agreement.
(2) No person shall place in a woman—
  (a) an embryo other than a permitted embryo (as defined by section 3ZA (see Statute Box 21.3)), or
  (b) any gametes other than permitted eggs or permitted sperm (as so defined).
(3) A licence cannot authorise—
  (a) keeping or using an embryo after the appearance of the primitive streak,
  (b) placing an embryo in any animal, or
  (c) keeping or using an embryo in any circumstances in which regulations prohibit its keeping or use.
(4) For the purposes of subsection (3)(a) above, the primitive streak is to be taken to have appeared in an embryo not later than the end of the period of 14 days beginning with the day on which the process of creating the embryo began, not counting any time during which the embryo is stored.

3A Prohibitions in connection with germ cells

(1) No person shall, for the purpose of providing fertility services for any woman, use female germ cells taken or derived from an embryo or a fetus or use embryos created by using such cells.
(2) In this section – 'female germ cells' means cells of the female germ line and includes such cells at any stage of maturity and accordingly includes eggs; and 'fertility services' means medical, surgical or obstetric services provided for the purpose of assisting women to carry children.

4 Prohibitions in connection with gametes

(1) No person shall—
  (a) store any gametes, or
  (b) in the course of providing treatment services for any woman, use—
    (i) any sperm, other than partner-donated sperm which has been neither processed nor stored,
    (ii) the woman's eggs after processing or storage, or
    (iii) the eggs of any other woman, except in pursuance of a licence.
1(A) No person shall procure, test, process or distribute any gametes intended for human application except in pursuance of a licence or a third party agreement.
(2) A licence cannot authorise storing or using gametes in any circumstances in which regulations prohibit their storage or use.

(3) No person shall place sperm and eggs in a woman in any circumstances specified in regulations except in pursuance of a licence.

(4) Regulations made by virtue of subsection (3) above may provide that, in relation to licences only to place sperm and eggs in a woman in such circumstances, sections 12 to 22 of this Act shall have effect with such modifications as may be specified in the regulations.

(5) Activities regulated by this section or section 3 or 4A of this Act are referred to in this Act as 'activities governed by this Act'.

4A Prohibitions in connection with genetic material not of human origin

(1) No person shall place in a woman—
  (a) a human admixed embryo,
  (b) any other embryo that is not a human embryo, or
  (c) any gametes other than human gametes.

(2) No person shall—
  (a) mix human gametes with animal gametes,
  (b) bring about the creation of a human admixed embryo, or
  (c) keep or use a human admixed embryo, except in pursuance of a licence.

(3) A licence cannot authorise keeping or using a human admixed embryo after the earliest of the following—
  (a) the appearance of the primitive streak, or
  (b) the end of the period of 14 days beginning with the day on which the process of creating the human admixed embryo began, but not counting any time during which the human admixed embryo is stored.

(4) A licence cannot authorise placing a human admixed embryo in an animal.

(5) A licence cannot authorise keeping or using a human admixed embryo in any circumstances in which regulations prohibit its keeping or use.

(6) For the purposes of this Act a human admixed embryo is—
  (a) an embryo created by replacing the nucleus of an animal egg or of an animal cell, or two animal pronuclei, with (i) two human pronuclei, (ii) one nucleus of a human gamete or of any other human cell, or (iii) one human gamete or other human cell,
  (b) any other embryo created by using – (i) human gametes and animal gametes, or (ii) one human pronucleus and one animal pronucleus,
  (c) a human embryo that has been altered by the introduction of any sequence of nuclear or mitochondrial DNA of an animal into one or more cells of the embryo,
  (d) a human embryo that has been altered by the introduction of one or more animal cells, or
  (e) any embryo not falling within paragraphs (a) to (d) which contains both nuclear or mitochondrial DNA of a human and nuclear or mitochondrial DNA of an animal ('animal DNA') but in which the animal DNA is not predominant.

(7) In subsection (6)—
  (a) references to animal cells are to cells of an animal or of an animal embryo, and
  (b) references to human cells are to cells of a human or of a human embryo.
(8) For the purposes of this section an 'animal' is an animal other than man.
(9) In this section 'embryo' means a live embryo, including an egg that is in the process of fertilisation or is undergoing any other process capable of resulting in an embryo.
(10) In this section—
  (a) references to eggs are to live eggs, including cells of the female germ line at any stage of maturity, but (except in subsection (9)) not including eggs that are in the process of fertilisation or are undergoing any other process capable of resulting in an embryo, and
  (b) references to gametes are to eggs (as so defined) or to live sperm, including cells of the male germ line at any stage of maturity.
(11) If it appears to the Secretary of State necessary or desirable to do so in the light of developments in science or medicine, regulations may—
  (a) amend (but not repeal) paragraphs (a) to (e) of subsection (6),
  (b) provide that in this section 'embryo', 'eggs' or 'gametes' includes things specified in the regulations which would not otherwise fall within the definition.
(12) Regulations made by virtue of subsection (11)(a) may make any amendment of subsection (7) that appears to the Secretary of State to be appropriate in consequence of any amendment of subsection (6).

The definition of permitted eggs, sperm and embryos is shown in Statute Box 21.3.

Statute 21.3
Definition of permitted eggs, sperm and embryos – section 3ZA

(1) This section has effect for the interpretation of section 3(2).
(2) A permitted egg is one—
  (a) which has been produced by or extracted from the ovaries of a woman, and
  (b) whose nuclear or mitochondrial DNA has not been altered.
(3) Permitted sperm are sperm—
  (a) which have been produced by or extracted from the testes of a man, and
  (b) whose nuclear or mitochondrial DNA has not been altered.
(4) An embryo is a permitted embryo if—
  (a) it has been created by the fertilisation of a permitted egg by permitted sperm,
  (b) no nuclear or mitochondrial DNA of any cell of the embryo has been altered, and
  (c) no cell has been added to it other than by division of the embryo's own cells.

> (5) Regulations may provide that—
>   (a) an egg can be a permitted egg, or
>   (b) an embryo can be a permitted embryo, even though the egg or embryo has had applied to it in prescribed circumstances a prescribed process designed to prevent the transmission of serious mitochondrial disease.
> (6) In this section—
>   (a) 'woman' and 'man' include respectively a girl and a boy (from birth), and
>   (b) 'prescribed' means prescribed by regulations.

In vitro fertilisation (IVF)

The Human Fertilisation and Embryology Act 1990 (as amended) provides a framework for the control of the external fertilisation of an egg, extracted from the ovary, with semen. It covers the disposal of unwanted embryos, their ownership, authorisation to undertake research on these embryos, embryo donation to another woman or genetic engineering to prevent hereditary disorders or to create a superhuman. It also covers human admixed embryos. Fertilisation outside the body coupled with transfer of the embryo into the uterus is, in its most simple form, a means of overcoming a fertility problem in a married couple. However, because of the possibility of egg and semen donation and subsequent transfer to a woman other than the provider of the egg, a complex situation can arise. In addition, it can be coupled with a surrogacy arrangement whereby a couple for whom the woman is unable to carry a child arrange for an embryo created from their egg and semen to be inserted into a host woman who will return the child to the genetic parents after birth. The surrogacy arrangements are considered below. This part will deal with IVF and ET (embryo transfer) to the uterus.

The majority of the Warnock Committee recommended a time limit of 14 days on research on an embryo because at about the 15th day after conception the formation of the primitive streak can be identified. This is the first of several identifiable features that develop in and from the embryonic disc during the succeeding days. Information about the process of approving research proposals can be obtained from the HFEA website. It involves five stages: contacting HFEA; applying for a licence or renewal; undergoing peer review; inspection; and presentation to the research licence committee. Regulations relating to the disclosure of protected information for the purposes of research came into force on 6 April 2010.[24] The HFEA decided to publish details of the success rates of individual IVF clinics on an improved website. Couples are able to assess the 'predicted chance' of a live birth after treatment at individual clinics.[25]

Refusal to permit IVF

In a case in 1987[26] the High Court refused an application for judicial review of decisions by consultants who decided that a woman should be refused IVF treatment, on the grounds of past convictions and her prostitution. Section 13(5) of the 1990 Act made it a condition of any licence that treatment services are not to be provided unless account had been taken of the welfare of the child who may be born as a result of the treatment (including the need of that child for a father) and of any other child who may be affected by the birth. The 2008 Act amended this provision to substitute 'supportive parenting' for 'father'. The Code of Practice issued by the

HFEA gives further advice on how the licensed centres should assess these welfare issues and its guidance was updated in 2010.[27] HFEA issued new guidance in 2013 on how clinics should make an assessment of the welfare of any child who may be born as a result of treatment services.[28] In 1994 a 37-year-old woman was refused IVF treatment through the NHS on the grounds of her age.[29] Her application to the High Court to quash the health authority's decision failed on the grounds that, in the light of its limited resources, a health authority policy to set an age limit was not unreasonable. The HFEA Code of Practice does not stipulate any age limitation and paragraph 8.7 advises centres to assess applicants in a non-discriminatory way and not discriminate on the grounds of gender, race, disability, sexual orientation, religious belief or age. However, under the amended section 13(5) of the Act, cited above, it could be decided that the welfare of the child would be adversely affected by an elderly applicant.

The Court of Appeal overturned the decision of the High Court in a case where a couple had agreed to have IVF treatment that was unsuccessful on the first attempt. The couple then separated, but the woman did not tell the clinic and then, on the next attempt, became pregnant. Her former partner sought a declaration that he was the child's legal father and wished to establish contact. The High Court ruled that he was the legal father of the three-year-old girl. However, the woman's appeal succeeded. The Court of Appeal held that the wording of the 1990 Act meant that the partner of a woman receiving treatment with donor sperm will be the father of any resulting child only if the couple are receiving that treatment together, at the time that the sperm or embryo is placed in the womb. The House of Lords dismissed the appeal.[30]

A summary of the provisions of the Human Fertilisation and Embryology Act 1990 as amended by the 2008 Act on IVF is set out in Statute Box 21.1.

On 20 July 1994, the HFEA ruled that eggs from aborted fetuses could not be used in fertility treatment, but they could be used in research. The same ruling applies to the eggs of a dead woman, even though she is carrying a donor card. Guidance on the donation of sperm, eggs and embryos was published by the HFEA in January 2006 and implemented on 1 April 2006.[31] The report of the Sperm, Egg and Embryo Donation (SEED) review covers the adoption of professional standards for donor screening, greater clarity around the number of families that may be created using each donor and new guidance to help centres avoid exceeding this limit, new directions on the reimbursement of donors' expenses and compensation for loss of earnings, guidance on egg sharing and HFEA's policy on authorising imports and exports of gametes and embryos. The SEED Report can be downloaded from the HFEA website.[32]

In 2010 the HFEA commenced a review on many of its policies, including:

- the number of families to which donors can donate;
- expenses and compensation that donors can receive for donation;
- donation between family members; and
- the restrictions which donors can place on the use of their gametes or embryos.

A new edition of the HFEA Code of Practice was published in 2010 following the implementation of the Human Fertilisation and Embryology Act 2008 and was updated in October 2019 and revised in October 2023 to reflect recent developments.[33]

An infertile man who attempted to become a legal father to a sperm-donor baby simply by signing his partner's IVF consent form failed when the Court of Appeal overruled a paternity declaration in his favour by a High Court judge.[34]

Obtaining fertility treatment within the NHS has varied from health authority to health authority, with some couples having to pay as much as £3000 to obtain each private fertility treatment, while others are able to obtain the treatment on the NHS. In November 2000 the

Secretary of State for Health asked NICE (see chapter 5) to review the various fertility treatments with a view to ending the postcode lottery and to draw up national guidelines for the provision of fertility treatment within the NHS. NICE reported in August 2003 and recommended that women between 23 and 29 should be entitled to free IVF treatment under the NHS. NICE guidelines on IVF were published in February 2004 and recommended that all women between the ages of 23 and 39 should be offered three cycles of IVF. Following this, the Department of Health recommended that initially women under 40 years who had been unable to conceive after two years should have one course of IVF treatment, if appropriate, under the NHS. In its response to the Joint Committee scrutiny of the draft Human Tissue and Embryos Bill, the government stated that legislation was not an option to enforce NICE guidelines covering IVF treatment on primary care trusts and foundation trusts but the DH was funding a three-year programme of work that aimed to reduce inequalities in the provision of IVF. In 2009 NICE reported an increase in the number of centres which were offering the recommended three cycles of IVF. New guidance was issued by NICE in 2013 which suggests that women aged under 40 years should be offered three full cycles of IVF, women over 40 years one full cycle.[35] However, in July 2014 Mid Essex CCG stated that financial problems had resulted in IVF treatments only being available to HIV positive men and cancer patients (see chapter 5). The RCN published a policy briefing on the provision of infertility treatment in England.[36] It noted that around one in six couples in the UK have problems conceiving and over three million babies have been born worldwide as a result of IVF. This policy briefing states that full implementation of the NICE guidelines on IVF treatment would help many couples who are unable to conceive naturally. The briefing discusses how patient safety would be improved by implementing the NICE guidelines. It also highlights the key role that specialist nurses play in IVF, as they care for and inform the patient during what can be a highly emotional and stressful treatment. A lesbian couple won the right to have IVF on the NHS following a legal fight.[37] They were supported by the Equality and Human Rights Commission.

A new cheaper method of IVF known as the 'Alka-Seltzer IVF' is being promoted and is thought to be able to end the postcode lottery which currently exists in the NHS over obtaining IVF treatment.[38] Recent scientific developments have improved the chances of IVF succeeding.[39]

Embryos

The 1990 Act prohibits certain actions in relation to the use of embryos (see Statute Box 21.2). However, there were doubts as to whether the Act and therefore the HFEA prevented the use of embryos for stem cell research or human cloning. The definition of embryo has been the subject of dispute. Section 1 of the 1990 Act stated that '(a) an embryo means a live human embryo where fertilisation is complete and (b) references to an embryo include an egg in the process of fertilisation'. The House of Lords held that organisms created by cell nuclear replacement (CNR) came within the definition of 'embryo' in section 1(1) of the 1990 Act and accordingly were subject to regulation by the HFEA.[40] In the High Court[41] it had been held that live human embryos created outside the body by CNR were not 'embryos' within section 1 and accordingly were not subject to regulation under the Act. The Court of Appeal[42] allowed the appeal against this decision and the House of Lords dismissed the appeal against the decision of the Court of Appeal. In the light of the High Court decision (which meant that embryos created by CNR were not subject to the 1990 Act and therefore could be cloned) the Human Reproductive Cloning Act 2001 was passed and came into force on 4 December 2001 to prohibit the placing in a woman of a human embryo which has been created otherwise than by fertilisation. Proceedings could only be brought with the consent of the Director of Public Prosecutions. The 2001 Act was repealed by the 2008 Act since it was superseded by the provisions of section 3. Regulations to enable research on stem cells to take place within the provisions of the 1990 Act[43] were enacted and subsequently re-enacted in the 2008 Act. These enabled a licence to be issued for research for the purposes of increasing the knowledge about the development of embryos, increasing knowledge about serious disease or enabling any such knowledge to be applied in developing treatments for serious disease. The UK Stem Cell Bank has issued a Code of Practice on the use of stem cells but this has no legal force. Proposals to prevent research using hybrid embryos (formed from human and animal cells) which were to be included in new legislation were dropped following pressure from the scientific community.

A new section 3A was added to the 1990 Act (by the Criminal Justice and Public Order Act 1994) which prohibited the use of female germ cells derived from an embryo or fetus for the provision of treatment services for any woman.

Three-parent embryos

Regulations were published by the HFEA in December 2016 to enable the procedure whereby diseased mitochondria is removed from one egg and replaced by healthy mitochondria from another egg and then fertilised and implanted in the woman who carries the genetic mitochondrial defect. The HFEA granted their first license to Newcastle University in March 2017. On 6 February 2018, two women who were carrying mitochondrial mutations received licenses to undergo mitochondrial replacement therapy (MRT).

Criminal offences and civil wrongs relating to embryos

There have been several cases where mistakes have been made in the implantation of embryos. In one case a woman was told that her embryo had been thawed and unfortunately implanted in another woman's womb.[44] When the other woman found out that the embryo was not hers, she had an abortion. The Cardiff and Vale NHS Trust paid out compensation. In another case at the same hospital an embryo was lost when the tube and needle transferring them to the woman's womb became disconnected.[45] The Court had to rule in a case where, at the assisted conception unit of Leeds General Infirmary, eggs were inadvertently fertilised by the wrong man's sperm and as a result mixed race twins were born to white parents, Mr and Mrs A. Both couples, Mr and Mrs A and Mr and Mrs B, were having IVF treatment. The biological father Mr B wished to be declared the legal father of the twins. Dame Elizabeth Butler-Sloss, President of the Family Division, held that Mr B was the twins' legal father. The husband of a mother whose child is born after treatment with another man's sperm is the child's legal father, providing the husband consented to the treatment. Although Mr A had consented to his wife's treatment, he had not consented to the use of another man's sperm. The judge held that the twins' rights to respect for their family life with their mother and Mr A could be met by appropriate family or adoption orders and those orders would be proportionate to the infringements of those rights.[46] Another mishap occurred in Bristol when frozen sperm from 28 cancer patients whose treatment may have left them sterile was destroyed when a freezer unit broke down. An inquiry was set up[47] and subsequently six patients were successful in a claim against the North Bristol NHS Trust. The Court of Appeal allowed the appeal against the dismissal of the case holding that the sperm was property belonging to the men and they had a claim in tort and bailment and could recover for psychiatric injury or mental distress.[48] In a criminal case an embryologist was jailed for 18 months for deceiving couples by giving them test tubes containing saline solution instead of embryos.[49]

In July 2014 the HFEA admitted that about 550 incidents a year were reported, less than 1 per cent of the 60,000 cycles of IVF carried out. Of these only three fell into category A: the most serious. These included a family being given the wrong donor sperm, frozen sperm being destroyed and the third involved 11 embryos contaminated with cellular debris.[50]

Could donors be sued for any reason? A donor-conceived person born with an abnormality could sue their donor for damages if it is proven that the donor had not told the clinic relevant facts about their or their families' medical history when they donated.

Human Fertilisation and Embryology Authority (HFEA)

The HFEA was established under the provisions of the 1990 Act. It has the power to issue licences for centres to carry out IVF treatment and inspect them. It also issues a Code of Practice for the centres and provides guidance to the government on new areas for litigation and control.[51] The Human Genetics Advisory Commission (HGAC) operated from December 1996 to December 1999, providing the government with independent advice on issues arising from developments in human genetics. It published papers on: insurance and genetic testing (December 1997); cloning (December 1998); and employment and genetic testing (July 1999). It was replaced by the Human Genetics Commission (HGC) in December 1999, which also replaced the Advisory Committee on Genetic Testing and the Advisory Group on Scientific Advances in Genetics. The HGC had the remit of advising on necessary changes to the advisory and regulatory framework, of providing information and guidance to the minister on general issues in human genetics. Other non-statutory bodies advising in this area were: Gene Therapy Advisory Committee; Genetics and Insurance Committee; and the Nuffield Council on Bioethics, an independent body established by the trustees of the Nuffield Foundation in 1991 to consider the ethical issues arising from developments in medicine and biology.

The powers of the HFEA to refuse to authorise the implantation of more than three embryos in a particular patient were challenged by a clinic.[52] The court refused the application, holding that the court had no authority to intervene to quash the decision of the HFEA in circumstances where careful and thorough consideration had been given to the matter and opinion provided that was plainly rational. While the decisions of the authority were open to judicial review, they were only amenable to such scrutiny in circumstances where the authority had either exceeded or abused its powers. The Expert Group of the HFEA published the *One Child at a Time* report in October 2006, following which HFEA issued a public consultation on the issue of multiple births after IVF in October 2007. Following the consultation, the HFEA decided to adopt an outcome-based policy, which allowed centres the flexibility to develop their own elective single embryo transfer (eSET) strategy that is appropriate for them and the patients they treat. In 2009 (Year 1) the maximum multiple birth rate was 24 per cent (the national average at the time). This meant that no more than 24 per cent of a centre's annual live birth rate should be multiple births. In Year 2 from 6 April 2010 no more than 20 per cent of a centre's annual live birth rate from treatment started from this date should be multiples. The overall aim is to reduce the UK IVF multiple birth rate to 10 per cent in stages over a period of years. However, from 1 January 2014 HFEA no longer requires IVF clinics to keep their multiple birth rate below the HFEA target as one of the conditions for their licence. The decision followed a legal challenge by two clinics and a reduction of multiple births from one in four to one in six.[53] The HFEA has set up a 'One at a time' website, warning of the dangers of multiple births.[54]

Consent provisions for retrieval, storage and use of human gametes under the human fertilisation and embryology acts 1990 and 2008

Diane Blood was refused permission by the HFEA to use the stored sperm from her dead husband on the grounds that the husband had not given written consent for this use as required by the 1990 Act. She brought a case seeking judicial review of the Authority's refusal to license the infertility treatment. The sperm had been taken from her husband as he lay in a coma as a result of meningitis. The Court of Appeal[55] held that, as a result of the restrictions under the 1990 Act, she could not be lawfully treated with the sperm in this country. However, she would be permitted to receive treatment in Belgium according to Article 59 of the EC Treaty. She subsequently became pregnant and gave birth. Following this case, the Minister of Health appointed a committee under the chairmanship of Professor Sheila McLean to review the consent provisions in the Human Fertilisation and Embryology Act 1990. The committee sent out a questionnaire for public consultation and published its report in December 1998. In August 2000, the government published its response to the McLean Report.[56] It accepted all the recommendations of the report and went further, suggesting a retrospective effect.

1. The father's name should be allowed to appear on birth certificates where his sperm has been used after his death.
2. The legal position on consent and removal of gametes should remain unchanged: gametes can be taken from an incapacitated person who is likely to recover, if the removal of gametes is in their best interests.
3. The HFEA should have the power to permit the storage of gametes where consent has not been given, so long as the gametes have been lawfully removed. This will also benefit children who are about to undergo treatment that will affect their future fertility.
4. Families will be able to make these birth certificate changes retrospectively.
5. The best practice is for written consent to be obtained, since this most clearly constitutes effective consent. Where there is doubt over whether an effective consent has been obtained, this should be a matter for the courts.

Subsequently, Diane Blood won her claim to have her late husband legally recognised as the father of her two sons, when the Department of Health dropped its opposition.[57] The judge accepted that her inability to name her deceased husband as the father of her children was contrary to her human rights and he ordered the Department of Health to pay Mrs Blood's £20,000 legal costs. The Human Fertilisation and Embryology (Deceased Fathers) Act 2003, which came into force on 1 December 2003, specifies the circumstances in which a deceased father can be recorded on the birth certificate. The father must have given a written consent before his death. The 2008 Act replaced the provisions in the 1990 Act by section 39. Where a man's sperm is used after his death, the man may be treated as THE child's father, for the purposes of birth registration only, if various conditions are met. The man must have consented, in writing, to the use of the sperm or embryo after his death and to being treated as the child's father for the purposes of birth registration. The woman must elect that he should be treated in this way within 42 days (or 21 days in Scotland) of the child's birth.

The strict wording of the 1990 Act in relation to consent by both parties to the use of the gametes was applied by the High Court in a case[58] where couples who had agreed that embryos could be created and stored then disagreed over their later disposal. One woman placed six frozen embryos into storage before she had cancer treatment. The judge held that the court had no power to override the unconditional statutory right of either party to withdraw or vary consent to the use of embryos in connection with *in vitro* fertilisation treatment at any time before the fertilised embryo was implanted in the woman. In addition, where consent for treatment had originally been given for treatment together with a named partner, that consent remained neither effective nor valid once the parties ceased to be together. Ms Evans lost her appeal to the Court of Appeal in June 2004.[59] Her application to the ECHR for breach of Articles 2, 8 and 14 failed but a dissenting judgment held that there had been a breach of Article 8 and Article 14 in conjunction with Article 8.[60]

In another case,[61] a woman appealed against the decision of the High Court that sperm of her deceased husband should be allowed to perish or be destroyed. The Court of Appeal held, in applying the provisions relating to consent to the storage and use of gametes under sections 4(1)(a) and 11 and Schedule 3 of the 1990 Act, that the centre was entitled to rely on a form that gave consent to the perishing of the sperm and embryos in the event of death or mental incapacities. The Court of Appeal held that there was no evidence of undue influence by the centre and, without an effective consent by the husband, the continued storage and later use of his sperm by the centre would be unlawful. The husband had initially agreed that the sperm could be used after his death, but subsequently withdrew this consent at the request of a specialist nursing sister.

The 2008 Act extended the storage period for embryos from five to ten years. The provision came into force in October 2009. This would have been too late for some women whose embryos had to be destroyed and amendments were made to allow these embryos to be retained.[62]

In a recent case, Beth Warren challenged the deadline of April 2015 after which her dead husband's sperm would be destroyed.[63] The husband, who had died of a brain tumour, had agreed that his sperm could be used after his death but he signed a two-year cut-off clause. The HFEA had informed the widow that it had no power to extend the storage period beyond that to which her husband had given written consent. The High Court held on 6 March 2014 that it was her human right under Article 3 and 8 to be allowed to store his sperm for the next 55 years. She criticised the Care Fertility Clinic in Northampton for not ensuring that the necessary consent arrangements were in place. HFEA decided not to appeal against the ruling because the likelihood of future problems was not strong enough to warrant appealing in this case. The husband's wishes were clearly set out and if it weren't for the clinic's failings Mrs Warren would not have needed to seek a declaration from the court.[64]

Another recent case is that of AB whose husband was in a vegetative state but was given an emergency order for sperm to be removed. The Family Court ruled in the week beginning 16 January 2014 that that order should not have been granted.[65] It was reported that AB was appealing against this and the case was due to be heard in February 2014.[66] However, she has subsequently abandoned the case.

Counselling and consent

The provisions of the 1990 Act in relation to counselling and consent were extended by the 2008 Act. The requirement under the 1990 Act that a woman may not be provided with any treatment services involving donated gametes or embryos, or the use of an embryo which has been created *in vitro*, unless she and any man with whom she is being treated have been provided with relevant information and offered counselling is now extended to same-sex couples.

Before proceeding with embryo transfer or donor insemination, clinics are required to offer counselling and provide relevant information to couples who have given notice that they consent to the intended mother's partner being treated as the parent of a child who is conceived using donor sperm. In 2008 a new Schedule 3ZA (see Statute Box 21.4) was added to the 1990 Act to cover the circumstances in which the offer of counselling is required as a condition of a licence to provide treatment.

Statute 21.4

Schedule 3ZA Circumstances in Which Offer of Counselling Required as Condition of Licence for Treatment

Part 1: Kinds of treatment in relation to which counselling must be offered

1. The treatment services involve the use of the gametes of any person and that person's consent is required under paragraph 5 of Schedule 3 for the use in question.
2. The treatment services involve the use of any embryo the creation of which was brought about in vitro.
3. The treatment services involve the use of an embryo taken from a woman and the consent of the woman from whom the embryo was taken was required under paragraph 7 of Schedule 3 for the use in question.

Part 2: Events in connection with which counselling must be offered

1. A man gives the person responsible a notice under paragraph (a) of subsection (1) of section 37 of the Human Fertilisation and Embryology Act 2008 (agreed fatherhood conditions) in a case where the woman for whom the treatment services are provided has previously given a notice under paragraph (b) of that subsection referring to the man.
2. The woman for whom the treatment services are provided gives the person responsible a notice under paragraph (b) of that subsection in a case where the man to whom the notice relates has previously given a notice under paragraph (a) of that subsection.
3. A woman gives the person responsible notice under paragraph (a) of subsection (1) of section 44 of that Act (agreed female parenthood conditions) in a case where the woman for whom the treatment services are provided has previously given a notice under paragraph (b) of that subsection referring to her.
4. The woman for whom the treatment services are provided gives the person responsible a notice under paragraph (b) of that subsection in a case where the other woman to whom the notice relates has previously given a notice under paragraph (a) of that subsection.

Confidentiality

Section 33 of the 1990 Act placed tight restrictions on the disclosure of information held by the HFEA or a licensing authority. The few exceptions to these restrictions were considered to be inadequate and the Human Fertilisation and Embryology (Disclosure of Information) Act 1992 was passed, amending section 33 as follows: to enable the patient to give specific and general consent to disclosure; for information to be disclosed by a clinician to his legal adviser in relation to legal proceedings (the 1990 Act had permitted disclosures only in relation to action under the Congenital Disabilities (Civil Liability) Act 1976); and for a couple to obtain information about the legal parentage of a child born to a surrogate mother. The 1992 Act was repealed by the Human Fertilisation and Embryology Act 2008 and its provisions incorporated into the 2008 Act in a revised section 33A.

The following sections in the 1990 Act as amended by the 2008 Act cover the keeping and disclosing of information.

Register of information

31ZA. Request for information as to genetic parentage, etc.

31ZB. Request for information as to intended spouse, etc.

31ZC. Power of Authority to inform donor of request for information

31ZD. Provision to donor of information about resulting children

31ZE. Provision of information about donor-conceived genetic siblings

31ZF. Power of Authority to keep voluntary contact register

31ZG. Financial assistance for person setting up or keeping voluntary contact register

31A. The Authority's register of licences

31B. The Authority's register of serious adverse events and serious adverse reactions Information to be provided to Registrar General

33A. Disclosure of information

33B. Power to provide for additional exceptions from section 33A(1)

33C. Disclosure for the purposes of medical or other research

34. Disclosure in interests of justice

35. Disclosure in interests of justice: congenital disabilities, etc.

Section 33A prevents the disclosure of information specified in section 31(2) (identifiable treatment services, gametes, embryos, etc.) unless it comes under one of the exceptions set out in sections 31ZA–E. The legislation can be downloaded from the legislation website.[67]

A person of 18 or over has the right to obtain information from the HFEA if that person was born in consequence of treatment services, but an opportunity for proper counselling must be provided before disclosure. Section 31ZA inserted by the 2008 Act enables those over 16 to obtain non-identifying information from the HFEA.

Surrogacy

This might be thought, like IVF, to be a result of the recent developments in medical technology. However, the biblical story of Abraham resorting to the servant who could bear a child for him because Sarah was barren is an early example of one form of surrogacy. The possibility of embryo implantation has, however, increased the number of ways in which surrogacy can take place. The child that is born might have no genetic relationship with the ultimate parents, but be the natural child of the bearing mother or even an embryo from two donors. More likely, however, is the situation where the child is genetically related to the father as a result of artificial insemination, but not to the adopting mother. Prior to the Warnock Report, the only legislation that covered a surrogacy situation was the childcare legislation and rules relating to adoption. Section 50, for example, of the Adoption Act 1958 prohibits any payment in connection with adoption. Such surrogate cases as Baby Cotton[68] revealed the gaps in the law and the uncertainties surrounding basic questions. Is a contract for surrogacy enforceable by either party, neither party or only by the mother? What are the legal implications if the child is handicapped? What controls do the contracting couple have over the standard of life of the mother during the pregnancy, e.g. what if she smokes or drinks heavily? If she changes her mind and has an abortion, are damages then payable?

Case 21.1 *In re An Adoption (Surrogacy)* [1987]

A surrogacy dispute[69]

Mr and Mrs A were unable to have children and, because of their age, had been refused as adoptive parents. They entered into a surrogacy arrangement with Mrs B who wished to help the childless couple. Under the arrangement, it was agreed that Mr and Mrs A would pay £10,000 to Mrs B who would give up her job to have the child. In due course, a child was conceived, but in the event Mrs B accepted only £5000 and refused the balance. It was clear that the amount did not cover Mrs B's loss of earnings and expenses. After the birth, Mr and Mrs A applied to court for an adoption order. The question arose (a) whether the payment of money had been a payment of reward for adoption within the meaning of the Adoption Act section 50(1) and (b) if there had been a contravention of the section, whether the court could make a retrospective authorisation in respect of the payment under section 50(3) of the Act and grant an adoption order.

In Case 21.1 it was held that a payment to the mother in a surrogacy arrangement did not contravene the Act if payments made by those others to the natural mother did not include an element of profit or financial reward. Even if they were made for reward, the court had a discretion under the Act to authorise the payments retrospectively. The court granted the adoption order.

The Surrogacy Arrangements Act 1985 prohibits the making of surrogacy arrangements on a commercial basis. Those companies that had come over from the USA and started to arrange surrogacy contracts were thus forced out of business in the UK. This approach had been recommended by the Warnock Committee, whose recommendations, however, went further and suggested that both profit- and non-profit-making organisations should be made illegal and also that any professional who knowingly assisted in the establishment of a surrogacy pregnancy should be criminally liable. They recommended that all surrogacy arrangements should be held illegal and unenforceable in the courts. Section 36(i) of the Human Fertilisation and Embryology Act 1990 amended the 1985 Act to make a surrogacy arrangement unenforceable. It did not make it illegal.

The 1990 Act section 30 enabled a court to order a child to be treated as a child to the parties of the marriage where another woman has acted as surrogate, provided that certain conditions are met. In a case in 1996,[70] a couple applied under section 30 for a parental order in respect of a child who was born following a surrogacy arrangement. It was agreed that the unmarried woman would receive £8280 to cover her expenses and loss of earnings. The High Court judge was satisfied that the requirements of section 30 were met. In particular, the mother had given consent (although she admitted to tearing her copy in half) and the payments were reasonable and could be granted retrospectively. In this case, there was no man who was to be treated as the father and whose consent was required. Section 30 of the 1990 Act was repealed by the 2008 Act since its provisions were incorporated in sections 54, 55 and Schedule 6 (see below, Parental orders and surrogacy). In a case in 2007 a couple, Mr and Mrs J, agreed a surrogacy arrangement whereby Mrs P was fertilised by Mr J's sperm. However, Mrs P refused to hand over the child and brought him up as her own child. At the time of the hearing the child was 17 months old. The court awarded custody to the couple and ordered Mrs P to hand over the boy to them. The judge found that Mrs P was motivated by a compulsive desire to bear further children and never intended to let Mr J have the child. The Court of Appeal dismissed Mrs P's appeal. A collection order was made by the Court of Appeal empowering High Court staff to travel to Bristol with Mr J to oversee the handover of the child.[71] (See also the case of *Re T* where it was feared that harm would be caused to the child.)[72]

In 1997, Professor Margaret Brazier was appointed by the Department of Health to review the existing law relating to surrogacy arrangements. The terms of reference included whether payments for expenses should continue to be allowed; whether there was a case for the regulation of surrogacy arrangements through a recognised body and to advise on whether any changes were necessary to the 1985 Act and section 30 of the Human Fertilisation and Embryology Act 1990. An extensive consultation exercise was undertaken and subsequently the Brazier Report recommended that the Surrogacy Arrangements Act 1985 and section 30 of the 1990 Act should be replaced by new legislation and a code of practice on surrogacy should be drawn up by the Department of Health.

The Joint Parliamentary Scrutiny Committee reviewing the draft HFEA Bill recommended that it be amended to bring the regulation of surrogacy within the remit of the HFEA. Eventually the 1985 Act was retained but significant changes were made to the laws relating to surrogacy by section 59 of the 2008 Act. Not-for-profit bodies are permitted to receive payment for carrying out activities in initiating negotiations with a view to the making of a surrogacy arrangement and in compiling information about surrogacy on that basis. However, only reasonable payment can be made (i.e. it does not exceed the costs reasonably attributed to the activity). Not-for-profit bodies will not be permitted to receive payment for offering to negotiate a surrogacy arrangement or for taking part in negotiations about a surrogacy arrangement. These activities are not unlawful if there is no charge. Section 59 also makes changes in relation to advertising by non-profit-making bodies. Under the 1985 Act, it is an offence to publish or distribute an advertisement that someone may be willing to enter into a surrogacy arrangement, or that anyone is looking for a surrogate mother, or that anyone is willing to facilitate or negotiate such an arrangement. This is amended to enable a non-profit-making body to advertise about activities which may legally be undertaken on a commercial basis: for example, that it keeps a list of people seeking surrogate mothers.

Parental orders and surrogacy

Section 54 of the 2008 Act replaces section 30 of the 1990 Act and maintains the same criteria for a parental order as section 30 of the 1990 Act with the exception of the eligibility criteria that now permits civil partners and couples in an enduring family relationship to apply for a parental order, in addition to married couples.

Under section 55 of the 2008 Act regulations have been drawn up which enable specified adoption legislation to be applied, with modifications, to parental orders[73] which came into force on 6 April 2010. For England, Schedule 1 of the regulations apply (with modifications) to the Adoption and Children Act 2002 to a parental order. Thus, principles such as the welfare of the child is the paramount consideration and a checklist for determining the welfare of the child will apply to a parental order.

Compensation amounts and surrogacy

In a case in 2000,[74] a woman claimed compensation as a result of medical negligence that led to a stillborn child and a subtotal hysterectomy. The defendant health authority accepted liability, but damages were disputed. She claimed in addition to damages for pain, suffering and loss of amenity, compensation for the post-traumatic stress disorder as a result of the stillbirth and hysterectomy, loss of earnings and the cost of surrogacy. The court held that she would be awarded £66,000 for the infertility and the accompanying psychological condition. It refused, however, to compensate her for loss of earnings, since it held that regardless of the stillbirth and hysterectomy, she would not have been able to start her training as a teacher earlier. The court also refused the cost of surrogacy, which the claimant was arranging in the USA. The judge held that, under the present UK law, surrogacy arrangements were unenforceable and, if commercial, illegal. It would therefore be wrong, and contrary to public policy, that damages should be awarded to enable an unenforceable and unlawful contract to be entered into. The judge did not conclude that it would always be wrong to award damages for the cost of surrogacy, but in the claimant's particular circumstances, she could not succeed.

The law relating to surrogacy is as follows:

- The surrogate has the legal right to keep the child, even if it is not genetically related to her (unless she would pose a risk to the child).
- Surrogacy arrangements are not legally enforceable, even if a contract has been signed and the expenses of the surrogate have been paid.
- The surrogate will be the legal mother of the child unless or until parenthood is transferred to the intended mother through a parental order or adoption after the birth of the child.
- The surrogate has the legal right to change her mind and keep the child, even when the baby she gave birth to is not genetically related to her.
- The child's legal father or second parent is the surrogate's husband, civil partner (unless it is shown that husband/civil partner did not consent to the treatment) or partner (if the partner consented to being the father/second parent).
- If treatment was performed in a licensed clinic and the surrogate mother has no partner, the child will have no legal father or second parent.
- If the intended parents wish to become the legal parents of the child, they may either apply to adopt the child, or apply for a parental order. A parental order transfers the rights and obligations of parentage to the intended parents, providing certain conditions are met (section 54 of the 2008 Act).
- Applications for a parental order must generally be made to the court within six months of the birth of the child.
- To obtain a parental order, at least one of the commissioning couple must be genetically related to the baby, i.e. be the egg or sperm provider. Couples must be husband and wife, civil partners or two persons who are living as partners.

- If the commissioning couple cannot apply for a parental order because neither of them are genetically related to the baby (i.e. donor egg and donor sperm or donor embryos were used), then adoption of the baby is the only option available to them.
- A registered adoption agency must be involved in the surrogacy process if adoption is required.

The dangers of informal surrogacy arrangements were highlighted in March 2014 when a High Court judge held that turkey baster-style insemination left a mother with no parental rights over the baby. The judge warned against illegal private surrogacy arrangements. The woman had done a deal with a friend who was artificially inseminated with her husband's sperm. The marriage broke down shortly after the birth of the boy but the woman, being neither the boy's legal or biological parent had no parental rights. The birth certificate contained the names of the boy's father and the surrogate mother. The judge granted the woman a residency order to care for the child. The surrogate mother was banned from exercising her parental rights without permission from the court.[75]

In August 2013[76] the HFEA amended its requirements to allow one of the intended parents commissioning a surrogacy arrangement to be recognised as the legal parent when the child is born, if certain conditions are met and the relevant consents are in place.

Conscientious objection

The nurse's personal moral beliefs are taken into account by section 38 of the Human Fertilisation and Embryology Act 1990, which provides a conscientious objection clause as follows:

1. No person who has a conscientious objection to participating in any activity governed by this Act shall be under any duty, however arising, to do so.
2. In any legal proceedings, the burden of proof of conscientious objection shall rest on the person claiming to rely on it.
3. In any proceedings before a court in Scotland, a statement on oath by any person to the effect that he has a conscientious objection to participating in a particular activity governed by the Act shall be sufficient evidence of that fact for the purpose of discharging the burden of proof imposed by subsection (2) above.

Genetics

Considerable progress has been made in the science of gene identification. The Human Genome Project was an international collaboration by the US government and the Wellcome Trust that started in 1990. It aimed to identify every gene in the human body. At the same time, a private company, Celera Genomics Corp., headed by Craig Venter, was pursuing the same object. The project was completed on 26 July 2000 when a dead heat was claimed between the two rival organisations. The mapping of the human genome was declared complete in April 2003, two years ahead of schedule,[77] producing a 'book of life' containing 2.9 billion 'letters' of human DNA. Genes linked with some specific hereditary diseases have now been identified. One of the first genes to be linked with a specific disease was that of cystic fibrosis. Subsequently, there have been claims of genetic links with a wide range of medical conditions and human qualities and characteristics. For example, claims have been made for genetic links for sleeplessness,[78] for heart disease,[79] for dyslexia,[80, 81] for hibernation,[82] for diseases of old age,[83] for autism,[84] for early menopause,[85] for asthma[86] and many other disorders and characteristics. These discoveries present many ethical and legal issues: to what extent should parents have the right to modify the genetic inheritance of their children? What controls should there be over individuals purchasing commercial testing kits? Should insurers have the right to compel those seeking insurance to be tested? Baroness Kennedy was appointed by the government to head an inquiry into the implications of the mapping of the human genetic code and a White Paper on genetics was published in June 2003.[87] Its aim was to set out a vision of how patients could benefit in future from advances in genetics in healthcare. It presented a comprehensive plan for preparing the NHS, including the investment of £50 million over three years, to realise the benefits of genetics in healthcare. Initiatives included the upgrading of laboratories and increase in the numbers of health professionals involved in genetics, including counsellors, consultants and scientists; a new genetics education and development centre and new research programmes in pharmacogenetics, gene therapy and health services research. The Human Genetics Commission (HGC) and the National Screening Committee studied the ethical, social, scientific, economic and practical considerations of screening, and its report[88] *Choosing the Future* was published in 2004. In November 2007 the HGC began preparation for a citizen's inquiry into the use of DNA, details of which are available on its website. In August 2010 the HGC published a new Code of Practice. It expressed concerns about parental consent for DNA testing of their children. Such tests should be confined to cases where there is an immediate and compelling medical reason.[89] The HGC stated that such tests could infringe the rights of the child to take health decisions for themselves when they are adults. The HGC Code of Practice is for guidance only. It recommended that counselling should be offered before and after tests for serious genetic mutations such as those causing Huntington's disease and some forms of breast cancer. (See chapter 8 for discussion on DNA databases and acquittals in the criminal courts.) Following a review of quangos, the HGC published its final paper in 2012. It has been reconstituted as a Departmental Expert Committee.

Genetic testing for pregnant women

Which pregnant women should be offered genetic testing? The HGC[90] has issued guidance for consultation on behalf of the former Advisory Committee on Genetic Testing, whose work it has taken over. The guidance suggests that a woman should have access to prenatal genetic tests and the expertise she requires appropriate to her risk. There should be resources in primary care and hospitals for referral and subsequent care of the patient. Prenatal genetic testing for rare disorders should be arranged on a supra-regional or national level.

Gene therapy and genetic diagnosis

The Clothier Committee[91] recommended that research should continue for somatic cell gene therapy where treatment is given to an individual patient to alleviate disease (e.g. cystic fibrosis). However, germ-line gene therapy, where future generations are affected, should not as yet be lawful. It recommended the establishment of a supervisory body, the Gene Therapy Advisory Committee (GTAC). In its ninth annual report (which is available online)[92] the GTAC reviewed the use of gene therapy in treating children with X-linked severe combined immunodeficiency (leukaemia had developed in two of the children treated with gene therapy) and recommended that recruitment into the trials should only be on a case-by-case basis. The United Kingdom Ethics Committee Authority recognised GTAC as the UK research ethics committee for all gene trials under the new legislation governing clinical trials. The GTAC issued guidance in 2004 on gene therapy. It must be approved by GTAC, must not interfere with the germ-line and must not put patients at disproportionate risk.[93] In its 13th annual report it stated that it considered 14 applications for gene therapy clinical trials and they were all approved or conditionally approved. Around 1300 patients had been enrolled on to UK gene therapy trials by December 2006. GTAC has worked with the Department of Health, along with other regulators of stem cell research, to develop an online resource for researchers called the 'UK stem cell tool kit'. The website allows stem cell researchers to build a customised map outlining all of the regulatory steps to take their ideas for a new treatment from the laboratory to patients. In October 2010 the government announced that, following the Advisory Non-Departmental Public Bodies (ANDPB) Review, GTAC no longer needed to report and provide advice directly to Ministers, and that responsibility for supporting its Research Ethics Committee (REC) statutory functions should be transferred to the National Research Ethics Service (NRES) (see chapter 17).

Pre-implantation genetic diagnosis (PGD)

The HFEA and the Advisory Committee on Genetic Testing established in 1998 a joint working group to prepare a consultation paper on pre-implantation genetic diagnosis (PGD). This paper was published in November 1999.[94] PGD refers to the two-stage process in which IVF is used to create embryos that are then tested for a particular genetic disorder or to establish their sex (where the disorder is sex-linked). Embryos that do not carry the genetic disorder or are not of the potentially affected sex can then be transferred to the uterus in the hope that a pregnancy of a child without the hereditary condition will develop. Four centres in the UK are licensed to carry out PGD. Testing for cystic fibrosis is the most common reason for PGD for a single gene defect. However, there were concerns about the range of conditions for which PGD should be licensed, at the seriousness of the condition to be checked for, whether the late onset of a condition should be taken into account and what the nature of the regulation should be.

PGD has also been used in circumstances where parents wish to have a child who would be compatible with and therefore of life-saving assistance for a sibling who is suffering from a genetic disease. Several cases have been contested.

In a case that contrasts with Case 21.2, the HFEA turned down the application from the Witakers to use IVF techniques to select a baby who would be a perfect tissue match for Charlie,

Case 21.2   R (Quintavalle) v HFEA [2002–5]

Tissue typing for the benefit of a sibling[95]

Raj and Shahana Hashmi wished to bear a child who would be free of the genetic blood disorder, beta thalassaemia major, and whose tissue type would match that of their young son Zain, who suffered from the life-threatening disorder. They hoped that stem cells from blood taken from the umbilical cord of a newborn baby with matching tissue would cure their son. They applied to the HFEA for a licence for PGD. HFEA decided that tissue typing would only be permitted where PGD was already necessary to avoid the passing on of a serious genetic disorder and that licences would be granted on a case-by-case basis and on certain conditions. HFEA granted a licence permitting PGD and tissue typing as part of the couple's *in vitro* fertilisation treatment. The granting of the licence was challenged by Josephine Quintavalle on behalf of Comment on Reproductive Ethics who succeeded in an application for judicial review of the lawfulness of HFEA actions. HFEA appealed to the Court of Appeal.

The Court of Appeal held that the HFEA had the power to grant a licence to permit simultaneous tests to be carried out on an embryo for the purpose not only of identifying genetic defects in the embryo but also of ascertaining whether the tissue type of the embryo would match that of an existing child. The House of Lords dismissed the appeal against the Court of Appeal ruling and held that HFEA's discretion to award a licence for tissue typing of an embryo was not limited to its testing for defects in the embryo.

---

aged 3, who had a rare blood disorder and required a bone marrow transplant. The HFEA refused the application because embryos may be screened only if they might carry a serious genetic risk.[96] The Witakers subsequently obtained treatment in the USA.

These issues were the subject of an extensive consultation by the HFEA, which published its report in July 2004.[97] It concluded that balancing the likely benefit of pre-implantation tissue typing – to the sick sibling, the new baby and the family as a whole – against a better understanding of the possible physical and psychological risk to the child to be born, pre-implantation tissue typing should be available subject to appropriate safeguards, in cases in which there is a genuine need for potential life-saving tissue and a likelihood of therapeutic benefit for an affected child. In January 2006 the Human Genetics Commission published *Making Babies*,[98] an overview of reproductive decisions and genetic technologies. One of its many significant recommendations and conclusions was that the anxiety that PGD lies on the slippery slope leading to the possibility of a wide range of potential enhancements, such as intelligence or beauty, is misplaced. The HFEA has published a list of over 100 conditions which could justify the fertility clinic, using PGD, to screen out without seeking special permission. These include conditions which are not life-threatening[99] and are therefore controversial. Using PGD to reveal the sex of the embryo is not permissible unless it is related to a genetic disease (e.g. haemophilia). A New York clinic is offering sex prediction services on embryos to couples from the UK.[100] Since 2009 PGD can be used by families with a history of a genetic disorder to select unaffected embryos for IVF. PGD can be used for some later onset diseases, for example breast cancer.[101]

Embryo testing for genetic disease or sex selection now comes under Schedule 2 of the 2008 Act: activities which may be licensed under the 1990 Act. Under section 1ZA of Schedule 2 a licence cannot authorise the testing of an embryo except for one or more specified purposes. These purposes include establishing whether there is a genetic abnormality, establishing the sex where there is a particular risk that the child be seriously physically or mentally ill as a result of a gender-related abnormality. The purposes also include a situation where a sibling suffers from a serious medical condition which could be treated by umbilical cord blood stem cells, bone marrow or other tissue of any resulting child, establishing whether the tissue of any resulting child would be compatible with that of the sibling.

Gender selection

To what extent should parents be able to select the sex of their children? Certainly in some cultures, parental selection could lead to an oversupply of boys and very few girls, but there may be justification for it when hereditary diseases, such as haemophilia, are sex-linked. A commercial organisation has been set up to assist couples in obtaining the gender of their choice for their child. Where this does not involve gametes of other persons, it does not come under the provision of the 1990 Act as amended. Some consider, however, that there should be controls in this field. A public consultation paper was issued by the HFEA in January 1993.[102] In November 2003 the HFEA announced its recommendations on sex selection.[103] It found from its survey that public opposition to sex selection for non-medical reasons was clear and consistent. As a result of the Tissue and Cells Directive, which came into force in July 2007,[104] sperm-sorting services are now subject to regulation. Schedule 2 as amended covers the testing of embryos for sex selection and is shown in Statute Box 21.5.

Statute 21.5
Schedule 2 Activities that may be licensed under the 1990 Act

Sex selection

(1) A licence under paragraph 1 cannot authorise any practice designed to secure that any resulting child will be of one sex rather than the other.
(2) Sub-paragraph (1) does not prevent the authorisation of any testing of embryos that is capable of being authorised under paragraph 1ZA.
(3) Sub-paragraph (1) does not prevent the authorisation of any other practices designed to secure that any resulting child will be of one sex rather than the other in a case where there is a particular risk that a woman will give birth to a child who will have or develop—
   (a) a gender-related serious physical or mental disability,
   (b) a gender-related serious illness, or
   (c) any other gender-related serious medical condition.
(4) For the purposes of sub-paragraph (3), a physical or mental disability, illness or other medical condition is gender-related if the Authority is satisfied that—
   (a) it affects only one sex, or
   (b) it affects one sex significantly more than the other.

Genetic screening and testing

Concern at the possibility that insurers and employers would require compulsory genetic screening led to the Nuffield Council on Bioethics reporting on the ethical issues involved in genetic screening. It recommended safeguards in relation to consent, confidentiality and monitoring of genetic screening programmes.[105] A moratorium has been agreed between the government and the Association of British Insurers (ABI) on the use of predictive genetic test results.

Commercial screening kits

Do-it-yourself genetic screening test kits are now available and have raised considerable ethical concerns. *A Code of Practice and Guidance on Human Genetic Testing* was published on 23 September 1997 by the health departments of the United Kingdom.[106] It was put forward by the Advisory Committee on Genetic Testing (ACGT) on the basis of proposals prepared by a subgroup (chaired by Professor Marcus Pembrey). It recommended that a voluntary system of compliance and monitoring should be established rather than a statutory scheme. The Code of Practice and Guidance was intended to be used by those who supply genetic testing services direct to the public. The Code itself covered the following areas: testing laboratories, equipment and reagents; confidentiality and storage of samples and records; proposed tests should be cleared with the ACGT and comply with the Code; tests should not be available to those under 16 years or to those unable to make a competent decision regarding testing; specified information should be provided to the customer; pre- and post-test genetic consultation should be available without additional charge; and the involvement of medical practitioners. This voluntary code could work, given suppliers who have goodwill and purchasers who are well informed, without the necessity of statutory controls and criminal sanctions. The ACGT required companies selling the kits to submit them for prior approval, but it had no statutory powers and its guidelines were not enforceable. The ACGT was subsumed into the HGC in December 1999 and the HCG was replaced by an expert committee in 2012. On 20 January 2014 the *Daily Mail* announced that there were 38 British websites offering home testing kits costing up to £300; the most popular of which were paternity and genetic tests, while requests for tests to reveal genetic vulnerability to diseases were increasing.

Code of Practice on genetic tests from the insurers

The ABI published a Code of Practice in 1997. It made further revisions to it in 1999.[107] It is a voluntary code for insurers over genetic tests and gives the following guidance:

1. It should not require a person to take a genetic test to obtain insurance cover.
2. If the results of a genetic test are in a person's medical records, they can be taken into account only if they apply to one of seven conditions for which the tests are deemed reliable. (These conditions include breast cancer, Alzheimer's and Huntington's chorea.)
3. If the test is later found to be unreliable, the person is entitled to a refund of overpaid premiums and cheaper future payments.
4. A person is obliged to tell an insurance company if he has had a genetic test and disclose the results.
5. Anyone refused insurance cover or who wishes to complain can contact the ABI.[108]

Some evidence emerged that, contrary to the assertion of the ABI, some people were being refused insurance cover on the grounds that they have a genetic disorder.[109, 110] It was thought that either statutory intervention or some form of state insurance cover may be necessary to protect those who are vulnerable. In October 2000, new guidelines were recommended by a genetics and insurance committee established by the Department of Health.[111] The committee recommended that the reliability and relevance of the genetic test for Huntington's chorea is sufficient for insurance companies to use the result when assessing applications for life insurance. Insurers will not be able to require prospective clients to take the test, but they will be able to ask clients if they have taken tests for Huntington's chorea and to ask for the results to be given. The recommendations have been criticised, for example by the National Consumer Council, on the grounds that they will create a genetic underclass and will dissuade people from taking the tests.[112] In addition, scientists are fearful that potential volunteers for genetic tests will refuse to cooperate in this country. Thus, many scientists would have no option but to work outside this country, where potential research subjects would not have to disclose results to insurance companies.[113] The HGC has endorsed a regime of self-regulation for companies supplying genetic tests to the public, but their recommendations were criticised by Human Genetics Alert and GeneWatch UK.[114] In April 2003 the HGC issued a report saying that direct sales of such tests raised serious questions and that a 'robust but flexible' regulatory system needed to be established to control them. The HGC did not recommend an outright ban as people have the right to information about themselves, but they did want to ensure proper protection. They recommended that genetic tests should be carried out under the supervision of a doctor within the NHS.[115]

In 2005 the Department of Health and the ABI agreed a moratorium on the use of predictive genetic test results (unless the test has been approved), which has been extended to 2014. The moratorium applies to life insurance policies up to £500,000 and critical illness, long-term care and income protection up to £300,000. The only test which has been approved and would therefore have to be disclosed is that for Huntington's disease. The House of Lords Scientific and Technology Committee recommended that the moratorium should be kept until 2014 but should be tightened to make it clear that people who have had tests do not have to inform insurers. It also recommended that a White Paper on genomics should be prepared.[116] The moratorium was subsequently extended to 2017, and further extended to 2019. The ABI stated that it had proved to work well, enabling people to insure themselves and their families, even if they have had an adverse result from a predictive genetic test.[117] There are reviews at three-year intervals.

Genetics and confidentiality

The identification of genes linked to disabilities has raised serious legal and ethical issues, as Practical Dilemma 21.1 illustrates.

Practical dilemma 21.1 — Concealing information

Lisa undergoes a genetic test and discovers that she is carrying a gene that is linked with Huntington's chorea. Her sister, Rachel, has just got married and Lisa knows her sister intends having children and that both her sister and any children could be at risk of suffering from that disease. Lisa decides that she will keep this information to herself.

In this situation, the ordinary laws of confidentiality (see chapter 8) apply. There are no specific statutes that require the testers to disclose the results to any members of the family. If Rachel were unaware that there is a family risk of Huntington's chorea, she would not have the grounds to have herself tested or to seek a disclosure of the results of the test on Lisa. By the time Rachel has had her children and maybe finds that she is suffering from or is a carrier

> **Box 21.2** **GMC guidelines on confidentiality, paragraphs 73–75**
>
> **Disclosing genetic and other shared information**
>
> 73 Genetic and some other information about your patient might also be information about others with whom the patient shares genetic or other links. The diagnosis of a patient's illness might, for example, point to the certainty or likelihood of the same illness in a blood relative. 74 Most patients will readily share information about their own health with their children and other relatives, particularly if they are told it might help those relatives to:
>
> (a) get prophylaxis or other preventative treatments or interventions;
>
> (b) make use of increased surveillance or other investigations; and
>
> (c) prepare for potential health problems.
>
> 75 If a patient refuses to consent to information being disclosed that would benefit others, disclosure might still be justified in the public interest if failure to disclose the information leaves others at risk of death or serious harm (see paragraphs 63–70). If a patient refuses consent to disclosure, you will need to balance your duty to make the care of your patient your first concern against your duty to help protect the other person from serious harm.

of the disease, it is too late to take preventive action. Had she known of the risk, she could have opted for the testing of embryos before implantation. New guidance from the GMC published in 2017[118] (see Box 21.2) suggests that there may be circumstances where the confidentiality of patients with genetic diseases may not be kept in order to protect their families.

Huntington's disease is the only predictive genetic test which has to be reported to insurers under the terms of the moratorium outlined above.

Cloning

In 1997 Dolly the sheep became the first vertebrate cloned from a cell of an adult animal. Because of the immense significance of this scientific development, the Human Genetics Advisory Commission set up a working group and held a consultation exercise on cloning. It issued a consultation paper in 1998.[119] Following this exercise, HFEA recommended that research should continue into creating cloned tissue that can be transplanted, but that cloning for reproductive purposes should continue to be illegal.[120]

Following the report of the Chief Medical Officer's expert group on therapeutic cloning,[121] the government accepted its recommendations (press announcement, 16 August 2000) and agreed that:

1. The currently permitted grounds for embryo research will include treatment for a range of human diseases and research on human embryonic stem cells should be permitted. (At present research on embryos is restricted to the first 14 days and is permitted for five specific purposes relating to infertility, congenital disease, gene or chromosomal abnormalities, miscarriage or contraception. Additional purposes can be added by Statutory Instrument.)

2. Research involving cell nuclear replacement (so-called 'therapeutic cloning') should be allowed to help understand the biological mechanisms involved in the growth and development of human cells.

3. Specific consent must be given before early embryos can be donated for stem cell research.

On 19 December 2000 the House of Commons passed secondary legislation legalising research on the stem cells of embryos and the House of Lords approved the changes in 2001. A Statutory Instrument was enacted in 2001.[122] (This was subsequently repealed and replaced by Schedule 2 of the 2008 Act.) This means that it is possible for stem cells to be used in the research for illnesses such as cancer, Parkinson's disease, diabetes, osteoporosis, spinal cord injuries, Alzheimer's, leukaemia and multiple sclerosis. A licence is required from the HFEA and the cloning of human beings for reproductive purposes remains illegal.

Human cloning has been used to create embryonic stem cells from adult skin cells which could be used to grow new tissues or even organs that would be genetically identical to a patient's own cells thus overcoming the risk of rejection.[122]

Children over 16 years can give stem cells and in November it was reported that a girl of 17 had made medical history by giving stem cells to a stranger. She had signed up to the Anthony Nolan Register.[124, 125] See Code of Practice No 6 on the donation of allogeneic bone marrow and peripheral blood stem cells for transplantation issued by the Human Tissue Authority.[126]

The United Nations voted in November 2003 not to ban all forms of cloning. This led to a statement by the Department of Health[127] that welcomed the United Nations' decision, seeing it as a victory for the UK position. The UK is firmly against reproductive cloning but it believed that therapeutic cloning research offers enormous potential to develop cures for serious diseases such as Alzheimer's, Parkinson's and heart disease, and this therapeutic cloning is strictly controlled under licence from the HFEA. In January 2004 a claim was made by Dr Zavos, an American scientist, that he had implanted a cloned embryo in a woman's womb. This led to the president of the Royal Society and other top scientists appealing for a worldwide ban on human reproductive cloning.[128] Under the 2008 Act the use of inter-species embryos for research is permitted, with the HFEA having the power to authorise or refuse licences.

Personalised medication

The sequencing of the human genome has enabled an entire genetic code to be profiled with an ever-decreasing cost (now about £3000). Saudi Arabia has announced that it is to sequence the genomes of 100,000 citizens to facilitate personalised medicine which should prove more effective and cheaper.[129] The Royal Marsden Hospital is looking at dangerous mutations of 100 genes covering many types of cancer in order to provide the most suitable drugs to cancer patients.[130] The 100,000 Genomes Project was announced by the Prime Minister on 31 July 2014. The project will sequence the genomes of 75,000 sick children and their parents in order to target medicines and is due to last three years.[131]

The speed in the identification of disease-related genes would suggest that personalised medication will develop extensively, for instance: it is suggested that children should be tested for the ovarian cancer gene;[132] the possibilities of a genetic treatment for Down's syndrome are now known;[133] cold sores have been blamed on a mutant gene;[134] survival rates of leukaemia have improved greatly as a result of new treatment which genetically modifies the patient's own white blood cells;[135] a gene linked to intelligence which may assist in the treatment and diagnosis of schizophrenia and autism has been identified;[136] and it has been found that using a gene present in babies, but which is later switched off, may assist burns victims.[137]

The Personal Genome Project UK was launched on 7 November 2013 seeking 100,000 volunteers who agree to undergo genetic screening to identify their genome sequence. The aim is to assist in the development of personalised treatments. It cautions that there is no promise of confidentiality.[138]

Conclusions

It is inevitable that as science progresses further, amendments to legislation in this field will be required. However, for the time being the 2008 Act has filled a gap. Many issues are still ongoing. The decision not to amalgamate the Human Fertilisation and Embryology Authority with the Human Tissue Authority has now been revised as a result of the arm's-length bodies review.[139] The review suggests that while both the HFEA and HTA should initially be retained, eventually their research licensing functions should be transferred to a new research regulator, their inspection and control functions should be transferred to the Care Quality Commission, and their information and collection functions to the Social Care Information Centre. The new regulations relating to the three-parent child, which came into force at the end of 2015 indicate the extent to which changes to the law are required to keep pace with new technology in this field.

The government stated in response to the House of Lords Science and Technology Committee Inquiry into Regenerative Medicine that it remains committed to the field of regenerative medicine which is recognised as one of the UK's Eight Great Technologies and is supporting ongoing research through funding and the National Institute for Health Research which funds infrastructure in the NHS for translational research in regenerative medicine.[140]

Reflection questions

1. Where a child is born as the result of a surrogacy arrangement so that an embryo from a woman and her husband is transplanted into the uterus of another woman, what legal rights do you believe that the woman giving birth to the child should have over the genetic mother? What legal rights does she have?
2. To what extent do you think that couples should have the legal right to obtain treatment for their infertility?
3. Can experimentation on an embryo and its replacement in the uterus to develop as a human being be justified?

Further exercises

1. Look at the daily papers and journals over the next month and collect details on the cases, debates and articles on the topics discussed in this chapter.
2. To what extent do you think the law is an appropriate machinery to determine the choices of parents and professionals in the topics discussed in this chapter?

References

[1] Committee of Inquiry into Human Fertilisation and Embryology chaired by Baroness Warnock 1984, Cmnd 9314, HMSO, London, 1984
[2] White Paper, Review of the Human Fertilisation and Embryology Act: Proposals for revised legislation, Cm 6989, DH, December 2006
[3] Secretary of State for Health, Government response to the report from the Joint Committee, Cm 7209, DH, October 2007
[4] Committee of Inquiry into Human Fertilisation and Embryology chaired by Baroness Warnock 1984, Cmnd 9314, HMSO, London, 1984
[5] The Human Fertilisation and Embryology (Quality and Safety) Regulations SI 2007/1522 implementing European Union Tissue and Cells 2004/23/EC
[6] *Dickson and Another* v *United Kingdom*, The Times Law Report, 21 December 2007
[7] *A* v *C* [1978] 8 Fam Law 170
[8] Frances Gibb, Gay father wins case over baby of lesbian, *The Times*, 7 May 2002
[9] *Re D (Contact and PR: Lesbian mothers and known father) No. 2* [2006] EWHC 2 Fam
[10] Rosemary Bennett, Lesbian mother and gay father in court fight over children, *The Times*, 9 November 2010
[11] News item, Lesbian must let 'sperm donor' lover see his son, *The Times*, 22 February 2014
[12] *Re G (Shared residence order: biological mother of donor egg)* [2014] EWCA Civ 336
[13] *M* v *F and H (Legal Paternity)* [2013] EWHC 1901
[14] Alexandra Frean, Donor children should be able to find fathers, *The Times*, 27 July 2002
[15] Department of Health press release 2004/0023, Anonymity to be removed from future sperm, egg and embryo donors, 2004
[16] HFEA (Disclosure of Donor Information) Regulations, SI 2004/1511
[17] HFEA, Disclosure of information relating to gamete donation, CH(04)07
[18] [1] Jonathan Leake, Egg and sperm donors may get £800 payment, *The Sunday Times*, 22 August 2010
[19] Human Tissue (Quality and Safety) Regulations, SI 2007/1522; Human Tissue (Quality and Safety for Human Applications) Regulations, SI 2007/1523
[20] 2004/23/EC Tissues and Cells Directive
[21] Lois Rogers, IVF doctors to raffle human egg, *The Sunday Times*, 14 March 2010
[22] Jean McHale, Raffles, human eggs and the market place in human material, *British Journal of Nursing*, 19(6):388–9, 2010
[23] Committee of Inquiry into Human Fertilisation and Embryology chaired by Baroness Warnock 1984, Cmnd 9314, HMSO, London, 1984
[24] The Human Fertilisation and Embryology (Disclosure of Information for Research Purposes) Regulations 2010 SI 2010/995
[25] David Rose, IVF clinics are to be rated on probability that patients will have a healthy baby, *The Times*, 30 September 2009

26 *R v Ethical Committee of St Mary's Hospital ex parte Harriot*, The Times Law Report, 27 October 1987; [1988] 1 FLR 512
27 Human Fertilisation and Embryology Authority, *Code of Practice*, 8th edn, 2010, HFEA
28 HFEA Code of Practice 8, Welfare of the Child revised 2013
29 *R v Sheffield HA ex parte Seale* (1994) 25 BMLR 1
30 *Re D (A Child)* [2003] EWCA Civ 182; [2005] UKHL 33
31 HFEA, Sperm, Egg and Embryo Donation Review (SEED), January 2006
32 www.hfea.gov.uk/
33 Human Fertilisation and Embryology Authority, *Code of Practice*, 8th edn, 2017, HFEA
34 *Re R (A child)* [2003] EWCA 182
35 NICE, Fertility: assessment and treatment for people with fertility problems, CG 156, 2013
36 Royal College of Nursing, Infertility provision in England, Policy Briefing 003571, RCN, 2009
37 Sarah-Kate Templeton, Lesbian couple win fight for IVF on the NHS, *Sunday Times*, 19 July 2009
38 Chris Smyth, 'Alka-Seltzer IVF' is cut-price alternative, *The Times*, 9 July 2013
39 Hannah Devlin, New IVF technique could give 78 per cent chance of success, *The Times*, 17 May 2013
40 *R (Quintavalle) v Secretary of State for Health*, The Times Law Report, 14 March 2003; [2003] 2 WLR 692 HL
41 Ibid. 5 December 2001; [2001] 4 All ER 1013
42 Ibid. 25 January 2002; [2002] 2 WLR 550; [2003] UKHL 13
43 Human Fertilisation and Embryology (Research Purposes) Regulations 2001, SI 2001/188
44 Sarah-Kate Templeton, Someone else got my IVF baby, *The Sunday Times*, 14 June 2009
45 Lucy Bannerman, Fertility clinic apologises for second calamity, *The Times*, 18 June 2009
46 *Leeds Teaching Hospitals NHS Trust v Mr A, Mrs A, YA and ZA (by their litigation friend the Official Solicitor), the Human Fertilisation and Embryology Authority, Mr B and Mrs B* [2003] Lloyd's Rep Med 3 151
47 News item, *The Times*, 20 July 2003
48 *Jonathan Yearworth and others v North Bristol NHS Trust* [2009] EWCA Civ 37
49 Lewis Smith, Despicable conman jailed for IVF fraud, *The Times*, 16 January 2003
50 Chris Smyth, Woman given wrong sperm by IVF clinic, *The Times*, 8 July 2014
51 Human Fertilisation and Embryology Authority Code of Practice, HFEA, London, 1995
52 *R (on the application of Assisted Reproduction and Gynaecology Centre) v Human Fertilisation and Embryology Authority* [2002] EWCA Civ 20; *Independent*, 6 February 2002; [2003] 1 FCR 266 CA
53 *Assisted Reproduction and Gynaecology Centre and Anor v Human Fertilisation and Embryology Authority* [2013] EWHC 3087
54 www.oneatatime.org.uk
55 *R v Human Fertilisation and Embryology Authority ex p Blood* [1997] 2 WLR 806
56 Department of Health press announcement, 25 August 2000
57 Helen Rumbelow, Victory for Mrs Blood changes law of paternity, *The Times*, 1 March 2003
58 *Evans v Amicus Healthcare Ltd and Others; Hadley v Midland Fertility Services Ltd and Others*, The Times Law Report, 2 October 2003; [2003] EWHC 2161; [2007] ECHR 264 (Application No. 6339/05)

[59] *Evans* v *Amicus Healthcare* [2004] EWCA 727
[60] *Evans* v *United Kingdom* [2007] ECHR 264 (Application No. 6339/05)
[61] *Mrs U* v *Centre for Reproductive Medicine* [2002] Lloyd's Law Rep Med 259 CA
[62] David Rose, What a difference a day makes in embryo campaign, *The Times*, 10 September 2009
[63] *Elizabeth Warren* v *Care Fertility (Northampton)* Ltd and other [2014] EWHC 602 Fam
[64] www.hfea.gov.uk
[65] *Re (On the application of AB)* v *HFEA*, [2014]; www.nataliegambleassociates.co.uk
[66] Hannah Devlin, Woman fights to have baby of stricken fiancé, *The Times*, 17 January 2014
[67] www.legislation.gov.uk
[68] *Re C (A minor: wardship: Surrogacy)* [1985] FLR 846 (the father was able to obtain a wardship summons in order to obtain custody of the baby)
[69] *In re An Adoption (surrogacy)* [1987] 2 All ER 826
[70] *Re Q (Parental Order)* [1996] 1 FLR 369
[71] Nicola Woodcock, Couple win toddler from mother who broke surrogacy agreement, *The Times*, 27 July 2007
[72] *Re T (A child) (Surrogacy: Residence Order)* [2011] EWHC 33
[73] The Human Fertilisation and Embryology (Parental Orders) Regulations 2010 SI 2010/985
[74] *Briody* v *St Helen's and Knowsley HA* (2000), *The Times*, 1 March 2000; [2001] EWCA Civ 1010
[75] *JP* v *LP and Ors* [2014] EWHC 595 Fam
[76] HFEA Chair's letters CH(13)01
[77] Department of Health, NHS update, 22 April 2003
[78] Nigel Hawkes, Uncontrollable sleepers and hope in gene clue, *The Times*, 6 August 1999
[79] A correspondent, Heart gene discovered, *The Times*, 8 November 1999
[80] Ian Murray, Genetic link to dyslexia is found, *The Times*, 7 September 1999
[81] Mark Henderson, Gene fault clue to tackling dyslexia, *The Times*, 28 August 2003
[82] Roger Dobson, Found: the hibernating gene that could send man to the stars, *The Sunday Times*, 6 February 2000
[83] Nigel Hawkes, Gene discovery may reduce diseases linked to old age, *The Times*, 11 April 2000
[84] Mark Henderson, Clue to why men suffer more from autism, *The Times*, 10 September 2003
[85] Mark Henderson, Genetic clue to early menopause found, *The Times*, 11 July 2003
[86] Mark Henderson, Asthma could be stopped in its tracts, *The Times*, 19 May 2003
[87] Department of Health, White Paper, Our Inheritance, Our Future: realising the potential of genetics in the NHS, Cm 5791, Stationery Office, London, June 2003
[88] HGC, Choosing the Future: genetic and reproductive decision making, 2004
[89] Mark Henderson, DNA tests may threaten your child's rights, *The Times*, 4 August 2010
[90] www.dh.gov.uk
[91] Clothier Committee, HMSO, London, January 1992
[92] Department of Health www.gov.uk
[93] Gene Therapy Advisory Committee 2004, Operational Procedures for the Gene Therapy Advisory Committee in its role as the National Ethics Committee for Gene Therapy Clinical Trials, DH, 2004
[94] Human Fertilisation and Embryology Authority and Advisory Committee on Genetic Testing Consultation Document on Pre-implantation Genetic Diagnosis, HFEA and ACGT, London, 1999

[95] *R (Quintavalle)* v *Human Fertilisation and Embryology Authority* [2002] EWHC 3000; [2003] EWCA Civ 667; [2005] UKHL 28
[96] Laura Peek, Couple lose fight for designer baby, *The Times*, 2 August 2002
[97] HFEA, Report on pre-implantation tissue typing policy review, July 2004
[98] HGC, Making Babies: reproductive decisions and genetic technologies, January 2006
[99] Lois Rogers, Embryos destroyed for 'minor conditions', *The Sunday Times*, 24 January 2010
[100] Alice Fishburn, Pink or blue booties? No need to guess, *The Times*, 22 August 2009101 The Parliamentary Office of Science and Technology (2013) 101 The Parliamentary Office of Science and Technology (2013) https://researchbriefings.files.parliament.uk/documents/POST-PN-445/POST-PN-445.pdf
[101] The Parliamentary Office of Science and Technology (2013) https://researchbriefings.files.parliament.uk/documents/POST-PN-445/POST-PN-445.pdf
[102] Human Fertilisation and Embryology Authority, Public Consultation on Sex Selection, HFEA, London, January 1993
[103] Human Fertilisation and Embryology Authority, Sex Selection Report and Summary Document, HFEA, London, November 2003; www.hfea.gov.uk
[104] 2004/23/EC Tissues and Cells Directive
[105] A citizens' jury on the topic was held in November 1997 at the University of Glamorgan. For further information on the report of the jury's recommendations contact Marcus Longley of the Welsh Institute of Health and Social Care, University of Glamorgan; Tel. 01443 483070
[106] Advisory Committee on Genetic Testing, Code of Practice and Guidance on Human Genetic Testing, Health Departments of the United Kingdom, 23 September 1997
[107] Association of British Insurers, Code of Practice for Genetic Testing, 1999
[108] Association of British Insurers; Tel. 0207 600 3333
[109] News item, Insurers ignore genetics code, *The Sunday Times*, 13 December 1998
[110] Robert Winnett, Medical underclass fears insurance blacklisting, *The Sunday Times*, 26 March 2000
[111] Department of Health, Committee on Genetics and Insurance Report, DH, October 2000
[112] Mark Henderson, Insurers to check for genetic illness, *The Times*, 13 October 2000
[113] Mark Henderson, Scientists attack gene test ruling, *The Times*, 27 November 2000
[114] Nigel Hawkes, Alarm over unregulated DIY genetic health test, *The Times*, 3 February 2003
[115] Nigel Hawkes, Genetic tests must not go on public sale, government told, *The Times*, 10 April 2003
[116] House of Lords Scientific and Technology Committee, 2nd Report, Genomic Medicine Session 2008/9 HL 107, Stationery Office
[117] www.abi.org.uk
[118] General Medical Council, Confidentiality, 2017, GMC, London
[119] Human Genetics Advisory Commission (HGAC) and Human Fertilisation and Embryology Authority, Consultation Document on Cloning Issues in Reproduction, Science and Medicine, HGAC, London, 1998
[120] Human Fertilisation and Embryology Authority and Human Genetic Advisory Commission, Cloning Issues in Reproduction, Science and Medicine, HFEA/HGAC, London, December 1998
[121] Chief Medical Officer's Expert Group on Therapeutic Cloning, Stem Cell Research: medical progress with responsibility, DH, August 2000
[122] Human Fertilisation and Embryology (Research Purposes) Regulations 2001, SI 2001/188

[123] Hannah Devlin, Human cloning advance raised hope of medical treatment, *The Times*, 16 May 2013
[124] Tom Knowles, Girl, 17, makes medical history by giving stem cells to stranger, *The Times*, 25 November 2013
[125] www.anthonynolan.org
[126] www.hta.gov.uk
[127] Department of Health press release 2003/0429, Statement from the Department of Health
[128] Mark Henderson, Top scientists want 'cowboy cloning' banned, *The Times*, 21 January 2004
[129] News item, Personalised therapy gets a step closer, *The Times*, 9 December 2013
[130] Chris Smyth, Fast gene test will aid cancer patient, *The Times*, 21 May 2013
[131] Chris Smyth, DNA maps to revolutionise cancer care, *The Times*, 1 August 2014
[132] Kate Gibbons, Call to test children for the ovarian cancer gene, *The Times*, 16 September 2013
[133] Hannah Devlin, Scientists close in on genetic treatment for Down's, *The Times*, 18 July 2013
[134] Michael Glackin, Blame those cold sores on a mutant gene, *The Times*, 17 September 2013
[135] Hannah Devlin, GM cell therapy hailed as leukaemia breakthrough, *The Times*, 20 February 2014
[136] News item, Scientists find the gene linked to intelligence, *The Times*, 12 February 2014
[137] Hannah Devlin, Babies' healing gene may help burns victims, *The Times*, 8 November 2014
[138] www.personalgenomes.org.uk
[139] Department of Health, Liberating the NHS: report of the arm's-length bodies, London, Crown, 2010
[140] Government Response to the House of Lords Science and Technology Committee Inquiry into Regenerative Medicine, Cm 8713, October 2013

Chapter 22

Community and Primary Care Nursing

This chapter discusses

- NHS and social services provision
- Funding of long-term care
- Care Act 2014
- Human rights and care homes
- Delayed discharges
- Carers
- Negligence
- Safety of the community professional
- Consent to treatment
- Protection of property
- Disclosure of information
- Criminal suspicion
- Standards: care homes
- Community matrons
- The specialist community public health nurse
- The school nurse
- The clinic nurse
- The practice nurse
- Developments in technology and structure

Introduction

This chapter covers the law relating to nurses who work in the community and in primary care, including community/district nurses, health visitors, practice nurses and specialist nurses. Community psychiatric nurses (CPNs) will also find chapter 19 on mental healthcare of relevance, and for health visitors and school nurses chapter 25 provides information on the law relating to public health.

The development of community care and the earlier establishment of primary care trusts (PCTs) meant that the focus for many health professionals switched from the institution to the community and to primary care, and those who have always been community workers, such as the health visitor and the district nurse, felt the increased pressure from the implications of the policy to transfer patients from the institution to the community. Recent developments have seen an increase in specialist posts in the community. Community nurses for those with learning disabilities and CPNs are increasing in number and specialist posts for stoma care, incontinence, asthma, diabetes, terminal illness and other specialist areas have been established. Many liaison nurses are now seeking specialist training. There are increased appointments in the community for occupational therapists, physiotherapists and paediatricians. These organisational changes have continued with the creation of clinical commissioning groups (see chapter 5) under the Health and Social Care Act 2012. Box 22.1 illustrates some of the particular difficulties with which these workers are faced.

Box 22.1 Difficulties faced by the nurse in the community

1. Isolation
2. Vulnerability
3. Sole responsibility
4. Pressure to go beyond job description: definitions of the scope of professional practice
5. Health and safety hazard and occupier's liability
6. Variable facilities and resources

NHS and social services provision

Considerable problems have arisen in the provision of a seamless service between NHS and social services because NHS care is free at the point of delivery whereas most social services provision is means tested. The NHS and Community Care Act 1990 placed responsibility upon local authorities for funding, on a means-tested basis, the residential care costs of its residents. Local criteria for the eligibility for NHS continuing care were drawn up in each area and those who disagreed with the decisions could use the complaints procedures established by the strategic health authority and local authority. From 2010 there has been a uniform complaints procedure between health and social services (see chapter 26).

Disputes over eligibility for continuing care have been the concern of the Parliamentary and Health Service Ombudsman. Cases 22.1, 22.2 and 22.3 illustrate concerns about the system of means testing for those in residential care.

The Court of Appeal held that nursing care for the chronically sick was not always the sole responsibility of the NHS, but could, in appropriate circumstances, be provided by a local authority as a social service and the patient could, depending on her means, be liable to meet the

| Case 22.1 | *R v N and E Devon Health Authority ex parte Coughlan* [2000] |

NHS or means-tested care?[1]

Pamela Coughlan brought an action against the health authority in 1999 when she was told that she would have to leave the nursing home she was living in at NHS expense and move to another home that would be means-tested. She had been grievously injured in a road traffic accident in 1971. She was tetraplegic, doubly incontinent and partially paralysed in the respiratory tract. She had been promised by the health authority that she would be able to stay in Mardon House for life, the costs of her care being met by the NHS.

cost of that care. However, there was no overriding public interest in the health authority breaking its promise to her that she could stay in that home for her life.

There was no appeal against the Court of Appeal's decision. Pamela Coughlan was able to continue to have NHS funding of her care, but the court had accepted the principle that nursing care did not always have to be funded by the NHS, so in that sense both parties won their case. However, the principle that nursing and other personal care should be funded by the NHS was put forward by the majority recommendations in the Royal Commission Report on the long-term care of the elderly.[2] The National Framework for continuing care is considered below.

Following the Coughlan judgment,[3] the Ombudsman issued a report on continuing care on 20 February 2003 after which the Department of Health issued instructions[4] that the then strategic health authorities should agree with local councils one set of criteria for continuing care in keeping with the Coughlan judgment.

Subsequently, in 2007, the DH announced that a National Framework for continuing care would be implemented in October 2007. Assessments for continuing NHS care were to be carried out by a multidisciplinary team using the concept of 'a primary health' need as the criteria for the receipt of continuing healthcare.[5] This initiative was intended to resolve the issues which were raised by the High Court decision in the Grogan case[6] (see Case 22.3).

A dispute arose in relation to the provision of services to disabled people under the Chronic Sick and Disabled Persons Act 1970 and the extent to which the local authority could take into account its financial resources.

| Case 22.2 | *R v Gloucester CC and Another ex parte Barry* [1997] |

Assessment of disabled persons[7]

A man of 79 with severe disabilities brought an action in Gloucester when the local authority informed him that it was going to withdraw his cleaning and laundry services. He obtained judicial review of the local authority's decision on the grounds that they had not reassessed his needs prior to withdrawing the services. The High

Court judge refused to grant a declaration that, in carrying out the reassessment, the local authority was not entitled to take into account the resources available to it. The Court of Appeal allowed his appeal, on the grounds that the local authority was not entitled to take into account the resources available to it. The local authority appealed to the House of Lords.

The House of Lords allowed the appeal holding that, for the purposes of section 2(1) of the 1970 Act, a chronically sick or disabled person's needs were to be assessed in the context of, and by reference to, the provision of certain types of assistance for promoting the welfare of disabled people using eligibility criteria. These criteria had to be set taking into account current acceptable standards of living, the nature and extent of the disability and the relative cost balanced against the relative benefit and the relative need for that benefit. Its impact on its resources had to be evaluated and therefore its financial position was relevant. The authority could not make the decision in a vacuum from which all considerations of costs were expelled. In another significant court decision, the Court of Appeal[8] allowed the application for judicial review and held that Sefton Borough Council had behaved unlawfully[9] when it set up a scheme whereby those who were entitled to be provided with accommodation under section 21 could have their capital taken into account unless it was or fell below £1500 (this figure was chosen since it would usually leave sufficient for a funeral). Subsequently the Community Care (Residential Accommodation) Act 1998 was passed to put the decision of the Court of Appeal on a statutory basis. Section 1 of the 1998 Act states that in determining whether care and attention are otherwise available to a person, a local authority shall disregard so much of the person's capital as does not exceed the capital limit for the purposes of section 22 of the National Assistance Act 1948. The regulations on capital disregard must be followed by local authorities in means testing.[10]

In July 2001 the Department of Health published a consultation document, 'Guidance on Fair Access to Care Services', to ensure greater consistency in the use of eligibility criteria for access to care services.

Case 22.3 *R (on the application of Grogan) v Bexley NHS care trust* [2006]

Continuing care[11]

G applied for judicial review of a decision by an NHS trust that she did not qualify for continuing NHS healthcare. If the NHS provided care, it would be free; if it were the social services, she would be means tested. The High Court held that an NHS trust should apply a primary health need test to determine whether accommodation should be provided by the NHS or social services. The criteria of the NHS trust for determining whether the patient had continuing care needs were fatally flawed and it failed to give reasons why it considered that the patient's continuing care needs were neither complex nor intense. The Court ordered the trust's decision to be set aside and remitted for fresh consideration.

Following the decision in the Grogan case the DH announced that a national framework for continuing care would be implemented in October 2007 and gave interim guidance.[12]

Assessments for continuing NHS care were to be carried out by a multidisciplinary team using the concept of 'a primary health' need as the criteria for the receipt of continuing healthcare.[13]

The *National Framework for NHS Continuing Healthcare and NHS-funded Nursing Care*, published in October 2007[14] revised in 2009 and 2012 and updated in 2013, set out the national framework, the legal framework, the primary health need, core values, and principles, eligibility considerations, links to other policies, care planning and provision, review, dispute resolution and governance. It stated that primary health need should be assessed by looking at all of the care needs and relating them to four key indicators:

- **Nature** – the type of condition or treatment required and its quality and quantity;
- **Complexity** – symptoms that interact, making them difficult to manage or control;
- **Intensity** – one or more needs which are so severe that they require regular interventions; and
- **Unpredictability** – unexpected changes in condition that are difficult to manage and present a risk to the patient or to others.

To be eligible for continuing healthcare the person must be assessed as having a primary health need and have a complex medical condition and substantial and ongoing care needs.[15]

The NHS would make decisions on eligibility for NHS continuing healthcare in collaboration with the local authority through a multidisciplinary team and with the full and active involvement of the patient and carers. Further information on the national framework on continuing care is available on the government website. Answers to frequently asked questions on continuing care are also incorporated in the guidance.

Information on the right to receive continuing healthcare can be found online at: NHS Continuing Healthcare (CHC) Checklist; Decision Support Tool for NHS CHC; and *National Framework for NHS Continuing Healthcare and NHS-funded Nursing Care*.

In 2008 the government initiated a consultation on the future of care and support. It set up a care and support website (now archived)[16] which could be accessed to take part in the debate. It pointed out that given the longer life expectancy, the cost of disability benefits could increase by 50 per cent in the next 20 years and there could be a £6 billion funding gap for social care. Since the proportion of people of working age in the population would decline, the government would not be able to raise enough money through tax alone to meet the costs of care and support. A new insurance-based system was seen as a means of funding care for the elderly which was forecast to reach £4 billion in the next 20 years. Feedback was invited in its efforts to find an affordable, fair and sustainable way of delivering and funding a first-class care and support system for the twenty-first century. In a letter to *The Times*[17] from representatives of 12 organisations involved with the care of older and disabled people and their carers, it was highlighted that disabled and older people were being forced to end their support services because they could not afford them, and they called on the government to conduct a thorough review of the impact of care charges and for these issues to be addressed in adult care reform.

There was also concern and inconsistency about relatives paying top-up fees.[18] Councils should only ask for top-up fees from relatives if the family has requested a particular care home for their relative other than the one chosen by the local authority. Otherwise the local authority should pay the fees in full where the assets of the old person are less than £13,500. Where the elderly person has assets of between £13,500 and £22,250 then there is a sliding scale of contribution.

In August 2009 the NHS was ordered to pay £100,000 to the family of an Alzheimer's sufferer to cover care home fees which the local NHS trust had refused to pay. Judith Roe died aged 74 in October 2008. The NHS trust had ruled that she did not qualify for NHS funding because her condition was deemed to be a social rather than a health problem. The Ombudsman said that the fees should have been met by Worcester PCT and ordered NHS Worcestershire (which replaced the PCT) to pay the family more than £100,000. Disputes have also arisen between local authorities over the responsibility to fund an individual's community care package. In one case in 2009 the Court of Appeal held that once the Secretary of State had determined that a person was ordinarily resident in a particular area then that local authority had a responsibility to fund a care package, even though another local authority had set up the package.[19]

Rationing care

Many local authorities have tightened their criteria for providing social care and are offering help only in critical cases. A legal challenge was brought against Harrow Council by several claimants, who were in receipt of community care services. Harrow had proposed that owing to financial constraints it would limit provision of care services to people with need categorised as critical under the Fair Access to Care Services guidance issued by the Secretary of State. The judge decided that there was a general duty under section 49A of the Disability Discrimination Act 1995 to have due regard to considerations listed therein. Those were important duties which included the need to promote equality of opportunity and to take account of disabilities, even where that involved treating the disabled more favourably than others. There was no evidence that the legal duty and its implications were drawn to the attention of the decision makers who should have been informed, not just of the disabled as an issue, but of the particular obligations that the law imposed. Harrow Council's decision-making process had not complied with section 49A of the Act.[20]

Funding of long-term care

With Respect to Old Age,[21] the Royal Commission's 1999 report into long-term care, made radical recommendations for the future care of older people. It suggested that:

> **The costs of long-term care should be split between living costs, housing costs and personal care. Personal care should be available after assessment, according to need and paid for from general taxation; the rest should be subject to a co-payment according to means.**

A minority of two members of the Royal Commission, in a note of dissent, stated that they could not support the majority view that personal care should be provided free of charge, paid for from general taxation, on the basis of need. The government did not accept the Royal Commission's recommendation that personal care should be met from public funds, although it made various recommendations to reduce the hardship of means-tested payment of fees. The disputes between the demarcation of NHS-funded care (and therefore free at the point of delivery) and means-tested social services care continued to give rise to many concerns and complaints.

The Court of Appeal held that a local authority was entitled to consider what an individual's needs were as the starting point for the calculation of a personal budget and had to give reasons for its decision.[22]

Green paper on the funding of long-term care in the future

In July 2009 the long-awaited Green Paper[23] was published. It identified six features that everyone was entitled to expect. These were:

1. The right support to help you stay independent and well for as long as possible and to stop your care and support needs getting worse.
2. Wherever you are in England, you will have the right to have your care and support needs assessed in the same way and you will have a right to have the same proportion of your care and support costs paid for wherever you live.
3. All the services that you need will work together smoothly, particularly when your needs are assessed . . . You will only need to have one assessment of your needs to gain access to a whole range of care and support services.
4. You can understand and find your way through the care and support system easily.
5. The services you use will be based on your personal circumstances and need. Your care and support will be designed and delivered around your individual needs. As part of your care and support plan, you will have much greater choice over how and where you receive support, and the possibility of controlling your own budget wherever appropriate.
6. Your money will be spent wisely and everyone who qualifies for care and support from the state will get some help meeting the cost of care and support needs.

The aim was to build a National Care Service that was fair, simple and affordable. Everyone who qualified for care and support from the state should get some help with paying for it. Any new system must therefore be

- fair;
- simple and easy to understand;
- affordable;
- universal, underpinned by national rights and entitlements, and helping everyone who needs care to pay for it; and
- personalised to individual needs, and flexible enough to support people to live their lives in the ways in which they want.

Three funding options were put forward for consultation:

1. Partnership – in this system, everyone who qualified for care and support from the state would be entitled to have a set proportion – for example, a quarter or a third – of their basic care and support costs paid for by the state. People who were less well-off would have more care and support paid for – for example, two-thirds – while the least well-off people would continue to get all their care and support for free.
2. Insurance – in this system, everyone would be entitled to have a share of their care and support costs met, just as in the Partnership model. But this system would go further to help people cover the additional costs of their care and support through insurance, if they wanted to.
3. Comprehensive – in this system, everyone over retirement age who had the resources to do so would be required to pay into a state insurance scheme. Everyone who was able to pay would pay their contribution, and then everyone whose needs meant that they qualified for care and support from the state would get all of their basic care and support for free when they needed it.

Three systems were ruled out.

1. The current system with some getting their social care paid for but others receiving no help at all.
2. A tax funded system where people would pay tax throughout their lives, which would be used to pay for all the people who currently need care. When, in turn, people needed care themselves, they would get all their basic care free. This option was ruled out because it places a heavy burden on people of working age.
3. Pay for Yourself – in which everybody would be responsible for paying for their own basic care and support, when they needed it; they could take out insurance to cover some of these costs, or use their income and savings. This was ruled out because it would leave many people without the care and support they need, and is fundamentally unfair because people cannot predict what care and support they will need.

Following the Green Paper a White Paper was published in March 2010.

White Paper on social care[24]

The White Paper recommended a National Care Service which would be free at the point of delivery to be set up within five years. There would be three stages:

1. free care at home for the elderly and the infirm with critical needs;
2. a guarantee by 2014 that residential care will be free after the first two years; and
3. a universal system free at the point of delivery with the necessary legislative changes contained in a Personal Care at Home Bill.

Criticisms of the White Paper included the absence of a clear plan on meeting the costs and timescale.[25] The Personal Care at Home Act 2010 was passed and was seen as the first stage in the development towards a National Care Service. It would have amended the Community Care (Delayed Discharges) Act of 2003 to include the provision of free personal care at home and would have provided free personal care for 280,000 people with the highest needs – including those with serious dementia or Parkinson's disease. However, the coalition government stated on 20 May 2010 that it did not intend to implement the provision of free personal care and instead appointed Andrew Dilnot to chair a Commission to review the funding of care for the elderly.

The Dilnot Report on Social Care[26]

In 2011 the Independent Commission chaired by Andrew Dilnot reported on the funding of social care. It found that the current system is confusing, unfair and unsustainable and made the following recommendations:

- Capping lifetime individual contributions to care at £35,000;
- Providing free care for those who develop needs before they reach 40;
- Raising the means-tested threshold for savings below which people become eligible for state-funded residential care from £23,250 to £100,000;
- Standardising contributions to board and lodging costs in residential care at between £7,000 to £10,000 a year;

- Introducing a national system of assessment and eligibility, initially set at substantial need; and
- Giving free state support to people who enter adulthood with a care and support need immediately rather than being subjected to a means test.

In December 2013 research by the London School of Economics showed that nearly half a million elderly and disabled people had been denied social care due to a squeeze on council funding over the past five years.[27] The LSE found that 86 per cent of English councils responsible for social services offered care to only those with needs deemed 'critical' or 'substantial'. The Care and Support Minister Norman Lamb stated that from 2015 a new minimum eligibility threshold would provide clarity and consistency on whether a person was eligible for care and support. He also stated that the government was investing £3.8 million through the Better Care Fund to join up health and social services so that people can live as independently as possible. Concerns over the repercussions of this transfer on NHS funding led to a modified plan with at least £1 billion of the Better Care Fund having to be spent on the NHS.[28]

A daughter won her case against Worcester County Council which wished to assess the family home to pay for her mother's care home fees. She claimed that she rented a property and regarded her mother's home as her only real home and she intended to retire to it. The Court held that the council had erred in law by

1. conflating the concept of occupation of a home with that of permanent residence, and
2. wrongly considering that the application of the exemption could only be determined on a once-and-for-all basis at the time of the resident's admission into care.[29]

Caring for our future: reforming care and support

A White Paper[30] on social care and funding was published by the government in 2012. It can be accessed on the government website[31] and sets out the key actions which it intended to take to reform the provision and payment for social care. The Law Commission, which had conducted a three-year review into adult social care law, published its final report in May 2011[32] (accessible on the Law Commission website[33]). It recommended a single, clear, modern statute and code of practice paving the way for a coherent social care system. The government response was published in July 2012.[34] The Care and Support Bill (enacted in 2014 as the Care Act) was published to implement the White Paper recommendations, (including modified Dilnot recommendations), those of the Law Commission and also some of the recommendations of the Francis Inquiry into Mid Staffordshire NHS Trust (see chapter 5). The Dilnot cap was raised to £75,000 but led to controversy over the deferred payment scheme, since people would not be eligible for a deferred payment if they had more than £23,000 in assets excluding the value of their home. The deferred payment scheme required LAs to pay care fees up front, to be reimbursed later from the estate, thus freeing families from the burden of paying care home fees until after their loved ones had died. As a result of the Care Act 2014, in April 2016 the threshold for self-funding was to increase to £118,000 and lifetime care costs would have been capped at £72,000. However, the government has delayed this for a further four years (to 2020). At present in England if a person has capital more than £23,250 they will have to meet the full cost of care home fees. In Wales, the figure is £40,000, and in Scotland the lower and upper capital limits are £17,000 and £27,250 (April 2018), however people over 65 can claim personal care payments, which are currently £174 per week for personal care, £79 per week for nursing care and £253 per week for personal and nursing care.[35]

Care Act 2014

The Act has been described as the most significant reform of care and support in more than 60 years. Earlier legislation is repealed for England including section 47 of the National Assistance Act 1948 (which gave local authorities the power to remove a person in need of care to a place of safety). The Care Act 2014 is in the main focused on England since social care is a devolved matter. However, there are exceptions to this and the explanatory memorandum to the Act (available on the legislation website[36]) provides fuller information on territorial extent. In Wales, the Social Services and Wellbeing (Wales) Act 2014 has similar provisions to the Care Act in England.

Statute Box 22.1 sets out the main provisions of the Care Act 2014.

The following are some of the Act's key features:

1. The local authority has a statutory duty to promote people's well-being not only of the users of the services but also of the carers. Well-being includes physical, mental and emotional needs. Users and carers have a right to receive support once it has been determined that they have eligible needs (sections 1, 18 and 20) (see Statute Box 22.2).

2. A local authority also has a statutory duty to provide preventative services to maintain people's health (section 2) (see Statute Box 22.3).

3. A local authority has a statutory duty to ensure the integration of care and support provision with health provision and health-related provision in performing its functions (section 3) (see Statute Box 22.4). This is comparable to the reciprocal duty placed upon NHS England and the clinical commissioning groups under sections 13N and 14Z1 of the amended NHS Act 2006.

4. A minimum eligibility threshold is introduced – a set of criteria that makes it clear when local authorities have to provide support (section 13).

5. People can appeal against council decisions on eligibility and funding for care and support (section 72 and regulations).

6. Local authorities will be required to provide information and advice (section 4). A new website for NHS Choices will give information on provider profiles to help people choose, compare and comment on care homes and other care services.

7. All those receiving care and support, whether in residential care or home, are now covered by the Human Rights Act, except those who pay for their own care (section 73).

8. There will be a cap of £72,000 (although as previously mentioned this cap has been delayed by the government until at least April 2020, and there is some debate as to whether the cap will ever be implemented) on reasonable care costs and financial support (not including accommodation) enabling people to plan their finances. Councils must offer a deferred payment scheme so that people do not have to sell their home in their lifetime (sections 24–30 and 34–36).

9. Legal right for those with a care and support plan to have a personal budget which can be received as a direct payment (sections 28 and 31–33).

10. Moving to a different authority will not lead to loss of care and support (section 37 and 38).

11. Greater independence for the CQC (see chapter 5).

12. Health Education England to be the first ever non-departmental public body with responsibility for training and education of staff in the NHS (sections 96–102) (see chapter 17).

13. A duty of candour on healthcare organisations to be introduced through regulations (section 81) (see chapter 5).

A memorandum of understanding sent by the government to every council in England in May 2014 recommended that each council should appoint a senior responsible officer (SRO) to be accountable for local implementation of the Act. Each local authority is required to agree a completed Better Care Fund plan (pooling health and social care funds) with its partner Clinical Commissioning Group and the plan must be signed off by the local Health and Wellbeing Board.

Statute 22.1

Care Act 2014

Part 1 Care and Support

General responsibilities of local authorities

1. Promoting individual well-being
2. Preventing needs for care and support
3. Promoting integration of care and support with health services, etc.
4. Providing information and advice
5. Promoting diversity and quality in provision of services
6. Cooperating generally
7. Cooperating in specific cases

Meeting needs for care, etc.

8. How to meet needs

Assessing needs

9. Assessment of an adult's needs for care and support
10. Assessment of a carer's needs for support
11. Refusal of assessment
12. Assessments under sections 9 and 10: further provision
13. The eligibility criteria

Charging and assessing financial resources

14. Power of local authority to charge
15. Cap on care costs
16. Cap on care costs: annual adjustment
17. Assessment of financial resources

Duties and powers to meet needs

18. Duty to meet needs for care and support
19. Power to meet needs for care and support
20. Duty and power to meet a carer's needs for support

21 Exception for persons subject to immigration control
22 Exception for provision of health services
23 Exception for provision of housing, etc.

Next steps after assessments

24 The steps for the local authority to take
25 Care and support plan, support plan
26 Personal budget
27 Review of care and support plan or of support plan
28 Independent personal budget
29 Care account
30 Cases where adult expresses preference for particular accommodation

Direct payments

31 Adults with capacity to request direct payments
32 Adults without capacity to request direct payments
33 Direct payments: further provision

Deferred payment agreements, etc.

34 Deferred payment agreements and loans
35 Deferred payment agreements and loans: further provision
36 Alternative financial arrangements

Continuity of care and support when adult moves

37 Notification, assessment, etc.
38 Case where assessments not complete on day of move

Establishing where a person lives, etc.

39 Where a person's ordinary residence is
40 Disputes about ordinary residence or continuity of care
41 Financial adjustments between local authorities

Safeguarding adults at risk of abuse or neglect

42 Enquiry by local authority
43 Safeguarding Adults Boards
44 Safeguarding adults reviews
45 Supply of information
46 Abolition of local authority's power to remove persons in need of care
47 Protecting property of adults being cared for away from home

48–80   Provider Failure; market oversight; transition for children to adult care; independent advocacy and miscellaneous

Part 2 Care standards

Part 3 Health [Health Education England and Health Research Authority]

Part 4 Health and social care [Better Care Fund established]

Part 5 General

The general responsibilities of local authorities are shown in Statute Box 22.2.

Statute 22.2
General responsibilities of local authorities under the Care Act 2014 Section 1

Promoting individual well-being

1(1) The general duty of a local authority, in exercising a function under this Part in the case of an individual, is to promote that individual's well-being.

(2) 'Well-being', in relation to an individual, means that individual's well-being so far as relating to any of the following—

  (a) personal dignity (including treatment of the individual with respect);
  (b) physical and mental health and emotional well-being;
  (c) protection from abuse and neglect;
  (d) control by the individual over day-to-day life (including over care and support, or support, provided to the individual and the way in which it is provided);
  (e) participation in work, education, training or recreation;
  (f) social and economic well-being;
  (g) domestic, family and personal relationships;
  (h) suitability of living accommodation;
  (i) the individual's contribution to society.

(3) In exercising a function under this Part in the case of an individual, a local authority must have regard to the following matters in particular—

  (a) the importance of beginning with the assumption that the individual is best-placed to judge the individual's well-being;
  (b) the individual's views, wishes, feelings and beliefs;
  (c) the importance of preventing or delaying the development of needs for care and support or needs for support and the importance of reducing needs of either kind that already exist;

(d) the need to ensure that decisions about the individual are made having regard to all the individual's circumstances (and are not based only on the individual's age or appearance or any condition of the individual's or aspect of the individual's behaviour which might lead others to make unjustified assumptions about the individual's well-being);

(e) the importance of the individual participating as fully as possible in decisions relating to the exercise of the function concerned and being provided with the information and support necessary to enable the individual to participate;

(f) the importance of achieving a balance between the individual's well-being and that of any friends or relatives who are involved in caring for the individual;

(g) the need to protect people from abuse and neglect;

(h) the need to ensure that any restriction on the individual's rights or freedom of action that is involved in the exercise of the function is kept to the minimum necessary for achieving the purpose for which the function is being exercised.

Statute 22.3

General responsibilities of local authorities under the Care Act 2014 section 2

Preventing needs for care and support

2(1) A local authority must provide or arrange for the provision of services, facilities or resources, or take other steps, which it considers will—

(a) contribute towards preventing or delaying the development by adults in its area of needs for care and support;

(b) contribute towards preventing or delaying the development by carers in its area of needs for support;

(c) reduce the needs for care and support of adults in its area;

(d) reduce the needs for support of carers in its area.

2 In performing that duty, a local authority must have regard to—

(a) the importance of identifying services, facilities and resources already available in the authority's area and the extent to which the authority could involve or make use of them in performing that duty;

(b) the importance of identifying adults in the authority's area with needs for care and support which are not being met (by the authority or otherwise);

(c) the importance of identifying carers in the authority's area with needs for support which are not being met (by the authority or otherwise).

Statute 22.4

Care Act 2014 section 3

Promoting integration of care and support with health services, etc.

(3)1 A local authority must exercise its functions under this Part with a view to ensuring the integration of care and support provision with health provision and health-related provision where it considers that this would—

 (a) promote the well-being of adults in its area with needs for care and support and the well-being of carers in its area,

 (b) contribute to the prevention or delay of the development by adults in its area of needs for care and support or the development by carers in its area of needs for support, or

 (c) improve the quality of care and support for adults, and of support for carers, provided in its area (including the outcomes that are achieved from such provision).

Care and support provision means provision to meet adults' needs, carers' needs and provision of services, facilities or resources, or the taking of other steps, under section 2 (see Statute Box 22.3).

The local authority also has a duty to ensure that it establishes and maintains a service for giving advice and information (section 4), promotes diversity and equality in the provision of services (section 5), and cooperates both generally and specifically with the relevant partners as defined in the Act (sections 6 and 7). Under section 8, examples are given as to how it meets the needs under sections 18 and 19. They are shown in Statute Box 22.5.

Statute 22.5

Care Act 2014 section 8

How to meet needs

(8)1 The following are examples of what may be provided to meet needs under sections 18 to 20—

 (a) accommodation in a care home or in premises of some other type;

 (b) care and support at home or in the community;

 (c) counselling and other types of social work;

 (d) goods and facilities;

 (e) information, advice and advocacy.

> (2) The following are examples of the ways in which a local authority may meet needs under sections 18 to 20—
>
> (a) by arranging for a person other than it to provide a service;
> (b) by itself providing a service;
> (c) by making direct payments.

Sections 9 and 10 set out details for making an assessment of the person and of the carer. If the person refuses an assessment then section 11 relieves the LA from carrying out that assessment, but if (a) the adult lacks capacity to refuse the assessment and the authority is satisfied that carrying out the assessment would be in the adult's best interests, or (b) the adult is experiencing, or is at risk of, abuse or neglect, then the assessment must be carried out. Regulations are to make further provisions for assessments for both clients and carers. The LA is required to give a written record of the assessment to the adult, the carer and any other person to whom the adult requests a copy to be given.

Eligibility criteria

Under section 13 where a local authority is satisfied on the basis of a needs or carer's assessment that an adult has needs for care and support or that a carer has needs for support, it must determine whether any of the needs meet the eligibility criteria. The provisions of section 13 are shown in Statute Box 22.6.

Statute 22.6
Care Act 2014 section 13
Eligibility criteria

> (1) Where a local authority is satisfied on the basis of a needs or carer's assessment that an adult has needs for care and support or that a carer has needs for support, it must determine whether any of the needs meet the eligibility criteria (see subsection (7)).
> (2) Having made a determination under subsection (1), the local authority must give the adult concerned a written record of the determination and the reasons for it.
> (3) Where at least some of an adult's needs for care and support meet the eligibility criteria, the local authority must—
>
> (a) consider what could be done to meet those needs that do,
> (b) ascertain whether the adult wants to have those needs met by the local authority in accordance with this Part, and
> (c) establish whether the adult is ordinarily resident in the local authority's area.
>
> (4) Where at least some of a carer's needs for support meet the eligibility criteria, the local authority must—
>
> (a) consider what could be done to meet those needs that do, and

(b) establish whether the adult needing care is ordinarily resident in the local authority's area.

(5) Where none of the needs of the adult concerned meet the eligibility criteria, the local authority must give him or her written advice and information about—

(a) what can be done to meet or reduce the needs;

(b) what can be done to prevent or delay the development of needs for care and support, or the development of needs for support, in the future.

(6) Regulations may make provision about the making of the determination under subsection (1).

(7) Needs meet the eligibility criteria if—

(a) they are of a description specified in regulations, or

(b) they form part of a combination of needs of a description so specified.

(8) The regulations may, in particular, describe needs by reference to—

(a) the effect that the needs have on the adult concerned;

(b) the adult's circumstances.

Section 18 and 19 set out the duty (s. 18) and power (s. 19) of the LA to meet the needs for care and support. Section 20 sets out the LA duty and power to meet the needs for support for a carer.

At the time of writing, regulations on eligibility criteria were under consultation.

The next steps for the local authority to take

Care and support plan

Statute Box 22.7 sets out the provisions of section 24 and the steps a local authority must take in relation to the preparation of a care and support plan which is defined in section 25 as shown in Statute Box 22.8.

Statute 22.7
Care Act 2014 section 24

The steps for the local authority to take

(1) Where a local authority is required to meet needs under section 18 or 20(1), or decides to do so under section 19(1) or (2) or 20(6), it must—

(a) prepare a care and support plan or a support plan for the adult concerned,

(b) tell the adult which (if any) of the needs that it is going to meet may be met by direct payments, and

(c) help the adult with deciding how to have the needs met.

(2) Where a local authority has carried out a needs or carer's assessment but is not required to meet needs under section 18 or 20(1), and does not decide to do so under section 19(1) or (2) or 20(6), it must give the adult concerned—

(a) its written reasons for not meeting the needs, and

(b) (unless it has already done so under section 13(5)) advice and information about—
- (i) what can be done to meet or reduce the needs;
- (ii) what can be done to prevent or delay the development by the adult concerned of needs for care and support or of needs for support in the future.

(3) Where a local authority is not going to meet an adult's needs for care and support, it must nonetheless prepare an independent personal budget for the adult (see section 28) if—
- (a) the needs meet the eligibility criteria,
- (b) at least some of the needs are not being met by a carer, and
- (c) the adult is ordinarily resident in the authority's area or is present in its area but of no settled residence.

Statute 22.8
Care Act 2014 section 25

Care and support plan

(1) A care and support plan or, in the case of a carer, a support plan is a document prepared by a local authority which—
- (a) specifies the needs identified by the needs assessment or carer's assessment,
- (b) specifies whether, and if so to what extent, the needs meet the eligibility criteria,
- (c) specifies the needs that the local authority is going to meet and how it is going to meet them,
- (d) specifies to which of the matters referred to in section 9(4) the provision of care and support could be relevant or to which of the matters referred to in section 10(5) and (6) the provision of support could be relevant,
- (e) includes the personal budget for the adult concerned (see section 26), and
- (f) includes advice and information about—
  - (i) what can be done to meet or reduce the needs in question;
  - (ii) what can be done to prevent or delay the development of needs for care and support or of needs for support in the future.

(2) Where some or all of the needs are to be met by making direct payments, the plan must also specify—
- (a) the needs which are to be so met, and
- (b) the amount and frequency of the direct payments.

(3) In preparing a care and support plan, the local authority must involve—
- (a) the adult for whom it is being prepared,

(b) any carer that the adult has, and

(c) any person whom the adult asks the authority to involve or, where the adult lacks capacity to ask the authority to do that, any person who appears to the authority to be interested in the adult's welfare.

(4) In preparing a support plan, the local authority must involve—

(a) the carer for whom it is being prepared,

(b) the adult needing care, if the carer asks the authority to do so, and

(c) any other person whom the carer asks the authority to involve.

(5) In performing the duty under subsection (3)(a) or (4)(a), the local authority must take all reasonable steps to reach agreement with the adult or carer for whom the plan is being prepared about how the authority should meet the needs in question.

(6) In seeking to ensure that the plan is proportionate to the needs to be met, the local authority must have regard in particular—

(a) in the case of a care and support plan, to the matters referred to in section 9(4),

(b) in the case of a support plan, to the matters referred to in section 10(5) and (6).

(7) The local authority may authorise a person (including the person for whom the plan is to be prepared) to prepare the plan jointly with the authority.

(8) The local authority may do things to facilitate the preparation of the plan in a case within subsection (7); it may, for example, provide a person authorised under that subsection with—

(a) in the case of a care and support plan, information about the adult for whom the plan is being prepared;

(b) in the case of a support plan, information about the carer and the adult needing care;

(c) in either case, whatever resources, or access to whatever facilities, the authority thinks are required to prepare the plan.

(9) The local authority must give a copy of a care and support plan to—

(a) the adult for whom it has been prepared,

(b) any carer that the adult has, if the adult asks the authority to do so, and

(c) any other person to whom the adult asks the authority to give a copy.

(10) The local authority must give a copy of a support plan to—

(a) the carer for whom it has been prepared,

(b) the adult needing care, if the carer asks the authority to do so, and

(c) any other person to whom the carer asks the authority to give a copy.

(11) A local authority may combine a care and support plan or a support plan with a plan (whether or not prepared by it and whether or not under this Part) relating to another person only if the adult for whom the care and support plan or the support plan is being prepared agrees and—

(a) where the combination would include a plan prepared for another adult, that other adult agrees;

> (b) where the combination would include a plan prepared for a child (including a young carer), the consent condition is met in relation to the child.
>
> (12) The consent condition is met in relation to a child if—
>
>   (a) the child has capacity or is competent to agree to the plans being combined and does so agree, or
>
>   (b) the child lacks capacity or is not competent so to agree but the local authority is satisfied that the combining the plans would be in the child's best interests.
>
> (13) Regulations may specify cases or circumstances in which such of paragraphs (a) to (f) of subsection (1) and paragraphs (a) and (b) of subsection (2) as are specified do not apply.
>
> (14) The regulations may in particular specify that the paragraphs in question do not apply as regards specified needs or matters.

Deferred payments

Sections 35 to 37 of the Care Act 2014 set out the terms of the 'deferred payment agreement' under which a local authority agrees not to require payment until the specified time. Regulations may, in such cases or circumstances and subject to such conditions as may be specified, require or permit a local authority to enter into a deferred payment agreement with an adult. The regulations may, in particular, prohibit a local authority from entering into, or permit it to refuse to enter into, a deferred payment agreement unless it obtains adequate security (as defined in the regulations) for the payment of the adult's deferred amount. The regulations will also specify interest, costs and other payments which have to be made. 'Alternative financial arrangements' can also be set up which equate in substance to a deferred payment agreement but achieve a similar effect to an agreement of the kind in question without including provision for the payment of interest.

Criticism of the new scheme for deferred payments was made in a study by the Institute and Faculty of Actuaries which found that the average pensioner will spend an average of £140,000 of their own savings on the cost of elderly care. Only 1 in 10 of those entering care in 2016 would have reached the new cap designed to prevent older people from being forced to sell their homes to fund the cost of care. The cap which would have come into force in 2016 was set at £72,000, however it would only have applied to care costs set by local authorities. It would not have included the cost of housing and living expenses.[37]

Independent advocate

Under section 67(4) of the Care Act 2014 the local authority is required to ensure that an independent advocate is appointed to speak on behalf of a person where, in the absence of such an advocate, the individual would experience substantial difficulty in doing one or more of the following:

(a) understanding relevant information,

(b) retaining that information,

(c) using or weighing that information as part of the process of being involved, and

(d) communicating the individual's views, wishes or feelings (whether by talking, using sign language or any other means).

This applies where the LA is:

- carrying out needs assessment (section 9(5)(a) and (b)),
- carrying out carer's assessment (section 10(7)(a)),
- preparing a care and support plan (section 25(3)(a) and (b)),
- preparing a support plan (section 25(4)(a) and (b)),
- revising the care and support plan (section 27(2)(b)(i) and (ii)),
- revising the support plan (section 27(3)(b)(i) and (ii)),
- carrying out child's needs assessment (section 59(2)(a) and (b)),
- carrying out child's carer's assessment (section 61(3)(a)), and
- carrying out young carer's assessment (section 64(3)(a) and (b)).

Community equipment

In 2000 the Audit Commission published its findings on the provision of equipment for older and disabled people.[38] It found that users were not asked basic questions about the sort of help they needed; they had to wait for long periods of time for their equipment; the equipment was not always suitable or of a high quality; and the current organisation of equipment services is a recipe for inequality and inefficiency. Among its many significant recommendations are suggestions for involving users, restructuring of mobility services, the integration of health and social services provision for community equipment under the powers of the Health Act 1999, and the introduction of policy reviews and dissemination of good practice. Care trusts have now been set up to ensure integration of health and social service provision. Brian Donnelly has carried out an independent review of the delivery of community equipment services across England and Wales.[39] He estimated that there are approximately 10 million pieces of community equipment delivered to 3.5 million clients every year in England and Wales. He proposed National Minimum Standards to reduce risks, improve quality and safety, and save public funds.[40] The CQC has published details of the Community Equipment Code of Practice Scheme (CECOPS), which is a social enterprise set up to manage registration, training and accreditation of users of the code of practice for community equipment. The Code sets out a quality framework for procurement and provision of services. CECOPS aims to assist all public and private sector providers and commissioners. Further details can be found on the CQC website.[41]

Human rights and care homes

The Human Rights Act 1998 applies to public authorities and organisations exercising functions of a public nature. How far does it apply to the private sector? In a case brought against the Leonard Cheshire Foundation,[42] the Court of Appeal held that on the particular facts before it (the redevelopment of the home), the charity had not carried out the functions of a public authority. In June 2007 the House of Lords held in a majority decision (in keeping with an earlier decision by the Court of Appeal)[43] that a private care home, which was under contract with a local authority to provide care and accommodation for elderly persons, was not an organisation exercising functions of a public nature.[44] An 84-year-old resident who suffered from Alzheimer's disease was therefore unable to make a claim under Article 8 of the European Convention on Human Rights in respect of her removal from the care home. This decision led to a campaign for legislation to bring private care homes under the auspices of the Human Rights Act 1998. The campaign was given added momentum following the report of the Parliamentary Joint Committee on Human Rights in August 2007.[45] This report found that more than a fifth of care homes have been found to be failing basic standards of care for privacy and dignity. The report considered that elder abuse is a serious and severe human rights abuse which is perpetrated on vulnerable older people who often depend on their abusers to provide them with care. The Joint Committee criticised the Department of Health and Ministry of Justice for failing to provide proper leadership and guidance on the Human Rights Act to providers of health and residential care. It recommended that care standards regulations should be amended so that all care homes are brought under the Human Rights Act and that eventually the Human Rights Act should be amended to ensure that private care homes came under its remit. It also recognised the importance of the role of staff in protecting human rights and made specific recommendation on the training of staff and suggested that there should be a duty specified in the care standards requiring staff to report abuse, with protection for whistleblowing and confidentiality.

As a consequence of the reaction to these court decisions, section 145 of the Health and Social Care Act 2008 was enacted to define the provision of certain social care as a public function. Section 145 states that:

(1) A person ('P') who provides accommodation, together with nursing or personal care, in a care home for an individual under arrangements made with P under the relevant statutory provisions is to be taken for the purposes of subsection (3)(b) of section 6 of the Human Rights Act 1998 (c. 42) (acts of public authorities) to be exercising a function of a public nature in doing so.

(2) The 'relevant statutory provisions' are–

   (a) in relation to England and Wales, sections 21(1)(a) and 26 of the National Assistance Act 1948 (c. 29),

   (b) in relation to Scotland, section 12 or 13A of the Social Work (Scotland) Act 1968 (c. 49), and

   (c) in relation to Northern Ireland, Articles 15 and 36 of the Health and Personal Social Services (Northern Ireland) Order 1972 (SI 1972/1265 (NI 14)).

This provision is not retrospective and does not apply to cases prior to the coming into force of section 145.

Section 73 of the Care Act 2014 extends this provision so that the provider of care and support is exercising functions of a public nature if:

(a) the care or support is arranged by an authority specified in the Act, and

(b) the authority arranges or pays for the care or support under specified legislation.

For England the specified authorities are local authorities (under s. 2, 18, 19, 20, 38 and 48 of the Care Act 2014) and Health and Social Care Trusts (under s. 51 of the Care Act 2014). The provision extends across the UK.

Those funding their own care cannot claim the protection of the Human Rights Act, although they may be able to seek redress via a breach of contract between themselves and the home/care centre.

An allegation that a local authority was in breach of Article 5 of the European Convention on Human Rights succeeded in 2006.[46] The local authority had placed the claimant's husband in a care home, justifying the placement on grounds that any restriction on his liberty was in his best interests and he was not being deprived of his liberty within the meaning of Article 5. The court held that the crucial issue was whether the person was free to leave and concluded that he was not. Since October 2007 the provisions of the Mental Capacity Act 2005 would apply to this situation – see the Deprivation of Liberty Safeguards (DoLS) and the Supreme Court judgment in the Cheshire case[47] (see chapter 16).

In another successful action alleging a breach of Article 8, the claimant, who was blind, suffered from diabetes and had suffered several strokes, obtained judicial review of a primary care trust's refusal to provide 24-hour nursing care in her own home (her parents ceasing to be able to provide hands-on care). The court held that removing her from her home into residential care would interfere with her right to respect for her family life within Article 8.[48]

In contrast with the previous two cases, the challenge of a wife whose husband was transferred from a nursing home to a hospital because of his health and behavioural problems failed in her claim.[49] The judge held that the without notice application for the transfer by the local authority was justified and there was no breach of Article 8. The injunctions to forbid the wife to interfere with her husband's transfer or his care at the hospital or attempting to see him at the hospital except as agreed and supervised by the local authority were justified.

Case 22.4 R (McDonald) v Kensington and Chelsea Royal London Borough Council (ECHR) [2014][50]

The Supreme Court[51] had held that there was no breach of Article 8 rights when an LA withdrew the provision of a night-time carer to assist a disabled person to use a commode when required and instead provided her with incontinence pads to wear at night (Baroness Hale dissented). The ECHR held that there was a breach of Article 8 for part of the time. However, where the withdrawal had been made after a proper assessment, the interference with her right to respect for her private life had been both proportionate and justified as necessary in a democratic society and there was no breach of Article 8.

The implications of this ECHR decision is that failure by the local authority to carry out an appropriate assessment before removing any assistance from or refusing to provide a service to a community client could be seen as a breach of Article 8 rights.

In 2013 a strengthened CQC announced that it would consider using CCTV in care homes to check whether there was abuse. Details of the new regime of inspections introduced from 2012 are available from the CQC website.[52] In July 2014 the CQC chief inspector for adult social care announced that from 2015 the CQC would introduce placing non-performing care homes in special measures as part of a new inspection system for care home and care agencies, comparable to the special measures used for hospitals. The CQC was recruiting a team of 700 inspectors.[53]

A serious case review into the deaths of five elderly people at Orchid View in West Sussex was highly critical of the role of the CQC in failing to alert prospective residents and families to concern about conditions at the home. It called for more stringent regulation. After reviewing the deaths of 19 residents between 2009 and 2011 the coroner concluded that all had suffered from sub-optimal care and five had died from natural causes contributed to by neglect.[54] The CQC's chief inspector of adult social care promised an overhaul into how care homes are inspected.[55]

A cosmetic surgeon who used a basement to carry out cosmetic surgery was held to be in breach of the registration provisions since he had carried on an independent hospital without being registered. He failed in his appeal.[56]

In March 2014 the House of Lords published its post-legislative scrutiny on the Mental Capacity Act 2005[57] which stated that patients were being drugged or locked up and deprived of their liberty without protection of the law. See also the case of Steven Neary[58] which illustrated the problems in using the Deprivation of Liberty Safeguards (see chapter 16).

Delayed discharges

Problems in bed blocking because accommodation was not found in the community for patients ready for discharge from NHS beds were met by the Community Care (Delayed Discharges etc.) Act 2003, which made provision for social services authorities to make payments in cases where the discharge of patients is delayed for reasons relating to the provision of community care services or services for carers. Regulations published in 2003 made provisions for the details of the delayed discharges scheme.[59] They set out the type of care which a patient must be receiving to come within the provisions of the Act; set out the details of the notice which the relevant NHS body must give to the local social services authority to inform it that there is a patient who is likely to need community care services on discharge and also set the time limits for notice and the amounts which the local authority must pay. The regulations also provide for resolution of a dispute. Failure by the social services authority to comply with these statutory duties can lead to the authority being liable to make a payment of the amount prescribed in the regulations for each day of the delayed discharge.

Where a patient refuses to be discharged to a residential care home and no longer requires medical or nursing care in hospital, the patient is not entitled to occupy the bed and the NHS trust is entitled to reclaim possession of its hospital premises from the patient.[60] More recently an NHS trust was granted possession of a bedroom in a hospital care unit which a patient had continued to occupy for many months despite having no medical reason to do so. The woman had suffered a fractured femur and had had a number of operations on her knee. She had been admitted to the rehabilitation facility in August 2015 after surgery. She now no longer had any need to take up a bedroom in the unit. She was assessed as having the same mobility level as before the surgery, and as being able to live at home, albeit with some help from social services. She could not use stairs but with a walking frame could walk 40 metres. She had not required a nurse since November 2015 and had declined all therapy. The Court held that the trust had clearly established the right to possession of the bedroom. It had attempted to engage with the patient but she had refused to communicate with it or the local authority and had refused to provide them with relevant details such as financial information which might have enabled other care arrangements to be made. On the medical evidence, there was no reason why she could not return home, and the trust was granted possession and awarded £8000 in costs.[61]

In 2012 the government launched the Hospital 2 Home resource pack designed to support older people who are returning to their homes after a stay in hospital. The pack indicates that the

NHS spends about £600 million each year treating people in healthcare settings when they are well enough to go home but poor housing delays their discharge.[62] The pack contains information, suggestions for action, case studies and checklists for considering older patients' housing situations in hospital discharge and transfer of care. In June 2013 £1 billion was transferred from the NHS budget to social care to enable frail elderly to be looked after better in their own homes. It was part of a £3.8 billion pot in 2015/16 to be used for schemes commissioned jointly by local health and social care policy makers.[63] The Better Care Fund was established to allow CCGs and local authorities to commission joint service provision through arrangements made under the Care Act 2014, section 75. In 2018/19 the budget for the Better Care Fund will be £5.617 billion.

In October 2013 the Department of Health issued Directions[64] requiring NHS trusts to take reasonable steps to ensure that an assessment of eligibility for NHS Continuing Healthcare is carried out in all cases where it appears to the trust that the patient may have a need for such care, in consultation, where appropriate, with the relevant local social services authority. The Directions are accessible on the government website.[65]

Duty of local authority on discharge of hospital patients with care and support needs

The Care Act 2014 has re-enacted the provisions of the Community Care (Delayed Discharges etc.) Act 2003. Statute Box 22.9 shows the provisions under Schedule 3 of the Care Act (brought into effect by section 74).

Statute 22.9
Care Act 2014 Schedule 3

Cases where hospital patient is likely to have care and support needs after discharge

1. Where the NHS body responsible for a hospital patient considers that it is not likely to be safe to discharge the patient unless arrangements for meeting the patient's needs for care and support are in place, the body must give notice to—
   (a) the local authority in whose area the patient is ordinarily resident, or
   (b) if it appears to the body that the patient is of no settled residence, the local authority in whose area the hospital is situated.
2. A notice under sub-paragraph (1) is referred to in this Schedule as an 'assessment notice'; and the local authority to which an assessment notice is given is referred to in this Schedule as 'the relevant authority'.
3. An assessment notice—
   (a) must describe itself as such, and
   (b) may not be given more than seven days before the day on which the patient is expected to be admitted to hospital.
4. Before giving an assessment notice, the NHS body responsible for the patient must consult—
   (a) the patient, and
   (b) where it is feasible to do so, any carer that the patient has.

5   An assessment notice remains in force until—
    (a) the patient is discharged (whether by the NHS body responsible for the patient or by the patient himself or herself),
    (b) the patient dies, or
    (c) the NHS body responsible for the patient withdraws the notice by giving a notice (a 'withdrawal notice') to the relevant authority.
6   A reference in this paragraph to a hospital patient includes a reference to a person who it is reasonable to expect is about to become one.

Assessment notice given by responsible NHS body to local authority

1   The NHS body responsible for a hospital patient, having given the relevant authority an assessment notice, must—
    (a) consult the authority before deciding what it will do for the patient in order for discharge to be safe, and
    (b) give the authority notice of the day on which it proposes to discharge the patient.
2   A notice under sub-paragraph (1)(b) is referred to in this Schedule as a 'discharge notice'.
3   A discharge notice must specify—
    (a) whether the NHS body responsible for the patient will be providing or arranging for the provision of services under the National Health Service Act 2006 to the patient after discharge, and
    (b) if it will, what those services are.
4   A discharge notice remains in force until—
    (a) the end of the relevant day, or
    (b) the NHS body responsible for the patient withdraws the notice by giving a withdrawal notice to the relevant authority.
5   The 'relevant day' is the later of—
    (a) the day specified in the discharge notice, and
    (b) the last day of such period as regulations may specify.
6   A period specified under sub-paragraph (5)(b) must—
    (a) begin with the day after that on which the assessment notice is given, and
    (b) last for a period of at least two days.

Assessment notice given by responsible NHS body to local authority

1   The relevant authority, having received an assessment notice and having in light of it carried out a needs assessment and (where applicable) a carer's assessment, must inform the NHS body responsible for the patient—
    (a) whether the patient has needs for care and support,

(b) (where applicable) whether a carer has needs for support,

(c) whether any of the needs referred to in paragraphs (a) and (b) meet the eligibility criteria, and

(d) how the authority plans to meet such of those needs as meet the eligibility criteria.

2 Where, having carried out a needs assessment or carer's assessment in a case within section 27(4), the relevant authority considers that the patient's needs for care and support or (as the case may be) the carer's needs for support have changed, it must inform the NHS body responsible for the patient of the change.

Cases where discharge of the patient is delayed

4(1) If the relevant authority, having received an assessment notice and a discharge notice, has not carried out a needs or (where applicable) carer's assessment and the patient has not been discharged by the end of the relevant day, the NHS body responsible for the patient may require the relevant authority to pay the specified amount for each day of the specified period.

(2) If the relevant authority has not put in place arrangements for meeting some or all of those of the needs under sections 18 to 20 [Care Act 2014] that it proposes to meet in the case of the patient or (where applicable) a carer, and the patient has for that reason alone not been discharged by the end of the relevant day, the NHS body responsible for the patient may require the relevant authority to pay the specified amount for each day of the specified period.

Carers

According to the Carers Trust (2018) it has been estimated that Great Britain has 7 million carers and 1 in 10 households contains a carer.[66] The Carers (Recognition and Services) Act 1995 required local authorities to carry out an assessment of the carer's ability to provide and to continue to provide care for the person receiving community care services, but it did not give local authorities the power to offer carers services to support them in their caring role.

In 1999 the government published a Carer's National Strategy Document[67] highlighting the need for legislation to enable local authorities to provide services direct to carers. The Carers and Disabled Children Act 2000 had four main purposes:

1. It gave local authorities the power to supply certain services direct to carers.

2. It enabled local authorities to make direct payments to carers, including 16- and 17-year-olds, to persons with parental responsibility for disabled children and to the disabled children. These direct payments can then be used for a provider for those services chosen by the carer.

3. Local authorities could provide short-term break voucher schemes, which would give carers flexibility in the timing and choice of breaks.

4. The local authorities were given power to charge carers for the services they receive. In its assessment, the LA can take into account any assessment made under the 1995 Act. The

2000 Act does not apply if the carer is an employee or a volunteer for a voluntary organisation. The LA must consider the assessment and decide:

- whether the carer has needs in relation to the care that they provide or intend to provide,
- if so, whether they could be satisfied (wholly or partly) by services which the LA may provide, and
- if they could be so satisfied, whether or not to provide services to the carer.

Direct payments are considered in chapter 16.

Under the Care Act 2014 the local authority has a duty to assess a carer's needs for support (section 10) and a duty and power to meet those needs.

Liability of client for carer

A carer won a payout from a widower who had employed her to care for his wife. Following the death of his wife the widower cut her hours from 30 to 16 a week and the carer, Jayne Wakefield, claimed that she had been unfairly dismissed and was awarded, by the employment appeal tribunal, £3569 for constructive and unfair dismissal and breach of contract.[68]

Negligence

Standard of care

In Practical Dilemma 22.1 it is possible that the relatives will be present and probably represented by a solicitor or barrister at the inquest. The inquest might well be followed by a civil claim against the

Practical Dilemma 22.1 — Key worker

The Roger Park Community NHS Trust set up a series of location managers and teams of multidisciplinary professionals for clients. Each client was assigned a key worker who would discuss with the team that particular client's difficulties and try to resolve them as far as possible on his own, thus preventing the client from being visited by a whole host of different professionals. This key worker could be any one of a variety of professionals, but as far as possible it was one whose training was most relevant to the client's needs. Margaret Downs lived on her own and was recovering from a stroke. With the help of the physiotherapist she was making good progress and the community nurse, Angela Hide, was visiting her twice a week to dress a leg ulcer and also to give her a bath. The community nurse was Margaret's key worker. After a few weeks, Angela decided that Margaret would be able to manage to bath herself on her own if she had a bath rail and support. She got in touch with the local authority department that provided home aids and ordered the appropriate devices to be fitted. She told Margaret that once they were installed she would not need any assistance to bathe, but that if she got into any difficulties she should let Angela know. A few days later Margaret, who had not been seen by neighbours for a few days, was found dead in the bath. A post mortem showed that she had slipped while trying to get out of the bath, that the handrail was not in a suitable position and that she had probably died of exposure. The coroner held an inquest and Angela was asked to provide a statement, as was the occupational therapist in the team, since the task of assessment for bath aids was normally that of the occupational therapist.

NHS trust on the basis of its direct liability for the death of Margaret in failing to lay down an appropriate procedure for caring for patients in the community and also on the basis of its indirect or vicarious liability for Angela's negligence. Was Angela negligent? Obviously, there are very few facts given here on which the answer to such a question could be determined, but at the heart of the negligence action will be the question: did Angela follow the accepted approved practice in making those recommendations about the bath aids? Or, if she did not follow the approved practice, was there justification for her not doing so and would that justification be supported by competent professional opinion? The question of whether such a decision was within her competence or whether she should have brought in the occupational therapist, whose training includes that type of assessment, will be crucial. It does not, of course, follow that the mere fact that Angela strayed outside her competence will automatically mean that she failed to follow a reasonable standard of care. In addition, the relatives will also have to establish that there was a causal link between the breach of duty by Angela and the harm caused to Margaret and that that harm was reasonably foreseeable.

The most important feature in any team approach and key worker system is that each should know the limits of their competence and the point at which the patient's safety demands that another person be brought in to advise. In the Wilsher case (considered in detail in chapter 4), the court has held that there is no concept of team liability. It is a question of individual liability and/or the liability of the NHS trust. (The legal issues arising from the scope of professional practice are considered in chapter 23.) A salutary lesson on the importance of training individual nurses is seen in the account of a tetraplegic patient dependent on a ventilator at home whose agency nurse accidentally switched off his life support, causing him to suffer serious brain damage.[69] His family indicated their intention to sue the PCT, which had carried out an investigation which found that the nurse was not qualified in the use of ventilators even though that was one of the requirements for the job. The patient had complained of poor standards of care and set up a camera which recorded the incident.

To whom is the nurse responsible?

Practical Dilemma 22.2, in which there is a clash between what the nurse is told to do and what she feels is her duty to the patient, is not unusual, neither is it confined to the community. Other situations, for example where the nurse is told not to take patients in her car or where she is given instructions about lifting that she cannot carry out because the facilities or staff are not available, place the nurse in a dilemma. Is she to fulfil what she believes to be her duty to the

Practical Dilemma 22.2   A clash of duties

Community nurses in the Roger Park Unit had been given instructions that they should not carry drugs in their cars, neither should they personally arrange for drugs on prescriptions to be collected from the chemists. Ruth Green was caring for a terminally ill patient who was being nursed by her husband at home. The GP had left a prescription on his last visit and the husband asked her if she would be kind enough to bring the drugs back from the chemist. He said that he did not have any transport or any neighbours who could help and he did not want to leave his wife on her own. Ruth said that she was not allowed to collect drugs from the chemist for patients. He was clearly distressed and offered to come with her if she could provide the transport, but it would still mean leaving his wife on her own. She agreed to this and took him to the chemist and then home again – a round trip of about seven miles that took 20 minutes. The husband could not understand why he had to go with her, leaving his wife for such a long time and obviously in danger. Ruth herself felt that the rules were not appropriate to that situation and wondered whether there was any law that covered her duties.

---

patient or should she obey the NHS trust's or nurse manager's instructions? The clash can be seen as a conflict between the Code set down by the NMC[70] and her employer's orders. She has a contractual duty to obey the latter, since it is an implied term of her contract of employment that she obey the reasonable orders of her employer; contrariwise, she has a professional duty to follow the Code. If provisions of the Code are included in the contract of employment, then there should in theory be no clash between the two. Instructions by the employer must be reasonable and it can be argued that any instructions that clash with the professional obligations of the registered practitioner cannot be reasonable.

The first task for Ruth Green in a situation like this is for the nurse management to be given the full facts of any potential hardship suffered by the patient as a result of their instructions and procedures. Examples of the difficulties that have and will arise from following these instructions must be provided in detail. It may so happen that, when presented with this evidence, management might well feel that either the whole policy should be revised or that certain exceptions can be made in circumstances where the patient is likely to suffer harm.

Alternatively, it may be possible for other arrangements to be made that will ensure the safety and well-being of the patient. For example, in rural areas, pharmacists sometimes provide a home delivery service for medicines and oxygen. If the management is adamant that the procedures must be followed without any exception, the nurse has a duty to undertake those unless there is likely to be such harm to the patient that it is clearly contrary to her duty of care to the patient. In such a situation, her records would have to be very comprehensive to justify her action. In serious situations, the nurse should raise concerns with senior levels of management in accordance with the Public Interest Disclosure Act (see chapter 4).

In the following case, the fact that a GP relied heavily upon the role of community nurses was the subject of disciplinary action.

Case 22.5   R v FHS Appeal Authority ex p Muralidhar [1999]

Medical treatment: reasonableness of doctor relying on nurses[71]

A GP applied for judicial review of a finding by the chief executive of a family health services authority that he was in breach of his terms of service by relying on district nurses who had visited the patient daily to treat a patient's bedsores. The patient suffered from senile dementia, incontinence and was bedridden. The doctor visited her, prescribed antibiotics for infected bedsores, leaving instructions with staff that he should be contacted if there were any deterioration. He was not contacted, but subsequently the patient was removed to hospital where criticism of her previous nursing care was made. The judge, in granting the application, held that the chief executive had failed to consider whether the doctor had behaved in accordance with his terms of service and had taken irrelevant considerations into account. There was also procedural unfairness in that the chief executive had not alerted the doctor to the importance he attached to these considerations so that the doctor could make relevant representations.

There are clear lessons for nursing staff from this case. If they are concerned about a patient's condition they should ensure that the doctor is called in to examine the patient.

Examples of serious breaches of the duty of care

It was reported that two council workers (a social worker and a team leader) were suspended after the death of an elderly woman who was left alone for nine days after her care agency was shut.[72] Carefirst 24 was contracted to care for her and provide daily visits.

Abele View Ltd which ran a care home near Stourbridge was fined £133,000 and ordered to pay £122,412 in costs following the death of a resident in the garden. The resident died of hypothermia and his disappearance went unnoticed. The prosecution was brought under health and safety legislation[73] (see chapter 12).

Three staff were suspended from an old people's home after a local authority started an investigation into standards at the Bupa-owned St Mark's Nursing Centre, Maidenhead.[74]

Giving advice

One of the most important tasks of many registered practitioners, and in particular the specialist community public health nurse (SCPHN), is giving advice to clients, young and old, on all aspects of their health and ways of keeping healthy. For example, one of the vexed questions these days is the extent to which the SCPHN should encourage a mother to have her child vaccinated and the possibility of the SCPHN themselves being held liable for giving advice that turns out to cause harm. The topic of liability for communications was discussed in chapter 4. If a health visitor, knowing that a child has a history of convulsions, fails to take this into account in advising the mother to have the child vaccinated and also fails to ensure that the doctor is advised of this fact, the health visitor may well share some responsibility for any harm that befalls the child as a result of undergoing the vaccination. (Vaccinations are considered in chapter 25.)

Safety of the community professional

Entering other people's homes can be dangerous. Unlike the NHS trust, the occupiers have no obligations under the Health and Safety at Work Act 1974, but they do have obligations under the Occupiers' Liability Act 1957. This is discussed in detail in chapter 12. The community worker faces problems in relation to both the standard of the structure and the fixtures and fittings. In addition, they might find difficulties caused by the client or the relatives.

This particular situation may be unique but it represents the many dangers with which a community worker is faced.

What are the practicalities of obtaining compensation? Is the NHS trust liable? The answer is probably no, unless it can be shown that it was aware of the danger that an employee was in

> **Practical Dilemma 22.3** **Defective premises**
>
> Pam Hughes, a health visitor, had a large caseload in one of the poorer parts of the city. In one council house, conditions were very bad: the wallpaper was peeling off the walls and there were piles of empty milk bottles in the kitchen and a miscellaneous assortment of carpet pieces on the concrete floor. The local authority had been notified of certain defects to the roof and the fittings, but had said that, because of the backlog of maintenance work and staff cuts, it would be several weeks before they could repair the property. The occupiers, Mr and Mrs James and their seven children, could not cope with the situation. Mr James was unemployed and attempted to rectify some of the defects, including putting a new piece of glass in the front door to replace the pane that had been broken when the door was slammed shut. The door had swollen owing to the guttering leaking onto it. Pam Hughes was well used to the family and had been visiting regularly because of her concern over the two youngest children. After one visit, she let herself out – as was her usual custom – and had to pull hard on the front door to open it. As she pulled, the new pane fell out onto her hand, cutting her severely across the wrist. After medical treatment and the advice of a specialist, it appeared that the tendons were severed and she would have very little movement in the four fingers of her right hand. It is certainly questionable whether she will be able to continue her work as a health visitor. Since she is unmarried, and the sole breadwinner, caring for her elderly mother, she is frightened at the prospect of losing her job. She is therefore anxious to recover financial compensation for the injuries.

and failed to take reasonable precautions to safeguard her. There is no evidence that this was so in this case. However, the employers may be prepared to ensure that compensation is paid to her on an ex gratia basis since she was injured in the course of her employment. Mr and Mrs James are possibly liable. As occupiers, they failed to ensure that the premises were safe for the visitor. Mr James may well have repaired the door negligently. However, unless they are insured, the question is academic, since they are unlikely to be able to pay any compensation.

Since it is a council house, it may be that Pam could establish a case against the council in its capacity as landlord and therefore occupier of the building. However, to succeed it would be important to show that, from the obligations under the lease, the landlord had a duty to carry out repairs and his failure to do so had reasonably foreseeably caused the injury to Pam's arm. However, Mr James's repair work makes a break in this chain of causation. If Pam fails against all three potential defendants, then all she can do is fall back on her own insurance cover. Some household insurance schemes also cover for personal injuries or she may have her own personal accident cover. If not, she is unlikely to obtain any compensation other than the usual statutory sick pay scheme and the DSS injury benefits, which are considerably smaller than the level of compensation awarded in the civil courts.

The lesson is clear: because of the dangers of working in variable conditions, it is probably essential that community workers have some form of insurance cover for personal accidents. Some local authorities, professional associations and trade unions have negotiated group schemes of cover. It is, however, the policy of the NHS not to take out insurance cover. If the professional is working on NHS trust premises all the time, then the authority as occupier has a duty to ensure that she is safe, and if it fails in this duty then it could be held liable under the Occupiers' Liability Act.

Case 22.6   *R v Hillingdon Health Authority ex parte Wyatt* [1977]

Aggression in the community[75]

Mrs Wyatt suffered from multiple sclerosis, could do nothing for herself and needed nursing assistance. The health authority had the duty to provide a home nursing service under section 25 of the NHS Act 1946 (as amended by the 1973 Reorganisation Act). The husband, who was also an invalid, abused the nursing staff when they visited his wife and was aggressive and threatening. He was asked to give an assurance that he would cease to behave so, but he refused. The authority told Mrs Wyatt's solicitors that because of Mr Wyatt's behaviour they could not continue the nursing service.

The Court of Appeal held that the authority was doing all that could be reasonably expected of it and the application to compel the authority to provide the service would be dismissed.

The principle established in the Wyatt case can be applied to other situations, including the dangerous nature of the premises. However, before any service can be justifiably withdrawn, the threat to the safety of the community worker must have reached a serious level and every possible precaution must have been taken. For example, it might be necessary for some nurses to be sent in pairs to clients where they face danger. One question that a community nurse sometimes asks is: Can I refuse to go if I consider that I am in personal danger? If the employer's instruction to go to a particular place is unreasonable with regard to the danger with which the worker is faced and the lack of precautions that the employer has taken for the employee's safety, then the employee can refuse to obey them. What is meant by unreasonable? This is a matter of balancing all the options available, including other precautions that it is reasonable for the employer to take against the risks involved and the needs of the client. Where the danger to the professional is the neighbourhood itself, it might, for example, be reasonable for the employer to arrange for an alarm/warning system to be carried by the employee or to ensure that they visit homes in pairs. Where the danger comes from aggressive clients or their relatives, then it might be sufficient if a senior nurse accompanies the nurse to ensure their safety. A similar situation of a conflict between patients/carers and the health professionals has arisen in manual handling, where the patient refuses to be lifted by a hoist. This issue is considered in chapter 12. The Health and Safety Executive (HSE) has developed a pack for violence management training in healthcare settings which could be applied to work in the community.[76]

Practical Dilemma 22.4   Community dangers

Mark was a man of 32 with learning disabilities who had been living in a community home for about six weeks. He had settled down well and, provided that he took his medication, he coped quite well, taking his share of the household chores. He was due for an injection, but to the surprise of the community nurse, he said that he was not going to take it. She pleaded with him, but to no avail. She said she would return that night, but he again refused the injection. She offered to provide it in tablet form, but he said that he would not take it in any form. The nurse tried to give the injection to him again, but he lost his temper, striking out and severely injuring her.

Several problems emerge from this: one is the issue of consent to treatment in the community, to which we shall return later; the other is the question of the safety of community nurses for the mentally ill and those with learning disabilities.

It is the employer's duty to take reasonable care of the health, safety and welfare of his employee. If it is known that a particular patient is a danger to nursing staff, then the employer has a duty to take reasonable precautions to see that they will be safe. These precautions might mean ensuring that a female nurse never visits the patient on her own. There is quite likely to be a need for refuge to be provided so that, if a client is particularly disturbed, he can leave the community or family house and make use of a respite bed, i.e. providing respite for the family. In the situation above, in deciding whether the NHS trust is liable for the injuries suffered by the community nurse, account would have to be taken of whether it was known that the patient was aggressive and, if so, whether the appropriate precautions had been taken, whether the community nurse followed approved accepted practice in her dealings with the patient or whether she provoked the patient by what she did and was therefore, to some extent, to blame for what happened. (See further discussion on health and safety in chapter 12.)

Official advice on violence

The Health and Safety Commission (now merged with the Health and Safety Executive) published guidance on the assessment and management of risks of violence and aggression to staff in health services.[77] This includes, in Appendix 3, a home visiting checklist. The three Vs of visiting are 'vet – verify – vigilance'. The checklist for staff is shown in Box 22.2. Another checklist is provided for managers.

Box 22.2 **Checklist for staff who make home visits**

Have you:

- had all the relevant training about violence to staff?
- a sound grasp of your unit's safety policy for visitors?
- a clear idea about the area into which you are going?
- carefully previewed today's cases? Any 'PVs' (potentially violent clients/patients)?
- asked to double up, take an escort or use a taxi if unsure?
- made appointments?
- left your itinerary and expected departure/arrival times?
- told colleagues, manager about possible changes of plans?
- arranged for contact if your return is overdue?

Do you have:

- forms on which to record and report incidents?
- a personal alarm or radio? Does it work? Is it handy?

- a bag/briefcase, wear an outer uniform or car stickers that suggest you have money or drugs with you? Is this wise where you are going today/tonight?
- out of hours telephone numbers to summon help?

Can you:

- be certain your attitudes, body language, etc. won't cause trouble?
- defuse potential problems and manage aggression?

Consent to treatment

Mental capacity

If a person is mentally capable, he or she is entitled to make their own decisions.[78] A person who has the necessary mental capacity can refuse treatment for a good reason, a bad reason or no reason at all.[79,80] (This is considered further in chapter 7.) However, it is essential that the capacity of the individual to make decisions is assessed by the health professional since if the person lacks the mental capacity then action has to be taken in their best interests.[81,82] The Mental Capacity Act 2005 applies where a person lacks the requisite mental capacity to make decisions (see chapters 7 and 16). In Practical Dilemma 22.4 it may be that Mark lacks the mental capacity to decide whether or not to take his medication and therefore action must be taken in his best interests in accordance with the Mental Capacity Act 2005. The principles and basic provisions of the Act are considered in chapter 7 and the provisions relating to the loss of liberty for those incapable of giving consent, but who are not detained under the Mental Health Act 1983 (known as the Deprivation of Liberty Safeguards (DoLS)), are considered in chapter 16. Alternatively, if the treatment is for mental disorder, then the provisions of the Mental Health Act 1983 as amended may apply (see chapter 19).

Mental disorders

In chapter 19, which deals with the psychiatric nurse, the problem of giving drugs in the community is discussed. Medication can only be given without consent if it comes within the provisions of the Mental Health Act 1983 as amended by the Mental Health Act 2007 or under the provisions of the Mental Capacity Act 2005 where a person lacks the requisite mental capacity and action is taken in his or her best interests. The Mental Health Act 2007 has introduced a new community treatment order which replaces the provision for aftercare under supervision. In Practical Dilemma 22.4, if the treatment is for mental disorder and Mark continues to refuse to take it, he could be admitted to a mental hospital as an inpatient in order to be treated compulsorily.

Forcible entry

Another point that often concerns the community nurse and the health visitor is whether they have any rights of entry. As far as the statutory law is concerned, the answer is no. There may be a power of entry at common law where it is feared that an old person is in need of help, but it exists only in an emergency to save life.

> **Practical Dilemma 22.5**   **A row of bottles**
>
> Neighbours drew the attention of the community nurse to a row of bottles outside the house of an elderly recluse. They feared for her safety and suggested that they should break into the house to check that all was well. The community nurse was hesitant.

In a case like this, it is preferable from the practical, as well as the theoretical, point of view for the police to be summoned. Their involvement would provide legal justification (under the Police and Criminal Evidence Act 1984 s. 17(e)) as well as facilitating physical entry to the premises. Social workers have statutory powers of entry under specific conditions, but health workers do not.

Compulsory removal

Under the Mental Health Act 1983

As a community nurse, Laura has no power to enter the house. However, powers do exist: under section 115 of the Mental Health Act 1983 as amended by the Mental Health Act 2007, an

> **Practical Dilemma 22.6**   **Refusal to leave**
>
> Laura Thomas, a community nurse for the mentally ill, was notified that two sisters who were regarded as recluses had not been seen for several days. Neighbours reported that a number of cats were howling around their home and that the curtains had not been drawn for three days. Laura was also informed that of the two sisters, Annie, the younger one, was considered to be suffering from bipolar disorder. Laura went to the house and the door was answered by Agnes. She was abrupt and unwelcoming. When asked about her sister, she said they did not want nosey parkers and they were quite happy. From the doorway, Laura could see that the house was in a dirty condition and Agnes herself was in a dishevelled state. She feared for the physical and mental well-being of Annie. What could she do?

approved mental health professional (AMHP) (replacing the approved social worker under the 1983 Act) may, at all reasonable times after producing, if asked to do so, some duly authenticated document showing that he is such an AMHP, enter and inspect any premises (not being a hospital) in the area of that authority in which a mentally disordered patient is living, if they have reasonable cause to believe that the patient is not receiving care. This power enables the AMHP to inspect premises, other than hospitals, where a mentally disordered person is living. It does not, however, give the right to enforce entry, but refusal to permit the inspection could constitute an offence under section 129 of the Mental Health Act 1983. Premises are not defined, but could include private premises, provided a mentally disordered person is living there and provided there is reasonable cause to believe the patient is not under proper care. Laura would therefore have to arrange for an AMHP to visit the home. If entry were obstructed under section 115, the AMHP would have to make use of their power to apply to the Justice of the Peace for a warrant to search and remove patients under section 135. The AMHP would have to give information on oath that there is reasonable cause to suspect that a person believed to be suffering from mental disorder:

(a) has been, or is being, ill-treated, neglected, or kept otherwise than under proper control, in any place within the jurisdiction of the justice; or

(b) being unable to care for themselves, is living alone in any such place.

The justice may then issue a warrant authorising any constable to enter, if need be by force, any premises specified in the warrant in which that person is believed to be and if it is thought fit to remove him to a place of safety with a view to the making of an application for his care and treatment. An AMHP must accompany a constable. If it is thought fit, Annie could be removed to a place of safety and kept there for up to 24 hours under section 135(3ZA). (See chapter 19.) Prior to 11 December 2017, a person could be detained under section 136 for up to 72 hours. However this was felt to be too long, so the government amended section 135 of the Mental Health Act through the Policing and Crime Act 2017.[83]

Under the National Assistance Act 1948

The provision of the Mental Health Act described in the last paragraph can be used only in the case of a person believed within the meaning of the Act to be suffering from mental disorder. There are occasionally cases where those powers are not appropriate. In the above situation, it may well be that, although Annie suffers from learning disabilities and may well come within the definition of suffering from mental disorder, Agnes might not, but she might equally be in need of help.

Section 47 of the 1948 Act which authorised the removal to suitable premises of persons in need of care and control to secure the necessary care and attention is abolished for England by section 46 of the Care Act 2014. The Law Commission which had recommended the repeal also suggested that the situation should be reviewed to see if any statutory emergency powers were required.[84]

The coroner urged the government to issue new guidelines on how to interpret legislation. Mayan Coomeraswamy, a 51-year-old suffering from schizophrenia, was found dead in a damp, freezing, squalid flat, with mould growing on the floor and exposed electrical wires. The bathroom ceiling had collapsed, the boiler broken down and neighbours were complaining about the smell. The LA staff felt that they had to respect his right of choice because he was considered to have sufficient mental capacity.[85] The case illustrates the apparent conflict between human rights legislation and the powers under section 135 of the Mental Health Act 1983 and section 47 of the National Assistance Act 1948 (now repealed under section 46 of the Care Act 2014).

The Social Care Institute for Excellence (SCIE) has published guidance on the options available to nurses and other care staff who are being prevented from entering a person's home where they nurse reasonably suspects the person is a vulnerable adult at risk.[86]

Protection of property

If both Annie and Agnes were removed from the house, what happens to their home?

Under section 48 of the National Assistance Act 1948, the council had a duty to provide temporary protection for the property of persons admitted to hospitals. This section is now replaced by section 47 of Care Act 2014 which places upon the local authority a duty in relation to the property of those transferred to hospital or residential care home. The care of patients' and residents' property is considered in chapter 24.

Disclosure of information

This topic is discussed in chapter 8 where an example of the problems faced by community staff is considered (see Practical Dilemma 8.6). The specialist community public health nurse is more likely to be required to give evidence in court than any other community worker and should refer to chapter 9 on giving evidence in court. The policy that she should wait to be subpoenaed before giving evidence in cases involving children has changed because of her duty to the child under the Children Act 1989.

Criminal suspicion

Community nurses often work alone and if they are charged with theft it is one professional's word against that of the client or relative. In a case like Practical Dilemma 22.7, Kate could well have been accused of theft by the old lady herself if she was at all absent-minded and had forgotten what she had done. The safest rule is therefore never to accept gifts, even though this might distress the client.

If the client is insistent and wishes to make a generous gift, then a health service manager could be called in to give advice, but the client should be represented, since if there were any evidence of undue influence the gift would be voidable.

The NMC's Code (2015) does not forbid nurses from accepting any gifts. Rather it requires, under standard 21, that nurses uphold their position as a registered nurse by:

- refusing all but the most trivial gifts, favours or hospitality as accepting them could be interpreted as an attempt to gain preferential treatment,
- never asking for or accepting loans from anyone in their care or anyone close to them, and
- acting with honesty and integrity in any financial dealings they have with everyone they have a professional relationship with, including people in their care.

The legal issue of gifts and favours is considered in chapter 24.

Practical Dilemma 22.7 — Suspected

Kate Giles was a community nurse who had long been visiting an elderly widow who appeared to have no family apart from two grandchildren, who rarely visited, and few other visitors. One of Kate's tasks was to dress the client's leg. On one occasion, the client was anxious to point out some of her treasures to Kate. They included some very fine pieces of bone china. It was suggested to Kate that she might like to have a tiny cat as a small gift. Kate protested that she was not allowed to receive gifts from clients. Her protests were ignored and the old lady wrapped the gift up in an old paper bag and gave it to Kate. Kate forgot to mention it to her nursing officer the next day and after that it seemed too small a matter to be of any concern. Shortly after this the old lady died. The grandchildren discovered that a piece of Spode was missing. They made some enquiries and Kate stated that she had been given it by the elderly lady, but that they would, of course, be entitled to have it back. Kate was severely reprimanded and the grandchildren said they did not believe her story, since the old lady had never been known to give anything away; they suggested that Kate had, in fact, stolen the china.

Standards: care homes

The Health and Social Care Act 2008 and Health and Social Care Act Regulations 2009 amended the Care Standards Act 2000 so that from April 2010 regulated health and from October 2010 adult social care providers have been required to register with the Care Quality Commission and comply with their fundamental standards. From April 2011 GP and dental health practices have also been required to register with the CQC. The CQC has issued guidance which makes the registration requirements clear to providers. The guidance signals an important shift away from measuring systems and processes towards measuring outcomes for people who use services. The CQC can enforce compliance with the registration requirements and the guidance by imposing conditions on the registration, fines and ultimately cancellation of the registration. Further information can be obtained from the CQC website.[87] See also chapter 5.

It was reported in March 2014 that the NHS was investigating claims that GPs were charging residential homes for visits to their clients which should be free. Ministers are working with CQC and NHS England to prevent abuses.

Prosecutions against care home managers and owners can also be brought under section 44(2) of the Mental Capacity Act 2005 which came into force in April 2007 and which creates a criminal offence of ill-treating or wilfully neglecting a person who lacks capacity. Cases brought under section 44(2) are discussed in chapter 18.[88]

In May 2010 the manager of a care home was jailed for 10 years after the death of an elderly resident.[89] She was found guilty of manslaughter. Evidence showed that she had stolen patients' drugs, forged medical records and lied to investigators who were investigating suspicious deaths at the care home.

In 2013 the Chief Inspector of Social Care stated that care services will have to satisfy a test of 'good enough for my Mum' and announced that inspections by the CQC will be done by specialist inspectors and accompanied by residents and carers. Every home and agency will be graded on a four-point rating system.[90]

A report from the International Longevity Centre and Anchor in February 2014 suggested that a million extra care workers will be needed to meet the needs of the ageing population by 2025 and more men must be prepared to work in the care sector.[91]

A narrative verdict was recorded by a coroner holding an inquest into the death of a woman who died of malnutrition a day after being admitted to hospital from a care home. The coroner said that he would write to the local health authorities and police to raise his concerns about the care that Mrs Willits, who had been categorised as a high-risk patient, received at Ashbourne Nursing Home in Rochdale.

NICE methods and processes are to be used by the NICE Collaborating Centre for Social Care to develop social care quality standards.

Case 22.7 illustrates the duty the local authority has to make an assessment of community care needs.

Case 22.7 R (on the Application of Ireneschild) v Lambeth [2006]

Rehousing request refused[92]

A claimant, X, succeeded in an application for judicial review of a community care assessment by Lambeth LBC which had refused a rehousing request. X was incontinent and unable to stand or walk unsupported following an accident and lived in a flat. An assessment in 1999 noted that there were concerns about her accommodation and in 2003 an occupational therapist recommended that she be rehoused. However, in 2006 an assessment held that there was no eligible need arising from her accommodation. The judge held that the local authority had failed to take into account the history of her falls and issues relating to manual handling in her two sons, her carers, having to take her upstairs; had failed to follow the relevant guidance; and had failed to give her an opportunity to participate in the assessment process.

Community matrons

The NHS Improvement Plan for 2004 envisaged the use of community matrons (England only) to provide case management of people with long-term conditions. Community matrons would be experienced, skilled nurses who would have the following functions:

- Use data to actively seek out patients who will benefit from the case management approach;
- Combine high-level assessment of physical, mental and social care needs;
- Review medication and prescribe medicine via independent and supplementary prescribing arrangements;
- Provide clinical care and health-promoting interventions;
- Coordinate inputs from all other agencies, ensuring all needs are met;
- Teach and educate patients and their carers about warning signs of complications or crises;
- Provide information so patients and families can make choices about current and future care needs;
- Are highly visible to patients, and their families and carers and are seen by them as being in charge of their care; and
- Are seen by colleagues across all agencies as having the key role for patients with very high-intensity needs.

The result of the employment of community matrons was expected to be the prevention of unnecessary admissions to hospital, a reduction in the length of stay in hospital, improved outcomes for patients, the integration of all elements of care, an improvement in patients' ability to function and their quality of life, helping patients and their families plan for the future, increase choice for patients, enable patients to remain in their home and communities and improve end-of-life care.[93] Best practice guidance was issued by the Department of Health in April 2006 to provide a framework for commissioners and providers of education and training for community matrons and case managers.[94] A report on nurses as case managers in primary care and their contribution to chronic disease management for the National Institute for Health Research in 2010 found that while their role was extremely significant it was undermined by continued organisational experimentation.

The specialist community public health nurse

The specialist community public health nurse (SCPHN) has been defined by the specialist community public health nursing committee as follows:

> Specialist Community Public Health nursing aims to reduce health inequalities by working with individuals, families, and communities promoting health, preventing ill health and in the protection of health. The emphasis is on partnership working that cuts across disciplinary, professional and organisational boundaries that impact on organised social and political policy to influence the determinants of health and promote the health of whole populations.

Standards were set for SCPHNs by the NMC in 2004 and can be downloaded from the NMC website. Guidance has also been issued for nurses working in public health or as school nurses and occupational health nurses for them to qualify as SCPHNs.[95] In 2012 the NMC published clarification of admission criteria to SCPHN programmes.[96] Entrants to the SCPHN programmes must be a first-level nurse or midwife before being accepted onto a SCPHN programme.

In May 2022, the NMC approved new standards of proficiency for specialist community health nurses, and there were based around 6 spheres of influences:

1. Sphere of influence A: Being an autonomous specialist community public health nuring practitioner
2. Sphere of influence B: Transforming specialist community public health practice: evidence, research, evaluation and translation
3. Sphere of influence C: Promoting human rights and addressing inequalities: assessment, surveillance and intervention
4. Sphere of influence D: Population of health: enabling, supporting and improving health outcomes of people across the life course
5. Sphere of influence E: Advancing public health services and promoting healthy places, environments and cultures
6. Sphere of influence F: Leading and collaborating: from investment to action and dissemination

The school nurse

The traditional role of one school nurse per school with a wide job description has generally been replaced by a nurse with responsibility for several schools, but having an advisory and teaching role rather than seeing children individually and with no direct involvement in first aid for pupils. They may be employed by the NHS (but increasingly now by local authorities), but work within an educational environment, which could cause tension, as the discussion on Case 22.8 shows. The Department of Health stated that in March 2006 there were 2409 school nurses in England and it was the intention of the joint strategy of the Department for Education and Skills (now the DE) and the Department of Health to increase these numbers. The aim of the strategy was that there should be at least one full-time qualified nurse working with every cluster of primary schools and their related secondary schools by 2010. *Looking for a School Nurse*[97] was published by the government in 2006, aimed at head teachers and setting out the advantages and practical considerations of employing a school nurse. Although the number of school nurses rose to 2987 as a result of these initiatives, the transfer of responsibility for public health to local authorities in England under the Health and Social Care Act 2012 and the impact of austerity measures on local authority budgets saw that number fall to 2433 full-time posts by 2017,[98] and even further to 1,945 by 2022.[99]

Extent of duty

In this tragic situation, many different questions arise. There is no mention of a school nurse but, if one had been appointed, what should have been their role? Are they on call for the whole time in school hours, waiting for such an emergency to arise? Many would say no, but it does depend, of course, on the individual employment contract and job description. The role the school nurse plays as far as teaching is concerned also varies from school to school. In some, they might take on the task of teaching such subjects as personal hygiene, health education, sex education, biology, etc. Where they are undertaking this role, it can hardly be expected that they will be fulfilling an emergency first aid role as well. There would appear to be failure by the school and the education authority to provide a basic first aid training for staff, especially when it would have been known that the boy was asthmatic, and to provide a system for dealing with such emergencies.

> **Case 22.8   An asthma attack [2010]**
>
> ## An asthma attack[100] [2010]
>
> A boy suffering from asthma had been left to wait in a hallway while having an attack. The emergency services were not called. The inquest jury found that staff had failed to implement the asthma policy, were not sufficiently trained to deal with asthma and that a healthcare plan was not in place. The jury found that the boy had died of natural causes but that neglect at an individual and systemic level had been a significant contributory factor. The headmistress and four school staff were suspended.

Details of a school nurse practice development resource pack (updated in 2006), a health visitor and school nurse development programme and primary school/primary health links projects operating with the Health Schools Standard are available from the Department of Health website.[101] This was followed in 2012 by a DH publication *Getting it right for children, young people and families* which provided school nursing with a framework of the services it could provide. To complement this framework, the RCN developed in 2013 a comprehensive tool kit for school nurses.[102] In 2012 the RCN published a UK-wide position statement on school nursing.[103] In 2014 Public Health England produced several documents on school nursing and public health services covering a variety of issues: maximising the school nursing team contribution to the public health of school-aged children; promoting emotional well-being and positive mental health; developing strong relationships and supporting positive sexual health; and supporting the health and well-being of young carers. They are designed to support effective commissioning of school nursing services to provide public health for school-aged children and are obtainable on the government website.[104] School nurses, like health visitors, are now increasingly employed by local authorities which have responsibility for public health. (See chapter 25.)

Use of car

Like any community worker, a school nurse must ensure that they have the appropriate insurance policy to cover all the uses that they are likely to make of a car for work purposes.

> **Practical Dilemma 22.8** **Car insurance**
>
> A child, Mary Pugh, cut her head very badly in the gymnasium. The children had been told to trot around like ponies with their heads up high. Mary trotted straight into the teeth of another child. Blood gushed from the wound. Audrey, the school nurse, realised the importance of getting her to the A&E department for stitches. She put the child in her own car and rushed to the local hospital. In her haste, she came out of a side road too quickly and crashed into a motorcyclist coming along the main road. She got out of the car to see what could be done and, seeing that other people had gathered around, she decided that it was her duty to get Mary to hospital. Subsequently, she was notified that the police were charging her with failing to report an accident and having no adequate insurance cover. Relatives of the motorcyclist were also intending to sue her for causing the accident and failing to provide assistance, since the ambulance had taken 20 minutes to arrive and the cyclist had bled to death.

Any employee who does not usually use their car for work, other than going to and from work, would be well advised to ensure that insurance cover is provided for the exceptional circumstance when a car might be needed. Clinic nurses other than peripatetic nurses, school nurses or outpatient nurses might all find that on very rare occasions they need to use their car for work purposes and then they are not covered. The effect is that, although the insurance company may pay out compensation to the victim, it has the right to claim this money back from the person whose insurance did not cover this use. (If the company refuses to pay out compensation, compensation for physical injuries may be payable by the Motors Insurance Bureau.) If exceptional use of a car is foreseeable, it is wiser for the nurse to ensure that her insurance company is notified of this possibility.

As far as the failure to report the accident is concerned, it is a duty under the Road Traffic Act 1988 as amended to ensure that the police are notified of any accident in which personal injuries are caused. Audrey's failure to ensure that this was done could lead to a successful prosecution. Her failure to stop and help the cyclist is a difficult question. On the one hand there is no legal obligation to volunteer help, but the NMC considers that a professional duty exists at all times (see chapter 3). In this case Audrey caused the harm and is under a legal obligation to mitigate it as far as possible but she also has a duty to Mary and it is a question of assessing who is in most need. From the facts given here, it would appear that the cyclist was in more danger and Audrey should have checked that there was nothing she could do before she went away.

The clinic nurse

Clinic nurses may spend their time in one clinic assisting at mother and baby clinics, be attached to specialist clinics such as family planning clinics or travel from school to school, assisting the school doctors in provision of medical, eye and other examinations for schoolchildren.

Obtaining consent

There are two separate issues here: the one is the consent of the parents; the other is the timing of the vaccination. As far as consent is concerned, the basic principles are that parents have the

> **Practical Dilemma 22.9**   **Consent to rubella vaccinations**
>
> Brenda West provided nursing assistance to the medical team that carried out the school medical examinations. One of their tasks was to offer the Year 8 girls a rubella vaccination. Letters were sent to the parents in advance, advising them of the service and asking for their consent. Unfortunately, Brenda failed to notice that the parents of Rachel Tyne had not signed the consent form and Rachel was given an injection by the school doctor. Shortly afterwards, Rachel came out in an all-over rash. Investigations were made and it appeared that Rachel had recently had a variety of drugs in anticipation of a holiday to Morocco and these had reacted with the rubella vaccination. The parents were threatening to sue since they did not want Rachel to have the vaccination as she had had German measles a few years before. They also felt that the doctor and nurse should have checked with them before they gave the vaccination to ensure that there were no contraindications.

right to consent to treatment for their children. As far as school health is concerned, it could be argued that under the Education Acts the school can provide the care as long as the parents do not object. This may well cover medical examinations, but is unlikely to cover the giving of injections. Some schools rely on a passive consent. A letter is sent saying: 'We intend to examine and give your child X on . . . If you do not consent, please contact . . . '

However, if the vaccination is to proceed, it is essential that actual consent should be obtained, that any potential contraindications are identified and that the parents advise the school of any recent events in the child's medical history that suggest that a vaccination would be inappropriate at that particular time or, indeed, at any time. Because of the importance of this, it is advisable for the parents to give positive consent to the vaccination and reassure the staff about the non-existence of any contraindications. A child who is Gillick-competent (see chapter 13) could give a valid consent to treatment which is in her or his best interests. The government has prepared a consent form for HPV for the parent and requiring their signature, which can be downloaded from its website.[105]

As far as responsibility between the nurse and the doctor is concerned, much depends on the local policy in relation to who has the duty of ensuring that the parents' consent has been obtained. In some authorities, this would fall on the doctor. However, this does not necessarily mean that the nurse is free of all liability.

Minors

Several issues arise here. One is the question of the nurse's personal knowledge and the extent to which she should inform the doctor of this. The other is the question of the law relating to an under-16-year-old in this context (see chapter 13). From the House of Lords' decision in the Gillick case, it can be seen that treatment and advice can be given to a girl under 16 without the parents being involved, provided that she has the requisite competence to give consent.

As far as the first issue is concerned, it could be argued that even though the nurse has acquired information about the patient from a different source, if this is relevant to the doctor's care and treatment of the patient, then it should be disclosed, i.e. her duty of care to the patient would require her to tell the doctor that the girl was 15. Similarly, if she knew that the girl suffered from epilepsy, even though the girl had not told the doctor this, the nurse should pass on the information. It could be argued that this principle applies only to information that is relevant

> **Practical Dilemma 22.10** **Family planning and the under-16-year-old**
>
> Maureen was working as a clinic nurse in the family planning clinic. She recognised one of the patients, Emily Wright, as a friend of her eldest daughter, aged 15. She completed the forms and the girl told her she was 17. Maureen knew that this was a lie. She was uncertain whether to tell the doctor and decided against this. The doctor prescribed the pill and asked Emily the name of her family doctor. Emily said she did not have one. She said she did not want any communication with her family and the doctor said that would not be necessary if she was over 16.

to the care of the child. Thus, if she by chance knew that the girl had been charged by the police for shoplifting, this need not be passed on.

The Children Act 1989 requires decisions relating to children to take into account the wishes of the child where the child has the capacity.

The practice nurse

The legal situation of the practice nurse can vary, especially as far as employment rights are concerned. Some practice nurses may be employed by a single-handed or group general practitioner; others are employed by clinical commissioning groups (CCGs). Practice nurses employed by CCGs are more likely to be part of a nursing hierarchy and to receive guidance and policies from the employer. Recent years have seen a considerable growth in the educational and management support provided to practice nurses. In many areas, a practice liaison nurse is appointed to provide assistance and professional advice across the CGT area(s). A dedicated website for practice nurses[106] provides a forum for exchanging information. The RCN also has a Practice Nurses' Association[107] providing updates on the significance of the Francis and CQC reports (see chapter 5) and gives information about the Winston Churchill Memorial Trust's Travelling Fellowships.

Scope of professional practice and the practice nurse

Like other nurses, practice nurses are finding that their scope of professional practice is expanding as they are required to undertake a wider range of responsibilities. While practice nurses were not identified in the First Crown Report on nurse prescribing as one of the groups able to prescribe in the community, they were, together with nurses working in walk-in centres, added to the list of nurses who could prescribe in February 2000. The Final Crown Report envisaged that many different health professionals would be recognised as dependent or independent prescribers. With a new nursing curriculum coming into place in September 2020, the NMC are requiring nurses to be prescriber ready. (This is discussed further in chapter 27. Legal issues relating to the scope of professional practice are considered in chapter 23.)

Cervical screening

The practice nurse may be required to undertake cervical screening. It is essential that they have appropriate approved training. A practice nurse in Birmingham, who had been taught by her GP to undertake cervical screening, was discovered to be using the spatula by the wrong end and her failure to take the correct samples led to non-diagnosis of several women with cervical cancer.

The standard required in cervical screening came before the courts when East Kent Health Authority was alleged to have been liable for the negligent examination of cervical smears, as explained in Case 22.9.

Case 22.9 Penney, Palmer and Cannon v E Kent Health Authority [2000]

Cervical screening[108]

The claimants brought an action on the grounds that their cervical smears were negligently examined and reported as negative between 1989 and 1992. As a consequence, they were deprived of the opportunity of obtaining early treatment that would have prevented the development of endocervical carcinoma. Screening was carried out by qualified biomedical scientists or by qualified cytology screeners. They were not qualified to diagnose; their only function was to report what, using their expertise, they were able to see. If the screener detected an abnormality in the smear or was in doubt whether what he saw was abnormal, he had to pass the smear on to a senior screener known as a checker. The cervical screening programme guidelines required an absolute confidence test. The trial judge decided that this absolute confidence test had not been complied with and found for the claimants.

The judge preferred the views of the claimants' experts as to whether, in the light of what the cytoscreeners saw, it was negligent to fail either to classify the smears as borderline or to refer the smears to the checker and/or to the pathologist. The Bolam principle did not apply because the Bolam Test was concerned with acceptable and unacceptable practice, whereas no question of acceptable practice arose in the instant case because the cytoscreeners were wrong in their classification of the smears. Even if the Bolam principle were relevant, the defendant's experts' views did not stand up to logical analysis because the cytoscreeners did not have the ability to draw a distinction between benign and pre-cancerous cells and so should have classified the smears as borderline.

The Court of Appeal dismissed the appeal and upheld the finding that the health authority was liable. It held that the Bolam Test was appropriate where the exercise of skill and judgement of the screener was being questioned. In this case, however, the Bolam Test did not apply since the screeners were not expected to exercise judgement.

It was announced in 2000 that the government was to introduce a pilot study of a new form of cervical screening, liquid-based cytology (LBC), together with tests for the virus HPV that causes cervical cancer. The National Institute for Health and Care Excellence has suggested that LBC could increase the sensitivity of the slides, reduce the number of badly taken smears and improve the speed and accuracy with which cytoscreeners can read the slides.[109] The Department of Health has established a website for information on cancer screening.[110] See also information on specialised websites.[111]

Staffing concerns

Concerns about nurse and general practitioner numbers are growing. The Queen's Nursing Institute has called for the government to act to stem the decline in district nurse numbers, which fell by some 46 per cent between 2010 and 2017.[112] This was despite the Department of Health in its 2013 Report[113] seeing district nurses as key professionals in the delivery of care closer to home. Their significance in the present strategy of shifting patients from hospital to the community for treatment is undeniable. The RCN has provided guidance on their role.[114] The Queen's Nursing Institute has also painted a picture of the skills necessary and the tasks faced by district nurses.[115] At least 50 per cent of nurses will do community placements during their training to encourage them to work in local clinics rather than hospitals.[116] The Department of Health has given instructions to Health Education England that half of all medical students should train to become GPs so that there are 2000 more family doctors by 2018 while more than 100,000 NHS staff will have more training on treating people with dementia. In June 2013 the Academy of Royal Colleges, the NHS Confederation and the patient group National Voices all agreed that resources must be transferred from hospitals to GP surgeries, health centres and district nurses. This was the only way the NHS could survive and meet the demographic changes ahead.[117] A survey by the National Nursing Research Unit at King's College London found that many district nurses did not have time to answer patients' questions, talk about their condition or offer emotional support.[118]

Developments in technology and structure

Major developments are also taking place in technology which could have significant implications for professional practice. For example, NHS North East Essex has launched a fully-fledged tele-health service in partnership with Tunstall Healthcare. Over six months the average number of GP visits made by patients had fallen by 66 per cent, the average number of patient hospital attendances or 999 call-outs was down 44 per cent and the average number of home visits required had dropped by 19 per cent. Increased use of electronic tablet devices are changing the methods of communication and have considerable implications for the record keeping of community staff.

Social enterprise groups

We are also seeing a development, especially in the community, where staff are taking over the running of certain services on a cooperative basis. For example, in Central Surrey Healthcare 700 nurses have taken over the community services across most of the county. They each own a 1p share in the not-for-profit company which provides £26 million of services each year. The buildings, equipment and pensions remain the responsibility of the NHS; the co-owners are in charge of running the services.[119] Such schemes increased following the implementation of the White Paper published in 2010 and the Health and Social Care Act 2012.

Social Enterprise UK[120] is collaborating with CCGs in Building Health Partnerships programmes between CCGs and local voluntary and community and social enterprise organisations to improve health in local communities. One example given is that of a social prescribing project in City and Hackney to improve the health of isolated over-50s and people with type 2 diabetes. However it must be noted that these are generally England-only initiatives, and in Scotland,

Wales and Northern Ireland there is still considerable political opposition to not-for-profit organisations delivering mainstream healthcare.

Conclusions

The Care Act 2014 represents a major development in the law relating to care in community implementing the Law Commission's recommendations[121] of a single statute on adult social care supported by regulations and guidance. Care however remains a topical issue, and at the 2017 General Election the Conservative Party's manifesto included a pledge to remove pensioners' triple lock and winter fuel payments, as well as seeing wealthier pensioners being asked to pay more for their care, dubbed by the Labour Party as a dementia tax. However, the proposed changes were not popular and may in part be an explanation for the failure of the party to achieve a working majority in the House of Commons.

Care and how it is delivered and funded remains a notable concern for many people and in an ageing population will remain a prominent topic for some time to come.

Reflection questions

1. You break an ornament while visiting a patient. The ornament is valued at £5000. You are personally unable to meet the costs of replacing it. What remedies are available to the owner of the ornament? (See also chapter 24.)
2. What special concerns does the community professional have in relation to health and safety and what specific precautions should be taken to protect them? (Refer also to chapter 12.)
3. What difficulties, if any, arise from the fact that the school nurse is now employed by the local authority but works with education authority staff as a health professional? Could the school nurse refuse to undertake tasks allocated by the head teacher? What are the likely implications?
4. What differences exist in law between the clinic nurse who spends all their time in a clinic and the nurse who visits patients in their own homes?
5. Consider the expanded-role activities that are sometimes undertaken by the practice nurse or community nurse and outline the legal requirements. (See chapter 23.)

Further exercises

1. As a community nurse, you visit a patient who appears to you to be incapable of caring for herself. What action would you take? Outline a procedure to cover the situation if the patient shows extreme reluctance to move from their home and there are no relatives to care for them.
2. What procedures would you follow in assessing a patient for community care? What criteria are used to decide if the patient is entitled to long-term NHS care?

3. What are the implications of the Care Act 2014 for your work as a community nurse? In what way do the provisions of the Act affect your professional practice and the quality of care provided to the patient?
4. Access the CQC website and find out its powers in relation to the registration and inspection of residential care homes.

References

[1] *R v North and East Devon Health Authority ex parte Coughlan* [2000] 3 All ER 850; [2000] 2 WLR 622
[2] Royal Commission, Report on the Long-Term Care of the Elderly, with Respect to Old Age, Stationery Office, London, 1999
[3] *R v North and East Devon Health Authority ex parte Coughlan* [2000] 3 All ER 850; [2000] 2 WLR 622
[4] DH response to the Ombudsman's report on continuing care, last modified February 2007
[5] DH, The National Framework for NHS Continuing Healthcare and NHS-funded Nursing Care, June 2007
[6] *R (Grogan) v Bexley NHS Care Trust* [2006] EWHC 44; (2006) 9 CCL 188
[7] *R v Gloucester County Council and Another ex parte Barry* [1997] 2 All ER 1 HL
[8] *R v Sefton Metropolitan Borough Council ex parte Help the Aged* [1997] 3 FCR 573 CA
[9] LASSL(97)13 Responsibilities of Local Authority Social Services Departments: implications of recent legal judgments
[10] LAC(98)19 Community Care (Residential Accommodation) Act 1998
[11] *R (on the application of Grogan) v Bexley NHS Care Trust* [2006] EWHC 44; (2006) 9 CCL 188
[12] Department of Health, NHS Continuing Care: Action following the Grogan Case, DH, 2006
[13] Department of Health, The National Framework for NHS Continuing Healthcare and NHS-funded Nursing Care, DH, June 2007, revised 2009
[14] Ibid., revised 2009 and 2012 and updated in 2013; www.gov.uk
[15] www.nhs.uk
[16] www.gov.uk/careandsupport
[17] Adult Care Reform, Letter to the Editor, *The Times*, 5 June 2008 from Mencap, Age Concern and others
[18] Rosemary Bennett, Councils demand care home top-ups from old people, *The Times*, 17 January 2009
[19] *R (Manchester City Council) v St Helens Metropolitan Borough Council*, The Times Law Report, 13 November 2009
[20] *R (On the application of Chavda) v Harrow LBC* [2007] EWHC 3064 Admin; (2008) 11 CCL Rep 187
[21] Royal Commission, With Respect to Old Age, Stationery Office, London, March 1999
[22] *R (Savva) v Kensington and Chelsea Royal LBC*, The Times Law Report, 15 November 2010
[23] Department of Health, Shaping the Future of Care Together, Cm 7673, Stationery Office, London, 2009
[24] HM Government, White Paper, Building the National Care Service, Cmnd 7854, March 2010, Stationery Office, London

25. Sam Lister, Free care for elderly – just don't ask how or when, *The Times*, 31 March 2010
26. Dilnot Report, Fairer Care Funding, 2011
27. Jill Sherman, 500,000 old and vulnerable hit by loss of homecare, *The Times*, 16 December 2013
28. Chris Smyth, Overhaul for NHS care scheme after hospital cash warning, *The Times*, 10 July 2014.
29. *R (Miss Glen Walford)* v *Worcestershire County Council, Secretary of State for Health intervening* [2014] EWHC 234
30. White Paper: Caring for our future: reforming care and support, July 2012, CM 8378, Stationery Office
31. www.gov.uk
32. Law Commission Adult Social Care Report, No. 326, Stationery Office, May 2011
33. www.lawcom.gov.uk
34. Department of Health, Reforming the law for adult care and support, July 2012
35. www.moneyadviceservice.org
36. www.legislation.gov.uk
37. Laura Pital, Your old age will set you back £140,000, *The Times*, 12 May 2014
38. Audit Commission Report, Fully Equipped: the provision of equipment to older or disabled people by the NHS and social services in England and Wales, AC, March 2000
39. B. Donnelly, Community Equipment Services England and Wales 2009, The Need for National Minimum Standards, www.communityequipment.org.uk
40. Brian Donnelly, Minimum standards for equipment services, *British Journal of Healthcare Management*, 16(4):180–5, 2010
41. www.cqc.org.uk
42. *R (on the application of Heather)* v *Leonard Cheshire Foundation* [2002] EWCA Civ 366; The Times Law Report, 8 April 2002
43. *R (on the application of Johnson)* v *Havering LBC* [2007] EWCA 26; The Times Law Report, 2 February 2007
44. *YL* v *Birmingham City Council and others* [2007] UKHL 22; The Times Law Report, 21 June 2007
45. House of Lords and House of Commons Joint Committee on Human Rights of Older People in Healthcare, 18th Session 2006–7, HL 156–1/HC 378–1, August 2007
46. *JE* v *DE*; Sub nom *DE, Re* [2006] EWHC 3459 (Fam)
47. *P (by his litigation friend the Official Solicitor)* v *Cheshire West and Cheshire Council and Anor* [2014] UKSC 19
48. *R (on the application of Gunter)* v *SouthWestern Staffordshire Primary Care Trust* [2005] EWHC 1894
49. *B Borough Council* v *S* [2006] EWHC 2584
50. *McDonald* v *UK (Application no 4241/12) European Court of Human Rights*, The Times Law Report, 13 June 2014; *McDonald* v *UK Chamber judgement* [2014] ECHR 492
51. *R (McDonald)* v *Kensington and Chelsea Royal London Borough Council* [2011] UKSC 11
52. www.cqc.org.uk
53. Chris Smyth, Care homes to shape up or shut down, *The Times*, 17 July 2014
54. Rosemary Bennett, Call to regulate care homes like hospitals, *The Times*, 10 June 2014
55. Chris Smyth, Institutionalised abuse led to five deaths at care home, *The Times*, 19 October 2013
56. *Waghorn* v *Care Quality Commission* [2012] EWHC 1816

57 House of Lords Select Committee Mental Capacity Act 2005: post-legislative scrutiny HL Paper 139, March 2014
58 *London Borough of Hillingdon* v *Neary and another* [2011] EWCOP 1377
59 Delayed Discharges (England) Regulations 2003, SI 2003/2277
60 *Barnet Primary Care Trust* v *X* [2006] EWHC 787; (2006) BMLR 17
61 *Sussex Community NHS Foundation Trust* v *Price* [2016] EWHC 3167
62 Department of Health, Hospital 2 Home resource pack 2012; www.housinglin.org.uk
63 Chris Smyth, Chancellor 'raids' NHS to find £1bn to improve pensioners' social care, *The Times*, 27 June 2013
64 The Delayed Discharges (Continuing Care) Directions 2013
65 www.gov.uk
66 https://carers.org/key-facts-about-carers-and-people-they-care
67 Carer's National Strategy Document, Caring about Carers, Stationery Office, London, 8 February 1999
68 Tom Knowles, Carer wins payout from widower who cut hours, *The Times*, 24 October 2013
69 Sam Lister, Simon de Bruxelles, Nurse switched off life support by accident, *The Times*, 26 October 2010
70 Nursing and Midwifery Council (2015) The Code: Professional standards of practice and behaviour for nurses and midwives, NMC, London
71 *R* v *Family Health Services Appeal Authority ex p Muralidhar* [1999] COD 80
72 News item, Care agency failings after woman, 81, dies, *The Times*, 17 September 2013
73 News item, *The Times*, 9 November 2013
74 News item, *The Times*, 2 November 2013
75 *R* v *Hillingdon Health Authority ex parte Wyatt*, The Times Law Report, 20 December 1977 CA
76 Health and Safety Executive, RR495, Violence management training: the development of effective trainers in the delivery of violence management training in healthcare settings, HSE, 2006
77 Health and Safety Commission, Violence and aggression to staff in health services, HSE Books, 1997
78 *Re C (An Adult: refusal of medical treatment)* [1994] 1 All ER 819
79 *Re MB (Adult: medical treatment)* [1997] 2 FLR 426
80 *St George's Healthcare NHS Trust* v *S* [1998] 3 All ER 673
81 *Re T* [1992] 4 All ER 649
82 *F* v *Berkshire HA* [1989] 2 All ER 545
83 Policing and Crime Act 2017; www.legilslation.uk
84 Law Commission, Adult Social Care Report No. 326 (HC 941), May 2011
85 Eleanor Harding, Intervening behind closed doors, *Guardian*, 31 March 2010
86 Social Care Institute for Excellence (2014) Gaining access to an adult suspected to be at risk of neglect or abuse: a guide for social workers and their managers in England, SCIE, London
87 www.cqc.org.uk
88 Rosemary Bennett, Women convicted of wilful neglect at filthy care home for the elderly, *The Times*, 7 August 2010
89 News item, Home manager jailed over resident's death, *The Times*, 22 May 2010
90 Chris Smyth, Care homes face the 'good enough for my Mum' test, *The Times*, 15 October 2013
91 Rosemary Bennett, A million care staff needed (and most should be men), *The Times*, 25 February 2014
92 *R (On the application of Ireneschild)* v *Lambeth LBC* [2006] EWHC 2354

93 Department of Health, Community Matrons, DH, May 2007
94 Department of Health, Best Practice Guidance Framework for commissioners and providers of education and training for community matrons and case managers, DH, April 2006
95 Nursing and Midwifery Council, Information packs for public health nurses (October 2006); for school and occupational health nurses (December 2006)
96 Circular 02/2012
97 DfES, Looking for a School Nurse, DfES, 2006
98 David Connett, School nurse shortage 'putting children's lives at risk', *The Guardian*, 25 August 2017
99 Church, E (2023) School nurses face 'perfect storm' as numbers dwindle, Nursing Times (Online) https://www.nursingtimes.net/news/public-health/school-nurses-face-perfect-storm-as-numbers-dwindle-13-04-2023/#:~:text=NHS%20England%20recently%20released%20its,as%20%22qualified%20school%20nurses%22
100 Joanna Sugden, Headmistress and four school staff are suspended over boy's asthma death, *The Times*, 25 March 2010
101 www.dh.gov.uk
102 RCN, Tool kit for school nurses, 003233, RCN, 2013
103 www.rcn.org.uk
104 www.gov.uk
105 www.gov.uk
106 www.practicenursing.co.uk
107 www.rcn.org.uk
108 *Penney, Palmer and Cannon* v *East Kent Health Authority* [2000] Lloyd's Rep Med 41 CA
109 Dr Thomas Stuttaford, New screening should cut smear errors, *The Times*, 3 August 2000
110 www.cancerscreening.nhs.uk
111 www.cancerresearchuk.org and www.nhs.uk/conditions/cancer-of-the-cervix
112 Alice Harrold, Call for Government action after district nurse numbers halve in seven years, *Nursing in Practice*, 21 November 2017
113 Department of Health, Care in Local Communities: a new vision and model of district nursing, London, 2013
114 Royal College of Nursing, District Nursing – Harnessing the potential: the RCN's UK position on district nursing, London, 2013
115 The Queen's Nursing Institute, Nursing People at Home: the issues, the stories the actions, London, 2011
116 Chris Smyth, More flexible NHS to favour GPs over hospital specialists, *The Times*, 28 May 2013
117 Editorial, Hospital Pass, *The Times*, 5 June 2013
118 Chris Smyth, District nurses may be driven to extinction, *The Times*, 17 June 2014
119 Jill Sherman, Workers can take over hospitals, schools and prisons under Big Society scheme, *The Times*, 18 November 2010
120 www.socialenterprise.org.uk
121 Law Commission, Adult Social Care Report No. 326 (HC 941), May 2011

Chapter 23

Scope of Professional Practice, Clinical Nurse Specialist and Consultant Nurse

This chapter discusses

- Scope of professional practice
- Delegation and supervision
- Nurse consultants
- Clinical nurse specialists and specialist nurses
- Concerns about developments in scope of professional practice
- Scope of professional practice in primary care
- Scope of professional practice in theatre nursing
- Scope of professional practice in emergency nursing
- Scope of professional practice and X-rays
- NHS 111 (formerly NHS Direct) and walk-in clinics
- Modern matrons
- Agency nurses
- Healthcare support workers

Introduction

The government's plans for the NHS as shown in the White Paper in 1997,[1] in the document *Making a Difference*[2] and in the NHS Plan[3] relied heavily on a widened scope of practice for the nurse. NHS 111 (formerly NHS Direct) and walk-in clinics are run by nurses and provide an increasingly extensive and popular service. As a consequence of these developments, the role of the nurse has changed and is changing radically and these changes have major legal implications. This chapter considers the background to the scope of professional practice and the

NMC advice, the role of the consultant nurse and clinical nurse specialist. One development in the scope of professional practice is the change in nurse prescribing and this is considered in chapter 27.

Scope of professional practice

In June 1992, the UKCC (the predecessor to the NMC) published the *Scope of Professional Practice*. It marked a major development in the thinking underlying professional practice. Previously, the concept of the extended role highlighted the distinction between the basic training that the practitioner received in order to become a registered professional and post-registration training. Under 'the extended role', professional development was seen as incremental, task-oriented and often delegated from other professionals (usually medical). A circular in 1977 (CHC (77)22) gave advice on extended role tasks. This advice has now been superseded by subsequent developments on the scope of professional practice.

In 1986, a working party was set up by the Standing Medical Advisory Committee and the Standing Nursing and Midwifery Committee to review the extended role of the nurse. Its report was circulated under cover of a DHSS letter from the Chief Nursing Officer, dated 26 September 1989, and it paved the way for the publication of the UKCC's *Scope of Professional Practice*.

The UKCC emphasised that professional practice must be sensitive, relevant and responsive to the needs of individual patients and clients and have the capacity to adjust, where and when appropriate, to changing circumstances (paragraph 1). It set out principles that should govern adjustment to the scope of professional practice (paragraph 9). These are laid out in Box 23.1. The *Scope of Professional Practice* should be seen in the light of the revised NMC Code.[4] This requires, at standard 6, that nurses:

Always practise in line with the best available evidence
To achieve this, [nurses] must:

- make sure that any information or advice given is evidence-based, including information relating to using any healthcare products or services, and
- maintain the knowledge and skills [they] need for safe and effective practice.

Standard 13 of the Code requires that nurses:

Recognise and work within the limits of [their] competence
To achieve this, [nurses] must:

- accurately assess signs of normal or worsening physical and mental health in the person receiving care,
- make a timely and appropriate referral to another practitioner when it is in the best interests of the individual needing any action, care or treatment,
- ask for help from a suitably qualified and experienced healthcare professional to carry out any action or procedure that is beyond the limits of [their] competence,
- take account of personal safety as well as the safety of people in your care, and
- complete the necessary training before carrying out a new role.

> **Box 23.1** **Principles for adjusting the scope of professional practice**
>
> The registered nurse, midwife or health visitor:
>
> 1. must be satisfied that each aspect of practice is directed to meeting the needs and serving the interests of the patient or client
> 2. must endeavour always to achieve, maintain and develop knowledge, skill and competence to respond to those needs and interests
> 3. must honestly acknowledge any limits of personal knowledge and skill and take steps to remedy any relevant deficits in order effectively and appropriately to meet the needs of patients and clients
> 4. must ensure that any enlargement or adjustment of the scope of personal professional practice must be achieved without compromising or fragmenting existing aspects of professional practice and care and that requirements of the Council's Code of Professional Conduct are satisfied throughout the whole area of practice
> 5. must recognise and honour the direct or indirect personal accountability borne for all aspects of professional practice
> 6. must, in serving the interests of patients and clients and the wider interests of society, avoid any inappropriate delegation to others that compromises those interests

Where an aspect of practice is beyond the practitioner's level of competence or outside one's area of registration, then the registered professional must seek help and supervision from a competent practitioner, until the practitioner and her employer consider that the requisite knowledge and skill have been acquired. The NMC also recognises a duty for the practitioner to facilitate students and others to develop their competence.

Revalidation was introduced by the NMC from April 2016. Revalidation is a process that all nurses and midwives in the UK need to follow to maintain their registration with the NMC. It encourages reflection on the role of the Code in practice and demonstrates that nurses are 'living' the standards set out within it. Revalidation replaces the post-registration education and practice (PREP) requirements, and nurses have to revalidate every three years to renew registration. The requirements of revalidation are shown in Box 23.2.

The NHS Plan,[6] published in July 2000, envisaged that within the reformed NHS there would be radical changes in the ways in which staff work. The NHS Modernisation Agency (set up by the government to plan and implement the changes) led a major drive to ensure that protocol-based care took hold throughout the NHS. A statement on the future direction of the NHS Modernisation Agency was published by the DH in 2005 which envisaged the original organisation being replaced by a new central organisation smaller than the Modernisation Agency with a focus on innovation and an emphasis on local implementation. The NHS Quality Board is part of the DH Measuring for Quality Improvement initiative which identifies and develops quality indicators. Two hundred indicators were initially published. The 2010 annual report of the NHS Quality Board is available on the NHS England website. Reference should also be made to the Department of Health's essence of care benchmarks which were first published in 2001[7] and updated in 2010 (see chapter 3).

> **Box 23.2 Revalidation: the requirements**
>
> - 450 practice hours, or 900 if renewing as both a nurse and midwife
> - 35 hours of CPD including 20 hours of participatory learning
> - Five pieces of practice-related feedback
> - Five written reflective accounts
> - Reflective discussion
> - Health and character declaration
> - Professional indemnity arrangement
> - Confirmation[5]

The new approach to the scope of professional practice shattered old demarcations that have held back staff and slowed down care. NHS employers are required to empower appropriately qualified nurses, midwives and therapists to undertake a wider range of clinical tasks, including the right to make and receive referrals, admit and discharge patients, order investigations and diagnostic tests, run clinics and prescribe drugs. The inclusion of the suitably experienced nurse with the consultant and GP in identifying those responsible for making decisions on cardiopulmonary resuscitation[8] (see chapter 28) is a natural development of the scope of professional

> **Box 23.3 Ten key roles for nurses in the NHS Plan**
>
> 1. To order diagnostic investigations such as pathology tests and X-rays
> 2. To make and receive referrals direct, say, to a therapist or pain consultant
> 3. To admit and discharge patients for specified conditions and within agreed protocols
> 4. To manage patient caseloads, say for diabetes or rheumatology
> 5. To run clinics, say for ophthalmology or dermatology
> 6. To prescribe medicines and treatments
> 7. To carry out a wide range of resuscitation procedures, including defibrillation
> 8. To perform minor surgery and outpatient procedures
> 9. To triage patients using the latest IT to the most appropriate health professional
> 10. To take a lead in the way local health services are both organised and run

practice of the registered nurse. It is the responsibility of the individual nurse to ensure that they have the requisite competence to make such a decision.

The 10 key roles identified for the nurse by the Chief Nursing Officer and set out in the NHS Plan are shown in Box 23.3.

Delegation and supervision

The scope of professional practice of individual health professionals cannot be expanded unless there is either an increase in those registered professionals or activities are delegated to others such as healthcare assistants or support workers. The Bolam Test (see chapter 3) applies to the delegation of activities. It is the personal and professional responsibility of each practitioner who delegates activities to ensure that the person to carry out that activity is trained, competent and has the necessary experience to undertake the activity safely. The delegating practitioner must also ensure that the appropriate level of supervision is provided.

Standard 11 of the NMC Code requires that nurses:

Be accountable for [their] decisions to delegate tasks and duties to other people
To achieve this, [nurses] must:

- only delegate tasks and duties that are within the other person's scope of competence, making sure that they fully understand your instructions,
- make sure that everyone you delegate tasks to is adequately supervised and supported so they can provide safe and compassionate care, and
- confirm that the outcome of any task you have delegated to someone else meets the required standard.

It has also updated its A to Z guidance[9] (now replaced by guidance leaflets) which defines delegation as:

Delegation – the transfer to a competent individual, [of] the authority to perform a specific task in a specified situation that can be carried out in the absence of that nurse or midwife and without direct supervision.

The guidance considers the accountability and responsibility of the delegator, the documentation required and the principles which apply to delegation. It sets out 10 principles for nurses and midwives to follow when delegating to non-regulated healthcare staff. These principles are as follows:

1. The delegation of nursing or midwifery care must always take place in the best interests of the patient or client and the decision to delegate must always be based on an assessment of the individual patient or client's needs.
2. Where a registrant has authority to delegate tasks to another, they will retain responsibility and accountability for that delegation.
3. A registrant may only delegate an aspect of care to a person whom they deem competent to perform the task and they should assure themselves that the person to whom they have delegated fully understands the nature of the delegated task and what is required of them.
4. Where another, such as an employer, has the authority to delegate an aspect of care, the employer becomes accountable for that delegation. The registrant will, however, continue to carry responsibility to intervene if she feels that the proposed delegation is inappropriate or unsafe.

5. The decision whether or not to delegate an aspect of care and to transfer and/or to rescind delegation is the sole responsibility of the registrant and is based on their professional judgement.
6. The registrant has the right to refuse to delegate if they believe that it would be unsafe to do so or is unable to provide or ensure adequate supervision.
7. It is essential that those delegating care, and those employees undertaking delegated duties, do so within a robust local employment policy framework to protect the public and support safe practice.
8. The decision to delegate is either made by the registrant or the employer and it is the decision maker who is accountable for it.
9. Healthcare can sometimes be unpredictable. It is important that the person to whom aspects of care are being delegated understands their limitations and when not to proceed should the circumstances within which the task has been delegated change.
10. No one should feel pressurised into either delegating or accepting a delegated task. In such circumstances, advice should be sought, in the first instance, from the registrant's professional line manager and then, if necessary, the NMC.

The RCN has provided guidance on delegation to the scrub nurse[10] and in 2011 published a document setting out the principles of accountability and delegation for nurses, students, healthcare assistants and assistant practitioners.[11] The role of the healthcare support worker is discussed below.

Delegate tasks and duties that are within the other person's scope of competence

It is essential that nurses ensure the person they delegate to is competent to undertake the task and fully understands the instructions given. This might require the delegating nurse to provide further explanation and in some cases demonstration and training to ensure the task is carried out correctly and safely.

A coroner criticised a district nursing service as being unfit for purpose, and its staff as unprofessional, following the death of a patient in a care home. District nurses failed to delegate safely to care home staff and failed to ensure the care home staff understood their instructions.

The case concerned an 82-year-old woman who died from a stroke but the coroner ruled that bedsores she developed after district nurses failed to tell care assistants how to prevent them, contributed to her death (Robinson 2016).

The inquest heard that the deceased suffered from dementia. When her condition deteriorated staff at the care home sought help from the district nurse team who made several visits to the woman.

The coroner held that the district nursing service was aware the woman had rapidly deteriorating dementia, was immobile, had poor nutrition, poor hydration, and was doubly incontinent, and was therefore at significant risk factors of develop of pressure sores.

However, there were no indications in the district nurse records of:

- a completed pressure sore risk assessment
- a plan for managing the woman's pressure sore risk
- any information relating to the care of the deceased was communicated and safely delegated to the care home

This led the coroner to raise concerns about the unprofessional behaviour of the district nurse service.

In response to these criticisms the district nurse manager, in evidence, claimed that the district nursing service was too busy to write records and that all of their interactions with residential and care homes were verbal as they did not have time to do anything else.

The coroner held that failing to meet the standards on recordkeeping and delegation compromised patient care, communication of care and continuity of care. The outcome was that the patient did not have a preventative care plan to manage the high risk of developing pressure sores (Robinson 2016).

The coroner was confident that care home staff would have followed any care plan drawn up by nursing staff to prevent pressure sores from developing. In its absence, the untrained care staff were unaware that blisters the deceased developed indicated that she was likely to suffer from sores in the future.

The coroner was sufficiently concerned that the failings of the district nursing service would result in further deaths that he issued a report to the director of nursing at the trust, the chief executive, medical director, and the Care Quality Commission (CQC) stating that, from the evidence the care provided is unfit for service. Coroners have the authority to take action to prevent further deaths under the Coroners and Justice Act 2009, schedule 5, paragraph 7.

Confirm that the outcome of any task you have delegated to someone else meets the required standard

Registered nurses must ensure that the task and duty they have delegated has been carried out to the required standard and make a note that they have undertaken that check. In addition, where registered nurses delegate a task to support staff, students, or relatives, then they may also be required to exercise their professional judgement by evaluating the significance of the finding. When delegating risk assessments and monitoring assessments, such as completing vital signs, NEWS charts or pressure sore assessments, it is the registered nurses role to come to a conclusion on the significance of the assessment and take further action if necessary in accordance with standard 3 of the NMC Code (2018) which places a professional duty on nurse to ensure that peoples, physical, social and psychological needs are assessed and responded to.

A registered nurse's legal duty of care may be breached, and the nurse found liable in negligence if their failure to evaluate the outcome of a delegated task results in harm to the patient.

In *XM* v *Leicestershire Partnership Trust* [2020] a health visitor was held negligent for failing to follow a head circumference measurement they had delegated to a nursery nurse. The child had a rare and benign brain tumour that caused an accumulation of cerebrospinal fluid that caused the brain to grow abnormally fast. When the nursery nurse undertook the head circumference measurement it was recorded as being on the 99.6^{th} centile, but the reading was not checked by the health visitor and no evaluation was made of the significance of the reading. By the time the tumour was discovered permanent brain damage had occurred but it was accepted that had action been taken before the reading crossed the 99.6^{th} centile no permanent disability would have occurred.

The Court held that the health visitor was negligent for not following up the delegation by checking the reading and coming to a professional judgement on its significance. On the role of the nursery nurse, the court found that they were not negligence. The nursery nurse was not in their breach of duty by failing to appreciate that XM's head was disproportionately large. The standard of care expected of a nursery nurse was different from that expected of a health visitor. Although they performed certain delegated health visitor tasks, nursery nurses were not qualified nurses, were not trained to take or interpret head circumference measurements and would not look at head measurement charts.

Delegation of a task or duty does not end at the point of delegation. The registered nurse who initiated the delegation must follow up, check the task has been completed properly and safely and come to a professional judgement on any measurement or assessments that have been completed.[12]

Nurse consultants

Clinical nurse specialists and consultant nurses are seen as having a major role to play in providing an improved service for patients. The NHS Plan envisaged that there would be 1000 nurse consultants and therapist consultants would also be appointed. The key features of the consultant nurse as envisaged in the Department of Health's *Making a Difference*,[13] are shown in Box 23.4.

Box 23.4 Key features of the consultant nurse

1. Expert practice
2. Professional leadership and consultancy
3. Education and development
4. Practice and service development linked to research and evaluation

It was envisaged that at least 50 per cent of the time of nurse consultants will be spent on clinical work with career opportunities. NHS trusts were required to agree the posts with regional offices of the DH. Nurse consultant posts are advertised on the website for NHS careers.[14] The RCN has published a report on becoming and being a nurse consultant.[15] This resulted from two years' research into the role of the nurse consultant which aimed at enabling nurse consultants and aspiring nurse consultants to become effective through a programme of support.

Clinical nurse specialists and specialist nurses

In addition, clinical nurse specialists have taken on a wide range of expanded duties, often working within protocols agreed with medical staff. They may also have managerial responsibilities. Other specialist nurses may or may not come within the category of clinical nurse specialists, but are increasingly taking on expanded-role functions. It would be impossible in a book of this type to explore the wide range of specialties covered by nurses, often functioning within a multidisciplinary team, but making many decisions on their own. They include continence care, stoma care, pain management, diabetic and A&E nurse practitioners.

A checklist published by the RCN that applies to all expanded-role tasks covers the following questions for extending roles:

- Is this new skill/role consistent with nursing practice?
- Is it consistent with my current job description?
- Does it fit current priorities – nursing and organisational?
- What changes will it entail?
- Will I need to stop some parts of my current care?
- Do I need accreditation?
- How will I get it?
- Do I need additional skills?
- How will I get them?
- Do I need a training period before I take on the new responsibility?
- Do I have a mentor for this change?
- How will I evaluate my performance in the new role?
- Have I got clinical supervision?[16]

Clinical Nurse Specialists and Consultant Nurses and Clinical Guidelines

It has been emphasised that when a clinical nurse specialist or consultant nurse takes on an expanded role they must provide the same standard of care which would have been provided by the health professional who would originally have performed that activity. Thus an A&E clinical specialist nurse undertaking activities that would in the past have been performed by doctors would be expected to provide the reasonable standard of care of a doctor. Jo Wilson[17] has suggested that guidelines can be very useful in role expansion and assist the expanded-role practitioner in delivering a higher standard of care that reflects: additional training and regular updates; additional competency and expertise; skills required for the activity. She lists the considerations that should be taken into account in drafting guidelines:

- description and limitations to the activity being performed;
- degree of supervision required;
- audit, evaluation and outcome data;
- making the status of the treating nurse known to patient;
- obtaining the patient's consent; and
- regular education/training updates.

(Further consideration on the legal significance of guidelines, procedures and protocols can be found in chapter 3.) The RCN has provided guidance on clinical nurse specialists in the context of rheumatology[18] in stoma care[19] and dementia care.[20]

Concerns about developments in scope of professional practice

Practitioners have concerns, however, as a result of the move away from certified tasks and the rapid development in the scope of professional practice, which include the following:

1. How do I know if I am competent?
2. How does my employer know if I am competent?
3. What happens if I undertake an activity that is outside my field of competence?
4. Where do I stand if a doctor/senior manager/other professional ignores my refusal to undertake an activity because I have not sufficient competence or experience to undertake that activity?
5. How can I ensure that I receive the appropriate training for my expanded role?

Some situations will be considered that highlight these dilemmas.

Practical dilemma 23.1   Scope of professional practice (1)

Mavis, a staff nurse, was asked by the registrar to do the intravenous infusions. The registrar rushed away before she had the chance to explain to him that she had not developed the skills, competence and knowledge to undertake that activity safely. However, she decided that she would carry out his instructions as best she could. Unfortunately, when she was adding a drug to Jimmy Price's intravenous infusion, she failed to set the speed of his drip correctly and as a result Jimmy became very ill. Where do Mavis and the registrar stand in relation to the responsibility for the harm to Jimmy?

As far as Mavis was concerned, she was at fault in failing to mention her lack of competence for that activity to the registrar. No nurse should work outside her range of competence and skill unless a dire emergency arises when the risks in failing to act are greater than the risks in acting. There is no suggestion that this was an emergency. The nurse ignored a fundamental principle of the Code quoted above. The failure of Mavis to notify the doctor that she was not competent in this area and the resulting mistake that caused harm to the patient could result in a civil action being brought against her employer because of its vicarious liability for the negligent actions of an employee acting in the course of employment (see pages 73–8). Mavis herself may be subject to fitness to practise proceedings before the NMC Conduct and Competence Committee. Were Jimmy to die, she might also face criminal proceedings. Her employer, of course, would commence its own disciplinary inquiry and proceedings.

What of the registrar? Is he also at fault? If the addition of drugs to intravenous transfusions were seen as a task delegated by a doctor to a nurse practitioner, he would be liable as delegator in failing to ensure that he was delegating to a competent person. However, under the scope of professional practice, such activities are not seen as 'delegated tasks' and the duty is incumbent on the individual nurse practitioner to ensure that, if she herself was not competent, another practitioner, whether medical or nursing, who was competent, performed the activity. The standard of care that the patient is entitled to expect does not depend on which professional is undertaking a particular activity. The reasonable standard of care will be required of any professional carrying out an extended role: if that activity were formerly carried out by a doctor, then a nurse undertaking that activity will be expected to provide the reasonable standard that a doctor would have provided. The Bolam Test is used to define the reasonable standard (see chapter 3). The managerial responsibilities in ensuring appropriate supervision and allocation of activities are discussed in chapter 4.

Can a nurse refuse to undertake training in new areas of competency?

It was a principle under the concept of the 'extended role' that nurses could refuse to undertake a new task or activity. However, this approach is no longer appropriate in relation to the scope of professional practice. The Code requires nurses to 'maintain the knowledge and skills you need for safe and effective practice'.

It would be entirely inappropriate for a practitioner to refuse to develop their professional practice beyond the level they reached when they became registered. They would be contractually entitled to receive from their employer the necessary training to ensure that they were competent in the new range of activities. It is a contractual requirement of the employer to ensure that staff are competent to perform the work they are asked to perform.

There are other contractual considerations. In an interview for a job, for example, a nurse might be told that a contractual requirement for that particular post is that the nurse is competent in a specified area. If the nurse agrees to this condition, then they are contractually bound to develop, with support from the employer, the appropriate skills, knowledge and competence. If they refuse the condition, they will probably not get the post.

Scope of professional practice in primary care

Practical dilemma 23.2 Liability and the scope of professional practice (2)

Practice Nurse Jenny Brown was asked by the GP, her employer, to make a primary visit to a child whose mother had reported him too ill to come to surgery. Jenny Brown visited the child, took his temperature and blood pressure and examined him. She told the mother that she thought he was suffering from the flu that was going round at present, to keep him warm with lots of drinks and, if he worsened or failed to improve within a few days, to let the surgery know. She reported the results of the visit to the GP, who approved of her action. Unfortunately, that same night an emergency call was made by the mother to the out-of-hours service and the boy was rushed to hospital, where he was diagnosed as suffering from meningitis. He eventually died. The mother is now demanding that action be taken against both the nurse and the doctor. What is the responsibility of the nurse and the doctor?

If the nurse had acted outside her competence, been negligent and caused harm as a consequence, then she will be liable. The doctor or clinical commissioning group will be vicariously liable for the actions of a negligent nurse employed by the doctor or clinical commissioning group. In this case, there would be an investigation to establish the tests undertaken by the nurse and the advice that she gave to the mother and whether her actions satisfied the standard of the reasonable medical practitioner. The competence of a nurse in making a primary visit has become of increasing importance with the expansion of nurse prescribing. In any case, even when the doctor is not the employer of the nurse, where there is delegation of a task that is normally performed by a doctor, the doctor will remain liable in civil law for that task unless he has delegated it to a competent, trained person and provides the requisite supervision for the task to be done safely. Here one might question whether it was a suitable case for the practice nurse to undertake. Had she the necessary training and skills to detect whether the patient was suffering from mumps or another condition? Once she had visited the patient, should she not have arranged for the GP to attend or ensured that a closer eye was kept on him? Did she make all the appropriate tests and checks when she visited the boy? If these questions are answered in such a way that the nurse is shown to be at fault, then the GP could well be liable for any harm that has consequentially befallen the boy (there may, in fact, be no harm suffered, since the short delay in diagnosis may have had no effect) and the nurse would also be liable for undertaking a task that she was not competent to perform. In either event, the nurse would be held professionally accountable before the NMC for her actions. Even had there been no negligence on the part of the GP, he, as her employer, would be vicariously liable for the practice nurse's negligence. The White Paper of 2010[21] envisaged that commissioning responsibilities would be devolved to GPs. Subsequently, the Health and Social Care Act 2012 has created clinical commissioning groups which may lead to further expansion in the scope of the primary care nurse (see chapters 5 and 22).

Scope of professional practice in theatre nursing

Practical dilemma 23.3 Scope of professional practice and theatres

Myra Jones had worked in theatre for over 20 years and was an extremely experienced nurse. She had asked for training in acting as a first assistant, but the surgeons had stated that this was not a role that should be performed by nurses. One day, she was asked by the registrar to assist in an appendectomy because there was a shortage of junior doctors. She knew that she could do the work competently, but was hesitant. What is the legal situation?

Should she refuse on the grounds that she has not been trained to fulfil this role? What if this request comes at night when there is only a registrar on his own and it is an emergency case? The basic principle is that, whatever duties she is called on to perform, she should undertake no work that she is not competent to undertake.

In an emergency situation, when the harm to the patient of her acting is outweighed by the harm to the patient of her not acting, the balance might be in favour of her acting as assistant (but these occasions are likely to be rare). To refuse to perform certain tasks is not pleasant for the nurse, but it is her duty both in civil law and also as part of the Code of Professional Conduct of her profession. Only in this way can the safety of the patient be ensured. If such situations arise where the nurse is expected to undertake tasks for which she is not trained, this must ultimately be referred to nurse management. If this proves ineffective, then the nurse may need to take advantage of the whistleblower's protection (discussed in chapter 4).

In Practical Dilemma 23.3 the Royal College of Surgeons (RCS) has the responsibility of recognising the extent to which nurses can play a significant role in theatre. In 2005 the RCS published *Modern Surgical Workforce* (available on its website[22]) which considered the move from the role of the individual consultant to multidisciplinary team working. It recognised the increasing role for non-medically qualified practitioners (NMQP) which would lead to a wider role for the theatre nurse. Julie Quick[23] has analysed the role of the surgical care practitioner (SCP) within the surgical team, showing that the surgeons interviewed considered the addition of the SCP to the surgical team brought benefits to the patient, the members of the surgical team, the practitioner and the employing organisation. Dimond (1994) stated that 'Where activities normally undertaken by doctors are delegated to nursing staff they [sic] would be expected to meet the standards that would be required from a doctor were the doctor to perform the task,' further adding 'The patient is entitled to expect to have the same approved standard of care whether the task is undertaken by a doctor or by a nurse'.[24]

Scope of professional practice in emergency nursing

A joint report by the RCN and the DH[25] attempted to dispel the myths about what nurses and other health professionals may or are entitled to do in emergency care. The booklet aimed to show directors of nursing how they could empower staff to take responsibility for change and to show managers to use it to support staff in developing their roles. It is available from the DH website.[26] Fact sheets cover the myths about the legal and professional framework, clinical governance, the emergency services collaboration, coronary heart disease and primary care collaboratives. (See chapter 20 for further discussion on the emergency care practitioner.)

Scope of professional practice and X-rays

The ordering of X-rays may constitute an expanded role for the nurses, but they should be aware of the rules relating to this. The Ionising Radiation (Medical Exposure) Regulations 2017[27] were enacted, together with the Ionising Radiations Regulations 2017,[28] to comply with European Directive 97/43/Euratom.[29] This Directive lays down:

- basic measures for the health protection of individuals against dangers of ionising radiation in relation to medical exposure;

- duties on those responsible for administering ionising radiation; and
- the need to protect persons undergoing medical exposure whether as part of their own medical diagnosis or treatment or of occupational health surveillance, health screening, voluntary participation in research or medicolegal procedures.

The regulations do not specify that any specified health professional must be a referrer (i.e. the person ordering the X-ray) but require that the referrer must be entitled in accordance with the employer's procedures to refer individuals for medical exposure to a practitioner. Regulation 6 prohibits any medical exposure from being carried out that has not been justified and authorised and sets out matters to be taken into account for justification.

The referrer has a duty to supply the practitioner with sufficient medical data relevant to the medical exposure requested by the referrer to enable the practitioner to decide whether there is sufficient net benefit as required by regulations 10(5) and 11(1)(b). Applying these requirements to nurses: this means that nurses may be referrers, i.e. order X-rays, but they must have the training and competence which enables them to provide the medical data to enable the radiographer to decide whether the patient should be exposed to the X-rays.[30] Guidance has been provided by the Department of Health on the regulations and is available on the internet.[31] The fact sheet provided within the publication *Freedom to Practise: dispelling the myths*[32] points out that nurses requesting radiological examinations can be referrers under the Ionising Regulations, provided that they have the competence, conferred by training and experience, to provide the medical data required to enable the practitioner (usually a radiologist) to decide whether there is net benefit to the patient from the exposure. The nurse would require the consent of the employer who would specify the type or range of conditions for which the nurse can be the referrer. The RCN has provided guidance for non-medically qualified persons on clinical imaging requests which also sets out the law relating to ionising radiation regulations.[33] The scope of professional practice of the nurse is extended by their ability to refer patients for X-rays and, by their wider remit in the X-ray department.

NHS 111 (formerly NHS Direct) and walk-in clinics

NHS 111 (formerly NHS Direct) and walk-in clinics (see chapter 5) depend heavily on nursing staff, who are the main group employed in these areas. Nurses have to be sure that they work within the scope of their professional competence.

Practical dilemma 23.4 Scope of professional practice (3)

A nurse employed by NHS 111 received a phone call from a woman of 28 who said she was suffering from severe indigestion and asked what was recommended. The nurse failed to clarify whether the woman was pregnant and suggested that she should take some indigestion pills. Subsequently, the woman was admitted in an emergency to hospital with hypertension. The family are now wishing to sue the NHS.

In this situation, there would probably be a protocol the nurse should have followed and ascertaining the possibility of pregnancy would have been an essential question to ask.

There would appear to be *prima facie* evidence of negligence. Clearly, the safest advice to be given by any nurse answering calls on the NHS 111 Service is for the patient to seek an appointment with his or her general practitioner. However, this might reduce the value of the service.

From 2013 NHS Direct was replaced by locally commissioned services using the NHS 111 number. The 111 service is provided by a range of providers such as Ambulance Service Trusts or GP's out-of-hours service.

Similar problems beset the nurse providing the services in walk-in clinics, since the majority are nurse-led. It is essential that nurse practitioners have the appropriate training to run such clinics competently and to be aware of the limits of their knowledge and have the confidence to be firm on what they do not know. Minor injuries can probably be dealt with on a one-off basis, such as suturing or bandaging a sprain. However, there may be a need to refer to X-ray, to arrange for further diagnostic tests or to seek specialist advice, and the nurse needs to be confident when this is required and when they need to refer the patient on for medical advice. In February 2000 practice nurses and nurses who work in walk-in centres were given statutory powers to prescribe from a limited list, as do community nurses and health visitors.[34] Subsequently, the new developments in nurse prescribing enable any nurse who has had the appropriate training to prescribe medications within their competence (see chapter 27). These powers increase the dangers of a nurse working outside their competence. (For further discussion on NHS 111 and walk-in centres, see chapter 5.)

Modern matrons

The role of matron was reintroduced into the NHS as part of the NHS Plan. It was intended that matrons should provide strong leadership on wards and be highly visible and accessible to patients; that they should set an example in driving up standards of clinical care and empowering nurses to take on a greater range of clinical tasks to help improve patient care. A report was published in April 2003 on progress in these appointments and the Chief Nursing Officer of the Department of Health set out the plans to extend the role of modern matrons in A&E departments to improve patient experience of NHS emergency care. Each matron in charge of an A&E department was to have a £10,000 budget to help bring these improvements about. A progress report was provided in February 2004 that gave examples of how the monies had been spent.[35] The function of modern matrons in A&E departments includes: clinical leadership; improving patient experience; improving the clinical and patient environment; and managing the ward/departmental environment budget. The intention to appoint 3000 community matrons was announced in June 2004. In September 2007 the DH announced that it was placing responsibility for the cleanliness of wards and departments upon nurses who would have the right of appealing to the chief management if their recommendations were not accepted. This further emphasises the importance of the role of the matron. By 2008 over 5000 matrons had been appointed but, interestingly, whether or not they had made a difference was questioned in an article in the *Nursing Times*.[36] Increasingly matrons have been appointed from the ranks of health professions other than nurses. They are paid, like consultant nurses on band 8a–c.

The basic principles which apply to the scope of professional practice are shown in Box 23.5.

> ### Box 23.5　Basic principles that apply to the scope of professional practice
>
> 1. Always work within the scope of your professional practice
> 2. Identify any training or supervised practice needs and take steps to ensure that these are met
> 3. Be aware that the law does not accept a principle of team liability; each individual practitioner is personally and professionally accountable for their own actions
> 4. Do not obey orders, except in an extreme emergency, unless you are satisfied that they constitute reasonable professional practice
> 5. Be prepared to refuse to undertake any activity unless it is within your competence
> 6. Do not accept an undertaking that someone else will accept responsibility for what you do (I'll take responsibility!)
> 7. Ensure that any development in your professional practice takes place in the context of multidisciplinary discussions, with full management support and an awareness of the need to educate the patient and others to the new situation

Agency nurses

In recent years the shortage in the number of nurses has led to the growth in the use of agencies for the provision of nurse staffing. Many nurses, too, find working for an agency suits their practical needs of combining family and work by giving them greater flexibility and control over their time. Nursing agencies have to register with the CQC and complete an annual quality assurance assessment. Further information is on the CQC website.[37]

Nurses working for an agency should be clear over the legal implications of their status when they are allocated to an NHS trust. Do they become employees of the trust or are they employees of the agency or are they classified as self-employed practitioners? Their employment status has considerable repercussions for both their legal liability and also for their entitlements to statutory provisions for the employee (see chapter 10). The RCN has provided guidance on agency nurse induction for employers, nursing agencies and nursing staff.[38] The European Union issued a Directive[39] giving new rights for temporary workers, including workers hired through agencies which came into force in the UK in 2010 (see chapter 10).

Healthcare support workers

Essential to the development of enhanced professional practice of the registered nurse is a trained competent body of nursing auxiliaries/healthcare support workers who are able to undertake those activities delegated to them. Although there have been discussions over the registration of such support workers, with the NMC and the Health and Care Professions Council (HCPC) both being contenders for the role of registration authority, no action has as yet been taken.

Indeed, there is evidence that such workers are not even being trained in some of the activities they are expected to undertake. *The Sunday Times* published an alarmist article on the fact that support workers were undertaking technical nursing tasks with limited, if any, training.[40] Peter Carter, the then RCN General Secretary, recommended that healthcare assistants should receive a substantial minimum training period as well as being subjected to a code of conduct. In July 2010 the NMC published the findings of research it had commissioned into the regulation of healthcare support workers. It is available on the NMC website.

There has been considerable pressure for the registration and training of support workers. The Mid-Staffordshire Inquiry[41] (see chapter 5) made several recommendations on this topic.

> Recommendation 209: healthcare support workers should be registered and no unregistered person should be permitted to provide for reward direct physical care to patients currently under the care and treatment of a doctor or nurse (or who are dependent on such care by reason of disability or infirmity) in a hospital or care home setting. The system should apply to healthcare support workers whether they are working for the NHS or independent healthcare providers, in the community, for agencies or as independent agents. (Exemptions should be made for persons caring for members of their own family or those with whom they have a genuine social relationship.)
>
> Recommendation 210: there should be a national code of conduct for healthcare support workers.
>
> Recommendation 211: there should be a common set of national standards for the education and training of healthcare support workers.
>
> Recommendation 212: the NMC should be responsible for the preparation of the code of conduct, education and training standards and requirements for registration of healthcare support workers.

The report led to demands for basic skills training and testing of healthcare assistants. The Health Secretary has ruled out full registration but a review conducted by Camilla Cavendish, the *Sunday Times* columnist, concluded that all support workers should be required to have a certificate of fundamental care without which they would not be allowed to care for patients.[42]

The Care Minister announced in October 2013 that all healthcare assistants and social care support workers would, before starting work, have to be certified in a skills and values test. The Care Certificate will provide clear evidence to employers, patients and service users that the person in front of them has been trained to a specific set of standards. Section 95 of the Care Act 2014 adds a new subsection to section 20 to the Health and Social Care Act 2008 to enable the Secretary of State to specify persons to set the standards which persons undergoing training in regulated activities must attain. Under section 98 of the Care Act 2014 Health Education England (see chapter 17) must ensure that a sufficient number of persons with the skills and training to work as healthcare workers is available throughout England. To many these reforms do not go far enough, with the RCN recommending mandatory regulations for all healthcare support workers.[43] However, until the regulations are published it is impossible to say how effective this provision will be in setting and improving standards for healthcare assistants.

Karen Barker[44] considers that perhaps registration would allow HCAs to feel more valued and access the training to help them do the job they want to do to a high standard.

A report in 2014 by Baroness Kingsmill criticised the fact that the 1.8 million of care workers for the elderly were under-qualified, under-trained and paid below the minimum wage which led to the frail and the elderly not receiving the help they required.[45] She recommended a licence to practice for care managers and a register for all care workers with zero hours contracts being banned and minimum wage laws rigorously enforced.

In May 2014 the NMC and Health Education England commissioned a review into nurse and healthcare assistant education and training in England to be led by Lord Willis of Knaresborough.

In the light of the concern about the lack of regulation of healthcare support workers it is interesting that proposals are being put forward for a new grade of physician assistant: science graduates with an intensive two-year training. Known as 'physician associates' they will not be registered with the GMC or any other regulator, except possibly have entry onto a voluntary register. The concept has proved popular in the USA where they have existed for over 50 years and now number over 80,000.[46] Critics say the scheme is a means of getting doctors on the cheap and could be dangerous for patients. However, the President of the UK Association for Physician Associates[47] stated that patients are in safer hands with them than with junior doctors.[48]

Conclusions

The scope of professional practice of the nurse, midwife and specialist community public health nurse has continued to develop and it is clear that the initial pre-registration training is the foundation upon which an expanded professional role can take place. Registered practitioners must work within their competence and ensure that they have the training and supervision to develop their practice in new areas. The most extensive area of expansion has been in the field of prescribing and these developments are considered in chapter 27. However, other traditional areas of clinical practice such as surgery are opening up to nurses. The repercussions of such developments are significant not just for the individual registered practitioner, but also for the culture and interrelationships of professionals within health and social care. The 'Freedom to Practise: dispelling the myths' template has paved the way for further professional development but there is still much further to go. There are very few Acts of Parliament which require certain activities to be carried out by a member of a specified registered health profession, which means that the law enables an expansion of the professional role of the registered nurse and midwife across almost the whole field of health and social care.

Reflection questions

1. You have been working as a clinical nurse specialist in the diabetic clinic and have now been asked if you would wish to seek a post of consultant nurse in the same department. What differences would you anticipate there would be between your present post and the post of consultant nurse? What legal implications would there be if you were to obtain the new post?

2. You are aware that your expanded scope of professional practice includes several activities that were originally performed by doctors. In what ways could you assure patients that you are competent to perform these activities?

3. You have been asked to undertake training to be able to act as a clinical supervisor. What are the legal implications of this role?

4. What documentation should be kept in respect of clinical supervision?

Further exercises

1. Study a copy of your NHS trust's policy on the scope of professional practice duties and the principles contained therein. In what ways do you consider that your professional practice could develop? What are the barriers to such development and how could these barriers be overcome?

References

[1] Department of Health, The New NHS – modern, dependable, HMSO, London, 1997
[2] Department of Health, Making a Difference: the new NHS, DH, July 1999
[3] Secretary of State for Health, The NHS Plan, Cm 4818–1, Stationery Office, London, July 2000
[4] Nursing and Midwifery Council, The Code: Professional standards of practice and behaviour for nurses and midwives, NMC, London, 2015
[5] http://revalidation.nmc.org.uk
[6] Secretary of State for Health, The NHS Plan, Cm 4818–1, Stationery Office, London, July 2000
[7] Department of Health, Essence of Care, 2010, Stationery Office
[8] British Medical Association, Resuscitation Council (UK) and the Royal College of Nursing, Decisions Relating to Cardiopulmonary Resuscitation, BMA, October 2007, Paragraph 13, p. 19
[9] Nursing and Midwifery Council, A to Z: Delegation, updated 2008
[10] Royal College of Nursing, Delegation: the support worker in the scrub role, 003 149, RCN, London, February 2007
[11] Royal College of Nursing, Principles of accountability and delegation for nurses, students, health care assistants and assistant practitioners, 003 942, RCN, October 2011
[12] Robinson J. (2016) Coroner brands district nursing team 'unfit for service' after they fail to care for dying woman, 82, and reports supervisor for 'smiling and chuckling' through the inquest available on the Mailonline Website at http://www.dailymail.co.uk/news/article-3559891/Coroner-brands-district-nursing-team-unfit-service-fail-care-dying-woman-82-reports-supervisor-smiling-chuckling-inquest.html *XM* v *Leicestershire Partnership Trust* [2020] EWHC 3102
[13] Department of Health, Making a Difference: the new NHS, DH, July 1999
[14] www.nhscareers.nhs.uk
[15] Royal College of Nursing, Becoming and being a nurse consultant, RCN, 2012
[16] Royal College of Nursing, Developing Roles: nurses working in breast care, Order No. 001 957, RCN, May 1999
[17] Jo Wilson, Why Clinical Guidelines? A nursing perspective, in John Tingle and Charles Foster (eds) *Clinical Guidelines: Law, Policy and Practice*, Cavendish Publishing, London, 2002
[18] Royal College of Nursing, Clinical Nurse Specialists: adding value to care – an executive summary, 003 598, RCN, London, May 2010
[19] Royal College of Nursing, Clinical Nurse Specialists: stoma care, 003 520, RCN, London, October 2009

20. Royal College of Nursing, Scoping the role of the dementia nurse specialist in acute care, 004 429, RCN, London 2013
21. Department of Health, Equity and Excellence: Liberating the NHS, White Paper Cm 7881, Stationery Office, 2010
22. www.rcseng.ac.uk
23. Julie Quick, The role of the surgical care practitioner within the surgical team, *British Journal of Nursing*, 22(13):759–765, 2013
24. B. Dimond, Legal Aspects of Role Expansion, in Hunt, G. and Wainwright, P. (eds) *Expanding the Role of the Nurse*, Blackwell Scientific Publications, Oxford, 1994
25. Royal College of Nursing and Department of Health, Freedom to Practise: dispelling the myths, RCN and DH, 2003
26. Ibid.
27. Ionising Radiation (Medical Exposure) Regulations 2017 SI 2017/1322
28. Ionising Radiations Regulations 2017 SI 2017/1075
29. European Directive 97/43/Euratom (OJ No. L180, 9.7.97, p. 22)
30. See B. Dimond, *Legal Aspects of Radiography and Radiology* (Chapter 16), Blackwell Scientific Publications, Oxford, 2002
31. Department of Health www.gov.uk
32. Department of Health and Royal College of Nursing, Freedom to Practise: dispelling the myths, November 2003
33. Royal College of Nursing, Clinical imaging requests from non-medically qualified professionals, 003 101, RCN, London, March 2008
34. The National Health Service (Pharmaceutical Services) Amendment Regulations 2000, SI 2000/121
35. Department of Health press release 2004/0047, Health Minister urges A&E Matrons to Claim their £10,000
36. Helen Mooney, Are modern matrons making a difference? *Nursing Times*, 17 June 2008
37. www.cqc.org.uk
38. Royal College of Nursing, Agency nurse induction guidelines. RCN guidance for employers, nursing agencies and nursing staff; www.rcn.org.uk/get-help/rcn-advice/agency-workers
39. Directive 2008/104/EC
40. Sarah-Kate Templeton, Novices do nurses' job after week's training, *The Sunday Times*, 30 August 2009
41. Report of the Mid Staffordshire NHS Foundation Trust Public Inquiry, HC 947, February 2013, Stationery Office; www.midstaffspublicinquiry.com
42. Chris Smyth, Healthcare assistants must pass basic skills test under shake-up, *The Times*, 10 July 2013
43. Chris Smyth, Care assistants to take skills test before helping on wards, *The Times*, 31 October 2013
44. Karen Barker, Support of the health-care assistant, *British Journal of Midwifery*, 21(8):538, August 2013
45. Baroness Denise Kingsmill, Taking Care: review of exploitation in the care sector, May 2014
46. Chris Smyth, Fears over new medics trained for 2 years, *The Times*, 22 August 2014
47. www.ukapa.co.uk
48. Chris Smyth, Patients in safer hands with assistants than junior doctors, *The Times*, 23 August 2014

Part III
General Areas

Chapter 24

Legal Aspects of Property

This chapter discusses

- Principles of liability
- Administrative failures
- Exclusion of liability
- Property of the mentally incapacitated patient
- Mental Capacity Act 2005
- Day-to-day care of money
- Power of attorney
- Court of Protection
- Protecting patients from relatives
- Returning the patient's property
- Staff property
- Gifts

Introduction

The nurse may have many concerns about property. He or she may wonder if they are liable if the patient's property is lost. This becomes of particular concern in those situations where the patient is incompetent to take care of their own possessions. What are the legal requirements? The nurse may also be concerned for their own property. Does the NHS trust as an employer have any duty to make arrangements to care for the nurse's property? What happens if the nurse's car is damaged in the hospital car park? Does it make any difference to the liability of the employer if a patient damages the car?

Principles of liability

Practical Dilemma 24.1 Seen on X-ray

Janice was rushing to get to a party when she felt faint and collapsed in the street. She was unconscious and was taken in an ambulance to hospital. On admission she was X-rayed and then admitted to the emergency ward. She recovered consciousness and asked to have her necklace returned. The ward staff told her that she was not wearing a necklace and showed her a plastic patient's property bag into which had been placed everything that she had with her on admission. She checked and there was no necklace in the bag. She asked for the loss of the necklace to be investigated. Subsequently it was found that the X-ray showed that she was wearing a necklace. Janice is now claiming that the hospital is responsible for its loss which she estimates to be over £10,000.

In Practical Dilemma 24.1, the first issue that arises is: can it be said that the NHS trust is liable for the missing property and is anyone personally liable? In general, a person does not become liable for another person's property unless he or she can be shown to have assumed some responsibility for it. The person who undertakes to look after the property of another person is known as a *bailee*. The person who owns the property is known as the *bailor*. Thus, if a patient were to give a gold watch to the ward manager, the manager on behalf of the NHS trust acts as bailee of that property entrusted to it by the patient, the bailor. It is the duty of the bailee to carry out the instructions of the bailor and to surrender the property of the bailor when requested to do so or as previously agreed. In most circumstances, the relationship of bailor/bailee is a voluntary one and one person cannot force another into being the bailee of one's property. When the person agrees to act as bailee (and there may be no reward for doing so), a transfer of possession takes place so that the bailee then becomes liable. In contrast with the usual principles of negligence, once the existence of the bailment is established, it is not for the bailor to establish negligence by the bailee, but for the bailee to show that he or she exercised all reasonable care for the goods and was not negligent. This is a reversal of the usual burdens of proof.

In the context of hospital care, another duty arises under the law of negligence. If an unconscious patient is brought into the A&E department, the NHS trust and the professionals have a duty to care for the patient and this would include caring for his or her property if they are unable to look after it. This is known as involuntary bailment. Looking at Janice's situation, could it be said that the NHS trust became an involuntary bailee of her property and had a duty of care in relation to it? The answer is that in the street when she was unconscious and was unable to look after her property herself, first the ambulance staff had a duty of care and then when she was transferred to the A&E staff the latter then assumed the duty of care of both herself and her property. Were it not for the evidence of the X-ray there would be doubt as to whether someone in the street or the ambulance staff had removed and kept the necklace. However, the X-ray shows clearly that Janice was still wearing the necklace when she came to hospital and it was 'lost' after that. There would have to be an inquiry to find out at what point Janice was not wearing the necklace and who had the opportunity of taking the necklace after the X-ray.

The fact that Janice had not personally entrusted the necklace to the care of the hospital could not be used as a defence in the involuntary bailment situation. The burden would be on the hospital to establish that it took good care of Janice and her property.

The trust would probably be advised to offer an *ex gratia* payment to Janice (i.e. an offer in which liability is not admitted but a sum of money is offered to dispose of the case quickly (see chapter 3)). There is likely to be difficulty in establishing the value of the missing necklace, unless Janice has a receipt and can prove that it was the receipted item which can be seen in the X-ray.

Administrative failures

When property, which has not been entrusted to the care of hospital staff, is lost, there is unlikely to be litigation, since it would be difficult to establish the responsibility of the hospital. The loss is more likely to be the subject of a complaint about the administrative procedures. For example, there may have been a failure by staff to point out to the patient and to the relatives the procedures for dealing with property. Complaints of this kind, though they may not lead to a court action, may result in the NHS trust making an *ex gratia* payment to the patient or relatives. This is not an admission of liability, but an attempt to appease the relatives and make up for administrative shortcomings. Under the current complaints scheme, any complaint of missing property would be investigated at a local level and an attempt made to resolve it. If the complainant is not satisfied with the outcome, then they can apply to the Parliamentary and Health Service Ombudsman for an independent review (see chapter 26).

Practical Dilemma 24.2 A lost engagement ring

Louise was admitted for an appendectomy and was expecting to stay in hospital only for a few days. She took very little cash in with her, but did take her engagement ring. When she was using the wash basin in the toilets, she took off her ring, placing it on the side and then forgot to put it back on. She had been back in the ward only a short time when she realised what she had done and rushed back to fetch it, but unfortunately it was gone. She knows that someone must have stolen it. Can she recover compensation from the trust?

There is no legal right for Louise to obtain compensation from the trust. She did not entrust her property to the trust employees, and at the time that it was lost she was responsible for it. However, she may be able to show that there were administrative failings. For example, it might not have been pointed out to her that she brings her property into the hospital at her own risk. While, therefore, there may be no legal basis for a claim, she may be able to use the complaints procedure to raise concerns and, depending on the results, the trust may make an *ex gratia* payment to her. Contrariwise, if the trust explained the situation about patient's property and a notice pointing out that the trust did not accept liability was shown to her, she would probably be unable to obtain any compensation.

Exclusion of liability

What is the legal significance of the notice absolving the NHS trust or PCT of all responsibility for the patient's property? Under the Unfair Contract Terms Act 1977 (see chapter 6, Statute Box 6.2), such an exemption or exclusion notice is effective in relation to the loss or damage of property, provided that it is reasonable to exclude liability for the negligence that has led to such loss or damage. (Liability for negligence that leads to personal injury or death cannot be excluded.) How is reasonableness defined? The requirement of reasonableness is defined in Statute Box 24.1.

> **Statute 24.1**
> **Definition of Reasonableness in Section 11 of the Unfair Contract Terms Act 1977**
>
> [I]t should be fair and reasonable to allow reliance upon it, having regard to all the circumstances obtaining when the liability arose or [but for the Notice] would have arisen (section 11(3)).
>
> It is for the party claiming that a contract term or notice satisfies the requirement of reasonableness to show that it does (section 11(5)).

If in Practical Dilemma 24.1, a notice had been displayed on the wall, and if it could be argued that the NHS trust's employees had been negligent in relation to her property, then the NHS trust might claim to rely on the notice to avoid liability. It would then have to show that it was reasonable for them to rely on it. This would be difficult since Janice, being unconscious and incapable of reading the notice, would not have been aware of the exclusion of liability. In contrast, in Practical Dilemma 24.2 Louise would have been able to read such an exemption notice, and exclusion of liability by the trust would be more likely to succeed.

Patients should be advised not to bring valuable property into hospital. If they do, then it can be recommended to them that the property should be taken into safekeeping by the nursing

> **Box 24.1 Patients' property: form of notice disclaiming liability**
>
> I acknowledge that the opportunity has been given to me to hand over my personal property to be placed in safekeeping, that I have been advised to do so and that I have declined the offer of safekeeping of my personal property.
>
> Signature of patient
> Witnessed by
> (Member of staff)
> Designation
> Date
> To be filed in patient's case notes folder

staff. If they are unwilling to part with the property, then they can be asked to sign a form whereby they accept responsibility for the care of the property which has the added advantage of impressing upon the patient the dangers of having valuable property in hospital, as in Box 24.1.

Property of the mentally incapacitated patient

What about the property of those who are unconscious or who have learning disabilities or who are mentally unwell, and have capacity issues?

Temporary Incapacity

Practical Dilemma 24.3 | Lost teeth

Arthur Brown was rushed into hospital one night with a cardiac arrest. He survived following a six-hour operation. When he recovered from the operation, he was told that it was touch and go as to whether he would pull through. A few days later, he discovered that his set of teeth was missing. He told the staff nurse who said that a search would be started, but they were not found. What remedies does he have?

In this situation, it is clear that Arthur was incapable of taking care of his personal property on admission and it is likely that his teeth were removed preoperatively. (There would have to be a check to see if they were removed pre-admission or by the ambulance crew.) If following investigations it appears that the hospital staff did remove them and failed to take reasonable care, the trust would be seen as the bailee of the property and responsible for their loss. It would be advisable for the trust to admit liability and make Arthur a speedy offer of an *ex gratia* payment. Some staff may feel that, in view of the fact that staff saved Arthur's life, it is unreasonable of Arthur to complain. However, if there were a justified complaint, the fact that a patient's life has been saved would not be a successful defence.

Permanent Incapacity

In other situations of long-term mental incapacity, there may be tensions between attempting to develop the autonomy of a person and the care of personal property as the following situation indicates.

Practical Dilemma 24.4 | Pocket money

James Jones, an adult of 24 with learning disabilities, lived in a community home with others of a similar condition. He regularly earned himself significant amounts of money from doing odd jobs around the home and thus accumulated over £100. The staff in the home attempted to encourage James to put this in the bank. However, he could not be persuaded and there were rumours that he slept with it under his pillow at night. One morning, he screamed with distress and it appeared that all his money had been stolen from under his bed. A search revealed nothing and there was no hint as to where it had gone. Is the organisation which ran the home liable for the loss?

In Practical Dilemma 24.4 there was no transfer of possession from James to the care home owners or managers, so that the latter is not *prima facie* liable. However, much depends on James's mental competence and whether sufficient effort was made to persuade him to allow it to be taken for safekeeping. A system of tokens can sometimes be devised to protect patients' property, although care must be taken not to limit their purchasing power and to ensure that the funds are available for them when they want them. In addition, in this case, it could be argued that the care home had a duty of care in relation to the security of the home.

Mental Capacity Act 2005

The Mental Capacity Act 2005 established a new Court of Protection whose jurisdiction covers both personal welfare and property and affairs for those over 16. The Court has the power to make orders in respect of those under 16 if there is reasonable belief that their incapacity will continue beyond 16. The Court can make declarations and/or it can appoint a deputy to make decisions on behalf of those lacking mental capacity. In addition, a person, over 18, when mentally competent can draw up a lasting power of attorney (LPA) which gives the power to make decisions to another person over 18 on both personal welfare and property and affairs. The LPA must be registered with the Office of Public Guardian. The LPA over personal welfare can only take effect when the donor loses the requisite mental capacity. Where small amounts of money are involved the present system whereby appointees can collect Department for Work and Pensions moneys on behalf of those incapacitated continues.

Day-to-day care of money

Practical Dilemma 24.5 Shopping

At the heart of the philosophy of community care of those with learning disabilities or severe mental health problems is the principle of autonomy. Clients are encouraged to shop and take part in community activities and realise as much of their potential as possible. In these circumstances, moneys might be entrusted to staff to guide clients in making small purchases. On one such shopping expedition, Gary White, the team leader at a community home for those with learning disabilities, took three residents to the shops. Two were able to manage their own purchases, but the third, Leonard, needed some guidance and Gary aided him in purchasing several small items – toiletries, sweets, etc. On their return, Leonard complained to another resident that Gary had spent all his money. This came to the attention of the home manager who asked Gary for an immediate explanation. Gary showed how the money had been spent, but was unable to produce any receipts or supporting evidence. Neither was he able to remember exactly where the money had gone.

In a situation like this, the member of staff is like a trustee for the resident's property and should be able to account for it in detail with supporting receipts. Of course, the receipts do not in themselves show that the money was spent on the patient but, together with evidence from other witnesses, it should be possible to record exactly how the money was spent and that it was spent in the interests of the resident. In a case like this, the home manager would discipline Gary for his failure to follow the correct procedure.

In the community, many residents may have considerable sums to spend and the staff are therefore vulnerable to an accusation that they have spent the money on themselves. Under the Health and Social Care Act 2008 the Care Quality Commission (CQC) is responsible for the regulatory system for care homes (see chapter 22) which require that there should be accurate records kept of residents' property. It is essential that staff be trained in good practices of book-keeping and that there should be, as far as possible, witnesses to give evidence as to how the money has been spent. The ultimate aim is, of course, that the resident should be the watchdog for his own funds, but many residents/clients may never get beyond the stage of entrusting all such matters to others. As the registration authority and the inspector of care homes, the Care Quality Commission is responsible for ensuring that regulations relating to patients'/clients' property are observed.

It was reported in December 2013 that the Royal Mencap Society had paid out more that £60,000 to five severely disabled clients at one home after carers spent their money on hundreds of unauthorised purchases.[1] These included the purchase of a karaoke machine for a resident who could not speak. The sister of one resident set up a company Finacare to safeguard the finances of at-risk adults and her brother was threatened with the loss of his place in the home. Mencap subsequently retracted the threat. Mencap stated that it was confident that it had appropriate financial procedures in place across its 128 registered care homes to prevent financial abuse. The CQC had carried out eight inspections in the home since 2010 and none of them apart from the most recent one raised financial abuse. The CQC said that it had the power to check financial processes but could not carry out restrospective investigations on financial abuse.[2]

Local Authority and Duties in Relation to Financial Abuse and Care of Property

Under section 42 of the Care Act 2014 the local authority has a duty to make whatever enquiries it thinks necessary to enable it to decide whether any action should be taken in the adult's case where (among other situations) an adult is experiencing, or is at risk of, abuse or neglect.

'Abuse' includes financial abuse; and for that purpose 'financial abuse' includes:

(a) having money or other property stolen,

(b) being defrauded,

(c) being put under pressure in relation to money or other property, and

(d) having money or other property misused.

Under section 47 of the Care Act 2014 the local authority has a duty to protect the property of adults being cared for away from home. The section is shown in Statute Box 24.2.

> ## Statute 24.2
> ### Care of Property under Section 47 Care Act 2014
>
> 1. This section applies where
>   (a) an adult is having needs for care and support met under section 18 or 19 in a way that involves the provision of accommodation, or is admitted to hospital (or both), and
>   (b) it appears to a local authority that there is a danger of loss or damage to movable property of the adult's in the authority's area because—
>   (i) the adult is unable (whether permanently or temporarily) to protect or deal with the property, and
>   (ii) no suitable arrangements have been or are being made.
> 2. the local authority must take reasonable steps to prevent or mitigate the loss or damage.
> 3. For the purpose of performing that duty, the local authority—
>   (a) may at all reasonable times and on reasonable notice enter any premises which the adult was living in immediately before being provided with accommodation or admitted to hospital, and
>   (b) may deal with any of the adult's movable property in any way which is reasonably necessary for preventing or mitigating loss or damage.
> 4. A local authority may not exercise the power under subsection (3)(a) unless—
>   (a) it has obtained the consent of the adult concerned or, where the adult lacks capacity to give consent, the consent of a person authorised under the Mental Capacity Act 2005 to give it on the adult's behalf, or
>   (b) where the adult lacks capacity to give consent and there is no person so authorised, the local authority is satisfied that exercising the power would be in the adult's best interests.
> 5. Where a local authority is proposing to exercise the power under subsection (3)(a), the officer it authorises to do so must, if required, produce valid documentation setting out the authorisation to do so.
> 6. A person who, without reasonable excuse, obstructs the exercise of the power under subsection (3)(a)—
>   (a) commits an offence, and
>   (b) is liable on summary conviction to a fine not exceeding level 4 on the standard scale.
> 7. A local authority may recover from an adult whatever reasonable expenses the authority incurs under this section in the adult's case.

Power of attorney

Patients who have the necessary mental capacity can grant a power of attorney. Under the Powers of Attorney Act 1971 this power was revoked (i.e. withdrawn) if the person granting it became mentally incapable. However, since this is often the very occasion when it would be useful to exercise the power on behalf of the patient, an Enduring Power of Attorney Act 1985 was passed, which came into effect in 1986. The enduring power of attorney came into existence only if the person wished the power to continue after the time at which he became incapable; he or she had to sign to this effect and indicate that they were aware of the significance of the enduring element. From 1 October 2007 it is no longer possible to create an enduring power of attorney. Instead, as the result of the Mental Capacity Act 2005, a lasting power of attorney can be set up. Different forms are completed and registered for an LPA covering personal welfare and one covering property and affairs. Existing enduring powers of attorney continue to be valid, and if the donor still retains the requisite mental capacity could be replaced by an LPA. Box 24.2 sets out some of the requirements for and the characteristics of an LPA.

Box 24.2 Lasting powers of attorney

1. Lasting powers of attorney can be set up in respect of personal welfare and property and affairs. The LPA in respect of personal welfare only comes into force when the donor lacks the requisite mental capacity. The LPA in respect of property and affairs can come into effect even though the donor still has the requisite mental capacity.
2. The LPA must be in the exact form prescribed in the Regulations.[3]
3. The LPA may give: a general power – which authorises the attorney to carry out any transactions or make personal welfare decisions on behalf of the donor, or a specific power – which authorises the attorney to deal only with those aspects of the donor's affairs that are specified in the power or make specific personal welfare decisions.
4. The donor can revoke or cancel the lasting power at any time while she/he remains mentally capable, but the power cannot be cancelled or revoked once it has been registered, unless the Office of Public Guardian confirms the revocation.
5. When the donor becomes mentally incapable, the attorney must notify the Office of Public Guardian.
6. Once registered, the attorney has the power to act on behalf of the donor – either general or specific.

Court of Protection

In October 2007 a new Court of Protection was established under the Mental Capacity Act 2005.[4] The Court has considerable jurisdiction in relation to both personal welfare and property and affairs of those who lack the requisite mental capacity. It can also determine whether capacity is lacking. Ordinary hearings take place in private but an application can be made for the hearing to be held in public on specified conditions.[5] The Court of Protection is consulting on allowing the public to sit in on hearings and is seeking greater openness while at the same time protecting the anonymity of those needing its protection.

Where there is no enduring or lasting power of attorney in existence and the person is incapable of managing his affairs, an application can be made to the Court of Protection for the appointment of a deputy to manage the affairs. There is a short procedure that can be used where the assets are small. A relative, or perhaps an NHS organisation or social services organisation, could apply for a deputy to be appointed to manage the patient's affairs and to allow money to be spent on the patient. The powers of the Court of Protection are considerable. The applicant will have to pay in to the court a sum of money as a *recognisance*. Notice of the application is given to the patient, who has the opportunity of opposing it. Medical evidence will also be required to show that the patient lacks the requisite mental capacity (as defined in the Mental Capacity Act sections 2 and 3 (see chapter 7)) to be capable of handling his affairs. This medical evidence can be challenged by the patient. The Court of Protection has the power of making a will in the name of the incompetent person and can arrange for sums to be paid to other persons who would have been dependent on the patient or would have looked to him for help, even though these obligations would not have been legally enforceable. Obviously, there is a power to pay all debts. The powers given to the Court of Protection under Part 7 of the Mental Health Act 1983 have been replaced by those given under the Mental Capacity Act 2005. In Scotland the Adults with Incapacity (Scotland) Act 2000 has been in force since 2001. Further information can be obtained from the Office of Public Guardian website.[6]

Protecting patients from relatives

Practical Dilemma 24.6 Grasping relatives

Mary Bennet was visited regularly by her daughter, Jean, and each week the ward manager noticed that Jean brought the pension book in for her mother to sign. However, it was noticeable that Mary never seemed to have any money for purchases from the ward trolley and if the ward had not supplied her with squash, tissues and soap, she would not have had any of those items. Janice, the ward manager, mentioned it to Jean, who flushed a little and said that she did not have anything to do with her mother's money and by the time she had personally paid for the bus fare to the hospital, she did not have any funds for such purchases and, anyway, the hospital provided that, did they not?

Many nurses would recognise this type of situation and the dilemma that arises for them is this: to what extent is the nurse a protector of the patient, even when she has to protect the patient from his own relatives? In one sense, this type of situation will not continue for very long since certain benefits are reduced and ultimately end after several weeks. However, the same issue can arise in other circumstances, for example, the signing of wills (considered in chapter 28). In the above situation, there is little that the ward sister can do. In any event, she cannot be sure that the money is not being used to meet Mary's bills at home and the sum is, of course, far too small to consider taking out a Court of Protection order. However, the fact that the relatives are aware of her concern might be of some small influence.[7] The Department for Work and Pensions (DWP)[8] can appoint someone (an appointee) to claim and spend benefits on a person's behalf if that person lacks the requisite mental capacity.[9] The DWP has a responsibility to visit the claimant and see if an appointee is needed and to supervise the situation. Any concerns about misappropriation could be reported to the DWP.

(The law relating to the care of a patient's property on the death of a patient and the making of wills is considered in chapter 28.)

Returning the patient's property

Practical Dilemma 24.7 Weekend property problems

It was the accepted practice at Roger Park General Hospital for the money on any patients who were admitted in an emergency to be retained by the general office for safekeeping during their stay. On discharge, they were then able to obtain a cheque representing that amount of money from the general office. Most patients, except those with no bank accounts, accepted the system. Problems, however, arose at weekends when no general office staff were on duty or when discharge was sudden and the cheques could not be made available in time. On such occasions, patients complained that the actual cash that was taken from them was not returned and, since not all banks were open on Saturday, they could not change the cheques and some had no cash with which to return home. What is the legal position?

The legal position depends to a certain extent on the circumstances of the money being taken by the NHS trust. If the patient is fully conscious when the money is handed over, he should be told that he will be given a cheque for this amount on discharge. If he refuses to agree to this, then it is open to him to ask relatives to look after his money or to take the risk of keeping that sum on his person. If, however, the money has been taken from the unconscious patient after an emergency admission, then there is no chance of the terms of the bailment being agreed with him. In such circumstances, the hospital holds the money as part of its duty of care to look after the patient. It could be argued that this duty requires the hospital to return to the patient exactly the same coins and notes that were taken from him. Alternatively, it could be said that the hospital carries out its duty of care by giving the patient the equivalent of what was taken in the form of a cheque. Unfortunately, there is no decided case to clarify the position in law. As far as administrative practice is concerned, possibly the best solution is to discuss with the patient as soon as he is conscious and capable of handling his affairs what the patient would prefer and, if the patient is unhappy at receiving a cheque for the entire amount, to consider the possibility of providing part in cash for immediate needs. Where the discharge is contemplated for a weekend, then either the cheque should be prepared in advance or there should be an emergency scheme to provide the patient with a cash advance. Where the patient has no bank account, the hospital should be able to make special arrangements either for the cheque to be cleared at a local branch or for the cash to be made available.

Staff property

Practical Dilemma 24.8 Lost handbag

Ben Jarvis, a staff nurse, was going straight from work to a travel company to pay for his holiday to Greece. He was holidaying with a friend and had £500 in cash to pay for both of them. The money was contained in a wallet inside his rucksack. At the hospital, all nursing staff were provided with a locker in a staffroom in their ward or department. The lockers were fitted with a padlock and key. Ben locked his locker and carried the key around for the whole shift. Several people knew that he was going to the travel agent after work. At the end of the shift, when he went to his locker, he found that it had been broken into: the small padlock had been forced open and the money was missing from the wallet. The police were summoned, but despite intensive questioning and a search the money was never recovered or the thief discovered. Ben feels that the NHS trust should pay for the missing money since, he argued, the padlock was inadequate and a far tougher system should have been provided for taking care of staff property. Is he right in law?

Unfortunately for Ben, it is highly unlikely that he would win in a court action against the NHS trust. The NHS trust is not the bailee of Ben's cash; he has not transferred it for its safekeeping. He has, so to speak, brought the property into the hospital at his own risk. If, of course, he had gone to the general office and said, 'Please take care of this for me since I have to go to the travel agent straight after work', and it had done so, the situation would have been very different. In that case, the NHS trust would have become a bailee of his money and would be accountable to him for its return. What about the argument that the locker should have been stronger? The locker should be as strong as is compatible with the value of property that is reasonable to be kept in there. There must be few who would think that attempting to keep £500 is reasonable. Anyone who brings valuable goods to work and keeps them there cannot expect the NHS trust to be held responsible for their loss, unless, of course, it is a requirement of the job that such items are brought to work, or unless the employer has assumed responsibility for the property. The employer can, through the contract of employment, take on a wider responsibility for the property of employees, although this would be unusual. The courts are unlikely to imply a term that the employer has a duty to take care of the property of the employee. There would have to be an explicit undertaking to that effect.

Practical Dilemma 24.9 Staff car park

Jean Jones, a staff nurse in the outpatients department, parked her car in the hospital car park, paying the daily fee of £3.00. When she came back, she found that her car had been broken into and the radio/DVD player taken. A pathology laboratory technician whose office overlooked the car park came up to her as she was looking at the damage and said that he had seen the whole incident. He had seen two youths break into the car who were then chased by the car park attendant. When car park charges were introduced, staff had been assured that there would be better protection for their cars. Could Jean Jones hold the security firm or the NHS trust responsible for the damage?

There are two possible causes of action: one against the security firm and the other against the trust. If it were the responsibility of the security firm to protect the vehicles in the car park on a 24-hour basis, then they have failed to fulfil that responsibility. There may be a contractual right against them by the NHS trust, but it depends on the terms of the contract. Although the trust has a right of action in contract, Jean Jones does not have a right of action, unless she can make use of the Contracts (Rights of Third Parties) Act 1999, which enables a person not a party to the contract to sue for benefits under it. In addition, it may be argued that the security firm owed a duty of care in the law of negligence to each employee or user of the car park. This might be difficult to establish. Any liability of the trust depends on Jean's being able to establish that it owed Jean a duty of care in respect of her car and had not excluded any liability by an exemption notice. This would depend on the actual facts. The likelihood is that Jean will be unable to obtain compensation from either the security firm or her employers and will be dependent on any insurance cover she has for theft.

Gifts

It is extremely important that NMC guidance and local policies relating to gifts from patients/clients are closely followed to prevent any accusations of theft or bribery. The NMC in its Code (2015)[10] under the heading 'Promote professionalism and trust', states:

> **refuse all but the most trivial gifts, favours or hospitality as accepting them could be interpreted as an attempt to gain preferential treatment.**

As a consequence of their ability to prescribe, nurses may be offered inducements by medicine companies. Therefore in its Practice Standard 21 on gifts and benefits in its Guidance on nurse prescribing[11] the NMC states:

> 21.1 You must make your choice of medicinal product for the patient/client, based on clinical suitability and cost effectiveness
> 21.2 You must maintain a 'register of interests' within your own personal portfolio, which may be produced on request if required for audit purposes
> 21.3 You should adhere to local corporate policy when maintaining a 'register of interests'.

The NMC points out that:

> **Personal gifts are prohibited and it is an offence to solicit or accept a gift or inducement. Companies may offer hospitality for a professional/scientific meeting, but such hospitality must be reasonable in level, and subordinate to, the main purpose of the meeting.**

If a grateful patient wishes to express thanks in some tangible way it is preferable to refer the patient to the manager to ensure that the patient is appropriately represented and that any element of undue influence can be prevented. This may be significant where the patient makes a gift to the hospital in a will (see chapter 28). Even where smaller gifts such as boxes of chocolates are made, the line manager should be notified about the gift. In July 2014 a nurse who used donations to buy drinks for patients and pay for staff parties was cleared of misconduct by the NMC after she admitted accepting money from four patients' families and failing to record them. Her employers demoted her and gave her a warning. She was acquitted at Edinburgh Sheriff Court, where it was held that although she broke hospital accounting rules, she was not dishonest.[12]

In determining whether a gift has been made and no theft has taken place, the court would consider the mental capacity of the owner of the property. For example, the House of Lords held in the case of *R v Hinks*[13] that the main carer of a man with limited intelligence who gave her about £60,000 in small amounts over a six-month period had in fact stolen the money. She was convicted of theft, the jury considering her to have dishonestly appropriated the money, applying the test of the standards of reasonable and honest people. The House of Lords upheld the conviction.

Conclusions

The Mental Capacity Act 2005, in establishing a new Court of Protection, an Office of Public Guardian and the concept of the lasting power of attorney is having a major impact on the property and affairs of those lacking the requisite mental capacity to make decisions. A Code of Practice[14] has been prepared to assist those responsible for the property of others, and help and information on the Mental Capacity Act is available from the Ministry of Justice.[15] Local policies should be in place relating to the protection of patient property, exclusion of liability and receipt of gifts.

Reflection questions

1. Consider the liability of the NHS trust, if any, for the loss of a patient's pyjamas. It appears that they were removed when the patient was given a bath and probably placed with the sheets in the laundry bag. The laundry has denied any knowledge of them.
2. Examine the procedure followed in relation to property when patients are admitted to hospital.
3. You are working at a psychiatric hospital and one of the patients drags a nail along the side of your new car. Is the NHS trust responsible? Would it make any difference if there were a notice by the car park exempting the NHS trust from loss or damage to staff cars parked there?
4. The Court of Protection has been appointed to manage the property of one of the patients on your ward. What powers does it have and who will administer the property?

Further exercises

1. How many disclaimer notices or exclusion notices do you see around the hospital? Consider the extent to which reliance on each notice would be reasonable to exclude liability for damage or loss of property caused by the negligence of the NHS trust or its staff.
2. The relative of a patient in your medical wards asks you if you would witness a power of attorney so that the relative can manage the patient's affairs on his behalf. You know that the patient is mentally disordered but is reputed to be quite wealthy. What advice would you give to the relative?

References

1. Alexi Mostrous, Care staff 'financially abused' the vunerable, *The Times*, 23 December 2013
2. Alexi Mostrous, Staff at care home 'too scared to tell of financial deceit', *The Times*, 24 December 2013
3. The Lasting Powers of Attorney, Enduring Powers of Attorney and Public Guardian Regulations 2007, SI 2007/1253
4. Ministry of Justice; www.gov.uk
5. *Independent News and Media Ltd and Others* v *A*, The Times Law Report, 17 November 2009; [2009] EWHC 2858
6. www.publicguardian.gov.uk
7. B. Dimond, *Legal Aspects of Mental Capacity*, Blackwell Scientific Publishing, Oxford, 2007
8. www.dwp.gov.uk
9. www.gov.uk/become-appointee-for-someone-claiming-benefits
10. Nursing and Midwifery Council, The Code: Professional standards of practice and behaviour for nurses and midwives, NMC, London, 2015
11. Nursing and Midwifery Council, Standards for prescribing, NMC, London, 2006
12. News item, *The Times*, 14 July 2014
13. *R* v *Hinks* [2001] 2 AC 241
14. Code of Practice, Mental Capacity Act 2005, Department for Constitutional Affairs, February 2007, paragraph 7.21
15. Ministry of Justice; www.gov.uk

Chapter 25
Legal Aspects of Public Health

This chapter discusses

- Public health legislation
- Notifiable diseases
- Cross-infection control
- Health and Social Care Act 2008
- Health Protection Agency (now Public Health England)
- Public Health England
- Tuberculosis (TB)
- Hepatitis
- HIV-infected persons and AIDS patients
- Vaccination
- Blood donors
- Confidentiality

Introduction

Significant changes have taken place in the management of public health., for example the establishment of Public Health England (now referred to as the UK Health Security Agency (UKHSA) and transfer of responsibility from health service organisations to local authorities. The challenge of hospital acquired infections, though still present, is slowly coming under control and the legal issues relating to AIDs and HIV no longer hold such a prominent position in public health management. The worldwide threat from diseases such as Ebola and Covid-19 and the concern about antibiotic-resistant diseases means that public health law will have a prominent place in health professional practice.

Public health legislation

Our public health legislation has developed piecemeal from the Public Health (Control of Diseases) Act 1984 and subsequent legislation. Notification provisions revised in 2010 require information to be given about specified infectious diseases and considerable powers are given to Justices of the Peace to protect public health. In 2005 the Law Commission[1] recommended that significant changes should be made to the 1984 Act to strengthen the response to infectious diseases and contamination by chemicals and radiation. These recommendations have been enacted in the Health and Social Care Act 2008 together with three sets of regulations (2010/657, 2010/658 and 2010/659). Information on diseases which must be notified is available on the Health Protection Agency (HPA) website;[2] the HPA is now absorbed into Public Health England. The Health Protection (Notification) Regulations 2010 (SI 2010/659) can be accessed on the legislation website[3] and are shown together with the other two sets of regulations in Statute Boxes 25.1, 25.2 and 25.3.

Statute 25.1
Local authority powers (SI 2010/657)

The requirement to keep a child away from school
The requirement to provide details of children attending school
Disinfection or decontamination of things:

- on the request of the owner
- on the request of person with custody or control
- on premises on request of tenant

Requests for cooperation for health protection purposes
Restriction of contact with dead bodies
Restriction of access to dead bodies
Relocation of dead bodies

Statute 25.2
Part 2A Orders (i.e. Application to Justice of the Peace) (SI 2010/658)

Duty of local authorities to give notice of Part 2A applications
Evidence required for a Part 2A application
Period for which Part 2A order in relation to persons may be in force
Affected persons in relation to Part 2A orders in relation to persons and dead bodies or human remains
Discretionary power for local authorities to charge in connection with Part 2A order in relation to things and premises

> Duty on local authorities to provide information in relation to Part 2A order in relation to persons
> Duty on local authorities to have regard to welfare following a Part 2A order in relation to persons
> Duty on local authorities to report Part 2A applications to the Health Protection Agency
> Duty on local authorities to report variations or revocations of Part 2A orders to the Health Protection Agency (now Public Health England)

Statute 25.3
Notification provisions (SI 2010/659)

Promoting individual well-being

> Duty to notify suspected disease, infection or contamination in patients
> Duty to notify suspected disease, infection or contamination in dead persons
> Duty of notify causative agents found in human samples
> Duty to provide information to the Health Protection Agency (now Public Health England)
> Duty on the relevant local authority to disclose notification to others.
>
> Schedule 1 lists the notifiable diseases and Schedule 2 the causative agents.

The Health Protection Agency was abolished by the Health and Social Care Act 2012 and its functions have been transferred to the Secretary of State and Public Health England – an executive agency of the Department of Health – which came into being in April 2013.

The role of Healthwatch England and the local healthwatch is considered in chapter 26.

Powers of the Justice of the Peace

The Justice of the Peace (JP) has considerable powers in relation to the protection of public health. The powers were set out in Public Health (Control of Disease) Act 1984 which has been substantially amended by the Health and Social Care Act 2008 by the insertion of a new Part 2A to the 1984 Act. The powers of the JP to order health measures in relation to persons are set out in s. 45G; to order health measures in relation to things in s. 45H; to order health measures in relation to premises in s. 45I; and to make these orders in relation to groups of people, things or premises in s. 45J.

Under s. 18 of the 2012 Health and Social Care Act, regulations may require a local authority to exercise any of the public health functions of the Secretary of State (so far as relating to the health of the public in the authority's area) by taking such steps as may be prescribed.

Notifiable diseases

Diseases that are notifiable are shown in Statute Box 25.4.

Statute 25.4
Notifiable diseases

Schedule 1 of the 2010 Regulations:

acute encephalitis, acute meningitis, acute poliomyelitis, acute infectious hepatitis, anthrax, botulism, brucellosis, cholera, covid-19, diphtheria, enteric fever (typhoid or paratyphoid fever), food poisoning, haemolytic uraemic syndrome (HUS), infectious bloody diarrhoea, invasive group A streptococcal disease and scarlet fever, legionnaire's disease, leprosy, malaria, measles, meningococcal septicaemia, mumps, plague, rabies, rubella, SARS, smallpox, tetanus, tuberculosis, typhus, viral haemorrhagic fever (VHF), whooping cough, yellow fever.

Schedule 2 Causative Agents:

Bacillus anthracis, Bacillus cereus (only if associated with food poisoning), *Bordetella pertussis, Borrelia* spp., *Brucella* spp., *Burkholderia mallei, Burkholderia pseudomallei, Campylobacter* spp., Chikungunya virus, *Chlamydophila psittaci, Clostridium botulinum, Clostridium perfringens* (only if associated with food poisoning), *Clostridium tetani, Corynebacterium diphtheriae, Corynebacterium ulcerans, Coxiella burnetii,* Crimean–Congo haemorrhagic fever virus, *Cryptosporidium* spp., dengue virus, Ebola virus, *Entamoeba histolytica, Francisella tularensis, Giardia lamblia,* Guanarito virus *Haemophilus influenzae* (invasive), hantavirus hepatitis A, B, C, delta and E viruses, influenza virus, Junin virus, Kyasanur Forest disease virus, Lassa virus, *Legionella* spp., *Leptospira interrogans, Listeria monocytogenes,* Machupo virus, Marburg virus, measles virus, mumps virus, *Mycobacterium tuberculosis* complex, *Neisseria meningitidis,* Omsk haemorrhagic fever virus, *Plasmodium falciparum, p. vivax, p. ovale, p. malariae, p. knowlesi,* polio virus (wild or vaccine types), rabies virus (classical rabies and rabies-related lyssaviruses), *Rickettsia* spp., Rift Valley fever virus, rubella virus, Sabia virus, *Salmonella* spp., SARS coronavirus, *Shigella* spp., *Streptococcus pneumoniae* (invasive), *Streptococcus pyogenes* (invasive), varicella zoster virus, variola virus, verocytotoxigenic *Escherichia coli* (including *E. coli* O157), *Vibrio cholerae,* West Nile virus, yellow fever virus, *Yersinia pestis.*

Schedule 1 covers those notifiable diseases that come under the notification procedure set out in Regulation 2 (see Statute Box 25.5). Schedule 2 covers those diseases which must be reported by diagnostic laboratories to the Health Protection Authority under Regulation 4 of the Health Protection (Notification) Regulations 2010.[4]

Procedure for Notification

Under section 11 of the 1984 Act, a registered medical practitioner has a duty to notify the proper office of the local authority if he becomes aware, or suspects, that a patient whom he is attending within the district of a local authority is suffering from a notifiable disease or from food poisoning. The duty does not apply if he believes, and has reasonable grounds for believing, that some other registered medical practitioner has complied with the duty. See Statute Box 25.5.

Statute 25.5

Notification procedure (Regulations 2010/659, Regulation 2)

2(1) A registered medical practitioner (R) must notify the proper officer of the relevant local authority where R has reasonable grounds for suspecting that a patient (P) whom R is attending—

(a) has a notifiable disease;

(b) has an infection which, in the view of R, presents or could present significant harm to human health; or

(c) is contaminated in a manner which, in the view of R, presents or could present significant harm to human health.

What Information must be Notified?

Statute Box 25.6 shows the information that must be notified.[5]

Statute 25.6

Notification Regulations 2010

Information that must be notified

Regulation 2(2) The notification must include the following information insofar as it is known to R—

(a) P's name, date of birth and sex;
(b) P's home address including postcode;
(c) P's current residence (if not home address);
(d) P's telephone number;
(e) P's NHS number;
(f) P's occupation (if R considers it relevant);
(g) the name, address and postcode of P's place of work or education (if R considers it relevant);
(h) P's relevant overseas travel history;
(i) P's ethnicity;
(j) contact details for a parent of P (where P is a child);
(k) the disease or infection which P has or is suspected of having or the nature of P's contamination or suspected contamination;
(l) the date of onset of P's symptoms;
(m) the date of R's diagnosis; and
(n) R's name, address and telephone number.

> (3) The notification must be provided in writing within 3 days beginning with the day on which R forms a suspicion under paragraph (1).
>
> (4) Without prejudice to paragraph (3), if R considers that the case is urgent, notification must be provided orally as soon as reasonably practicable.
>
> (5) In determining whether the case is urgent, R must have regard to—
>   (a) the nature of the suspected disease, infection or contamination;
>   (b) the ease of spread of that disease, infection or contamination;
>   (c) the ways in which the spread of the disease, infection or contamination can be prevented or controlled;
>   (d) P's circumstances (including age, sex and occupation).
>
> (NB: Public Health (Control of Disease) Act 1984 section 11(4) imposes a criminal sanction on a person who fails to comply with an obligation imposed on him under the provisions set out above.)

Regulation 3 extends the obligation set out in Statute Box 25.6 to cover notification of a suspected disease, infection or contamination in a dead body.

Cross-infection control

The last two decades have seen major concerns about the level of hospital-acquired infection (HAI). A report by the National Audit Office (NAO)[6] in 2000 raised concerns about the level of HAI suggesting that HAI could be the main or a contributory cause in 20,000 or 4 per cent of deaths a year in the UK and that there are at least about 100,000 cases of HAI with an estimated cost to the NHS of £1 billion. The NAO made recommendations on the strategic management of HAI.

The government responded to this report by announcing a multi-pronged initiative to tackle HAI. Among the initiatives planned were an antimicrobial strategy, including a clampdown on inappropriate antibiotic use and better infection control measures.[7] The Audit Commission and Commission for Health Improvement (now the Care Quality Commission) were to assume the responsibility of independent inspection of wards and had the right to seek information on HAI and to publish it.[8] Numerous initiatives have followed since then, with the emphasis on different types of infections changing. The Secretary of State for Health admitted in 2001 that methicillin-resistant Staphylococcus aureus (MRSA) was endemic in England's hospitals.[9] The role of 'Matron' was reintroduced with responsibilities for hygiene and standards of cleanliness. The NMC provided advice to registrants on infection control.[10] The RCN has also provided guidance on good practice in infection prevention and control.[11]

Clostridium difficile (*C. difficile*) was described by the HPA in 2007 as the most important cause of hospital-acquired diarrhoea. Further information, including the findings and recommendations from a review of epidemiology by the Directors of Infection Prevention and Control in England,[12] can be found on the HPA website[13] and the DH website.[14] In 2007 one of the first acts of the then new Secretary of State, Alan Johnson, was to give £50 million to tackle MRSA and *C. difficile* by doubling the size of the DH's infection improvement team who advise NHS trusts on developing plans to cut infections. In July 2007 the Healthcare Commission published a national study into healthcare-associated infection. To reduce the risk of infections the report recommended that trusts should develop a culture of safety, have a good system of corporate and clinical governance, review performance, manage risk and communicate with patients and the public. A report by the Healthcare Commission in October 2007 into Maidstone and Tunbridge Wells Trust revealed that up to 90 patients had died between 2004 and 2006 after being infected with *C. difficile*. The Minister of Health responded by announcing plans for a new super-regulator to be established in April 2009, i.e. the Care Quality Commission, combining the Healthcare Commission, Mental Health Act Commission and the Commission for Social Care Inspection, with powers to close NHS and private hospitals and residential care homes. The new powers under the Corporate Manslaughter and Corporate Homicide Act may be used against NHS trusts which fail to control HAI. It was reported on 17 January 2007 that Lesley Ash, an actress, received a £5 million settlement after she caught MRSA at the Chelsea and Westminster Hospital. It caused her devastating disabilities and meant that she would never again be able to play an active role as an actress.

The Chief Medical Officer in December 2013 issued an international blueprint to fight antibiotic resistance which included a proposal to use vaccinations against common bacteria and hospital superbugs.[15] In July 2014 the Prime Minister urged global action to find new antibiotics and he appointed an economist to lead the challenge to encourage pharmaceutical companies to undertake more research.

Further information on the levels of infection and the most common infections can be found on website of Public Health England and the Cochrane Library website.[16]

Practical Dilemma 25.1   Cross-infection nurse

Joan was appointed as the hospital infection control nurse. Immediately on starting her new post, she undertook an audit of existing practices on infection control. She found that basic standards, including handwashing, were extremely lax, particularly among junior doctors. However, her attempts to raise standards appeared to be thwarted. What is the legal situation?

When Joan was appointed, she should have been notified of the organisational support that would be given to her post. This would include such details as to whom she reported, who was her immediate line manager, the resources available to her and the strategy of the organisation in setting down and complying with the standards issued by the government. There should be in place a committee for infection control. She would need to prepare a report on her findings, giving her conclusions in a clear, unemotional report with constructive recommendations on the action that could be taken. If there is no follow-up action from her report, then she may have justification in following the procedures set up under the Public Interest Disclosure Act 1998 (see chapter 4) to ensure that action is taken.

In 2014 the Ebola outbreak in West Africa was declared an international emergency as over 1000 people had died from the disease. Ethical and legal issues were raised in the discussion over whether to give untested drugs to sufferers. The World Health Organization (WHO) panel ruled that the severity of the outbreak meant that it was ethically acceptable to give the drugs to patients. Informed consent by the patient was essential.[17] Fortunately early indications suggested that the untested drug was effective.

Health and Social Care Act 2008

Provision was made in the Health and Social Care Act 2008 to strengthen measures to protect the public health from infection and contamination. Under section 20 the Secretary of State is given power to make regulations in respect of regulated activities which include:

> the prevention and control of health care associated infections and may include such provision as the Secretary of State considers appropriate for the purpose of safeguarding individuals (whether receiving health or social care or otherwise) from the risk, or any increased risk, of being exposed to health care associated infections or of being made susceptible, or more susceptible, to them (s. 20(5)).

Under section 21(1) the Secretary of State may issue a code of practice about compliance with any requirements of regulations under section 20 which relate to the prevention or control of healthcare-associated infections.

Under section 21(3) the Secretary of State must keep the code under review and may from time to time—

(a) revise the whole or any part of the code, and
(b) issue a revised code.

Prior to the issue of the code the Secretary of State is obliged to consult with such persons as he considers appropriate. The code of practice is to be taken into account by the Care Quality Commission in making decisions under the Act and it is admissible in evidence in civil and criminal proceedings, but a failure to observe any provision of a code of practice under section 21 does not of itself make a person liable to any criminal or civil proceedings (s. 25(3)).

The Health and Social Care Act 2008 section 129 also inserted a new Part 2A into the Public Health (Control of Disease) Act 1984 which gives greater powers to make regulations controlling contamination and the spread of disease. For example, a new section 45C to the Public Health (Control of Diseases) Act 1984 covers domestic health protection regulations and is shown in Statute Box 25.7.

Statute 25.7

Domestic health protection regulations – Section 45C of 1984 Act (Inserted by Health and Social Care Act 2008)

1. The appropriate Minister may by regulations make provision for the purpose of preventing, protecting against, controlling or providing a public health response to the incidence or spread of infection or contamination in England and Wales (whether from risks originating there or elsewhere).
2. The power in subsection (1) may be exercised—
    (a) in relation to infection or contamination generally or in relation to particular forms of infection or contamination, and

> (b) so as to make provision of a general nature, to make contingent provision or to make specific provision in response to a particular set of circumstances.
>
> 3. Regulations under subsection (1) may in particular include provision—
>   (a) imposing duties on registered medical practitioners or other persons to record and notify cases or suspected cases of infection or contamination,
>   (b) conferring on local authorities or other persons functions in relation to the monitoring of public health risks, and
>   (c) imposing or enabling the imposition of restrictions or requirements on or in relation to persons, things or premises in the event of, or in response to, a threat to public health.
>
> 4. The restrictions or requirements mentioned in subsection (3)(c) include in particular—
>   (a) a requirement that a child is to be kept away from school,
>   (b) a prohibition or restriction relating to the holding of an event or gathering,
>   (c) a restriction or requirement relating to the handling, transport, burial or cremation of dead bodies or the handling, transport or disposal of human remains, and
>   (d) a special restriction or requirement.

The power to make the regulations shown in Statute Box 25.7 is subject to restrictions set out in s. 45D which requires that the restriction or requirement is proportionate to what is sought to be achieved by imposing it. Special restrictions or requirements cannot be imposed unless (a) the regulations are made in response to a serious and imminent threat to public health, or (b) imposition of the restriction or requirement is expressed to be contingent on there being such a threat at the time when it is imposed.

1. Under section 45G a Justice of the Peace may make an order under subsection 2 if satisfied that—
   (a) P is or may be infected or contaminated,
   (b) the infection or contamination is one which presents or could present significant harm to human health,
   (c) there is a risk that P might infect or contaminate others, and
   (d) it is necessary to make the order in order to remove or reduce that risk.

2. The order may impose on or in relation to P one or more of the following restrictions or requirements—
   (a) that P submit to medical examination;
   (b) that P be removed to a hospital or other suitable establishment;
   (c) that P be detained in a hospital or other suitable establishment;
   (d) that P be kept in isolation or quarantine;
   (e) that P be disinfected or decontaminated;
   (f) that P wear protective clothing;
   (g) that P provide information or answer questions about P's health or other circumstances;
   (h) that P's health be monitored and the results reported;
   (i) that P attend training or advice sessions on how to reduce the risk of infecting or contaminating others;
   (j) that P be subject to restrictions on where P goes or with whom P has contact;
   (k) that P abstain from working or trading.

3. A Justice of the Peace may make an order under subsection (4) in relation to a person ('P') if the justice is satisfied that—
   (a) P is or may be infected or contaminated,
   (b) the infection or contamination is one which presents or could present significant harm to human health,
   (c) there is a risk that a related party might infect or contaminate others, and
   (d) it is necessary to make the order in order to remove or reduce that risk.
4. The order may impose on or in relation to P a requirement that P provide information or answer questions about P's health or other circumstances (including, in particular, information or questions about the identity of a related party).

The World Health Organization warned in May 2013 that a virus similar to Sars, called coronavirus, has killed more than half of the people it has infected and is a threat to the entire world.[18] In its August 2018 update the WHO reported that Middle East respiratory syndrome coronavirus remained a worldwide public health threat. From 2012–18 there have been 2229 laboratory-confirmed cases resulting in some 791 deaths. However, thanks to improved infection prevention and control practices in hospitals the numbers of hospital acquired cases had dropped significantly since 2015.[19]

European Union and Patient Safety

In 2009 the Council of the European Union made recommendations on patient safety[20] which included recommendations relating to education and training of healthcare workers and national strategies, and long-term priorities for the control and prevention of healthcare-associated infections.

Health Protection Agency (now UK Health Security Agency)

In April 2003 the HPA was created to provide a coordinated approach to health protection and reduce the impact of infectious diseases, poisons, chemicals, biological and radiation hazards. It was set up in the light of the Chief Medical Officer of Health's report *Getting Ahead of the Curve*,[21] which recognised the need to bring together in one organisation the skills and expertise in a number of organisations to work in a more coordinated way, to reduce the burden and consequences of health protection threats or disease with the aim of providing a more comprehensive and effective response to threats to the public's health. The HPA brought together the following organisations into the one body:

- Public Health Laboratory Service (including the Communicable Disease Surveillance Centre and Central Public Health Laboratory);
- Centre for Applied Microbiology and Research;
- National Focus for Chemical Incidents;
- Regional service provider units that support the management of chemical incidents;
- National Poisons Information Service;
- NHS public health staff responsible for infectious disease control, emergency planning and other protection support; and
- National Radiological Protection Board (NRPB) (incorporated into the Health Protection Agency in April 2005).

The HPA was established as a special health authority under section 11 of the National Health Service Act 1977 but under the Health Protection Agency Act 2004 it became a non-departmental public body.

However, with a budget of £175 million a year, it had to be accountable and this was initially to the Department of Health and parliamentary monitoring.

The HPA was one of the quangos that was identified for closure, with its functions being reallocated to save costs. The review of arm's-length bodies recommended the abolition of the HPA and the National Treatment Agency (see chapter 27) as statutory organisations and the transfer of their functions to the Secretary of State as part of the new Public Health Service in 2012.[22]

Public Health England

As envisaged in the Public Health White Paper *Healthy Lives, Healthy People – our strategy for public health in England* (November 2010), the Health Protection Agency was abolished by the Health and Social Care Act 2012. Its functions were transferred to the Secretary of State and Public Health England – an executive agency of the Department of Health – and came into being in April 2013. At local level, local authorities now have responsibility for improving the health of their local populations and must employ a director of public health, and publish annual reports. LAs coordinate the work done by the NHS, social care, housing, environmental health, leisure and transport services. In 2021 Public Health England was dissolved and its functions taken over by the UK Health Security Agency. Public Health Scotland and Public Health Wales have similar responsibilities as the UKHSA. In Northern Ireland public health is coordinated by the Public Health Agency.

Care Quality Commission

In April 2013 Public Health England signed a memorandum of understanding with the Care Quality Commission. The Care Quality Commission (CQC) (formerly the Healthcare Commission) also has powers under the Health and Social Care (Community Health and Standards) Act 2003 section 53A (as added by the Health Act 2006 section 16) to issue improvement notices in respect of hygiene failings.

Tuberculosis (TB)

TB was once thought to have been eradicated. However, there is evidence that poor housing conditions, poverty and malnourishment are leading to an increase in TB levels, often particularly associated with the refugee population. Public Health England in cooperation with the DH is aiming to eliminate TB within England in accordance with the action plan published by the Chief Medical Officer of Health in 2004.[23] In May 2005 more than 700 patients who had been treated at the Lister Hospital Stevenage were sent letters urging them to be alert to TB symptoms after an unnamed health worker had been diagnosed with the disease.[24]

Public Health England report that cases of reported TB increased year-on-year until 2011 when some 8919 cases were reported. Since then there has been a drop in cases year-on-year, with the figure for 2016 standing at 6175.[25]

Hepatitis

The BMA called for all children in Britain to be immunised against hepatitis B since transmission rates were rising and it was 50 to 100 times more infectious than the AIDS virus.[26] In 2004 the Department of Health issued revised guidance on prevention and testing in children and HIV which also covers advice about hepatitis B and C.[27] The British HIV Association has published guidelines for the management of HIV infection in pregnant women.[28] Sharon Wilson describes the challenges for midwives in facing HIV-positive pregnant woman.[29]

Practical advice for midwives in suggesting tests for sexually transmitted infections in pregnancy is given by Julie Williams.[30] In January 2004 NICE approved new treatment for those suffering from hepatitis C. It suggested that the drug pegylated interferon should be prescribed on the NHS along with another drug, ribavirin.[31]

Hepatitis B vaccination is now routinely available for babies at 8, 12 and 16 weeks of age. It is also offered to those at increased risk of hepatitis B, with a full list available on the NHS Choices website.[32]

HIV-infected persons and AIDS patients

Significant progress has been made in the past 30 years in the treatment and prevention of AIDS and attitudes to those who are HIV-infected. A diagnosis of HIV-positive now means long-term antiretroviral drugs, but no automatic full-blown AIDS. In November 2013 it was reported that research was to commence on a potential cure for HIV[33] and in January 2014 the European Commission gave approval to a once a day pill to control HIV developed by GlaxoSmithKline.[34] Gone is the hysteria which once surrounded the condition, so that any healthcare worker who worked with exposure-prone procedures would lose their job if he or she was HIV-infected. The Department of Health lifted the ban on health workers with HIV performing surgery and dentistry, and self-testing kits for HIV were to be made legal from April 2014 and are available on the internet.[35]

Government Policy on Testing

In December 1998 the government launched a campaign to encourage all pregnant women to have an HIV test. The press release stated that only 30 per cent of women who are HIV-positive are aware that they are infected. If a pregnant woman is known to be HIV-positive, then the risk of passing on HIV to the fetus can be reduced by arranging for delivery to be by Caesarean section. Avoiding breastfeeding also removes the risk of passing on the virus through the milk. However, the law has not been changed and a test for HIV still requires the consent of the woman. The government set a national target to achieve an 80 per cent reduction by December 2002 in the number of children who acquire HIV from their mothers.[36] In their HIV/AIDS Services 2000/01 allocation and strategy, NHS organisations were instructed that part of the HIV-prevention budget was to be used to support antenatal services in recommending an HIV test to all pregnant women. A research project to estimate the cost-effectiveness of a universal, voluntary HIV screening programme suggested that it is effective and should be implemented in the London area, with other areas being considered for screening.[37] For further information on guidelines for the management of HIV infections in pregnant women see the article by Lyall[38] and guidance from the Department of Health.[39] The Expert Advisory Group on AIDS published guidelines which were updated in 2002 and are available on its website.[40] It points out that all women in England are now offered and recommended an HIV test as part of their antenatal care and it sets out the pre-test discussions which should take place. Named testing should only take place with the consent of the person.

A GP who carried out secret HIV tests on five patients he suspected were indulging in risky sex was given a serious reprimand by the GMC. One of the patients had found out about the test when he applied for a life insurance policy and he notified the GMC. The disciplinary committee of the GMC noted that the GP believed that he was acting in the patients' best interests, but concluded that 'such a benevolent, paternalistic attitude has no place in modern medicine'.[41]

In Case 25.1, an HIV-positive mother refused to allow her baby to be tested for HIV.

Case 25.1 Re C (HIV test) [1999]

Refusal of HIV test[42]

The local authority applied for a specific issue order that a baby born to an HIV-positive mother be tested for HIV. The mother was sceptical of the conventional treatment for HIV and AIDS, had refused medication during the pregnancy and intended to continue breastfeeding until the child was about 2 years old. The judge found that there was a 20–25 per cent chance that the baby was infected with HIV; the risk had been increased with the breastfeeding. The judge held that the views of the parents were important factors in the decision and any court invited to overrule parental wishes had to move extremely cautiously. He concluded that in the present circumstances the arguments for overruling the wishes of the parents and for testing the baby were overwhelming. The baby had rights of her own, recognised in national and international law; the baby's welfare was paramount and in the baby's interests the test should take place. The parents appealed, but did not attend court on the date their application was due to be heard, having disappeared from their home, taking the child with them. The Court of Appeal refused permission to appeal: the question whether the child should or should not be tested was a matter relating to the welfare of the child, not the rights of the parents, and it was clearly not in the child's best interests for either the parents or the health professionals to remain ignorant of her state of health.

The Royal College of Paediatrics and Child Health published an update report on reducing mother-to-child transmission of HIV infection in the UK in 2006.[43] It recommended the development of networks for sharing expertise and facilities, the improvement of case management, the evolution in the management of HIV disease (through the use of antiretroviral treatment, Caesarean section and avoidance of breastfeeding) and the long-term follow-up of infants exposed to antiretroviral drugs. Annex E of the Expert Advisory Group Report considers the special circumstances of pregnancy and the use of HIV post-exposure prophylaxis (PEP).[44] Guidelines on good practice for pupils living with HIV were published by the National Children's Bureau and the Children and Young People HIV Network[45] which give advice to schools on supporting children infected or affected by HIV. The guidance was updated in 2010 and is available on its website.[46]

The Aids Control Act 1987 was repealed by the Health and Social Care Act 2012. It required district health authorities to report matters set out in a schedule and other such relevant information as the Secretary of State may direct. The schedule included information on the number of people known to have AIDS and the timing of the diagnosis; the particulars of facilities and services provided by each authority; the numbers of people employed by the authority in providing such facilities and future provision over the next 12 months. A subsequent statutory instrument extended the information required to include HIV-positive persons.[47]

The HIV Testing Kits and Services Regulations[48] – which made it an offence to advertise HIV testing kits, services or components, or to sell or supply such kits without an accompanying warning note, and to provide HIV testing services which were not provided or directed by a registered medical practitioner – were repealed in 2014.[49]

Criminal Law and HIV/AIDS

In the first successful prosecution for sexually transmitting HIV in England, a man was convicted of inflicting 'biological' grievous bodily harm on two women and sentenced to four and a half years' imprisonment.[50] The Court of Appeal set out the basic provisions which apply to this criminal offence in the case of Konzani.[51] A man who had known for three years that he was HIV-positive was sentenced to nine years' imprisonment for having unprotected sex with a woman to whom he did not disclose his HIV status.[52] In September 2010 a man was jailed for one year for infecting a woman with HIV.[53]

Human Rights and HIV/AIDS

In a case brought against the Swedish government, an HIV patient argued that there had been a breach of his human rights under Article 5(1) of the European Convention on Human Rights when he had been compulsorily isolated for periods amounting to one and a half years over a seven-year period. The European Court of Human Rights held that the authorities had failed to strike a fair balance between the need to ensure that HIV did not spread and the applicant's right to liberty.[54] In contrast, the House of Lords held that there was no breach of Article 3 rights when a Ugandan woman was refused asylum even though she was suffering from full-blown AIDS and needed the retroviral drugs available in the UK to stay alive. Article 3 could not be interpreted as requiring contracting states to admit and treat AIDS sufferers from all over the world for the rest of their lives. They came to their unanimous decision despite their considerable sympathy for the woman.[55]

Under the Equality Act 2010 paragraph 6 of Schedule 1 defines certain medical conditions as a disability: cancer, HIV infection and multiple sclerosis. HIV infection is defined as an infection by a virus capable of causing the Acquired Immune Deficiency Syndrome. Therefore anyone diagnosed with HIV would be entitled to the same protection against discrimination in employment, getting goods and services, education, trade union membership and accommodation as other protected categories. (See chapter 10.)

Confidentiality and Identifying Patients Who may be at Risk

In one case,[56] the claimant was working as a healthcare worker when he was diagnosed as HIV-positive. He informed the health authority and ceased working immediately. The health authority wanted to conduct a 'look back' exercise that involved contacting various patients of the claimant's who were thought to be potentially at risk of infection. The claimant did not believe that his patients were at sufficient risk to justify that exercise and sought a declaration that the look back exercise was unlawful on the grounds that it breached clinical confidentiality. He also sought an order restraining the authority from making use of the patient records and from doing anything that might directly or indirectly reveal his identity. An order was in force stating that the parties were only to be identified by initials. A newspaper wished to publish the story and the claimant sought an order to prevent its revealing his identity. The injunction was issued but was subsequently varied on the application of the newspaper so that it could name the health authority, the claimant's specialty and the date of his diagnosis as HIV-positive. The Court of Appeal held that it was appropriate for the health authority and claimant to be identified by initials, for the claimant's specialty to be identified, and ordered the claimant to make available to the health authority such patient records as were reasonably required on the understanding that they would not be disclosed without either the permission of the claimant or the court.

The Department of Health initiated a consultation on confidentiality and sexually transmitted diseases in 2006 in the light of a High Court case where claimants sought a declaration relating to the common law on disclosure, the Human Rights Act and the legislation relating to disclosure and sexually transmitted diseases.

HIV-infected Healthcare Workers

The Department of Health has updated its guidance on HIV-infected healthcare workers[57] and it is now incorporated in the report of the Expert Advisory Group on AIDS[58] and its advice on HIV post-exposure prophylaxis should be followed. It makes it clear that, because of the very low risk of infection, there is no longer a requirement to notify all patients, but whether notification is necessary should be assessed on a case-by-case basis using risk assessment.

In 2011 a report by the tripartite working group on the management of HIV-infected healthcare workers recommended they could perform exposure-prone procedures (EPP) provided they satisfied certain conditions and were under the supervision of a consultant in occupational health.[59]

Announcing the ending of restrictions, the Chief Medical Officer of Health Dame Sally Davis stated that it was more likely that someone would be struck down by lightning than infected by an HIV-infected healthcare worker. In addition the restriction on the purchase of HIV home testing kits was lifted, enabling people to find out their HIV status.[60]

Vaccination

Compensation for vaccine damage can be obtained in two ways. First, there is a statutory scheme of compensation under the Vaccine Damage Payments Act 1979. Under this scheme, £120,000[61] is payable to a person who can establish that they have been severely disabled as a result of a vaccination against the specified diseases of diphtheria, tetanus, whooping cough, poliomyelitis, measles, mumps, rubella, tuberculosis, smallpox (up to August 1971), *Haemophilus influenza* type b infection (HIB), meningococcal group C and pneumococcal infection and any other disease specified by the Secretary of State. Human papillomavirus was added in 2008.[62] Subsequent regulations[63] have reduced the severity of the disability, which must be proved to 60 per cent. Whether the disability has been caused by the vaccination shall be established on a balance of probabilities. The claim must be made before whichever is the later of the date on which the disabled person attains the age of 21 years (or, where they have died, would have attained that age) and the end of a period of six years, beginning on the date of the vaccination against the disease to which the claim relates. The person need not be under 18 at the time of vaccination, neither need there be an outbreak of the disease.[64]

This statutory scheme does not prevent a claim being made in the civil courts for negligence in relation to damage caused by vaccine. Clearly, if such a case could succeed, far more than £120,000 would be payable for severely disabled persons. However, civil action faces a further difficulty, as well as having to establish a causal link between the vaccine and the disability. The claimant must also show that the disability occurred as a result of negligence by the defendant; for example, the professionals failed to take account of the person's present health condition or previous history and the vaccine was contraindicated for that person. A claim could also be brought against the drug company if there were some defect in the vaccine and this claim could now come under the Consumer Protection Act (considered in chapter 12), under which it is not necessary to show negligence by a manufacturer, but simply that there was a defect in the product. This would be extremely difficult if the victim was the only one from a particular batch who suffered harm. The civil cases so far have not overcome the problems of proving causation (see Case 25.2) apart from a case in Ireland.

In November 2013 a mother whose son died of Creutzfeldt-Jakob disease (CJD) refused £120,000 in compensation and warned that the illness remains a ticking time bomb in Britain.[65]

It was reported in August 2010 that the mother of a Cheshire teenager who was left severely brain-damaged by the MMR vaccine won a compensation award from the government. Robert Fletcher, 18, from Warrington, suffered a fit 10 days after he had the vaccination when he was 13 months old. His mother Jackie received a £90,000 pay-out from a medical assessment panel. The family successfully appealed after their application for compensation was originally turned down in 1997. The tribunal specifically stated that the finding that his brain damage was caused by the MMR jab is not relevant to the claims of a link between the jab and autism.[66] It was reported in November 2013 that more than 1000 families who wished to claim compensation following MMR vaccines are now due to sue their lawyers. A class action on behalf of the families was dropped in 2003 during the Andrew Wakefield controversy, but some of the families are now suing their lawyers on the grounds that their action should have been based on a faulty batch of vaccines used between 1988 and 1992 and not the Wakefield dispute.[67] They alleged that the time limit of bringing the action within 10 years from the date of supply of the vaccine from the manufacturers was breached.[68]

It is estimated that 60 people will share in a £60 million payout because they suffered brain damage caused by swine flu vaccine. The compensation will be paid by GlaxoSmithKline (GSK) who will reclaim the cost from the government.[69] (GSK obtained an indemnity from the government against any claim for side effects.)

The Sunday Times used a Freedom of Information request to establish that 40 children are suspected of having died as a result of receiving routine vaccinations over a period of seven years.[70]

The judge held that on a balance of probabilities the claimant had failed to show that pertussis vaccine could cause permanent brain damage in young children. The case therefore failed on this point of causation. The judge also said that even if he had found in favour of the claimant on this preliminary point, the claimant would still face insuperable difficulties in establishing negligence on the part of the doctor or nurse who administered the vaccine. Such a claim would have to be based on the ground that the vaccination had been given in spite of the presence of certain contraindications.

> **Case 25.2** *Loveday v Renton and Another* [1988]
>
> ## Vaccine damage[71]
>
> Susan Loveday was vaccinated for whooping cough in 1970 and 1971, following which she suffered permanent brain damage. She claimed compensation from the Wellcome Foundation, which made the vaccine, and from the doctor who administered it.

In a case in Ireland brought against the Wellcome Foundation,[72] £2.75 million was awarded in respect of brain damage following a vaccination. It was established that a particular batch of vaccine was below standard and should not have been released on to the market.

In another case an appeal by a GP against a finding of negligent advice in respect of a polio vaccine succeeded. The Court of Appeal held that the trial judge had wrongly found the GP to be in breach of his duty of care when he advised parents that there was no reason to postpone a polio vaccination because the child had an abscess on his buttocks. Subsequently the child contracted polio. The Court of Appeal held it was not reasonably foreseeable that the GP could have foreseen the results of his failure to explain his advice to the parents. His reasoning was based on possible pain to the child, not the possibility of polio being contracted.[73]

Further information on compensation for vaccine damage is available from the government website.[74] Payments can be claimed and forms can be downloaded from a dedicated vaccine payments website.[75] The Department of Health publishes the *Green Book* giving information on vaccines and preventable infectious diseases which is updated on a regular basis and available on the government website.

In March 2014 it was announced that a vaccine for meningitis B would be made available. This reverses an earlier decision of the Joint Committee on Vaccination and Immunisation which said it would not be cost-effective to make it part of the routine child immunisation programme.[76] In 2015 meningitis B vaccine was added to the routine UK immunisation schedule with children being offered the vaccine at 8 weeks, 16 weeks and 1 year alongside other routine vaccinations.[77]

The Mesothelioma Act 2014

This legislation allows for a package of support, funded by insurance firms, to pay in excess of 800 eligible people in 2014 and 300 every year after that until 2024. Payments are increased to around £123,000 plus £7000 towards legal fees. The scheme applies to those diagnosed with mesothelioma since 25 July 2012. Further information is available on the government website[78] and from the Asbestos Victims Support Group Forum.[79]

The MMR dispute

Concern about MMR was raised in 1995[80] by Dr Wakefield of the Royal Free Hospital, London, who published claims of a link between the measles vaccination and the inflammatory bowel condition known as Crohn's disease. He subsequently published a second study that showed that some children who had developed the bowel condition also developed autism. The study was too small to demonstrate a causal connection with MMR, but it was suggested by Dr Wakefield that, pending further research, MMR should be temporarily abandoned and single doses of the different vaccines should be given. Subsequently, there was considerable disquiet over whether it was safe for health professionals to recommend MMR and many parents opted for the single dose that is not available on the NHS. The government attempted to induce confidence in MMR. For example, on 13 December 2001 a Department of Health press release[81] announced the publication of a report commissioned by the Department of Health and carried out by the Medical Research Council that there was no evidence to link autism with the measles, mumps and rubella vaccine. The apparent increase in prevalence of autism spectrum disorders (ASDs) was likely to have resulted from better diagnosis and clearer definition as well as increased awareness. In January 2004 the Department of Health published an MMR information pack for parents setting out the reasons why MMR is recommended, and providing seven information sheets.[82] Further information on supplies and the administration of MMR was issued in May 2005[83] and an assessment of the press coverage of the MMR vaccine was published by the Department of Health two days earlier.[84]

The issue came to the attention of the courts when a dispute arose between two sets of parents over whether the children should be given the MMR vaccine; in each case the mother was against the triple vaccine and the father wanted it given. The High Court ruled that it was in the best interest of the children to have the MMR. The Court of Appeal dismissed the appeal on the grounds that the judge had decided the applications by reference to the paramount consideration of the welfare of the two children, in accordance with section 1 of the Children Act 1989.[85] A practice direction was issued in July 2003 on MMR/MR vaccine litigation, which required such actions to commence in the Royal Courts of Justice and those that have commenced in the county court or district registry must be transferred. The actions had been allocated to the multi-track and came under the Civil Procedure Rules.[86] The independence of Dr Wakefield's research was subsequently criticised and the safety of MMR reaffirmed. Following three years of investigations, the GMC found Dr Wakefield guilty of serious professional misconduct and he was struck off the Register.[87] In 2007 an increase in measles was held to be directly linked with the failure in uptake of the MMR vaccine as a result of the controversy, and figures published in January 2010 show that there were 1348 cases of measles in 2008 compared with 56 in 1998.[88] A similar outbreak took place in Swansea, South Wales in 2013. Fears that a time bomb of babies being born deaf and blind as a result of teenagers not receiving the MMR jab have been expressed by Professor Colin Blakemore.[89]

The MMR controversy is explored in a book by Tammy Boyce.[90] In September 2014 the Texan state appeals court ruled that Mr Wakefield could not sue for defamation against the *BMJ* and its editor, and Brian Deer, a freelance writer for *The Sunday Times*, in Texas because the state did not have jurisdiction to hear the case.

In 2013 Mrs Justice Theis ruled that two girls of 15 and 11 could be given the MMR vaccine despite the opposition from them both and their mother. Their divorced father brought the case having originally been opposed to MMR but having changed his mind after the link between the vaccination and autism was discredited.[91]

Coronavirus

At the end of 2019 a new public health emergency emerged worldwide, beginning in China and quickly spreading across the world to cover almost all nations, including the UK. This emergency was referred to as SARS-CoV-2, that caused the disease COVID-19, a respiratory virus. For some time no vaccine was available, so from 2020 lockdown of the population was imposed by most nations to safeguard the public. (The first vaccine was given in December 2020). The Covid pandemic led to emergency legislation in the UK. The Coronavirus Act 2020 legally allowed the government to impose lockdowns, to restrict movements of people, and to restrict gatherings. The act did give considerable freedom to the devolved nations to manage the pandemic in their own ways, which led to a great deal of divergence amongst the UK governments. Covid-19 has moved from the pandemic stage to the endemic stage, however it demonstrates how the government can and is willing to impose protection measures if needed in a major public health emergency.[92]

Blood donors

The present practice is for blood donors to be asked to agree that their blood can be tested for HIV and a leaflet is given to them to sign as to whether they are in any of the high-risk groups and which asks them not to give blood if they are. The donors should not, of course, run any risk of contracting HIV as a result of giving blood. In October 2009 a review suggested that the ban on gay men donating blood could be lifted in 2010.[93] The NHS Blood and Transplant Agency had called for an increase of 50 per cent in blood donors and it was felt that the ban was no longer necessary.[94] The guidance was modified in 2011 to allow gay men to donate blood if they had abstained from intercourse for a year. In 2017 the guidance was updated in line with improved testing to three months after having sex. On 14 June 2021, gay, bisexual and other men can donate blood without any waiting period if they declare that hey have met legibility for blood donation via a legally binding statutory declaration, as is the case with any other donor.

Haemophiliacs and Recipients of Blood

The compensation available to those who received contaminated blood together with the Archer Report (the Skipton and Caxton Funds) is discussed in chapter 15.

Confidentiality

Practical Dilemma 25.2   A justified disclosure?

Dr Jones, a general practitioner, was treating Ben James for an undiagnosed condition. He thought initially that it could be glandular fever. However, the blood tests revealed that he was suffering from AIDS. Dr Jones was uncertain as to who he could inform about this result. Ben was anxious that no one be told and that the information should be kept from his wife until much later on. Dr Jones wondered if the practice nurse and others working in the health centre who were likely to come into contact with Ben should be notified.

One of the exceptions to the duty of confidentiality was where disclosure was justified on grounds of the public interest (see chapter 8). This is one of the most difficult exceptions, since there is no clear judicial or statutory definition over what are the limits and extent of the term 'public interest' in this context. In the story of Ben in Practical Dilemma 25.2, if Dr Jones also treats Ben's wife, it could be argued that he is not fulfilling his duty of care to her if he fails to inform her that she is at risk of contracting AIDS and, even if she is not his patient, he should inform her GP (unless, of course, he can persuade Ben to tell her). This breach in the duty of confidentiality owed to Ben is therefore justifiable on the grounds of the public interest. The same argument could be applied to informing any person in the health centre who is likely to be at risk from infection from Ben. Thus there may be justification in informing the practice nurse, but not the receptionist, since the latter is not likely to acquire the disease from Ben. The fact that the law is uncertain makes for considerable difficulties and ultimately it is up to individual practitioners to decide whether, in the specific circumstances of an individual case, there should be disclosure. The balance between an action for breach of confidentiality and an action for breach of a duty to care for the safety of a fellow employee is a very fine one.

In contrast to the case of X v Y (see Case 25.3), the Court of Appeal allowed an order of disclosure of the person who had informed the press about an Ashworth patient. Subsequently a later Court of Appeal decided that the journalist did not have to identify his source.[95]

Case 25.3 X v Y [1988]

Order of disclosure and non-disclosure under contempt of court[96]

The High Court held that public interest did not justify a newspaper publishing or using information disclosed by a health authority employee in breach of contract who admitted to a journalist that two identified doctors were being treated for AIDS at an identified hospital. The newspaper was fined £10,000 for contempt of a court order. However, the health authority was not able to obtain disclosure of the name of the informant employee, even though he or she was clearly in breach of the duty of employment, because this was not one of the occasions on which the press were obliged to disclose the source of their information under the contempt of court legislation.

Conclusions

In recent years the focus in infectious diseases has moved away from that of AIDS/HIV infection to that of MRSA/*Clostridium difficile*. However, the continuing increase in the numbers infected with HIV leaves no room for complacency. There are suggestions that AIDS could be under control worldwide imminently.[97] There are signs that a reduction of hospital-acquired infections is at last being achieved as a result of the work of the Health Protection Agency and the Care Quality Commission. The figures for *C. difficile* and other superbugs show a declining rate with infections down 70 per cent over recent years. However, research suggests that there may be underreporting with one in two doctors believing that hospitals underreport superbug cases in order to avoid paying heavy fines.[98]

It is clear that improvements in the safety of hospitals and the reduction of deaths through hospital-acquired infections rests with individual standards of personal hygiene. It remains to be seen whether the provision made in the Health and Social Care Act 2008 for amending the Public Health (Control of Disease) Act 1984 to provide a more effective and proportionate response to infectious disease is effective in controlling outbreaks. There is uncertainty too over the effect of a new public health service which has seen the abolition of the Health Protection Agency and the National Treatment Agency. Local authorities have now taken over responsibilities for public health and it is as yet too soon to evaluate the effects of this.

A dispute has arisen over the value of the NHS Health Check programme with the Nordic Cochrane Centre in Copenhagen arguing that they could find no beneficial effects and that they were likely to lead to unnecessary diagnoses and treatments.[99] The tests were defended by Public Health England on the grounds that the precautionary principle justified efforts to spot risk factors for disease.[100] Public Health will continue to be a controversial area.

Reflection questions

1. What is meant by 'reasonably practical precautions to safeguard the safety of other employees'? To what extent do you consider your present practice meets this requirement in relation to the dangers of infection from infections? (See also chapter 12.)
2. Many regard the hepatitis B virus as an even greater danger to health service staff than AIDS. What are the main differences in the law (if any) relating to AIDS and to hepatitis?
3. Look again at the laws relating to the notification of infectious diseases. To what extent do you consider they could impinge on your professional practice?
4. What is meant by the duty of confidentiality in relation to those suffering from infections? Are any exceptions to the duty justified? To what extent do you consider that the duty is carried out and what suggestions would you make for improvements for all staff to observe this duty? (See also chapter 8.)

Further exercises

1. Obtain a copy of the Secretary of State's Code of Practice relating to infection control and discuss the extent to which this is fully implemented in your organisation.
2. Study the figures of your organisation on the cross-infection of patients following admission. What improvements could be made in cross-infection control?
3. What role do you consider that the individual nurse should play in ensuring that hospitals and other health premises are clean and hygienic?

References

[1] Law Commission, Ninth Programme of Law Reform, March 2005 HC 535, Stationery Office, London
[2] www.hpa.org.uk/Topics/InfectiousDiseases

[3] www.legislation.gov.uk
[4] The Health Protection (Notification) Regulations 2010, SI 2010/659
[5] Public Health (Control of Disease) Act 1984 Section 11 as amended by The Health Protection (Notification) Regulations 2010, SI 2010/659
[6] National Audit Office, The Management and Control of Hospital Acquired Infection in Acute NHS Trusts in England, Stationery Office, London, 2000
[7] www.dh.gov.uk
[8] Department of Health press release 12 June 2000; Jill Sherman, Infections caught in hospital to be exposed, *The Times*, 13 June 2000
[9] David Charter, Milburn admits superbug is endemic, *The Times*, 8 January 2001
[10] Nursing and Midwifery Council, A–Z advice sheet: Infection control, March 2006
[11] Royal College of Nursing, Good practice in infection prevention and control, RCN, 2006 updated 2010
[12] Directors of Infection Prevention and Control in England, *Clostridium difficile*: findings and recommendations from a review of epidemiology and a survey, HPA, July 2006
[13] www.hpa.org.uk/infections/topics_az/clostridium_difficile
[14] www.gov.uk
[15] Report from Conference Antimicrobial Resistance: In Search of a Collaborative Solution, 2013 World Innovation Summit for Health; www.wish-qatar.org
[16] www.thecochranelibrary.com
[17] Jerome Starkey, Ebola patients to be given untested drugs, *The Times*, 13 August 2014
[18] John Simpson, Killer virus 'threatens world', *The Times*, 30 May 2013
[19] www.who.int/emergencies/mers-cov/en
[20] Council of the European Union, Council recommendation on patient safety including prevention and control of healthcare associated infections, *Official Journal of the European Union*, 2009/C 151/01 5 June 2009
[21] Chief Medical Officer of Health, Getting Ahead of the Curve, DH, London, January 2002
[22] Department of Health, Liberating the NHS: Report of the arm's-length bodies, London, Crown, 2010
[23] Chief Medical Officer of Health, Stopping Tuberculosis in England, October 2004
[24] News item, *The Times*, 11 May 2005
[25] www.gov.uk/government/collections/tuberculosis-and-other-mycobacterial-diseases-diagnosis-screening-management-and-data
[26] News item, Doctors issue hepatitis alert, *The Times*, 10 May 2005
[27] Department of Health, Children in Need and Bloodborne Viruses: HIV and hepatitis, 5 November 2004
[28] British HIV Association, Guidelines for the Management of HIV infection in pregnant women, London, BHIVA, 2008
[29] Wilson, HIV and pregnancy: challenges in practice, *Practising Midwife*, 14(3):16–18, March 2011
[30] Williams, Testing for sexually transmitted infections in pregnancy, *Practising Midwife*, 14(2):36–41, February 2011
[31] www.nice.org.uk
[32] www.nhs.uk/conditions/vaccinations/hepatitis-b-vaccine
[33] Chris Smyth, UK trials hope to put HIV patients into remission, *The Times*, 26 November 2013
[34] Andrew Clark, Glaxo's once-a-day HIV pill given go-ahead in Brussels, *The Times*, 22 January 2014
[35] Tom Whipple, HIV-positive surgeons are cleared to operate, *The Times*, 15 August 2013

[36] HSC 1999/183
[37] M.J. Postma et al., Universal HIV screening of pregnant women in England: cost-effectiveness analysis, *BMJ*, 318:1656–60, 19 June 1999
[38] E.G. Lyall et al., Guidelines for the management of HIV infections in pregnant women in prevention of mother to baby transmission, *HIV Medicine*, 2(4):314–34, 2001
[39] Department of Health, Reducing Mother to Baby Transmission of HIV, HSC 1999/183, DH
[40] Department of Health www.gov.uk
[41] News item, HIV test reprimand, *The Times*, 6 January 2000
[42] *Re C (HIV Test)* [1999] 2 FLR 1004
[43] Royal College of Paediatrics and Child Health, Reducing mother to child transmission of HIV in the United Kingdom, July 2006
[44] Report of Expert Advisory Group on AIDS HIV Post-Exposure Prophylaxis, DH, London, 2008
[45] National Children's Bureau, HIV in schools: good practice to supporting children infected or affected by HIV, 2005
[46] www.ncb.org.uk
[47] Aids (Control) (Contents of Reports) (No. 2) Order 1988, SI 1988/1047
[48] The HIV Testing Kits and Services Regulations 1992 SI 1992/460
[49] The HIV Testing Kits and Services Regulations 2014 SI 2014/451
[50] *R v Dica [2004] EWCA Crim 1103*; Michael Horsnell, Lover convicted after infecting women with HIV, The Times Law Report, 15 October 2003
[51] *R v Konzani* [2005] EWCA Crim 706
[52] Michael Horsnell, HIV chef who recklessly infected his lover is jailed for nine years, *The Times*, 6 April 2007, p. 26
[53] News item, *The Times*, 1 September 2010
[54] *Enhorn v Sweden* [2005] ECHR 56529
[55] *N v Secretary of State for the Home Department* [2005] UKHL 31
[56] *H (A Healthcare Worker) v Associated Newspapers Ltd; H (A Healthcare Worker) v N (A Health Authority)* [2002] Civ 195; [2002] Lloyd's Rep Med 210 CA
[57] Department of Health, AIDS/HIV Infected Health Care Workers: guidance on the management of infected health care workers and patient notification, DH, London, 1999, updated July 2005 and 2008
[58] Report of Expert Advisory Group on AIDS HIV Post-Exposure Prophylaxis, DH, London, 2008
[59] Department of Health, Management of HIV-infected Healthcare Workers, April 2011
[60] Sarah Boseley, Restrictions on health workers with HIV lifted as 'outdated' ban ends, *The Guardian*, 15 August 2013
[61] Vaccine Damage Payments Act 1979, Statutory Sum Order 2007, SI 2007/1931
[62] Vaccine Damages Payments (Specific Diseases) Order 2008, SI 2008/2103
[63] Regulatory Reform (Vaccine Damage Payments Act 1979) Order 2002, SI 2002/1592
[64] Vaccine Damages Payments (Specific Diseases) Order 2001, SI 2002/1652; 2008 SI 2008/2103
[65] Emily Cope and James Gillespie, Victim's mother warns of CJD 'timebomb', *The Sunday Times*, 24 November 2013
[66] Sarah-Kate Templeton, Mother wins MMR payout after 18 years, *The Sunday Times*, 29 August 2010
[67] Frances Gibb, MMR Vaccine families to sue lawyers for negligence, *The Times*, 23 November 2013
[68] Frances Gibb, MMR families sue their legal aid lawyers, *The Times*, 26 June 2014
[69] Lois Rogers, Victims of swine flu jab to get £60m payout, *The Sunday Times*, 2 February 2014

70 Sarah-Kate Templeton, 40 deaths linked to child vaccines over seven years, *The Sunday Times*, 24 October 2010
71 *Loveday* v *Renton and Another*, *The Times*, 31 March 1988
72 *Best* v *Wellcome Foundation, Dr O'Keefe, the Southern Health Board, the Minister for Health of Ireland and the Attorney General* [1994] 5 Med LR 81
73 *Thompson* v *Bradford* [2005] EWCA 1439
74 www.direct.gov.uk/disability-vdp
75 www.gov.uk/vaccine-damage-payment
76 News item, *The Times*, 21 March 2014
77 https://assets.publishing.service.gov.uk/government/uploads/system/uploads/attachment_data/file/554011/Green_Book_Chapter_22.pdf
78 www.gov.uk
79 www.asbestosforum.org.uk
80 Nigel Hawkes, A lone doctor's fear set parents against experts, *The Times*, 7 February 2002
81 Department of Health, Medical Research Council Autism Review Report, 2001/0615, 13 December 2001
82 Department of Health, MMR Information Pack, January 2004, Gateway reference 2004
83 Department of Health, Further Information on Supplies and Administration of MMR, May 2005
84 Department of Health, Measles, Mumps and Rubella (MMR) Vaccine: assessment of press coverage, May 2005
85 *In re C (A Child: immunisation: parental rights) and Others* [2003] 3 FCR 156 CA
86 www.courtservice.gov.uk/cms/7731.html
87 David Rose, Doctor in MMR scare to challenge striking-off order, *The Times*, 25 May 2010
88 Brian Deer, Callous, unethical and dishonest, *The Times*, 31 January 2010
89 Chris Smyth, Babies at risk from MMR jab time bomb, *The Times*, 30 May 2013
90 Tammy Boyce, *Health, Risk and News: The MMR Vaccine and the Media*, Peter Lang Publ Inc, 2007
91 *F* v *F* [2013] EWHC 2683 (Fam)
92 Dowie I (2021) Understanding the legal considerations of consent in nursing practice. *Nursing Standard* 36 (12) 29-34.
93 David Rose, Ban on homosexual blood donors could be lifted next year, *The Times*, 27 October 2009
94 Ibid.
95 *Mersey Care NHS Trust* v *Ackroyd* [2007] EWCA 101
96 *X* v *Y and Another* [1988] 2 All ER 648
97 Mark Henderson, Aids could be under control worldwide in five years, *The Times*, 2 February 2010
98 Chris Smyth, Big fines may make hospitals reluctant to report superbug, *The Times*, 8 November 2013
99 Lasse Krogsboll T, Letter to the Editor, *The Times*, 20 August 2013
100 Chris Smyth, NHS checks on over-40s condemned as 'useless', *The Times*, 20 August 2013

Chapter 26

Handling Complaints

This chapter discusses

- Methods of complaining
- Handling complaints
- Hospital Complaints Procedure Act 1985 and the Wilson Report
- Complaints procedure 2004
- Complaints procedure 2004 and 2006
- Complaints procedure 2009
- The Health Service and Parliamentary Ombudsman (HSC)
- The House of Commons Select Committee
- Healthwatch England
- Local Healthwatch (formerly LINKS)
- Independent Complaints Advocacy Service (ICAS)
- Patient Advice and Liaison Services (PALS)
- Other quality assurance methods
- Complaints relating to detained patients
- Secretary of State inquiries
- The NHS Constitution
- Review of NHS complaints system

Introduction

It is highly likely that at some time in their career a nurse will be involved in a complaint, either in relation to their own conduct or in handling a complaint about someone else's. There is no doubt that there is an increase in the number of complaints made about the NHS. To some, this is a very bad sign and is indicative of a growing discontent with the health services.

However, others see this as a positive and valuable sign – an opportunity to improve the service and at the same time a sign that patients are more prepared to raise their voices over their concerns.

Certainly, the current emphasis on customer and consumer relations is encouraging patients, through consumer satisfaction surveys, to make their views known so that the service can be improved. Feedback from the patient is essential if the quality of care is to be improved. There are now statutory duties for the NHS Commissioning Board (NHS England) and the clinical commissioning groups to involve patients in decision-making processes and to ensure that they have the requisite information. Unfortunately, as the reports of the Health Service Commissioner show only too frequently, whether or not a complaint is initially justified, the way in which the complaint is handled can itself become a cause for complaint. Patients' charters, the Human Rights Act 1998, National Service Frameworks and reports from the Care Quality Commission, other bodies and the NHS Constitution may also encourage patients to criticise the services they have received in comparison with the standards they were led to expect and their rights as laid down in the European Convention on Human Rights (see chapter 1 and the website for this book). This section will review the procedures for handling complaints and discuss the legal powers of those statutory bodies that can represent or investigate the grievances of the patient.

Methods of complaining

Figure 26.1 shows the variety of ways of making a complaint about the NHS. Private hospitals have their own system for handling complaints and these tend to be on an individual hospital basis.

Many different motives exist behind a complaint. Some of the reasons why patients complain are shown in Figure 26.2 and the outcomes that they are seeking are shown in Box 26.1. However, it should be appreciated that, for many people, to make a formal complaint requires considerable courage and there are many reasons why justifiable grievances are not brought to the attention of management (see Box 26.2). It is very difficult for patients who are suffering from chronic conditions where they are dependent on the continued support of a particular department to make a formal complaint.

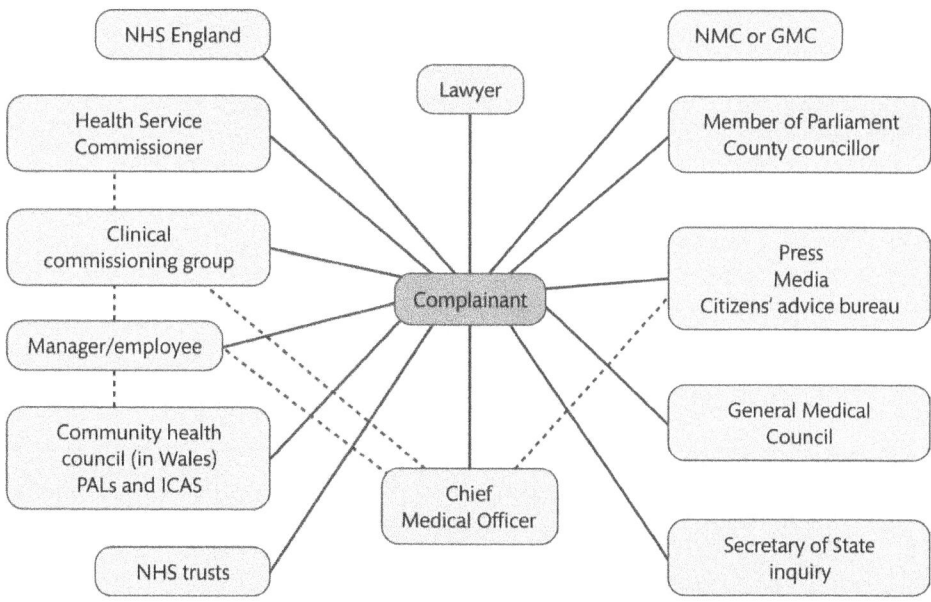

Figure 26.1

Various ways of making a complaint

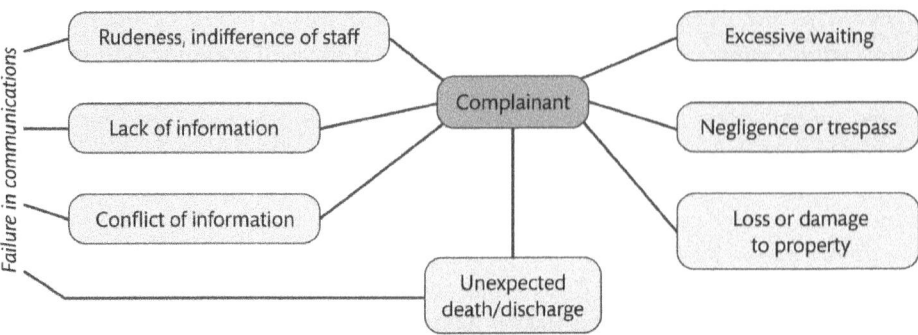

Figure 26.2 Why do people complain?

Box 26.1 What do complainants seek?

Apology
Explanation
Improvement
Prevention of similar occurrences
Compensation
Punishment:
  discipline
  dismissal
  striking off
Criminal proceedings

In the Review conducted by Ann Clwyd MP and Professor Tricia Hart the following actions were sought by complainants: information and accessibility; freedom from fear; sensitivity; responsiveness; prompt and clear process; seamless service; support (through the process of complaining) effectiveness and independence.

Box 26.2 Why do people *not* complain?

1. No reason to complain
2. No perceived reason to complain
3. There is a perceived reason *but*:
   - Positive reasons:
     (i) sympathy with staff
     (ii) immediate apology/explanation offered
     (iii) promise of rectification/improvement
     (iv) immediate interview with consultant/senior manager.
   - Negative reasons:
     (i) apathy/indifference
     (ii) ignorance of how to complain
     (iii) acceptance that errors/inefficiency are inevitable
     (iv) useless to complain – no point
     (v) fear of retribution

A typical letter of complaint will be considered to illustrate how it should be handled and the role of the nurse.

Handling complaints

Practical Dilemma 26.1 Dear Sir

Dear Sir

I was furious at the way my daughter was treated when we went to the diabetic clinic the other day. We waited two hours to be seen and then we saw a foreign doctor who could barely speak English and who changed her drugs. Since then she has had a diabetic coma and the GP has said that the dose should never have been changed. I think that that doctor should be prevented from practising again.

Yours sincerely
Valerie Machin

This type of complaint is typical since, like many, it covers several different complaints, some of which relate to clinical matters and others to non-clinical matters, and often a lack of communication underlies the problem. This complaint is not directly concerned with nursing matters, but the nurses in the clinic may well be asked to provide a statement as to what took place in the clinic and whether the parents complained at the time and what was done.

The complaint raises the following issues:

- waiting time in an outpatient department clinic;
- communication between doctor and patient;
- clinical practice of the doctor; and
- patient's current clinical condition.

The normal procedure would be for a letter of this kind to be referred to the hospital complaints manager acting on behalf of the chief executive. Many complainants are not always aware of the procedure and the letter could be sent to anyone. Staff should be aware of a procedure that ensures the letter is received by the complaints manager, who can follow it up to ensure that the correct procedure is followed and an acknowledgement, and later a report, are sent to the complainant by the chief executive.

The designated complaints manager would be responsible for ensuring that every point raised by the complainant is investigated and reported on satisfactorily. The chief executive officer would be expected to sign letters to a complainant personally:

1. The first task would be to refer the last two points listed above urgently to the consultant in charge of the patient to assess: it may be necessary for the consultant to discuss her present condition urgently with the GP to ensure that she is now on the appropriate medication.
2. Once her present clinical condition is satisfactory, the complaints relating to clinical matters would be investigated according to the appropriate procedure, which is considered below.

3. An investigation into the waiting times would be initiated by asking the director of nursing services for a report and also asking for a report from the medical records officer or any administrative officer in charge of that department. There should be a system in place for recording the times of the patients' arrival and departure and a system for pinpointing unreasonable delays. Some clinics do not operate an appointments system and block booking can often create unacceptable waiting times. Nursing staff will be required to provide information as to the usual way in which the diabetic clinic functioned, whether this could be improved and whether there were any extenuating circumstances on that occasion.

4. The consultant and director of nursing services would also be asked to report on the level of communication of the doctor in question, and whether his English was of an acceptable level. (Knowledge of English is a requirement for a licence to practice medicine in England.[1]) It may be that that aspect of the complaint could be due to some form of racial prejudice, but it should never be assumed that the complaint is without foundation. A full inquiry must always be held.

The usual practice would be for the Director of Nursing Services or his/her assistant to arrange for any individual nurse who was present at the time of the clinic visit to make a statement on what occurred. It is essential that the nurse receives guidance in preparing such a report and also checks with all the available documentation on the ward or department. (Guidance is given in chapter 9 on preparing statements.) The nurse should never submit the statement unless he or she is 100 per cent satisfied with the contents and that they have, where possible, checked its accuracy. The report that is sent to the complainant will be based on what the nurse has said and if there are any inaccuracies in this which are not spotted by other hospital personnel, then the nurse could, if the complainant took the complaint further, be questioned in an investigation by the Parliamentary and Health Service Ombudsman and criticism could be made of them.

When the complaints manager has received all the relevant reports, including at this stage the report by the consultant on the clinical complaints, a response will be sent to the complainant. This might be just a letter or it might be an invitation to attend a meeting or both. It is vital that every single point raised by the complainant is answered fully and honestly. This might at this stage mean apologising for some shortcoming that has been revealed in the service.

In serious cases, the NHS trust might decide to set up an inquiry into the complaint. Such inquiries will come under the recommendations set out by the DH in 2001, *Building a Safer NHS for Patients*, and the statutory complaints regulations.

Hospital Complaints Procedure Act 1985 and the Wilson Report

Under the Hospital Complaints Act 1985 each health authority was required to establish a complaints procedure. Guidance also required authorities to establish a procedure in relation to community health services. Following a review chaired by Professor Alan Wilson into the handling of hospital complaints, a consultation document was published.[2] The Department of Health accepted the principal recommendations of the Wilson Report and published guidance and directions for its implementation by NHS trusts and health service authorities.[3]

The Wilson Report found the system for dealing with complaints relating to health services to be confusing, bureaucratic, slow and inefficient. The Report reviewed the current situation and set objectives for any effective complaints system. The principles it saw for any effective complaints system are set out in Box 26.3.

The Report recommended that these principles should be incorporated into an NHS complaints system. On 1 April 1996 a new complaints procedure came into effect that implemented the majority of recommendations contained in the Wilson Report.

> **Box 26.3 Key elements in a complaints procedure**
>
> 1. Responsiveness
> 2. Quality enhancement
> 3. Cost-effectiveness
> 4. Accessibility
> 5. Impartiality
> 6. Simplicity
> 7. Speed
> 8. Confidentiality
> 9. Accountability

Complaints procedure 2004

Research into the Complaints System

The Department of Health commissioned an investigation into the effectiveness of the complaints procedure established following the Wilson Report. In its publication, *NHS Complaints Reform: making things right*,[4] the Department of Health noted that criticisms of the existing complaints procedure were that:

- It is unclear how, and difficult, to pursue complaints and concerns;
- There is often delay in responding when concerns arise;
- Too often there is a negative attitude to concerns expressed;
- Complaints seem not to get a fair hearing;
- Patients do not get the support they need when they want to complain;
- The independent review stage does not have the credibility it needs;
- The process does not provide the redress the patients want; and
- There does not seem to be any systematic processes for using feedback from complaints to drive improvements in services.

The aims of the reforms to the complaints procedure were to establish clear national standards and accountabilities, devolution to clinicians and managers backed up by independent scrutiny, flexibility and ensuring that patients can choose how they wish to pursue their concerns and have the support they need to help them do so.

The Department of Health recommended that there be:

- Increasing support and information for people who make complaints through local patient advice and liaison services and independent complaints and advice services.
- Patient feedback and customer care and training for NHS staff, including board members, to improve the way people are dealt with to help resolve complaints quickly.
- Subject to legislation, responsibility for independent complaints review placed with the Commission for Healthcare Audit and Inspection (CHAI) (The Healthcare Commission). (This was abolished in April 2009 and replaced by the Care Quality Commission which does not act as a second stage in the complaints system. Instead, dissatisfied complainants can apply to the Parliamentary and Health Service Ombudsman.)

Complaints procedure 2004 and 2006

The Health and Social Care (Community Health and Standards) Act 2003 Part 2 Chapter 9 gave power to the Secretary of State to make regulations on the handling of complaints about healthcare (s. 113), social services (s. 114), and section 115 set out topics that could be covered by regulations. Under the Department of Health's complaints procedure in 2004 there were still three stages: local resolution, independent review, Health Service Commissioner (Ombudsman), but there were significant changes to each stage and the support provided to patients. On 30 July 2004 regulations[5] on the new complaints system came into force with the Healthcare Commission acting as the independent second stage.

NHS and Social Services Complaints: a Single Comprehensive Procedure

Regulations relating to social services complaints[6] came into force on 1 September 2006. They impose time limits on making complaints, new timescales for handling stages of the process and provide greater independence at the final review panel stage. They can be downloaded from the Office of Public Sector Information.[7] The NHS complaints regulations were amended[8] following the White Paper commitment to develop a single comprehensive complaints procedure across health and social care by 2009. The amendments are intended to make the system more responsive and give better links with the arrangements for responding to social care complaints.

Criticisms by the Healthcare Commission

In October 2007 the Healthcare Commission published its first audit on how NHS trusts handled complaints, which is available on the website of its successor, the CQC.[9] It found considerable variation in how complaints were handled across the country. Its report highlighted the issues shown in Box 26.4.

> **Box 26.4** **Issues raised by Healthcare Commission on complaints handling (2007)**
>
> - More needs to be done to make the complaints system open and accessible, especially for those with learning disabilities and from ethnic communities
> - People who complain should be confident that their care will not suffer
> - Trusts should use complaints data to inform decision making
> - While there is no one-size-fits-all approach to investigating complaints, a common approach would improve risk management of complaints and manage the expectations of complainants
> - There are no nationally available standard tools and resources such as case studies, checklists and training aids for staff

Complaints procedure 2009

Since 2009 there has been a simplified two-stage complaints procedure in the NHS. The first stage is local resolution and the second is an application to the Ombudsman (Parliamentary and Health Service Commissioner). The procedure is described by the NHS website as follows:

> Since April 2009, the NHS has run a simple complaints process, which has two stages. Ask your hospital or trust for a copy of its complaints procedure, which will explain how to proceed. Your first step will normally be to raise the matter (in writing or by speaking to them) with the practitioner, e.g. the nurse or doctor concerned, or with their organisation, which will have a complaints manager. This is called local resolution, and most cases are resolved at this stage.
>
> If you're still unhappy, you can refer the matter to the Parliamentary and Health Service Ombudsman, who is independent of the NHS and government.

The DH then gives reference details for the Ombudsman, PALS and ICAS.

The 2009 regulations[10] which came into force in April 2009 place a duty on each responsible body (local authority, NHS body, primary care provider and independent provider) to make arrangements for handling and consideration of complaints so as to ensure that:

(a) complaints are dealt with efficiently;
(b) complaints are properly investigated;
(c) complainants are treated with respect and courtesy;
(d) complainants receive, so far as is reasonably practical—
  (i) assistance to enable them to understand the procedure in relation to complaints; or
  (ii) advice on where they may obtain such assistance;

(e) complainants receive a timely and appropriate response;

(f) complainants are told the outcome of the investigation of their complaint; and

(g) action is taken if necessary in the light of the outcome of a complaint.

The responsible body must identify a person (the chief executive) to be responsible for compliance with the regulations and a complaints manager responsible for managing the complaints procedures and hearing the complaints.

Excluded from the complaints procedure are the following:

(a) a complaint by a responsible body;

(b) a complaint by an employee of a local authority or NHS body about any matter relating to that employment;

(c) a complaint which—
  (i) is made orally; and
  (ii) is resolved to the complainant's satisfaction not later than the next working day after the day on which the complaint was made;

(d) a complaint the subject matter of which is the same as that of a complaint that has previously been made and resolved in accordance with sub-paragraph (c);

(e) a complaint the subject matter of which has previously been investigated under—
  (i) these Regulations;
  (ii) the 2004 Regulations, in relation to a complaint made under those Regulations before 1 April 2009;
  (iii) the 2006 Regulations, in relation to a complaint made under those Regulations before 1 April 2009; or
  (iv) a relevant complaints procedure in relation to a complaint made under such a procedure before 1 April 2009;

(f) a complaint the subject matter of which is being or has been investigated by—
  (i) a Local Commissioner under the Local Government Act 1974(a); or
  (ii) a Health Service Commissioner under the 1993 Act;

(g) a complaint arising out of the alleged failure by a responsible body to comply with a request for information under the Freedom of Information Act 2000(b); and

(h) a complaint which relates to any scheme established under section 10 (superannuation of persons engaged in health services, etc.) or section 24 (compensation for loss of office, etc.) of the Superannuation Act 1972(c), or to the administration of those schemes.

The complainant must be notified if his/her complaint comes under the above exclusions. A complaint must not be made later than 12 months after the date that the matter which is the subject of the complaint occurred or from when the complainant had knowledge of the matter. This time can be extended if the responsible body is satisfied that (a) the complainant had good reasons for not making the complaint within that time limit; and that (b) notwithstanding the delay, it is still possible to investigate the complaint effectively and fairly.

Para. 13 of the regulations lays down the procedures which the responsible body must comply with and is shown in Box 26.5.

> **Box 26.5** **Procedure for handling complaints from April 2009 (Regulation 13)**
>
> 1. A complaint may be made orally, in writing or electronically.
> 2. Where a complaint is made orally, the responsible body to which the complaint is made must—
>   (a) make a written record of the complaint; and
>   (b) provide a copy of the written record to the complainant.
> 3. Except where Regulation 6(5) (where the complaint is referred to another responsible body) or 7(1) (primary care trust complaint) applies in relation to a complaint, the responsible body must acknowledge the complaint not later than 3 working days after the day on which it receives the complaint.
> 4. Where paragraph (5) of Regulation 6 applies, and a responsible body ('the recipient body') receives a complaint sent to it by another responsible body in accordance with that paragraph, the complaint must be acknowledged by the recipient body not later than 3 working days after the day on which it receives the complaint.
> 5. Where Regulation 7(1) applies to a complaint—
>   (a) the primary care trust which receives the complaint must acknowledge the complaint not later than 3 working days after the day on which it receives it; and
>   (b) where a responsible body receives notification given to it under Regulation 7(5)(a), it must acknowledge the complaint not later than 3 working days after the day on which it receives the notification.
> 6. The acknowledgement may be made orally or in writing.
> 7. At the time it acknowledges the complaint, the responsible body must offer to discuss with the complainant, at a time to be agreed with the complainant—
>   (a) the manner in which the complaint is to be handled; and
>   (b) the period ('the response period') within which—
>   (i) the investigation of the complaint is likely to be completed; and
>   (ii) the response required by Regulation 14(2) is likely to be sent to the complainant.
> 8. If the complainant does not accept the offer of a discussion under paragraph (7), the responsible body must—
>   (a) determine the response period specified in paragraph (7)(b); and
>   (b) notify the complainant in writing of that period.

The 2009 regulations which set out the requirements and the process for handling complaints are shown in Boxes 26.6–26.10.

Box 26.6 Requirements for investigation and response (Regulation 14)

1. A responsible body to which a complaint is made must—
   (a) investigate the complaint in a manner appropriate to resolve it speedily and efficiently; and
   (b) during the investigation, keep the complainant informed, as far as reasonably practicable, as to the progress of the investigation.
2. As soon as reasonably practicable after completing the investigation, the responsible body must send the complainant in writing a response, signed by the responsible person, which includes—
   (a) a report which includes the following matters—
      (i) an explanation of how the complaint has been considered; and
      (ii) the conclusions reached in relation to the complaint, including any matters for which the complaint specifies, or the responsible body considers, that remedial action is needed; and
   (b) confirmation as to whether the responsible body is satisfied that any action needed in consequence of the complaint has been taken or is proposed to be taken;
   (c) where the complaint relates wholly or in part to the functions of a local authority, details of the complainant's right to take their complaint to a Local Commissioner under the Local Government Act 1974(a); and
   (d) except where the complaint relates only to the functions of a local authority, details of the complainant's right to take their complaint to the Health Service Commissioner under the 1993 Act.
3. In Paragraph (4), 'relevant period' means the period of 6 months commencing on the day on which the complaint was received, or such longer period as may be agreed before the expiry of that period by the complainant and the responsible body.
4. If the responsible body does not send the complainant a response in accordance with Paragraph (2) within the relevant period, the responsible body must—
   (a) notify the complainant in writing accordingly and explain the reason why; and
   (b) send the complainant in writing a response in accordance with Paragraph (2) as soon as reasonably practicable after the relevant period.

Box 26.7 Form of communications (Regulation 15)

Any communication which is required by these Regulations to be made to a complainant may be sent to the complainant electronically where the complainant—

(a) has consented in writing or electronically; and
(b) has not withdrawn such consent in writing or electronically.

Any requirement in these regulations for a document to be signed by a person is satisfied, in the case of a document which is sent electronically in accordance with these regulations, by the individual who is authorised to sign the document typing their name or producing their name using a computer or other electronic means.

Box 26.8 Publicity (Regulation 16)

Each responsible body must make information available to the public as to—

(a) its arrangements for dealing with complaints; and
(b) how further information about those arrangements may be obtained.

Box 26.9 Monitoring (Regulation 17)

For the purpose of monitoring the arrangements under these Regulations each responsible body must maintain a record of the following matters—

(a) each complaint received;
(b) the subject matter and outcome of each complaint; and
(c) where the responsible body informed the complainant of—
    (i) the response period specified in Regulation 13(7)(b); or
    (ii) any amendment to that period,
    whether a report of the outcome of the investigation was sent to the complainant within that period or any amended period.

Box 26.10 Annual reports (Regulation 18)

1. Each responsible body must prepare an annual report for each year which must—
   (a) specify the number of complaints which the responsible body received;
   (b) specify the number of complaints which the responsible body decided were well-founded;
   (c) specify the number of complaints which the responsible body has been informed have been referred to—
       (i) the Health Service Commissioner to consider under the 1993 Act; or
       (ii) the Local Commissioner to consider under the Local Government Act 1974; and
   (d) summarise—
       (i) the subject matter of complaints that the responsible body received;
       (ii) any matters of general importance arising out of those complaints, or the way in which the complaints were handled;

> (iii) any matters where action has been or is to be taken to improve services as a consequence of those complaints.
>
> 2. In paragraph (1), 'year' means a period of 12 months ending with 31 March.
> 3. Each responsible body must ensure that its annual report is available to any person on request.
> 4. This paragraph applies to a responsible body which is—
>   (a) an NHS body other than a primary care trust; or
>   (b) a primary care provider or an independent provider,
>
>   and which in any year provides, or agrees to provide, services under arrangements with a primary care trust.
> 5. Where paragraph (4) applies to a responsible body, the responsible body must send a copy of its annual report to the primary care trust which arranged for the provision of the services by the responsible body.
> 6. Each primary care trust must send a copy of its annual report to the strategic health authority whose area includes any part of the area of the primary care trust.
> 7. The copy of the annual report required to be sent in accordance with paragraph (5) or (6) must be sent as soon as reasonably practicable after the end of the year to which the report relates.

Statutory Feedback from Patients

From April 2013 all acute NHS trusts are required to ask both inpatients and emergency department patients one standard question known as the Friends and Family Test introduced by NHS England. Further information about the test including the feedback from patients for individual hospitals can be found on the NHS England website.[11] The question is 'How likely are you to recommend our ward/emergency department to friends and family if they needed similar care or treatment?' Fuller feedback is also being sought from every patient visiting a GP, hospital or dentist. The Family and Friends Test undertook a development project during the summer of 2018 to continue improving the Family and Friends Test, for example to:

- Explore a more effective question, and
- Support the best possible use of the data.

The Health Service and Parliamentary Ombudsman (HSC)

Since 2009 the only independent review for unresolved complaints is recourse to the Ombudsman.[12] Its jurisdiction derives from the Health Service Commissioners Act 1993 (as amended). (Northern Ireland has its own Health Service Ombudsman and the Scottish Public Services Ombudsman has had jurisdiction over complaints about the NHS in Scotland since 2002 and the Public Services Ombudsman for Wales has had jurisdiction over complaints about the NHS in Wales since 2005.)

If a complainant is not satisfied with the response of the authority to a complaint, he can apply to the Ombudsman for further investigation: the Parliamentary and Health Service Ombudsman in respect of complaints about the NHS and the Local Authority Commissioner Ombudsman in respect of complaints about local authority services. As a result of legislation in 1996 the Health Service Commissioner's (HSC) jurisdiction was extended to cover matters relating to family practitioner services, independent providers of NHS services and matters of clinical judgement. Disciplinary matters were not included in its jurisdiction (see Box 26.11 below). The HSC has a duty to prepare a report that is submitted to Parliament, under section 14(4) of the Health Service Commissioners Act 1993. These reports are available on the HSC website and can be a very useful source of information. For example, its second report for 2008/09 was concerned with the provision of services for people with learning disabilities which it had investigated following complaints by the families of six people with learning disabilities whose complaints were taken up by Mencap.[13] The Select Committee of the House of Commons has the power to investigate further any complaint reported by the HSC, if necessary summoning witnesses to London for questioning (see below). The HSC is completely independent of the NHS and the government and has the jurisdiction to investigate complaints against any part of the NHS, as shown in Box 26.11. It was held in a case heard in 2006 that the HSC had exceeded their statutory powers by going outside the remit of the complaint. The complaint concerned the discontinuation by a trust of a specialist vitamin unit which a father had found benefited his son who had epilepsy and learning and communication difficulties. The Court found that the HSC had not confined herself to the investigation of the complaint but had expanded the ambit of the investigation beyond the scope of the original complaint and had therefore exceeded her statutory powers.[14] Further information can be found on its website.[15]

Box 26.11 Jurisdiction of the Health Service Ombudsman

The Health Service Ombudsman's jurisdiction covers:

1. A failure in service;
2. A failure to purchase or provide a service one is entitled to receive; or
3. Maladministration (administrative affairs); or
4. Matters of clinical judgement.

The following are excluded from his investigation:

1. Actions where there is already an existing remedy in law (but there is a discretion to hear such matters if the Ombudsman is satisfied that it is not reasonable to expect the complainant to resort to this);
2. Personnel matters or contractual matters to do with the NHS;
3. Out-of-time complaints – although there is discretion to extend this; and
4. Complaints that have not yet been referred to the organisation for dealing through the complaints procedure.

The House of Commons Select Committee

A final possibility in the complaints process (and this can be very effective) is for an inquiry to be set up by the Select Committee of the House of Commons, to whom the Health Service Ombudsman reports. This Committee has the power to investigate a matter further by summoning witnesses to appear before it and if, in the report of the Ombudsman, it is clear that an authority has ignored its recommendations, the Committee can ask the authority to explain itself – an experience that few witnesses who have appeared before it will ever forget. There is no secrecy. All these cases are fully reported and the proceedings of the Select Committee are themselves published and may also be televised. There is no doubt that the fact that eventually an authority might have to explain how it dealt with any complaint is an important factor in ensuring that the complaint is properly, speedily and effectively dealt with.

Healthwatch England

The Commission for Patient and Public Involvement in Health (CPPIH), envisaged in the NHS Plan,[16] was established under section 20 of the NHS Reform and Health Care Professions Act 2002 in January 2003. Its functions set out in section 20(2) of the 2002 Act, included advising the Secretary of State about arrangements for public involvement in and consultation about matters relating to the health service in England and the provision of independent advocacy services. It was abolished in 2008 when the Local Government and Public Involvement in Health Act 2007 was enacted and LINKS replacing the patient forums were established.

Healthwatch England was established as a Statutory Committee of the Care Quality Commission under section 181 of the 2012 Act amending the Health and Social Care Act 2008 by adding sections 45A, B and C to that Act.

The purpose of Healthwatch England is to:

provide the Commission or other persons with advice, information or other assistance in accordance with provision made by or under this or any other Act.

Specific functions are set out as follows:

- It must provide local Healthwatch organisations with general advice and assistance in relation to their activities under section 221 of the Local Government and Public Involvement in Health Act 2007.
- It can give written notice to a local authority of its concern about a failure to carry out its functions.
- It must provide (a) the Secretary of State; (b) the National Health Service Commissioning Board; (c) Monitor; and (d) English local authorities with information and advice on—
    - **(a)** the views of people who use health or social care services and of other members of the public on their needs for and experiences of health and social care services, and
    - **(b)** the views of local Healthwatch organisations and of other persons on the standard of provision of health and social care services and on whether or how the standard could or should be improved.

A person provided with such advice must inform the Healthwatch England committee in writing of its response or proposed response to the advice.

The Healthwatch England committee may provide the Commission with information and advice on the matters mentioned above and the Commission must inform the committee in writing of its response or proposed response to the advice.

In performing functions under this section, the Healthwatch England committee must have regard to such aspects of government policy as the Secretary of State may direct.

The Healthwatch England committee is obliged to publish an annual report to the Care Quality Commission as soon as possible after the end of each financial year, covering topics specified. It must lay the report before Parliament and give a copy to the Secretary of State and the local Healthwatch organisations. It can also publish other reports at such times and on such matters relating to health or social care, as it thinks appropriate. Its annual report for 2012/13 is available on its website.[17]

Local Healthwatch (formerly LINKS)

Various organisations established to ensure local involvement and input into the organisation and standards of local services have been established. Patient Forums were set up under the NHS Reform and Health Care Professions Act 2002. There were over 400 patient and public involvement forums, one for each NHS trust in England, supported by the Commission for Patient and Public Involvement in Health (CPPIH).

The House of Commons Select Health Committee published a report on patient and public involvement in the NHS in April 2007.[18] As a consequence of its recommendations significant changes were proposed to the arrangements for the involvement of the public in healthcare and incorporated in the Local Government and Public Involvement in Health Act 2007. Local involvement networks (LINKS) replaced patients' forums and the Commission for Patient and Public Involvement in Health was abolished. The changes came into force in 2008.

LINKS have now been replaced by local Healthwatch organisations.

Sections 182 to 189 of the Health and Social Care Act 2012 makes provision for the local Healthwatch organisations building on the statutory provision for LINKS and section 221 of the Local Government and Public Involvement in Health Act 2007. Local Healthwatch organisations can be found on the Healthwatch website.[19]

Local Healthwatch organisations are independent, able to employ their own staff and involve volunteers with the aim of giving citizens and communities a stronger voice to influence and challenge how health and social care services are provided within the locality. It has a role in promoting public health, health improvements and in tackling health inequalities. Each local Healthwatch group will have a seat on the Health and Wellbeing Board. It will enable people to share views and concerns about local health and social care services and can alert Healthwatch England to concerns about specific care providers. Funded by LAs they are held to account for their ability to operate effectively and be value for money. Regulations relating to their right of entry to premises for public health purposes were enacted in 2013.[20]

Independent Complaints Advocacy Service (ICAS)

Under section 12 of the Health and Social Care Act 2001, the Secretary of State has a responsibility to provide independent advocacy services to assist patients in making complaints against the NHS. ICAS[21] was available nationally from September 2003. A consultation paper,

'Involving Patients and the Public in Healthcare',[22] was issued by the Department of Health in September 2001 for consultation on proposals for greater public representation to replace the community health councils (CHCs).

ICAS focused on helping individuals to pursue complaints about NHS services. It aimed to ensure that complainants have access to the support they need to articulate their concerns and navigate the complaints system, maximising the chances of their complaint being resolved more quickly and effectively. ICAS worked alongside the trust-based patients' forums (subsequently abolished) and patient advocacy and liaison services. It was announced in January 2006 that following a rigorous exercise, the DH awarded contracts to three organisations to deliver a new and improved ICAS from 1 April 2006. However, since 1 April 2013, commissioning of NHS complaints advocacy services transferred to individual local authorities. Section 185 of the Health and Social Care Act 2012 added section 223A to the Local Government and Public Involvement in Health Act 2007 requiring each local authority to make provision of independent advocacy services (defined as services providing assistance (by way of representation or otherwise) to persons making a complaint). Section 223A (2) a–g lists the complaints in its jurisdiction.

Patient Advice and Liaison Services (PALS)

A significant proposal in the NHS Plan[23] was the Patient Advice and Liaison Services (PALS). The Plan envisaged that by 2002 PALS would be established in every major hospital, with an annual national budget of around £10 million. Their core functions are:

- To provide on-the-spot help and speedy resolution of problems;
- To act as a gateway to independent advice and advocacy services;
- To provide accurate information about the trust's services and other related services;
- As a key source of feedback to the trust, to act as a catalyst for change and improvement; and
- To support staff in the development of a responsive, listening culture.

Special provision is made in respect of patient and advocacy services for the purposes of the Mental Health Act 1983 and section 134, which concerns the withholding of correspondence. Under regulations of 2003, correspondence with a PALS is exempt from the provisions of section 134.[24]

All NHS trusts were required to establish a PALS service by April 2002. A national evaluation of PALS was conducted from January 2005 to January 2007 and a report on the key messages published in October 2006 by the Department of Health is available on its website. Patients can contact their local PALS by phoning the local hospital, clinic, GP surgery or health centre, phoning NHS 111 or searching the Department of Health and Social Care website. The local PALS can also be found through the NHS website.[25]

Complaints and Litigation

Under the complaints procedure which was based on the Wilson Report, if the complainant indicated that he or she wished to pursue a legal remedy, the complaints procedure would be halted. The proposals for a new compensation scheme for clinical negligence claims, 'Making Amends' (discussed in chapter 6), recommended that complaints handling and early investigation of a potential legal action be combined. This recommendation was not included in the NHS redress scheme and the NHS complaints regulations exclude from its procedure a complaint where the complainant has stated in writing that he intends to take legal proceedings. In contrast, in Wales regulations were implemented to enable complainants to obtain compensation in an NHS redress scheme.

The Nurse and Complaints

It is in the interests of all health professionals to ensure that any complaints by patients or relatives relating to the provision of health services are resolved as speedily as possible informally, without requiring the complainant to make use of the formal procedure. Nurses should have the confidence to realise that complaints can be a useful way of monitoring and improving the services to patients, that it takes courage to make a complaint, especially where the patient suffers from a chronic condition, and that improvements can be made if clients are prepared to discuss with the health professionals ways in which the services could be enhanced.

Other quality assurance methods

Individuals who have complaints against the services provided in the NHS do not have any contractual right to bring an action before the court for breach of contract. If harm has been suffered as a result of a failure or omission, they may have a successful claim in the law of negligence (see chapter 3) or, if a service has not been provided, they may be able to bring a case of breach of statutory duty for failure to provide that service (see chapter 5). Otherwise, they must rely on the complaints procedure. They could apply for judicial review to the High Court if the principles of natural justice have not been followed, but they would be expected to exhaust appeals procedures within the NHS complaints system first. There are, however, many other mechanisms to ensure the maintenance of high standards of healthcare that cannot be directly utilised by the patient. The White Paper on the NHS in 1997 put forward a strategy for improving quality assurance and its mechanisms which was implemented in the Health Act 1999. These mechanisms included a National Institute for Health and Care Excellence (NICE), a Healthcare Commission (now the CQC) and a framework for national standards. The establishment of clinical governance whereby chief executives of trusts are held accountable for the clinical performance of their organisations provides more evidence to the patient about the standards of care locally. These innovations are discussed in chapter 5.

Complaints relating to detained patients

Under the 1983 Mental Health Act, there was a statutory duty placed on the Mental Health Act Commission to investigate complaints by detained patients. The jurisdiction could be extended to cover informal patients. Under section 52 of the Health and Social Care Act 2008 the functions of the Secretary of State and of the Mental Health Act Commission (MHAC) under the Mental Health Act were transferred to the Care Quality Commission (CQC) in England and the Welsh Ministers in Wales. The CQC can also investigate complaints of a detained patient on both clinical and non-clinical matters. A high proportion of the complaints that the MHAC has investigated were concerned with clinical matters such as medication, medical and nursing care. There is no power to subpoena witnesses or to take evidence on oath and the CQC is itself one of the bodies whose administrative function can be investigated by the Parliamentary and Health Service

Ombudsman. From the biennial reports of the MHAC, it was clear that the number and variety of the complaints that it had investigated were considerable. The CQC, like its MHAC predecessor, has complete discretion over how the complaints are to be investigated – methods range from a word to a ward sister to a full-scale investigation by commissioners. It is also apparent that, while its terms of reference are so far only to cover the detained patient, many of its recommendations are wider and affect the care of the informal patient. For example, the MHAC procedure on the consent to treatment of the mentally disordered outside the provisions of Part 4 of the 1983 Act had major implications for the care of the informal patient. In addition, the Code of Practice on the Mental Health Act provides advice about procedures and precautions to take if informal patients are detained in locked wards. The CQC has been given the responsibility of monitoring the operation of the Deprivation of Liberty Safeguards (see chapter 16) under the Mental Capacity Act 2005. Through this function, CQC seeks to ensure that the safeguards are working properly, highlight where they are not and, where necessary, require remedial action to be taken. CQC visits hospitals and care homes and, where necessary, interviews any patients who are deprived of their liberty and ask to see the relevant records. CQC reports once a year to the Secretary of State, summarising its activities and findings in relation to these safeguards.[26] Further information can be obtained on the CQC website[27] (see also chapters 5 and 19).

Secretary of State inquiries

Statutory powers are given in the NHS legislation for the Secretary of State to set up an inquiry into any case 'where he deems it advisable to do so in connection with any matter arising under this Act'.[28] The powers of such an inquiry are extensive and include the power to summon witnesses and order the production of documents and the taking of evidence on oath. Any person who refuses to give evidence or attend or destroys documents is guilty of a criminal offence.

A public inquiry of this nature is kept for the most serious of complaints with very serious implications. One example is the inquiry into Stafford Hospital which was chaired by Robert Francis QC (see chapter 5).[29]

The Secretary of State can also make an intervention order in relation to an NHS body other than NHS foundation trusts where he considers that the NHS body is not performing one or more of its functions adequately or at all or that there are significant failings in the way the body is being run, and he is satisfied that it is appropriate for him to intervene.[30] The effect of an intervention order is that he can remove all or any members from the board of the NHS body and appoint replacements or suspend any members.[31] Under the Health and Social Care Act 2012, Monitor (now NHS Improvement) has powers to withdraw the licence of any provider which is failing to perform (see chapter 5).

The NHS Constitution

The Health Act 2009 put the NHS Constitution and the accompanying Handbook on to a statutory basis. It can be seen on the website of this book. It identifies the rights of the patient and staff and sets out pledges which the NHS will endeavour to fulfil. The NHS Constitution sets out seven key principles to guide the NHS in all it does. These were amended in 2013 (see chapter 5 Box 5.2).

The seven key principles in the NHS Constitution are underpinned by core NHS values which have been derived from extensive discussions with staff, patients and the public.

The values are: respect and dignity; commitment to quality of care; compassion; improving lives; working together for patients; and everyone counts.

The NHS Constitution sets out the rights of the patient in respect of any complaint and redress and says (as amended in 2013):

Complaint and redress:
> You have the right to have any complaint you make about NHS services acknowledged within three working days and to have it properly investigated.
>
> You have the right to discuss the manner in which the complaint is to be handled, and to know the period within which the investigation is likely to be completed and the response sent.
>
> You have the right to be kept informed of the progress and to know the outcome of any investigation into your complaint, including an explanation of the conclusions and confirmation that any action needed in consequence of the complaint has been taken or is proposed to be taken.
>
> You have the right to take your complaint to the independent Parliamentary and Health Service Ombudsman, if you are not satisfied with the way your complaint has been dealt with by the NHS.
>
> You have the right to make a claim for judicial review if you think you have been directly affected by an unlawful act or decision of an NHS body.
>
> You have the right to compensation where you have been harmed by negligent treatment.

It does not specify any additional remedies provided by the NHS Constitution itself, and, any complainant will have to rely upon the existing complaints procedures.

Review of NHS complaints system

In the wake of the Francis Report on Mid Staffordshire the Prime Minister and Health Secretary commissioned Ann Clwyd MP and Professor Tricia Hart, the Chief Executive of South Tees Hospitals NHS Foundation Trust, to carry out a review of the NHS complaints system. The negative personal experience of Ann Clwyd following the alleged mistreatment and death of her husband was reinforced by 2500 letters about hospital neglect and poor care. The Report was published on 28 October 2013.[32]

The recommendations revolved around the following areas and those responsible for implementation were identified:

- improving the quality of care;
- improvements in the way complaints are handled; and
- greater perceived and actual independence in the complaints process and whistleblowing.

Several drivers for change were identified:

- consumer power;
- a champion for complaints reform (the CQC with its Chief Inspector of Hospitals); and
- concrete commitments or pledges to act by major NHS players.

Those organisations who had pledged to take action included: the NMC; the RCN; NHS Trust Development Authority (NHSTDA); Health Education England (HEE); Local Government

Association (LGA); NHS Confederation; NHS Employers; General Medical Council; Monitor; Care Quality Commission; NHS England and the Parliamentary and Health Service Ombudsman. The Report set out the action which each organisation was pledged to take.

The Report also highlighted good work in the NHS such as the critical friend at the Central Manchester University Hospitals NHS Foundation Trust and the customer focus at Birmingham Heartlands Hospital.

The President of the Royal College of Physicians, Sir Richard Thompson, who had made suggestions to the working party which led to the Review, wrote to the editor of *The Times*[33] on 2 November 2013 making more fundamental proposals including:

- the discussion of complaints within annual appraisals of staff with appraisers bringing these concerns to the attention of the management;
- a doctor from the medical staff elected to the Trust Board responsible for overseeing concerns;
- patients to be asked by ward/clinic staff when leaving if they have any concerns which would be collated by the ward/clinic nursing sister and the responsible named consultant and ward sister would handle the complaint face to face with the complainant or in writing, and if necessary they should be responsible for following the complaint through the Trust management system with the consultant signing off the reply not the chief executive.

He also suggested that professional groups should discuss concerns and make suggestions to management, that more attention should be given to the views and experience of junior doctors, and that the professional bodies should provide confidential support for whistleblowers who fail to get satisfaction.

The NMC has also issued guidance on raising concerns about a nurse or midwife (available on its website[34]) which sets out:

- the standards to expect from a nurse or midwife;
- the action which can be taken if care is unsatisfactory;
- where advice can be obtained; and
- the action the NMC can take.

Conclusions

Establishing an effective and efficient system of handling patients' complaints is proving an intractable problem for the NHS. The procedure set up following the Wilson Report proved too cumbersome and ineffective. Yet its replacement in 2004 has not been any more successful. The second stage of independent review has now been removed, with the Parliamentary and Health Services Commissioner or Ombudsman being the only independent review stage. The defects reported by the Health Commission and shown in Box 26.4 have still not been remedied. Nor has local representation within the NHS run smoothly. In 2008, patients' forums were replaced by local involvement networks (LINKS), and the Commission for Patient and Public Involvement in Health was also abolished. Local Healthwatch organisations have taken over from LINKS. Yet the successful implementation of an NHS Constitution depends to a considerable extent on the effectiveness and efficiency of a complaints procedure which can speedily rectify failures to implement the rights and responsibilities recognised in the Charter. The White Paper on the NHS published by the Coalition government declares that patients will be put at the heart of the

NHS and will have access to information, can make choices about their care and have increased control over their own records. It also states that:

> **We will strengthen the collective voice of patients and the public through arrangements led by local authorities, and at national level, through a powerful new consumer champion, HealthWatch England, located in the Care Quality Commission.**

However, the only means of enforcing such rights will be through an effective complaints procedure and the NHS has over the past 30 years been singularly unsuccessful in establishing one. The new devolved system of complaints hearings established in 2009 was assessed by the Health Service Ombudsman in the report of its first year.[35] The two most common grounds for complaints were: failings in care and treatment, and the attitude of staff. A poor explanation or an incomplete response were the most common reasons given for people's dissatisfaction with the NHS complaint handling. The Ombudsman held that poor quality or inconsistent information about complaints and their outcomes makes it more difficult for the NHS to learn lessons.

The Francis Report (see chapter 5) shows the weaknesses of our current system for handling complaints and the need for a radical overview has been promoted by Ann Clwyd. Hopefully there will be improvements. In July 2014 the Health and Social Care Information Centre initiated a consultation on NHS written complaints which may lead to changes to the data collection.

Nurses have a professional responsibility to respond appropriately to both informal and formal complaints, and should ensure that their documentation reflects the required standard of professional practice.

Reflection questions

1. What do you consider to be the most appropriate system for recording informal complaints?
2. Complaints are one means of obtaining feedback from patients about their stay. Consider other means of a more positive nature to obtain information relating to patient satisfaction and consider the possibility of implementing them.
3. You are a staff nurse on a medical ward. A patient complains to you that he thinks that he is suffering from the side effects of medication. How would you deal with this complaint? (See also chapter 27.)

Further exercises

1. Obtain a copy of the complaints procedure of your NHS trust or employer and familiarise yourself with it.
2. Ask the complaints manager in your organisation if you may see the complaints book and, if you can, see how an individual complaint has been followed up. (Remember the duty of confidentiality.)
3. Access the reports of the Health Service Commissioner on its investigations of NHS complaints and consider the extent to which any of its recommendations could apply in your organisation.

References

1. The Medical Act 1983 (Amendment) (Knowledge of English) Order 2014 SI 2014/1101
2. Being Heard: The Report of a Review Committee chaired by Professor Wilson on NHS complaints procedures, DH, London, 1994
3. NHS Executive, Guidance on the Implementation of the NHS Complaints Procedure, London, DH, March 1996; EL(96)19 Directions to NHS Trusts, Health Authorities and Special Health Authorities for Special Hospitals on Hospital Complaints Procedures; Directions to Health Authorities on Dealing with Complaints about Family Health Services Practitioners; Miscellaneous Directions to Health Authorities for Dealing with Complaints, DH, London, March 1996
4. Department of Health, NHS Complaints Reform: making things right, DH, London, 2003
5. The National Health Service (Complaints) Regulations 2004, SI 2004/1768
6. The Local Authority Social Services Complaints (England) Regulations 2006, SI 2006/1681
7. www.opsi.gov.uk
8. The National Health Service (Complaints) Amendment Regulations 2006, SI 2006/2084
9. www.cqc.org.uk
10. The Local Authority Social Services, National Health Services Complaints (England) Regulations 2009, SI 2009/309
11. www.nhs.uk
12. www.ombudsman.org.uk
13. Health Service Commissioner, Six Lives: the provision of public services to people with learning disabilities HC 203-1, 2009, Stationery Office, London
14. *R (on the application of Cavanagh, Bhatt and Redmond)* v *Health Service Commissioner* [2005] EWCA Civ 1578; [2006] 3 All ER 543
15. www.ombudsman.org.uk; customer help line 0345 015 4033
16. Department of Health, The NHS Plan, Cm 4818–1, DH, London, 1 July 2000 (Chapter 10)
17. www.healthwatch.co.uk
18. House of Commons Health Committee, Patient and Public Involvement in the NHS: Third Report of Session 2006–7, HC 278–1, 20 April 2007
19. www.healthwatch.co.uk
20. The Local Authorities (Public Health functions and entry to premises by local health-watch representatives) Regulations 2013 SI 2013/351
21. Information on ICAS is available from the DH website at www.gov.uk
22. Department of Health, Involving Patients and the Public in Healthcare, DH, London, September 2001
23. Department of Health, The NHS Plan: a plan for investment, a plan for reform, Cm 4818–1, DH, London, 2000
24. Mental Health (Correspondence of Patients, Patient Advocacy and Liaison Services) Regulations 2003, SI 2003/2042
25. www.nhs.uk
26. Care Quality Commission, Enforcement Policy 2009, CQC, London
27. www.cqc.org.uk
28. Section 84 National Health Service Act 1977
29. Report of the Mid Staffordshire NHS Foundation Trust Public Inquiry, HC 947, Stationery Office, February 2013; www.midstaffspublicinquiry.com
30. Section 66 National Health Service Act 2006 (as re-enacted)

[31] Section 67 National Health Service Act 2006 (as re-enacted)
[32] Clwyd Ann and Hart Tricia, A Review of the NHS Hospitals Complaints System: Putting Patients Back in the Picture, DH, October 2013; www.gov.uk
[33] Letter to the Editor, *The Times*, 2 November 2013
[34] www.nmc.org.uk
[35] Health Service Ombudsman's review of complaint handling by the NHS in England 2009–10, Stationery Office, London, 2010

Chapter 27

Legal Aspects of Medicines

This chapter discusses

- General principles
- Controlled drugs
- Problems in the administration of medicine
- Management of errors or incidents in the administration of medicines
- Self-administration by patients
- Covert administration of medicines
- Nurse as prescriber
- Group protocols or patient group directions
- Nurse prescribing: independent and dependent (subsequently known as supplementary) prescribers
- Role of the pharmacist
- Safety of medicines
- Product liability and drugs
- Misuse of drugs
- National Prescribing Centre
- Availability of medicines within the NHS

Introduction

The main legislation controlling the supply, storage and administration of medicines is the Medicines Act 1968 and the Misuse of Drugs Act 1971 and many subsequent statutory instruments. Of particular importance were the Misuse of Drugs Regulations 2001.[1] This legislation has now been consolidated in the 2012 regulations (as amended in 2013 and 2014).[2] The Medicines Act 1968 set up a comprehensive system of medicine controls (as can be seen on pages 676 and 694–6). The Medicines Control Agency was absorbed into the Medicines and Healthcare Products Regulatory Agency (MHRA) in April 2003 and information on the regulation of medicines can be accessed via the MHRA website.[3] The main provisions of the Misuse of Drugs Act 1971 are set out in Statute Box 27.1 and the 2001 regulations in Statute Box 27.2.

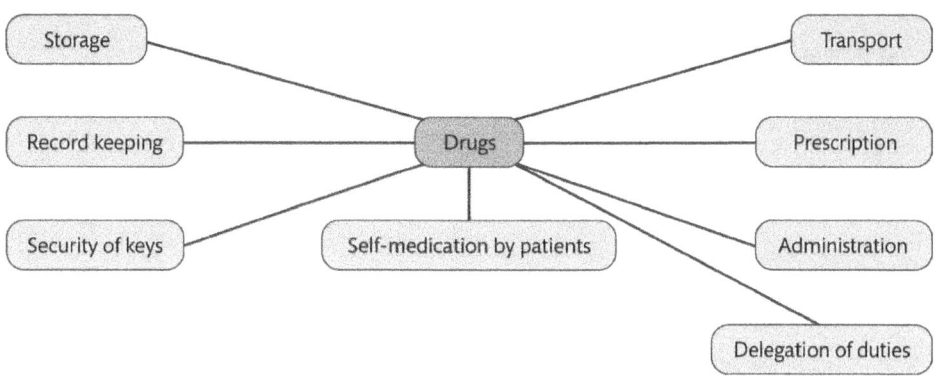

Figure 27.1 Areas that concern the nurse

Charges for prescriptions were the first charges to be introduced in the NHS and have grown steadily over the years with an increasing number of persons exempt. Wales abolished prescription charges in 2007 but the number of prescriptions issued in Wales has risen from £59.1 million to £80 million between 2007 and 2017. Wales dispensed the highest number of prescription items per head in 2017 at 25.8 compared with 20.0 in England.[4]

Figure 27.1 illustrates the main areas of control of drugs that are the concern of the nurse. Any local policy must, of course, comply with the statutory framework. Further information on medicines, medicines management and related issues can be obtained from the Royal Pharmaceutical Society,[5] which ceased to be the registration body for pharmacists with the establishment of the General Pharmaceutical Council in 2010.[6]

General principles

Under the Medicines Act, drugs are divided into categories for the purposes of supply to the public. The Part III regulations cover the following:

1. *Pharmacy-only products* (P) i.e. these can be sold or supplied retail only by someone conducting a retail pharmacy business when the product must be sold from a registered pharmacy by or under the supervision of a pharmacist.
2. *General sales list* (GSL) i.e. medicinal products that may be sold other than from a retail pharmacy, as long as provisions relating to section 53 of the Medicines Act are complied with, i.e. the place of sale must be the premises where the business is carried out; they must be capable of excluding the public; the medicines must have been made up elsewhere and the contents must not have been opened since make-up.
3. *Prescription-only list* (POM) i.e. these medicines are available only on a practitioner's prescription. Schedule 1 of the subsequent regulations lists the prescription-only products and Part II of the schedule lists the prescription-only products that are covered by the Misuse of Drugs Act. Hospitals are exempt from these prescription-only provisions, as are midwives.

The Misuse of Drugs Act and the 2001 regulations make provision for the classification of controlled drugs and their possession, supply and manufacture.

Statute 27.1
Misuse of Drugs Act 1971

1. Lists and classifies controlled drugs
2. Creates criminal offences in relation to the manufacture, supply and possession of controlled drugs
3. Gives the Secretary of State power to make regulations and directions to prevent misuse of controlled drugs
4. Creates advisory council on misuse of drugs
5. Gives powers of search, arrest and forfeiture

Statute 27.2
Medicines Acts 1968 and 1971

The Acts set up a comprehensive system of medicine controls covering:

1. administrative system
2. licensing system
3. sale and supply of medicines to the public:
   - pharmacy-only products
   - general sales list
   - prescription-only list
4. retail pharmacies
5. packing and labelling of medicinal products
6. British pharmacopoeia

NB: Exception to Part III regulations on sale and supply of medicines to the public:
- Hospitals: 'Prescription medicines may be sold or supplied by a hospital, provided they are in accordance with the written instructions of a doctor, although these instructions need not be contained in a formal prescription.'

Administration of drugs

Box 27.1 shows a checklist that a nurse should go through before a drug is administered to a patient. There is no team liability for negligence, as was seen in the Wilsher case (chapter 4, Case 4.3). Each professional must ensure that they fulfil their duties according to the approved standard of practice expected. If something goes wrong, they are accountable in the criminal courts, the civil courts, before their employer and before the Conduct and Competence Committee of the NMC for their activities and would have to show that they followed the approved accepted

Box 27.1 Checklist for the administration of drugs

1. *The correct patient. Consent?*
   Capacity to consent:
   child
   mentally ill or lacking mental capacity
   Pre-existing disability or contraindications
   Warnings about side effects, drowsiness, etc.

2. *Correct drug*
   Side effects
   Timing
   Special precautions
   Any contraindications
   Expiry date

3. *Correct dose*
   Type of patient
   Physique of patient
   Allergy frequency

4. *Correct site and method of administration*
   Injection: skin, muscular, vein, artery, site on body

5. *Correct procedure*
   Level of competence of nurse
   Skill, training
   Appropriate delegation
   Safe equipment, sound sterile procedure
   Correct gauge of needle, form of drug and transport

6. *Correct record keeping of dose, time, drug and method*

practice. Prescription-only medicines can be administered without the direction of a doctor where the situation is an emergency for the purpose of saving a life. For example, a parent or teacher who needed to administer adrenalin when a child has suffered anaphylactic shock would be covered for such actions.

Controlled drugs

The classification of controlled drugs by the Misuse of Drugs Regulations 2001 is shown in the Statute Box 27.3. Examples only are given here of the different schedules. The full list can be found in the *British National Formulary*. The nurse should be familiar with the procedure for access to the controlled drugs stock and the record keeping, the way in which any destruction of the drugs is recorded and the changes resulting from the Fourth Shipman Report. As a consequence of the Fourth Shipman Inquiry, the Health Act 2006 sections 17 to 25 introduced new laws in relation to the safe custody,[7] the supervision of management and use of controlled drugs, and regulations strengthened the governance and monitoring arrangements for controlled drugs.[8] These 2006 regulations were subsequently replaced by regulations in 2013.[9] An Accountable Officer must now be appointed within each trust to have responsibility for the safe use and management of controlled drugs. The guidance built on the safe and secure handling of medicines (known as the revised Duthie Report, March 2005). In addition, amendments to the Misuse of Drugs Regulations enabled all details on prescriptions for controlled drugs, except the signature, to be computer-generated and the computerisation of controlled drugs registers for drugs listed in Schedules 2 and 3. The final changes to record-keeping requirements can be obtained from the DH.[10] Powers were given to a constable or other authorised person to enter and inspect premises and stocks and records of controlled drugs. In May 2007 the Department of Health and the Royal Pharmaceutical Society of Great Britain published a paper on the safer management of controlled drugs.[11] In 2010 the Court of Appeal held that a person in possession of controlled drugs who intended to supply them outside the jurisdiction did not commit an offence under the Misuse of Drugs Act 1971 sections 4(1) and 5(3).[12] In April 2013 the 2006 regulations were revoked by new regulations.[13] The provisions of these regulations are set out in Statute Box 27.3.

Statute 27.3
Misuse of Drugs Regulations 2001[14]

Drugs are divided into five schedules, each specifying the requirements governing the import, export, production, supply, possession, prescribing and record keeping.

Schedule 1 e.g. cannabis, lysergide. Possession and supply prohibited except in accordance with Home Office authority.

Schedule 2 e.g. diamorphine, morphine, pethidine, glutethimide, amphetamine – subject to full controlled drug requirements relating to prescriptions, safe custody, the need to keep registers.

Schedule 3 e.g. barbiturates, diethylpropion, mazindol – subject to special prescription requirements but not safe custody requirements (except for diethylpropion) or to the need to keep registers.

Schedule 4 includes 33 benzodiazepines that are subject to minimal control. In particular, controlled drug prescription requirements do *not* apply and they are *not* subject to safe custody.

Schedule 5 preparations that, because of their strength, are exempt from most controlled drug requirements, other than retention of invoices for two years.

Makes provision for:

1. Certain exemptions from the Misuse of Drugs Act 1971 in relation to the production, importation, exportation, possession and supply of controlled drugs.
2. Prescriptions, records and furnishing of information concerning controlled drugs and for the supervision of the destruction of such drugs.

Examples of the Regulations

1. *Persons entitled* to have controlled drugs in their *possession* include under paragraph 6(7)(f): a person engaged in conveying the drug to a person who may lawfully have that drug in his possession.
2. *Administration of drugs* in Schedules 2, 3, 4 and 5, paragraph 7(3): any person other than a doctor or dentist may administer to a patient, in accordance with the direction of a doctor or dentist, any drug specified in Schedules 2, 3 and 4.

Production and supply of drugs

Paragraph 8(2)(e)

In the case of Schedule 2 and 5 drugs supplied to her by a person responsible for the dispensing and supply of medicines at the hospital or nursing home, the sister or acting sister for the time being in charge of a ward, theatre or other department in such a hospital or nursing home as aforesaid . . . may, when acting in her capacity as such, supply, or offer to supply any drug specified in Schedule 2 or 5 to any person who may lawfully have that drug in his possession, provided that nothing in the paragraph authorises:

(a) . . .
(b) a sister or acting sister for the time being in charge of a ward, theatre, or other department to supply any drug otherwise than for the administration to a patient in that ward, theatre or department in accordance with the directions of a doctor or dentist.

The CQC has been asked to monitor progress on the implementation of the 2013 regulations and overall compliance with the requirements. See Statute Box 27.4 below. Further information on the impact of these regulations and the role of the Controlled Drugs Accountable Officer (CDAO) is given in the Department of Health information guide.[15]

Statute 27.4
Regulations on supervision and management of controlled drugs

The 2013 Regulations:

designate a number of healthcare providers that are required to appoint CDAOs;
set out who may be appointed to the CDAO role and under what circumstances they should be removed from this role;
set out the registration requirements for CDAOs;
set out the core duties and functions of the CDAO including the scrutiny of the relevant staff prescribing CDs;
set out the duties of the NHS Commissioning Board in appointing CDAOs to taken the lead in establishing Local Involvement Networks (LINs) for a particular area.

Regulation 6 sets out the bodies which can provide members for LINs.

Problems in the administration of medicine

Conflict with prescriber

Practical Dilemma 27.1 — Challenging the doctor

Staff Nurse Johnson was a children's nurse with some two years' experience. One evening, a child was admitted with suspected meningitis. The house officer on call wrote the child up for antibiotics after having given an injection. Staff Nurse Johnson was surprised at the dosage and queried this with the house officer who was furious to find his treatment questioned by a nurse and confirmed that the nurse should administer that drug at the prescribed dose and at the intervals set out. Since Staff Nurse Johnson had not had many years' experience in paediatrics, she was uncertain what to do since she knew that the child was seriously ill and that a higher dose than usual might be justified in the circumstances. She also knew that it was imperative that there were no delays in administering the drug. She was in charge of the ward.

The nurse is personally accountable for their actions in administering any drug. Only in the most serious emergency where speed is of the essence could Staff Nurse Johnson rely on the fact that a doctor ordered her to give the drug and she did not have the opportunity to question the dosage because of the seriousness of the situation. In any case, where the nurse is not satisfied with some aspect of the drug they are instructed to administer, they must ensure the prescription is checked. They would have to do this despite considerable pressure brought by a junior doctor. The difficulties for Staff Nurse Johnson are that, at night, she may have to get someone in to check. She would inform her immediate nurse manager of her concern and would ask the registrar, and, if necessary, the consultant, to confirm that the medication, dosage, frequency and route are correct. If possible, she could obtain the advice of the pharmacist. In extreme circumstances, she is entitled to tell the doctor that she is refusing to administer the drug and the doctor then has the option of administering it or of rethinking the position. Staff Nurse Johnson, of course, risks disciplinary action for her refusal, but if she has good grounds for her belief that the drug or dosage is inappropriate, she should have the support of her management.

Sources of information

The nurse should also be familiar with the *British National Formulary*. There should be an up-to-date copy on the ward and they should have easy access to it. There is some useful information at the beginning, giving guidance on prescribing. The NMC withdrew their guidance on medicines management in 2018 and now advise nurses to take note of the Royal Pharmaceutical Society's guidance on *The Safe and Secure Handling of Medicines* that was revised in 2018.

Illegible writing

Nurses often complain that they are unable to read the doctors' writing on the drug charts. If they have any doubt about the drug prescribed, they should not administer it unless they have checked it with the doctor who wrote it, the doctor's superior or, in certain circumstances, the pharmacist. If the nurse fails to double-check illegible writing, they could become liable, as the following case illustrates.

Case 27.1   *Prendergast* v Sam Dee Ltd and Others [1989]

Illegible writing[16]

One of three items on a prescription was for 21 Amoxil tablets. The pharmacist misread this as Daonil. The patient suffered hypoglycaemia and sustained permanent brain damage. The pharmacist said that he had read the 'A' for a 'D' and the 'x' for an 'n'. There were other indications from which the pharmacist should have realised that his interpretation was for the wrong drug, i.e. the other drugs that were prescribed, the dosage and the fact that the patient paid for his prescription. (Daonil is a drug used by diabetic patients, who do not have to pay prescription charges.) Both doctor and pharmacist were held liable for the harm that befell the patient. The doctor was held 25 per cent liable. Damages totalled £137,547.

In a case where a woman was prescribed a top-up epidural following a hysterectomy in a private hospital, the junior doctor mistook a dose of 3 ml of diamorphine for 30 ml. The woman collapsed following its administration and the doctor was unable to use the resuscitation equipment, as he had not had the necessary training. Although the consultant was able to revive her, she died a few days later.[17]

The CQC criticised the Manchester Children's Hospital in its inspection in December 2013 because 'we found that many entries in the medical notes were illegible'.[18]

Bad maths

The UKCC (now NMC) advised in 2000 that student nurses should be given more mathematics training following claims that drug calculation errors could be putting patients at risk. Professor Bryn Davis, a UKCC member, stated that the GCSE maths exam, which is a compulsory entry requirement for training, is failing to prepare nurses for complex drug calculations.[19] An example of the fatal effects of miswriting decimals was seen in October 2000 when it was alleged that a baby in a neonatal unit died when a decimal point in a drug prescription was entered in the wrong place.[20] The death had been reported to the coroner. The issue of numeracy rose again in 2014 when it was reported that the NHS was rejecting 1 in 3 university-trained nurses because they were unable to do simple sums such as to calculate how many 15 mg tablets are required to make up 30 mg. University College London Hospitals NHS Foundation Trust found that 15 per cent of nursing applicants failed similar drug calculation tests.[21]

Management of errors or incidents in the administration of medicines

The NMC emphasises the importance of reporting errors speedily through the local risk management systems.

In 2004 the Department of Health published a new guide to improve safety in the prescribing, dispensing and administration of medicines.[22] The guide examines the causes and frequency of medication errors, highlights drugs and clinical settings that carry particular risks and identifies models of good practice for health professionals and NHS organisations.

The National Patient Safety Agency (NPSA) in its annual report for 2006/07 stated that in partnership with the DH and the Welsh Assembly it had initiated a safe medication practice work programme for 2007/08 which aimed to improve the safe use of medicines in the NHS. Patient safety alerts cover five distinct areas of medicines management: anticoagulant medicines management; liquid medicines administered via oral and other enteral routes; injectable medicines; epidural injections and infusions; and paediatric intravenous infusions. In March 2007 the NPSA published *Safety in Doses: improving the use of medicines in the NHS*. It is also looking at preventing medication errors by improving the packaging design. These reports are available on the NPSA website.[23] The NPSA graded patient safety incidents in terms of no harm (including where the incident has been prevented and where it has not been prevented), low harm where the incident required extra observation or minor treatment, moderate harm, severe harm and death. In 2009 the NPSA stated that at least 100 patients are dying or suffering serious harm each year after healthcare workers give them the wrong medication. The number of alerts relating to errors or near misses in the supply or prescription of medicines had more than doubled in two years, with 86,000 incidents regarding medication being reported in 2007. Of the cases, 96 per cent were cases of no or low harm. Causes of the mistakes were workload pressures, long hours, fatigue and reduced staff levels. The figures are based on the voluntary reporting of incidents, but it is thought that probably only about 10 per cent of incidents were being reported, so the actual figure of errors could be vastly more – perhaps 860,000. Over 82 per cent of the incidents occurred in the administration or dispensing of medicines by nurses or pharmacists. Of the deaths, 41 were caused in the administration of drugs to patients by nurses and 32 were due to prescribing.[24]

In June 2009 the NPSA published its first report into health and safety incidents involving children and stated that 61,000 alerts related to patients under 18 years with 18,200 involving babies under 1 month. A quarter of the cases were the result of misuse of medication with some patients being given 10 times too much of a drug owing to a dose miscalculation. More than 2800 alerts involved a wrong or unclear dose or strength, and children under the age of 4 were particularly affected.[25] The most frequently reported types of medication incidents involved: wrong dose, omitted or delayed medicines and wrong medicine.[26] In August 2009 it was reported that an out-of-hours GP administered six times the correct dosage of diamorphine to two patients during the same shift, killing one and causing the other to stop breathing.[27] He was given a suspended sentence for manslaughter in Germany and appeared before the GMC which removed him from its Register on the grounds that his fitness to practise was impaired because of his misconduct.[28] An article in the *British Journal of Nursing* analyses medication errors by nursing staff and suggests ways in which nursing practice can be improved to prevent their occurrence.[29] NICE together with the National Reporting and Learning Service published guidance on medicines reconciliation to ensure that patients on admission were prescribed medicines which corresponded to those the patients were taking before admission.[30] Alerts on the safety of medicines and medicinal products are published by the Medicines and Healthcare Products Regulatory Agency (MHRA).[31] In 2014 the MHRA and NHS England worked together to simplify adverse incident reporting. Further information on patient safety alert on improving medication error incident reporting and learning can be found on the website.[32]

The Department of Health publishes a list of 'never events', i.e. incidents which are considered unacceptable and eminently preventable (see page 402). The list for 2016/17 obtainable on the NHS Improvement website[33] contains 445 such events, 12 per cent of which relate to the administration of medicines, e.g. wrongly prepared high-risk injectable medication, maladministration of potassium-containing solutions, wrong route administration of chemotherapy, and intravenous administration of epidural medication.

NICE in its guidance in May 2014 on hospital staffing levels suggested that when nurses forget to give patients medication it should be seen as a 'red flag' that a ward is dangerously understaffed (see chapter 4). In 2014 the Secretary of State initiated a 'Sign up to Safety' campaign for trusts to identify serious mistakes and take action to halve the incidence. In February 2018 the Health and Social Care Secretary announced new measures to tackle medication errors that are estimated to contribute to some 22,000 deaths each year.[34] Details of the measures are set out in the report of the Short Life Working Group on reducing medication-related harm.[35]

Shared liability

It may happen that several different practitioners are involved in an incident that causes harm to a patient. The court has to determine the respective responsibility of each person and their employer (if any). Under the Civil Liability (Contribution) Act 1978, a successful claimant can obtain compensation from any one of several defendants and that defendant can then claim from the other defendants reimbursement according to their responsibility for the harm. An example of this is given in Case 27.2. The case does not involve a nurse, but if the situation were in a hospital context rather than in the home, one can imagine a nurse being involved.

Case 27.2 *Dwyer v Roderick* [1984]

Over-prescribing[36]

It was alleged by Mrs Dwyer that Dr Roderick prescribed a particular drug (Migril) and was negligent in choosing the number and frequency with which the relevant tablets should be taken, so that within a relatively short time she had received a dangerous overdose. The manufacturers had warned that not more than four tablets should be taken for any one attack of migraine and that no more than 12 tablets should be taken in the course of 1 week. Dr Roderick's prescription was for two tablets to be taken every 4 hours as necessary. He prescribed a total of 60 tablets. Dr Roderick admitted that this was utterly wrong: 'I have no satisfactory explanation. It was a mental aberration.' When the prescription was taken for dispensing, there were two qualified pharmacists in the shop, neither of whom noticed the error and simply repeated Dr Roderick's instructions on the label. They in turn accepted some liability. Over the next six days, Mrs Dwyer took 36 Migril tablets. As a result of this overdose, she suffered serious personal injuries, i.e. irreversible ergotamine poisoning which resulted in constriction of the blood vessels and gangrene of her toes and lower limbs. As well as suing the chemists and Dr Roderick, Mrs Dwyer sued as second defendant Dr Roderick's partner, Dr Jackson, who saw her three days after the prescription had been given and who failed to discover the fact that his partner had over-prescribed the drug and failed to stop her taking it.

In Case 27.2, the trial judge decided that each defendant was liable: Dr Roderick was 45 per cent liable, Dr Jackson was 15 per cent liable and the pharmacists were 40 per cent liable. The Court of Appeal held by a majority that Dr Jackson was not negligent. It accepted his evidence that it was his usual practice to enquire what medication a patient was on. Liability was thus divided between Dr Roderick and the pharmacists. Mrs Dwyer received £92,000 compensation.

One particularly interesting aspect of this case is that the incident occurred in November 1973, but did not come to court until 1982. Thus the actual evidence of what happened was scanty and undoubtedly made Mrs Dwyer's case against Dr Jackson very difficult. The court commented adversely on the delay and suggested that the time might be ripe for changes designed to enable the court and the judiciary to play a greater part in encouraging the parties and their advisers to speed up the process of litigation. These changes have now taken place (known as the Woolf Reforms) and are discussed in chapter 6. Cases may still commence many years after an incident (see chapter 6 on limitation of time) and therefore nurses must be aware of the importance of record keeping (see chapter 9). In any such incident, the nurse is likely to have very little personal recall, but will be heavily dependent on the clarity and comprehensiveness of the records.

Fitness to practise case

Case 27.3 Fitness to practise[37]

A registered general nurse who was employed first as the lead nurse in an ophthalmology department, then on a care of the elderly ward, faced allegations that she put an instruction to 'dilate both eyes' on a patient's notes without medical authorisation, that she administered a drug via the wrong route and while she was not competent to do so, and made a false entry on a patient's fluid balance chart relating to that drug error. The nurse admitted all the charges except that of making the false entry.

In hearing Case 27.3 the Professional Conduct Committee of the NMC found the facts proved and were convinced by the evidence that the nurse had added the letters SC (subcutaneous) at a later date. It found that the proved facts of all the charges amounted to misconduct. It decided that the nurse's name should be removed from the Register.

PRN medication

PRN medication (*pro re nata* – 'as required, whenever necessary') enables a doctor to write the patient up for medication, but leaves to the nurse the discretion as to when, if at all, the drug should be administered, depending on the patient's condition.

The value of this system is that it allows the patient to have a drug when necessary, without calling the doctor for the specific purpose of prescribing the drug for it to be administered immediately. Thus pain relief drugs, sleeping tablets and indigestion drugs can be prescribed in case the patient might need such help. Unfortunately, the doctor does not always ensure that sufficient information is given on the drugs sheet. He or she might, for instance, fail to give the maximum amount that can be given in any 24-hour period. He or she might also fail to specify the dose and the intervals at which it can be given. The hospital pharmacist should check the drugs sheets regularly to ensure that all the relevant information is present and the nurse should not administer these drugs without first checking the limitations. It is also essential that every drug that is administered PRN should be recorded when given, as overdoses could easily occur if a record is not kept. Each hospital should have a policy relating to PRN medication.

Infusion therapy

Since 1968 there have been many cases of inadvertent intrathecal injection of the vinca alkaloid drug vincristine reported around the world (and around half of these have been in England). One of the targets of the National Patient Safety Agency (see chapter 12) was to reduce the number of patients dying or being paralysed by maladministered spinal injections to zero by the end of 2001. A junior doctor in Nottingham pleaded guilty to manslaughter following the administration of a chemotherapy drug by epidural rather than IV to a patient suffering from leukaemia (see chapter 2). The RCN published guidance for administering IV drugs in the community to children.[38] Guidance on standards for infusion therapy in hospitals and the community was published by the RCN in 2003.[39] These provide information on standards on:

- infection control;
- most appropriate infusion devices and infusion-related equipment;
- infusion-related complications;
- infusion therapies, including chemotherapy, analgesia, transfusion and epidural; and
- placement, care and maintenance of vascular access devices.

The RCN has subsequently provided guidance for community nurses on advance preparation of insulin syringes for patients to administer at home.[40] This aims to assist elderly patients to manage their insulin injections. Further publications from the RCN include *Guidance on Competences: an education and training competency framework for administering medicines intravenously to children and young people*[41] and *Right Blood, Right Patients, Right Time. RCN guidance for improving transfusion practice*.[42]

Updated national guidance on the safe administration of intrathecal chemotherapy was issued by the Department of Health in 2003 and updated in 2008.[43] The guidance contained in the annexe to the circular was to be fully complied with by NHS trusts by 30 November 2003. A training toolkit and video were issued to support local induction and training programmes. Under the guidance, the chief executive of a trust is required to identify a designated lead to oversee compliance within the trust; trusts that undertake fewer than ten procedures a year (low-volume trusts) should carry out a risk assessment to decide if they should continue to provide the service; high-volume trusts (500+ procedures a year) should carry out a risk assessment to check the capacity and safety of the service; a written local protocol should be drawn up and a register established to identify personnel who have been trained and are authorised to prescribe, dispense, issue, check or administer; automatic inclusion in a hospital's register on the transfer of staff should not occur. There should be annual reviews of competence and a certificate or other written confirmation of competence should be issued. The guidance also includes advice on those eligible to prescribe, documentation, storage, administration of intrathecal chemotherapy after intravenous chemotherapy has been administered, an area should be designated for the administration of intrathecal chemotherapy and it should only be administered in normal working hours. Guidance on waivers is also given.

Instructions by telephone and remote assessment and prescribing

The situation highlighted in Practical Dilemma 27.2 is not uncommon.

Practical Dilemma 27.2 — Night orders

Ward Sister Dury was the night sister at a small hospital that was served by GPs. One night she was very worried about the condition of a frail patient whose blood pressure and temperature were raised. She telephoned the duty GP and expressed her anxieties to him. He was of the opinion that she need not be concerned and suggested that the patient should be given paracetamol. She was reluctant to take instructions over the telephone, but decided that, since he would not visit, there was little else she could do for the patient. She gave the dose of paracetamol, but unfortunately the patient's condition deteriorated and she again telephoned the GP, who did not visit until 9.00 a.m. the next day, by which time the patient had died.

What is the position of the ward sister? Should she have taken instructions over the telephone?

Practice Standard 20 of the NMC standards of proficiency for nurse and midwife prescribers covers remote prescribing via telephone, email, fax, video link or website and states:

20.1 From time to time it may be appropriate to use a telephone or other non face-to-face medium to prescribe medicines and treatment for patient/clients. Such situations may occur where:
 (a) You have responsibility for the care of the patient/client;
 (b) You are working in remote and rural areas;
 (c) You have prior knowledge and understanding of the patient/client's condition and medical history; [and]
 (d) You have authority to access the patient/client's records and you are working within the scope of a supplementary prescriber, but the doctor/dentist required to authorise the clinical management plan works at a distance.

20.2 In all circumstances, you must ensure that you:
 (a) Establish the patient/client's current medical conditions, history and concurrent or recent use of other medications including non-prescription medicines;
 (b) Carry out an adequate assessment of the patient/client's condition (in line with Practice Standard 3);
 (c) Identify the likely cause of the patient/client's condition;
 (d) Ensure that there is sufficient justification to prescribe the medicines or treatment proposed. Where appropriate you should discuss other treatment options with the patient/client;
 (e) Ensure that the treatment and/or medicine is not contra-indicated for the patient/client;
 (f) Make a clear, accurate, legible and contemporaneous record of all medicines prescribed; [and]
 (g) Are competent to make a prescribing decision.

20.3 Where you cannot meet all of these requirements you must not use remote means to prescribe medicine for a patient/client.

The NMC set out its position on remote assessment and prescribing in 2008.[44] It sets out its support of the use of remote assessment and prescribing and lays down the procedure which should be followed.

It would now be possible for patient group directions to be drawn up so that, following appropriate training, the ward sister could prescribe and administer against an agreed protocol.

Self-administration by patients

The involvement of the patient in his or her own medication is increasingly being adopted as a form of rehabilitation and as a move towards discharge and the assumption by the patient of responsibility for their own health and care.

The nurse must ensure that the patient is able to open the medicine containers or is offered assistance, e.g. compliance aid.

Although the nurse has a duty of care towards all patients, the registrant is not liable if a patient makes a mistake self-administering as long as the assessment was completed as the local policy describes and appropriate actions were taken to prevent re-occurrence of the incident.

Guidance has been published by the Royal Pharmaceutical Society of Great Britain on medicines management during patient admission to the ward, which includes guidance on the self-administration of medicines.[45] The Care Quality Commission published a report in 2009 on the management of patients' medicines after discharge from hospital[46] raising many concerns, including the fact that of those researched only 14 per cent of GPs gave information on medicines which should be stopped. In 47 per cent of the GP practices visited, discharge summaries from hospitals were not received in enough time to be useful and 81 per cent of practices reported that details of prescribed medicines were incomplete or inaccurate all the time or most of the time.

Covert administration of medicines

It is a basic principle of law that the consent of an adult to treatment including medication is required. However, problems can arise when an adult lacks the mental capacity to give consent. The UKCC published a position statement in 2001[47] on the covert administration of medicines disguised in food or drink. The guidance was republished by the NMC in the form of a position statement within its A–Z advice sheets.[48] (These A–Z sheets are no longer in use.) The advice was updated in 2007.[49] It makes clear that covert administration would not apply to a patient who had the mental capacity to make his or her own decisions even in a life-saving situation and could only be justified where the patient lacked the mental capacity to make his or her own decisions and the administration of medicines in this way was in the best interests of the patient. The NMC stated:

> **The covert administration of medicines is only likely to be necessary or appropriate in the case of patients or clients who actively refuse medication but who are judged not to have the capacity to understand the consequences of their refusal.**

The NMC recommends that any local policies on covert administration should be revised in the light of its statement.

A review carried out for the Department of Health in November 2009[50] found that over 144,000 patients suffering from dementia were being given anti-psychotic drugs unnecessarily. It estimated that only 36,000 of the 180,000 people being given the drugs derive any benefit from them. The drugs are misused as a chemical cosh to suppress the anxiety and distress common in people with dementia.[51] (See also chapter 18.)

The United Kingdom Supreme Court's judgment in *Cheshire West and Chester Council* v *P* [2014][52] has had a huge impact on the promotion of human rights of vulnerable patients. The ruling emphasises the positive duty on the state and its organisations, such as the NHS, to have in place procedures that independently confirm that the human rights of vulnerable patients in hospitals and other care settings are being applied in the same way as any other human being. The Supreme Court ensured that the state was obliged to independently verify the care arrangements of vulnerable incapable adults.

The European Court of Human Rights requires three elements be considered when identifying a deprivation of liberty:

1. Objective element, i.e. the person is confined in a particular restricted space for a not negligible length of time.
2. Subjective element, i.e. the person has not consented to the restrictions.
3. Deprivation of liberty is one for which state is responsible (e.g. *HL* v *United Kingdom (45508/99)* (2005)[53]).

When considering the objective element, the Supreme Court in *Cheshire West* held that the key acid test was that the patient was under continuous supervision and control and was not free to leave. All three parts of the test must be present for the objective element to be satisfied.

Objective deprivation of liberty and covert administration

Covert administration of medicines usually means disguising medication by administering it in food or drink so that the person takes the drug unknowingly.[54] Nurses sometimes resort to this method of administration where a patient who lacks capacity has refused to take medication when offered and treatment is in the best interests of the person's physical or mental health. The Nursing and Midwifery Council (NMC) takes a general view that disguising medication in food or drink is not good practice. The NMC nevertheless accepts that covert administration may be acceptable as a last resort measure where doing so is in the best interests of the patient but emphasise that the nurse is accountable for their decision.[55] The National Institute for Health and Care Excellence (NICE)[56] also argue that the covert administration of medicines should only be used in exceptional circumstances when and where a management plan is in place following a formal best interest meeting attended by nursing staff, the prescriber and pharmacist and a person who can communicate the views and interests of the patient such as a family member, friend or independent mental capacity advocate.

A decision by the Court of Protection has held that the use of covert administration of medicines with adults who lack decision-making capacity is a serious interference with a person's right to liberty and a private life under articles 5 and 8 of the European Convention of Human Rights.[57] The use of medication covertly whether for physical health or for mental health always calls for close scrutiny that, for vulnerable, incapable patients in hospital, can be achieved by obtaining a Deprivation of Liberty Safeguard standard authorisation under the Mental Capacity Act 2005, Schedule A1.

In *AG* v *BMBC & SNH* [2016][58] the Court of Protection was hearing an appeal against the issuing of a standard authorisation of the deprivation of liberty of a 92-year-old woman. When reviewing the evidence it became clear that the woman's care involved the covert administration of sedative medication in the form of promethazine and then diazepam. The judge was concerned that proper consideration was not given to the initial covert use of promethazine and the use of covert medication was not subject to proper reviews or safeguards. He was also concerned that a decision to then administer diazepam covertly after a standard authorisation of a deprivation of liberty was in place was not communicated to the supervisory body or to the relevant person's representative (RPR). The best interest decision-making process for the covert use of diazepam did not involve family members or RPR. There was also no provision for reviewing the decision to administer medication covertly even though the evidence of the managing authority suggested that NICE guidelines were being followed.

The judge held that covert medication is an interference with the right to respect for private life under Article 8 of the European Convention on Human Rights and a restriction that contributes to the finding that the patient is being subject to continuous supervision and control that are relevant to the existence of a deprivation of liberty. Such a serious interference with a vulnerable person's human rights requires evidence-based objective justification and further safeguards by way of independent review of the decision to covertly administer medicines.

Managing authorities, currently hospitals and care homes, have a duty to seek a standard authorisation where they believe the restrictions in a patient's care plan, including the covert use of medication, amounts to a deprivation of liberty (Mental Capacity Act 2005, schedule A1, para 24). Managing authorities also have a duty to keep the authorisation under review and seek a prompt reassessment from the supervisory body should the nature of the restriction change (Mental Capacity Act 2005, schedule A1, para 103). In *AG* v *BMBC & SNH* [2016] the court held that administering newly prescribed medication covertly was one such reason for a request to review a standard authorisation.

Court of Protection guidance

The Court (*AG* v *BMBC & SNH* [2016] (District Judge Bellamy)) issued the following guidance to assist in cases of covert administration of medicine and deprivation of liberty:

- Where there is a covert medication policy in place to decide on the use of covert administration it must include full consultation between healthcare professionals and family.
- Administering medication covertly must be clearly identified within the care plan, assessment of deprivation of liberty and authorisation of a deprivation of liberty.
- If the standard authorisation is for longer than six months there should be clear provision for regular, monthly, reviews of the care plan.
- There should also be regular reviews involving the family, RPR and healthcare professionals.
- Any change of medication or treatment regime should trigger a review where the medication is covertly administered.
- Supervisory bodies and best interests assessors should consider placing appropriate conditions to the standard authorisation that ensure these guidelines are complied with.

Nurse as prescriber

There have been major developments in the scope of professional practice of the nurse, which are considered in chapter 23. Of these developments, one of the most significant ones is nurse prescribing. This section looks at the current situation in relation to nurse prescribing following the Crown Report.

Community nurse prescribing

Prescribing by community nurses was recommended by the Cumberlege Report in 1986[59] and these conclusions were supported in the report of the advisory group on nurse prescribing (known as the First Crown Report) to the Department of Health in December 1989. Legislation was passed to give specified practitioners the power to prescribe specified medicines (Medicinal Products (Prescription by Nurses) Act 1992). Health visitors and community nurses who had had the requisite training could prescribe in the community from a nursing formulary. In February 2000,[60] prescribing powers were given to nurses employed by a doctor on the medical list (i.e. GP) and also to nurses working in walk-in centres, defined in the regulations as 'A centre at which information and treatment for minor conditions is provided to the public under arrangements made by or on behalf of the Secretary of State'.

Practical Dilemma 27.3 — Holding stocks in the community

Brenda was a community nurse who was eligible to prescribe medicines in the community. Often patients would, when the treatment had ended, offer her dressings and other medicines that they had been prescribed and were left over. She was happy to take them since to dispose of them would be a waste. She thus built up a considerable stock, which she kept in the boot of her car, and would issue to new patients before their prescriptions had been dispensed. She is now concerned to know the legality of what she is doing.

There are considerable dangers in the practice followed by Brenda. In the first place, the medicinal products obtained on prescription for one patient should be used for that patient and not for others. Second, by supplying these medicinal products to others, she could be seen as the supplier under the Consumer Protection Act 1987 (see chapter 12) and become liable for any defects. In addition, there is the security and safety aspect of keeping such products in the boot of her car. To ensure that a safe practice is followed, she should discuss with her manager and the pharmacist the possibility of the pharmacist taking the unwanted goods back into stock.

Supplying medicines in hospital and primary care

The legal changes permitting nurse prescribing in the community brought into focus the situation in hospitals and family practitioner centres where supplying medicines by nurses was taking place according to protocols or written instructions signed by the delegating doctor. The anomalies raised by this quasi-legal situation led the government to appoint Dr June Crown to review the position on prescribing, supply and administration of medicines and make recommendations (First Crown Report).[61]

Group protocols or patient group directions

The Crown Committee first considered the arrangements for and legality of group protocols and reported in March 1998 and recommended legislation to ensure that their legal validity was clarified. The criteria against which any group protocol should be tested were set out in the Report. It recommended that certain products should be excluded from group protocols. These included:

1. new drugs under intensive monitoring and subject to special adverse reaction reporting requirements (the Black Triangle scheme)[62];
2. unlicensed medicines;
3. medicines used outside their licensed indications; and
4. medicines being used in clinical trials.

As a consequence of the Crown Report on group protocols, new regulations came into force on 9 August 2000.[63] These provided for patient group directions to be drawn up to make provision for the sale or supply of a prescription-only medicine in hospitals in accordance with the written direction of a doctor or dentist. To be lawful, the patient group direction must cover the particulars that are set out in Part I of Schedule 7 of the Statutory Instrument. These particulars are shown in Box 27.2.

The classes of individuals by whom supplies may be made are set out in Part III of Schedule 7 and include the following:

1. ambulance paramedics (who are registered or hold a certificate of proficiency),
2. pharmacists,
3. registered health visitors,
4. registered midwives,
5. registered nurses,
6. registered ophthalmic opticians,
7. state registered chiropodists/podiatrists,
8. state registered orthoptists,
9. state registered physiotherapists, and
10. state registered radiographers.

The person who is to supply or administer the medicine must be designated in writing on behalf of the authorising person for the purpose of the patient group direction. In addition to compliance with the particulars set out in Box 27.2, a patient group direction must be signed on behalf of the authorising person. The Department of Health has developed patient group directions for certain chemical and biological countermeasures in emergency situations, such as atropine, and these can be downloaded from its website[64] The Royal Pharmaceutical Society of Great Britain updated in 2008 a resource pack for pharmacists on patient group directions which would also be of interest to NMC-registered practitioners and this is available on its website. In 2009 the NMC published guidance for student nurses and student midwives on the patient group directions (PGDs) making it clear that these students could not administer medicines using PGDs even if under direct supervision.[65] Guidance is also available from the Medicines and Healthcare Products Regulatory Authority and the National Prescribing Centre (now in NICE).

Box 27.2 Particulars for patient group direction

- Period during which the direction shall have effect.
- Description or class of prescription-only medicines to which the direction relates.
- Whether there are any restrictions on the quantity of medicine which may be supplied on any one occasion and, if so, what restrictions.
- Clinical situations that prescription-only medicines of that description or class may be used to treat.
- Clinical criteria under which a person shall be eligible for treatment.
- Whether any class of person is excluded from treatment under the direction and, if so, what class of person.
- Whether there are circumstances in which further advice should be sought from a doctor or dentist and, if so, what circumstances.
- Pharmaceutical form or forms in which prescription-only medicines of that description or class are to be administered.
- Strength, or maximum strength, at which prescription-only medicines of that description or class are to be administered.
- Applicable dosage or maximum dosage.
- Route of administration.
- Frequency of administration.
- Any minimum or maximum period of administration applicable to prescription-only medicines of that description or class.
- Whether there are any relevant warnings to note and, if so, what warnings.
- Whether there is any follow-up action to be taken in any circumstances and, if so, what action and in what circumstances.
- Arrangements for referral for medical advice.
- Details of the records to be kept of the supply or the administration of medicines under the direction.

Nurse prescribing: independent and dependent (subsequently known as supplementary) prescribers

In March 1999 the Final Crown Report was published.[66] Its terms of reference included the requirements:

1. to develop a consistent policy framework to guide judgements on the circumstances in which health professionals might undertake new responsibilities with regard to prescribing, supply and administration of medicines;
2. to advise on the likely impact of any proposed changes; and
3. to consider possible implications for legislation, professional training and standards.

Its most significant recommendation was that there should be two types of prescriber:

- The *independent prescriber* who is defined as the person who is responsible for the assessment of patients with undiagnosed conditions and for decisions about the clinical management required, including prescribing. This group would include doctors, dentists and certain nurses who are already legally authorised prescribers. Other health professionals may also become newly legally authorised independent prescribers.
- The *dependent prescriber* (now known as the *supplementary prescriber*) who is defined as the person who is responsible for the continuing care of patients who have been clinically assessed by an independent practitioner. The continuing care can include prescribing that will be informed by clinical guidelines and will be consistent with individual treatment plans. Dependent prescribers may also be involved in continuing established treatments by issuing repeat prescriptions, with authority to adjust the dose or dosage form according to patients' needs. There should be provision for regular clinical review by the assessing clinician.

Nurse independent prescribing

Legislation implementing the Final Crown Report recommendations was contained in section 63 of the Health and Social Care Act 2001, which amended the Medicines Act 1968 and enabled the Secretary of State to draw up regulations to lay down the conditions on which prescribing powers can be extended to specified health professionals. A nurse independent prescriber means a person (a) who is a registered nurse or registered midwife and (b) against whom is recorded in the professional register an annotation signifying that she is qualified to order drugs, medicines and appliances as a nurse independent prescriber or a nurse independent/supplementary prescriber. A qualified nurse, independent prescribers are now able to prescribe any licensed medicine for any medical condition within their competence, including some controlled drugs.

Nurse independent prescribers were only able to prescribe or administer a limited range of controlled drugs as set out in Schedule 3A of the Statutory Instrument. However, this was extended in 2012 when the Department of Health announced changes to nurse and pharmacist independent prescribing. As a result of changes to the Misuse of Drugs Regulations appropriately qualified nurses and pharmacists are able to prescribe, supply, offer to supply and administer controlled drugs like morphine, diamorphine and prescription strength co-codamol. (This does not apply to the supply to people addicted to cocaine, diamorphine or dipipanone to addicts otherwise than for the purpose of treating organic disease or injury.) Changes include the authority to mix drugs listed in Schedules 2–5. In addition, nurses and pharmacists working under a PGD can supply or administer diamorphine and morphine where administration of such drugs is required for the immediate and necessary treatment of sick and injured persons (excluding the treatment of addiction). (Previously a nurse could only supply diamorphine under a PGD for the treatment of cardiac pain in patients admitted to a coronary care unit or A&E department of a hospital.)[67]

The NMC has issued guidance on disclosure barring service checks, and the educational and training requirements for independent prescribing and for specialist community public health nursing programmes.[68]

Additional criteria for eligibility to become an independent nurse prescriber

In its guidance on implementation the Department of Health has advised that, in addition to fulfilling the legal criteria, applicants for the prescribing preparation will need:

- the ability to study at level 3 (degree level);
- at least three years' post-registration clinical nursing experience (or part-time equivalent): nominees will usually be at band 6 or above;
- a medical prescriber willing to contribute and to supervise the nurse's twelve-day learning in the practice element of preparation; and
- the support of the employer and confirmation of certain conditions.

The three key principles to prioritise potential applicants for training as independent nurse prescribers are seen by the DH as being:

- patient safety;
- maximum benefit to patients in terms of quicker and more efficient access to medicines for patients; and
- better use of nurses' skills.

Supplementary prescribing

This is defined by the NMC as:

> A voluntary partnership between an independent prescriber (doctor/dentist) and a supplementary prescriber, to implement an agreed patient/client-specific clinical management plan with the patient/client's agreement.

Following the recommendations of the Final Crown Report in 1999 the Department of Health[69] in April 2002 announced its intention of introducing supplementary prescribing by a nurse or pharmacist in 2003. The aim was to enable the pharmacists and nurses to work in partnership with doctors and help treat such conditions as asthma, diabetes, high blood pressure and arthritis. The doctor would draw up a plan with the patient's agreement – known as the clinical management plan – laying out the range of medicines that may be prescribed and when to refer back to the doctor. This early announcement was followed by a press release in

November 2002,[70] which gave further details of the patient conditions and the medicinal products that would be the subject of supplementary prescribing. In April 2005 chiropodists and podiatrists, physiotherapists and radiographers were added to the list of those who could become supplementary prescribers, and restrictions on their prescribing controlled drugs or unlicensed medicines were removed.[71]

The clinical management plan must be agreed with the patient in relation to specified conditions. It must state the name of the patient, the condition being treated, the class or description of medical products that can be prescribed or administered and the circumstances in which the supplementary prescriber should refer back to the independent prescriber.

NMC guidance on prescribing

The NMC has published Standards of *Proficiency for Nurse and Midwife Prescribers*.[72] Sections cover:

- **the educational and training provision to prepare nurses and midwives to prescribe;**
- **standards for prescribing practice;**
- **additional guidance; and**
- **annexe 2 sets out the principal areas, knowledge, skills and competencies required to underpin prescribing practice.**

The guidance sets down 21 Practice Standards which cover such topics as accountability, consent, communication, record keeping, prescribing and dispensing, clinical management plans for supplementary prescribing, evidence-based prescribing and continuing professional development. The document can be downloaded from the NMC website.

Implications of nurse prescribing for the scope of professional practice

The Crown Report and subsequent developments have, in a sense, given approval to a controlled development of professional competence in areas formerly the sole preserve of medical staff. However, clear checks are in place to ensure that these developments take place with well-defined precautions to secure patient safety and also to secure efficient use of resources. While nurses are likely to be the most numerous group to develop prescribing skills, other professionals, such as physiotherapists, radiographers, orthoptists, dietitians, speech therapists and many others, have found that the new legislation has facilitated professional development or at the minimum validated activities already taking place. The need to obtain a doctor's personal attendance on a patient in order that a specific drug could be prescribed has placed an unnecessary obstacle in the advancement of professional practice for many health professionals and this has now been lifted. (Issues relating to the scope of professional practice and the role of the clinical nurse specialist and the consultant nurse are discussed in chapter 23.)

Perhaps the most important of the recommendations in the final Crown Report is that to individual practitioners:

> All legally authorised prescribers should take personal responsibility for maintaining and updating their knowledge and practice related to prescribing, including taking part in clinical audit, and should never prescribe in situations beyond their professional competence.

Electronic prescriptions

Regulations were enacted in 2001 to allow the use of an electronic signature for the electronic transmission of prescriptions in pilot studies and this is extended to CCGs to facilitate the use of electronic prescriptions.[73] The system allows the patient's prescription to be sent electronically from their GP to a pharmacy. Further information on the current stage of the initiative can be obtained from the Department of Health website or from the Health and Social Care Information Centre (which took over the functions of Connecting for Health in March 2013.)[74]

Mixing of medicines prior to administration

Following the recommendations of the Commission on Human Medicine regulations were amended[75] to enable doctors and other prescribers to mix medicines themselves and to direct (in writing) others to mix medicines (mixing is seen as manufacturing which is closely regulated). The Department of Health issued guidance in May 2010.[76] The NMC has also provided advice for its registrants.[77]

Role of the pharmacist

In January 2014 heads of 23 health groups including the Royal College of Nursing and the Royal College of GPs urged patients to seek advice from pharmacists instead of going to the GP.[78] Professor Darracott of Pharmacy Voice estimated that 51 million GP visits could have been dealt with at a pharmacy. As a consequence of the changes made by the Human Medicines Regulations in 2012[79] pharmacists are able to make changes to prescriptions in the exercise of their professional skill and judgement if they believe it appropriate to do so, including the name of the product or its common name, the directions for use of the product and precautions relating to the use of the product.

Safety of medicines

The Committee on Safety of Medicines was one committee set up under section 4 of the Medicines Act on the advice of the Medicines Commission to the Minister. It is regulated under Schedule 1 of the Medicines Act and under Statutory Instrument.[80] It can in turn set up its own subcommittees. Like all other section 4 committees and the Medicines Commission itself, it must submit an annual report about its work to ministers. The Medicines Control Agency was the licensing authority under the Medicines Act and the European Regulations and had the function of monitoring the safety and quality of medicines. It operated a Defective Medicines Report Centre. On 1 April 2003 the Medicines Control Agency was amalgamated with the Medical Devices Agency to form the Medicines and Healthcare Products Regulatory Agency (MHRA). The MHRA and the Committee on the Safety of Medicines publish a drug safety update bulletin which provides information on adverse drug reactions. For example doctors were advised by the MHRA not to prescribe codeine for children under 12 years.[81] The MHRA has the responsibility of pharmacovigilance (safety of medicines) in accordance with Directives from the EU[82] and supervises the yellow card adverse drug reaction scheme. Directive 2012/26/EU of the European Parliament amending regulations on pharmacovigilance were incorporated into UK law by regulations which came into force on 11 November 2013.[83]

The yellow card scheme

A yellow card adverse drug reaction (ADR) reporting scheme is a voluntary scheme, through which doctors, dentists, coroners and pharmacists notify the Medicines Control Agency (MCA)/Committee on Safety of Medicines (CSM) of suspected adverse drug reactions. The yellow cards for completion can be found at the back of the *British National Formulary (BNF)/Nurse Prescribers' Formulary (NPF)*. The MCA/CSM encourage the reporting of all suspected adverse drug reactions to newly licensed medicines that are under intensive monitoring (identified by a Δ symbol both on the product information for the drug and in the *BNF* and *MIMS*), and all serious suspected adverse drug reactions to all other established drugs. Serious reactions include those that are fatal, life-threatening, disabling, incapacitating or which result in or prolong hospitalisation and/or are medically significant. The yellow card reporting scheme was extended to nurses, midwives and health visitors in 2002. At the same time an electronic reporting system was introduced to enable quicker and easier submission of reports. Patients are able to report adverse medicinal reactions (NHS 111). In 2013 the Chief Nursing Officer issued a bulletin emphasising the importance of nurses reporting adverse drug reactions.[84] A Freedom of Information inquiry by *The Times* found that figures for the reporting of adverse drug reactions had dropped, with the Chair of the Royal College of GPs suggesting that family doctors found it difficult to make time to use the yellow card scheme.[85] In 2013 there were 116,348 reports of suspected adverse reactions with 2715 from the public and 13,633 from healthcare professionals. (See also chapter 12 and the role of the National Patient Safety Agency.) Rules relating to the sale of herbal medicines and recent EU Directives are considered in chapter 29.

Product liability and drugs

The case brought against the manufacturers of Opren has shown the difficulties and expense of suing a company for harm caused by medication. Initially, a judge decided that a class action could not be brought on behalf of all those who claimed to have suffered side effects, but each person claiming compensation would have to sue individually and contribute his share to the total costs. This led to a demand for changes in the procedure in respect of such actions involving thousands of litigants. Class actions have now been initiated in respect of several drug products.

Under the present laws of negligence it is in any case difficult to show that a firm failed to take all reasonable care in testing and manufacturing its products. The victims of thalidomide did not establish negligence by the Distillers Company in this country, but agreed an *ex gratia* settlement, which was subsequently increased. It is possible that the Consumer Protection Act 1987 Part I, which is applicable to damage suffered after the Act came into force, will make any action for liability by someone harmed by drugs easier on the basis that, provided the patient can prove that he has suffered injury as a result of a defect in a particular drug, it is then up to the manufacturer to show that one of the many defences open to him under the Act was present. (This is further discussed in chapter 12.)

Misuse of drugs

Nurses may sometimes encounter patients in their work who are addicted to various substances. They should know the law relating to such persons and how it affects their own position. In the past, there was a requirement that doctors should send to the Home Office particulars of drug addicts. However, this requirement was revoked by the Misuse of Drugs (Supply to Addicts) Regulations 1997 in May 1997.[86] Doctors are now expected to report on a standard form cases of drug misuse to their local Drug Misuse Database (DMD). Phone numbers are set out in the *BNF*. The notification to the DMD should be made when a patient first presents with a drug problem or re-presents after a gap of six months or more. All types of problem drug misuse should be reported, including opioid, benzo-diazepine and CNS stimulant misuse. The data held on the databases is anonymised, so it cannot be used to check on multiple prescribing. Under the Misuse of Drugs (Supply to Addicts) Regulations 1997, only medical practitioners who hold a special licence issued by the Home Secretary may prescribe, administer or supply diamorphine, Diconal or cocaine in the treatment of drug addiction. Other practitioners must refer any addict who requires these drugs to a treatment centre. Guidance on notification is provided in the *BNF*. The Crime and Justice Act 2013 amends the Road Traffic Act 1985 by adding section 5A to make it an offence to drive or be in charge of a motor vehicle with concentrations of specific controlled drugs above set limits. It is a defence if the drug had been prescribed for medical or dental purposes, but the defence fails if the person had been warned not to drive.

A National Treatment Agency (NTA)[87] for substance abuse was established in 2001 as a special health authority to exercise on behalf of the Secretary of State such functions in connection with the treatment of drug misusers and such other functions as he may direct it to perform.[88] Its overall purpose was to improve the availability, capacity and effectiveness of treatment for drug misuse in England. Regulations relating to membership, termination of office and the appointment of committees and the duty to furnish reports and certain other information to the Secretary of State have been passed.[89] It became part of Public Health England in 2013.[90] In 2004 the change of status of cannabis from a Class B to a Class C drug was implemented despite considerable pressure from organisations such as the British Medical Association and others alleging a link between cannabis usage and psychosis. The Advisory Council on the Misuse of Drugs had concluded that there was no evidence that cannabis caused mental illness.[91] The Home Office launched a £1 million campaign to explain to parents and young people the new law on the possession of cannabis. However, in 2008 legislation led to its reclassification as Category B.[92] The Department of Health has set up an A–Z guide on all its substance misuse guidance and publications which can be accessed via its website.

In September 2009 Jack Straw, then Minister of Justice, called for heroin to be made available on the NHS to addicts at regulated clinics on the grounds that this would reduce criminal behaviour.[93] His proposals led to considerable controversy on the grounds that this would not wean addicts off the drug, and there was no indication that the coalition government was inclined to support this development. In July 2010 the Centre for Social Justice recommended that the National Treatment Agency should be abolished and replaced by an Addiction Recovery Board with the aim of getting addicts off drugs altogether, and that methadone should only be used as part of a wider treatment programme aiming at abstinence.[94] In August 2010 DrugScope called for illicit substances to be decriminalised[95] and this is in line with a paper from the United Nations Office of Drugs and Crime which calls for a move from a sanction-based approach to a health-oriented one.

A White Paper published in December 2010 on *Drugs Strategy* and the White Paper in November 2010 *Healthy Lives, Health People* envisaged a locally led, recovery-oriented system under which most drugs and alcohol services would be commissioned by local authorities through Directors of Public Health supported by Health and Wellbeing Boards. The NTA was abolished as part of these developments and its functions transferred to the new national service Public Health England set up in April 2013 but information from website can still be accessed.[96]

The aim of the drugs strategy is:

To prevent drug taking, disrupt drug supply, strengthen enforcement and promote drug treatment with the focus on enabling people to become free of their addictions, including alcohol, to recover fully and contribute to society.

In response to the drug strategy consultation Lord Patel produced a report[97] on reducing drug-related crime and rehabilitating offenders. The report focuses on drug treatment and interventions for people in prison, people moving between prisons and the continuity of care for people on release from prison.

There have been several prosecutions of persons who have used cannabis to relieve symptoms of multiple sclerosis. In June 2010 the MHRA approved the use of the mouth spray Sativex which is licensed to treat involuntary spasms and cramps associated with MS and which contains active ingredients known as cannabinoids.[98]

Two charity workers were jailed for knowingly permitting or suffering the supply of a Class A drug on the premises.[99] Concerns about breach of confidentiality are considered in chapter 8. Nurses who remove illegal drugs from patients on admission and who ensure that these drugs are immediately handed into the pharmacy department should be protected from charges of illegal possession of drugs.

NICE published a quality standard for drug use disorders in November 2012 which is available on the NICE website.[100] The NHS website[101] offers advice for drug users and professionals. A free information phoneline named Frank[102] provides information about drugs and the different options available for help and support. The confidential helpline is open every day for 24 hours a day. It also runs a website.[103] In Scotland, Know the Score offers information and advice about drugs.[104] In Wales, Dan is a free and bilingual helpline[105] and Northern Ireland also offers online help and advice.[106]

Concern has been expressed about a sharp rise in the number of deaths from 'legal highs' with deaths from mephedrone and Spice rising from 29 to 52 in 2012.[107] In addition the number of deaths involving Tramadol rose to a record 175 more than double the number recorded in 2008. However, the overall number of deaths linked to drug misuse continue to show a long-term fall, down from 1941 in 2008 to 1496 in 2012, possibly in part due to a heroin drought in the UK and the provision of treatment. There have been calls for ketamine to be upgraded to a Class B drug because of an increase in the number of people going to hospital after taking it.[108] Baroness Meacher who chairs the House of Lords all-party group on drug policy called for the creation of a Class D category of legal regulated substances that could include weak cannabis and low-risk new highs.[109] She held that the war on drugs has failed. In December 2013 the Home Office announced a full review of the law regulating legal highs.[110] The Psychoactive Substances Act 2016 now prohibits the production, distribution, sale and supply of what were previously called legal highs.

The Advisory Council on the Misuse of Drugs was asked by the government in December 2013 to draw up an action plan to combat the addiction to prescription and over-the-counter drugs.[111] Prescription drug addiction is considered in a *Sunday Times* feature[112] warning of the dangers in particular of Tramadol. GPs have been given new guidance on how addicts can be weaned off prescription drugs such as benzodiazepines.[113] The Home Affairs Select Committee reported that GPs should collect information and draw up a list of patients who are suspected of being addicted to prescription drugs to prevent them 'doctor shopping' to get more supplies.[114]

In March 2014 the International Narcotics Control Board of the United Nations stated that moves to liberalise drug laws around the world including decriminalising cannabis use, pose a grave danger to public health.[115] It said that the commercial use of cannabis for medical reasons in Colorado had led to an increase in car accidents and in cannabis-related hospital admissions.

National Prescribing Centre

In 2011 the National Prescribing Centre[116] became part of NICE and works to integrate its products and services into the overall NICE programme. It published Patient Group Directions in December 2009 which is a practical guide and framework of competencies for all professionals using patient group directions. It has also published a single competency framework for all prescribers which has been incorporated into the medicines optimisation guideline published in February 2015.

Availability of medicines within the NHS

The National Institute for Health and Care Excellence has the function of gatekeeper to patient access to new medicines through the NHS and has been criticised for its slowness in approving new medicines. For example in August 2013 it rejected for use in the NHS the drug Xalkori (also known as crizotinib, and used to treat a rare form of lung cancer and costing from £37,512 for a course). It is one of a new generation of drugs tailored to specific genetic make-ups.[117] In 2013 the Public Accounts Committee expressed concern that drug companies were not publishing the full trial results, with favourable results more likely to be published than negative ones. It urged NICE to make sure it studied all the trial results in its review of medicines.[118]

In January 2014 the HSCIC published data on the use of NICE-appraised medicines in the NHS in England.[119] While it could not conclude that lower figures of observed against expected use indicated a failure to follow NICE guidelines, with further improvements to its data collection and with the requested feedback from readers, future reports will be useful in determining the extent to which NICE has removed the post code lottery from medicines prescribing. A dispute between the government and NICE over the evaluation of new medicines arose in February 2014 when it was proposed that NICE should take wider societal benefits into account when considering whether to pay for a drug. The head of NICE Sir Andrew Dillon expressed concern that this would tilt funding away from the old because younger patients had more time to gain from treatment and more to give back.[120] On 25 January 2014 the Chairman of NICE David Haslam is reported as urging patients to be more proactive in their treatment and learn more about the drugs on offer. 'When products have been approved for use by the NHS by NICE, patients have a legal right to those drugs – as long as they are clinically appropriate.'[121]

In May 2014 NICE said that it could not recommend abiraterone, a drug for prostate cancer, prior to chemotherapy, since there was not enough evidence that the £3,000 per month drug is cost-effective. Even though NICE has ruled not to recommend a specific drug, it may be available to patients through the Cancer Drugs Fund. For example NICE has ruled out Enzalutamide, a prostate cancer drug as not being value for money, yet it is available through the Fund. The Fund, which is worth £289 million a year, ends in 2016.

In June 2014 NICE recommended that doctors should stop prescribing aspirin for a heart condition since any benefit conferred by the drug could be cancelled by the increased risk of bleeding. In contrast in the same month a dispute broke out over NICE recommendations that statins should be prescribed to a wider group of the at risk population, leading to arguments that there is no real benefit in extending their use and the side effects are being ignored.

Figures produced in January 2014 on prescribing patterns across the NHS showed that there was a 29-fold difference in the likelihood of patients getting new drugs in different areas of the country suggesting that Britain is a slow adopter of new science.[122] The DH is to announce a scheme to cut the time lag between early clinical research and widespread use to as little as five years compared with the current industry average of 10 to 15 years. The scheme also includes plans to grant promising new drugs a special 'breakthrough' status.

Media campaigns have developed behind specific medicines: Michael Parkinson, for instance, supported the lifting of restrictions on a prostate cancer drug enzalutamide. NICE had decided that it should only be available for men who have not been prescribed abiraterone and who have stopped responding to other treatments.[123]

In February 2014 NICE stated that children should be taking part in clinical trials since it is an important factor that has contributed to improved survival rates on childhood cancers. NICE published new guidance on 27 February 2014.

In Scotland an initiative has given patients and doctors a greater say in which drugs will be approved for use in the NHS. The Scottish Medical Consortium (SMC) held a meeting with Patient and Clinical Engagement (PACE) to discuss which drugs would be approved. In addition, drugs companies can discuss prices if the SMC states that they are above an acceptable level.[124]

Conclusions

Following the implementation of the Crown Reports, prescribing by nurses has developed rapidly. The ability of nurses in hospitals and in primary care to issue prescriptions has a major impact on the development of their scope of professional practice. The regulatory impact assessment of the Statutory Instrument abolishing the extended formulary[125] stated that

> **enabling nurses to prescribe any licensed medicine for any condition subject to clinical competence will not be at the expense of endangering public health.**

This can only be achieved if the additional responsibilities are coupled with adequate resources and training. The significance of NICE rulings on medications and the availability of certain medications within the NHS continues to be a major concern (see chapter 5). Even where NICE has recommended a particular medicine as being effective there is evidence that these medicines are not universally available and the postcode lottery still exists.[126] A five-year agreement has been reached by drugs companies and the NHS whereby the cost of any drugs over a £12 billion annual cap will be paid back by the drug companies. They say that this should enable patients to get new drugs more quickly, and believe NICE will be under pressure to approve more new medicines. The legal right to healthcare is considered in chapter 5. The way forward on the control of illegal substances is uncertain, with some anxious to see the field reviewed and decriminalised, and others seeking to maintain the existing regime.

Reflection questions

1. A patient is concerned at the possibility of having suffered side effects from medication. What is the relevant law? (Refer also to the duty of care to inform the patient) (See chapter 7).
2. In your hospital, when a patient is admitted, any drugs that he brings from home are immediately taken from him and destroyed. One patient complains about this practice because it is wasteful and because he paid the prescription price for those drugs. What do you consider should be the correct practice?
3. What are the advantages and disadvantages of administering controlled drugs PRN?

Further exercises

1. Review your practice in the administration of drugs. Are there any ways in which you consider you might not be meeting the legal requirements? Consider any advice and guidance issued by the person in your trust identified as the Accountable Officer for the safe use and management of controlled drugs.
2. Design a policy for handling medicines to be learnt by a first-year student.
3. What safeguards do you consider should be laid down to protect the patient as nurse prescribing extends?

References

[1] Misuse of Drug Regulations 2001, SI 2001/3998
[2] Human Medicines Regulations 2012, SI 2012/1916
[3] www.mhra.gov.uk
[4] https://gov.wales/statistics-and-research/prescriptions-dispensed-community/?lang=en
[5] www.rpharms.com
[6] www.pharmacyregulation.org
[7] Misuse of Drugs (Safe Custody) Amendment Regulations 2007, SI 2007/2154
[8] Controlled Drugs (Supervision of Management and Use) Regulations 2006, SI 2006/3148
[9] Controlled Drugs (Supervision of Management and Use) Regulations 2013, SI 2013/373
[10] Department of Health, Safer Management of Controlled Drugs: changes to record keeping requirements, DH Gateway Ref. 7187, October 2006
[11] Department of Health and Royal Pharmaceutical Society of Great Britain, Safer Management of Controlled Drugs, May 2007
[12] *R v Hussian (Shabbir)*, The Times Law Report, 17 March 2010
[13] Controlled Drugs (Supervision of Management and Use) Regulations 2013, SI 2013/373

14. Misuse of Drug Regulations 2001 SI 2001/3988 as amended by SI 2012/973
15. Department of Health, Controlled Drugs (Supervision of Management and Use) Regulations 2013: information about the Regulations, DH, February 2013
16. *Prendergast v Sam Dee Ltd and Others*, The Times Law Report, 14 March 1989
17. Dominic Kennedy, Hospital blamed in report on overdose drug, *The Times*, 3 July 2000
18. www.cqc.org.uk
19. Rebecca Coombes, Nurses need a dose of maths, *Nursing Times*, 96(24):4–5, 15 June 1999
20. Greg Hurst, Baby dies after one decimal point drug dose error, *The Times*, 11 October 2000
21. News item, Poor maths mean graduate nurses can't add up drugs, *The Times*, 9 June 2014
22. Chief Pharmaceutical Officer, Department of Health, Building a safer NHS for patients – improving medication safety, DH, London, January 2004
23. www.npsa.nhs.uk
24. David Rose, Wrong medication kills or harms 100 a year and it may be a great many more, *The Times*, 4 September 2009
25. Sam Lister, NHS gives thousands of children wrong medicine dose, *The Times*, 18 June 2009
26. www.nrls.npsa.nhs.uk/resources/patient-safety-topics/medication-safety
27. Russell Jenkins, Doctor gave overdose of drugs to two patients on same day, *The Times*, 25 August 2009
28. David Rose, Doctor banned over fatal drug overdose, *The Times*, July 2010
29. Rebecca Agyemang, Esi Owusu and Alison White, Medication errors: types, causes and impact on nursing practice, *British Journal of Nursing*, 19(6):381–5, 2010
30. NICE, NPSA medicines reconciliation adults, Ref No. 1035, December 2007
31. www.mhra.gov.uk
32. www.england.nhs.uk
33. https://improvement.nhs.uk/documents/2347/Never_Events_1_April_2016_-_31_March_2017_FINAL_v2.pdf
34. www.manchester.ac.uk/discover/news/more-than-200-million-medication-errors-occur-in-nhs-per-year-say-researchers
35. https://assets.publishing.service.gov.uk/government/uploads/system/uploads/attachment_data/file/683430/short-life-working-group-report-on-medication-errors.pdf
36. *Dwyer v Roderick*, 20 June 1984, QBD
37. Nursing and Midwifery Council, Professional Conduct Annual Report, NMC, London, 2002–3, pp. 17–19
38. Royal College of Nursing, Administering intravenous therapy to children in the community: guidance for nursing staff 001 244, RCN, London, March 2003
39. Royal College of Nursing, Standards for infusion therapy, 002 179, RCN, London, October 2003
40. Royal College of Nursing, Advance preparation of insulin syringes for patients to administer at home – RCN guidance for community nurses, 003 066, RCN, London, October 2006
41. www.rcn.org.uk
42. Royal College of Nursing, Right blood, right patients, right time. RCN guidance for improving transfusion practice, 002 306, RCN, 2013
43. Department of Health, Updated National Guidance on the Safe Administration of Intrathecal Chemotherapy, HSC 2003/010, DH, London, October 2003; HSC 2008/001 August 2008

[44] Nursing and Midwifery Council, Remote assessment and prescribing, Circular 16/2008, NMC
[45] Royal Pharmaceutical Society of Great Britain, Medicines Management During Patient Admission to the Ward, RPSGB, London, 2003
[46] Care Quality Commission, National Study: managing patients' medication after discharge from hospital, 2009, CQC, London
[47] UKCC, Registrar's letter 26/2001, Position Statement on the Covert Administration of Medicines – disguising medicine in food and drink
[48] Nursing and Midwifery Council, A–Z Advice Sheet: Medicines Management, last updated March 2006
[49] Nursing and Midwifery Council, Covert Administration of Medicines: disguising medicine in food and drink, NMC, 2007
[50] Sube Banerjee, Report on the prescribing of anti-psychotic drugs to people with dementia, November 2009, DH
[51] David Rose, 'Chemical cosh' for dementia kills 1,800 a year, *The Times*, 13 November 2009
[52] *Cheshire West and Chester Council v P* [2014] UKSC 19
[53] *HL v United Kingdom (45508/99)* (2005) 40 EHRR 32
[54] Haw, C. and Stubbs, J. (2010) Covert administration of medication to older adults: a review of the literature and published studies, *Journal of Psychiatric and Mental Health Nursing* 17(9): 761–768
[55] Nursing and Midwifery Council (2010) Standards for medicines management, NMC, London
[56] National Institute for Health and Care Excellence (2015) Medicines management in care homes; retrieved from www.nice.org.uk/guidance/qs85/chapter/quality-statement-6-covert-medicines-administration
[57] Council of Europe (1950) European Convention on Fundamental Human Rights and Freedoms, Council of Europe, Rome
[58] *AG v BMBC & SNH* [2016] EWCOP 37
[59] Department of Health and Social Security, Neighbourhood Nursing: a focus for care, Stationery Office, London, 1986
[60] National Health Service (Pharmaceutical Services) Amendment Regulations 2000, SI 2000/121
[61] Department of Health, Report on the supply and administration of medicines under group protocols, First Crown Report, Stationery Office, London, 1998
[62] The Black Triangle scheme refers to newly introduced drugs, still subject to special monitoring for potential side effects by the Medicine Control Agency (so-called because they are identified by a black triangle symbol in the *British National Formulary*)
[63] Prescription-Only Medicines (Human Use) Amendment Order 2000, SI 2000/1917 (incorporated into the Human Medicines Regulations 2012 SI 2012/1916)
[64] www.dh.gov.uk
[65] NMC Circular 05/2009
[66] Department of Health, Review of Prescribing, Supply and Administration of Medicines, Final Crown Report, DH, London, March 1999
[67] Misuse of Drugs Regulations (Amendment No 2) (England, Wales and Scotland) Regulations 2012 SI 2012/973
[68] NMC circulars 29/2007; 30/2007 and 31/2007
[69] Department of Health press release 2002/0189, Groundbreaking new consultation aims to extend prescribing powers for pharmacists and nurses, 16 April 2002
[70] Department of Health press release 2002/0488, Pharmacists to prescribe for the first time; nurses will prescribe for chronic illness, 21 November 2002

71 The National Health Service (Primary Medical Services) (Miscellaneous Amendments) Regulations, SI 2005/893; The Medicines for Human Use (Prescribing) Order, SI 2005/765
72 Nursing and Midwifery Council, Standards of proficiency for nurse and midwife prescribers, NMC, 2006
73 The National Health Service (Primary Medical Services) (Miscellaneous Amendments) Regulations, SI 2005/893
74 www.hscic.gov.uk
75 Human Medicines Regulations 2012 SI 2012/1916
76 Gateway ref 14330 www.gov.uk
77 NMC, Mixing medicines prior to administration, June 2012
78 Chris Smyth, See the pharmacist not the GP 'key to survival of the health service', The Times, 15 January 2014
79 Human Medicines Regulations, 2012 SI 2012/1916
80 Committee on Safety of Medicines, 1970, SI 1970/1257
81 Chris Smyth, Doctors warned not to prescribe codeine for children under 12, The Times, 24 June 2013
82 Parliament and Council Regulation 1235/2010 EU amending Regulation EC No 726/2004
83 The Human Medicines (Amendment) (No 2) Regulations 2013 SI 2593
84 Department of Health, Chief Nursing Officer's Bulletin January 2013, MHRA's yellow care scheme and nursing colleagues: protecting public health, DH, London, 2013
85 Philip Nye, 'Overworked' GPs failing to report the side-effects of drugs, The Times, 6 January 2014
86 The Misuse of Drugs (Supply to Addicts) Regulations 1977 SI 1001 (amended SI 2005/2864 and 2012/2394)
87 www.gov.uk/government/organisations/national-treatment-agency-for-substance-misuse
88 National Treatment Agency (Establishment and Constitution) Order 2001, SI 2001/713; National Treatment Agency (Amendment) Regulations 2001, SI 2001/4044
89 National Treatment Agency Regulations 2001, SI 2001/715
90 www.gov.uk/government/organisations/public-health-england
91 Stewart Tendler, New drug law confuses the public, The Times, 16 January 2004
92 Misuse of Drugs Act 1971 (Amendment) Order 2008, SI 2008/3130
93 News item, Jack Straw wants a quick heroin fix, Sunday Times, 20 September 2009
94 Rosemary Bennett, Heroin users facing firmer action to cut drug addiction, The Times, 10 July 2010
95 Richard Ford, Decriminalise drug use and call it a health problem say the experts, The Times, 24 August 2010
96 www.gov.uk/government/organisations/public-health-england
97 Professor Lord Patel of Bradford, Reducing drug-related crime and rehabilitating offenders, DH, 2010
98 Catherine Boyle, Thousands of MS sufferers to benefit as cannabis-based medicine wins UK licence, The Times, 22 June 2010
99 Alan Simpson, What price confidentiality? Nursing Times, 96(9):35, 2 March 2000
100 www.nice.org.uk
101 www.nhs.uk/Livewell/drugs
102 0300 123 6600
103 www.talktofrank.com/
104 www.knowthescore.info or 0800 5875879
105 www.dan247.org.uk or 0808 808 2234
106 www.nidirect.gov.uk/getting-help-with-drug-or-alcohol-problems

107. Richard Ford, Sharp rise in number of deaths from 'legal highs', *The Times*, 29 August 2013
108. Richard Ford, Harsher penalties urged for ketamine, *The Times*, 11 December 2013
109. Lucy Fisher, Call for a new drug category to cover 'low risk' legal highs, *The Times*, 25 November 2013
110. Richard Ford, Drugs laws under new scrutiny in battle against 'legal highs', *The Times*, 12 December 2014
111. Marie Woolf, Drug experts on high alert over prescription pills, *The Sunday Times*, 15 December 2013
112. Jon Ungoed-Thomas, A nation of pill poppers, *The Sunday Times*, 8 September 2013
113. Chris Smyth, GPs given more power to help addicts come off prescription drugs, *The Times*, 18 November 2013
114. Richard Ford, GPs urged to get drugs data on addict patients, *The Times*, 20 December 2013
115. Richard Ford, Legalising cannabis a mistake UN says, *The Times*, 6 March 2014
116. www.nice.org.uk/about/nice-communities/medicines-and-prescribing
117. News item, *The Times*, 16 August 2013
118. Chris Smyth, Secrecy by drug giants could put patients at risks, say PS, *The Times*, 3 January 2014
119. Health and Social Care Information Centre, Use of NICE appraised medicines in the NHS in England – 2012, experimental statistics, HSCIC, January 2014
120. Chris Smyth, Hard-nosed drugs policy would write off elderly, *The Times*, 17 February 2014
121. News item, Patients must demand more says watchdog, *The Times*, 25 January 2014
122. Andrew Clark, Industry hits out at 'slow adoption of drugs' by the NHS, *The Times*, 22 January 2014
123. Sarah-Kate Templeton, Parkinson wants ban on prostate cancer drug lifted, *The Sunday Times*, 2 February 2014
124. Lindsay McIntosh, Drugs access review speeds help for Scots, *The Times*, 1 February 2014.
125. Medicines for Human Use (Prescribing) (Miscellaneous Amendments) Order, SI 2006/915, Explanatory memorandum and regulatory impact assessment, available on www.opsi.gov.uk/legislation
126. Lois Rogers, Dying cancer patients are denied approved drugs, *The Sunday Times*, 25 April 2010

Chapter 28
End-of-life Care and Death

This chapter discusses

- End-of-life care
- Definition of death
- Importance of exact time of death
- Legality of switching machines off
- Not for resuscitation
- Patients refusing treatment
- Relatives and treatment of the patient
- Advance decisions to refuse treatment (living wills)
- Certification and registration of death
- Disposal of the body
- Post-mortems
- Deaths that have to be reported to the coroner
- Inquests
- Recommendations of the Shipman Inquiry
- The Coroners and Justice Act 2009: overview
- Property of the deceased
- Wills

Introduction

Nurses inevitably encounter death in their work. It can be a distressing time and uncertainties surrounding legal issues and numerous questions from troubled relatives can add to the nurse's difficulties. It is important that nurses should have confidence in their knowledge and be well acquainted with the procedures and the law so that they can answer questions or know from where further information is available. This chapter looks at issues arising from end-of-life care, the definition of death, the difference between killing and letting die and the provisions of the Mental Capacity Act 2005 in relation to advance decisions. Significant recommendations on the certification of and procedures following death have been made by the inquiry set up following the conviction of Dr Shipman which have led to the changes contained in the Coroners and Justice Act 2009, and these are also considered.

End-of-life care

Palliative care nurses may work in the community visiting patients in their own homes or in a hospice/hospital or both. Issues relating to resuscitation and DNAR (do not attempt resuscitation) instructions and the distinction between killing and letting die are considered in this chapter. In the case of Bodkin Adams, where an Eastbourne doctor was prosecuted for the death of the patient on the grounds that he had prescribed an overdose of morphine, the judge, in directing the jury on the law that applied to the case, said:

> **There has been a good deal of discussion about the circumstances in which a doctor might be justified in giving drugs which would shorten life in cases of severe pain. It is my duty to tell you that the law knows no special defence of this character. But that does not mean that a doctor aiding the sick or dying has to calculate in minutes or hours, or perhaps in days or weeks, the effect on a patient's life of the medicines which he administers.**
>
> **If the first purpose of medicine – the restoration of health – can no longer be achieved, there is still much for the doctor to do, and he is entitled to do all that is proper and necessary to relieve pain and suffering even if the measures he takes may incidentally shorten life ... It remains a fact, and remains a law, that no doctor has the right to cut off life deliberately ... [the defence counsel] was saying that the treatment given by the doctor was designed to promote comfort; and if it was the right and proper treatment of the case, the fact that incidentally it shortened life does not give any grounds for convicting him of murder.[1]**

Dr Adams was found not guilty of murder.

To prescribe medication to control pain is not an offence. However, the level of prescribing must be consistent with the reasonable practice of a competent medical practitioner and any nurse who was concerned about the levels of analgesics given to a patient could check the prescription with another registered medical practitioner or ask a pharmacist for advice in the light of the previous medicinal history of the patient. There have been disputes over the use of end-of-life care pathways, particularly the one known as the Liverpool Care Pathway (LCP).[2,3] Some have argued that sedation of dying patients was being used inappropriately and the LCP encouraged a tick box approach to patient care and dehydration of the patient. Further criticism of the LCP in 2013 was made in an independent review chaired by Baroness Neuberger which found that in too many cases the LCP was so badly implemented that it became a byword for negligence.[4] It recommended that the LCP should be phased out and replaced with an individual end-of-life care plan.[5] As a consequence of the review the government decided to scrap the pathway and to move towards a more personalised end-of-life care plan in which decisions about treatment rest with senior clinicians, in consultation with relatives. Incentive payments for use of an end-of-life plan were withdrawn. Further research reported in *The Times*[6] suggested that the Liverpool Care Pathway provides little better than standard care for cancer patients in hospital. The LCP was phased out by 14 July 2014.

In its place, NHS England published five new priorities for care, which was based on the work of the Leadership Alliance for the Care of Dying People.[7] The priorities are:

1. the possibility that a person may die within the coming days and hours is recognised and communicated clearly and decisions about are made in accordance with the person's needs and wishes and these are reviewed and revised regularly;

2. sensitive communication takes place between staff and the person who is dying and those important to them;

3. the dying person, and those identified as important to them, are involved in decisions about treatment and care;

4. the people important to the dying person are listened to and their needs respected;

5. care is tailored to the individual and delivered with compassion – with an individual care plan in place.

The NMC has incorporated its fundamental care standards into the revised Code for nurses.[8] An audit carried out by the Marie Curie Palliative Care Institute in Liverpool and the Royal College of Physicians found that 1 in 4 families are not informed when doctors decide that a patient in hospital is dying.[9] End-of-life care was the cause of more than half of the NHS complaints about acute hospital care between 2004 and 2006. A study by the National Council for Palliative Care later found that 300,000 people died each year without receiving the specialist care and pain management which they needed.[10] A website has been set up by a clinical nurse specialist in pain management to provide a forum for information giving and discussion on pain management.[11] Revised guidance[12] was issued in October 2007 by the BMA, the Resuscitation Council (UK)[13] and the RCN on resuscitation, which envisaged that a registered nurse could be the responsible clinician making the decision over cardiopulmonary resuscitation (CPR) (see p. 712). A Palliative Care Bill introduced by Baroness Finley into the House of Lords in 2007 received its third reading but failed to progress. In 2013 Lord Falconer tabled a Bill on assisted suicide following the report of his Commission on Assisted Dying.

The government's ten-year End-of-Life Care Strategy (2008) aimed to shift public attitudes to death and dying, invest in local workforce training and create 'rapid response' nursing teams to provide care and support to those who wish to die in a hospice or at home. Extra funds were provided in 2008 as part of this strategy to help people who wanted to die in their own homes. However, a year later, because the funds were not ring-fenced, they could not be traced as having been spent on palliative care.[14] Furthermore, research by the charity Macmillan Cancer Support showed that shortage of nursing staff meant that patients were not able to choose to die at home.[15] A Freedom of Information inquiry by Macmillan in November 2010 found only 58 per cent of PCTs had a system in place to record people's wishes about where they wanted to die.[16] Guidelines from the National Audit Office (NAO) and from NICE advised that all patients should have access to 24-hour nursing services, but the NAO reported in 2008 that only just over half (53.2 per cent) of local health authorities provided such a service to all patients seven days a week and the situation had not improved by 2014.[17] Coalition government plans published on 18 October 2010 recommended that everyone should be given a choice over their place of death with the appropriate support, and that patients should be in control and involved as much as they want to be. There are clearly concerns that, in a time of budget deficits and public expenditure cuts, palliative care services are likely to suffer and the End-of-Life Care Strategy will not be implemented.

The Gosport Independent Panel (2018), set up to address concerns raised by families about the care and deaths of patients in Gosport War Memorial Hospital, delivered its report in June 2018. The panel found that in some 456 cases there was evidence that opioids were used without clinical indication resulting in the shortening of the lives of those people as a result of the pattern of prescribing and administering those drugs.

Nurses use controlled drugs, including opioids, for their contribution to the care of patients especially those in intractable pain or receiving palliative care. Such care often requires the dose to be increased in response to greater pain and suffering by the patient.

Intention to kill

Any care or treatment given to a patient that is motivated by a desire to bring about a patient's death is unlawful (Mental Capacity Act 2005, s. 4) and could result in prosecution for murder or attempted murder. In *R v Cox* [1992] a consultant rheumatologist was convicted of attempted murder after he admitted injecting a patient with potassium chloride to end her life and with it her pain and suffering.

Murder, in common with most criminal offences, requires two elements to be present in order to prove the offence has been committed. These elements are a blameworthy act – or the *actus reus* and the state of mind of the accused – the *mens rea*. Both must be present at the time of committing the offence. In murder the prosecution would need to prove that the accused intended to cause death or serious harm to the victim and did so through a blame worthy act. In *R v O* [2005] a man was convicted of murder when he killed the victim by striking him over the head with a wooden plank in a racially motivated attack. In this case the defendant directly intended to seriously harm or kill the victim.

Oblique intention for murder

The necessary intention for murder can also be made out through the less direct actions of a person. In *R v Woollin* [1999] a man was charged with murder when he killed his child by throwing it across a room towards a soft play pen. The child struck its head on the wooden arm of a chair and died. *Woollin* argued that he had not intended to kill or do serious harm to the child. The House of Lords considered how a judge should direct a jury in circumstances in which a defendant did an act which caused death without the purpose of killing or causing serious harm.

The House of Lords held that where a person foresees with virtual certainty that their actions will result in death or serious harm, the inference may be irresistible that they intended that result, however little they may have desired or wished it to happen (*R v Woollin* [1999] (Lord Steyn)).

The House of Lords opinion in *Woollin* would seem to suggest that if a nurse administered a very high dose of a controlled drug to a patient to relieve pain but foresaw serious harm or death as virtually certain, even though they did not wish it, because of the size of the dose being given then, it is possible a jury would conclude that there was an intention to murder the patient.

Principle of double effect

However, the Courts do differentiate between an intention to murder and an intention to relive pain. Ever since the case of *R v Bodkin Adams* [1957] the courts have recognised that increased doses of sedation and analgesia may be given to relieve pain even though the unwanted effect of such treatment is to shorten life under the principle of double effect. The courts accept that nobody should die in pain and effective palliative care can require what seems like very high doses of analgesia and sedation in the form of controlled drugs (*Airedale NHS Trust* v *Bland* [1993]).

In *Pretty* v *DPP* [2001] Lord Steyn held that, 'under the double effect principle medical treatment may be administered to a terminally ill person to alleviate pain although it may hasten death. This principle entails a distinction between foreseeing an outcome and intending it' (*Pretty* v *DPP* [2001] (per Lord Steyn at 65).

The apparent confusion by the courts over the precise status of the principle of double effect under English law has been compounded by the case of Harold Shipman after a jury accepted that his intention when administering high doses of analgesia in the form of controlled drugs to his patients was to kill not relieve pain (*R* v *Shipman* [2000]).

Such confusion has led to the prosecution of health professionals for murder or attempted murder where doubt about their intention to relieve pain arises. In *R* v *Moor* 2000 a well respected GP was charged with murder after a journalist published an article quoting him as saying that he had used high doses of controlled drug analgesia and sedation to help patients to a pain free death. At his trial the jury accepted that Dr Moor had used high doses of controlled drugs to relieve pain under the principle of double effect and that he was not motivated by a desire to kill his patients.

Dr Howard Martin was charged with murder and accused of giving his patients six times the normal dose of controlled drug. He was also acquitted of murder by a jury who accepted that he was administering the drugs under the principle of double effect (Strokes 2005).

However, where the motive of a health professional, including nurses, is seen to be hastening death instead of relieving intractable pain then a criminal prosecution will follow.

In *R* v *Salisbury* [2005] a ward sister was convicted of the attempted murder of two of her patients after the jury heard evidence that she had administered high doses of diamorphine and was overheard telling a patient to "give in, it is time to go".

The case and its subsequent appeal focused on whether Sister Salisbury's intention was to kill the patients by using diamorphine when it was not clinically indicated or whether the diamorphine has been prescribed and administered appropriately to relive pain.

The Court of Appeal heard that Sister Salisbury persuaded the ward consultant to prescribe diamorphine because a patient was in considerable pain even though other nurses gave evidence that the patient was unresponsive and the records consistently noted the absence of pain. In the case of a second patient the sister insisted he be nursed flat on his back in the hope that 'his lungs would fill and he would die (*R* v *Salisbury* [2005] at para 42). She again obtained a prescription for diamorphine for pain even though the other ward nurses noted an absence of pain in his case as well. The Court of Appeal agreed with the jury that the evidence showed there was no clinical indication for the use of diamorphine and accepted that the ward sister had administered controlled drugs to her patients with the intention of killing them.

The *Salisbury* case does show that where there is evidence that controlled drugs such as diamorphine and other opioids are prescribed and administered without clinical indication then this is against the law. The Gosport Independent Panel accepted that where it is necessary to control otherwise intolerable pain, appropriate escalation of the dose of an opioid where there may be a concomitant risk of respiratory arrest is both lawful and ethical. Increasing the dose simply to end life is unlawful.

The report shows that the principle of double effect can be wrongly applied leading to circumstances where opiates are prescribed to hasten death rather than to relive pain. In Gosport War memorial Hospital there was an institutionalised regime of prescribing and administering dangerous doses of a hazardous combination of medication not clinically indicated or justified, with patients and relatives powerless in their relationship with professional staff (Gosport Independent Panel 2018). The practice persisted from 1987 to 2001. Some nurses raised concerns in 1991 but their warnings went unheeded.

The principle of double effect has dignity and compassion at its heart. An acceptance by the courts that nobody should die in intractable pain even if the unintended consequence of administering the opioid at a high dose is a shortening of life.

The opaque nature of law means that it is difficult for nurses to be clear about the permitted use of controlled drugs under the principle of double effect (Corner 1997). How much would be too much in the eyes of the law? Both Dr Moor and Dr Martin gave six times the usual dose to combat the severe pain of the patient. Sister Salisbury gave what was prescribed. What they at the heart of the cases was the intention of the practitioners and whether the use of such a high dose was clinically indicated.

The real concern arising from the Gosport independent panel report and the cases of Sister Salisbury, Dr Moore and Dr Martin is that patient will not receive the analgesia in the doses needed to relive their pain.

Definition of death

There is no statutory definition of death, the courts rely on guidance issued by the professional bodies. The traditional method for the determination of whether life has ceased was to check whether breathing had stopped by checking the pulse, the heartbeat and placing a mirror in front of the mouth, i.e. the cessation of circulatory and respiratory functions as evidenced by an absence of heartbeat, pulse and respiration. For most cases, this was satisfactory. However, if the patient was on a ventilator where breathing was maintained artificially, this traditional definition was inappropriate. In addition, the advance in medical technology, particularly in transplant surgery, meant that it was essential to use the organs as soon as possible after respiration had ceased and, if there was likely to be a delay, to keep the body ventilated, i.e. artificially breathing, until such time as the organs required for transplant could be taken. In these cases, 'brain death' became the criterion for whether death had taken place. If the traditional definition of death was used, there was an 88 per cent incidence of postoperative renal failure in kidney transplants, whereas if the criterion of brain death was used on a patient maintained on a ventilator, the postoperative failure rate was 10–20 per cent. The same percentage occurs when kidneys from living donors are used.

What is Brain Death?

A conference of the Royal Colleges in 1976 set out the diagnostic tests to be used for the determination of brain death; these were circulated in 1978 and also included in the Code of Practice for the Removal of Cadaveric Organs for Transplantation, which was distributed to doctors in January 1980. The British Paediatric Association produced guidelines in 1991 on the diagnosis of brainstem death in infants and children. A definition of brainstem death was adopted by the Department of Health in 1998[18] which accepted that, while there was no statutory definition of death, 'irreversible loss of the capacity for consciousness, combined with irreversible loss of the capacity to breathe' should be regarded as the definition of death. A revised Code of Practice for the Diagnosis and Certification of Death was prepared by a working party on behalf of the Royal College of Anaesthetists in 2006. It sought to separate the diagnosis of death from any subsequent events, allowing patients in whatever situation to be diagnosed and treated appropriately. It also gave considerably more detail than the previous guidelines, in some areas, particularly in stating the relevant biochemical values and other data.[19] Subsequently, in 2008 the Academy of the Medical Royal Colleges prepared a Code of Practice for the diagnosis and confirmation of death.[20] The criteria it gives in respect of death following irreversible cessation of brainstem function are shown in Box 28.1.

In a case in 1992 where parents wished their child to be kept on a ventilator, the judge ruled that A, who had been certified as brainstem-dead, was for all legal as well as all medical purposes dead and that a doctor who disconnected the ventilator was not acting unlawfully.[21] Section 47 of the Human Tissue Act 2004 for the law relating to the ventilation of a body for organ transplant is relevant here.

Box 28.1 Diagnosis of death following irreversible cessation of brainstem function

Code of Practice of Academy of Medical Royal Colleges

6.1 Absence of brain-stem reflexes

- **6.1.1** The pupils are fixed and do not respond to sharp changes in the intensity of incident light
- **6.1.2** There is no corneal reflex – care should be taken to avoid damage to the cornea
- **6.1.3** The oculo-vestibular reflexes are absent. No eye movements are seen during or following the slow injection of at least 50 ml of ice cold water over one minute into each external auditory meatus in turn. Clear access to the tympanic membrane must be established by direct inspection and the head should be at 30° to the horizontal plane, unless this positioning is contraindicated by the presence of an unstable spinal injury. In the case of 6.1.1, 6.1.2 and 6.1.3, testing of these reflexes may be prevented on one or other side by local injury or disease but this does not invalidate the diagnosis of death as a result of cessation of brain-stem reflexes. In the case of bilateral injury or disease, ancillary testing should be considered
- **6.1.4** No motor responses within the cranial nerve distribution can be elicited by adequate stimulation of any somatic area. No motor response can be elicited within the cranial nerve or somatic distribution in response to supraorbital pressure
- **6.1.5** There is no cough reflex response to bronchial stimulation by a suction catheter placed down the trachea to the carina, or gag response to stimulation of the posterior pharynx with a spatula

The Code of Practice of the Academy of Medical Royal Colleges covers the diagnosis in many different circumstances and can be downloaded from its website.[22]

Case 28.1 — Re A [1992]

Definition of death[23]

An infant aged 19 months was placed on a ventilator following serious head injuries sustained at home. He showed no signs of recovery. The hospital followed the guidelines laid down by the Medical Research Council in carrying out various diagnostic tests and was satisfied that he was dead. It then applied to court for a declaration that the child could be removed from the ventilator. The Family Court judge, Judge Johnson, identified the results of the tests carried out by the doctors and stated that he had 'no hesitation at all in holding that A has been dead since Tuesday of last week, 21 January'. (It was then 27 January.)

Importance of exact time of death

The actual timing of death can be a significant feature in a variety of court actions. A few examples are set out in Box 28.2.

Box 28.2 — Causes of action where the time of death has considerable significance

Civil law

(A) Survivorship. The rules of inheritance depend on the order in which people die. If, therefore, there are incidents leading to multiple deaths, which victim died first can be very significant for inheritance. There are certain presumptions in law relating to the order of deaths in such circumstances, i.e. the oldest died first. However, if one of the victims is supported on a life support machine and kept 'alive' longer, the presumption would no longer operate.

(B) Insurance policies often require that where death follows an accident it must be established that the death occurred within a fixed time limit to claim under the policy.

(C) Where the machine is switched off this could lead to claims for compensation for negligence by professional staff, especially where organs are used for transplantation. (It used to be a requirement that to constitute the offence of murder, the victim had to die within a year and a day of the act leading to the death. This time limit was removed in 1996.)

Missing persons

The Presumption of Death Act 2013 introduces into the law for England and Wales a new court-based procedure enabling those left behind to obtain a declaration from the High Court that the missing person is deemed to have died. The court will make a declaration if it is satisfied that the missing person has died or has not been known to be alive for a period of at least seven years. The person's name will be listed on a new register of presumed deaths and property will pass to those entitled as if that person had died. The Act follows comparable provisions in Scotland (Presumption of Death (Scotland) Act 1977) and Northern Ireland (Presumption of Death (Northern Ireland) Act 2009).

Criminal law

In the past, to constitute murder the victim must have died within a year and a day of the act. In 1996, this time limit requirement was removed. However, issues of causation may still arise. If the victim is taken off the machine, is that the cause of death or is the cause of death the original assault on the victim? If he is kept on a machine for longer than that, is it murder? Several defendants have tried to argue that it was not.

Case 28.2   R v *Malcherek*; R v *Steel* [1981]

Causal link[24]

Malcherek was convicted of the murder of a victim of assault who had been connected to a life support machine that had been disconnected by medical practitioners. He was sentenced to life imprisonment. In a similar case, Steel was also convicted and sentenced to life imprisonment. Malcherek appealed against this decision and Steel applied for leave to put in further medical evidence as to the sufficiency and adequacy of tests by the doctors to determine brain death. They were both effectively challenging that there was a causal link between the assaults and the deaths of the victims. The judge in each case had withdrawn the issue of causation from the jury.

The Court of Appeal held that in each case it is clear that the initial assault was the cause of the grave head injuries in the one case and of the massive abdominal haemorrhage in the other. In each case, the initial assault was the reason for the medical treatment being necessary. In each case, the medical treatment given was normal and conventional. The court looked in detail at the tests carried out by the doctors and stated:

> It is not part of the task of this court to inquire whether the criteria, the royal colleges' confirmatory tests, are a satisfactory code of practice. It is not part of the task of this court to decide whether the doctors were, in either of these two cases, justified in omitting one or more of the so called 'confirmatory tests'. The doctors are not on trial: the applicant and the appellant were.

The Court of Appeal concluded that all the evidence suggested that at the time of death the original wound or injury was a continuing, operating and, indeed, substantial cause of death. The fact that the victim's life support treatment had been discontinued did not break the chain of causation between the initial injury and death. The issue of causation had therefore properly been withdrawn from the jury. The convictions were confirmed. Amendment to the defences to a charge of murder made by the Coroners and Justice Act are considered in chapter 2.

Legality of switching machines off

In an article by Ian Kennedy[25] three different circumstances are described where a professional might be concerned about the legality of switching off a life support machine. These are set out in Box 28.3 and modified in the light of the Ms B case where a mentally competent adult was held to be entitled in law to ask for her ventilator to be switched off. Kennedy also makes the point that there should be no difference in law between the legality of switching on the machine and of switching it off. The law does not expect a doctor to place every dying patient on a life support machine, only where there is a hope of recovery and the facilities exist.

Box 28.3 Switching off a life support machine

(A) The unconscious dying patient

1. The machine can be switched off if the patient is brain-dead.
2. If the patient can breathe without it but weakly, then the decision to put the patient back on the machine depends on the medical prognosis. If treatment is futile then there is unlikely to be an obligation to put the patient back on again.
3. Where the patient can breathe on his own and the respirator is not needed, then the machine can be switched off. If the patient needs to have assistance again and the prognosis is hopeless, then there is unlikely to be a legal obligation to reconnect the respirator.

(B) The chronically dependent patient such as a polio victim

1. If a mentally competent patient refuses to be ventilated, it would not be a criminal offence for anyone to disconnect it. (However, it would be necessary to seek a declaration of the court.) (See the case of Ms B[26] and chapter 7.)
2. If the machine is turned off against the wishes of the patient this would, of course, be murder.

(C) Temporarily dependent emergency patient

If the ultimate prognosis is recovery and improvement, then switching off the machine would be murder. However, if the ultimate prognosis is extremely poor and hopeless, then the considerations in A1 above would apply.

Where a person has the requisite mental capacity he or she is entitled to request that the artificial ventilation be switched off or to refuse any further life-saving treatment[27] (see chapter 7). Also, where a person has made an advance decision to refuse treatment, which complies with the requirements of the Mental Capacity Act 2005 in relation to the refusal of life-sustaining treatment, then that will be binding on health professionals, as Case 28.3 shows.

Case 28.3 — AK (Adult Patient: Medical Treatment: Consent) Re [2001]

Letting die[28]

The health authority responsible for the treatment of AK, a patient who suffered from motor neurone disease, sought a declaration that it would be lawful to comply with AK's request to discontinue, two weeks from the date that he lost the ability to communicate, the artificial ventilation and the artificial nutrition and hydration which was being provided to him. AK was able to communicate solely by the movement of one eyelid but this movement would shortly cease. In communicating his wish by this means to have the ventilator removed, he had been aware that such action would lead to his death. The court granted the declaration. It held that a patient's refusal to consent to medical treatment had to be observed where that patient was an adult of full capacity. An advance indication of a patient's wishes should be observed by those treating him, although care should be taken to ensure that such indication continued to be the wish of the patient. It was not an unlawful termination of life to cease invasive treatment; rather it would be unlawful to treat a patient in the face of a wish not to be treated. Care should be taken to ensure that the patient was of full capacity and that his wishes had been effectively communicated, particularly where communication was difficult. AK was of full capacity and had clearly communicated his wishes. It was therefore lawful to cease treating him in the event that he lost the ability to communicate. Nothing in the Human Rights Act 1998 was against such a conclusion.

Were the facts in Case 28.3 to reoccur, the situation would now be covered by the Mental Capacity Act 2005 in relation to living wills or advance decisions.

Persistent vegetative state

Case 28.4 — Airedale NHS Trust v Bland [1993]

Ending tube feeding[29]

Tony Bland was crushed in the Hillsborough football tragedy and for three and a half years was in a persistent vegetative state, being artificially fed but breathing unaided. He could not see, hear, taste, smell, speak or communicate in any way. The trust, in agreement with the parents, applied for the withdrawal of nasal-gastric tube feeding. The House of Lords held that medical treatment, including artificial feeding, could be withdrawn from a patient in a persistent vegetative state, if this were in the patient's best interests and it did not amount to a criminal act.

Another application to the courts in similar circumstances was made in January 1994 in respect of a patient in Bristol.[30] In 2007 an application by a hospital that it was in the best interests of a patient in a persistent vegetative state to be allowed to die was granted.[31] W had suffered profound brain damage in a cycling accident. The withdrawal of artificial hydration and nutrition involved no breach of her human rights. The decision was supported by her husband and family.

In a case where the parents objected to ending life support, because they had witnessed signs of awareness, the doctors all agreed that the patient who suffered from mitochondrial cytopathy was in a persistent vegetative state and the court granted the declaration sought, i.e. it was in the best interests of the patient to be allowed to die.[32]

Relatives appealed against a decision that life-sustaining medical treatment (including the insertion of a new line in his groin for haemofiltration) for X could be discontinued. The son argued that, as Muslims, they believed that discontinuing the treatment would be contrary to the principles of Islam and the patient's religious beliefs and therefore was not in his best interests. The Court of Appeal held that it was for the court ultimately to determine what was in the best interests of X, the judge had been correct in concluding that the key question was if there was any chance that X could recover a quality of life to justify his continued discomfort. The medical evidence for this was to the contrary and therefore it was difficult for the religious views of X and his family to overcome the fact that continued treatment was not in X's best interests. The judge had correctly considered the position of the son and the family and the religious beliefs, and the appeal was dismissed.[33]

These situations would now be covered by the Mental Capacity Act 2005 (MCA). Under the MCA, decisions must be made in the best interests of a person who lacked the requisite mental capacity. Extremely serious decisions such as whether life support should be ended would be referred to the Court of Protection to determine if this would be in the best interests of the patient (see chapter 7). In the case of *An NHS Trust* v *AW* who had suffered a severe intra-cerebral haemorrhage in July 2008[34] the judge made the following findings (on 23 January 2013): that AW was in a permanent vegetative state; there will be no change or improvement in her condition; there is no treatment available which could confer any benefit; and that accordingly her treatment regime is futile and the suffering caused by withdrawal of artificial nutrition and hydration will be managed by appropriate use of pain relief in accordance with the plan created for her. He then made the following declaration:

> **AW lacks capacity to litigate in these proceedings or make decisions about her medical treatment; it is lawful and in her best interests for life-sustaining treatment in the form of artificial nutrition and hydration to be withdrawn and it is AW's best interests to receive such treatment and nursing care as may be appropriate to ensure that she retains the greatest dignity until her life ends. (Judge Jackson)**

Minimally conscious state

In a case in 2011[35] the mother of a brain-damaged woman known as M applied for the withdrawal of her daughter's life-sustaining treatment. She was in a minimally conscious state (MCS). She had suffered from serious brain damage since 2003 when she was afflicted by encephalitis. Mr Justice Baker decided:

1. that it would not be in her best interests for artificial nutrition and hydration (ANH) to be withdrawn,
2. there should be a radical review of her care, and
3. the current DNR order should be continued.

> **Case 28.5** *An NHS Trust v DJ and others* [2012][36]
>
> Mr Justice Peter Jackson refused to grant a declaration that it is lawful and in DJ's best interests for certain specified treatments to be withheld in the event of clinical deterioration. The specified treatments included cardiopulmonary resuscitation, invasive support for circulatory problems, renal replacement therapy and IV antibiotics. DJ was a talented musician who had complications following cancer of the colon. He had multi-organ failure and was placed on a ventilator. He suffered deterioration of brain function and was considered to lack the mental capacity to make his own decisions. The judge felt that it would not be appropriate at that time to make the declarations sought, even though they have unanimous medical support and the backing of the Official Solicitor. The judge was not persuaded that the treatment would be futile or overly burdensome, or that there was no prospect of recovery.

Nurses are never justified in continuing life-sustaining treatment regardless of the risk and burdens inherent in the treatment or whatever the quality of life of the person thereafter. The courts agree that adopting such an absolutist approach is not correct in law. The courts require all decisions about the withholding of treatment to be based on a best interests approach.[37]

The determination of best interests is now set out under the provisions of the Mental Capacity Act 2005, s. 1(5) that requires all acts, or decisions made, under the Act for or on behalf of the person who lacks capacity be done, or made, in the person's best interests.

The Mental Capacity Act 2005, section 4 and its Code of Practice[38] set out the process for determining a patient's best interests. Nurses are required to consider all circumstances relevant to the case. This will include but is not limited to the risk, benefits and burdens of the care and treatment. They must then consider the person's past and present wishes, feelings, beliefs and values and consult with others about their views as to what care and treatment would be in the patient's best interests.

The UK Supreme Court has now ruled that a court order does not always need to be obtained before clinically assisted nutrition and hydration (CANH), which was keeping alive a person with a prolonged disorder of consciousness (PDOC), could be withdrawn.

In *NHS Trust v Y* [2018] a man suffering from PDOC required CANH to keep him alive. His doctor and nursing team concluded that even if he were to regain consciousness, he would have profound cognitive and physical disabilities. The man's family agreed with the clinical team that it would be in his best interests for CANH to be withdrawn. As this was his only source of sustenance its removal would result in the man's death.

In keeping with the request of the then judicial committee of the House of Lords (now the Supreme Court) in *Airedale NHS Trust v Bland* [1993] the NHS Trust caring for the man sought a declaration that it not be unlawful to withdraw CANH but they also sought a declaration that it was not mandatory, to seek the court's approval for the withdrawal of CANH in these circumstances.

The Official Solicitor, acting for the patient, argued that it was only by requiring judicial scrutiny in every case concerning the withdrawal of CANH from a patient suffering from PDOC that human life and dignity would be properly safeguarded.

The need to seek the approval of the court

In an earlier Supreme Court case, Lady Hale in *Aintree University Hospitals Foundation Trust* v *James* [2013] stressed the duty on health professionals, including nurses, to have regard to the Mental Capacity Act 2005 Code of Practice (2007) when making decisions for or on behalf of those who lack decision making capacity (Mental Capacity Act 2005, s. 42).

The Mental Capacity Act 2005 code of practice (Department for Constitutional Affairs 2007) states that before the Act came into force in 2007, the courts decided that some decisions relating to the provision of medical treatment were so serious that in each case, an application should be made to the court for a declaration that the proposed action was lawful before that action was taken. Cases requiring court approval included:

- decisions about the proposed withholding or withdrawal of artificial nutrition and hydration from patients in a permanent vegetative state (PVS), and
- other cases where there is a doubt or dispute about whether a particular treatment will be in a person's best interests.

A decade on the Court of Protection, High Court and now the Supreme Court have indicated that a declaration from a judge was never mandatory and not always necessary in cases where CANH is no longer in the best interests of a person with PDOC (*M* v *A Hospital* [2017]; *NHS Trust* v *Y* [2017]; *NHS Trust* v *Y* [2018]).

The Supreme Court in *NHS Trust* v *Y* [2018] held that the best interests test of the Mental Capacity Act, section 4 applied in cases concerning life-sustaining treatment, including CANH. The Mental Capacity Act 2005, section 5 set out the circumstances in which a nurse would avoid liability for acts done in connection with the care or treatment of a person who lacked capacity.

The 2005 Act did not stipulate that the best interests test had to be determined by the court in every case or that particular types of case had to be determined by the court, and it did not limit the protection afforded by section 5 to cases determined by the court. There was a statutory requirement for nurses to have regard to the code of practice (Department for Constitutional Affairs 2007), but the code did not create legal requirements independent of the Mental Capacity Act 2005.

An application should still be made to the court where the lawfulness of treatment was in doubt or where there was a disagreement, but an application is not mandatory in all cases.

Best interests and life-sustaining treatment

Nurses must be clear that under the Mental Capacity Act 2005 a determination of best interests with regard to life-sustaining treatment cannot be motivated by a desire to bring about a patient's death.

The 2005 Act does allow for the withholding or withdrawing of treatment necessary to sustain life where it is futile and it is no longer in the patient's best interests to receive it.[39]

When does continued treatment become futile?

The courts have long recognised that continued life-sustaining treatment to very sick or critically ill patients can be futile. In *Airedale NHS Trust* v *Bland* [1993] the House of Lords held that treatment is not appropriate or requisite simply to prolong a patient's life. So in *Bland* when treatment had no therapeutic purpose of any kind it was futile and could be withdrawn.

The test adopted by the House of Lords in *Bland* required treatment to have no therapeutic purpose of any kind before it could be regarded as futile.

The general presumption in law is that a patient's best interests requires the continuation of treatment to preserve life but this presumption is rebuttable.

Supreme Court Ruling

The Supreme Court set out the correct approach to making decisions about whether to give life-sustaining treatment in the case of persons lacking the capacity (*Aintree University Hospitals Foundation Trust v James* [2013][40]).

The Supreme Court held that the focus when making decisions in such cases must be whether it was in the patient's best interests to give treatment, rather than whether it was in the patient's best interests to withhold or withdraw it. If continued treatment is not in the patient's best interests then it would be lawful to withhold or withdraw that treatment. It would in fact be unlawful to continue with treatment and nurses who acted reasonably and without negligence in these circumstances would not be in breach of their duty towards the patient by withholding or withdrawing treatment.

Not for resuscitation

In intensive care units, where the patient has not made an advance decision to refuse treatment, it is usually the consultant who will decide whether it is in the best interests of a patient for a ventilator to be turned on or off. However, it is sometimes the practice for doctors to mark the patient's notes 'NFR' (not for resuscitation) or 'DNAR' (do not attempt resuscitation) and nurses are then in a quandary as to what they should do. They may feel that they are in an impossible, no-win situation: if they do not initiate resuscitation procedures following a collapse, they could possibly be criticised by relatives or even face criminal charges; if, contrariwise, they ignore the letters 'NFR' and start resuscitation procedures, they could be criticised by the medical staff and face disciplinary proceedings. It is vital in these circumstances that nurses are involved in the discussions over the patient's prognosis so that they can understand the likely outcome and the reasons for the doctor's decision. If they are in any doubt, they should seek expert advice and always err on the side of saving life. An example of the confusion that can arise is illustrated by a situation at the BMI Mount Alvernia private hospital in Surrey.[41] An emergency nurse stated that he was ordered to stop trying to revive a patient by a resident medical officer who could not produce a 'Do Not Resuscitate' (DNR) form. The form was only completed after the woman had died. The Consultant who had admitted the patient, and had discussed resuscitation with her stated that no forms were available. This incident followed a critical report by the Care Quality Commission into concerns over patient safety.

Lawfulness of a DNACPR Notice

The general lawfulness of a 'Do Not Attempt Cardiopulmonary Resuscitation' (DNACPR) notice was specifically considered by the courts in *R (adult: medical treatment)* [1996].[42] In this case a 23-year-old man born with a malformation of the brain and cerebral palsy had a signed direction headed 'Do not resuscitate' in his notes which was challenged on his behalf by the official solicitor. The court held that a do not resuscitate policy may be appropriate where CPR was unlikely to be successful. The Supreme Court recognise that there is no duty to provide treatment where doing so would be futile.[43]

Duty to provide treatment

In *R(Burke)* v *GMC* [2005][44] the Court of Appeal held that once a patient is accepted into hospital, staff come under a positive duty to care for the patient. A fundamental aspect of this positive duty of care is to take such steps as are reasonable to keep the patient alive.

In the case of cardiopulmonary resuscitation the initial presumption would therefore be in favour of attempting resuscitation. Cardiac nurses would normally be required to instigate CPR on patients in their care who required it.

Duty not to provide futile treatment

In *Aintree University Hospitals Foundation Trust* v *James* [2013] the Supreme Court held that it would be lawful to consider treatment futile if it was not in the patient's best interests to receive it. The ruling confirms the approach adopted in *R (adult: medical treatment)* [1996] that a DNACPR notice would be lawful where it was decided that it would not be in the patient's best interests to provide resuscitation.

Requirement to consult the patient

The decision to place a DNACPR notice on a patient's record is generally taken by the doctor in charge of the patient's care in consultation with other health professionals involved in the patient's care.

Controversy over the decision to issue a DNACPR notice often arises from patients and their families who were not consulted about the notice and were unaware that it had been issued.[45]

In *Tracey* v *Cambridge University Hospitals NHS Foundation Trust and others* [2014][46] a man sought judicial review of the decisions of an NHS trust concerning the treatment of his wife who had terminal lung cancer and had been admitted to hospital following a road traffic accident. The trust had placed a DNACPR notice on her medical file that was cancelled after three days when the family expressed concern about it. Three days later, her condition deteriorated and another notice was imposed after consultation with her family and she died two days later.

The family argued that:

- Neither the patient nor her family were consulted about the first DNACPR notice.
- A DNACPR decision engaged Article 8 of the European Convention on Human Rights (ECHR) 1950 and this required:
  - clinicians to involve the patient in a DNACPR decision, and
  - that NHS trusts should have a clear and accessible DNACPR policy that should be given to the patient as part of the DNACPR decision.

The Court of Appeal held that Article 8 is engaged by a DNACPR decision because it concerns how an individual chooses to pass the closing days and moments of their life and how they manage their death.[47]

Article 8: Respect for private and family life, home and correspondence

Article 8 concerns the everyday right of individuals to respect for their private and family life, home and correspondence. However, as a qualified right Article 8(2) allows scope for intrusion into this right on a variety of grounds including the denial of futile treatment.

The ECHR interprets the concept of private life very broadly. It includes the right to autonomy and self-determination and to psychological and physical integrity that includes personal dignity.[48]

Any intrusion with an Article 8 right must be in accordance with the law and be proportionate to the aim being achieved. This implies an obligation to have procedures in place to ensure effective respect for these rights. The ECHR guarantees rights that are practical and effective, not theoretical or illusory. Since a DNACPR decision is one that potentially deprives a patient of life-saving treatment there must be a presumption in favour of patient involvement, i.e. cardiac nurses and doctors must involve the patient in the DNACPR decision and there must be convincing reasons not to involve the patient (*Tracey* v *Cambridge University Hospitals NHS Foundation Trust and others* [2014][49]).

The Court of appeal in *Tracey* held that the courts should be slow to give general guidance as to the circumstances where it would not be appropriate to consult a patient in relation to a DNACPR decision. Nevertheless a nurse and doctor would be correct to consider it inappropriate and therefore not a requirement of Article 8 to involve the patient in the process if they consider that to do so is likely to cause the patient to suffer physical or psychological harm. However, nurses and doctors must be wary of being too ready to exclude patients from the process on the grounds that their involvement is likely to be distressful. The Court acknowledged that it was very likely that many patients would find it distressing to discuss the question of whether CPR should be withheld from them in the event of a cardiorespiratory arrest. Nurses who form the view that the patient will not suffer harm if consulted would not be justified in excluding that patient from the decision because they may find the topic distressing.

The decision in *Tracey* limited the right to be consulted about the placing of a DNACPR notice to patients with decision-making capacity.

Consulting the relatives of incapable patients

In *Winspear* v *City Hospitals Sunderland NHSFT* [2015][50] a mother claimed that an NHS trust had breached her son's rights under Article 8 of the ECHR by placing a DNACPR notice on his clinical record without consulting her.

Her son was 28 years old but suffered from various health conditions including cerebral palsy, epilepsy and spinal deformities. He lacked decision-making capacity under the Mental Capacity Act 2005. He had been admitted to hospital with a chest infection. During the early hours of the morning, a specialist registrar in cardiology had placed the notice on the son's record without consulting the mother or any person representing his interests. The registrar had not considered that there was an imminent risk of cardiac arrest, but made the decision because he considered that CPR would be futile should one occur.

The High Court held that although this case concerned a patient who did not have capacity and was unable to express any view on treatment, Article 8 of the ECHR was still engaged. His mother was clearly involved in the care of her son and was interested in his welfare. The concept of human dignity did not apply any less in the case of a patient without capacity. The core principle of prior consultation applied before a decision not to attempt CPR was put into place. In these circumstances the discussion should be with a person to be consulted as part of the best interests decision under section 4(7) of the Mental Capacity Act 2005 or an independent mental capacity advocate if such a person could not be identified.

Accessible and clear DNACPR policy

Any interference with an individual's right to a private life has to be in accordance with the law (European Convention on Human Rights, Article 8(2)). The Court of Appeal in *Tracey* and the High Court in *Winspear* held that this requires a DNACPR policy that describes the circumstances when it would be right to interfere with a patient's Article 8 rights by coming to a decision. Their Lordships further held that the DNACPR policy must be accessible and clear to be compatible with the ECHR, i.e. any interference in the right to a private life, as in the case of a DNACPR decision, must be:

- sufficiently accessible to the individual who is affected or their relatives, and
- sufficiently precise to enable them to understand its scope and foresee the consequences of this action.

The right to be consulted and notified about DNACPR decisions would be undermined if the patient or the relative of an incapable patient was not aware of the criteria by which the doctor reached the decision to complete a DNACPR notice.

Patients refusing treatment

Since the Suicide Act 1961, suicide has not been a crime, as set out in Statute Box 28.1.

Statute 28.1
Sections 1 and 2(1) of the Suicide Act 1961 as Amended by the Coroners and Justice Act 2009

Section 1 The rule of law whereby it is a crime for a person to commit suicide is hereby abrogated.

    (a) D does an act capable of encouraging or assisting the suicide or attempted suicide of another person, and

    (b) D's act was intended to encourage or assist suicide or an attempt at suicide.

2(1)(A) The person referred to in subsection (1)(a) need not be a specific person (or class of persons) known to, or identified by, D.

2(1)(B) D may commit an offence under this section whether or not a suicide, or an attempt at suicide, occurs.

2(1)(C) An offence under this section is triable on indictment and a person convicted of such an offence is liable to imprisonment for a term not exceeding 14 years.

> **2(2)** If on the trial of an indictment for murder or manslaughter of a person it is proved that the deceased person committed suicide, and the accused committed an offence under sub-section (1) in relation to that suicide, the jury may find the accused guilty of the offence under subsection (1).
>
> ### 2A Acts capable of encouraging or assisting
>
> **(1)** If D arranges for a person ('D2') to do an act that is capable of encouraging or assisting the suicide or attempted suicide of another person and D2 does that act, D is also to be treated for the purposes of this Act as having done it.
>
> **(2)** Where the facts are such that an act is not capable of encouraging or assisting suicide or attempted suicide, for the purposes of this Act it is to be treated as so capable if the act would have been so capable had the facts been as D believed them to be at the time of the act or had subsequent events happened in the manner D believed they would happen (or both).
>
> **(3)** A reference in this Act to a person ('P') doing an act that is capable of encouraging the suicide or attempted suicide of another person includes a reference to P doing so by threatening another person or otherwise putting pressure on another person to commit or attempt suicide.
>
> ### 2B Course of conduct
>
> A reference in this Act to an act includes a reference to a course of conduct, and a reference to doing an act is to be read accordingly.

While it is no longer a crime for a person to decide on and bring about their own death, it is still, however, a crime for anyone to encourage or assist in the suicide of another, as shown in section 2.

The effect of the changes made by the Coroners and Justice Act 2009 is to create a wider ambit for the offence of assisting a suicide so that persons giving advice to others over the internet could now be committing an offence under the Act.

Although the Debbie Purdy case (see Case 28.7) was being heard at the same time as the Coroners and Justice Bill was being debated in Parliament, Parliament did not clarify the law on whether escorting persons to a clinic in Switzerland to meet their deaths were guilty of a criminal offence under the Suicide Act 1961 and it was left to the Director of Public Prosecutions at the request of the House of Lords to clarify when a prosecution would be brought. Two people were found dead in a fume-filled car in September 2010, having met on the internet and agreed to commit suicide ('catch the bus' (ctb)). It was reported that the police were looking on websites for those who had encouraged the pair to commit suicide.[51]

The position is clear for professional staff. Even though they sympathise with a patient's wish to die, they are prohibited by the criminal law in taking any steps or giving any advice to the patient to help him carry out this wish. Where a patient is clearly refusing medication because of this desire, it is essential for staff to record detailed accounts of the patient's attitude, their level of competence, the advice given to them and, preferably, where the patient takes their own discharge contrary to professional advice, to obtain the patient's signature to that effect. In a case in 2004 the judge held that a woman, who had a degenerative brain condition, could not be prevented from travelling to Switzerland for her life to be ended, since she had the mental capacity to make that decision.[52] Clearly, however, anyone assisting such travel in this country is in danger of committing an offence under section 2(1) of the Suicide Act 1961 (see Statute Box 28.1). In 2013 it was estimated that 29 Britons travelled to the Swiss Dignitas clinic to end their lives. In a news item on 19 August 2013 it was stated that police had arrested a mother and her son after police suspected that they were planning to take the woman's 71-year-old husband to the Dignitas clinic to commit suicide. Police confirmed that the mental capacity of the man was being assessed.

Euthanasia is not recognised by law in this country. The courts recognised that in law there is a distinction between letting die and killing a person (see Case 28.4), even though this is not accepted by some philosophers. Decisions sometimes have to be made in special care baby units and in intensive care or renal dialysis units, or over transplants, on who may be treated. This effectively means that those not selected for treatment may eventually die. This is, however, a very different matter from taking an action that will bring about or assist in bringing about another person's death.

The House of Lords Select Committee on Medical Ethics in 1994[53] did not support any proposals to change the law that makes euthanasia illegal and several attempts to pass an Assisted Suicide law since then have failed. Supporters of euthanasia point to the situation in the Netherlands and Switzerland where assisted suicide is lawful. Lord Joffe has stated that, despite the failures of his attempts to change the law, he has not given up.

Relatives and treatment of the patient

Practical Dilemma 28.1   The relatives say 'no'

Katy Brown was 85 and just recovering from a particularly serious hiatus hernia operation. She was very weak and there was considerable likelihood that she would not survive. The relatives discussed her case with the doctors and asked that, in the possible event of a collapse, she should not be resuscitated since they did not want her to continue as an invalid and felt sure that this is what Katy would have wished. What is the doctor's position?

Where the patient is mentally incapacitated, the only criterion that can determine whether or not treatment should proceed is the best interests of the patient, unless the patient has created an advance decision or living will. There is a legal requirement under the Mental Capacity Act 2005 that in determining what are the best interests of the patient, the views of relatives and others should be obtained on what would have been the wishes of the patient. Nor can those making the decision about life-sustaining treatment be motivated by a desire to bring about the death in deciding what are the best interests (s. 4(5) of 2005 Act). In Practical Dilemma 28.1 it is not the wishes of Katy's relatives which should prevail, but the best interests of Katy and in determining these, consideration must be given to any wishes which she had expressed or statement she had made. Clearly, had Katy drawn up an advance decision which complied with the requirements of the Mental Capacity Act 2005 and was applicable to the situation, then that would prevail.

Practical Dilemma 28.2 — To let go

Harry Judd, aged 84, had told his daughter that if he became ill and suffered a cardiac arrest he did not want to be resuscitated. His wife had died two years before and he had become increasingly depressed and frail, with failing eyesight caused by his diabetes. He was still managing to cope on his own with a home help, but it was becoming more and more of a struggle. One day, the home help found him in a coma and he was rushed into hospital. He remained seriously ill for several days and then slowly improved. His consultant physician, Dr Jones, discussed Harry's prognosis with his daughter and son-in-law. It appeared unlikely that he would be able to manage on his own. The daughter reported Harry's views about not being resuscitated. The next evening, Harry suffered a cardiac arrest. The staff nurse summoned Dr Jones, who was unwilling to use resuscitative machinery. Is he obliged to do so?

From the above discussion, it will be evident that it is essential to clarify two issues: first, the mental capacity of Harry when he stated that he would not want to be resuscitated; and, second, the medical prognosis of Harry. In addition, since 1 October 2007 the provisions of the Mental Capacity Act 2005 in relation to advance decisions must be complied with. If Harry were mentally competent when he asked not to be resuscitated, his views should be respected. If, however, his wishes were the result of extreme depression caused by his bereavement and illness, then it may be concluded that he was not mentally capable when he made that request. He must then be treated according to his best interests. If it were absolutely clear that Harry's prognosis is hopeless, then there is no legal duty to resuscitate. If, however, there is any chance that Harry could recover and would have a reasonable prognosis, then Dr Jones's duty would require him to resuscitate him. If Harry is considered to lack the requisite mental capacity, the situation is covered by the Mental Capacity Act 2005. The BMA have issued guidelines on withdrawing treatment.[54] The GMC revised its guidelines in 2010.[55]

In 2013 the widow of a man who had died in December 2012 appealed against a decision of the Court of Appeal that it was in his best interests to have life-sustaining treatment withheld. The Supreme Court dismissed her appeal. It ruled that the focus should be on whether it was in the patient's best interests to give the treatment, rather than on whether it was in his best interests to withhold or withdraw it. In determining his best interests, decision makers had to look at his welfare in the widest sense, not just medical, but social and psychological. The guidance in the Mental Capacity Code of Practice and that given by the General Medical Council in its booklet 'Treatment and care towards the end of life: good practice in decision making' was applicable.[56]

Case 28.6 — Diane Pretty

Helping to die[57]

Diane Pretty, a sufferer of motor neurone disease, appealed to the House of Lords that her husband should be allowed to end her life, and not be prosecuted under the Suicide Act 1961. The House of Lords did not allow her appeal. It held that if there were to be any changes to the Suicide Act to legalise the killing of another person, then these changes should be made by Parliament. As the law stood, the Suicide Act made it a criminal offence to aid and abet the suicide of another person and the husband could not be granted immunity from prosecution were he to assist his wife to die. The House of Lords held that there was no conflict between the human rights of Mrs Pretty as set out in the European Convention on Human Rights.

Mrs Pretty then applied to the European Court of Human Rights in Strasbourg, but lost. The court held that there was no conflict between the Suicide Act 1961 and the European Convention on Human Rights. The Council of Europe issued a press release entitled 'Chamber judgment in the case of *Pretty* v *the United Kingdom*', published on 29 April 2002.[58]

Case 28.7 Debbie Purdy[59]

An MS sufferer, Debbie Purdy brought an action on the law on assisted suicide. She wished her husband to take her to a Belgian clinic or Switzerland to commit suicide if her condition became unbearably painful and wanted to ensure that he would not be prosecuted for aiding and abetting her suicide. The High Court dismissed her application for further guidance from the Director of Public Prosecutions as to when a prosecution for assisted suicide would be brought. She was given leave to appeal but the Court of Appeal dismissed her appeal.[60] It held that she was not entitled to have the specific guidance she was seeking, but that there were broad circumstances in which aiding and abetting suicide would not be prosecuted. She appealed to the House of Lords which heard the case on 3 June 2009 and gave its judgment on 30 July 2009.[61] The House of Lords unanimously held that the DPP should be required to promulgate a policy identifying the facts and circumstances he would take into account in considering whether to prosecute persons such as the claimant's husband for aiding and abetting an assisted suicide abroad. The lack of clarity on whether there would be a prosecution of relatives who took someone abroad to die was an infringement of Article 8 rights.

Director of Public Prosecutions guidance

As a consequence of the direction by the House of Lords, the DPP (after interim guidance and a consultation) issued final guidance in February 2010[62] clarifying the factors which should be taken into account in deciding whether or not there should be a prosecution under the Suicide Act 1961 as amended. The public interest factors for and against prosecutions are shown below.

Director of Public Prosecution policy on assisted suicide prosecutions

The public interest factors against prosecution

1. The victim had reached a voluntary, clear, settled and informed decision to commit suicide.
2. The suspect was wholly motivated by compassion.

3. The actions of the suspect, although sufficient to come within the definition of the offence, were of only minor encouragement or assistance.
4. The suspect had sought to dissuade the victim from taking the course of action which resulted in his or her suicide.
5. The actions of the suspect may be characterised as reluctant encouragement or assistance in the face of a determined wish on the part of the victim to commit suicide.
6. The suspect reported the victim's suicide to the police and fully assisted them in their enquiries into the circumstances of the suicide or the attempt and his or her part in providing encouragement or assistance.

The public interest factors which make prosecution more likely

In contrast, the public interest factors which mean a prosecution is more likely to be required are:

1. The victim was under 18 years of age.
2. The victim did not have the capacity (as defined by the Mental Capacity Act 2005) to reach an informed decision to commit suicide.
3. The victim had not reached a voluntary, clear, settled and informed decision to commit suicide.
4. The victim had not clearly and unequivocally communicated his or her decision to commit suicide to the suspect.
5. The victim did not seek the encouragement or assistance of the suspect personally or on his or her own initiative.
6. The suspect was not wholly motivated by compassion; for example, the suspect was motivated by the prospect that he or she or a person closely connected to him or her stood to gain in some way from the death of the victim.
7. The suspect pressured the victim to commit suicide.
8. The suspect did not take reasonable steps to ensure that any other person had not pressured the victim to commit suicide.
9. The suspect had a history of violence or abuse against the victim.
10. The victim was physically able to undertake the act that constituted the assistance to him or herself.
11. The suspect was unknown to the victim and encouraged or assisted the victim to commit or attempt to commit suicide by providing specific information via, for example, a website or publication.
12. The suspect gave encouragement or assistance to more than one victim who were not known to each other.
13. The suspect was paid by the victim or those close to the victim for his or her encouragement or assistance.
14. The suspect was acting in his or her capacity as a medical doctor, nurse, other healthcare professional, a professional carer (whether for payment or not), or as a person in authority, such as a prison officer, and the victim was in his or her care.
15. The suspect was aware that the victim intended to commit suicide in a public place where it was reasonable to think that members of the public may be present.

16. The suspect was acting in his or her capacity as a person involved in the management or as an employee (whether for payment or not) of an organisation or group, a purpose of which is to provide a physical environment (whether for payment or not) in which to allow another to commit suicide.

The guidance from the DPP does not change the law; assisted suicide or voluntary euthanasia is a criminal offence. In January 2010 Kay Gilderdale was found not guilty of the attempted murder of her daughter who suffered from myalgic encephalomyelitis (ME), but received a 12-month conditional discharge after admitting assisting an attempted suicide. She had given her daughter two syringes of morphine and then injected her with three syringes of air. In contrast, Frances Inglis was found guilty of the murder of her brain-damaged son when she injected him with a lethal dose of heroin.[63] In his summing up the judge said that there was in law no concept of mercy killing and it was still a killing 'no matter how kind the intention'. The mother's appeal to the Court of Appeal failed. It held that the law did not distinguish between murder committed for malevolent reasons and murder motivated by familial love. However, the factors relating to mercy killing could be taken into account in sentencing and the court reduced the minimum term from 9 to 5 years.[64] A man who watched his partner of 15 years (who was wheelchair bound after contracting Lyme's disease) die after taking tranquilisers purchased on the internet and who was arrested on suspicion of assisting a suicide and released on bail, killed himself by the same method.[65] In an inquest on the death of an elderly couple in a suicide pact, the coroner in a narrative verdict held that the daughter, who had a lethal drug from the internet and helped prepare it for her parents, 'was motivated by compassion and a genuine desire to carry out her parents' wishes'. The Crown Prosecution Service decided that it was not in the public interest to charge the daughter. (The father had become bed-ridden and the wife found out that she had dementia and they decided to end their lives.[66])

A 50-year-old man who pleaded guilty to the attempted murder of his terminally ill mother was sentenced to 2 years' imprisonment suspended for 18 months.[67] He had attempted suicide after her death and told a psychiatrist that he was consumed with guilt after killing his mother by suffocating her. The CPS said that it could not prove he had killed her, but his confession was the basis for a charge of attempted murder.

Three Tragic Cases

Tony Nicklinson (who suffered from locked-in syndrome following a stroke) sought declarations from the High Court[68] that

(a) It would not be unlawful on the grounds of necessity for a doctor to terminate his life,

(b) The current law of murder and assisted suicide was incompatible with Article 8 of the Human Rights Convention, and

(c) Existing domestic law and practice failed adequately to regulate the practice of active euthanasia in breach of Article 2.

He succeeded in being allowed to proceed in seeking the first declaration, but failed on the other two.

Subsequently, Tony Nicklinson and Martin (who also suffered from locked-in syndrome following a brain-stem stroke) sought judicial review from the High Court[69] which ruled in favour of Martin, but not of Nicklinson, holding that it could not give the doctors immunity from prosecution were they to assist him to die. It was for Parliament to change the law. Nicklinson died by starving himself after he heard that he had lost the case, but his widow vowed to continue the legal battle and appealed the decision. Martin sought a declaration that if doctors helped him to die, they would not be prosecuted. His wife was not prepared to take him to the Dignitas clinic in Switzerland, and he would therefore need the help of non-family members who would probably not be covered by the DPP guidelines. The High Court was not prepared to require the DPP to clarify further its guidelines, considered that only Parliament could change the law and refused the application for judicial review.

Paul Lamb who was paralysed after a car accident 24 years earlier also brought a case to seek the right of a doctor to end his life at the time of his choosing. The accident left him with only the slightest flicker of movement in the claw of his right hand, which was fading.[70]

Following Tony Nicklinson's death, his widow, Martin and Paul Lamb appealed to the Court of Appeal.[71] The Court of Appeal dismissed the appeals of Nicklinson and Lamb but allowed the appeal of Martin holding that the DPP failed to provide sufficient clarity as to its prosecution policy with respect to those persons who fall into what the court described as the class 2 category (i.e. those seeking help from persons with no close or emotional connection with the victim).

The Supreme Court in a majority judgment ruled that it was not yet prepared to grant a declaration that section 2 of the Suicide Act 1961 (as amended) was incompatible with Article 8 of the European Convention on Human Rights and therefore the appeals must fail. It urged Parliament to consider whether section 2 should be amended.[72] Two judges dissented: Lady Hale and Lord Kerr, while agreeing that Parliament was the appropriate forum in which the issue should be decided, were prepared to issue a declaration of incompatibility that the current law against assisted suicide was contrary to Article 8.

MPs overwhelmingly voted down an attempt to pass an Assisted Dying Bill into law in 2015.[73]

Advance decisions to refuse treatment (living wills)

In this country, the legality of a 'living will' (also known as an advance statement or an advance refusal or decision) was recognised at common law (i.e. judge-made law) and is now provided for in the Mental Capacity Act 2005. An 'advance decision to refuse treatment' means a decision made by a person (P), who is over 18 years and has the capacity to make the decision, that if at a later time and in such circumstances as they may specify, a specified treatment is proposed to be carried out or continued by a person providing healthcare for them, and at that time they lack the capacity to consent to the carrying out or continuation of the treatment, then the specified treatment is not to be carried out or continued.[74] The advance decision can be written in layman's language and no formalities are required unless it is intended to cover a situation where life-sustaining treatment is necessary. Where the advance decision is intended to apply to life-sustaining treatment, then P, the maker, of the advance decision must make it clear that the advance decision is intended to apply to life-sustaining treatment and also:

(a) it is in writing;

(b) it is signed by P or by another person in P's presence and by P's direction;

(c) the signature is made or acknowledged by P in the presence of a witness; and

(d) the witness signs it, or acknowledges their signature, in P's presence.

As long as the maker of the decision has the requisite mental capacity to make decisions, the advance decision remains inapplicable. Only where the maker lacks the mental capacity to make decisions will the advance decision become relevant. The effect of a valid advance decision which applies to the treatment in question is that any person who carried out the treatment contrary to the advance decision could be guilty of an offence or civil wrong. An advance decision can be withdrawn or altered without any formality unless it relates to life-sustaining treatment, when the statutory provisions set out above must be followed. The minimum age for being able to create an advance decision is 18 years because a young person under 18 years cannot refuse life-sustaining treatment if such treatment is in his or her best interests. If there are doubts as to the validity or relevance of an advance decision, then an application can be made to the Court of Protection to determine such questions. In the meantime, any necessary action can be taken to keep the person alive.

The validity of an advance decision drawn up by a person suffering from anorexia was considered in a case in 2012 set out in Case 28.8.

Case 28.8 Re E [2012][75]

The local authority brought a case seeking authority to feed, if necessary by force, a 34-year-old woman suffering from extremely severe anorexia and other chronic health conditions including alcohol dependence. The woman had made advance decisions refusing treatment.

The judge held that E lacked the capacity to make the advance decisions and to refuse treatment. He did not consider future treatment to be futile and the presumption in favour of life should not be displaced. He made a declaration that E lacked capacity and that it would be lawful and in E's best interests for her to be fed, forcibly if necessary.

Requirement of Treatment: The Burke case

It is not possible by means of a living will or advance decision to compel health service professionals to provide treatment at a later time when the patient lacks the mental capacity to make his or her own decisions. An advance decision can therefore only legally be a refusal of treatment. This is the ruling in the case brought by Mr Burke, who challenged the guidance provided by the GMC on withholding or withdrawing treatment in respect of a mentally incapacitated adult and claimed the right to insist that specific treatments were provided for him, even though it was contrary to the professional discretion of the medical staff.[76] The Court of Appeal upheld the GMC's appeal against the High Court decision. The result is that a person has no legal right to insist on specific treatment being given at a later time, when he lacks the requisite mental capacity. Although a person can refuse specific treatments, a person cannot insist on specific treatments being given (this does not of course apply to direct oral nutrition and hydration).

The Mental Capacity Act 2005 also provides for the creation of a lasting power of attorney (LPA) by which the donor can give powers for decisions to be made on his or her behalf covering either personal welfare or finance/property. An LPA creating powers of decision making in personal welfare matters can only be exercised by the donee when the donor lacks the requisite mental capacity (see chapter 18).

Certification and registration of death

Certification of death is a medical task. In contrast, verification of death can be carried out by those who have had the necessary training.

Here we consider the nurse's role and the procedures to be followed generally.

Practical Dilemma 28.3 — An expanded role?

Night porters at Roger Park Hospital had clear instructions that no body should be taken to the mortuary unless it had been certified dead. This resulted from an unfortunate incident some time before when a body was taken to the mortuary, but was seen to move and therefore quickly returned to the ward. An investigation revealed that the person had been certified dead by a nurse. The nurses were told always to call a doctor to certify death. However, junior doctors were not happy about being called out just to certify death and considerable pressure was put on the nursing staff. One night, it was clear that one patient was extremely ill. There were no immediate relatives, but a distant relative was notified of the situation. The patient died at 3 a.m. The nurse summoned the doctor, who said that he would not come down, but would see the patient in the mortuary and sign the certificate there in the morning. The nurse was asked by the bed bureau if she had a spare bed, as a GP had just phoned and was sending in an emergency case. The hospital had no spare beds at all, except the one occupied by the dead person. Could the nurse herself identify that death had occurred and arrange for the porters to remove the body?

The law at present requires a doctor to certify a death. Section 20 of the Coroners and Justice Act 2009 enables the Secretary of State to make regulations relating to the medical certification of death. The certification cannot be undertaken by nurses. However, a nurse may have had the training to be able to confirm that a patient has died, i.e. to verify a death. In certain parts of the country, the local medical committees have advised nursing homes and residential care homes that the nurse or manager in charge of the home should, where death is expected, confirm that death has taken place and the doctor would sign the certificate at a later time. If the nurse considers that she is unable to confirm that death has taken place, she should not give way to any pressure, however reasonable it might appear. Should the nurse feel unable, she may be able to obtain help from another nurse who is competent or from a doctor who is prepared to come to the ward and verify that the patient is dead.

Case 28.9   Fatal diagnosis[77]

The son of Mrs Maureen Jones summoned a GP when he found his mother collapsed in her bedroom. The GP said that she had died and advised the relatives to notify the police. The undertakers were summoned. A policeman called to the scene saw the woman's leg move and applied mouth-to-mouth resuscitation until the paramedics arrived. She then made a full recovery in hospital. She had been in a diabetic coma. A county court judge found the doctor negligent in making a diagnosis of death. Damages were agreed with the Medical Defence Union at £38,500. Following an investigation, the health authority agreed that the doctor could continue in practice, but was given an official reprimand, told to comply more closely with her terms of service and was required to undergo educational assessment and support.

Verification of death is seen as an expanded role activity and the RCN has provided a paper on verification of death by registered nurses.[78] The NMC, in its guidance on confirmation of death,[79] stated that:

> A nurse cannot legally certify death – this is one of the few activities required by law to be carried out by a registered medical practitioner. In the event of death, a registered nurse may confirm or verify when death has occurred, providing there is an explicit local policy or protocol in place to allow such an action, which includes guidance on when other authorities, e.g. the police or the coroner, should be informed prior to removal of the body.
>
> Nurses undertaking this responsibility must only do so providing they have received appropriate education and training and have been assessed as competent. The Code says
>
> - You must have the knowledge and skills for safe and effective practice when working without direct supervision;
> - You must recognise and work within the limits of your competence;
> - You must keep your knowledge and skills up to date throughout your working life; and
> - You must take part in appropriate learning and practice activities that maintain and develop your competence and performance. [You] must also be aware of [your] accountability when performing this role.

(Issues relating to the scope of professional practice and the expanded role of the nurse are considered in chapter 23.)

The general office of the hospital or the medical records department discusses with bereaved relatives the administrative details that must be dealt with. Sometimes there is a special office for dealing with the bereaved and during weekdays the relatives can be shown to this place. However, at night and during the weekends and bank holidays the nurse may have to deal with the administrative details. They should know the details relating to the registration of death and the disposal of the body. Box 28.4 sets out the procedure to be followed.

> **Box 28.4** **Procedures for dealing with death**
>
> The medical certificate should be taken by the next of kin or, if not available, by any relatives living in the district or present at the death to the Registrar for births, marriages and deaths within five days of the death. He will require the following information: the full name of the deceased; the last known address; date of birth; occupation; and whether the deceased was in receipt of a pension. The Registrar will give the person registering the death a certificate of disposal form which can be handed to the undertaker. If the death has been referred to the coroner, the relatives should be notified that they will not receive the certificate from the hospital. The coroner will issue his own disposal certificate.
>
> The relatives will receive from the Registrar, in addition to the certificate of disposal form, a certificate of registration of death. This may be required by the Benefits Agency to claim any entitlements. (The death grant is no longer payable but other benefits are available to those who are eligible.) This certificate may also be required to obtain transfer of any bank accounts, etc. and further copies are available from the Registrar on payment of a fee. New rules relating to cremation came into force in January 2009.[80] There are new statutory forms for cremation and for stillbirths and a confirmatory medical certificate is not required where the patient died in hospital as an inpatient.

Changes to certification and registration of death Under Coroners and Justice Act 2009

Under chapter 2 of the Act, amendments are made to the law relating to the certification and registration of death. Regulations may be made for the registered medical practitioner who attended the deceased before his or her death (an 'attending practitioner')—

(i) to prepare a certificate stating the cause of death to the best of the practitioner's knowledge and belief (an 'attending practitioner's certificate'), or

(ii) where the practitioner is unable to establish the cause of death, to refer the case to a senior coroner.

Each clinical commissioning group in England (in Wales the successors to the Local Health Boards) must appoint a medical examiner (a registered medical practitioner of at least five years' experience) who has the responsibility of receiving the death certificate from the attending doctor and is able to make whatever enquiries appear to be necessary to confirm or establish the cause of death. A medical examiner to whom a copy of an attending practitioner's certificate has been given can:

(i) confirm the cause of death stated on the certificate and notify a Registrar that the cause of death has been confirmed, or

(ii) where the examiner is unable to confirm the cause of death, refer the case to a senior coroner.

Once the cause of death has been confirmed, an attending practitioner's certificate can be given to a Registrar.

Where the senior coroner has referred a death to the medical examiner, he can issue a certificate stating the cause of death to the best of the examiner's knowledge and belief (a 'medical examiner's certificate') and notify a Registrar that the certificate has been issued, or where the examiner is unable to establish the cause of the death, to refer the case back to the coroner.

A medical examiner, if invited to do so by the Registrar, can issue a fresh medical examiner's certificate superseding the existing one.

In 2010 (updated in 2014) the Ministry of Justice published a Guide to Coroners which can be downloaded from the gov.uk website.[81]

New Coroners' Investigations Regulations in 2013[82] cover:

1. coroner availability, register of reported deaths, informing the deceased's next of kin or personal representative, delegation of admin functions, providing information to the registrar of births and deaths, interim certificate of fact of death, resumption of investigation;
2. post-mortem examinations;
3. transfer of investigations;
4. powers in relation to bodies;
5. disclosure and provision of information; and
6. action to prevent other deaths.

They can be downloaded from the legislation website.

In September 2024 a statutory medical examiner system rolls out across England and wales to provide independent scrutiny of deaths and aims to give bereaved people a voice. All deaths in any health setting, that is not investigated by the coroner will be reviewed by a medical examiner. Placing medical examiners on a statutory basis is part of the government's response to a number of concerns arising from the Shipman Inquiry, Mid Staffordshire NHS FT public inquiry, Morecambe Bay investigation, Gosport Independent Panel and the trails of Lucy Letby.[83]

The move to statutory medical examiners is part of a range of reforms of death certification which also includes a revised medical certificate of cause of death and a change to allow any doctor who has attended a patient in their lifetime to provide a medical certificate of cause of death when the patient dies.[84]

Disposal of the body

Different arrangements exist according to the local hospital facilities. Some hospital mortuaries also double up as the public mortuary and it is possible for the body to remain there until collected by the undertakers for the funeral. Before the body is taken from the ward, the nurse must ensure that it is properly labelled and that a receipt is signed and that any property on the body, e.g. rings, are carefully noted and signed for. Similar procedures to check identification and property on the body and the giving of receipts must also be followed when the body is handed over by the porters, administrators or even nurses to the undertakers. Unfortunately, mix-up between bodies still occurs and the wrong body is released.

A husband was given special planning permission by Gelding Council to bury his late wife in their front garden.[85]

Post-mortems

The coroner might require a post-mortem to ascertain the cause of death and can direct a legally qualified medical practitioner to carry out the post mortem. A post-mortem ordered by a coroner may or may not precede an inquest. If the coroner orders a post-mortem, then the person in possession of the body has no choice but to agree. Sometimes, however, medical staff may request the relative's permission to confirm the cause of death or for research purposes. They require the consent of the person in possession of the body (Human Tissue Act 2004). This can be a distressing request to make to relatives and the request should be put to them with sensitivity. Organs should not be retained by hospital doctors without the relatives' consent. (The issue of retention of organs and the provisions of the Human Tissue Act 2004 are considered in chapter 15.) Part 3 of the regulations published in 2013[86] cover the following topics: delay in post-mortem examinations to be avoided; post-mortem examination where homicide is suspected; notification of post-mortem examination; preservation or retention of material from a post-mortem examination; post-mortem examination report and discontinuance of investigation where cause of death is revealed by post-mortem examination.

Deaths that have to be reported to the coroner

These are shown in Box 28.5.

Box 28.5 Deaths that have to be reported to the coroner

1. Where there is reasonable cause to suspect a person has died a violent or unnatural death.
2. Where the cause of death is unknown.
3. Where the person has died in custody or otherwise in state detention.

Those causes of death which should be reported to the coroner include: abortions; accidents and injuries; alcoholism; anaesthetics and operations; crime or suspected crime; drugs; ill-treatment; industrial diseases; infant deaths if in any way obscure; pensioners where death might be connected with a pensionable disability; persons in legal custody; poisoning; septicaemias if originating from an injury; stillbirths where there may have been a possibility or suspicion that the child may have been born alive; and where the person who died was not visited by a doctor during their final illness or the doctor who signed the medical certificate had not seen the person who died within 14 days of the death.

If it is likely to be a coroner's case, no unofficial post-mortem should be undertaken without the coroner's approval. The coroner can order a post-mortem examination to be carried out before deciding to hold an inquest.

Inquests

The Coroners and Justice Act 2009 which repeals the Coroners Act 1988 covers the appointment of coroners, the holding of inquests, and post-mortem examination. A decision by the coroner not to hold an inquest can be the subject of an application to the High Court. For example, in one case where a mother had suffered from a cerebral haemorrhage soon after giving birth in circumstances that suggested that had her blood pressure been properly monitored immediately after the birth her death might have been avoided, the coroner concluded that she had suffered a natural death. The High Court decided that he had erred in deciding not to hold an inquest. The coroner appealed to the Court of Appeal, which dismissed the appeal. The Court of Appeal held that for the purposes of the Coroners Act 1988 section 8(1)(a) a death by natural causes was an 'unnatural death' where it was wholly unexpected and would not have occurred but for some culpable human failing.[87] A breach of Article 2 rights was claimed when a coroner refused to resume an adjourned hearing (adjourned pending criminal proceedings) into the death of a man who was stabbed and killed in May 2000 even though the death had occurred before the Human Rights Act 1998 came into force in October 2000. The victim's mother claimed that there were failures by the police and local housing authority in failing to avert the death. The Court of Appeal held that the inquest should be resumed and the Commissioner of Police appealed against this decision. The House of Lords found that the coroner's decision was lawful and allowed the appeal.[88]

The House of Lords laid down the implications of Article 2 on the state's obligations to protect life. It stated that Article 2 of the Convention imposed on the state a substantive obligation to establish a framework of laws, precautions, procedures and means of enforcement which would, to the greatest extent reasonably practicable protect life.[89] This ruling was followed in a case where the claimant sought judicial review of the failure to conduct an independent and immediate investigation following the suicide of his wife who was a patient detained in a psychiatric hospital under section 3 of the Mental Health Act 1983. The inquest (which found that the wife had not committed suicide but was the outcome from self-harming) met the minimum standards required of the state.[90] The Middleton ruling was also applied in another case where a 14-year-old boy died after drinking methadone. The local authority, which had been aware of his drinking, drugs and shoplifting for the previous nine months, succeeded in its application for judicial review of the coroner's decision to hold a Middleton inquest. The High Court identified three possible obligations under Article 2 a general duty to protect the right to life; an operational duty which arose when the authorities had known of a real and immediate risk to life and a procedural duty to investigate any arguable breaches of the general duty. There was no operational duty in place and there was no breach of the general duty.[91] A GP, who had prescribed Heminevrin to a patient who took an overdose, failed in his application for judicial review of the conduct of an inquest which returned a verdict of unlawful killing. The Court of Appeal held that his role in the deceased's death was crucial to the investigation and justified the coroner authorising a full investigation of his prescribing history and his system of using repeat prescriptions.[92]

In December 2007 the European Court of Human Rights held that failure by the state to investigate credible allegations about unlawful killings could amount to a breach of Article 2 and the right to life in relation to alleged failings by the Royal Ulster Constabulary.[93] In another Northern Ireland case, the European Court of Human Rights held that excessive delay in investigating the deaths of people at the hand of the security forces in Northern Ireland amounted to a violation of the procedural aspect of the right to life, guaranteed by Article 2.[94]

Practical Dilemma 28.4   An unexpected death

Bill Arthur was undergoing a stomach operation when the anaesthetist reported that his pulse was becoming very weak. Resuscitative procedures were undertaken, but unfortunately Bill died. The death was reported to the coroner who decided that an inquest should be held.

What is the Purpose of the Inquest?

The Coroners and Justice Act 2009 section 5(1) states that:

1. **The purpose of an investigation under this Part into a person's death is to ascertain—**
    (a) who the deceased was;
    (b) how, when and where the deceased came by his or her death;
    (c) the particulars (if any) required by the 1953 Act to be registered concerning the death.
2. Where necessary in order to avoid a breach of any Convention rights (within the meaning of the Human Rights Act 1998, the purpose mentioned in subsection (1)(b) is to be read as including the purpose of ascertaining in what circumstances the deceased came by his or her death).
3. Neither the senior coroner conducting an investigation under this Part into a person's death nor the jury (if there is one) may express any opinion on any matter other than—
    (a) the questions mentioned in subsection (1)(a) and (b) (read with subsection (2) where applicable);
    (b) the particulars mentioned in subsection (1)(c).

This is subject to Paragraph 7 of Schedule 5 which covers the duty of the senior coroner to report to a person he believes may have power to take action on a matter of concern that the circumstances creating a risk of other deaths will occur or continue to occur.

Section 10(2) of the Coroners and Justice Act 2009 specifically states that a determination of the jury may not be framed in such a way as to appear to determine any question of—

(a) criminal liability on the part of a named person,

(b) or civil liability.

The Coroners (Inquest) Rules 2013[95] set out the procedures to be followed and cover the formalities: disclosure, management of the inquest hearing, jury inquests and record. A Schedule covers the form for juror summons and the form for record of inquest. There are nine short form conclusions or a narrative verdict. The standard of proof required for unlawful killing or suicide is the criminal standard of proof. For all other short form conclusions and a narrative statement the standard of proof is the civil standard of proof.

Who should attend?

The coroner has a duty[96] to examine on oath all persons who tender evidence as to the facts of the death and all persons having knowledge of the facts whom the coroner considers it expedient to examine. Under the Coroners' Rules 2013[97] (which replace the 2008 Rules[98]) the coroner has considerable discretion in deciding who should attend. They must (Rule 9) notify the date, hour and place of an inquest (within one week of setting the date) to:

1. the next of kin or personal representative of the deceased whose name and address are known to the coroner; and
2. any other person who has made themselves known to the coroner.

The details must be made publicly before the hearing.

Examination of Witnesses

Any of the persons listed in the second point under 2 above are entitled to examine the witnesses either in person or through a solicitor or barrister. The coroner has the power to disallow any question that, in their opinion, is not relevant or is otherwise not a proper question (Rule 19).

The procedure is for any witness to be examined by the coroner first and then by any interested person and then if the witness is represented at the inquest, by the representative last. No witness is obliged to answer any question tending to incriminate themselves. Where it appears to the coroner that a witness has been asked such a question, the coroner must inform the witness that they may refuse to answer.

Nature of the Inquest

The coroner's inquest is very different from the hearings in the other courts of law in this country. It is an **inquisitorial** hearing as opposed to those in the civil and criminal courts, which are **accusatorial** or **adversarial**. This means that in an inquest there are not two opposing parties with the coroner sitting back and hearing them argue out a case, intervening only to ensure fair play. At an inquest, the coroner takes the lead and is in control. It is up to him or her to obtain answers to the questions set out above. He or she calls the witnesses and decides the order in which they are to give evidence and generally controls the court and hearing. Under section 7 of the Coroners and Justice Act an inquest should be held without a jury unless subsections 2 and 3 apply. These state that:

(2) An inquest into a death must be held with a jury if the senior coroner has reason to suspect—
  (a) that the deceased died while in custody or otherwise in state detention, and that either—
    (i) the death was a violent or unnatural one, or
    (ii) the cause of death is unknown,
  (b) that the death resulted from an act or omission of—
    (i) a police officer, or
    (ii) a member of a service police force, in the purported execution of the officer's or member's duty as such, or
  (c) that the death was caused by a notifiable accident, poisoning or disease.
(3) An inquest into a death may be held with a jury if the senior coroner thinks that there is sufficient reason for doing so.

The decision of the coroner in the inquest into the death of Princess Diana and her companion not to hold a jury was held by the High Court to be wrong.[99]

Returning to Practical Dilemma 28.4, the coroner's officer will have requested statements from relevant people who were present in theatre and who were concerned with Bill's treatment. It is helpful if those making a statement can keep a copy. (Refer to chapter 9 for the making of statements.) The coroner will probably have requested a post-mortem examination to ascertain the cause of death. They will decide which people they require to summon as witnesses. Clearly, in Bill's case, there will have to be evidence of identity and also of what took place in theatre. The surgeon, anaesthetist and the nurse are all likely to be called to give evidence. If detailed pathology laboratory results are not yet available, there could well be an adjournment until they are ready. Bill's family will obviously wish to be present in order that they can ask for the relevant questions to be put to prepare for a possible case of negligence in the civil courts. The coroner has the power to prevent any question that they do not consider relevant to the inquest. Schedule 5 Paragraph 7 of the Coroners and Justice Act 2009 requires the coroner to send a report to a person who could take action to prevent a similar death. Regulation 28 of the 2013 Investigation Regulations expands on this duty.[100] The recipient is required to give a written response. Regulation 28 reports can be obtained from the Chief Coroner's office.[101]

Preparation for the Theatre Nurse before Attending the Inquest

The theatre nurse has, one hopes, kept a copy of the statement that they made for the coroner. The statement should have followed those guidelines discussed in chapter 9. The nurse may be advised by a senior nursing officer who has had some experience in such matters on the sort of questions they can expect and how to cope. Preferably, they should be advised by the solicitor to the trust (see chapter 9). The importance of comprehensive, meaningful record keeping cannot, once again, be overstressed. Prior to the hearing, the solicitor to the trust should take the nurse through their evidence and answer any concerns that they have.

Recommendations of the Shipman Inquiry

Following the conviction of Dr Shipman for murder an inquiry was set up under the chairmanship of Dame Janet Smith DBE. The First Report[102] considered how many patients Shipman killed, the means employed and the period over which the killings took place. The Second Report examined the conduct of the police investigation into Shipman that took place in March 1998 and failed to uncover his crimes.[103] The Third Report[104] considered the present system for death and cremation certification and for the investigation of deaths by coroners, together with the conduct of those who had operated those systems in the aftermath of the deaths of Shipman's victims. The Report noted that the present system of death and cremation certification failed to detect that Shipman had killed any of his 215 victims. Even though many of the deaths occurred suddenly and unexpectedly and should under the present procedures have been reported to the coroner, Shipman managed to avoid any coronial investigation in all but two of the cases in which he had killed. He did this by claiming to be in a position to certify the cause of death and by persuading relatives that no autopsy (and therefore no referral to the coroner) was necessary. The present system failed to protect the public. This Third Report made extensive recommendations, which are summarised in Box 28.6. The inquiry took into account feedback to a consultation paper published by the Fundamental Review of Death Certification and the Coroner Services in England, Wales and Northern Ireland chaired by Mr Tom Luce and accepted the recommendations of the coroner's review on changes to the scope and conduct of inquests. The Fourth Shipman Report, which was published in July 2004,[105] considered the regulation of controlled drugs in the community (see chapter 27).

Box 28.6 Issues covered by the Shipman Inquiry into death and cremation certification and the role of the coroner

- Future of the coronial system
- Aim and purposes of the new coroner service
- Need for leadership, training and expertise in the coroner service
- Structure and organisation of the coroner service
- Death certification
- Registration
- Further investigation
- Pathology services
- Statutory duty to report concerns about a death
- Public education
- Audit and appeal
- Transitional arrangements
- The future

The Fifth Report of this inquiry was published in December 2004.[106] It considered the handling of complaints against GPs, the raising of concerns about GPs, the procedures of the General Medical Council and the revalidation of doctors, and made significant recommendations for the more effective regulation of GPs. Many of the detailed changes for GMC procedures recommended in the Fifth Shipman Report could also apply, where appropriate, to the NMC as could the results from a review carried out by the Chief Medical Officer. The Sixth and final Shipman Report considered how many patients Shipman killed during his career as a junior doctor at Pontefract General Infirmary and in his time at Hyde.[107]

The inquiry recommended that a new coronial system should be established that would provide an independent, cohesive system of death investigation and certification, readily accessible and understood by the public. It should seek to establish the cause of every death and to record the formal details accurately for the purposes of registration and the collection of mortality statistics. It should seek to meet the needs and expectations of the bereaved and its procedures should be designed to detect cases of homicide, medical error and neglect. It should provide a thorough and open investigation of all deaths giving rise to public concern. It should ensure that the knowledge gained from death investigation is applied for the prevention of avoidable death and injury in the future. The legal and medical functions of the coroner's office should be carried out respectively by a judicial and medical coroner who should be independent officeholders under the Crown. The Coroner Service should have a corps of trained investigators, who would be the mainstays of the new system. The Coroner Service should be an executive non-departmental public body, independent of the Department for Constitutional Affairs (now the Ministry of Justice) and the Department of Health. A board should govern the service and formulate policy, strategic direction and the promotion of public education of its work. Three members of the board would be the Chief Judicial Coroner, the Chief Medical Coroner and the Chief Coroner's Investigator. There should also be an advisory council.

Recommendations for death certification are that there should be one system for death certification for all deaths, whether death is to be followed by burial or cremation. Two forms will need to be completed: Form 1 would provide an official record of the fact and circumstances of death and be completed by a doctor, accredited nurse or paramedic or a trained and accredited coroner's investigator who confirmed that death had occurred; Form 2 would be completed by the doctor who had treated the deceased person during the last illness or if no doctor had treated the deceased person in the recent past, by the deceased's usual medical practitioner. Form 2 would contain a brief summary of the deceased person's recent medical history and the chain of events leading to death and the doctor could express an opinion as to the cause of death. There would be a statutory duty on doctors to complete the death certificate and the General Medical Council should impose a professional duty for doctors to cooperate with the death certification system.

All deaths would be reported to the Coroner Service, which would have responsibility for certification of death and decide if further investigation were necessary. Where Form 2 stated the doctor's opinion as to the cause of death, the coroner's investigator would consult with the deceased's family and decide if certification could proceed. There should be random and targeted checks to consider whether fuller investigation is required. A new certificate of cause of death should be completed by the coroner's investigator or, if an investigation has been undertaken, by the medical coroner. There should only be an inquest in a case in which the public interest requires a public investigation for reasons connected with the facts and circumstances of the individual case and decided by the judicial coroner. There would be a mandatory inquest in a few specified circumstances. Where an inquest was not held, a report of further investigations would be prepared by the medical and/or judicial coroner, explaining how and why the deceased died. Any recommendation of the medical or judicial coroner should be submitted to the Chief Coroners, who should take it forward. Statutory powers, including powers of entry, search and seizure of documents should be given to the coroners. The family should have the right to appeal against an autopsy being held or to make representations for one to be held. Detailed proposals are made for the investigations by the medical and judicial coroners. The relationship between criminal proceedings relating to a death and investigations by the Health and Safety Executive and the medical and judicial coroners are also spelt out. Deaths which were or might be caused or contributed to by medical error or neglect should be investigated by the Coroner Service, initially by the medical coroner and if after investigation it appears that the death might have been caused or contributed to by medical error or neglect, the case should be referred to the regional coroner's office for investigation by the regional medical coroner and judicial coroner. The recommended statutory duty to report concerns about a death should be placed on any 'qualified' or 'responsible' person. Employers should encourage employees to report any concerns relating to the cause or circumstances of a death and should pass on these reports to the appropriate quarter without delay and without any possibility of the reporter being subject to criticism or reprisal. The public should be educated about the functions of the Coroner Service and should be encouraged to report any concerns about a death. The Report also recommended that there should be a systematic audit of the Coroner Service and rights of appeal.

Following the Third Shipman Report, a position paper was published by the Home Office[108] in March 2004 and constituted the government's response to the *Fundamental Review of Death Certification and Coroner Services*[109] and the Shipman Inquiry. In February 2006 the Minister of State for Constitutional Affairs announced the implementation of the first set of reforms: those relating to the Coroner Service.[110] Six key reforms were to be introduced:

- Bereaved people will have a right to contribute to coroners' investigations. They will be able to bring their concerns to coroners even where a death certificate has been issued. A coroners' charter will set out the service bereaved people can expect. (A draft was published in 2006 and revised in 2008.)

- A Chief Coroner (accountable to the government) and an advisory Coronial Council would be introduced to provide national leadership, guidance and support. Coroners would continue to be appointed and funded by their local councils and served by coroners' officers drawn from the local police or local authority. The Chief Coroner will have the power to commission audits and inspections and will be responsible for monitoring the coroners' charter for bereaved people. The Chief Coroner will also have power to appoint judges in complex cases. The Coronial Council will include independent lay members and representatives of voluntary groups. It will act as a further check on standards and will advise the Chief Coroner on what service and strategic issues may need further scrutiny.

- A body of full-time coroners would be created and current boundaries would be reshaped to create a smaller number of coroner jurisdictions. The full-time coroners would be supported by a pool of assistant coroners to act in their absence. All new appointments to the service will be required to have a legal qualification.

- The investigation and inquest processes would be modernised and coroners would be given new powers to obtain information to help their investigations.

- In limited and specific cases, such as some suicides and child deaths, coroners will have a new discretion to complete their investigations and decide on the facts without holding inquests, where no public interest is served by doing so.

- A Chief Medical Adviser will be appointed to support the Chief Coroner to give advice on medical best practice and medical issues related to coroners' investigations.

In addition:

- At local level funding will be provided to coroners to ensure appropriate local medical advice to support their investigation.

- Coroners will no longer have the task of determining whether a particular find should be classified as treasure. A new national coroner for treasure will be appointed to take on the work currently undertaken by coroners at local level.

A draft Coroner's Bill, together with a draft charter for the bereaved, was published in June 2006 to enable pre-legislative scrutiny to be undertaken by the Select Committee for the Department of Constitutional Affairs. The draft Bill was scrutinised by the DCA Select Committee[111] which made strong criticisms about the fact that many of the proposals contained in the Shipman Report and in the position paper were omitted from the Bill, in particular the changes to the death certification system and a national system for the office of coroner. The Select Committee was also concerned that there was inadequate resourcing of the coronial service. The government responded to these recommendations in November 2006.[112] It did not accept the recommendation that all deaths should be reported to the coroner, since this could lead to unnecessary delays for families in preparing the funeral. It did accept the recommendation that there should be a positive statutory duty for doctors to refer certain categories of death to the coroner and suitable guidance and training to improve doctors' knowledge of death certificate requirements should take place with the GMC and the General Register Office.

The Coroners and Justice Act 2009: overview

The Coroners and Justice Act 2009 received royal assent on 12 November 2009 and included measures to:

- Reform and clarify the law on homicide, in particular to the partial defences (see chapter 2);
- Update the language of the offence of assisting suicide;
- Establish a new Sentencing Council for England and Wales, with a strengthened remit to promote consistency in sentencing practice;
- Create a new national coroner service, led by a new chief coroner;
- Create a new system of secondary certification of deaths that are not referred to the coroner, covering burials and cremations;
- Enable the courts to pass an indeterminate sentence for public protection for certain terrorist offences;
- Prevent criminals from profiting from publications about their crimes;
- Amend the Data Protection Act to strengthen the Information Commissioner's inspection powers;
- Re-enact the provisions of the emergency Criminal Evidence (Witness Anonymity) Act 2008 so that the courts may continue to grant anonymity to vulnerable or intimidated witnesses where this is consistent with a defendant's right to a fair trial;
- Allow the courts to grant Investigative Witness Anonymity Orders in certain gun and knife crime cases; and
- Extend the use of special measures in criminal proceedings, such as live video links and screens around the witness box, so vulnerable and intimidated witnesses give their best evidence.

The full Act can be accessed on the legislation website.[113]

Peter Thornton was appointed as Chief Coroner in 2012 and set out his focus of driving up standards and tackling delays.[114] Changes include the formulations of new rules and regulations which will speed up inquests and families will receive information earlier and have greater access to documents and evidence; coroners will be able to release bodies earlier for burial and cremation with the overall number of inquests being reduced. There is to be compulsory training courses for coroners and their officers and for local authorities, police, pathologists, lawyers, charities and others. Changes are also being made to the appointment system to ensure a more open, transparent and fair system. There will be a retirement age of 70 and coroners cannot appoint their spouses and partners as assistant coroners. Guidance is being provided to coroners on the appointment of coroners, location of inquests, recording hearings, a cadre for service deaths, reports to prevent future deaths, post-mortem imaging and oaths and robes.

Guidance and law sheets including Regulation 28 reports can be obtained from the Chief Coroner's office.[115]

Property of the deceased

When a patient has died, there is an obligation on the staff to ensure that the property is listed and accounted for. Usually, the next of kin will arrange for clothes and small personal items to be taken away. However, any property that looks as though it might be of some value should be handed over to the executor or personal representative only on production of the grant of probate or letters of administration relating to the estate. A form of indemnity may be required to protect the NHS trust. This is the only way in which the NHS trust can defend itself if it is challenged for handing the property over to the wrong person. (See chapter 24 on property.)

Case 28.10 Property of the deceased[116]

A patient was brought into hospital following a heart attack at a garden centre and was found to be dead on arrival. His widow realised that he was carrying the house keys in his pocket and asked for them so that she could return home. The nursing sister stated that the keys had to be left in the safe until after the post-mortem, even though the widow told her that she would not be able to get into her house without them. She returned to the house with her daughter, but was unable to get in and had to hire a locksmith the next day.

Even though the hospital was probably following the set procedure for handling property following an unexpected death which was reported to the coroner, there would appear to be reasonable grounds for permitting the widow to receive the keys, perhaps on receipt of an indemnity. There were no suspicious circumstances relating to the death and the hospital could have safeguarded its position by obtaining the consent of the coroner to the handing over of the keys.

Wills

The best advice to nursing staff in relation to the drawing up or signing of wills for patients is: *do not get involved*. Ideally, if a patient makes it known that he or she wishes to make their will (the person making a will is known as the *testator*), the unit manager should be advised and the patient's solicitor called. The nurse should not be involved. If there is likely to be any dispute as to the patient's competence to make a will, medical opinion should be obtained to confirm that the patient is mentally competent, since one of the grounds for challenging a will's validity is that the patient lacked the competence to sign it, since they were unaware of the implications of their act. Another ground on which its provisions can be challenged is that the patient was subjected to undue influence at the time of signing it so that its provisions do not represent their real intent. Nursing and medical evidence thus becomes crucial in any such legal dispute. If there is a statement in the medical records that the patient signed their will on such and such a day and that their state of mind was rational, clear and unconfused, while that is not in itself evidence of the truth of what is stated, it should at least contain sufficient information to assist professionals in the recall of events, should they be subjected to cross-examination on the patient's competence or independent state of mind.

Practical Dilemma 28.5 — Execution at night

Florence Evans was convinced that she was dying. She fretted that she had not made her will and asked the night sister if she would sign a piece of paper declaring how she would like her property disposed of. The night sister was very reluctant to become involved, although she knew that Florence was, in fact, very ill. Florence showed her the paper on which everything was written and asked her to sign it with the auxiliary as a witness. Just to settle Florence, the night sister agreed and she and the nursing auxiliary together watched Florence sign the piece of paper and then they signed their own names. Florence died that same week.

A few weeks later the sister was told that Florence's daughter was disputing the will which left everything to her two brothers and nothing to her. She said that the formalities were not complied with and that it was not a proper will.

Practical Dilemma 28.5 gives an example of one reason why nursing staff are advised not to become involved with will making. Hospitals should provide advice on what staff should do in this situation. In some hospitals, it would be possible for a sister in this situation to summon the on-call manager to take care of Florence's will. The actual signing and witnessing of the will is known as the *execution* of the will and strict rules are in force in relation to the validity of the process. These have been eased slightly since 1982, but the revised procedures must be strictly followed. Any irregularity in the execution of the will may lead to the will being declared invalid. There are no special forms to be used although these are available. The legal requirements are set out in Statute Box 28.2.

Statute 28.2
Administration of Justice Act 1982 section 17 amending section 9 of the Wills Act 1837

No will shall be valid unless:

- It is in writing and signed by the testator, or by some other person in his presence and by his direction.
- It appears that the testator intended by his signature to give effect to the will.
- The signature is made or acknowledged by the testator in the presence of two or more witnesses present at the same time.
- Each witness either:
    (i) attests and signs the will, or
    (ii) acknowledges his signature in the presence of the testator (but not necessarily in the presence of any other witness), but no form of attestation shall be necessary.

Additional requirements:

- the testator must be over 18 (unless in the armed forces or the merchant navy),
- the testator must have the required mental competence at the time he signs the will.

Any person who signs the will as a witness is prevented from being a beneficiary under the will and this applies to the spouse as well. (In one case where the solicitor allowed the beneficiary's spouse to sign the will, the solicitor was liable for the lost inheritance.) If the testator intends leaving a gift to the NHS trust or its staff, then no one from the NHS trust should be involved in the drawing up or signing of the will, otherwise the gift could be invalidated on the grounds of undue influence. The Supreme Court allowed the rectification of a will when it was discovered that wills signed by husband and wife had been signed by the wrong spouse. The error had not been noticed when the wife died, but was realised when the husband died. The Supreme Court held that this was a clerical error capable of rectification and those who would have inherited on intestacy lost.[117]

The Court upheld the Vegetarian Society's claim that the deceased had testamentary capacity when he left his substantial estate to the Society rather than to his sister. The deceased suffered from schizophrenia but the court accepted expert evidence that he was able to comprehend what was required of him when making a will.[118] In contrast, claimants who alleged that the deceased lacked the requisite competence when she made two wills and sought a declaration that she died intestate succeeded. Evidence from care home staff and expert and other evidence suggested progressive dementia.[119]

In Practical Dilemma 28.5, where the sister and the nursing auxiliary witnessed the will, it is unlikely that the will could be declared invalid on the grounds of its actual execution even though it might be challenged on other grounds (the lack of mental competence, undue influence, etc.). However, the possibility of involvement in litigation does illustrate the advantages of nursing staff ensuring that, where possible, the experts are involved.

Conclusions

The government's End-of-Life Care Strategy is likely to suffer from the cuts in public expenditure, and palliative care nurses will continue to face many resource challenges. Parliament has resisted any change in the law to permit voluntary euthanasia. The guidance provided by the DPP on when there is likely to be a prosecution following assisted suicide has not resolved all the uncertainties, and cases demanding further clarity are likely to continue to arise. The implications of the Coroners and Justice Act 2009 have still to be seen and it is possible that more radical changes to the system of certification and coroners' inquests may eventually be made. Certification by registered nurses is still not an option at present but training in verification of death as an expanded role is likely to increase. Controversy over the right to receive assistance in a suicide attempt is likely to continue even if legislation is enacted. In September 2013 Stephen Hawking joined the ranks of the proponents of assisted suicide, arguing from his own experience of motor neurone disease, that those who help the terminally ill to die should not be prosecuted.[120]

Reflection questions

1. What is meant by brain death? What problems arise from recognising this as opposed to the traditional definition of death?
2. A patient who is being ventilated asks you to switch off the machine. What is the legal position?
3. Consider any patient whose death you have witnessed and whose relatives you have had to comfort and assist. Was there any information of which you were ignorant? Could you answer all their questions?
4. In what ways would an inquest differ from a hearing in the criminal or civil courts?

Further exercises

1. Obtain a copy of the local policy and guidelines on end-of-life care and compare it with the government's strategy. To what extent has it been implemented?
2. In what circumstances would an advance decision drawn up by a patient be applicable and relevant? What are the statutory requirements for its validity?
3. Draft a procedure for preparing a nurse who has been asked to give evidence at an inquest.
4. Obtain a copy of your NHS trust's leaflet for the guidance of patients on the care of property. Does it consider the procedure to be followed at the death of a patient? What precautions would you as a ward sister take to ensure that the property of the deceased was cared for?

References

[1] *R v Bodkin Adams* [1957] Crim LR 365
[2] Helen Brookes, Fatal decisions, *The Sunday Times*, 6 September 2009
[3] Katherine Murphy and Rob George, Do palliative care rules let patients down? *The Times*, 18 September 2009
[4] Editor's Leader, *The Times*, 16 July 2013
[5] Department of Health, Review of Liverpool Care Pathway for dying patients, DH, July 2013
[6] Chris Smyth, Study prompts rethink on care of the dying, *The Times*, 16 October 2013
[7] NHS England, More Care, Less Pathway, 2014
[8] Nursing and Midwifery Council (2015) The Code: Professional standards of practice and behaviour for nurses and midwives, NMC, London
[9] David Rose, Families 'kept in dark' as doctors make life or death decisions, *The Times*, 24 September 2009
[10] David Rose, Doctors practise 'slow euthanasia' on dying patients, *The Times*, 28 October 2009
[11] email Glenn Bruce (site manager) info@pain-talk.co.uk; www.pain-talk.co.uk
[12] British Medical Association, Resuscitation Council (UK) and the Royal College of Nursing, Decisions Relating to Cardiopulmonary Resuscitation, BMA, October 2007, Paragraph 13, p. 19

[13] www.resus.org.uk
[14] David Rose, NHS 'loses' £286m intended to ease last days of dying patients, *The Times*, 25 July 2009
[15] David Rose, Nursing shortfall threatens right to die at home, *The Times*, 1 March 2010
[16] Chris Smyth, Doctors failing to provide 'good death', *The Times*, 13 November 2010
[17] News item, *The Times*, 15 May 2014
[18] Department of Health, Code of Practice for the Diagnosis of Brain Stem Death, DH, March 1998
[19] Royal College of Anaesthetists, Letter dated 14 May 2006, Code of Practice for Diagnosis and Certification of Death and Guidelines for the Management of Potential Organ and Tissue Donors, 2006
[20] Academy of Medical Royal Colleges, Code of Practice for the Diagnosis and Confirmation of Death, AMRC, 2008
[21] *Re A* [1992] 3 Med LR 303
[22] www.aomrc.org.uk
[23] *Re A* [1992] 3 Med LR 303
[24] *R v Malcherek; R v Steel* [1981] 2 All ER 422 CA
[25] Criminal Law Report, 1977, p. 443
[26] *B (re) (Consent to treatment: capacity)*, The Times Law Report, 26 March 2002, [2002] 2 All ER 449
[27] Ibid.
[28] *AK (Adult Patient: medical treatment: consent) Re* [2001] 1 FLR 129
[29] *Airedale NHS Trust v Bland* [1993] 1 All ER 821
[30] *Frenchay NHS Trust v S*, The Times Law Report, 19 January 1994 CA
[31] *A Hospital v W; sub nom A Hospital v SW* [2007] EWHC 425
[32] *An NHS Trust v D* [2005] EWHC 2439, [2006] 1 FLR 638
[33] *An NHS Trust v X* [2005] EWCA 1145; [2006] Lloyd's Rep Med 29
[34] *NHS Trust v AW* [2013] EWHC 78 COP
[35] *W v M and others* [2011] EWCOP 2443
[36] *NHS Trust v DJ and others* [2012] EWHC 3524 CoP
[37] *Re J* [2000] 1 FLR 571 (Fam)
[38] Department for Constitutional Affairs (2007) Mental Capacity Act 2005 Code of Practice, TSO, London
[39] *An NHS Trust v Mr and Mrs H* [2012] EWHC B18 (Fam)
[40] *Aintree University Hospitals Foundation Trust v James* [2013] UKSC 67
[41] Martin Barrow, Hospital filled in 'Do Not Resuscitate' form after doctor ordered nurse to let woman die, *The Times*, 3 May 2013
[42] *R (adult: medical treatment)* [1996] 2 FLR 99
[43] *Aintree University Hospitals Foundation Trust v James* [2013] UKSC 67
[44] *R (On The Application Of Oliver Leslie Burke) (Respondent) v General Medical Council (Appellant) & The Disability Rights Commission & 8 Others (Interveners)* [2005] EWCA Civ 1003
[45] Ibid.
[46] *Tracey v Cambridge University Hospitals NHS Foundation Trust and others* [2014] EWCA Civ 822
[47] *Pretty v United Kingdom* [2002] 2 FLR 45
[48] Ibid.
[49] Op cit
[50] *Winspear v City Hospitals Sunderland NHSFT* [2015] EWHC 3250
[51] David Brown, Hunt for people who urged on suicide pair, *The Times*, 23 September 2010
[52] *Re Z* [2004] EWHC 2817

53 House of Lords Select Committee on Medical Ethics, HL Paper No. 21, 1, HMSO, London, 1994
54 British Medical Association, Withholding and Withdrawing Life-prolonging Treatment Guidelines, BMA, updated March 2007
55 General Medical Council, End of Life Treatment and Care, GMC, 2010
56 *Aintree University Hospitals NHS Foundation Trust v James* [2013] UKSC 67
57 *R (on the application of Pretty) v DPP* [2001] UKHL 61, [2001] 3 WLR 1598
58 *Pretty v United Kingdom* [2002] ECHR 427
59 *R (on the application of Purdy) v DPP* [2008], The Times Law Report, 17 November 2008
60 *R (Purdy) v Director of Public Prosecutions*, The Times Law Report, 24 February 2009
61 *R (Purdy) v Director of Public Prosecutions*, The Times Law Report, 31 July 2009, HL
62 Director of Public Prosecutions, Policy for prosecutors in respect of cases of encouraging or assisting suicide, DPP, February 2010
63 Lucy Bannerman, Jury heckled over murder verdict for mother who 'acted out of love', *The Times*, 21 January 2010
64 *R v Inglis*, The Times Law Report, 22 November 2010
65 News item, Man killed himself after his arrest for helping partner die, *The Times*, 4 December 2013
66 Alexi Mostrous, Daughter watched parents die after buying suicide drug, *The Times*, 16 January 2014
67 News item, *The Times*, 21 March 2014.
68 *Nicklinson v Ministry of Justice and others* [2012] EWHC 304
69 *Nicklinson, R (on the application of) v Ministry of Justice* [2012] EWHC 2381
70 Lucy Bannerman, Life is cruel, says man taking on campaign for right to die, *The Times*, 20 April 2013
71 *Nicklinson and Anor, R (on the application of) v Ministry of Justice* [2013] EWCA Civ 961
72 *R (Nicklinson) v Ministry of Justice; R (AM) v Director of Public Prosecutions*, The Times Law Report, 26 June 2014 SC; *Nicklinson and Anor R (on the application of) (Rev1)* [2014] UKSC 38
73 Rowena Mason, Assisted dying bill overwhelmingly rejected by MPs, *The Guardian*, 12 September 2015
74 Mental Capacity Act 2005 Section 24(1)
75 *Re E (Medical Treatment Anorexia)* [2012] EWCOP 1639
76 *R (on the application of Burke) v General Medical Council and Disability Rights Commission and the Official Solicitor to the Supreme Court* [2004] EWHC 1879, [2004] Lloyd's Rep Med 451
77 Paul Wilkinson, £38,500 for woman given up for dead, *The Times*, 27 September 2000
78 Royal College of Nursing, Confirmation (Verification) of Death by a Registered Nurse, Order No. 000594, RCN, May 1996 updated 2013
79 Nursing and Midwifery Council, Confirmation of Death for Registered Nurses, 2013
80 The Cremation (England and Wales) Regulations 2008 SI 2008/2841
81 www.gov.uk
82 Coroners (Investigations) Regulations 2013 SI 2013/1629
83 The Shipman Inquiry (2003) *Third Report Death Certification and the Investigation of Deaths by Coroners*, Cm 5854 London: TSO House of Commons (2013) *Report of the Mid Staffordshire NHS Foundation Trust Public Inquiry (Chair Robert Francis QC)* HC947 London: The Stationery Office Kirkup B. (2015) Report of the Morecambe Bay Investigation available on the UK Government Website at https://assets.publishing.service.gov.uk/media/5a7f3d7240f0b62305b85efb/47487_MBI_Accessible_v0.1.pdf Gosport Independent Panel (2018) *Gosport War Memorial Hospital, Report of the Gosport Independent Panel* retrived from Gosport Independent Panel website https://www.gosportpanel.independent.gov.uk/
84 The Medical Certificate of cause of Death Regulations 2024

[85] News item, *The Times*, 23 November 2013
[86] Coroners (Investigations) Regulations 2013 SI 2013/1629
[87] *R (on the application of Touche) v HM Coroner for Inner North London District* [2001] EWCA Civ 383; [2001] QB 1206 CA
[88] *R (on the application of Hurst) v London Northern District Coroner* [2007] UKHL 13; [2007] 2 All ER 1025
[89] *R (on the application of Middleton) v HM Coroner for Western Somerset* [2004] UKHL 10
[90] *R (on the application of Antoniou) v Central and North West London NHS Foundation Trust* [2013] EWHC 3055
[91] *R (on the application of Kent CC) v HM Coroner for Kent (North West District)* [2012] EWHC 2768
[92] *R (on the application of Sreedharan) v HM Coroner for the County of Greater Manchester* [2013] EWCA Civ 181
[93] *Brecknell v United Kingdom*, Application No. 32457/04 (and 4 other applications), The Times Law Report, 7 December 2007
[94] *McCaughey and others v United Kingdom*, The Times Law Report, 4 October 2013 ECHR
[95] Coroners (Inquests) Rules 2013 SI No. 1616
[96] Section 6 Coroners and Justice Act 2009
[97] Coroners (Inquests) Rules 2013 SI 2013/1616
[98] Coroners (Amendment) Rules 2008, SI 2008/1652
[99] *R (on the application of Paul and others) v Deputy Coroner of the Queen's Household and Assistant Deputy Coroner for Surrey* [2007] EWHC 408; [2007] 2 All ER 509
[100] Coroners (Investigations) Regulations 2013 SI 2013/1629
[101] www.judiciary.gov.uk
[102] Shipman Inquiry First Report: Death Disguised, 19 July 2002
[103] Shipman Inquiry Second Report: The Police Investigation of March 1998, 14 July 2003
[104] Shipman Inquiry Third Report: Death and Cremation Certification, 14 July 2003
[105] Shipman Inquiry Fourth Report: The Regulation of Controlled Drugs in the Community, 15 July 2004, Cm 6249, Stationery Office
[106] Shipman Inquiry Fifth Report: Safeguarding Patients: Lessons from the Past – Proposals for the Future, Command Paper Cm 6394, December 2004, Stationery Office
[107] Shipman Inquiry Sixth Report: The Final Report, January 2005, Stationery Office
[108] Home Office, Reforming the Coroner and Death Certification Service. A Position Paper, Cm 6159, March 2004, Stationery Office
[109] Tom Luce, Chair, Fundamental Review of Death Certification and the Coroner Services in England, Wales and Northern Ireland, Home Office, 2003
[110] Department for Constitutional Affairs, Coroners' Service Reform, Briefing Note, February 2006, DCA
[111] Department for Constitutional Affairs, Select Committee's Report on the Reform of the Coroners' System and Death Certification, DCA, 2006
[112] Government Response to the Report by the Constitutional Affairs Select Committee (Cm 6943, Session 2005–6), November 2006
[113] www.legislation.gov.uk
[114] Peter Thornton, Bereaved families are focus of reforms to update coroners' courts, *The Times*, 19 September 2013
[115] www.judiciary.gov.uk
[116] Oliver Wright, Widow forced to break into home, *The Times*, 28 August 2000
[117] *Marley v Rawlings and another*, The Times Law Report, 28 January 2014 Supreme Court
[118] *Vegetarian Society v Scott* [2013] EWHC 4097
[119] *Fischer v Diffley* [2013] EWHC 4567
[120] Rosemary Bennett, Hawking in favour of assisted suicide, *The Times*, 18 September 2013

Chapter 29

Complementary and Alternative Therapies

This chapter discusses

- Definitions of complementary and alternative therapies
- The NMC practitioner as a complementary therapist
- Liability for using complementary therapy at work
- Patients receiving complementary therapies
- House of Lords Select Committee
- Herbal medicines and acupuncture
- Complementary and Natural Healthcare Council (CNHC)

Introduction

Complementary and alternative therapies have enjoyed considerable growth over the past 20 years and it is estimated that one in every five adults has tried such therapies, spending about £1.6 billion on them.[1] Information in relation to the use of complementary therapies in the NHS is provided on the NHS England website. Increasingly, the focus has been on the proven effectiveness of such therapies and the extent to which the NHS would provide free access to them. More recently, there have been moves to encourage national registration for the practitioners to ensure that the public obtained greater protection.

This chapter looks at the legal implications of complementary therapy practice for nurses and midwives in two respects: one as a practitioner of a complementary therapy alongside the skills for which they are registered with the NMC; the other as a carer of patients who may be receiving complementary therapies as well as care from orthodox medicine. For more detailed information on the legal aspects of complementary therapies, see Bridgit Dimond's work.[2] Reference should also be made to the many books written by nurses about individual complementary therapies. Further information can be obtained from the website of the Complementary Healthcare Information Service.[3]

Definitions of complementary and alternative therapies

It is perhaps easier to define complementary and alternative therapy negatively in the sense that it is treatment for which health-giving or disease-repelling properties are claimed that are not yet accepted by those who practise orthodox medicine. If this definition is used, it could be argued that chiropractic and osteopathy were once, but are no longer, complementary therapies, but by becoming state-registered professions are now accepted as part of orthodox medicine and there are referrals funded by the NHS. If this definition is used, it would also follow that homeopathy has long been part of orthodox medicine; since the Faculty of Homeopathy was established in 1848, five schools of homeopathy have been established and both the schools and the hospitals receive state support. The Cochrane Collaboration defines complementary and alternative medicine as:

> A broad domain of healing resources that encompasses all health systems, modalities and practices and their accompanying theories and beliefs, other than those intrinsic to the politically dominant health systems of a particular society or culture in a given historical period.[4]

The term 'complementary and alternative therapy' covers a wide range of practices, from the well-established field of homeopathy to claims in respect of dowsing, radionics and astrology.

The NMC practitioner as a complementary therapist

Section 18 of the NMC Code (2015) asks all registrants to:

> Advise on, prescribe, supply, dispense or administer medicines within the limits of your training and competence, the law, our guidance and other relevant policies, guidance and regulations.

The Code makes no explicit reference to complementary therapies.

In the NMC's standards of proficiency for nurse and midwife prescribers,[5] paragraph 3.5 on complementary medicinal products requires the following of its registered practitioners:

> Nurses and midwives need to be familiar with a range of complementary medicinal products that their patient or clients may be using, or may wish to be used, in their treatment. These include homeopathic remedies, herbal remedies, aromatherapy oils, flower essences and the broad area of vitamin and mineral supplements. Nurses should not prescribe any complementary medicinal products unless they have undertaken appropriate recognised training to do so. Where a nurse or midwife considers that complementary medicinal products could be a substitute for, or a complement to, conventional medication then patient or clients should be referred to appropriately qualified practitioners to receive such treatment.

Standard 23 of its standards for medicines management[6] states:

> Registrants must have successfully undertaken training and be competent to practise the administration of complementary and alternative therapies.

An NMC practitioner who has been trained in a complementary therapy may wish to use it for the benefit of their NHS patients. The practitioner may, for example, have acquired skills in aromatherapy, reflexology or acupuncture and believe that these may be more effective in reducing pain or relaxing the patient than medication. What restrictions would there be on them practising their additional skills?

The NMC suggested[7] that employers may wish to establish local policies to provide a framework for the use of complementary therapies by nurses and midwives in their employment.

Employers would need to have information about insurance cover, and complementary and alternative medicine (CAM) practitioners should notify their employers about their qualifications and membership of the relevant associations. Unfortunately, there are considerable variations in the standards of training required and many therapies do not have a single overall professional body that sets standards. The consent of the employer must be obtained by any employee wishing to use CAM therapies, as the following situation indicates.

Practical Dilemma 29.1 Aromatherapy without consent

Brenda was an ITU nurse who had undertaken a course in aromatherapy. She knew that it would be relaxing and beneficial to the ventilated patients she was caring for and wished to use aromatherapy oils on them. Her employers were prepared to give consent to her using aromatherapy, but their policy on the use of complementary and alternative therapies required employees to obtain the consent of patients before initiating any treatment. Since most of Brenda's adult patients were unconscious and relatives could not give a valid consent on their behalf, she was thwarted in her plans. What is the law?

It is entirely reasonable for the employer to lay down instructions and protocols for the use of non-orthodox treatments. The requirement of the patient's consent is also consistent with the legal situation. Brenda, therefore, has to accept that until such time, if ever, aromatherapy becomes a recognised part of traditional nursing and medicine and could therefore be used in the best interests of a mentally incompetent patient, she would be unable to use it in ITU, unless she has the patient's consent when mentally capable.

Liability for using complementary therapy at work

If consent is not obtained from the employer but the nurse practises their complementary therapy skills during their work, there could be serious consequences for the nurse. On the one hand, the nurse has disobeyed the reasonable instructions of the employer and therefore faces disciplinary action, including dismissal. On the other hand, if the nurse causes harm to the patient, they may face personal liability for the harm that has been caused, since the employer might deny that it is vicariously liable for an employee who is disobeying reasonable instructions and who is not therefore acting in the course of employment (see chapter 4). Even if this argument by the employer did not succeed, since it could be held that the employee is still acting in the employer's interests, the employer might claim from the employee an indemnity for any compensation that it has to pay to the injured patient.

In contrast, if the employee *has* obtained consent from the employer and is working within the guidelines set by the employer, not only would there be no justification for disciplinary action for working outside the nurse's job description, but if harm were to occur to the patient as the result of negligence by the practitioner, the employer would be vicariously liable for that harm.

Different issues arise if the practitioner wishes to use their complementary therapy skills out of working hours but on the employer's premises, as the following case shows.

Case 29.1   *Watling* v *Gloucester County Council* [1995]

Private practice in working hours[8]

An occupational therapist was dismissed when he saw private patients for alternative therapy during working hours. His application for unfair dismissal failed. He had been warned by his employers not to conduct his private business during his working hours and that lunchtimes were for a break, not for private work.

It may be that as the clinical effectiveness of certain therapies is established, then employers will fund study leave for practitioners to develop these new skills as part of the scope of their professional practice (see chapter 23). At this point, some of these therapies might be seen as part of the reasonable standard of care to be provided to a patient and could then be given to mentally incapacitated adults in their best interests.

Notifying the Patients of Risks of Complementary Therapy

There appears to be a common fallacy that complementary and alternative therapies, being natural, can do only good and not harm and that there are no risks attached. However, this is not correct, as some of the cases reported in the author's work show.[9] Any significant risks, which reasonable professional practice would suggest should be made known to the patient, must be explained to the patient before consent is obtained. Exactly the same principles apply in complementary therapies to the obtaining of consent and the information to be given to a patient as apply in orthodox medicine (see chapter 7). If, for example, a patient were to be given acupuncture and suffered harm, it would be a defence if the defendant could show that there was no negligence on the part of the practitioner, that the patient had given a valid consent and that information about significant risks of substantial harm had been notified by the practitioner to the patient. There are obviously advantages if this information could be conveyed both in writing as well as by word of mouth. The Bolam Test[10] standard would apply as to what information should be given. It may, however, be more difficult to establish this in non-orthodox medicine.

Could liability for harm in complementary therapies be excluded by reference to a notice? The Unfair Contract Terms Act 1977 would prevent any exclusion of liability if negligence by the therapist caused personal injury or death (see chapter 6).

Patients receiving complementary therapies

If it is found that the patient, in addition to being treated by orthodox medicine, is also in receipt of complementary and alternative therapies, then care must be taken to ensure that there are no contraindications between the two treatments and as much information as possible is obtained about the other treatment. The patient may agree to give the name of the complementary therapist who could be contacted for details of their treatment and treatment plan. It may be, for example, that the patient is given conflicting advice: in such a situation, good communication is essential between the orthodox practitioners and the complementary therapist. There are considerable advantages in NMC practitioners obtaining a good understanding of the complementary therapies that their patients are most likely to be using, so that the practitioner can understand the implications for orthodox medicine and know where to obtain further advice and information.[11] The RCN provided guidance to its members on complementary therapies in 2003, updated in 2007 and 2013.[12] A study of pregnant women in Switzerland showed that none of the women had requested acupuncture during labour but accepted it when offered it by the midwife, confirming similar results in Germany.[13] There is no recent updated advice regarding the use of complementary therapies from the NMC or the RCN as it is expected that all registered practitioners if using a therapy are doing so safely, and using the principles of foreseeability to ensure avoidable harm does not occur. Likewise, in keeping with the Montgomery judgment, all side effects and risks of the treatment are disclosed.

The consent of the client must be obtained, as the following situation indicates.

Practical Dilemma 29.2 | Herbal medicine

Daphne asked a patient about the various bottles that she saw on her bedside locker. The patient explained that she was receiving herbal medicine for her arthritis. Daphne asked for details about what she was taking, but the patient said it was nothing to do with Daphne or her stay in hospital because she was being treated for a heart condition. Where does Daphne stand in law?

There are clear dangers here, since it could be that the herbal preparations could react against any medication given for the patient's heart condition or could even exacerbate the condition. Daphne should ensure that the medical staff are aware of the situation and it might be advisable to arrange for the pharmacist to see the patient and try to persuade her to disclose sufficient details about the herbal preparations and the herbalist advising the patient so that any necessary action can be taken to ensure that the patient is safe.

The NMC reported in its news service in January 2004[14] that cancer patients may be risking dangerous side effects by taking herbal remedies or supplements alongside their conventional treatment. A study at the Royal Marsden Hospital in London found that more than half the 300 patients studied took some form of complementary medicine. The NMC reminded practitioners of their Code of Professional Conduct, which requires practitioners to ensure that the use of complementary and alternative therapies is safe and in the interests of patients and clients, and referred them to more detailed guidance in the advice section on its website.[15] Researchers in America found that certain herbal remedies could work against drugs prescribed for heart disease. Patients did not always tell their doctors they were taking herbal supplements and doctors did not always ask.[16]

Further information should be sought from the Medicines and Healthcare Products Regulatory Agency[17] which publishes adverse warnings on medicines and healthcare products.

Although the NMC has since dispensed with formal guidance in relation to complementary therapies in either the Code (2015) or its website, it would still expect that any administration or prescribing of complementary therapies is done with the full consent of the patient, and that the patient is fully informed of all the treatment options available to them. Nurses cannot use their own personal preferences to place undue duress upon a patient to accept or reject complementary therapies. To do so would render any consent or refusal potentially invalid in law.

Case 29.2 *Shakoor (Deceased)* v *Situ* [2000]

Standard of care of a complementary therapist[18]

S, who was suffering from a skin condition, consulted a practitioner of traditional Chinese herbal medicine. After taking nine doses of the herbal remedy, S became ill and later died of acute liver failure, which was attributable to a rare and unpredictable reaction to the remedy. His widow brought proceedings against the practitioner, but failed. The High Court held that on the evidence before it the actions of the practitioner had been consistent with the standard of care appropriate to traditional Chinese herbal medicine in accordance with established requirements.

The mother of a boy, Neon Roberts, who had a cancerous brain tumour, lost her battle to refuse radiotherapy. She wanted time to research alternative therapies for him. The father had agreed to the boy having radiotherapy.[19]

Case 29.3 Criminal proceedings against a retailer of Chinese herbal medicines

Criminal proceedings were commenced against a Chinese herbalist who sold dangerous pills to a woman who then developed kidney failure and cancer.

Ying 'Susan' Wu pleaded guilty to selling pills that contained a banned substance and was given a 2-year conditional discharge.[20] The pills which the victim took to resolve a skin complaint were described as 'safe and natural' but contained aristolochic acid which should only have been given under prescription and was subsequently banned. The judge, in sentencing, stated that it was unfortunate that there was no system in this country to regulate Chinese herbal medicine retailers with an appropriate professional body or trade association. Such a registration would mean that retailers would be alerted to regulations. A registration system has been in force since May 2011 (see page 745, MRHA).

Case 29.4 — Professional Conduct proceedings against a GP practising ozone therapy

A retired GP Dr Jack, faced proceedings before the Medical Practitioners' Tribunal Service in Manchester following his administration of ozone therapy to a patient with a rare form of non-Hodgkin's Lymphoma. In more than 120 consultations he treated for 80 or 90 times the patient by taking out blood, mixing it with ozone and then reinjecting it into the vein. The treatment has not been subjected to any peer-reviewed papers. A spokesman for the GMC stated that the procedure exposed the patient to the risk of fatal septicaemia.[21] A hearing before the Medical Practitioners Tribunal Service found that his treatment amounted to misconduct. It may lead to a striking off order by the GMC.

House of Lords Select Committee

In November 2000, the Science and Technology Committee of the House of Lords[22] reported that there should be regulations of complementary and alternative medicines (CAM) and there should be further research to evaluate their effectiveness.

The Select Committee of the House of Lords considered that some remedies such as acupuncture and aromatherapy should be available on the NHS, and that NHS patients should have wider access to osteopathy and chiropractic. The implementation of these recommendations led to the establishment of working groups by the Department of Health.

Herbal medicines and acupuncture

Working groups established by the Department of Health to consider the regulation of herbal medicine practitioners and acupuncturists[23] put forward proposals that herbalists will have to register with a new governing body to be eligible to practise and some herbal treatments will only be available from licensed practitioners.[24] However, to date (2018) there is no statutory requirement for registration, and registration occurs on a voluntary basis.

The Health and Care Professions Council (from 2009)

The Health Professions Council, which replaced the Council for the Professions Supplementary to Medicine in 2002 and became the Health and Care Professions Council in 2009, had the capacity to recognise new registered professions. The HPC published guidelines setting criteria on opening new parts of the register.[25] Each applicant organisation must:

- cover a discrete area of activity displaying some homogeneity;
- apply a defined body of knowledge;
- practise based on evidence of efficacy;
- have at least one established professional body which accounts for a significant proportion of that occupational group;

- operate a voluntary register;
- have defined routes of entry to the profession;
- have independently assessed entry qualifications;
- have standards in relation to conduct, performance and ethics;
- have fitness to practise procedures to enforce those standards; be committed to continuous professional development.

Over 53 organisations sought statutory registration from the HCPC, including the Acupuncture Regulatory Working Group, the British Society of Clinical Hypnosis and the Craniosacral Therapy Association of the UK. Once the Council approved an application, an HCPC recommendation and an accompanying report to regulate the profession was submitted to the Secretary of State. If the Secretary of State agreed with the application, an order was drawn up under section 60 of the Health Act 1999, submitted for consultation, if necessary amended and then placed before Parliament. The establishment of the Complementary and Natural Healthcare Council (CNHC) reduced the role of the HCPC as the registration body for CAMs. The CNHC register complementary practitioners from 16 complementary therapy professions.

Medicine and Healthcare Products Regulatory Agency (MHRA)

State registration is not the only form of regulation and where medicinal and other healthcare products are concerned the MHRA is the enforcement agency. It carried out a public consultation on the regulation of herbal medicines at the same time as the Department of Health[26] and warned in September 2004 of the dangers because of the quality of traditional Chinese medicines. A European Directive on Traditional Herbal Medicinal Products[27] setting out the safety and quality of over-the-counter traditional herbal medicines[28] was implemented in October 2005.[29] Further details of the implications and the regulations on trademarks can be obtained from the website of the MHRA. In February 2007 a Chinese woman was prosecuted for selling customers bear bile, antelope and rare orchids as Chinese cures.[30] (See also Case 29.3 and chapter 27.) Since 2011 each EU state has been required to set up a traditional herbal registration scheme for manufactured herbal medicines that are suitable for use without medical supervision.[31]

Concern was expressed about hidden dangers to consumers because of adulterated herbal ingredients.[32] The Medicines and Healthcare Products Regulatory Agency stated that it was imposing a deadline of December 2013 for companies to meet the new EU quality standards, which requires companies to submit products for testing.

The Department of Health announced a new consolidated, multi-purpose, 'pick and mix' set of model byelaws that can be used for one, several or all types of skin-piercing/skin-colouring that are currently regulated.[33]

Complementary and Natural Healthcare Council (CNHC)

The Prince of Wales suggested the setting up of a group to consider the current positions of orthodox, complementary and alternative medicine in the UK and how far it would be appropriate and possible for them to work more closely together. Four working groups looking at research and development, education and training, regulation and delivery mechanisms were established under a steering group chaired by Dr Manon Williams, Assistant Private Secretary to HRH the Prince of Wales. It reported in 1997 and made extensive recommendations.[34] These included encouraging more research and the dissemination of its results; emphasising the common elements in the core curriculum of all healthcare workers, orthodox and CAM; establishing statutory self-regulatory bodies for those professions that could endanger patient safety; and identifying areas of conventional medicine and nursing that are not meeting patients' needs at present. It also recommended the establishment of an Independent Standards Commission for Complementary and Alternative Medicine.

In 2000 the House of Lords Select Committee on Science and Technology produced a report on complementary and alternative medicine (CAM)[35]. Following a 15-month enquiry the Committee's recommendations included a statement which said that the public interest would best be served by improved regulatory structures of many CAM professions.

The Lords grouped the therapies together into three categories. The first were therapies such as acupuncture and herbal medicine which the Lords described as claiming to have an individual diagnostic approach. The second group ('Group 2') were those '*therapies which are most often used to complement conventional medicine and do not purport to embrace diagnostic skills*[36]'. The third were those therapies which the Committee considered to be 'alternative' therapies and which included a diagnostic and treatment element'.

The Lords recommended a phased approach to statutory regulation for the Group 1 therapies that were not already regulated. For Groups 2 and 3 they recommended voluntary regulation and that associations group together to form a single body in each case. This led to the original aim of having single profession-specific registers for each therapy and the Prince's Foundation for Integrated Health (PFIH) initiated this work by bringing many of the professional therapy groups together to develop and agree standards. This goal was changed in 2006 after a report by Professor Julie Stone[37] which recommended that a federal (multi-registering) regulatory body would be the most effective model. Following a consultation held by PFIH in May 2006[38] which found support for that approach, a federal model was pursued.

In 2008 a Federal Working Group was set up. The group was chaired by Dame Professor Joan Higgins, then Chair of The Christie Hospital, Manchester. A huge amount of effort and work was undertaken during the year and the final report was produced in February 2008[39]. This report included a proposal to set up a single federal regulatory body to realise the following benefits as identified by the Federal Working Group:

- a single point of contact for the public;
- economies of scale, with the potential to keep costs to practitioners down;
- rationalisation of standards;
- accommodation of multi-disciplinary practitioners; and
- more weight in negotiations with other bodies.

The body which was set up became known as the Complementary and Natural Healthcare Council (CNHC) and the report provided the template for CNHC during its early work.

Department of Health Funding and Support

The Department of Health in England (in liaison with the devolved administrations) has been very supportive of complementary healthcare regulation. CNHC received three years' start-up funding from the Department which ended as planned at the end of March 2011: 2008/09

(£543,336); 2009/10 (£255,811); and 2009/10 (£31,397). Since April 2011 CNHC has been funded entirely from registrant fees.

The Department of Health also ensured that the principles underpinning professional regulation as set out in its White Paper, 'Trust, Assurance and Safety',[40] are implemented (see chapter 3).

CNHC Structure

It was realised very quickly that the structure proposed in the Federal Working Group report was exceedingly top heavy, expensive and unworkable in practice so this was simplified to an initial structure of:

- Federal Regulatory Board of nine lay (i.e. non CNHC registered) members;
- Professional Committees for Education & Standards; Registration; Finance; Conduct & Competence;
- To operate a robust process for handling complaints about registered practitioners; and
- Profession Specific Boards (representatives from the disciplines registered by CNHC).

In May 2009 the CHNC Board agreed to amalgamate the work of the Registration Committee with the Education and Standards Committee by the formation of a new Professional Standards Committee.

This structure was streamlined further during 2011 with the merging of the Professional Standards and Conduct & Competence Committees to become the Professional Committee. And in 2012 the functions of the Finance Committee were taken on by the CNHC Board.

The Professional Committee consists of experienced individuals who are called upon for Fitness to Practise activity or professional advice, as necessary, supported by the Profession Specific Boards.

From its inception, an essential component of the CNHC structure has been its links with the professions through the Profession Specific Boards (PSBs). There is one PSB for each discipline registered. The PSBs are the professional voice and advice route to and from the Board and the Professional Committee. Originally chosen by the professions themselves through a variety of processes, a new system of rolling elections for appointment, managed by CNHC, came into force in 2013.

CNHC's sole object is the protection of the public and it has four main functions:

- To establish and maintain a voluntary Register of complementary healthcare practitioners in the UK who meet its standards of competence and practice;
- To make the Register of practitioners available to the general public and to educate them about the CNHC quality mark as a quality standard;
- To operate a robust process for handling complaints about registered practitioners; and
- To work with professional bodies in the complementary healthcare field to further develop and improve standards of professional practice.

The CNHC describes its key function as follows:

> **Our key function is to enhance public protection, by setting standards for registration with CNHC. We anticipate that obtaining the CNHC 'quality mark' will swiftly be recognised as the hallmark of quality for the sector. Over time, the general public and those who commission the services of complementary healthcare practitioners will be able to choose with confidence, by looking for the CNHC quality mark.**

The CNHC describes itself as the UK voluntary regulator for complementary healthcare practitioners. The report recommended robust procedures for handling complaints and fitness to practise issues, along with a Code of Conduct and Ethics based on the code used by the Health Professions Council. The complementary healthcare professions that were part of the Foundation for Integrated Health's regulation programme worked with Skills for Health (the Sector Skills Council) to develop the competencies necessary for entry to the Register.

To be eligible to be admitted to the CNHC Register, a complementary therapist must:

- Have undertaken a programme of education and training which meets, as a minimum, the National Occupational Standards and the core curriculum for the complementary therapy/discipline concerned where a core curriculum has been agreed (*NB the requirement regarding the core curriculum was added in 2012*)

or

- Have achieved competency to the level of the National Occupational Standards for the complementary therapy/discipline concerned by means of relevant experience of at least three years and relevant training and been assessed by their peers as having met those standards

and

- Have provided an independent reference of their good character
- Have confirmed that they do not hold a criminal record (including cautions), or notified CNHC of any such record for consideration by the Registrar prior to acceptance
- Have confirmed that there are no health issues that have an impact on their ability to practise
- Have confirmed that they have not been the subject of any disciplinary or civil proceedings against them in relation to their practice or have notified CNHC of any such proceedings for consideration by the Registrar prior to acceptance
- Hold current professional indemnity insurance
- Have agreed to abide by:
  The CNHC Code of Conduct, Ethics and Performance
  CNHC's Continuing Professional Development (CPD) Policy
  CNHC's Data Protection Policy
  Terms of use of the CNHC Quality Mark and website

The Council's Register opened in January 2009 and currently it registers practitioners in the following professions

- Alexander Technique teaching
- aromatherapy
- Bowen Therapy
- colon hydrotherapy
- healing
- hypnotherapy
- microsystems acupuncture
- massage therapy

- craniosacral therapy
- naturopathy
- nutrional therapy
- reflexology
- reiki
- shiatsu
- sports therapy
- yoga therapy

Further information can be obtained from the CNHC website.[41]

The Register can be checked on the CNHC's website.[42] The overall intention is that the Council will provide enhanced consumer confidence and safety through a credible, robust and professional voluntary regulatory structure for the practice of complementary healthcare in the UK.

Registrants can display a certificate incorporating the CNHC quality mark, which provides an independent indication of quality to those wishing to use complementary and natural health services. The quality mark can also be used on websites, promotional literature and elsewhere as confirmation to the public that the CNHC registrant meets the standards set by the CNHC.

Clinical Effectiveness and CAMs

A petition to the government criticised the fact that CNHC registrants would use the certificate provided by the CNHC to imply efficacy and safety, yet the CNHC's approval of the therapy did not involve any actual evidence of efficacy and safety. The government responded to this petition by stating that:

> The CNHC does not promote the efficacy of disciplines practised by its registrants. The aim of the CNHC is protection of the public. Registration means that the practitioner has met certain entry standards (in terms of having an accredited qualification or relevant experience) and that they subscribe to a set of professional standards. The public will have the reassurance that the practitioner they choose meets these standards and will be subject to fitness to practise procedures should they behave inappropriately.
>
> Regulation, whether statutory or voluntary, is about protecting the public. For this reason, the Government fully supports the work of the CNHC. If patients choose to use complementary or alternative therapy, the Government's advice is to choose a practitioner registered with a reputable voluntary registration body such as the CNHC.

Registration with the CNHC does not therefore mean that a particular CAM is clinically effective other than through a placebo effect and there has been considerable discussion about the clinical effectiveness of many CAMs. Professor Ernst, Professor of Complementary Medicine at the University of Exeter, has been critical of the claims made by some alternative remedies such as homeopathy and chiropractic, and has asserted that his clash with the Prince of Wales's Private Secretary has led to the lack of funding support for his unit.[43] He retired in 2011. Criticisms by a science writer, Simon Singh, of chiropractic led to his being sued in a libel case. Although he won the case[44] he still stood to face £60,000 in legal costs.[45] The judgment of the Court of Appeal (which reversed a ruling in the High Court) noted that 'Scientific controversies must be settled by the methods of science rather than by the methods of litigation'. The law on defamation has now been changed to protect scientific research. (See also chapter 17.)

Conclusions

The establishment of the Complementary and Natural Healthcare Council marks a significant step in the protection of the public. As more and more therapies come under the umbrella of the CNHC, professional codes of practice and sanctions against those who fail to comply will become the norm. However, as the Department of Health noted in its reply to the criticism of the CNHC, the Council does not guarantee the clinical effectiveness of the therapies it regulates and there is likely to be continuing concern with their validity. Professor Ernst, Professor of Complementary Therapy at Exeter University, has challenged the value of chiropractic as a treatment option and voiced concern over the effectiveness of other therapies. It is essential that those involved in CAMs are prepared to answer such challenges with randomised controlled trials to establish their clinical effectiveness. The RCN published in 2007 guidance on the integration of complementary therapies into clinical practice.[46] Some of the concerns which it highlighted may gradually be resolved by the CNHC. There are likely to be increasing demands for CAM therapies to be available within the NHS, but their success will depend considerably on the extent to which research can show that there is clear clinical evidence to establish their effectiveness over orthodox medicine alternatives and their endorsement by NICE. In May 2007 it was reported that more than half of the PCTs in England were refusing to pay for homeopathy and other CAMs, on the grounds that their treatments are unproved or disproved.[47] From April 2013 clinical commissioning groups can determine their own policies in relation to the availability of complementary therapies for their patients. It remains to be seen whether there is an increase in their availability on the NHS. It is essential that all health professions registered with the NMC follow its guidance in the application of complementary and alternative therapies.

Reflection questions

1. You have decided that you would like to undertake training in aromatherapy and eventually use it as part of your practice as a clinical nurse specialist in intensive care. What actions would you take to ensure that your plans are compatible with your role as a registered nurse?
2. Identify the ways in which the knowledge that a patient was receiving complementary therapy treatment could affect the care that you give that person.

Further exercises

1. Do you consider that those complementary therapists who so wished should be permitted to have registered status under the Health and Care Professions Council or the Complementary and Natural Healthcare Council? What criteria would you lay down for a profession to receive registered status? (Refer also to chapter 11.)
2. Do you consider that patients should be under an obligation to inform their NHS carers if they are receiving complementary therapies?
3. Access the website of the Complementary and Natural Healthcare Council and consider the implications of its functions for your own professional development.

References

[1] David Rose, Alternative practitioners will need to prove training, *The Times*, 2 April 2010
[2] B.C. Dimond, *Legal Aspects of Complementary Therapy Practice*, Churchill Livingstone, Edinburgh, 1998
[3] www.chisuk.org.uk
[4] www.cochrane.org
[5] Nursing and Midwifery Council, Standards of proficiency for nurse and midwife prescribers, NMC, 2006
[6] Nursing and Midwifery Council, Standards for medicines management, NMC, updated 2012
[7] Nursing and Midwifery Council, Complementary alternative therapies and homeopathy, A–Z guides, NMC, 2008
[8] *Watling* v *Gloucester County Council* Employment Tribunal EAT/868/94, 17 March 1995, 23 November 1994, Lexis transcript
[9] B.C. Dimond, *Legal Aspects of Complementary Therapy Practice*, Churchill Livingstone, Edinburgh, 1998
[10] *Bolam* v *Friern Barnet HMC* [1957] 2 All ER 118
[11] Research Council for Complementary Medicine, www.rccm.org.uk; Institute for Complementary and Natural Medicine, icnm.org.uk; British Medical Association, bma.org.uk
[12] Royal College of Nursing, Complementary Therapies in Nursing, Midwifery and Health Visiting Practice, Order No. 002 204, RCN, October 2007 updated 2013
[13] Martina Gisin, Angela Poat, Katharina Fiez and Irena Anna Frie, Women's experience of acupuncture during labour, *British Journal of Midwifery*, 21(4):254–262, April 2013
[14] *Nursing and Midwifery Council News*, Herbal remedy warning for cancer patients, 21 January 2004
[15] www.nmc.org.uk
[16] David Rose, Herbal remedies 'can work against drugs prescribed for heart disease', *The Times*, 2 February 2010
[17] www.mhra.gov.uk
[18] *Shakoor (Deceased)* v *Situ* [2000] 4 All ER 181
[19] Neon Roberts, Mother loses radiotherapy court battle, BBC news, 21 December 2013
[20] David Rose, Herbalist's tablets caused 'terrible harm', *The Times*, 18 February 2010
[21] News item, GP accused of endangering patient with ozone therapy, *The Times*, 22 October 2013
[22] House of Lords Select Committee on Science and Technology, 6th Report: complementary and alternative medicine, Session 1999–2000, 21 November 2000
[23] Department of Health www.gov.uk
[24] Oliver Wright, Chris Johnston and Rosemary Bennett, Clampdown on alternative medicines, *The Times*, 20 September 2003
[25] www.hpc-uk.org
[26] www.mhra.gov.uk
[27] European Directive, Traditional Herbal Medicines, 2004/24/EC
[28] www.mhra.gov.uk
[29] Medicines (Traditional Herbal Medicinal Products for Human Use) Regulations 2005, SI 2005/2750
[30] Nicola Woolcock, Woman traded bear bile, antelope and rare orchids as Chinese cures, *The Times*, 15 February 2007, p. 3

31 EU directive 2004/24/EC
32 Hannah Devlin, Hidden dangers to consumers discovered in herbal remedies, *The Times*, 11 October 2013
33 Department of Health, Updated model byelaws for the regulation of acupuncture, tattooing, semi-permanent skin-colouring etc., DH, September 2006
34 Integrated Healthcare: a way forward for the next five years, Foundation for Integrated Medicine, 1997
35 2000, House of Lords Select Committee on Science & Technology Report, Complementary & Alternative Medicine
36 ibid
37 2005 Stone J Development of proposals for a future voluntary regulatory structure for complementary healthcare professions PFIH London
38 2006 Jack P *Exploring a Federal Approach to Voluntary Self Regulation of Complementary Healthcare: Consultation Document* PFIH London
39 2008 The Prince's Foundation for Integrated Health '*A Federal approach to Professionally-Led Voluntary Regulation for Complementary Healthcare*' PFIH London
40 Department of Health, Trust, Assurance and Safety: the regulation of health professionals in the 21st century, White Paper Cmnd 7013, 2007
41 www.cnhc.org.uk
42 www.cnhc.org.uk
43 Mark Henderson, Royal row 'threatens alternative medicine research', *The Times*, 3 March 2010
44 *British Chiropractice Association* v *Singh* [2009] EWHC 1101
45 Mark Henderson, Science writer faces a £60,000 bill after winning libel battle with chiropractors, *The Times*, 16 April 2010
46 Royal College of Nursing, Complementary Therapies in Nursing: midwifery and health visiting, Order No. 002 204, RCN, 2007; www.rcn.org.uk/direct
47 Mark Henderson, Hard-up NHS cuts back on homeopathy, *The Times*, 23 May 2007

Chapter 30

The Future

A challenge for any writer or editor in writing a legal textbook is that the law is an ever-changing beast, and any textbook is soon outdated. Yet it is important the law does change. Change is necessary to keep abreast of societal changes, and to respond to often tragic events to ensure greater protection of the society it is meant to serve. Health and nursing is no different. Nursing itself has undergone a period of change. Since 2020 there has been new nursing curriculum,[1] with a focus on advanced skills previously seen as being in the remit of the medical practitioner. Student nurses are also be expected to be prescriber-ready, thereby shortening the process taken to achieve postgraduate prescribing qualifications. In addition, nursing has seenthe advent of the Nursing Associate role in England (with a recommendation of introducing the role intp Wales), and there are already fears that this role may dilute the numbers of registered nurses in clinical practice.

All these changes will expand the legal accountability of the nurse. Further expanding the accountability of the nurse, the NMC has added the duty of candour into its 2015 code of practice for nurses, meaning that there should now be a more open and transparent process when mistakes occur, and also placing a professional responsibility upon nurses to escalate serious mistakes to senior managers. Public scrutiny of nursing will continue, and under the Criminal Justice and Courts Act 2015, nurses can be held criminally liable if they ill-treat or wilfully neglect their patients. Some nurses are serving custodial sentences as a result of very poor practice. While these examples are rare, it illustrates the increased accountability of all registered nurses, and also the consequences if nurses do not meet the standard expected of them.

There are going to be many opportunities and challenges ahead, but of course the greatest challenge or opportunity wasthe United Kingdom leaving the European Union in January 2020. Whilst a trade deal has been completed between the EU and the UK, recognition of professional qualifications is not a part of any deal, and EU nurses have been returning back to the EU, with an increasing reliance of nurses from other parts of the world being recruited to help with filling the many nursing vacancies across the NHS. EU regulations and directives in relation to medicines, safety, and even working hours are numerous to say the least, and while many of these are already written into UK law, it remains to be seen if these protections will continue or whether divergence begins to be seen. Today there continues to be much discussion about repealing or amending the Human Rights Act 1998, and even leaving the European Convention on Human Rights 1950. We have seen in chapter 22 how the Human Rights Act was extended to protect the rights of people in receipt of public money to pay for their costs in nursing and residential care, so tampering with legislation may weaken some of the rights that we all, including our patients, currently receive. However, since the election of the Labour government in July 2024, the likelihood of major constitutional changes in relation to Human Rights is reduced.

Other challenges include the continuing conflicts in Ukraine and Gaza, all of which increase inflationary pressures upon government and household budgets. In 2023 nurses took industrial action for more pay, and as recently as 2024 junior doctors have been on strike due to low pay. All of these challenges add to the pressures on the NHS, and due to inflation government spending on the NHS is in real terms lower than other before.

There continues to be expanding devolution within the UK. Wales, Scotland and Northern Ireland all have taken a different path in how they run the health service in those respective countries, and the COVID-19 pandemic illustrated how each of the home nations of the UK are content to pursue different approaches from central government While this book has often used English legislation as the focus, the reader must recognise that there are many laws in those countries that differ from England. For example the Care Act 2014 is in the main an English-only legislation. In Wales there are free prescriptions, and no hospital car parking charges, while in Scotland there is free personal care for people over the age of 65 if they need it. Northern Ireland is currently in a state of flux, with its assembly only just resumed after a long hiatus,, however it often legislates differently from England. You can also study to be a nurse for free in Wales and Scotland. England has removed the bursary and the funding of tuition fees, so student nurses in England now have to take out a student loan to cover costs. Already there are signals that this is affecting recruitment into the profession. However, waiting lists in Wales are higher than in England, and pressures upon the devolved nations to meet demands from the public are as acute as they are in England. The Reform party which saw considerable support during the 2024 election are even advocating major reforms to the NHS, including following a more insurance-based system.

Therefore, nurses cannot afford to be ignorant of the law. It is a part of everyday practice. With the challenges ahead there may be more pressures upon health service providers, especially financial and resource pressures. In the meantime the public will expect to receive a high quality service for their health care. The challenge for nurses is to maintain a reasonable standard of care, while managing an increasing workload. Having an understanding of the law can assist the nurse in making a sound decision. For example, if the nurse is struggling with workload, report and document it; if the manager is facing insurmountable challenges, escalate the matter to someone more senior and again document that you've done so. Ignoring the law will not help you, but working with the law can help you in your practice, and ultimately will help your patients too.

Finally the law is one matter, but ensuring a professional standard is met is an even greater challenge as it is often a lower bar to reach than the legal standard, so it is possible to not be held legally accountable but to be held professionally accountable for an alleged wrong doing The NMC is often viewed as an organisation to help nurses. It does so by providing guidance to all registrants mainly through the Code (2015)[2], but its prime purpose is to protect the public. Reading the Code will help you to understand what is expected of you as a registrant. Don't ignore it, but keep the Code close at hand.

It is hoped that an awareness of all the changes which have taken place over the past four years and the changes which are in progress will be of value to a nurse in understanding the changing legal context within which they practice.

The website to the book will provide an on-going update to these many changes.

References

[1] www.nursingtimes.net/news/education/nmc-confirms-new-midwife-education-standards-by-2020/7010918.article

[2] Nursing and Midwifery Council (2015) *The Code: Professional standards of practice and behaviour for nurses and midwives* London: NMC

Further Reading

Appelbe, G.E. Wingfield, J. and Taylor, L.M. (eds), *Dale and Appelbe's Pharmacy: Law and Ethics*, 10th ed., Pharmaceutical Press, 2013

Archbold, *Criminal Pleading, Evidence and Practice* (ed. P.J. Richardson), 62nd ed., Sweet & Maxwell, 2013

Atkinson, J., *Advance Directives in Mental Health – Theory, Practice and Ethics*, Jessica Kingsley Publications, 2007

Beale, H.G. (general editor), *Chitty on Contracts*, 3rd cumulative supplement to 32nd ed., Sweet & Maxwell, 2012

Beauchamp, T.L. and Childress, J.F., *Principles of Biomedical Ethics*, 7th ed., Oxford University Press, 2013

Benny, R., Jefferson, M. and Sargeant, M., *Employment Law 2014–15 Questions and Answers*, 6th ed., Oxford University Press, 2014

Blom-Cooper, L., Grounds, A. and Guinan, P. et al., *The Case of Jason Mitchell: Report of the Independent Panel of Inquiry*, Duckworth, 1996

Blom-Cooper, L., Hally, H. and Murphy, E., *The Falling Shadow – One Patient's Mental Health Care 1978–1993* (Report of an Inquiry into the Death of an Occupational Therapist at Edith Morgan Unit, Torbay 1993), Duckworth, 1996

Brazier, M., *Medicine, Patients and the Law*, 5th ed., Penguin, 2011

British Medical Association, *Medical Ethics Today*, BMJ Publishing, 1998

British Medical Association, *Consent, Rights and Choices in Health Care for Children and Young People*, BMJ Books, 2001

British Medical Association, *New Guide to Medicine and Drugs*, 8th ed., BMJ Publishing, 2011

Carey, P., *Data Protection – a practical guide to UK and EU law*, 3rd ed., Oxford University Press, 2009

Clarkson, C.M.V. and Keating, H.M., *Criminal Law Text and Materials*, 7th ed., Sweet & Maxwell, 2010

Clements, L., *Community Care and the Law*, 5th ed., Legal Action Group, 2011

Clerk, J.F., *Clerk and Lindsell on Torts*, 21st ed., Sweet & Maxwell, 2014

Committee of Experts Advisory Group on AIDS, *Guidance for Health Care Workers' Protection against Infection with HIV and Hepatitis*, HMSO, 1994

Connolly, M., *Discrimination Law*, 3rd ed., Thomson, Sweet & Maxwell, 2015

Deakin, S., Johnston, A. and Markensinis, B., *Markensinis and Deakin's Tort Law*, 7th ed., Clarendon Press, 2012

Denis, I.H., *The Law of Evidence*, 5th ed., Sweet & Maxwell, 2013

Department of Health, *AIDS/HIV Infected Health Care Workers*, DH, April 1993

Dimond, B.C., *Accountability and the Nurse*, Distance Learning Pack, South Bank University, 1992

Dimond, B.C., *Legal Aspects of Care in the Community*, Macmillan, 1997

Dimond, B.C., *Legal Aspects of Child Health Care*, Mosby, 1996

Dimond, B.C., *Legal Aspects of Complementary Therapy Practice*, Churchill Livingstone, 1998

Dimond, B.C., *Legal Aspects of Consent*, 2nd ed., Quay Publications/Mark Allen, 2009

Dimond, B.C., *Legal Aspects of Death*, Quay Publications/Mark Allen, 2008

Dimond, B.C., *Legal Aspects of Mental Capacity*, Blackwell Publishing, 2008

Dimond, B.C., *Legal Aspects of Midwifery*, 4th ed., Quay Publications/Mark Allen 2013

Dimond, B.C., *Legal Aspects of Occupational Therapy*, 3rd ed., Blackwell Scientific, 2010

Dimond, B.C., *Legal Aspects of Pain Management*, 2nd ed., Quay Publications/Mark Allen, 2010

Dimond, B.C., *Legal Aspects of Patient Confidentiality*, 2nd ed., Quay Publications/Mark Allen, 2010

Dimond, B.C., *Legal Aspects of Physiotherapy*, 2nd ed., Blackwell Science, 2009

Dimond, B.C., *Patients' Rights, Responsibilities and the Nurse*, 2nd ed., Central Health Studies, Quay Publications, 1999

Dimond, B.C. and Barker, F., *Mental Health Law for Nurses*, Blackwell Science, 1996

Eliot, C. and Quinn, F., *The English Legal System*, 14th ed., Pearson Education, 2013

Emir, A., *Selwyn's Law of Employment*, 17th ed., Butterworth, 2012

Ferguson, H. *Child Protection Practice*, Palgrave Macmillan, 2011

Glynn, J. and Gomez, D., *Regulation of Healthcare Professionals*, Sweet & Maxwell, 2012

Griffith, R., Tengah, C. and Patel, C., *Law and Professional Issues in Midwifery*, Learning Matters, 2010

Griffith, R. and Tengnah, C.A., *Law and Professional Issues in Nursing*, 3rd ed., 2014

Harris, D.J., *Cases and Materials on the European Convention on Human Rights*, 7th ed., Butterworth, 2010

Harris, P., *An Introduction to Law*, 7th ed., Cambridge, 2007

Health and Safety Commission, *Guidelines on Manual Handling in the Health Services*, HMSO, 1992

Health and Safety Commission, *Manual Handling Regulations: Approved Code of Practice*, HMSO, 1992

Health and Safety Commission, *Management of Health and Safety at Work Regulations: Approved Code of Practice*, HMSO, 1999

Hendrick, J., *Law and Ethics in Children's Nursing*, Wiley Blackwell, 2010

Herring, J., *Medical Law and Ethics*, Oxford University Press, 7th ed., 2018

Hoggett, B., *Mental Health Law*, 5th ed., Sweet & Maxwell, 2005

Holland, J. and Burnett, S., *Employment Law*, Oxford University Press, 2012

Howarth, D.R. and O'Sullivan, J.A., *Hepple, Howarth and Matthews' Tort: Cases and Materials*, 7th ed., Butterworth, 2015

Howells, G. and Weatherill, S., *Consumer Protection Law*, 2nd ed., Dartmouth, 2005

Humphreys, N., *Trade Union Law and Collective Employment Rights*, 2nd ed., Jordans, 2005

Hunt, G. and Wainwright, P. (eds) *Expanding the Role of the Nurse*, Blackwell Scientific, 1994

Hurwitz, B., *Clinical Guidelines and the Law*, Oxford Radcliffe Medical Press, 1998

Hurwitz, B. and Paquita, Z., *Everyday Ethics in Primary Care*, BMJ, 2006

Ingman, T., *The English Legal Process*, 13th ed., Oxford University Press, 2010

Jackson, E., *Medical Law*, 4th ed., Oxford University Press, 2016

Jay, R., *Data Protection Law and Practice*, 4th ed., Sweet & Maxwell, 2012

Jones, M.A., *Medical Negligence*, 5th ed., Sweet & Maxwell, 2013

Jones, M.A., *Textbook on Torts*, 9th ed., Oxford University Press, 2007

Jones, R., *Mental Capacity Act Manual*, 6th ed., Sweet & Maxwell, 2014

Jones, R., *Mental Health Act Manual*, 17th ed., Sweet & Maxwell, 2014

Kay, M., Sime, S. and French, D., *Blackstone's Civil Practice 2014*, revised ed., Oxford University Press, 2013

Keenan, D., *Smith and Keenan's English Law*, 17th ed., Pearson, 2013

Kennedy, I., Grubb, A., Laing, J. and McHale, J.V., *Principles of Medical Law*, 3rd ed., Oxford University Press, 2010

Kennedy, T., *Learning European Law*, Sweet & Maxwell, 1998

Kidner, R., *Blackstone's Statutes on Employment Law*, 2013–14, Oxford University Press, 2014

Kloss, D., *Occupational Health Law*, 5th ed., Wiley Blackwell, 2010

Leach, P., *Taking a Case to the European Court of Human Rights*, 3rd ed., Oxford University Press, 2011

Lee, R.G. and Morgan, D., *Human Fertilisation and Embryology*, Blackstone Press, 2001

Lewis, T., *Employment Law*, 10th ed., Legal Action Group, 2013

Lockton, D., *Employment Law*, 8th ed., Palgrave Mcmillan, 2011

Lynch J., *Health Records in Court*, Radcliffe Publishing Ltd, 2009

Macdonald, S. and Magil-Cuerden, J. (eds), *Mayes' Midwifery*, 14th ed., Balliere Tindall, 2011

Mahindra, R., *Medical Law Handbook*, Radcliffe Publishers Ltd, 2008

Mandelstam, M., *An A–Z of Community Care Law*, Jessica Kingsley, 1998

Mandelstam, M., *Community Care Practice and the Law*, 4th ed., Jessica Kingsley, 2005

Mandelstam, M., *Safeguarding Vulnerable Adults and the Law*, Jessica Kingsley, 2008

Mason, J.K. and Laurie, G.T., *Mason and McCall-Smith's, Law and Medical Ethics*, 9th ed., Oxford, 2014

McHale, J. and Fox, M., *Health Care Law*, 2nd ed., Sweet & Maxwell, 2007

McHale, J. and Tingle, J., *Law and Nursing*, 3rd ed., Butterworth–Heinemann Elsevier, 2007

McLean, S., *Impairment and Disability: Law and Ethics at the Beginning and End of Life*, Routledge-Cavendish, 2007

Miles, A., Hampton, J. and Hurwitz, B., *NICE, CHI and the NHS Reforms – Enabling Excellence or Imposing Control?*, Aesculapius, 2000

Morris, A.E. and Jones, M.A. *Blackstone's Statutes on Medical Law*, 9th ed., Oxford University Press, 2017

Murphy, J. and Witting, C., *Street on Torts*, 13th ed., Butterworth, 2012

O'Sullivan, J., Morgan, J., Tofaris, S. and Matthews, M., *Hepple and Matthews' Tort Law*, 7th ed., Hart Publishing, 2015

Painter, R.W. and Holmes, A.E.M., *Cases and Materials on Employment Law*, 9th ed., Oxford University Press, 2012

Pattinson, S.D., *Medical Law and Ethics*, 5th ed., Sweet & Maxwell, 2017

Pitt, G., *Employment Law*, 8th ed., Sweet & Maxwell, 2011

Pyne, R.H., *Professional Discipline in Nursing, Midwifery and Health Visiting*, 3rd ed., Blackwell Scientific, 1998

Rogers, W.V.H., *Winfield and Jolowicz on Tort*, 18th ed., Thomson, Sweet & Maxwell, 2010

Rowson, R., *An Introduction to Ethics for Nurses*, Scutari Press, 1990

Rowson, R., *Working Ethics – How to be Fair in a Culturally Complex World*, Jessica Kingsley, 2006

Rubenstein, M., *Discrimination. A Guide to the Relevant Case Law*, 19th ed., Eclipse Group, 2014

Rumbold, G., *Ethics in Nursing Practice*, 3rd ed., Baillière Tindall, 1999

Salvage, J., *Nurses at Risk: Guide to Health and Safety at Work*, 2nd ed., Heinemann, 1998

Sargeant, M., *Discrimination and the Law*, Routledge, 2013

Sellars, C., *Risk Assessment with People with Learning Disabilities*, Blackwell, 2011

Sharpley, D., *Criminal Litigation: Practice and Procedure CLP Legal Practice Guides*, College of Law, 2013

Silverton, L., *The Art and Science of Midwifery*, Pearson Education, 1998

Sime, S., *Practical Approach to Civil Procedure*, 15th ed., Blackstone Press, 2012

Skegg, P.D.G., *Law, Ethics and Medicine*, 2nd ed., Oxford University Press, 1998

Slapper, G. and Kelly, D., *The English Legal System, 2014–15*, 15th ed., Routledge-Cavendish, 2014

Smith, I. and Baker, A., *Smith and Wood's Employment Law*, 11th ed., Oxford University Press, 2013

Social Security Inspectorate, Department of Health, *No Longer Afraid: Safeguard of Older People in Domestic Settings*, HMSO, 1993

Stauch, M. and Wheat, K., *Text and Materials on Medical Law and Ethics*, 4th ed., Cavendish, 2011

Stevenson, K., Davies, A. and Gunn, M., *Blackstone's Guide to Sexual Offences Act 2003*, Oxford University Press, 2003

Stone, J. and Matthews, J., *Complementary Medicine and the Law*, Oxford University Press, 1996

Storch, J., *Towards a Moral Horizon: Nursing Ethics for Leadership and Practice*, Pearson Education, 2004

Symon, A., *Obstetric Litigation from A to Z*, Mark Allen Publishing, 2001

Taylor, S. and Emir, A., *Employment Law: An Introduction*, 3rd ed., Oxford University Press, 2012

Tilley, S. and Watson, R. (eds), *Accountability in Nursing and Midwifery*, 2nd ed., Blackwell Publishing, 2004

Tingle, J. and Cribb, A., *Nursing Law and Ethics*, 4th ed., Wiley Blackwell Publishers, 2013

Tingle, J. and Foster, C., *Clinical Guidelines: Law, Policy and Practice*, 2nd ed., Cavendish, 2006

Tolley's Health and Safety at Work Handbook 2017, 29th ed., Tolley, 2016

Tschudin, V., *Ethics in Nursing: The Caring Relationship*, 3rd ed., Butterworth–Heinemann, 2003

Vincent, C. (ed.), *Clinical Risk Management*, 2nd ed., BMJ Publishing, 2001

White, R. and Carr, P., *The Children Act in Practice*, Butterworth, 2008

Wild, C. and Weinstein, S., *Smith and Keenan's English Law*, 17th ed., Longman, 2013

Wilkinson, R. and Caulfield, H., *The Human Rights Act: A Practical Guide for Nurses*, Whurr Publishers, 2000

Woods, L. and Watson, P., *Steiner and Woods EU Law*, 12th ed., Oxford University Press, 2014

Zander, M., *Police and Criminal Evidence Act*, 6th ed., Sweet & Maxwell, 2013

Websites

39 Essex Chambers	www.39essex.com
Advisory, Conciliation and Arbitration Service	www.acas.org.uk
The Advocacy People (Independent Complaints Advocacy Service)	www.theadvocacypeople.org.uk
Age UK	www.ageuk.org.uk
Alzheimer's Society	www.alzheimers.org.uk
Anscombe Bioethics Centre (formerly Linacre Centre for Healthcare Ethics)	www.bioethics.org.uk
ASA (Advice Services Alliance)	www.asauk.org.uk
Association of Contentious Trust and Probate Specialists	www.actaps.com
Association of Lifetime Lawyers (formerly Solicitors for the Elderly)	https://sfe.legal
Bailii (case law and statute resource)	www.bailii.org
Bar Council	www.barcouncil.org.uk
Bipolar UK	www.bipolaruk.org
Care Quality Commission	www.cqc.org.uk
Care Rights UK (formerly Relatives and Residents Association)	www.carerightsuk.org
Carers Trust	www.carers.org
Carers UK	www.carersuk.org
Citizens' Advice Bureau	www.citizensadvice.org.uk
Civil Mediation Council	www.civilmediation.org
Civil Procedure Rules	www.justice.gov.uk/courts/procedure-rules/civil
Clinical Negligence Scheme for Trusts	https://resolution.nhs.uk/services/claims-management/clinical-schemes/clinical-negligence-scheme-for-trusts/
Criminal Injury Compensation Authority	www.gov.uk/government/organisations/criminal-injuries-compensation-authority
Community Legal Service Direct	www.clsdirect.org.uk
Complementary & Natural Healthcare Council	www.chnc.org.uk
Court Funds Office	www.gov.uk/contact-court-funds-office
Court of Protection	www.gov.uk/courts-tribunals/court-of-protection
Dementia UK	www.dementiauk.org
Department for Education	www.education.gov.uk
Department for Work and Pensions	www.dwp.gov.uk
Department of Health and Social Care	www.gov.uk/government/organisations/department-of-health-and-social-care
Dignity in Dying	www.dignityindying.org.uk
Disability Law Service	dls.org.uk
Down's Syndrome Association	www.downs-syndrome.org.uk
Equality and Human Rights Commission	www.equalityhumanrights.com
Family Carer Support Service	www.hft.org.uk/our-services/family-carer-support-service
Family Mediation Council	www.familymediationcouncil.org.uk
Foundation for People with Learning Disabilities	www.learningdisabilities.org.uk
General Medical Council	www.gmc-uk.org

Headway: The Brain Injury Association	www.headway.org.uk
Health and Safety Executive	www.hse.gov.uk
Health and Care Professions Council	www.hcpc-uk.org
Health Research Authority	www.hra.nhs.uk
His Majesty's Courts and Tribunal Service	www.gov.uk/government/organisations/hm-court-service
HF Trust (Learning Disability Allies)	www.hft.org.uk
Homecare Association	www.ukhca.co.uk
Hospice UK	www.hospiceuk.org
Hourglass (Action on Elder Abuse)	www.wearehourglass.org
Human Fertilisation and Embryology Authority	www.hfea.gov.uk
Independent Age	www.independentage.org
Independent Mental Capacity Advocate	www.scie.org.uk/publications/imca
Information Commissioner's Office	www.ico.org.uk
Law Centres Network	www.lawcentres.org.uk
Law Society	www.lawsociety.org.uk
Legislation	www.legislation.gov.uk
MedicAlert Foundation	www.medicalert.org.uk
Medicines and Healthcare Products Regulatory Agency	www.gov.uk/mhra
MENCAP	www.mencap.org.uk
Mental Health Foundation	www.mentalhealth.org.uk
Mental Health Lawyers Association	www.mhla.co.uk
Mental Health Matters	www.mhm.org.uk
Mind	www.mind.org.uk
Ministry of Justice	www.justice.gov.uk
Motor Neurone Disease Association	www.mndassociation.org
National Audit Office	www.nao.org.uk
National Autistic Society	www.autism.org.uk
National Care Association	www.nationalcareassociation.org.uk
National Domestic Abuse Helpline	www.nationaldahelpline.org.uk
National Institute for Health and Care Research	www.nihr.ac.uk
National Patient Safety Agency	www.npsa.org.uk
National Perinatal Epidemiology Unit	www.npeu.ox.ac.uk
NHS 111	https://111.nhs.uk
NHS Digital (data and information)	https://digital.nhs.uk
NHS Employers	www.nhsemployers.org
NHS Professionals	www.nhsprofessionals.nhs.uk
NHS Resolution	https://resolution.nhs.uk
NHS	www.nhs.uk
NICE	www.nice.org.uk
Northern Ireland Assembly	www.niassembly.gov.uk
Nursing and Midwifery Council	www.nmc.org.uk
Office for Health Improvement and Disparities	www.gov.uk/government/organisations/office-for-health-improvement-and-disparities
Office of the Public Guardian	www.gov.uk/government/organisations/office-of-the-public-guardian
Official Solicitor and Public Trustee	www.gov.uk/government/organisations/official-solicitor-and-public-trustee
Open Government	www.opengovernment.org.uk
Patients Association	www.patients-association.org.uk
Patients First	www.patientsfirst.org.uk
Prescription Pill Addictions	www.nhs.uk/live-well/addiction-support/drug-addiction-getting-help/
Public Sector Audit Appointments	www.psaa.co.uk
Re-engage (formerly Contact the Elderly)	www.reengage.org.uk
RESCARE (The Society for Children and Adults with Learning Disabilities and their Families)	www.rescare.org.uk
Respond	www.respond.org.uk
Rethink (formerly the National Schizophrenia Fellowship)	www.rethink.org
Royal College of Nursing	www.rcn.org.uk
Royal College of Paediatrics and Child Health	www.rcpch.ac.uk

Royal College of Psychiatrists	www.rcpsych.ac.uk
Royal College of Surgeons of England	www.rcseng.ac.uk
SANE	www.sane.org.uk
Scottish Government	www.gov.scot
Scope	www.scope.org.uk
Sense	www.sense.org.uk
Serious Fraud Office	www.sfo.gov.uk
Shipman Inquiry	https://webarchive.nationalarchives.gov.uk/ukgwa/timeline
	https://www.the-shipman-inquiry.org.uk
Skipton Fund	www.skiptonfund.org
Speak Up	www.speakup.org.uk
Stroke Association	www.stroke.org.uk
Together: for Mental Wellbeing	www.together-uk.org
Turning Point	www.turning-point.co.uk
UK Health Security Agency	www.gov.uk/government/organisations/uk-health-security-agency
UK Parliament	www.parliament.uk
United for Human Rights	www.humanrights.com
United Response	www.unitedresponse.org.uk
Veterans UK	www.gov.uk/government/organisations/veterans-uk
Welsh Government	https://gov.wales
World Medical Association	www.wma.net

Glossary

acceptance an agreement to the terms of an offer which leads to a binding legal obligation, i.e. a contract

acceptance

accusatorial a system of court proceedings where the two sides contest the issue (contrast with inquisitorial)

Act of Parliament, statute

action legal proceedings

actus reus essential element of a crime that must be proved to secure a conviction, as opposed to the mental state of the accused (mens rea)

adversarial approach adopted in an accusatorial system

advocates a person who pleads for another; it could be paid and professional, such as a barrister or solicitor, or it could be a lay advocate either paid or unpaid; a witness is not an advocate

alternative dispute resolution methods to resolve a dispute without going to court, such as mediation

approved mental health professional a person recognised under the Mental Health Act 1983 (as amended by the Mental Health Act 2007) as having responsibilities in relation to the admission and detention of persons under the Mental Health Act (replaces the *approved social worker*)

arrestable offence an offence defined in section 24 of the Police and Criminal Evidence Act 1984 that gives to the citizen the power of arrest in certain circumstances without a warrant

Assault a threat of unlawful contact (trespass to the person)

balance of probabilities standard of proof in civil proceedings

barristers a lawyer qualified to take a case in court

Battery an unlawful touching (see trespass to the person)

Bolam Test test laid down by Judge McNair in the case of Bolam v. Friern HMC on the standard of care expected of a professional in cases of alleged negligence

burden of proof duty of a party to litigation to establish the facts or, in criminal proceedings, the duty of the prosecution to establish both actus reus and mens rea

cause of action facts that entitle a person to sue

citation each case is reported in an official series of cases according to the following symbols: *Re F* (i.e. in the matter of F) or *F v. West Berkshire Health Authority* 1989 2 All ER 545 which means the year 1989 volume 2 of the All England Law Reports page 545. Each case can be cited by means of this reference system. In the case of *Whitehouse* v. *Jordan (Whitehouse* v. *Jordan* [1981] 1 All ER 267), Whitehouse is the claimant, Jordan the defendant and 'v.' stands for versus, i.e. against. Other law reports include: AC, Appeals Court; EWCA, England and Wales Court of Appeal; EWHC, England and Wales High Court; EWHL, England and Wales House of Lords; QB, Queens Bench Division; and WLR, Weekly Law Reports

civil action proceedings brought in the civil courts

civil wrongs An act or omission which can be pursued in the civil courts by the person who has suffered the wrong (see tort)

claimant person bringing a civil action (originally plaintiff)

committal proceedings hearings before the magistrates to decide if a person should be sent for trial in the Crown Court

Common law law derived from the decisions of judges, case law, judge-made law

conditional fee systems a system whereby client and lawyer can agree that payment of fees is dependent on the outcome of the court action, also known as 'no win, no fee'

conditions terms of a contract

constructive knowledge knowledge that can be obtained from the circumstances

continuous service length of service an employee must have served to be entitled to receive certain statutory or contractual rights

contract an agreement enforceable in law

contract for services an agreement enforceable in law whereby one party provides services, not being employment, in return for payment or other consideration from the other

contract of service a contract for employment

coroner a person appointed to hold an inquiry (inquest) into a death that occurred in unexpected or unusual circumstances

criminal an act or omission which can be pursued in the criminal courts

cross-examination questions asked of a witness by the lawyer for the opposing side; leading questions may be asked

damages a sum of money awarded by a court as compensation for a tort or breach of contract

declaration a ruling by the court setting out the legal situation

disclosure documents made available to the other party

dissenting judge a judge who disagrees with the decision of the majority of judges

distinguished (of cases) rules of precedent require judges to follow decisions of judges in previous cases, where these are binding on them. However, in some circumstances, it is possible to come to a different decision, because the facts of the earlier case are not comparable to the case now being heard and therefore the earlier decision can be 'distinguished'

Examination in chief witness is asked questions in court by the lawyer for the party that has asked the witness to attend; leading questions may not be asked

901

ex gratia as a matter of favour, e.g. without admission of liability, of payment offered to a client

expert witness evidence given by a person whose general opinion, based on training or experience, is relevant to some of the issues in dispute (contrast with witness of fact)

good character a person with no criminal convictions, cautions or professional sanctions on their record

good health the persons health does not present a risk of harm to patients or risk the public's confidence in the profession

guilty a finding in a criminal court of responsibility for a criminal offence

Hearsay evidence that has been learnt from another person

hierarchy recognised status of courts that results in lower courts following the decisions of higher courts (*see* **precedent**). Thus decisions of the Supreme Court must be followed by all lower courts unless they can be *distinguished*

indictment a written accusation against a person, charging him with a serious crime, triable by jury

informal not subject to a section, order or report detaining the person in hospital for the treatment of a mental disorder

injunction an discretionary (sometimes called an equitable) remedy in which a court orders a party to perform, or refrain from performing, a particular act.

inquisitorial a system of justice whereby the truth is revealed by an inquiry into the facts conducted by the judge, e.g. coroner's court

invitation to treat early stages in negotiating a contract, e.g. an advertisement or letter expressing interest. An invitation to treat will often precede an offer that, when accepted, leads to the formation of an agreement that, if there is consideration and an intention to create legal relations, will be binding

judicial review an application to the High Court for a judicial or administrative decision to be reviewed and an appropriate order made, e.g. declaration

Justice of the Peace a lay *magistrate*, i.e. not legally qualified, who hears *summary* (minor) *offences* and sometimes indictable (serious) offences in the magistrates' court in a group of three

King's Counsel a senior barrister, also known as a 'silk'

liability responsibility for the wrongdoing or harm in civil proceedings

litigation civil proceedings

magistrates a person (see Justice of the Peace) who hears summary (minor) offences or indictable offences that can be heard in the magistrates' court. A bench consists of three magistrates, known as Justices of the Peace, who sit in the magistrates' court

mandamus (we command) an order of the court requiring the defendant to take specified action

mens rea mental element in a crime (contrast with actus reus)

negligence civil *action* for compensation, also a failure to follow a reasonable standard of care

offer a proposal made by a party that, if accepted, can lead to a contract. It often follows an invitation to treat

Ombudsman a commissioner (e.g. health, local government) appointed by the government to hear complaints

payments into court an offer to settle a dispute at a particular sum, which is paid into court. The claimant's failure to accept the offer means that the claimant is liable to pay costs, if the final award is the same or less than the payment made

plaintiff term formerly used to describe one who brings an action in the civil courts. Now the term claimant is used

practice directions guidance issued by the head of the court to which they relate on the procedure to be followed

pre-action protocol rules of the Supreme Court that provide guidance on action to be taken before legal proceedings commence

precedents a decision that may have to be followed in a subsequent court hearing (*see hierarchy*)

prima facie at first sight; sufficient evidence brought by one party to require the other party to provide a defence

privilege in relation to evidence, being able to refuse to disclose it to the court

professional misconduct conduct of a registered health practitioner that could lead to conduct and competence proceedings by the registration body

proof evidence that secures the establishment of a claimant's, prosecution's or defendant's case

prosecution pursuing of criminal offences in court

quantum amount of compensation, or the monetary value of a claim

reasonable doubt to secure a conviction in criminal proceedings the prosecution must establish 'beyond reasonable doubt' the guilt of the accused

solicitor a lawyer who is qualified on the register held by the Law Society

specialist community public health nurse replaces the health visitor as a registered practitioner under the Nursing and Midwifery Council

statute law law made by Acts of Parliament

strict liability holding a individual or entity liable for damage or loss without having to prove carelessness

subpoena an order of the court requiring a person to appear as a witness (subpoena ad testificandum) or to bring records/documents (subpoena duces tecum)

summary judgment a procedure whereby the claimant can obtain judgment without the defendant being permitted to defend the action

summary offence a lesser offence that may only be heard by *magistrates*

torts a civil wrong, excluding breach of contract. It includes: negligence, trespass (to the person, goods or land), nuisance, breach of statutory duty and defamation

trespass to the person a wrongful direct interference with another person. Harm does not have to be proved

trial a court hearing before a judge

vicarious liability liability of an employer for wrongful acts of an employee committed while in the course of employment

volenti non fit injuria to the willing there is no wrong; voluntary assumption of risk

ward of court a minor placed under the protection of the High Court, which assumes responsibility for him or her and all decisions relating to his or her care must be made in accordance with the directions of the court

Wednesbury unreasonable a decision that is so unreasonable that it is irrational as no other reasonable person acting reasonably would have made it

without prejudice without detracting from or without disadvantage to. The use of the phrase prevents the other party using the information to the prejudice of the one providing it

witness of fact a person who gives evidence of what they saw, heard, did or failed to do (contrast with expert witness)

writ a form of written command, e.g. the document that used to commence civil proceedings. Now a claim form is served

Index

A

Abortion 437–452, 511
  being born alive 442
  challenge by putative father 444
  conscientious objection to participation 439–440
  consent by pregnant person under 16 years 449–450
  emergency provisions 439
  fetus, rights of 443
  future reforms of law 451–452
  general principles 437–439
  husband's attempt to stop 444–445
  illegal, confidentiality and 448
  illegal, when 442
  mental capacity, and 450–451
  negligence in failing to defect abnormality 443–444
  notification 448–449
  nurses' participation in prostaglandin abortions 441–442
  refused 445–447
  related offences 447–448
  right to 445–450
  termination one of multiple pregnancy 448
  whose choice 449
Acceptance 51
  of offer 268
Access to Medical Reports Act 1988 241
Accident and emergency (A&E) department 605–609
  aggravating factor, for serious offences 610
  assault on nurse 610
  assaults continue to rise 610–615
  clinical nurse specialist 614
  duty of care of GP, and 613
  emergency workers
    exercise of functions as 609
    legislation 609
  excessive waiting 615–617
  extent of duty of care 614
  giving information to patients 612–613
  local initiatives 608
  managing workload 606–608
  minor ailments 613
  mistaken identity 617
  National Audit Office Report 2013 608
  pressure of work - legal issues 611–612
  pressure to disclose confidential information 614–615
  road traffic accidents 615
  strategy 606
Accidents in the theatre 469–471
Accountability 5
  to employer 9
  professionalism, and 9
Acts of Parliament 9–10
Acupuncture 883–884
Acute care 465–489
  policies 467
  potential hazards in operating theatres 468
  practices 467
  professional liability 466–467
  theatre nurse and scope of professional practice 469
Adolescents 425–426
Advisory Committee on Genetic Testing (ACGT) 651
Advisory, Conciliation and Arbitration Service (ACAS) 284, 287, 290
Agency liability 87
Agency nurses 728
Agency Workers Regulations 2010 285
Agenda for Change 271
Airedale Inquiry Report 136
Allitt, Beverley 34, 136–137
Alternative dispute resolution 150
Amaro, Nurse 36

Ambulance services 612
Amputation of healthy limbs 188
Anti-smoking legislation 381–382
Apportioning responsibility 77
Approved mental health professional (AMHP) 580–581, 598, 696–697
Areas that concern the nurse 4
Arenas of accountability 5
Aromatherapy, without consent 879
Arrest, initial stages 24–26
Arrestable offence 232
Artificial insemination 626–629
  anonymity of donors 628–629
  donor, by 627–628
  husband, by 626–627
  safety of tissue and cells 629
Artificial insemination by donor (AID) 627–628
Artificial insemination by husband (AIH) 626–627
Assault 177
  on behalf of employer 82
Association of British Insurers (ABI) 651, 652
Association of the British Pharmaceutical Industry (ABPI) 536

B

Baby P 416–418
Balance of probabilities 154
Barristers 12
Battery 177
Blood
  compensation 474–475
  contamination 474–475
Blood donors 768
  haemophiliacs, and 768–769
Bolam Test 53, 94, 196, 203, 717, 723, 880
Bournewood Case 493–494

Brain death 836–838
British Chiropractic Association (BCA) 537
British Pregnancy Advisory Service (BPAS) 447
Bullying 378–380
Burden of proof 32

C

Caldicott Guardians 235–236
Caldicott Review 235–236
Care Act 2014 670–681
  care and support 671–673
  care and support plan 677–680
  community equipment 681
  deferred payments 680
  eligibility criteria 676–677
  how to meet needs 675–676
  independent advocate 680–681
  preventing needs for care and support 674
  promoting individual well-being 673–674
  promoting integration of care and support with health services 675
Care homes
  human rights, and 681–684
  standards 699–700
Care provider offence 140–141
  accidents and errors 142
  ill treatment 141
  wilful neglect 141
Care Quality Commission (CQC) 100, 105, 126–132, 204, 335–336, 343, 683–684, 699, 760, 791, 792
  first prosecution for failing to provide safe care and treatment 130–132
  functions 127
  matters to have regard 127–128

903

Care Quality Commission (*continued*)
  nursing the mentally disordered 600–601
  objectives 127
  registration with 129
  safe care and treatment 129–130
  statement on user involvement 128
Carers 499, 687–688
  Independent Mental Capacity Advocates 499
  liability of client for 688
  protection of autonomy of client 500–501
  refusal to grant accommodation 499
Care trusts 125
Case law *see* Common law
Causation 60–64
  blindness 61
  deafness 61
  factual 60–61
  loss of a chance 63–64
  reasonably foreseeable consequence 62
  taking one's claimant as one finds him 62
  thin skull rule 62–63
Cause of action 51, 239
Central Office for Research Ethics Committees (COREC) 531
Central sterile services department (CSSD) 354
Child abuse 411
  errors in identifying 420–421
  liability of local authorities for 419–420
Child protection 411–421
  Baby P 416–418
  Care Act 2014 413
  Children Act 1989 412
  Daniel Pelka 418–419
  Protection of Children Act 1999 421
  Working Together to Safeguard Children 413–416
Children and young persons 395–436
  adolescents 425–426
  anorexia nervosa 398
  blood transfusion 407
  children under sixteen years 400–401
  clash between parent and child 399, 404–406
  compulsory treatment for mental disorder 401
  consent to research 397–398

consent to treatment 396–397
deprivation of liberty 426–429
  authorising 429
  imputability of state 429
  inherent jurisdiction, of High Court 429–431
  local authorities 429
  minors 426
  objective 427–429
  restriction and 427–428
  subjective element 428
disciplining a child 423–425
dispute over treatment 405
DNA and parental consent 406
Down's syndrome 407
emergencies 398–399
Gillick case 402–404
letting die 408–409
National Deprivation of Liberty Court 429
no absolutist test 409–410
non-parents 401–402
parallel consent 399–400
permissive declarations 410–411
Protection of Children Act 1999 421
referring matter to court 410
refusal by fourteen-year-old Jehovah's Witness 403
refusal of blood by fifteen-year-old 400–401
refusal to have treatment 398
transplants and the interests of the child 406
withholding consent by parents 407–408
Children, contributory negligence and 162
Child sex abuse, mandatory reporting 419
CHRE 326–328
Civil actions 11–12
Civil and criminal law distinguished 11
Civil courts 8
Civil liability 8
Civil litigation, reforms to 172
Civil Procedure Rules 150, 151, 154
Civil proceedings 149–153
  case management 150–151
  claim form issued 152–153
  compensation for negligence 156–160
  calculating amount of compensation 159–160
  general damages 157–159
  non-pecuniary loss 157–158

pecuniary loss 158–159
special damages 157
defences 160–170
  contributory negligence 161–162
  denial of facts 160
  exemption from liability 164–166
  legal aid and conditional fees 169–170
  limitation of time 166
    delay 167
    extension 168
    judge's discretion to extend 168
    knowledge of harm 166–167
  missing element 160
  Unfair Contract Terms Act 1977 164–166
  volenti non fit injuria 163–164
  willing assumption of risk 163–164
disclosure and inspection of documents 152
early termination 152
fast track 151
hearing 154–155
  claimant's case 154
  cross-examination 154
  defendant's case 154–155
  examination in chief 154
  expert evidence 154
  judge's summing up 155
  re-examination 154
  res ipsa loquitur 155
mediation 150
multi track 152
payment into court 153
pre-action protocol 152
pre-trial review 153
service of claim form 153
small claims track 151
summary judgement 152
Civil wrongs 11
Claimant 8
Classification of offences 28
Clinical commissioning groups (CCGs) 114, 116–119, 705
  duties 118
  statutory duties 116–117
Clinical governance 125
Clinically assisted nutrition and hydration (CANH) 843
Clinical Negligence Scheme for Trusts (CNST) 90, 170–171

Clinic nurse 703–705
  consent, obtaining 703–704
  minors 704–705
  specialists 720–721
Cloning 653–655
  personalised medication 654–655
Closed material procedures (CMP) 19
Clothier Committee 647
Codes of practice 324
Commission for Patient and Public Involvement in Health (CPPIH) 788
Common law 10
Community and primary care nursing 661–712
  aggression in the community 693
  checklist for staff who make home visits 694–695
  community dangers 693
  consent to treatment 695–697
    compulsory removal 696–697
    forcible entry 695–696
    mental capacity 695
    mentally disordered 695
  continuing care 664
  criminal suspicion 698
  defective premises 692
  delayed discharges 684–687
  difficulties 662
  disabled persons, assessment of 663–664
  disclosure of information 698
  duty of local authority on discharge of hospital patients 685–687
  negligence 688–691
    examples of serious breaches of duty of care 691
    giving advice 691
    standard of care 688–689
    to whom nurse responsible 689–691
  NHS and social services provision 662–666
  official advice on violence 694
  protection of property 697
  rationing care 666
  safety of community professional 691–695
Community and primary care services 124–125
Community Equipment Code of Practice Scheme (CECOPS) 681
Community matrons 700

Community treatment order
    (CTO) 591–595
  treatment provisions for those
    on 595
Compensation payment to
    victim 44
Complaints 774–797
  criticisms by Healthcare
    Commission 780, 781
  detained patients 791–792
  handling 777–778
  Hospital Complaints Proce-
    dure Act 1985 778–779
  key elements in procedure 779
  and litigation 790–791
  methods 775–777
  NHS Constitution 792–793
  nurse and 791
  reasons for 775, 776
  research into system 779–780
  review of NHS system
    793–794
  what do complainants seek 776
  Wilson Report 778–779
Complaints procedure 2004
    779–780
Complaints procedure 2004 and
    2006 780–781
Complaints procedure 2009
    781–786
  annual reports 785–786
  form of communications
    784–785
  investigation and response 784
  monitoring 785
  procedure for handling 783
  publicity 785
  statutory feedback 786
Complementary and alternative
    therapies 877–891
  clinical effectiveness and
    CAMs 888
  CNHC 884–888
  criminal proceedings against
    retailer 882
  definitions 878
  House of Lords Select Com-
    mittee 883
  liability for using at work
    879–880
  MHRA 884
  NMC practitioner as com-
    plementary therapist
    878–879
  notifying patients of risks 880
  patients receiving 881–883
  professional conduct proceed-
    ings against GP practis-
    ing ozone therapy 883
  standard of care 882

Complementary and Natural
    Healthcare Council
    (CNHC) 884–888
  clinical effectiveness and
    CAMs 888
  Department of Health
    funding and support
    885–886
  structure 886–888
Conditional fee agreements
    (CFAs) 169
Conditional fees 169–170
Confidentiality 217–235,
    532–533, 768–769
  consent of patient 220–221
  court orders 222–225
  disclosure and Article
    8 rights 235
  disclosure before trial
    224–225
  disclosure in personal injury
    cases 224
  disclosure in the interests of
    the patient 222
  disclosure of information
    relating to mentally
    incapacitated adult 234
  disclosure on anonymous basis
    234–235
  disclosure refused by
    patient 221
  disclosure to press 221
  disclosure to registration body
    in public interest 229
  disclosure without consent
    227
  exceptions 219–220
  legal professional privilege
    223–224
  national data opt-out 219
  occupational health 228
  parents, disclosure to 234
  police, disclosure to 230–234
    criminal offence believed
      to have taken place 231
    Department of Health
      advice 231–232
    gas 233
    keeping patient until police
      arrive 232
    non-accidental injury 233
    patient's fitness for ques-
      tioning 232
    reporting crime 232–233
    suspected child abuse 233
    suspected stolen goods 233
    UKCC 233–234
  privilege on grounds of public
    interest 223
  professional standards 218

  psychotherapy, and 226–227
  public interest, and 226–229
  spouse 220
  statutory duty to disclose 225
  subpoena 222–223
  waiver 221
Consent in the theatre
  consent refused 472–473
  pre-medication, after
    471–472
Consent, research and 533–537
Consent to treatment 176–208
  anaesthesia 180
  basic principles 177
  forms of giving 177–178
  implied 180–181
  information to patient
    196–200
  Kennedy Report 178, 179
  legal professional privilege
    223–224
  Mental Health Act 1983 195
  non-therapeutic procedures
    200–201
  right to refuse treatment
    181–184
  risk of sterilisation failing 200
  Sidaway 197–200
  valid, requirements of 177
  word of mouth 180
  writing 178–180
Constructive dismissal 289–290
Constructive knowledge 168
Consumer Protection Act 1987
    352–356
  damage 355–356
  defect 352
  defences 355
  effect of product liability on
    nurse 354
  naming producer 354–355
  nurse as supplier 355
  product liability 352
  timing 354
Contestability 106
Continuing professional develop-
    ment (CPD) 325–326
Continuous service 277
Contract for services 87
Contract of employment 9,
    268–274
  breach 274
  changing 273–274
  content 270–272
  express terms 270, 271
  failure to declare particular
    medical condition
    or criminal record
    269–270
  formation 268–269

  implied terms 271–272
  pre-employment checks
    269–270
  right of employee to see or
    have 272–273
  statutory terms 271
  terms agreed at interview
    binding, whether 270
  terms resulting from custom
    and practice 272
  written statement of particu-
    lars 273
Contributory negligence
    161–162
  children, and 162
Controlled drugs 801–803
Controlled Drugs Accountable
    Officer (CDAO) 803
Control of Substances Hazardous
    to Health (COSHH)
    2002 359–360
Coping under pressure 94
Coronavirus see COVID-19
Coroners and Justice Act 2009
    869
Corporate Manslaughter and
    Corporate Homicide
    Act 2007 38, 360
Council for Healthcare
    Regulatory Excellence
    (CHRE) 326–328
Council for the Regulation of
    Health Care Professionals
    (CRHCP) 326–327
Court of Protection 195,
    501–502, 743–744
  appointment of deputy
    502–504
COVID-19 12, 750, 759,
    767–768, 893
CPD 325–326
Crime
  administration of drug by
    epidural instead of in-
    travenous injection 39
  defences 39–44
  definitions 33–34
  elements of 33–34
  mental and physical elements
    34
Crime and disorder reduction
    partnerships (CDRPs)
    365
Criminal courts 6
  overriding objective 27
Criminal injuries compensation
    44–45
Criminal Injuries Compensation
    Authority (CICA) 44
Criminal liability 5–7

Critical care services, review of 483–484
Cross-examination 32
Cross-examine witnesses 15
Cross-infection control 755–756
Crossing service provision boundaries 507
Crown Court proceedings 29–33
  sentencing 32, 33
Crown Prosecution Service (CPS) 26

D

Damages-Based Agreements (DBA) Regulations 169
Data protection 209–217 *see also* Confidentiality
  freedom of information legislation, and 238–239
  Information Commissioner 210
Day surgery 619–621
Death 831–876
  certification and registration 857–860
    changes under Coroners and Justice Act 2009 859–860
    fatal diagnosis 858
  coroner, report to 861
  definition 838
  diagnosis following irreversible cessation of brainstem function 837
  disposal of body 860
  exact time of 838
    criminal law 839–840
    missing persons 839
  legality of switching machines off 840–845
  procedures for dealing with 859
  property of deceased 870
Declaration 14
Defamation 261–263
  liability of references 262–263
  reports protected by privilege 262
Defences
  to civil action 160–170
    contributory negligence 161–162
    delay 167
    denial of facts 160
    exemption from liability 164–166
    extension 169
    judge's discretion to extend 168
    knowledge of harm 166–167
    legal aid and conditional fees 169–170
    limitation of time 166
    missing element 160
    Unfair Contract Terms Act 1977 164–166
    volenti non fit injuria 163–164
    willing assumption of risk 163–164
  trespass to the person 188–189
    patients lacking mental capacity 189
    unconscious patients 189–190
Defences to criminal offences 39–44
  absence of elements making up offence 39–40
  diminished responsibility 41
  duress 43
  infancy 40
  insanity 40–41
  loss of control 41–43
  mistake 43
  necessity 43
  self-defence 44
  superior orders 44
Delegation 717–718
  outcome of task 719–720
  tasks and duties, within other person's scope of competence 718–719
Dementia 553–557
  objectives of 555–556
  other legal issues, and 556–557
Department for Children, Schools and Families (DCSF) 415–416
Department for Constitutional Affairs (DCA) 14
Department for Work and Pensions (DWP) 744–745
Department of Health and Social Care (DHSC) 10, 113
Dependent nurse prescriber 817–819
Deprivation of Liberty Safeguards 195 *see also* DOLS
Deputies 195
Devolved law-making powers 19
Diminished responsibility 41
Direct liability, of employer 88–90
Director of Public Prosecutions (DPP) 18, 852–854
Direct payments for personal care 511–515
  health care 515
Disclosure and Barring Service (DBS) 7, 269, 276–277
Discrimination 294–305
  combined 300–301
  direct 300
  disability 295–296
  duty to make adjustments for disabled persons 301
  Equality Act 2010 295, 298–299, 301
  gender reassignment 296
  indirect 301
  male midwives 305
  nature of protection 297–300
  NHS, in 305
  positive action 303–304
  race 296
  religion 296–297
  sex 297
  sexual orientation 297
Dissenting judgment 18
DNA databases 240–241
Documentation, kept by police 25–26
DOLS 494–499
  application for authorisation 495–496
  appointment of representative 496
  assessments required 496
  authorisation granted 496
  procedures 495–499
  review and monitoring 496–499
  scope 495
Domestic violence 369–370
Domestic Violence Disclosure Scheme 370
Do Not Attempt Cardiopulmonary Resuscitation (DNACPR) 845–846
  accessible and clear policy 848
  consulting relatives of incapable patients 847–848
  duty not to provide futile treatment 846
  duty to provide treatment 846
  lawfulness 845–846
  requirement to consult patient 846–847
Drug Misuse Database (DMD) 822
Duress 43
Duty of care 49–53, 87–88
  duty of care arising, whether 52–53
  duty of nurse to volunteer help 51–52

E

East Sussex County Council (ESCC) 376–377
Electroconvulsive therapy (ECT) 585
Embryos 636–638
  civil wrongs 637–638
  criminal offences 637–638
  three-parent 637
Emergency, obeying orders in 79–80
Employer, direct liability of 88–90
Employer's Liability (Defective Equipment) Act 1969 355
Employment Appeal Tribunal (EAT) 285
Employment law 266–309, 526–527
  antenatal visits 280
  contract of employment 268–274
  contractual rights of lecturers 526–527
  dismissal and professional conduct and competence 286
  dismissal of maternity leave replacement 280
  dismissal on grounds of absenteeism or course failure 526
  flexible working 283
  maternity allowance 281
  maternity right to return to work 279–280
  paternal leave for caring for child 280
  paternity leave and pay 281
  practice learning opportunities 526
  pregnant employee, rights of 278–282
  Protection of Children Act 1999 275
  protection of vulnerable adults 275, 276
  right not unfairly dismissed, on grounds of pregnancy 279
  Safeguarding Vulnerable Groups Act 2006 276

Sexual Offences Act 1997 and 2003 275
sources of contract of 267
statutory maternity leave and pay 281
statutory provisions 274–286
statutory rights for employees 277–278
students 526
surveillance by employers 286
time off for dependants 282
time off provisions 281–282
End of life care 831–876
  Director of Public Prosecutions guidance 852
    policy on assisted suicide prosecutions 852–854
    public interest factors making prosecution more likely 853–854
  double effect, principle of 834–836
  intention to kill 834
  oblique intention for murder 834
  patients refusing treatment 848–850
  relatives and treatment of patient 850–855
  three tragic cases 854–855
Equality and Human Rights Commission (EHRC) 294
European Court of Human Rights (ECtHR) 10
European Court of Justice (ECJ) 10
European Union, patient safety and 759
Evidence in court 257–261
  cross-examination 260–261
  expert witness 259
  fears of giving 258
  preparation for court appearance 258–259
  witness of fact 259
Examination in chief 154
Ex gratia payment 49, 150, 164, 474, 737, 821
Expert witness 37, 54

F

Failure to call medical assistance 36
Family courts 12
Female circumcision 458–461

Fitness to Practice Committee (FtPC) 7, 8, 78, 81, 317–321
  action following reports received from medical examiner 322–323
  breach of the peace 320
  case examiners 322
  criminal misconduct 320–321
  hearing 318–319
  membership 321
  notice of referral 323
  outcomes 319
  panel 321
  procedure 322
  removal on grounds of health 321
  restoration to Register 323–324
  standard of proof 318–319
Freedom of Information Act 2000 19, 209, 235–240
  absolute exemptions 237
  access at common law 240
  codes of practice 239
  data protection, and 238–239
  exempt information 237
  records of deceased persons 239–240
Funding of long-term care 666–669
  Dilnot Report 668–669
  Green Paper 667–668
  White Paper 668, 669

G

Gender selection 650
General Data Protection Regulation (UK GDPR) 209–210, 532
  accountability 211–212
  breach 216
  consent 213–214
  data subject rights 214–215
  human rights 216–217
  Information Commissioner 210
  lawful basis for processing data 214
  legal processing 212–213
  nurse's duty of confidence 214
  personal data 210–211
  principles 211
  processing 211
  transparency 212
General Medical Council (GMC) 259
General sales list (GSL) 799

Gene therapy 647–649
Gene Therapy Advisory Committee (GTAC) 647–648
Genetic diagnosis 647–649
Genetics 646–647
  testing for pregnant women 647
Genetic screening and testing 650–653
  code of practice 651–652
  commercial screening kits 651
  confidentiality 652–653
Genito-urinary medicine 617–619
  confidentiality 617–618
  request for information by spouse 618
  tracing 618
  venereal disease regulations 619
Gifts 747–748
Gillick case 402
Gosport Independent Panel 137
Gosport War Memorial Hospital Enquiry 137
Gross negligence manslaughter 36–37
  redefining threshold 37–38

H

Harassment 302, 378–380
Harm 64–68
  delayed transfer 67
  nervous shock 65
  post-traumatic stress 65–68
  post-traumatic stress syndrome 65
Health and Care Professions Council (HCPC) 238, 883–884
Health and safety 332–392
  abolition of Crown immunity 334–335
  consultation with employee 338
  defective equipment 362–363
  duty of employer 360–361
  duty to review procedures 385
  failures by employer 361
  general duty of employer to non-employees 336
  Health and Safety at Work Act 1974 (HASWA) 332–334
    principles 332–333
    Section 2 333–334

Section 7 334
Section 8 338
Section 20 337–338
inspection initiative 385–386
inspectors 335–336
insurance by employer 362
liability of employer for work outside premises 364
powers of CQC 335–336
prosecution of individual nurse 336
protection of employees who report hazards 347
regulations 339
remedies 377
remedies available to injured employee 363–364
safety committees 338
safety representatives 338
Health and safety (consultation with employees) regulations 1996 338
Health and Safety Executive (HSE) 338
Health and Social Care Act 2008 757–759
Health and Social Care Act 2012 106–109, 113
  Monitor, and 120–124
Health Care and Associated Professions (Indemnity Arrangements) Order 2014 91
Healthcare professionals (HCPs) 202
Healthcare sharps injuries 382–386
  application of regulations to nurses 383
  duties under 2013 regulations 383
  duty to report 385
  health and safety law 382–383
  information and training 384–385
  preventing the recapping of needles 384
  prevention of exposure 384
  procedures for safe use and disposal 384
  sharps disposal containers 384
  specific regulations 383
  use of safer sharps 384
Healthcare support workers 728–730
Health Education England (HEE) 537–538
Health Protection Agency (HPA) 759–760
Health Research Authority (HRA) 531–532

Health Service and Parliamentary Ombudsman 786–787
Healthwatch England 788–789
Hearing 154–155, 318–319
  about unsound practices 525
  claimant's case 154
  cross-examination 154
  defendant's case 154–155
  examination in chief 154
  expert evidence 154
  judge's summing up 155
  re-examination 154
  res ipsa loquitur 155
Hearsay, avoidance of 256
Hepatitis 761
Herbal medicine 881, 883–884
HIV/AIDs 761–764
  confidentiality 763–764
  criminal law, and 763
  government policy on testing 761–763
  HIV-infected healthcare workers 764
  human rights, and 763
  identifying patients who may be at risk 763–764
Homicide Act 1957, amendments 41
House of Commons Select Committee 788
Human Fertilisation and Embryology Act 1990, as amended by 2008 Act 629–634
  confidentiality 642
  conscientious objection 646
  counselling and consent 640–641
  human gametes, consent provisions for retrieval, storage and use of 639–640
Human Fertilisation and Embryology Authority (HFEA) 625, 626, 638
Human gametes, consent provisions for retrieval, storage and use 639–640
Human Genetics Advisory Commission (HGAC) 638
Human Genetics Commission (HGC) 638, 647
Human rights 267–268
  care homes, and 681–684
  GDPR, and 216–217
  HIV/Aids, and 763
Human Rights Act 1998 13–19

Human Tissue and Embryos Bill 625–626
Hunger strikes 187–188

I

Ill-treatment 35–36
Ill-treatment or wilful neglect 139–141
  revised criminal offence 140
Implied consent 180–181
Indemnity from employee at fault 90–91
  professional indemnity insurance 91
Independent Complaints Advocacy Service (ICAS) 789–790
Independent contractors, duty of care and liability 87–88
Independent mental capacity advocate (IMCA) 194, 499
Independent mental health advocates (IMHA) 588
Independent nurse prescriber 817
Indictable offence 6, 27
Indictment 6
Inexperience 74–75
Infancy 40
Informal patients 575
Information Commissioner (IC) 210
Informing the patient 176–208
  no decision about me, without me 204–205
  notifying patient of negligence by colleague 203–204
  patient's rights 202–203
  relatives' rights 203
  terminally ill patient 201–202
Inherent jurisdiction, of High Court 429–431
Injunction 182
Inquests 862–865
  nature of 864–865
  preparation for theatre nurse before attending 865
  purpose 863
  who should attend 863–864
  witnesses, examination of 864
Inquisitorial hearing 864
Insanity 40–41
Intensive care units, resource pressures 482–483
Inter-departmental ministerial group (IDMG) 276

Internet 263–264
Investigating Committee 316–317
'Invitation to treat' 268
In vitro fertilisation 634–636
  refusal to permit 634–636

J

Judge-made law *see* Common law
Judicial review 7, 12
Jury, challenging 31
Justices of the peace (JP) 20, 752

K

Kennedy Report 99–101
  on Bristol paediatric heart surgery 204
  consent and 178, 179
King's Counsel (KC) 13

L

Lasting power of attorney (LPA) 194, 195, 565, 740, 857
Law-making powers 19
Learning disabilities 573
  property, and 511
  registration and inspections 515–516
  sexual relations, and 508–511
Ledward, Dr Rodney 137
Legal aid 169–170
Legal complaints 12–13
Legality of switching machines off 840–845
  best interests 844
  court approval 844
  futile continued treatment 844–845
  life-sustaining treatment 844
  minimally conscious state 842–843
  persistent vegetative state 841–842
  Supreme Court ruling 845
  switching off life support machine 840
Legal language 13
Legal personnel 12–13
Legal professional privilege 223–224
Legal Services Ombudsman 13
LETBs 538
Letby, Lucy 35
Letter before action 153

Liability
  in civil law 11
  for instructing others 524–525
Liberty protection safeguards 509
Lifting Operations and Lifting Equipment Regulations 1998 (LOLER) 375
Litigation 13
Liverpool Care Pathway (LCP) 832
Living wills 855–856
  requirement of treatment 856
Local authority (LA) 16
Local Education and Training Boards (LETBs) 538
Local Healthwatch (LINKS) 789
Local research ethics committee (LREC) 535, 536

M

Magistrates' courts 27–29
  course of hearing 28
Management of Health and Safety at Work Regulations 1999 339–342
  guidance 339
  recording 340
  risk assessment 340–341
  risk management 341–342
Mandamus 110
Manual handling 373–374
  court decisions 375–377
  enforcement of regulations 375
  remedies exist for compensation 377
  therapeutic handling 378
  training 377–378
Medical defence union (MDU) 5
Medicines 798–830
  administration of drugs 800–801
  areas that concern nurse 799
  availability within NHS 824–825
  bad maths 805
  community nurse prescribing 814
  conflict with prescriber 804
  covert administration 811–813
    Court of Protection guidance 813
    objective deprivation of liberty and 812–813
  electronic prescriptions 820
  general principles 799–801

group protocols 815–816
illegible writing 805
management of errors or incidents 806–811
  fitness to practise 808
  infusion therapy 809
  PRN medication 808–809
  remote assessment and prescribing 810–811
  shared liability 807–808
  telephone instructions 810–811
mixing prior to administration 820
NMC guidance on prescribing 819
nurse as prescriber 814–815, 817–820
  criteria for eligibility 818
  implications for scope of professional practice 819
patient group directions 815–816
pharmacist, role of 820
problems in administration 804–805
product liability and drugs 821
safety 820–821
self-administration by patients 811
sources of information 804
supplementary prescribing 818–819
supplying in hospital and primary care 814–815
yellow card scheme 820–821
Medicines Acts 1968 and 1971 800
Medicines and Healthcare Products Regulatory Agency (MHRA) 356–358, 820, 884
  adverse incident reporting procedures 358
  medical devices 356–358
  single-use items 358
Mental capacity
  abortion, and 450–451
  acting in best interests of adult 491–494
    Bournewood Case 493–494
    Mental Capacity Act 2005 492
    restraint 492–493
  definition 185–187
  patients lacking 189

Mental Capacity Act 2005 185–187, 190–195
  best interests 192–193
  Code of Practice 193–194
  definition of mental capacity 191
  independent mental capacity advocate 194
  lasting power of attorney 194
  principles 191
Mental disorder, definition 573
Mental Health Act Commission (MHAC) 791, 792
Mental health review tribunals, time limits 599
Mental Health Units (Use of Force) Act 201 599
Mesothelioma Act 2014 766
Mid Staffordshire NHS Foundation Trust Inquiry 138–142
Minimum practice income guarantee (MPIG) 119
Misuse of drugs 821–824
Misuse of Drugs Act 1971 800
Misuse of Drugs Regulations 2001 802–803
MMR dispute 766–767
Modern matrons 727–728
Monitor 120–125
  Health and Social Care Act 2012, and 120–124
  licensing 124
Multiple jeopardy 5

N

National Advisory Group on the Safety of Patients in England (2013) 140
National Audit Office 286
National Clinical Assessment Service (NCAS) 343
National Deprivation of Liberty Court 429
National Health Service (NHS) 104–148
  charges 144
  Commissioning Board 113–114
  constitution 142–143
  discrimination in 305
  distinction between statutory duties and guidance from Department of Health and Social Care 113

duty of quality 125–126
  enforcement of statutory duties 109–113
    bone marrow transplant postponed operation 111
    inadequate resources 110
    postponed operation 111
  foundation trusts 120
  Health and Social Care Act 2012 106–109
  mandate 119–120
  NHS 111 service 135–136
  principles 143
  private sector, and 143–144
  Trust Development Authority 124
  White Paper *Equity and Excellence: Liberating the NHS* 105–106
National Health Service Trust Development Authority (NHSTDA) 124
National Institute for Health and Care Excellence (NICE) 56, 57, 132–135
  duties 133
  quality standards 133–134
National Minimum Wage (NMW) Act 1998 284–285
National Patient Safety Agency (NPSA) 343, 558, 806
National Prescribing Centre 824
National Quality Board 136
National Research Ethics Service (NRES) 531
National Service Framework for long term conditions 2005 546
National Service Framework for Older People (NSFOP) 545
National Service Framework for long term conditions 2005 546
National Treatment Agency (NTA) 822
Nearest relative, definition and role of 579–580
Negligence 48–71
  causation 60–64
    blindness 61
    deafness 61
    factual 60–61
    loss of a chance 63–64
    reasonably foreseeable consequence 62

taking one's claimant as one finds him 62
    thin skull rule 62–63
  in communication 73
  compensation in civil proceedings 156–160
  crime as 36–38
  duty of care 49–53
    duty of care arising, whether 52–53
    duty of nurse to volunteer help 51–52
    examples of serious breaches of duty of care 691
    extent of liability 64
    giving advice 691
    harm 64–68
      delayed transfer 67
      nervous shock 65
      post-traumatic stress syndrome 65–68
    independent contractors 87–88
    inexperience 74–75
    instructions 524
    liability in civil court case 48–71
    notifying patient of 203–204
    standard of care 53–60, 688–689
      approved practice 53
      balancing risks 59–60
      benchmarks 56–58
      deviation from approved practice 54–55
      guidelines 56–58
      keeping up to date 59
      policies 56–58
      procedures 56–58
      protocol 56–58
      reasonable foreseeability 58
    volunteers 87
    to whom nurse responsible 689–691
Nervous shock 65
NHS 111 135–136, 609, 726–727
NHS and social services complaints, single comprehensive procedure 780
NHS and social services provision 662–666
NHS Blood and Transplant (NHSBT) 474
NHS complaints system, review of 793–794
NHS Constitution 792–793
NHS Digital 252
NHS England 113–114
  aims 114–116
  functions 115

NHS Improvement 120–125, 343
NHS Improving Quality
   (NHSIQ) 470
NHS Inquiries 136–137
NHS Litigation Authority
   (NHSLA) 90, 170–171
NHS Pay Review Body
   (NHSPRB) 271
NHS Plan 125
NHS Redress Act 2006 171–172
NHS website 823
NMC and standards in education 522
   good character and good health 522–523
No absolutist test 409–410
Non-therapeutic procedures 200–201
Not for resuscitation (NFR) 15, 845–848 *see also* DNACPR
Notifiable diseases 752–755
   information which must be displayed 754–755
   procedure for notification 753–754
Novus actus interveniens 62
NPSA 343
Nurse as manager 80
   delegation 80
   pressure on 80–82
   supervision 80
Nurse consultants 720
Nursing and Midwifery Council (NMC) 310–326
   background to establishment 310–311
   case examiners 315
   constitution 311–313
   education and training 324–325
   false representation 313–314
   Fitness to Practice Committee 317–321
      action following reports received from medical examiner 322–323
      breach of the peace 320
      case examiners 322
      criminal misconduct 320–321
      hearing 318–319
      membership 321
      notice of referral 323
      panel 321
      procedure 322
      removal on grounds of health 321
      restoration to Register 323–324
      standard of proof 318–319
   functions 312
   interim order 315
   practice committees 315, 316
   registration 313
   removal from Register 314
   removal on grounds of fitness to practise 315
   statutory committees 313
   suspension from Register 315
Nursing and Midwifery Council (NMC) Code 3, 214
Nursing associates 328
Nursing regulator 214
Nursing the mentally disordered 570–604
   Care Quality Commission 600–601
   community provisions 589–601
   compulsory admission 575–579
   compulsory detention of informal inpatient 575
   consent to treatment 583–589
      challenges to compulsory treatment 586
      ECT 585
      long-term detained patients 583–585
      physical illness 587–588
      role of nurse 585–586
      seclusion 586–587
      specified treatments 585
      urgent treatments 584
   definition and role of nearest relative 579–580
   European Convention on Human Rights 601
   failures in community 595–596
   guardianship 589–590
   holding power of nurse 573–575
   informal patients 571–572, 589
   informing patient 582–583
   informing relatives 583
   managers, role of 600
   mentally ill patients 601
   patients detained under mental health legislation 572
      fundamental principles 572–573
      mental disorder, definition 573
      role of approved mental health professional 580–581
   section 17 leave 590

section 117 aftercare services 590–591
section 135(1) removal to place of safety 596
section 136 removal of mentally disordered persons without warrant 597–599
   duration of detention 598
   Policing and Crime Act 2017 597–598
   protective searches 598–599
   short-term detained patients 589

O

Obeying orders, in emergency 79–80
Occupational health, confidentiality and 228
Occupational overuse syndrome (OOS) 380
'Occupiers' Liability Acts 1957 and 1984 347–352
   children 350
   general principles 347
   independent contractors 349
   nurse and premises in community 351–352
   occupier 347–348
   privatisation of cleaning and catering services 349
   slippery floor 348
   trespassers 351
   warning notice, effect 348–349
Offences, classification of 28
Office of Public Guardian 195
Older people, care of 542–569
   abuse 561–564
      code of practice 563
      legal protection 563–564
   bad practice 549–550
   consent to treatment 547–549
   continuing care 559–560
   control at night 551
   daily care 551–552
   decision making for mentally incapacitated adult 564–565
   force, restraint and assault 549
   intermediate care 546–547
   medication and the confused older patient 552–553
   Mental Capacity Act 2005 564–565
   pressure ulcers 558
   registered homes 560
   restless patients 550–551
   rights to care 543–544
   risk management 560
   standard of care 557–558
   winter crises 559
Openness and candour in the NHS 343–346
   duty to give explanation and apology 345
   guidance on duty 346
   notifiable patient safety incident 344
   professional duty 345–346
   statutory duty in Wales, Northern Ireland and Scotland 345
   statutory organisational duty 343–344
Operating department practitioners (ODPs) 469
Organ transplantation 475–482
   children, and 478–479
   consent by recipient 478–479
   deceased persons, from 475–476
   encouraging donors 480–481
   Human Bodies, Human Choices 482
   Human Tissue Act 2004 482
   keeping patient ventilated 476
   liability arising from 479–480
   living donors, from 476–478
   mental capacity, and 479
   retention of organs 481–482
Outpatients department 615–617

P

Parental care and the nurse 421–423
Part-time employees 285
Patel, Nurse 35
Patient Advice and Liaison Services (PALS) 790–791
Patient group directions (PGDs) 815–816, 818
Patient Information Advisory Group (PIAG) 532
Patient safety, European Union, and 759
Patient Safety Incident Response Framework (PSIRF) 48
Pelka, Daniel 418–419
Pharmacist, role of 820
Pharmacy-only products (P) 799
Plaintiff 13
Plea and case management hearing (PCMH) 6, 29, 32
Police
   disclosures to 230–234
   documentation kept by 25–26

Post-mortems 861
Post-registration revalidation 325–326
Post-traumatic stress syndrome 65–68
Power of attorney 742–743
Practice directions 27
Practice nurse 705–707
   cervical screening 705–706
   scope of practice 705
   staffing concerns 707
Pre-action protocol 152
Precedents 10
Pregnancy, failure to warn of risk 456–457
Pre-implementation genetic diagnosis (PGD) 648–649
Premature deaths of people with learning disability, confidential inquiry 506–507
Prescription-only list (POM) 799
Pressure from inadequate resources 91–96
   coping 94
   employer's responsibility 92–94
   failures by management 95–96
   general principles 92
   legal requirements on staffing 94–95
   manage risk 92
Pretty, Diane 851–852
Primary care trust (PCT) 112, 662
Private healthcare 457–458
Product Liability (Consumer Protection Act 1987) 355
Professional Conduct Committee (PCC) 86
Professional indemnity insurance 91
Professionalism 4–5
   accountability and 9
Professional liability 7–8
Professional misconduct proceedings 79
Professional Records Standards Body (PRSB) 252
Professional standards 324
Professional Standards Authority for Health and Social Care (PSA) 326–328
Professional Standards Authority (PSA) 345
Prolonged disorder of consciousness (PDOC) 843

Property 735–749
   administrative failures 737
   day-to-day care of money 740–742
   exclusion of liability 738–739
   local authority duties 741–742
   Mental Capacity Act 2005 740
   mentally incapacitated patient 739–740
   permanent incapacity 739–740
   temporary incapacity 739
   'patient's, returning 745
   principles of liability 736–737
Prosecution, initial stages 24–26
Protecting patients from relatives 744–745
Protection of vulnerable adults (POVA) 275, 276
Provision and Use of Work Equipment Regulations 1998 (PUWER) 374
Psychotherapy, confidentiality and 226–227
Public and private employees 294
Public Health England 760
Public health legislation 751–752
   powers of JPs 752
Public Interest Disclosure Act 1998 96–101
Public sector equality duty 304–305
Purdy, Debbie 852

Q

Qualifying disclosure 96
Quality assurance methods 791
Quantum 49

R

Record keeping 246–252
   abbreviations 249–250
   Care Quality Commission requirements 247–248
   clarity 249
   common errors 248–249
   comprehensiveness 249
   computerised records 251–252
   errors 250
   general principles 246–247
   legal document 250–251
   maintaining high standards 251

   by teachers 523–524
   use in court 250–251
   who should sign or write 250
Recovery room nursing 473–474
Recruitment and Retention of Staff in Critical Care 484
Redundancy 283
References, liability for 262–263
Refusal to obey orders 77–80
Repetitive strain injury (RSI) 380–381
Reporting of Injuries, Diseases and Dangerous Occurrences Regulations (RIDDOR) 342
Research
   consent and 533–537
      mentally incapacitated adult and 534–535
      statutory provisions 535
   fraud in 536
   health and safety 536–537
   publication and libel 537
   volunteers, liability for 535–536
Research Ethics Committees (RECs) 530–532
Research legal aspects 527–531
   control of research programme 529–530
Res ipsa loquitur 155
Retention of organs 481–482
Right not to be subjected to inhuman or degrading treatment 15–16
Right to a fair trial 17
Right to liberty and security 16
Right to life 14–15
Right to refuse treatment 181–184
   blood transfusion 184
   mental capacity 181–184
   patient's autonomy 182
   refusal to be ventilated 183
Right to respect for private and family life, home and correspondence 17–19
Risk management training 377–378
Robbie's Law 204
Royal College of Nursing (RCN) 56, 57
Royal College of Paediatrics and Child Health (RCPCH) 396

S

Safeguarding Adult Boards 276
Safeguarding vulnerable adults 507–508

Safety representatives 293
Safety representatives and safety committees regulations 1977 (SRSC) 338
School nurse 701–703
   extent of duty 702
   use of car 702–703
Scope of professional practice 714–716
   concerns about developments 722–723
   emergency nursing 725
   primary care 723–724
   principles for adjusting 715
   revalidation 716
   ten key roles 716
   theatre nursing 724–725
   X rays, and 725–726
Scottish Medical Consortium (SMC) 825
Secretary of State inquiries 792
Self-defence 44
Self-discharge 184–185
Sentencing, Crown Court 32, 33
Sexual harassment 378–380
Shipman Inquiry 137, 865–869
Sister Salisbury 34–35
Smoking 381–382
Social Care Institute for Excellence (SCIE) 697
Social media 263–264
Solicitors 12
Sources of law 9–10
Specialist community public health nurse (SCPHN) 311, 691, 700–701
Specialist nurses 720–721
Staff car park 746
Staffing, legal requirements 94–95
Staff property 746–747
Standard of care 53–60, 557–558
   approved practice 53
   balancing risks 59–60
   benchmarks 56–58
   continuing care 559–560
   deviation from approved practice 54–55
   guidelines 56–58
   keeping up to date 59
   policies 56–58
   pressure ulcers 558
   procedures 56–58
   protocol 56–58
   reasonable foreseeability 58
   registered homes 560
   winter crises 559

Statements 252–257
　accuracy 255–256
　clarity 257
　conciseness 256
　duty to make 254
　essential elements 255
　guidance 254–255
　hearsay, avoidance of 256
　keeping to facts 256
　legibility 257
　occasions when requested 252
　overall impact 257
　principles 255
　production in court 254
　purpose 254
　refusal to make 253
　relevance 256–257
　status as evidence 253–254
　writing 257
Statute law 10
Statutory instruments 9–10
Statutory maternity pay (SMP) 281
Statutory paternity pay (SPP) 281
Statutory sick pay (SSP) scheme 283
Sterilisation 452–454, 509–510
　adult with learning disabilities 452–453
　minor with learning disabilities 452
　spouse, rights of 458
　unsuccessful 453–454
Stress 370–373
Strict liability 536
Summary Care Record (SCR) 252
Summary offence 6
Supervision 717–718
Supplementary prescriber *see* Dependent prescriber
Surrogacy 642–646
　compensation amounts, and 645–646
　dispute 643
　parental orders, and 644–645

T

Taking instructions 77–80
Taking 'one's own discharge 184–185
Team liability 75–77
Technology developments 707–708
　social enterprise groups 707–708
Theft 24
Therapeutic handling 378
Thin skull rule 62–63
Torts 11
Trade union rights 292–293
Transfusions 474–475
Trespass to the person, defences 188–189
　patients lacking mental capacity 189
　unconscious patients 189–190
Triable either way offence 6, 28, 29
Tuberculosis 760

U

UKECA 531
Unfair dismissal 286–292
　automatically unfair 290–291
　compensation 288
　conditions for bringing action 287
　criteria for reasonableness of employer 292
　general principles 286–287
　hearing 291–292
　length of continuous service 288
　outcome 292
　procedure in application 290
　record keeping and 288
　statutory reasons to dismiss 291
United Kingdom Ethics Committee Authority (UKECA) 531
Unplanned pregnancies 454–456
Unsound practices, hearing about 525

V

Vaccination 764–767
Venereal disease regulations 619
Vicarious liability 79, 82–87
　activities incidental to work 84
　assault on behalf of employer 82
　course of employment 83–87
　interests of employer 83
　non-employees 86–87
　nurse off duty 86
　outside job description 84
　sexual abuse by warden 85
Victimisation 302–303
Violence 365–370
　criminal prosecution 367–368
　remedies following 366
　risk assessment 368–369
　self-defence 368
　suing NHS trust or employer 367
　suing the patient 367
　volenti non fit injuria 163–164
　zero tolerance 365–366
Volunteers, negligence of 87

W

Walk-in centres (WICs) 136
Walk-in clinics 135–136, 726–727
Wednesbury unreasonable 586
Whistleblowing 96–101
　disclosures relating to exceptionally serious failures 98
　gagging of employee 98
　Kennedy Report 99–101
　protected disclosure 96, 97
　protected disclosure bid 98–99
White Paper *Valuing People* 504–507
Wilful neglect 35–36
Wills 870–872
　execution at night 871
Wilson Report 778–779
Winterbourne View Hospital Report 136
Work equipment 374
Working Time Directive (WTD) 283–284
Writ 13